FERRI'S
NETTER PATIENT ADVISOR
2010-2011

Fred F. Ferri, MD, FACP

Clinical Professor
Department of Community Health
Alpert Medical School at Brown University
Providence, Rhode Island

Illustrations by **Frank H. Netter, MD**

Contributing Illustrators
Carlos A. G. Machado, MD
John A. Craig, MD

SAUNDERS

ELSEVIER

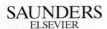

1600 John F. Kennedy Blvd.
Ste 1800
Philadelphia, PA 19103-2899

FERRI'S NETTER PATIENT ADVISOR 2010-2011   ISBN: 978-1-4160-6037-6

Notice

International Standard Serial Number (ISSN) 1943-9822

ISBN: 978-1-4160-6037-6

Acquisitions Editor: Elyse O'Grady
Developmental Editor: Marybeth Thiel
Publishing Services Manager: Linda Van Pelt
Project Manager: Sharon Lee
Design Direction: Louis Forgione
Director Netter Products and Services: Anne Lenehan
Netter Collection Specialist: Bob Gardler
Editorial Assistant: Julie Goolsby
Digital Asset Manager: Karen Oswald

Printed in China

Last digit is the print number: 9   8   7   6   5   4   3   2   1

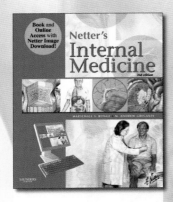
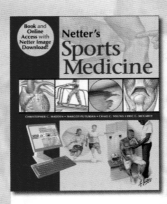
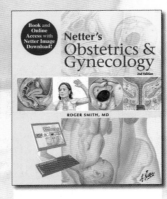
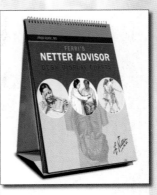
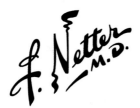
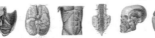

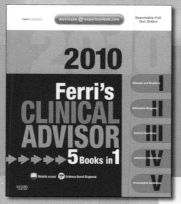 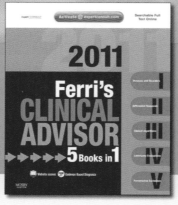 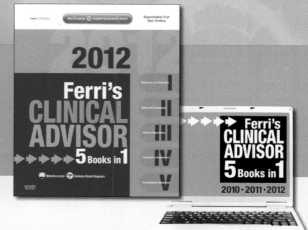
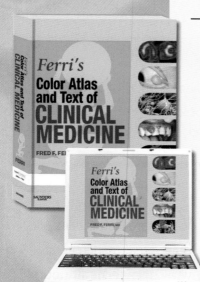

PREFACE

As a practicing primary care physician for the past 25 years, I am aware of the patient's needs for reliable, practical, and easy to understand medical information. The goal of this book is to be a comprehensive, current, and clinically relevant medical resource for the public.

This medical reference (book and online information) covers hundreds of topics, ranging from common disorders to rare diseases. Each section follows a similar format that consists of an initial description of the medical disorder and its causes, common signs and symptoms, diagnostic methods, recommended treatment, dos and don'ts in managing the specific disorder, and sources of additional information on each topic. Illustrations accompany each topic and facilitate its understanding. Visuals are the critical language of medical education. The old adage of "a picture is worth a thousand words" is certainly true in medicine. Recognition of disorders from illustrations remains crucial to early diagnosis and treatment, both of which are usually essential to improve prognosis. The use of thousands of illustrations from Dr. Frank Netter, an outstanding physician and perhaps the best medical illustrator of all time, makes this book unique amongst medical texts for the general public.

No book can replace the consultation and physical examination by a qualified physician; but by providing the reader with a better understanding of his or her medical condition, this medical guide is far ahead of its competitors and will certainly enhance communication between patients and physicians.

Knowledge is essential in maintaining good health. I hope that this book fulfills your every expectation and provides valuable learning support to your understanding of the numerous illnesses afflicting humanity.

Acknowledgment

This product represents a highly collaborative and dynamic effort between the Editor and Elsevier. I am greatly indebted to First-Consult for sharing some of their patient education material and to Drs. Frank Netter and Carlos Machado for their unparalleled illustrations. I also wish to thank Elsevier for their exceptional support and guidance in this project. Finally, I want to express my gratitude to the many authors of the Patient Teaching Guides in Ferri's Clinical Advisor, and Dr. Peter Petropoulos in particular, for their superb contributions and friendship.

Fred F. Ferri, MD, FACP
Clinical Professor
Alpert Medical School
Brown University
Providence, Rhode Island

CONTENTS

Endocrinology

Gastroenterology

Gynecology and Obstetrics

Hematology/Oncology

Infectious Diseases

Interdisciplinary Medicine

Nephrology

Neurology

Ophthalmology

Orthopedics

Otorhinolaryngology (ENT)

Pediatrics

Psychiatry

Pulmonary Disease

Rheumatology

Surgery, General

Urology

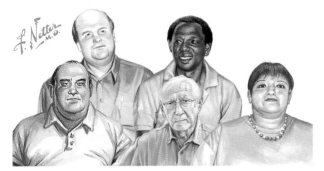

An abdominal aortic aneurysm is a bulging of the aorta, the largest artery in the body. This is dangerous because it may burst if untreated.

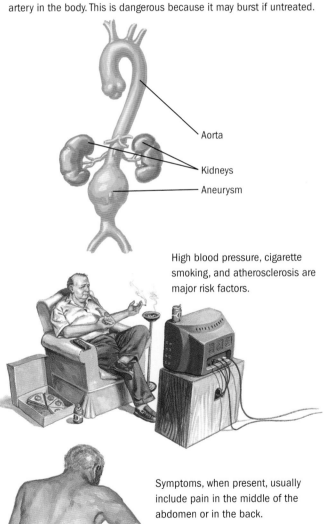

Aorta

Kidneys

Aneurysm

High blood pressure, cigarette smoking, and atherosclerosis are major risk factors.

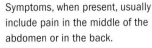

Symptoms, when present, usually include pain in the middle of the abdomen or in the back.

What Is an Abdominal Aortic Aneurysm?

An abdominal aortic aneurysm is a bulging of the aorta, the main blood vessel that takes blood from the heart to organs and tissues in the lower half of the body. The aorta is the largest artery in the body, and a bulge in the aorta is dangerous because it may split open (rupture) if not treated.

These aneurysms commonly occur in people older than 60 and affect men more than women. These ruptured aneurysms are the 10th leading cause of death in men older than 55 in the United States.

What Causes an Abdominal Aortic Aneurysm?

High blood pressure (which makes the aorta lining expand), cigarette smoking, and atherosclerosis (hardening of the arteries) are major risk factors. Others are trauma, infections, connective tissue disorders (e.g., Ehlers-Danlos syndrome), and aging.

What Are the Symptoms of an Abdominal Aortic Aneurysm?

Abdominal aortic aneurysms often don't produce symptoms. When present, symptoms usually include pain in the middle of the abdomen (belly) or back.

How Is an Abdominal Aortic Aneurysm Diagnosed?

Most aneurysms are found during routine physical examinations by doctors. A doctor can feel a large aneurysm pulsating over the middle of the abdomen.

If an aneurysm is suspected, the doctor will order abdominal ultrasound (sonogram) and computed tomography (CT). Ultrasound is nearly 100% accurate in finding an aneurysm and can estimate the size, but CT is more accurate in estimating size.

How Is an Abdominal Aortic Aneurysm Treated?

This aneurysm can be repaired if found early, before rupture. If it splits open suddenly, death is likely unless the rupture is treated immediately.

Treatment depends on aneurysm size and risk of rupture. If the aneurysm is small, no treatment may be needed, but regular check-ups (every 6 months to 1 year) are advised. A larger aneurysm or one causing symptoms is treated with drugs that lower blood pressure.

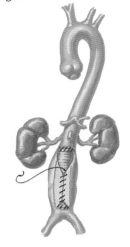

Surgery often involves putting a stent (synthetic tube) in the aorta to make it stronger.

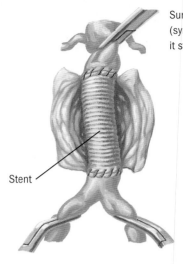

Stent

Surgery to fix aneurysms larger than 5 cm (2 inches) is usually recommended. The operation often involves putting a synthetic mesh tube (stent) in the aorta to make it stronger.

Treatment of aneurysms between 4 and 5 cm (1.6 and 2 inches) remains unclear. Some doctors recommend surgery and others just follow-up examinations.

DOs and DON'Ts in Managing Abdominal Aortic Aneurysm:

✔ **DO** make sure that you control your blood pressure.
✔ **DO** remember that the major complication of these aneurysms is rupture.
✔ **DO** call your doctor if you know you have an abdominal aneurysm and get new back or abdominal pain.
✔ **DO** call your doctor if you have pain, fever, or drainage from incision sites after surgery.

⊘ **DON'T** forget the numbers 4 cm and 5 cm (surgery for aneurysms larger than 5 cm, watching aneurysms smaller than 4 cm).
⊘ **DON'T** smoke. Cigarette smoking and high blood pressure are believed to be major risk factors for these aneurysms.

Don't smoke, and make sure your blood pressure is controlled.

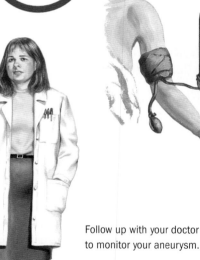

Follow up with your doctor on a regular basis to monitor your aneurysm.

FOR MORE INFORMATION

Contact the following sources:

- American Heart Association National Center
  7272 Greenville Avenue
  Dallas, TX 75231
  Tel: (800) 242-8721

- National Heart, Lung, and Blood Institute
  Tel: (301) 592-8573
  E-mail: NHLBIinfo@rover.nhlbi.nih.gov
  Website: http://www.nhlbi.nih.gov

- American College of Cardiology
  Tel: (800) 253-4636, (202) 375-6000
  Fax: (202) 375-7000
  Website: http://www.acc.org

- American College of Emergency Physicians
  Tel: (800) 798-1822, (972) 550-0911
  Fax: (972) 580-2816
  Website: http://www.acep.org

- American College of Surgeons
  Website: http://www.facs.org

FROM THE DESK OF

NOTES

MANAGING YOUR
ANGINA

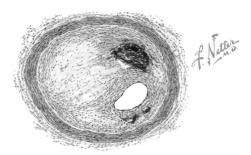

Atherosclerosis

Angina occurs when the heart doesn't get enough oxygen. The usual cause is narrowed blood vessels (from atherosclerosis).

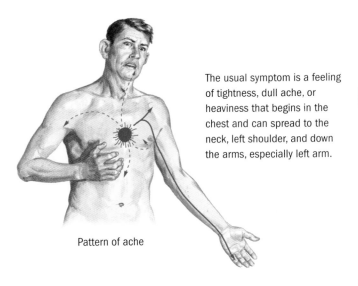

The usual symptom is a feeling of tightness, dull ache, or heaviness that begins in the chest and can spread to the neck, left shoulder, and down the arms, especially left arm.

Pattern of ache

The doctor makes a diagnosis by using an ECG and treadmill or exercise tests.

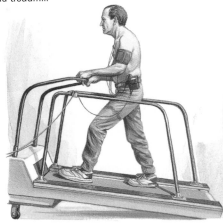

What Is Angina?

Angina is chest pain usually caused by narrowing of blood vessels in the heart. Less blood can reach the heart, so it has less oxygen for pumping blood. Angina may mean serious heart problems and needs immediate attention.

What Causes Angina?

Coronary artery disease from atherosclerosis (i.e., fatty deposits in blood vessels to the heart), abnormal heart rhythms (arrhythmias), fewer oxygen-carrying red blood cells (anemia), and spasms of the coronary arteries can reduce blood flow.

At increased risk for angina are men older than age 60, women after menopause, people with a family history of heart disease, people who eat high-fat high-cholesterol foods, people who don't exercise regularly, smokers, and people with diabetes, high blood pressure (hypertension), or high cholesterol levels.

What Are the Symptoms of Angina?

The primary symptom is a feeling of tightness, dull ache, or heaviness that begins in the chest and sometimes spreads to the back, neck, left shoulder, and down the arms (especially left arm). Pain may be dull or sharp or feel like heartburn or indigestion. Some people describe a smothering or crushing pain. It may begin slowly or be severe and sudden. Sweating, nausea, feeling faint or weak, dizziness, or shortness of breath may also occur.

How Is Angina Diagnosed?

The doctor makes a diagnosis by checking symptoms and doing examinations and laboratory and other tests. Tests include electrocardiograms (ECGs) and treadmill or exercise tests. A heart catheterization (checking the heart's blood flow by putting a device through an artery into the heart) may also be done if the initial tests show signs of blocked heart (coronary) arteries.

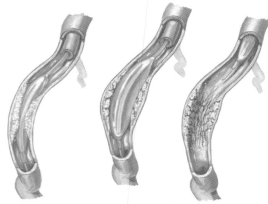

Severe angina that can't be treated with medicine may need angioplasty (opening clogged blood vessels with a balloonlike device).

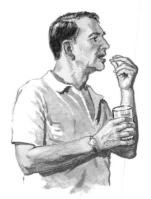

People with angina or heart disease should take aspirin daily unless told not to by a doctor.

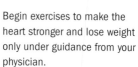

Begin exercises to make the heart stronger and lose weight only under guidance from your physician.

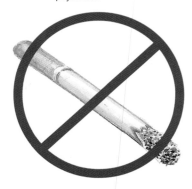

Don't drink alcohol in excess and don't smoke!

How Is Angina Treated?

The goal is to improve blood flow to the heart or to reduce the heart's work. Resting or reducing activity is the first treatment.

Aspirin improves blood flow. Nitrates such as nitroglycerin can also help blood flow. Other medications such as beta blockers slow down the heartbeat and the work done by the heart. Medicine for other diseases (e.g., hypertension, arrhythmias, diabetes, high cholesterol) may be given if these diseases are present.

Anyone with angina should take aspirin daily unless told not to by a doctor.

Lifestyle changes (exercise, diet, weight control, quitting smoking) are important.

If medicine doesn't work, surgery (angioplasty, an operation to open clogged blood vessels with a balloonlike device) may be needed. A small wire mesh tube, called a stent, is often inserted into the blocked artery after it has been opened to prevent it from narrowing again. Open heart surgery (coronary artery bypass graft, or CABG) may be necessary for severely blocked arteries.

DOs and DON'Ts in Managing Angina:

✔ **DO** change your diet and reduce weight to lower blood pressure and improve blood fat and sugar levels.
✔ **DO** begin an exercise program under the guidance of your physician to strengthen the heart and reduce weight, blood pressure, blood fat levels, and stress.
✔ **DO** stop smoking.
✔ **DO** take your medicines as directed.
✔ **DO** call your doctor if medicines don't control your pain.
✔ **DO** call 911 or get to the emergency room if you take nitroglycerin three times without symptom relief.
✔ **DO** call your doctor immediately if you have new or worsening symptoms that your medicine doesn't control.

⊘ **DON'T** do things that raise your blood pressure.
⊘ **DON'T** smoke, drink alcohol in excess, or eat salty or high-fat foods.
⊘ **DON'T** ignore your symptoms.
⊘ **DON'T** use Viagra®, Levitra®, or Cialis® if you take nitroglycerin.

FOR MORE INFORMATION

Contact the following sources:
- National Heart, Lung, and Blood Institute
  Tel: (301) 592-8573
  Website: http://www.nhlbi.nih.gov
- American Heart Association
  Heart and stroke information: (800) AHA-USA1 (242-8721)
  Women's health information: (888) MY HEART (694-3278)
  Website: http://www.americanheart.org

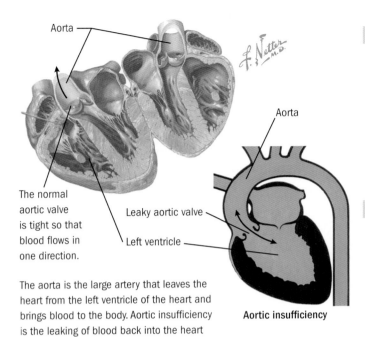

Aorta

The normal aortic valve is tight so that blood flows in one direction.

Aorta

Leaky aortic valve

Left ventricle

Aortic insufficiency

The aorta is the large artery that leaves the heart from the left ventricle of the heart and brings blood to the body. Aortic insufficiency is the leaking of blood back into the heart from the aorta.

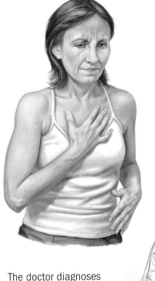

Symptoms, when present, include tiredness, chest pain, difficulty breathing, and coughing.

The doctor diagnoses aortic insufficiency by a physical examination and echocardiography.

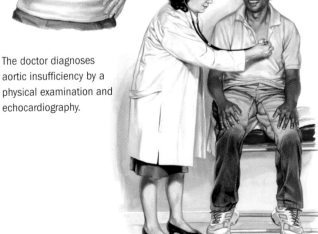

What Is Aortic Insufficiency?

The aorta is the large artery that leaves the heart from the left lower chamber (ventricle). The aortic valve is between the left ventricle and the aorta. Aortic insufficiency (or aortic regurgitation) is the leaking of blood from the aorta through the aortic valve into the left ventricle when the ventricle contracts.

Aortic insufficiency causes the left ventricle to get larger because of the extra blood in it.

What Causes Aortic Insufficiency?

The cause is a defective aortic valve or enlarged bottom part of the aorta. Infections such as rheumatic fever (usually from streptococcal infections) and endocarditis (bacterial infection in the heart) affect the valve. Congenital abnormalities such as bicuspid valve (two valve sections instead of three) are a common cause. Direct blunt injury (e.g., the chest hitting a steering wheel in an accident), connective tissue disorders such as Marfan's disease, and hypertension can lead to an enlarged aorta.

What Are the Symptoms of Aortic Insufficiency?

Most people have no symptoms. Symptoms when present are tiredness, chest pain, difficulty breathing (especially when lying down), coughing, and shortness of breath.

How Is Aortic Insufficiency Diagnosed?

The doctor makes a diagnosis from a physical examination. Blood flowing through the valve creates a heart murmur (extra or unusual sound during the heartbeat) that the doctor hears with the stethoscope. The doctor will recommend echocardiography (a test that uses ultrasound waves to give a picture of the heart).

For severe insufficiency with effects on the heart's function, the doctor may suggest cardiac catheterization. In catheterization a small tube (catheter) is inserted into a leg artery and passed into the heart to get pictures of the heart.

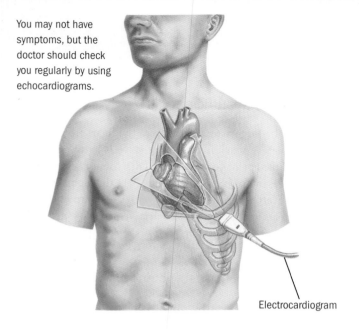

You may not have symptoms, but the doctor should check you regularly by using echocardiograms.

Electrocardiogram

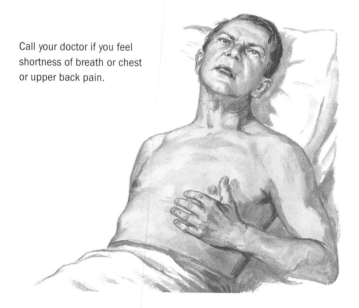

Call your doctor if you feel shortness of breath or chest or upper back pain.

How Is Aortic Insufficiency Treated?

For people without symptoms, the doctor may recommend regular check-ups including echocardiograms. If testing shows an enlarged heart, the doctor may suggest seeing a thoracic surgeon (a specialist who performs heart valve operations) to correct or replace the valve.

People with symptoms may take medicines to prevent fluid and pressure from building up in the heart. The doctor may also recommend referral to a thoracic surgeon.

DOs and DON'Ts in Managing Aortic Insufficiency:

✔ **DO** remember that you may not have symptoms but should be checked with echocardiograms to follow the valve disease.

✔ **DO** take antibiotics (if prescribed) before dental or surgical procedures if you had infectious endocarditis or heart surgery.

✔ **DO** go to see a cardiologist (a doctor who specializes in heart diseases) if you are having symptoms.

✔ **DO** call your doctor if you get shortness of breath, chest or upper back pain, palpitations or rapid heartbeat, or fainting.

⊘ **DON'T** do strenuous exercise if you have severe insufficiency.

⊘ **DON'T** forget that periodic checkups to monitor for aortic insufficiency and its effect on the heart are important.

FROM THE DESK OF

NOTES

FOR MORE INFORMATION
Contact the following sources:

• American Heart Association
Tel: (800) 242-8721
Website: http://www.americanheart.org

• American College of Cardiology
Tel: (800) 253-4636
Website: http://www.acc.org

• Heart Center Online
Website: http://www.heartcenteronline.com

MANAGING YOUR
AORTIC STENOSIS

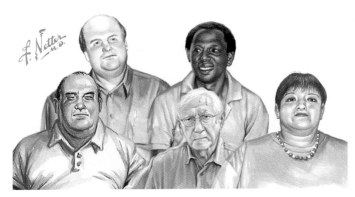

Aortic valve stenosis (AVS) is a disorder in which the opening of the aortic valve in the heart is too small or too stiff. The heart becomes big and weak. AVS occurs more often in men than women.

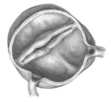
Two-sided valve

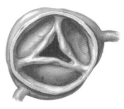
Three-sided valve

A valve is like a doorway. The normal aortic valve has three flaps (leaflets). Some people are born with a two-sided (bicuspid) valve instead of a normal, three-sided valve.

People with AVS will have a heart murmur, which is an extra or unusual sound of blood flow through the valve during the heartbeat.

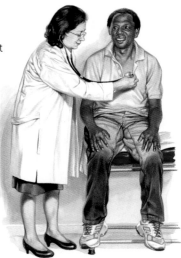

What Is Aortic Stenosis?

Aortic valve stenosis (AVS) is a disorder in which the opening of the aortic valve in the heart is too small or stiff. A valve is like a doorway, and the aortic valve is one of four valves controlling blood flow inside the heart. A normal aortic valve has three flaps (leaflets). The heart sends blood to the body through this valve. In AVS, the heart works harder to pump blood through the smaller opening. This extra effort can make the heart grow big and weak.

AVS occurs about three times more often in men than in women.

What Causes Aortic Stenosis?

Calcium and cholesterol deposits on the valve that occur with aging are the most common cause. Some people are born with damaged valves or have a two-sided (bicuspid), not three-sided, valve. Heart disease or rheumatic fever from childhood infections may also damage the valve.

What Are the Symptoms of Aortic Stenosis?

Most people at first have no symptoms. If the valve narrows enough, feeling tired, fainting with exercise, having chest pain with exercise or at rest, or having symptoms of left-sided heart failure (e.g., shortness of breath) may occur. Breathing problems during exercise may progress to problems at rest, or waking up at night unable to breathe.

How Is Aortic Stenosis Diagnosed?

The doctor will take a medical history and do a physical examination. The doctor may hear a heart murmur (an extra or unusual sound of blood flow through the valve during the heartbeat). If AVS is suspected, the doctor will order echocardiography (using sound waves to take heart pictures) to diagnose AVS.

Additional tests such as heart catheterization (uses x-rays and dye) may be done before surgery to replace the valve.

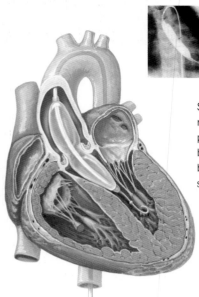

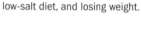

Surgical treatment involves replacing the valve. Young people may have a special balloon put in the valve and blown up, so the valve stretches open (valvuloplasty).

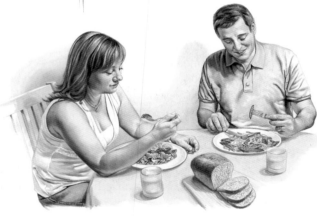

Ask your doctor about exercising, taking medicines, starting a low-salt diet, and losing weight.

Don't become dehydrated, which can make your symptoms worse.

FROM THE DESK OF

NOTES

How Is Aortic Stenosis Treated?

People without symptoms and with mild stenosis may not need treatment but should be monitored on a periodic basis by their doctor. For people with symptoms or severe disease, surgery to replace the valve is best.

Sometimes, a special balloon is put in the valve and blown up so the valve stretches (valvuloplasty). Valvuloplasty is often used in younger people who will get a replacement valve after they grow.

DOs and DON'Ts in Managing Aortic Stenosis:

✔ **DO** ask your doctor if you can exercise.
✔ **DO** stop smoking.
✔ **DO** start a low-salt diet and lose weight if you have congestive heart failure.
✔ **DO** take antibiotics before dental visits or surgery if your doctor prescribes them.
✔ **DO** call your doctor if, after you get a new valve, you have chest pain, shortness of breath, palpitations or rapid heart-beat, fainting, sudden weakness in an arm or leg, eyesight problems, fever, or blood from the surgery site.

⊘ **DON'T** become dehydrated. Dehydration will worsen aortic stenosis.
⊘ **DON'T** use any over-the-counter medicine without asking your doctor.
⊘ **DON'T** ignore worsening symptoms.

FOR MORE INFORMATION

Contact the following sources:

* American Heart Association
  Tel: (800) 242-8721
  Website: http://www.americanheart.org

* American College of Cardiology
  Tel: (800) 253-4636
  Website: http://www.acc.org

* Heart Center Online
  Website: http://www.heartcenteronline.com

MANAGING YOUR
ATRIAL FIBRILLATION

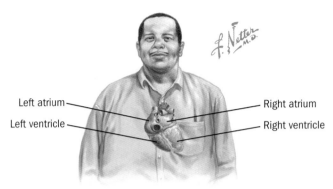

Left atrium

Left ventricle

Right atrium

Right ventricle

In atrial fibrillation, muscles in the wall of the upper heart chambers (left and right atrium) twitch abnormally. This causes the ventricles to work harder to get blood to the body, and heart failure may result.

Causes of and conditions related to atrial fibrillation

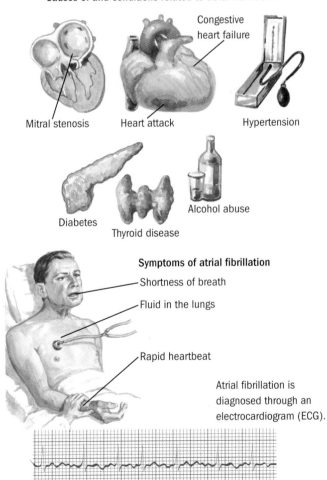

Mitral stenosis

Congestive heart failure

Heart attack

Hypertension

Diabetes

Thyroid disease

Alcohol abuse

Symptoms of atrial fibrillation

Shortness of breath

Fluid in the lungs

Rapid heartbeat

Atrial fibrillation is diagnosed through an electrocardiogram (ECG).

What Is Atrial Fibrillation?

An abnormal heart rhythm is called an *arrhythmia*. Atrial fibrillation is one type of abnormal rhythm. The muscle looks as if it is wiggling instead of squeezing (contracting).

What Happens During Atrial Fibrillation?

The human heart has four chambers. The upper ones are called atria; the lower ones, ventricles. All chambers must squeeze in a certain way to move the blood properly. A fibrillating atrium, however, has small, irregular, fast contractions. All the blood inside the atria is not pumped into ventricles, so blood pools. Pooled blood may clot, and clots can be pushed into the bloodstream and cause strokes. Ventricles work harder to get blood to the body, and heart failure may result.

What Causes Atrial Fibrillation?

Among the many causes, the most common is aging. Others are heart problems such as hypertension (high blood pressure), congestive heart failure (CHF), and mitral valve disease (mitral stenosis). Lung diseases, other illnesses (e.g., diabetes), and overactive thyroid are more causes. Caffeine, nicotine (cigarettes), and too much alcohol can cause it or make it worse.

What Are the Symptoms of Atrial Fibrillation?

Many people have atrial fibrillation and never feel it.

Symptoms often include the feeling of irregular or too fast (palpitations) heartbeats. Difficulty breathing, chest pain, or fainting may occur. Some people feel tired or cannot exercise.

Chest pain or signs of stroke must be checked immediately.

How Is Atrial Fibrillation Diagnosed?

The doctor looks for a certain pattern on an electrocardiogram (ECG), which shows the heart's electrical activity.

The doctor may check movements of the atria with an echocardiogram (using ultrasound to examine the heart).

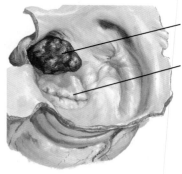

Blood clot (thrombus)

Abnormal mitral valve in the heart

Complications include valve abnormalities and blood clots, which can travel to other areas in the body, such as the brain (to cause stroke).

Treatments include using cardioversion and a dual-chamber pacemaker.

In cardioversion, an electrical shock causes the abnormal heartbeat to go back to normal.

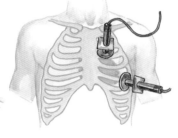

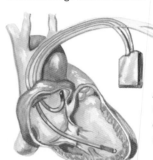

A dual-chamber pacemaker is placed under the skin of the chest and creates electrical pulses to keep the heart rate normal.

Ways to manage atrial fibrillation

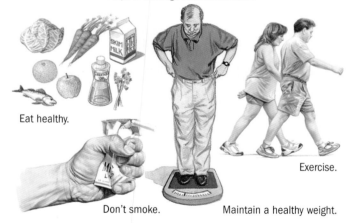

Eat healthy.

Don't smoke.

Maintain a healthy weight.

Exercise.

How Is Atrial Fibrillation Treated?

Treatment focuses on the cause. For example, if the person has thyroid disease, that illness is treated. If the cause is too much caffeine or excess alcohol, less should be used.

Controlling heart rhythm and the fibrillation rate with drugs is important. Sometimes atrial fibrillation stops on its own.

Clots are one complication of fibrillation. Blood thinners (anticoagulants) such as warfarin (e.g., Coumadin®) may be given for clots or to prevent them. This drug causes easy bruising or bleeding, so drug levels are checked regularly.

The abnormal rhythm can sometimes be shocked back to normal (called *cardioversion*). Chest pain, low blood pressure, CHF, or other serious symptoms may require emergency cardioversion. A dual chamber pacemaker may be placed. A heart catheter or surgery (maze procedure) may be used to destroy the part of the heart causing fibrillation.

DOs and DON'Ts in Managing Atrial Fibrillation:

✔ **DO** eat a heart-healthy diet (less fat and cholesterol).
✔ **DO** keep to an ideal body weight.
✔ **DO** reduce stress.
✔ **DO** exercise as much as you can if you are taking the proper drugs and have no symptoms.
✔ **DO** take your medicines as prescribed. Have blood drug levels checked.
✔ **DO** call your doctor if you have drug side effects or if you have new or worsening symptoms.

⊘ **DON'T** do activities that cause bruising if you are taking a blood thinner.
⊘ **DON'T** use tobacco.
⊘ **DON'T** drink too much alcohol or caffeine.

FROM THE DESK OF

NOTES

FOR MORE INFORMATION

Contact the following source:

• American Heart Association
  Tel: (800) 242-8721
  Website: http://www.americanheart.org

MANAGING YOUR
ATRIAL SEPTAL DEFECT

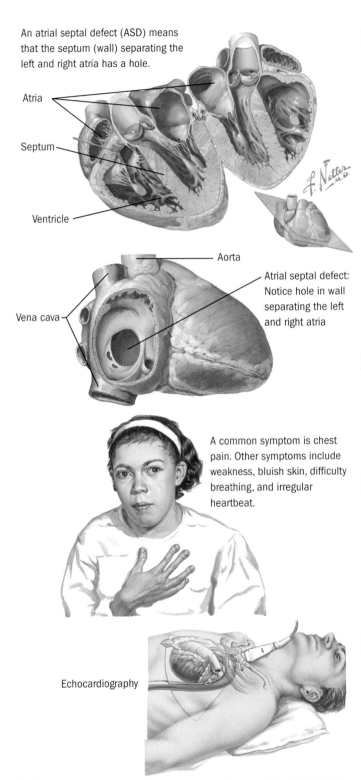

An atrial septal defect (ASD) means that the septum (wall) separating the left and right atria has a hole.

Atria

Septum

Ventricle

Aorta

Vena cava

Atrial septal defect: Notice hole in wall separating the left and right atria

A common symptom is chest pain. Other symptoms include weakness, bluish skin, difficulty breathing, and irregular heartbeat.

Echocardiography

To diagnose your problem, your doctor may want to do electrocardiography (ECG) and echocardiography (ultrasound of the heart) or send you to a heart specialist.

What Is Atrial Septal Defect?

The atria are the top chambers of the heart that send blood to the ventricles (bottom chambers). A septum is a wall separating the left and right sides of these chambers. An atrial septal defect (ASD) is an inborn (congenital) heart condition. It is a hole in the septum separating the left and right atria. The left side of the heart normally pumps under higher pressure than the right side. The defect produces a left-to-right shunt that allows blood from the two sides of the heart to mix. Blood with less oxygen is pumped to the body, and oxygenated blood travels back to the lungs. Abnormal circulation on the right side of the system causes increased pressure in the lungs (pulmonary hypertension).

ASD is more common in girls than boys. Some defects close as a child grows, but others may last into adulthood. ASD is the most common congenital heart defect diagnosed in adults. ASD cannot be prevented.

What Causes Atrial Septal Defect?

The cause is unknown. ASD develops before birth and may last into adulthood. ASD is more common in children with Down syndrome. The most common type of ASD, consisting of a small opening, is called a patent (open) foramen ovale (PFO).

What Are the Symptoms of Atrial Septal Defect?

Small defects may not cause a problem.

A large hole may produce weakness, breathing difficulties, chest pain, bluish skin color, and abnormal heartbeats (arrhythmias). Larger defects eventually overload the system controlled by the right side of the heart, possibly causing heart failure (inefficient pumping).

How Is Atrial Septal Defect Diagnosed?

The doctor may suspect the diagnosis on the basis of symptoms and findings at physical examination (heart murmur). An electrocardiogram (ECG) may show abnormalities. A chest x-ray may be abnormal, showing enlarged lung blood vessels and an enlarged heart. An echocardiogram (a test using ultrasound) can check the heart's structure and pumping and measure blood flow. The doctor may also recommend going to a cardiologist (a doctor who specializes in heart diseases) for more tests.

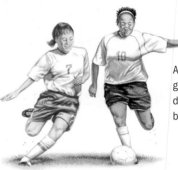

ASD is more common among girls than among boys. Some defects close as the child grows, but others may last into adulthood.

ASD is the most common congenital heart defect diagnosed among adults.

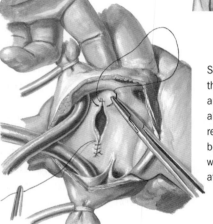

Surgery to fix the hole is the preferred treatment and is generally done at about the age of 4 years. A return to normal life can be expected in a few weeks to a few months after surgery.

People with ASD may be referred to a cardiologist.

Sometimes, people take medicine to treat symptoms.

FROM THE DESK OF

NOTES

How Is Atrial Septal Defect Treated?

People with very small defects or defects that close may never have symptoms and need no treatment. People who need treatment may be referred to a cardiologist. Medicine may also be given to treat symptoms. If the defect lasts, symptoms may develop that require treatment to correct the defect. Surgery is the preferred treatment and is usually done around the age of 4 years. If there is no other heart disease, correcting the defect usually allows a normal life span and lifestyle.

DOs and DON'Ts in Managing Atrial Septal Defect:

✔ **DO** take medicines as prescribed by your doctor.
✔ **DO** exercise, if your doctor says to do so.
✔ **DO** follow your doctor's advice to make sure you have full recovery and return to a normal life.
✔ **DO** call your doctor if you have such symptoms as shortness of breath, irregular heartbeat, chest pain, or bluish discoloration of your fingers.

⊘ **DON'T** ignore worsening symptoms. Get medical attention immediately.

FOR MORE INFORMATION

Contact the following sources:

* American Heart Association
  Tel: (800) 242-8721
  Website: http://www.americanheart.org

* Congenital Heart Information Network
  Tel: (215) 627-4034
  Fax: (215) 627-4036
  E-mail: mb@tchin.org
  Website: http://www.tchin.org

MANAGING YOUR
BUNDLE BRANCH BLOCK

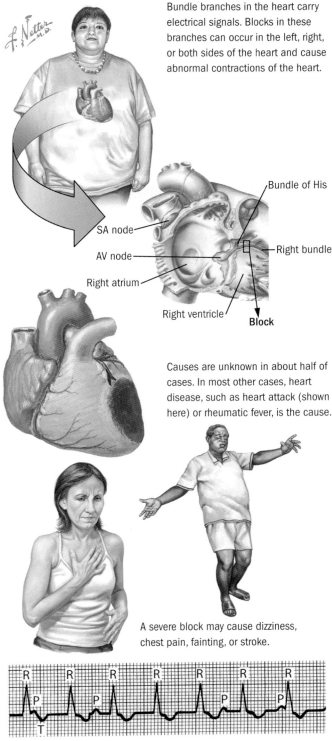

Bundle branches in the heart carry electrical signals. Blocks in these branches can occur in the left, right, or both sides of the heart and cause abnormal contractions of the heart.

Bundle of His

SA node

AV node

Right atrium

Right ventricle

Right bundle

Block

Causes are unknown in about half of cases. In most other cases, heart disease, such as heart attack (shown here) or rheumatic fever, is the cause.

A severe block may cause dizziness, chest pain, fainting, or stroke.

Your doctor will do a test called electrocardiography (ECG) to find out if you have a bundle block.

What Is Bundle Branch Block?

Many types of blocks of electrical signals occur in the heart. The heart has two bundle branches to carry electrical signals. The right and left bundles carry signals that cause the right and left ventricles (lower chambers of the heart) to contract. Signals start at the sinus (sinoatrial, or SA) node of the heart and spread through the atria (upper chambers) to the bundle of His and then to the bundle branches. Bundle branch block (BBB) is a delay of transmission of these signals from the atrium. These signals go through the bundle of His but are then blocked. The block can affect either the left or right side of the heart. The atria contract normally, but because the ventricles don't receive the signal. At the same time, the timing of contraction is affected.

BBB cannot be prevented.

What Causes BBB?

About half of cases have no known cause. Most people have some type of heart disease. They may have had damage to the heart from a heart attack (myocardial infarction), myocarditis (inflammation of heart muscle), or rheumatic fever (bacterial infection). Also, overdosing of certain medicines or congenital heart abnormality (present at birth) may be the cause.

What Are the Symptoms of BBB?

Most patients do not have any symptoms. Symptoms, when present, are related to not enough blood being pumped by the heart. Dizziness, fainting, angina (chest pain), or stroke (not enough blood flow to the brain) can occur in severe cases when there are other abnormalities present.

How Is BBB Diagnosed?

The doctor diagnoses BBB with electrocardiography (ECG), a test that measures the heart's electrical activity.

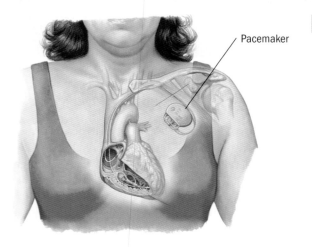

Pacemaker

Your doctor may recommend having a pacemaker inserted. A pacemaker is an electrical device that signals the heart to contract more regularly.

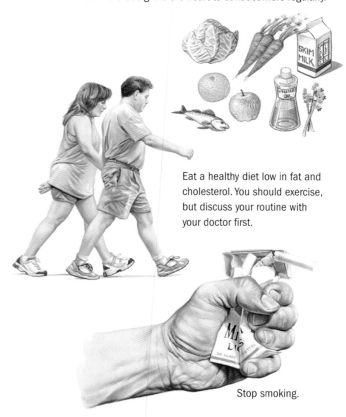

Eat a healthy diet low in fat and cholesterol. You should exercise, but discuss your routine with your doctor first.

Stop smoking.

How Is BBB Treated?

People without symptoms and heart disease need no treatment. People can exercise as tolerated (after checking with the doctor) and should have a healthy heart lifestyle.

People with symptoms and other heart rhythm abnormalities may have a pacemaker inserted. A pacemaker is an electrical device with a wire connected to the heart muscle to signal the ventricles to contract more regularly or faster (in response to more activity). Pacemakers can be outside the body, with the wire entering through a vein, or can be put inside the body. Newer pacemakers are safe and reliable. Still, strong magnetic or ultrasonic forces such as those used in physical therapy settings or airport security screening should be avoided.

DOs and DON'Ts in Managing BBB:

✔ **DO** take medicines as directed.
✔ **DO** eat a low-fat and low-cholesterol diet.
✔ **DO** lose weight.
✔ **DO** stop smoking.
✔ **DO** exercise as directed by your doctor if you have a pacemaker that will adjust to increased activity.
✔ **DO** call your doctor if you have dizziness, fainting, chest pain, or shortness of breath.

⊘ **DON'T** ignore worsening symptoms.

FROM THE DESK OF

NOTES

FOR MORE INFORMATION

Contact the following source:

• American Heart Association
Tel: (800) 242-8721
Website: http://www.americanheart.org

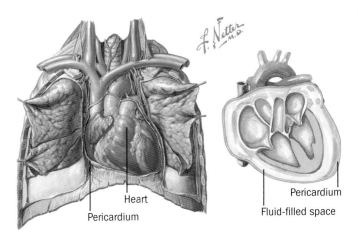

Heart

Pericardium

Pericardium

Fluid-filled space

The pericardium is a fluid-filled sac of tissue around the heart that keeps the heart in place and prevents it from rubbing against other body parts. If too much fluid pushes on the heart, it affects its pumping action. This is cardiac tamponade.

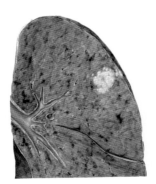

Lung cancer

Kidney failure

Chronic cardiac tamponade occurs slowly, because of cancer, kidney failure, underactive thyroid, or infection. Symptoms include shortness of breath and fast heartbeat.

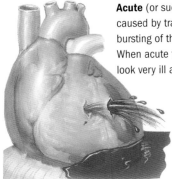

Acute (or sudden) cardiac tamponade is caused by trauma, such as a knife wound, or bursting of the heart muscle after a heart attack. When acute tamponade occurs, the person will look very ill and need immediate medical care.

What Is Cardiac Tamponade?

The heart really has one function: to pump blood. The heart is made up of muscle that contracts. A two-layered, fluid-filled sac of tissue, the pericardium, surrounds the heart. The pericardium keeps the heart in position and prevents the heart from moving too much or rubbing against other parts of the body.

Cardiac tamponade is a condition in which the heart is compressed by too much fluid in the pericardium, affecting its pumping action.

Cardiac tamponade can be life threatening. Prompt diagnosis and emergency treatment can be lifesaving. Intensive care monitoring is usually needed.

What Causes Cardiac Tamponade?

Tamponade can be chronic (occur slowly). The most common causes are cancers (lung, breast, lymphoma), kidney failure, underactive thyroid, and infections.

Tamponade can also be acute (sudden) and usually results from trauma, such as a penetrating knife wound or motor vehicle accident (when the chest hits the steering wheel and causes a tear of the main artery leaving the heart, called an aortic dissection).

Other causes of acute tamponade include bursting of the heart muscle after a heart attack and holes made in the heart during an operation (such as putting in a pacemaker).

What Are the Symptoms of Cardiac Tamponade?

People with chronic tamponade have shortness of breath, fast heartbeat, and possibly low blood pressure with abnormal heart sounds (friction rubs). Most people with acute tamponade are very ill and have low blood pressure with heart sounds that are hard to hear. Acute tamponade is a surgical emergency.

Chronic cardiac tamponade: Diagnosis and treatment

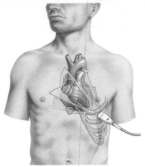

Echocardiography (ultrasound of the heart) can be used to see fluid in the sac.

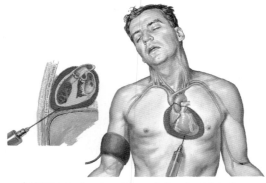

A needle can be placed through the chest, into the pericardium, to remove fluid for study and diagnosis.

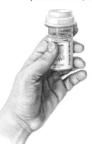

Your doctor may prescribe medicine depending on the cause of the tamponade.

Acute cardiac tamponade: Diagnosis and treatment

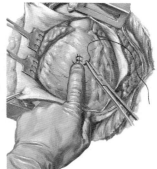

Acute tamponade is an emergency. A specialist called a cardiothoracic surgeon will likely be involved in care. Treatment will be based on the cause. For example, a tear in the pericardium will need to be sewn closed with stitches.

How Is Cardiac Tamponade Diagnosed?

The doctor may suspect cardiac tamponade by the person's symptoms and physical exam. Echocardiography (ultrasound of the heart) will confirm the diagnosis.

In people with life-threatening tamponade, a needle is put through the chest into the pericardium. This lets the doctor remove fluid as part of treatment and lets a doctor study the fluid under a microscope to determine the cause of the tamponade.

How Is Cardiac Tamponade Treated?

Treatment of chronic tamponade depends on the cause. In the case of cancer, drugs specific for the type of cancer will be suggested. Antibiotics or antifungal drugs can be used if the tamponade is due to a bacterial or fungal infection.

Acute tamponade is an emergency. A specialist called a cardiothoracic surgeon (who treats diseases of the heart and blood vessels) will likely be involved in care. Again, treatment depends on the specific cause of the tamponade.

DOs and DON'Ts in Managing Cardiac Tamponade:

✔ **DO** understand that cardiac tamponade affects the pumping action of the heart. This means that the heart cannot maintain blood pressure. Fluid must be removed very quickly to prevent shock and death.

✔ **DO** call your doctor if you are short of breath or have chest pain with fever, chills, and sweats.

⊘ **DON'T** forget that a cardiothoracic surgeon and a cardiologist (a medical doctor specializing in heart diseases) are best trained for treating cardiac tamponade.

⊘ **DON'T** miss your follow-up doctor appointments after you are discharged from the hospital. Pericardial fluid can sometimes build up again.

FROM THE DESK OF

NOTES

FOR MORE INFORMATION

Contact the following source:

• American Heart Association National Center
7272 Greenville Avenue
Dallas, TX 75231
Tel: (800) 242-8721

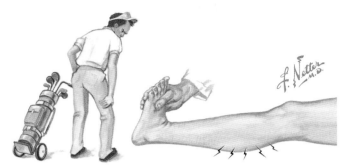

Poor circulation (also called claudication) is leg pain brought on by physical activity and relieved by rest. It affects mostly the calf muscle, but also feet, hips, thighs, and buttocks.

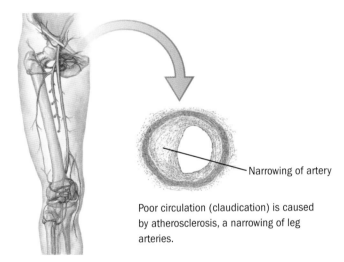

Narrowing of artery

Poor circulation (claudication) is caused by atherosclerosis, a narrowing of leg arteries.

Risk factors for getting atherosclerosis

 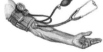

High cholesterol   High blood pressure   Tobacco use   Diabetes

The doctor diagnoses poor circulation by checking symptoms and ordering tests of blood vessels to check blood flow.

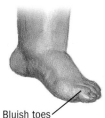 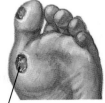 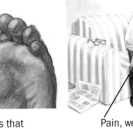

Bluish toes   Foot sores that don't heal   Pain, weakness, and limping

What Is Poor Circulation?

Poor circulation (also called claudication) refers to leg pain caused by exercise and relieved by rest. It is also called intermittent claudication, peripheral vascular disease (PVD), and poor circulation. The calf muscle is most likely affected, but feet, thighs, and buttocks can also be painful.

What Causes Poor Circulation?

The main cause is atherosclerosis, or narrowing of arteries that go to leg muscles. Risk factors leading to atherosclerosis are diabetes, high cholesterol level, high blood pressure, and smoking. Smoking tobacco is the major reason that disease worsens.

Claudication is not contagious or passed on from generation to generation.

What Are the Symptoms of Poor Circulation?

Symptoms are pain, muscle tension, weakness, and limping that occur after exercise and disappear after short rest. Other symptoms are cold feet at night, pain in the toe and foot, numbness of the leg, hair loss, brittle toenails, bluish toes, and foot sores that don't heal. Skin breakdown, ulcers, and gangrene can occur.

How Is Poor Circulation Diagnosed?

The doctor makes the diagnosis by checking symptoms and doing a physical exam. The doctor can order tests of blood vessels (including Doppler ultrasound) to find out about blood flow. If the tests show decreased circulation, angiography will be done before surgery. Angiography involves putting a catheter (small tube) into the artery of the leg and injecting dye to get a picture of the vessel.

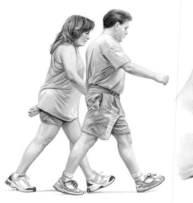
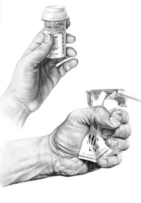

To relieve symptoms and prevent the condition from coming back, your doctor may suggest a healthier lifestyle, quitting smoking, and taking medicine to help blood circulate.

Sometimes an operation called angioplasty may be done. A balloon-tipped tube is inserted into the vessel and inflated to widen the vessel. Also, a stent (small mesh tube) may be put into the vessel to keep it open.

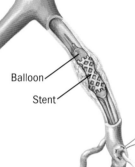

Balloon

Stent

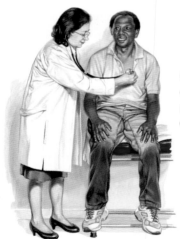

Get regular checkups so your doctor can check your blood pressure and blood sugar and cholesterol levels.

How Is Poor Circulation Treated?

The treatment goal is to relieve symptoms and prevent the condition from getting worse. Most people respond to lifestyle changes, including avoiding tobacco (the best treatment), losing weight, and changing the diet to control diabetes, hypertension, and high cholesterol. If symptoms remain, the doctor may prescribe medicine to help blood circulate better. A daily low dose of aspirin may be needed. Proper foot care is important to prevent infection.

If the blood flow is very reduced, a minor procedure called angioplasty may be advised to open up the blocked artery.

A balloon-tipped tube (catheter) is inserted into the narrowed vessel and inflated to widen the vessel. Also, a stent (small mesh tube) may be put into the vessel by angioplasty.

Sometimes, a tube of special material is joined to the vessel above and below where it is narrowed. This lets blood bypass the narrowed vessel.

People need surgery if they have ulcers that don't heal, their foot is cold and blue, the limb has gangrene, or they have severe pain at rest.

DOs and DON'Ts in Managing Poor Circulation:

✔ **DO** control risk factors of atherosclerosis (diabetes, high cholesterol, high blood pressure, smoking).

✔ **DO** exercise, control obesity, stop smoking, perform daily foot care, keep your blood pressure in check, and eat a low-fat diet.

✔ **DO** ask your doctor about your cholesterol, blood sugar, and blood pressure.

✔ **DO** call your doctor if you have calf, thigh, or buttock pain with walking.

✔ **DO** call your doctor if you have foot skin ulcers, a cold foot, or color changes in your feet.

🚫 **DON'T** smoke.

🚫 **DON'T** wear restrictive clothes on the legs, such as elastic stockings.

🚫 **DON'T** miss follow-up doctor appointments, especially to check on ulcer healing.

FROM THE DESK OF

NOTES

FOR MORE INFORMATION

Contact the following sources:

• National Heart, Lung, and Blood Institute
Tel: (301) 592-8573
Website: http://www.nhlb.nih.gov

• American Heart Association
Tel: (800) AHA-USA-1 (242-8721)
Website: http://www.americanheart.org

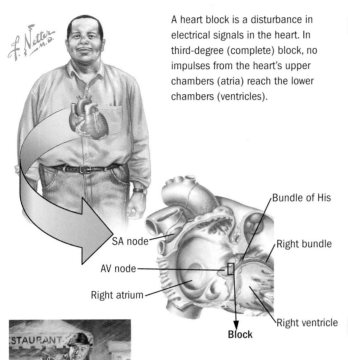

A heart block is a disturbance in electrical signals in the heart. In third-degree (complete) block, no impulses from the heart's upper chambers (atria) reach the lower chambers (ventricles).

SA node

AV node

Right atrium

Bundle of His

Right bundle

Right ventricle

Block

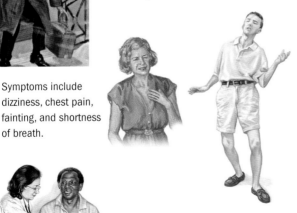

The cause is not always known. Heart conditions such as coronary artery disease and prior heart attacks can cause complete heart block.

Symptoms include dizziness, chest pain, fainting, and shortness of breath.

Your doctor may suspect a block if your pulse or heartbeat is slow during a regular examination. Tests such as an ECG are best for a certain diagnosis.

What Is Complete Heart Block?

The heart is a muscular pump with four chambers, two upper (left and right atria) and two lower (left and right ventricles). These contract and pump blood. Special tissue in the heart produces and sends electrical impulses to get the muscle to contract. Normal electrical signals start from the sinoatrial (SA) node in the wall of the right atrium. From there the signal goes to the left atrium and reaches the atrioventricular (AV) node between the atria and ventricles. The signal then goes to the left and right bundle branches and finally the ventricles. There it stimulates ventricles to contract.

Heart block refers to a disturbance of these impulses. Third-degree heart block, or complete heart block, is one of three types (first- and second-degree blocks are the others). In complete heart block, no impulses from the atria reach the ventricles. Signals are completely blocked at the AV node.

What Causes Complete Heart Block?

Complete heart block isn't contagious or passed from generation to generation. The exact cause is often unknown. It usually occurs in elderly people and may be the result of aging. Heart conditions including coronary artery disease, myocardial infarctions (heart attacks), heart valve disease, and congestive heart failure can cause complete heart block. Other causes are diseases, such as sarcoidosis, rheumatoid arthritis, or Lyme disease, and some medicines (e.g., digoxin, beta-blockers, and calcium channel blockers).

What Are the Symptoms of Complete Heart Block?

Symptoms can vary and include dizziness, lightheadedness, shortness of breath, chest pain, and fainting. Many people may have no symptoms.

How Is Complete Heart Block Diagnosed?

The doctor makes a diagnosis from the medical history and a very slow pulse at a physical examination.

The doctor will order electrocardiography (ECG) to measure the heart's electrical activity.

If additional tests are needed to confirm the diagnosis, a 24-hour recording of the heartbeat (Holter monitor) while following usual daily activities will be done. Sometimes, admission to a hospital is needed for constant monitoring.

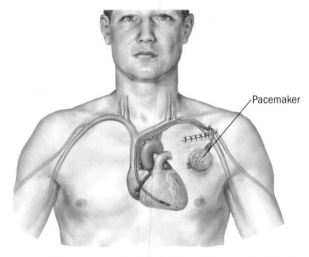

Pacemaker

Drugs cannot fix a complete heart block. The most common treatment is use of a pacemaker. A pacemaker is an electrical device that tells the heart to contract more regularly.

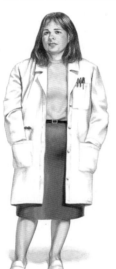

Talk to a specialist who treats heart diseases (cardiologist) about the different types of pacemakers available.

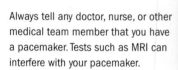

Always tell any doctor, nurse, or other medical team member that you have a pacemaker. Tests such as MRI can interfere with your pacemaker.

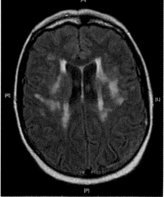

How Is Complete Heart Block Treated?

No drugs can treat complete heart block. If overdose of a drug is the cause, stopping the drug is required. The best treatment for complete heart block not caused by drugs is insertion of a pacemaker. Pacemakers are small, electrical devices put into the heart to tell it to beat to stimulate the heart to beat in a normal fashion.

DOs and DON'Ts in Managing Complete Heart Block:

✔ **DO** carry your pacemaker ID card. The card describes the type of pacemaker, insertion date, model, and serial number.

✔ **DO** call your doctor if you pass out with no warning, feel faint, or have chest pain or shortness of breath.

⊘ **DON'T** forget that certain devices such as cell phones and powerful magnets can make the pacemaker malfunction.

⊘ **DON'T** forget to tell doctors who suggest procedures such as magnetic resonance imaging (MRI) that you have a pacemaker.

FROM THE DESK OF

NOTES

FOR MORE INFORMATION

Contact the following source:

- American Heart Association
  Tel: (800) 242-8721
  Website: http://www.americanheart.org

MANAGING YOUR
CONGESTIVE HEART FAILURE (CHF)

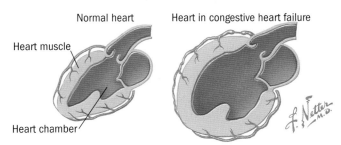

Normal heart   Heart in congestive heart failure

Heart muscle

Heart chamber

In CHF, the heart cannot pump enough blood to organs and tissues. Blood backs up in one side of the heart causing the other side to work harder.

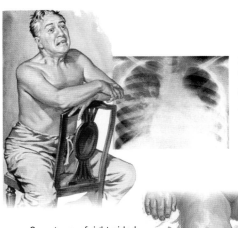

Symptoms of left-sided CHF include shortness of breath and fluid in lungs. Patients may feel better sitting up than lying down.

Symptoms of right-sided CHF include swelling of the legs and feet.

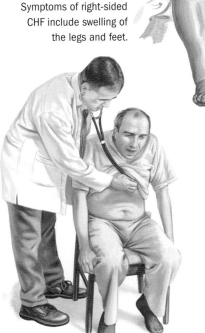

The doctor listens to the lungs for fluid buildup. Patients may be short of breath, and lips and nails may look blue.

What Is Congestive Heart Failure (CHF)?

CHF is a condition in which the heart cannot (fails to) pump enough blood to organs and tissues. One side of the heart (or both sides) cannot force enough blood out, so blood backs up. Congestion, or abnormal buildup of fluid, occurs in tissues or organs, and blood doesn't move well through the vascular system.

If the left side of the heart fails, the system on the right side becomes congested. The congested side of the heart must work harder and may also fail. The same thing can happen on the right side.

What Causes CHF?

Diseases that stress heart muscle can cause CHF. These conditions include high blood pressure, heart attack, heart muscle and valve diseases, infections, arrhythmias (abnormal heart rhythms), anemia, thyroid disease, pulmonary disease, and too much fluid in the body.

What Are the Symptoms of CHF?

When the left side of the heart fails, fluid leaks into the lungs. Fatigue (tiredness), difficulty breathing (especially at night when lying down), coughing, or shortness of breath can result.

In right-sided heart failure, the liver swells, which may cause pain in the abdomen (belly). Legs and feet may swell also.

How Is CHF Diagnosed?

A physical examination will show changes, such as swelling in the legs or crackling breath sounds, indicating excess fluid in the lungs.

A chest x-ray can show an enlarged heart and signs of fluid accumulation into the lungs. An echocardiogram (a test using sound waves to show the moving heart) can also reveal heart size and disease of the heart muscle or valve problems.

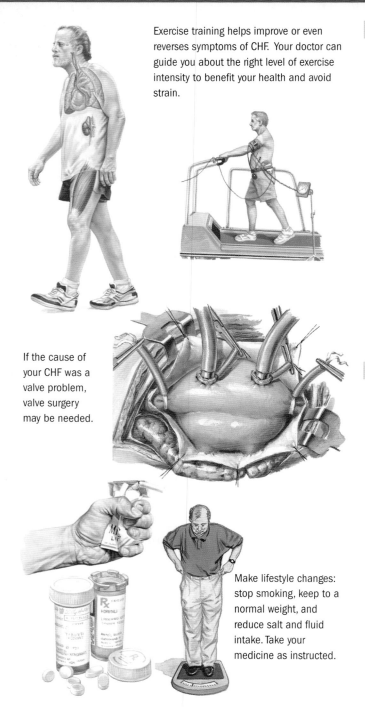

Exercise training helps improve or even reverses symptoms of CHF. Your doctor can guide you about the right level of exercise intensity to benefit your health and avoid strain.

If the cause of your CHF was a valve problem, valve surgery may be needed.

Make lifestyle changes: stop smoking, keep to a normal weight, and reduce salt and fluid intake. Take your medicine as instructed.

How Is CHF Treated?

Initial symptoms should be managed so the failing heart doesn't have to work as hard.

The cause of CHF also needs treatment. For example, if a heart valve problem is the cause, surgery may be needed to repair or replace the valve. Lifestyle changes will be needed. Smoking lowers the blood oxygen level and makes the heart work harder, so avoid tobacco. Less fluid and salt in the diet reduces fluid in the body. Also, losing weight will help. Dietitians and nutritionists can help plan a diet.

Oxygen may be given to reduce the workload on the lungs.

Medicines may be prescribed to reduce fluid in the body or help the ventricle contract better. Diuretics remove fluid. Nitrates open blood vessels so blood flows more easily. Angiotensin-converting enzyme (ACE) inhibitors help the ventricle contract. Beta-blockers help by slowing the heart rate. Other drugs reduce blood pressure. All may have side effects, including dehydration, cough, dizziness, fainting, and fatigue.

DOs and DON'Ts in Managing CHF:

✔ **DO** take your medicines properly.
✔ **DO** maintain your ideal body weight.
✔ **DO** reduce salt and extra fluid in your diet.
✔ **DO** get your family involved in your care, especially the needed lifestyle changes.
✔ **DO** call your doctor if you have side effects from your drugs or new or worsening symptoms, such as increasing shortness of breath, chest pain, or fainting.

⊘ **DON'T** forget to take all your medicines as directed.
⊘ **DON'T** smoke.
⊘ **DON'T** stop taking any medicines without telling your doctor.

FROM THE DESK OF

NOTES

FOR MORE INFORMATION

Contact the following source:

• American Heart Association
  Tel: (800) 242-8721
  Website: http://www.americanheart.org

MANAGING YOUR
CORONARY ARTERY DISEASE

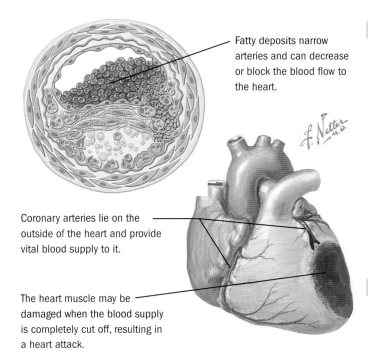

Fatty deposits narrow arteries and can decrease or block the blood flow to the heart.

Coronary arteries lie on the outside of the heart and provide vital blood supply to it.

The heart muscle may be damaged when the blood supply is completely cut off, resulting in a heart attack.

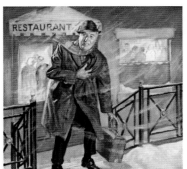

Cold weather, heavy meals, exertion, stress, and smoking can lead to chest pain (angina) in people with CAD. Left-sided chest pain is a classic symptom of angina.

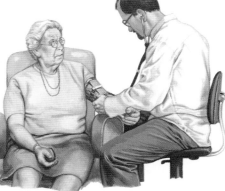

Coronary artery disease affects over 12 million Americans. You can help manage many of the risk factors in your lifestyle choices.

What Is Coronary Artery Disease (CAD)?

The heart pumps oxygen-rich blood through the huge network of arteries throughout the body. The blood carries oxygen and nutrients, especially sugar (glucose), needed by organs in the body. In coronary artery disease (CAD), or coronary heart disease, fatty deposits build up on inner layers of coronary arteries. These blood vessels are on the outside of the heart and take blood to the heart muscle itself. These fatty deposits, or plaque, may form in childhood and continue to thicken and enlarge throughout life. This thickening, called atherosclerosis, narrows the arteries and can reduce or block blood flow to the heart.

More than 12 million Americans have CAD, the number one killer of both men and women in the country.

What Are the Risk Factors for CAD?

Risk factors include high cholesterol levels in blood, high blood pressure (hypertension), inactivity, smoking, obesity, diabetes, and a family history of CAD.

What Are the Symptoms of CAD?

If too little oxygenated blood reaches the heart, chest pain called angina occurs. A complete block of the blood supply can cause a heart attack, with damage to the heart muscle. Symptoms of CAD depend on how severe the disease is. Some people with CAD have no symptoms, some have mild angina, and some have more severe angina. Other symptoms include feelings of heaviness, tightness, and pressure in the chest; pain in the arms, shoulders, jaw, neck, or back; shortness of breath; and nausea.

How Is CAD Diagnosed?

The doctor will take a complete medical history and do a physical examination and blood tests. Other tests include an electrocardiogram (ECG or EKG), which records the heart's electrical activity. A stress test (also called treadmill or exercise ECG) and coronary angiography (takes x-ray pictures of arteries) may be done. The doctor may also order nuclear scanning, which uses a radioactive dye to show healthy and damaged parts of the heart.

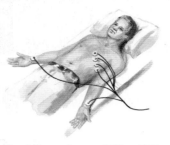
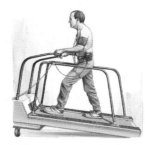

An electrocardiogram (ECG or EKG) or treadmill stress text may be done to diagnose CAD.

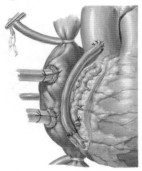
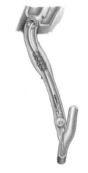

Graft   Stent

Have your blood pressure checked regularly. Medicines to help control your blood pressure may be prescribed by your doctor. Surgery (such as the graft or stent, pictured above) may be an option.

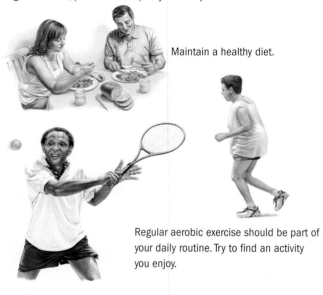

Maintain a healthy diet.

Regular aerobic exercise should be part of your daily routine. Try to find an activity you enjoy.

How Is Coronary Artery Disease Treated?

Controlling risk factors is crucial for preventing and treating CAD. Lifestyle changes include eating a low-fat diet and losing weight (if overweight), following a good exercise program, quitting smoking, controlling blood sugar (glucose) if diabetic, and reducing blood pressure.

Drugs are often prescribed to lower blood pressure, lower cholesterol, and increase coronary blood flow. More severe CAD may need coronary angioplasty, a procedure to widen arteries, which may include using a stent (special device to keep the artery open). The doctor may advise coronary artery bypass surgery, in which blood vessels from another part of the body (e.g., legs) are used to create a new route around blocked arteries.

DOs and DON'Ts in Managing Coronary Artery Disease:

✔ **DO** eat a healthy diet, rich in fruits, vegetables, and low-fat dairy products with less saturated and total fats.
✔ **DO** take your prescribed medicines.
✔ **DO** lower your dietary sodium (salt) intake to no more than 2400 mg per day.
✔ **DO** regular aerobic physical exercise, such as brisk walking (at least 30 minutes per day, most days of the week).
✔ **DO** keep to a normal body weight.

⊘ **DON'T** smoke or use tobacco products.
⊘ **DON'T** exert yourself too much, and avoid cold and stress.

FROM THE DESK OF

NOTES

FOR MORE INFORMATION

Contact the following sources:

- American Heart Association
  Tel: (800) 242-8721
  Website: http://www.americanheart.org

- National Heart, Lung, and Blood Institute
  Website: http://www.nhlbi.nih.gov

- American College of Cardiology
  Website: http://www.acc.org

MANAGING YOUR
DEEP VEIN THROMBOSIS

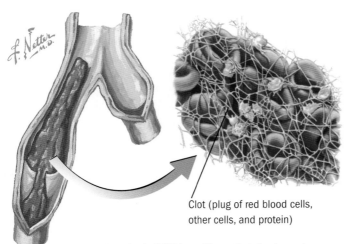

Clot (plug of red blood cells, other cells, and protein)

Deep vein thrombosis (DVT) is an illness that develops when blood clots in a vein. The clot causes blood flow to slow, resulting in pain and swelling. People who are physically inactive, elderly, or pregnant are at higher risk.

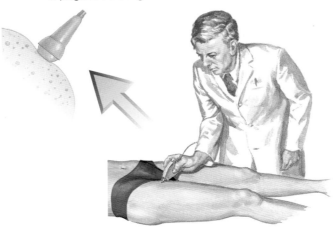

Your doctor may recommend ultrasound of the swollen leg or other part to measure blood flow in the area.

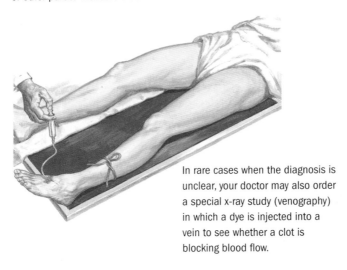

In rare cases when the diagnosis is unclear, your doctor may also order a special x-ray study (venography) in which a dye is injected into a vein to see whether a clot is blocking blood flow.

What Is Deep Vein Thrombosis?

Deep vein thrombosis (DVT) is an illness that develops when the blood clots in a vein. Affected veins are usually deep in leg muscles but can also be in other areas. The clot (thrombus) causes blood flow to slow. The area becomes swollen, red, and painful. If the clot moves to the lungs, a pulmonary embolism occurs and serious breathing problems can develop.

DVT most often affects people who are physically inactive, elderly, pregnant, or have blood disorders that increase the risk of blood clotting.

What Causes DVT?

Prolonged bed rest (more than 3 days), recent surgery (with anesthesia for more than 30 minutes), smoking, being overweight, air or car travel for prolonged periods, using certain oral contraceptives and estrogen replacement therapies, and family or personal history of blood clotting problems can increase the risk of DVT.

What Are the Symptoms of DVT?

Symptoms are pain, tenderness, warmth, swelling, and redness in the area.

How Is DVT Diagnosed?

The doctor will ask about symptoms and do an examination. If DVT is suspected, the doctor may recommend a sonogram (ultrasound) of the swollen leg or other part to measure blood flow in the area and a blood test (D-dimer). In rare cases when the diagnosis is suspected but sonogram and blood tests are inconclusive, the doctor may also order a special x-ray study (venography) in which a dye is injected into the vein to see whether a clot is blocking blood flow. Measuring clotting time of the blood may indicate a blood clot.

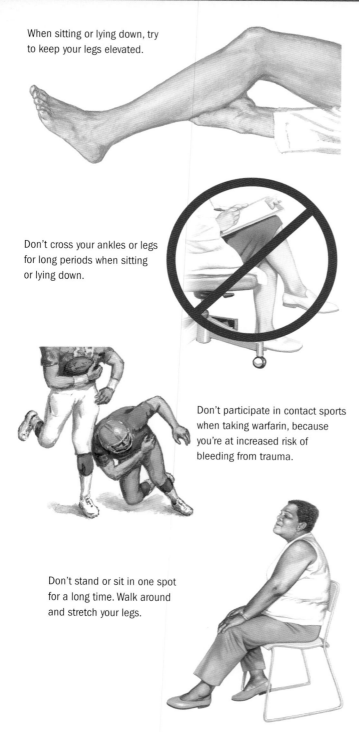

When sitting or lying down, try to keep your legs elevated.

Don't cross your ankles or legs for long periods when sitting or lying down.

Don't participate in contact sports when taking warfarin, because you're at increased risk of bleeding from trauma.

Don't stand or sit in one spot for a long time. Walk around and stretch your legs.

FROM THE DESK OF

NOTES

How Is DVT Treated?

Treatment is immediate injection of a blood thinner (heparin) to thin the blood and prevent growth of blood clots. Heparin can be given intravenously or injected under the skin (subcutaneously). Your doctor will decide which option is best for you. The doctor will also prescribe blood thinning pills (warfarin) to prevent the clot from enlarging and stop new ones from forming. For a few days, both heparin and warfarin are given. When warfarin reaches the desired level in blood, heparin will be stopped and warfarin will be continued, usually for 6 months, at times longer, depending on the cause of the DVT. Lifetime treatment may sometimes be needed. Blood tests to make sure that the warfarin dose is correct must be done.

The doctor may also recommend special stockings to control swelling in the legs. Overweight people should lose weight and become more active to prevent future clots.

DOs and DON'Ts in Managing DVT:

✔ **DO** take medicine and go for the blood tests (INR) as directed by your doctor to monitor the blood thinner level.
✔ **DO** follow your doctor's advice about losing weight and exercising more to lower your risk of recurrence of DVT.
✔ **DO** walk around and stretch your legs if you sit for long periods.
✔ **DO** call your doctor if your symptoms don't get better.
✔ **DO** call your doctor immediately if you have chest pain or cough up blood.
✔ **DO** call your doctor before you go on a long trip and ask your doctor about taking aspirin if you are no longer taking warfarin.
✔ **DO** try to keep your legs elevated when sitting or lying down.

⊘ **DON'T** stand or sit in one spot for a long time.
⊘ **DON'T** wear clothing that restricts blood flow in your legs.
⊘ **DON'T** cross your ankles or legs when sitting or lying down.
⊘ **DON'T** smoke.
⊘ **DON'T** participate in contact sports when taking warfarin, because you're at risk of bleeding from trauma.

FOR MORE INFORMATION

Contact the following sources:

• The Center for Outcome Research and the Venous Education Institute of North America (VEIN)
  Website: http://www.dvt.org

• The American Heart Association
  Tel: (800) 242-8721
  Website: http://www.americanheart.org

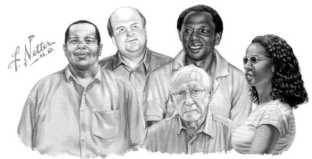

Dilated cardiomyopathy is a disease of the heart muscle. More men than women have it, and more African Americans than whites have it. Risk factors include obesity, family history of heart disease, and alcoholism.

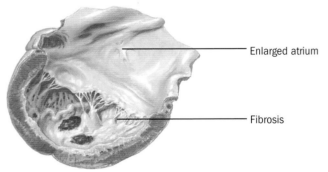

Enlarged atrium

Fibrosis

In cardiomyopathy, the heart can't pump enough blood to body organs. The heart weakens, heart muscle thickens, and the four heart chambers (top atria and bottom ventricles) get larger. Heart valves may be affected.

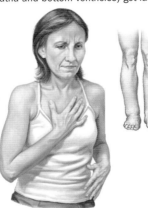

Symptoms include feeling tired and less able to exercise, shortness of breath, swelling of the legs or feet, chest pain, and heart palpitations.

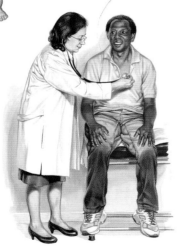

Your doctor will ask about symptoms, do a physical examination, and order tests such as ECG and chest x-rays.

What Is Dilated Cardiomyopathy?

Dilated cardiomyopathy is a disease of the heart muscle that prevents the muscle from producing the normal force of contraction. Therefore the heart cannot pump enough blood to the organs in the body. The heart becomes weaker and the four heart chambers get larger (dilate). These chambers are the atria (upper chambers) and ventricles (lower chambers). The heart muscle may thicken so that it can produce more force to keep blood pumping normally. The heart valves may also be affected as the heart chambers get large, which may worsen the flow of blood. The impaired heart action can affect lungs, liver, and other organs.

More men (about three times as many) than women have cardiomyopathy, and more African Americans (about three times) than whites.

What Causes Dilated Cardiomyopathy?

The cause is usually unknown. Factors that damage the heart muscle and lead to heart failure can cause it. These factors include coronary artery disease, poorly controlled diabetes, anemia, and valvular heart disease. Harmful chemicals (such as alcohol), infections, medications, cocaine, heroin, and some connective tissue diseases may also cause it. Cardiomyopathy cannot be prevented, but avoiding harmful chemicals such as alcohol may reduce the risk of getting it.

What Are the Symptoms of Dilated Cardiomyopathy?

Most people feel tired (fatigue), less able to exercise, or short of breath. Swelling of the legs or feet, chest pain, and palpitations (feeling that the heart beats too fast) may also occur.

How Is Dilated Cardiomyopathy Diagnosed?

The doctor will ask about symptoms, do a complete physical examination, and order tests. Electrocardiography (ECG) and chest x-rays, which can show an enlarged heart, will be done. The doctor will suggest seeing a heart specialist (cardiologist) for additional tests. Echocardiography (ultrasound examination of the heart) or angiography (special x-ray examination to check blood flow through the heart) may be done to determine how much damage is present.

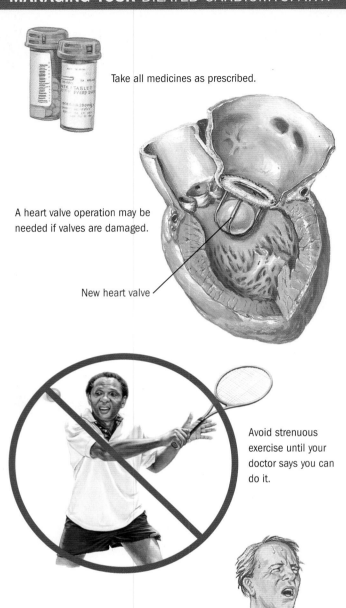

Take all medicines as prescribed.

A heart valve operation may be needed if valves are damaged.

New heart valve

Avoid strenuous exercise until your doctor says you can do it.

Call your doctor if you have new or worsening chest pain.

How Is Dilated Cardiomyopathy Treated?

Therapy is aimed at relieving symptoms and correcting abnormal heart rhythms (arrhythmias). Lowering salt intake and resting are important. A heart valve operation may be needed for damaged valves. If the cause of the cardiomyopathy is known, that condition is treated. The doctor may prescribe medicines to control the heart rhythm (antiarrhythmics) and dilate blood vessels (vasodilators), water pills (diuretics), and nutritional supplements. A cardioverter defibrillator may be inserted in the chest in people responding poorly to medications. If the heart's pumping action is seriously impaired and symptoms of heart failure get worse, heart transplantation can be considered for young people.

DOs and DON'Ts in Managing Dilated Cardiomyopathy:

✔ **DO** lower the amount of sodium (salt) and fluid in your diet.
✔ **DO** take all medicines as prescribed.
✔ **DO** call your doctor if you have new or worsening chest pain, shortness of breath, swelling in the legs, or fainting.

🚫 **DON'T** drink alcohol.
🚫 **DON'T** do strenuous exercise until your doctor says that you can.
🚫 **DON'T** abuse drugs. Cocaine, heroin, and organic solvents such as glue can cause dilated cardiomyopathy.

FROM THE DESK OF

NOTES

FOR MORE INFORMATION

Contact the following source:

• American Heart Association
 Tel: (800) 242-8721
 Website: http://www.americanheart.org

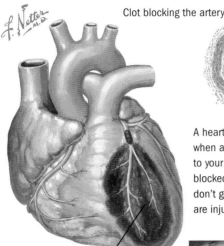

Clot blocking the artery

A heart attack, or MI, occurs when arteries carrying blood to your heart muscles are blocked. Then heart muscles don't get enough oxygen and are injured or die.

Dead muscle (infarct)

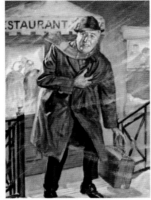

Chest pain is the most common symptom.

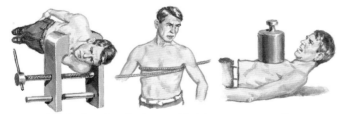

Pain is often described as crushing, heavy, or pressurelike.

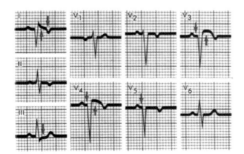

The doctor will examine you and take blood samples. The doctor will also order electrocardiography (ECG), which shows how much heart damage you have.

What Is a Heart Attack?

A heart attack, or myocardial infarction (MI), means that some heart muscles were injured or died because they didn't get enough oxygen. An MI occurs when arteries carrying blood to heart muscles (coronary arteries) are blocked.

What Causes a Heart Attack?

A heart attack occurs when a blood clot forms in a coronary artery and stops blood flow to the heart muscle, so the muscle is injured or dies. Smoking, high blood pressure, diabetes, high levels of cholesterol (a fatty substance), and a family history of heart disease and inflammation of the coronary arteries increase the risk of heart attacks.

What Are the Symptoms of a Heart Attack?

Chest pain, moderate to severe, is the most common symptom. Pain can also occur in the jaw, back, shoulders, or arms (especially the left arm). Pain is often described as crushing, heavy, or pressurelike. Some people have no pain. Sweating, shortness of breath, fast or irregular heartbeat, nausea, feeling of indigestion, and vomiting are other symptoms. Women and diabetics may have symptoms different from those in men, such as shortness of breath without chest pain.

How Is a Heart Attack Diagnosed?

The doctor will do an examination, take blood samples, and order electrocardiography (ECG) to see how well the heart beats.

How Is a Heart Attack Treated?

The treatment goal is to save as much heart muscle as possible. The choice of treatment depends on how much time has passed from the start of the heart attack and on the availability of special procedures at the hospital where you are treated. To salvage as much heart muscle as possible, medications to improve circulation and dissolve the clot blocking the artery are given, or a procedure called angioplasty may be done. Other medicine will control pain and blood pressure, and oxygen will help breathing. Other drugs, including aspirin and cholesterol-lowering drugs (statins), may be suggested.

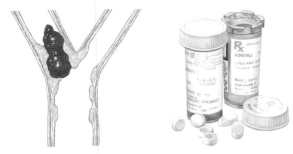

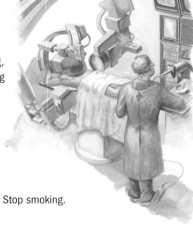

The blood clot that blocked the coronary artery is treated, usually first by clot-busting medicines. You may take other drugs, including aspirin and cholesterol-lowering drugs (statins).

Coronary angioplasty can open the blocked artery to allow blood to flow. In this procedure, a catheter (long, thin tube) is put into the leg and then into the blocked artery to open it.

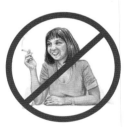

Stop smoking.

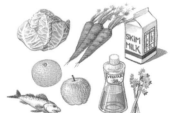

Eat a low-fat diet.

Try to maintain your ideal body weight.

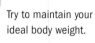

If angioplasty is done, a catheter (long plastic tube) is placed into a leg artery and passed to the heart to take pictures of coronary arteries. The blocked artery is opened with a small balloon on the tip of a catheter. A small metal wire mesh (stent) put into the blocked coronary artery will help keep the artery from blocking again. Medicine can also stop new blockage.

DOs and DON'Ts in Managing a Heart Attack:

✔ **DO** call 911 emergency if you have heart attack symptoms.
✔ **DO** understand that time is critical. The longer the blockage, the more heart damage.
✔ **DO** understand risk factors.
✔ **DO** stop smoking.
✔ **DO** take medicine as prescribed.
✔ **DO** have your cholesterol level checked regularly. Eat low-fat foods.
✔ **DO** try to maintain your ideal body weight.
✔ **DO** regular exercise, such as walking, if your doctor says it's OK.
✔ **DO** see your doctor regularly and call your doctor about changes in your condition, such as if you had a heart attack and develop shortness of breath when walking, and leg swelling or difficulty breathing when lying down.

🚫 **DON'T** forget to see a cardiologist (doctor specializing in heart diseases) for advice, both during and after a heart attack.
🚫 **DON'T** try to treat yourself or delay getting medical care.

FROM THE DESK OF

NOTES

FOR MORE INFORMATION

Contact the following sources:

- American Heart Association
  Tel: (800) 242-8721
  Website: http://www.americanheart.org
- National Heart, Lung, and Blood Institute
  Tel: (301) 592-8573
  Website: http://www.nhlbi.nih.gov
- American College of Cardiology
  Tel: (800) 253-4636
  Website: http://www.acc.org

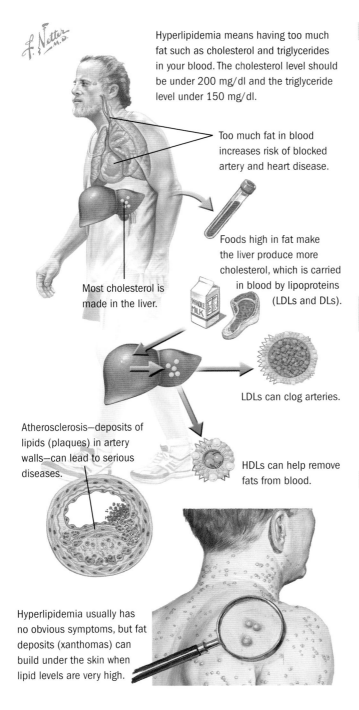

Hyperlipidemia means having too much fat such as cholesterol and triglycerides in your blood. The cholesterol level should be under 200 mg/dl and the triglyceride level under 150 mg/dl.

Too much fat in blood increases risk of blocked artery and heart disease.

Foods high in fat make the liver produce more cholesterol, which is carried in blood by lipoproteins (LDLs and DLs).

Most cholesterol is made in the liver.

LDLs can clog arteries.

Atherosclerosis—deposits of lipids (plaques) in artery walls—can lead to serious diseases.

HDLs can help remove fats from blood.

Hyperlipidemia usually has no obvious symptoms, but fat deposits (xanthomas) can build under the skin when lipid levels are very high.

What Is High Cholesterol?

Cholesterol is a lipid, or type of fat. It helps the body perform many normal functions. Cholesterol is made in the liver and carries fats in the bloodstream.

In the body, cholesterol forms fat-protein chemicals called lipoproteins. Lipoproteins are grouped as very low-density lipoproteins (VLDLs), low-density lipoproteins (LDLs), also known as "bad cholesterol," and high-density lipoproteins (HDLs). HDLs, "good cholesterol," help remove lipids from the bloodstream, so higher HDL levels are better.

VLDLs and LDLs can clog arteries. High levels of cholesterol, LDLs, and triglycerides (fatty substances) increase the risk for hardening of the arteries (atherosclerosis) and heart disease.

What Are the Causes and Symptoms of High Cholesterol?

Causes of hyperlipidemia include a family history, high-fat diet, being overweight, certain illnesses including diabetes, and some drugs.

Most people have no symptoms until their blood vessels are nearly closed or become clogged. Some people may have small fat deposits under the skin.

How Is High Cholesterol Diagnosed?

Blood levels of cholesterol, HDL, LDL, and triglycerides are measured. Preferred levels are less than 200 milligrams per deciliter (mg/dl) for cholesterol, less than 150 mg/dl for triglycerides, and over 40 mg/dl for HDLs. Recommended LDL levels are less than 130 mg/dl for most people but much lower (less than 70 mg/dl) for those with heart disease and diabetes.

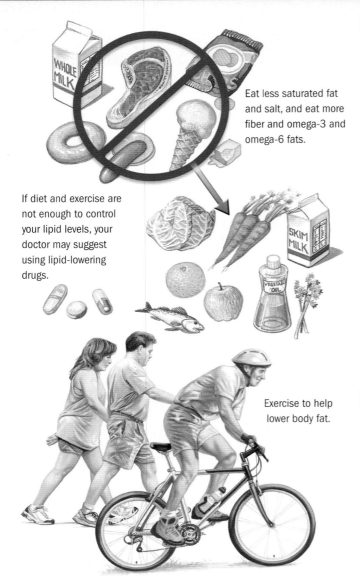

Eat less saturated fat and salt, and eat more fiber and omega-3 and omega-6 fats.

If diet and exercise are not enough to control your lipid levels, your doctor may suggest using lipid-lowering drugs.

Exercise to help lower body fat.

How Is High Cholesterol Treated?

Diet is the best way to reduce lipid levels. Lifestyle changes should reduce consumption of saturated fat to less than 7% of calories and cholesterol to less than 200 mg/day. Weight loss, exercise, and avoiding smoking are also important.

Lipid-lowering drugs are used when diet and exercise are not enough. The main classes of drugs include statins, fibrates, nicotinic acid, and omega-3 fatty acids.

Statins (e.g., simvastatin) reduce cholesterol and LDL production. They are effective, usually well tolerated, and preferred for higher cholesterol and LDL levels. They can have side effects such as muscle aches.

Fibrates (e.g., fenofibrate, gemfibrozil) help removal of VLDLs but have a small effect on cholesterol.

Nicotinic acid helps lower VLDL levels and increase HDL levels. Side effects (itching, facial flushing, liver problems) limit its use.

Omega-3 fatty acids (over-the-counter fish oil supplements) help patients with high triglyceride, low HDL, and moderate cholesterol levels.

DOs and DON'Ts in Managing High Cholesterol:

✔ **DO** exercise regularly.
✔ **DO** eat more fruits and vegetables and high-fiber foods such as oat bran. Cook with oils high in polyunsaturated fats such as safflower, sunflower, and corn oils (omega-6 fatty acids).
✔ **DO** eat fish (fish oils contain omega-3 fatty acids).
✔ **DO** stop smoking.
✔ **DO** lose weight by changing your diet and doing aerobic exercise such as walking, jogging, bicycling, or swimming. Exercise at least 30 minutes a day, 3 or 4 days a week.

⊘ **DON'T** forget to treat other medical conditions.
⊘ **DON'T** forget to take your usual medicines.
⊘ **DON'T** change your diet or medicines without your doctor's approval.

FROM THE DESK OF

NOTES

FOR MORE INFORMATION

Contact the following sources:

• American Heart Association
  Tel: (800) 242-8721
  Website: http://www.americanheart.org

• American College of Cardiology
  Tel: (800) 253-4636
  Website: http://www.acc.org

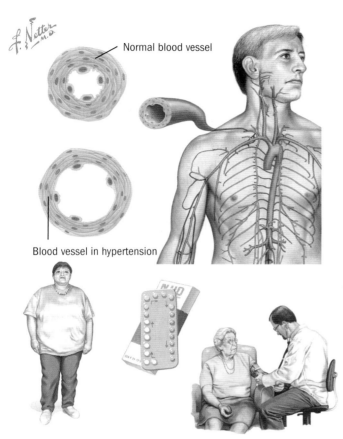

Normal blood vessel

Blood vessel in hypertension

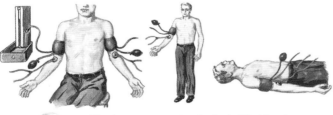

People with obesity and women taking oral contraceptives are at risk for hypertension. More than half of all Americans age 65 and older have high blood pressure (≥ 140/90 mm Hg)

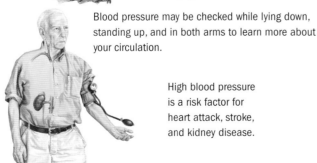

Blood pressure may be checked while lying down, standing up, and in both arms to learn more about your circulation.

High blood pressure is a risk factor for heart attack, stroke, and kidney disease.

What Is Hypertension?

Blood pressure is the force of the blood pushing against artery walls. Blood pressure is given as two numbers. The systolic pressure is the top number, and the diastolic pressure is the bottom number. Both are recorded as mm Hg (millimeters of mercury), which tells how high a column of mercury is raised by the pressure. Normal values are usually 120/80. The American Heart Association defines hypertension for adults as 140 mm Hg or higher systolic and/or 90 mm Hg or higher diastolic. These numbers should be used as a guide only.

What Causes Blood Pressure to Increase?

Being overweight, excessive salt (sodium) intake, some medications, and lack of physical activity contribute to hypertension.

What Are the Risk Factors for Hypertension?

More than half of all Americans age 65 and older have hypertension. People with obesity, diabetes, gout, or kidney disease; heavy drinkers of alcohol; and women taking birth control pills are at increased risk. African Americans (especially those living in southeastern United States) and people with parents or grandparents with hypertension have an increased risk.

What Are the Symptoms of Hypertension?

People usually have no or only mild vague symptoms. Severe hypertension can produce headaches, dizziness, blurred vision, nausea, ringing in the ears, confusion, and fatigue.

How Is Hypertension Diagnosed?

Hypertension is diagnosed only if blood pressure is high during at least three office visits. The doctor may check blood pressure in lying down and standing up positions, and in both arms.

What Are the Complications of Hypertension?

Untreated hypertension strains the heart and arteries and in time damages them. Hypertension is a key risk factor for heart failure, heart attack (myocardial infarction), stroke, and eye or kidney damage.

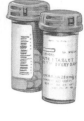

Your doctor may prescribe drugs to regulate the heart rate and contractions. These drugs include beta-blockers (e.g., propranolol) and calcium channel blockers (e.g., verapamil).

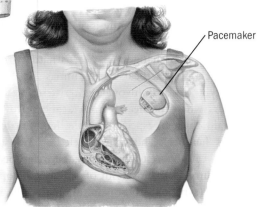

Pacemaker

If drugs aren't effective or cause severe side effects, implanting a pacemaker is possible.

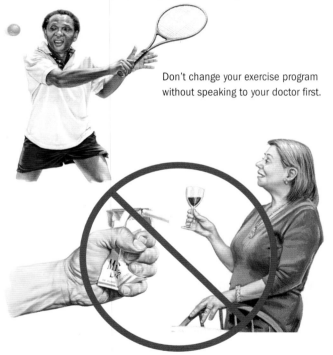

Don't change your exercise program without speaking to your doctor first.

Don't smoke or drink alcohol.

How Is Hypertrophic Cardiomyopathy Treated?

Treatment is aimed at controlling symptoms and slowing the disease progress by reducing excessive contractions of the ventricle. Symptoms of heart failure and arrhythmias are also treated. Drugs are usually prescribed to regulate the heart rate and strength of contractions. These drugs include beta-blockers (e.g., propranolol) and calcium channel blockers (e.g., verapamil). A pacemaker is an option to control the heartbeat. It is a small device that is put into the body during surgery. Surgery may also be done to remove part of the abnormal muscle and reduce the blockage of blood flow. Heart transplantation is possible for people who don't respond to other treatments.

DOs and DON'Ts in Managing Hypertrophic Cardiomyopathy:

✔ **DO** take medicine as prescribed by your doctor.
✔ **DO** tell your doctor if your symptoms get worse or don't improve with treatment.
✔ **DO** remember that family members should be checked for this disorder.
✔ **DO** call your doctor if you have new or worsening chest pain, shortness of breath, swelling in the legs, or fainting.

⊘ **DON'T** change your exercise program without telling your doctor first.
⊘ **DON'T** take over-the-counter drugs, foods, or herbal supplements before checking with your doctor because they may react with your heart medicine.
⊘ **DON'T** smoke.
⊘ **DON'T** drink alcohol.

FROM THE DESK OF

NOTES

FOR MORE INFORMATION

Contact the following sources:

- American Heart Association
  Tel: (800) 242-8721
  Website: http://www.americanheart.org
- American College of Cardiology
  Tel: (800) 253-4636
  Website: http://www.acc.org

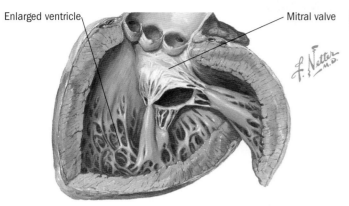

Enlarged ventricle

Mitral valve

The mitral valve is the valve in the heart that opens when the left atrium pumps blood into the left ventricle. Blood leaking back through the valve into the atrium from the ventricle is called mitral regurgitation.

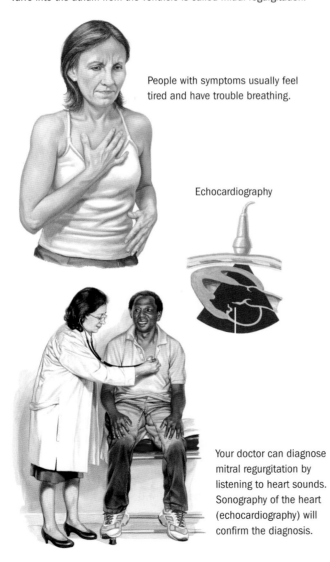

People with symptoms usually feel tired and have trouble breathing.

Echocardiography

Your doctor can diagnose mitral regurgitation by listening to heart sounds. Sonography of the heart (echocardiography) will confirm the diagnosis.

What Is Mitral Regurgitation?

The mitral valve in the heart is between the left atrium (a chamber in the top part of the heart) and left ventricle (a chamber in the bottom part). It opens when the atrium pumps blood into the ventricle. It closes when the ventricle pumps blood out into the body. Closing prevents the blood from going back into the atrium. Blood leaking back into the atrium from the ventricle is called regurgitation (or insufficiency or incompetence). Blood isn't pumped out of the heart properly, and the atrium cannot fill during the next cycle. Blood may back up in the right-sided system (to the lungs) and cause lungs to fill with fluid. The left ventricle then has to do more work to move blood. This extra work may later cause heart failure.

What Causes Mitral Regurgitation?

The cause is damage to the mitral valve. Damage may result from a congenital abnormality (present at birth) or a heart attack (or myocardial infarction, in which parts of the heart die because they don't have enough blood). Other causes are infections such as rheumatic fever (from streptococcal infections such as strep throat), connective tissue disorders such as lupus, and inherited conditions such as Marfan syndrome. Mitral valve prolapse also can lead to mitral regurgitation.

What Are the Symptoms of Mitral Regurgitation?

People often live for years without knowing that they have this condition. People with a small defect have no symptoms. Symptoms developing after a few years usually include tiredness and difficulty breathing.

How Is Mitral Regurgitation Diagnosed?

The doctor diagnoses mitral regurgitation by listening to heart sounds. Abnormal blood movement makes a sound called a murmur. The doctor hears the murmur through a stethoscope. The doctor may also order sonography of the heart (echocardiography), chest x-rays, and electrocardiography (ECG) to confirm the diagnosis. The x-rays often show a large left atrium. Abnormal heart rhythms (arrhythmias such as atrial fibrillation) can occur and may cause palpitations, or irregular heartbeat.

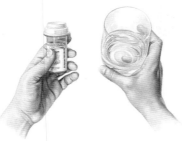

For a mild condition, medicines can prevent complications.

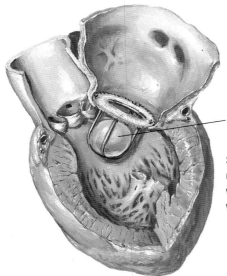

Replacement valve

Surgery (mitral valve replacement) is done when medicines don't work anymore.

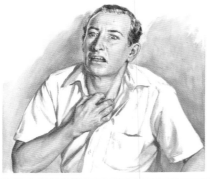

Exercise under the guidance of a physician.

Don't ignore worsening symptoms. Call your doctor.

How Is Mitral Regurgitation Treated?

For a mild condition, medicines are used to prevent complications. Surgery consisting of mitral valve replacement is done when regurgitation worsens and medicines don't work to control symptoms.

DOs and DON'Ts in Managing Mitral Regurgitation:

✔ **DO** take your medicines as directed.

✔ **DO** limit fluid and salt in your diet if you have symptoms of heart failure.

✔ **DO** exercise under the guidance of a physician.

✔ **DO** call your doctor if you have side effects from medicines or new or worsening symptoms, especially chest pain, shortness of breath, difficulty breathing at rest, light-headedness, palpitations (rapid heartbeat), or new swelling in your feet or legs.

⊘ **DON'T** ignore worsening symptoms.

FROM THE DESK OF

NOTES

FOR MORE INFORMATION

Contact the following sources:

- American College of Cardiology
  Tel: (800) 253-4636
  Website: http://www.acc.org

- American Heart Association
  Tel: (800) 242-8721
  Website: http://www.americanheart.org

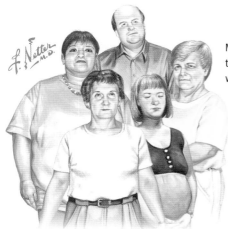

Mitral stenosis affects two to four times more women than men.

What Is Mitral Stenosis?

Mitral stenosis is abnormal narrowing or blocking of the mitral valve. The mitral valve lies between the left atrium (one of the upper chambers in the heart) and left ventricle (one of the lower chambers in the heart). A narrow valve means that the left atrium must pump harder to move blood into the left ventricle. If the left atrium cannot empty the blood properly, blood backs up into the right-sided heart system, and fluid leaks into the lungs. Mitral stenosis occurs two to four times more often in women than in men. It is a major cause of congestive heart failure.

When the mitral valve narrows, most often caused by scarring, the left atrium gets larger because it must work harder to pump blood into the left ventricle.

What Causes Mitral Stenosis?

The cause may be scarring of the valve from rheumatic fever that occurred earlier in life, usually in childhood. Rheumatic fever comes from a bacterial (streptococcus, or strep) infection. Other causes are congenital heart disease, calcium deposits, and infection.

What Are the Symptoms of Mitral Stenosis?

Symptoms include difficulty breathing (especially when lying down), swelling (edema) in legs, and tiredness. Other symptoms may be irregular heartbeat, coughing up blood, and chest pain. If an abnormal heartbeat called atrial fibrillation develops, the atrium doesn't contract normally, so blood pools in the atrium. Clots may form and move out of the heart to the brain and cause a stroke.

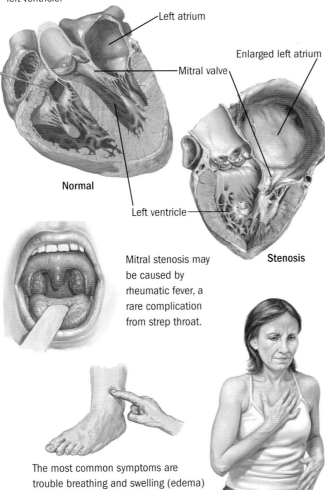

Left atrium

Enlarged left atrium

Mitral valve

Normal

Left ventricle

Stenosis

Mitral stenosis may be caused by rheumatic fever, a rare complication from strep throat.

The most common symptoms are trouble breathing and swelling (edema) in the legs.

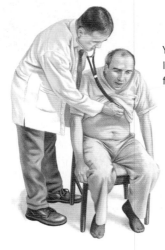

Your doctor will use a stethoscope to listen to your heart. Abnormal blood flow creates a sound called a murmur.

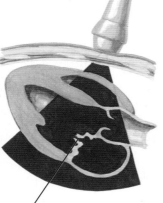

A sonogram of the heart may also be done for diagnosis.

Thickened, stenotic mitral valve

Your doctor may prescribe different medicines, depending on symptoms and their severity.

Surgery to widen or replace the mitral valve may be suggested if the narrowing is severe or medicines don't work.

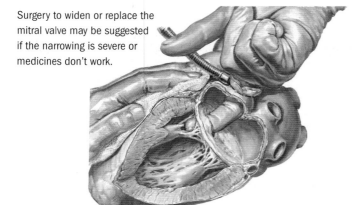

How Is Mitral Stenosis Diagnosed?

The doctor can make a diagnosis by listening to heart sounds. Blood moves abnormally through the mitral valve and causes a sound called a murmur. The doctor hears the murmur with a stethoscope. The timing and location of the murmur help the doctor tell which valve is affected. A sonogram of the heart (echocardiogram) can confirm the diagnosis. Other tests ordered may include a chest x-ray and electrocardiography (ECG).

How Is Mitral Stenosis Treated?

For a mild condition, attempts are made to prevent complications with medicines. When medicines cannot control symptoms any longer, an operation to have the mitral valve widened or replaced is usually performed.

DOs and DON'Ts in Managing Mitral Stenosis:

✔ **DO** take your medicine as directed.
✔ **DO** change your diet. Use moderate salt restriction (don't add salt to your food).
✔ **DO** call your doctor if you have side effects from your medicines.
✔ **DO** call your doctor if you have new or worsening symptoms, such as chest pain, shortness of breath, or swelling in the legs.
✔ **DO** call your doctor if you take anticoagulants and have a cut that doesn't stop bleeding.

⊘ **DON'T** ignore worsening symptoms.

FROM THE DESK OF

NOTES

FOR MORE INFORMATION

Contact the following sources:
- American College of Cardiology
  Tel: (800) 253-4636
  Website: http://www.acc.org
- American Heart Association
  Tel: (800) 242-8721
  Website: http://www.americanheart.org

MANAGING YOUR
MITRAL VALVE PROLAPSE

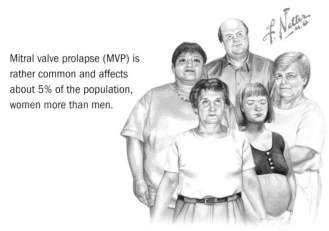

Mitral valve prolapse (MVP) is rather common and affects about 5% of the population, women more than men.

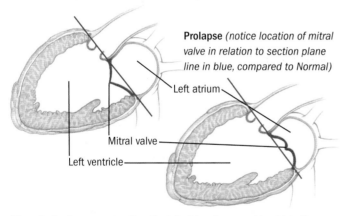

Normal *(notice location of mitral valve in relation to section plane line in blue)*

Prolapse *(notice location of mitral valve in relation to section plane line in blue, compared to Normal)*

Left atrium

Mitral valve

Left ventricle

The mitral valve opens to allow the left atrium to pump blood into the ventricle. MVP means that the valve, which is thickened, bulges back into the atrium.

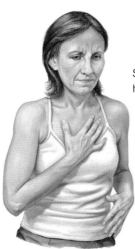

Symptoms include rapid or skipped heartbeat and chest pain.

What Is Mitral Valve Prolapse?

The mitral valve of the heart lies between the left atrium (one of the upper chambers in the heart) and left ventricle (one of the lower chambers in the heart). The mitral valve normally opens when the left atrium pumps blood into the ventricle. It closes to prevent blood from going back into the atrium as the ventricle pumps blood out of the heart. Mitral valve prolapse (MVP) means that the valve, which is thickened, bulges back into the atrium. Blood leaking back into the atrium from the ventricle is called regurgitation.

Prolapse can cause some degree of regurgitation. This means that the left ventricle must do more work to move the blood. Severe regurgitation occurs in about 15% of people with prolapse.

MVP is rather common and affects about 5% of the population, women more than men.

What Causes MVP?

Any damage to the mitral valve may cause MVP. Damage may result from a congenital abnormality (one present at birth) or heart attack. Other causes are infections such as rheumatic fever (from streptococcal infections, e.g., strep throat) and connective tissue disorders such as Marfan syndrome.

What Are the Symptoms of MVP?

People often live for years without knowing that they have this condition. People with a small defect usually do well and never have symptoms.

Symptoms when present may include rapid or skipped heartbeat (palpitations), chest pain, and rarely, difficulty breathing. Abnormal heart rhythms (arrhythmias) such as atrial fibrillation may occur if changes in the atrium affect the heart's electrical system.

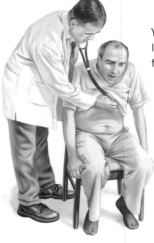

Your doctor will use a stethoscope to listen to your heart. Abnormal blood flow creates a sound called a murmur.

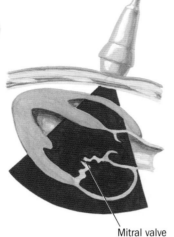

A sonogram of the heart may also be done for diagnosis.

Mitral valve

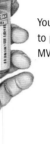

Your doctor may prescribe medicines to prevent or reduce complications if MVP is causing regurgitation.

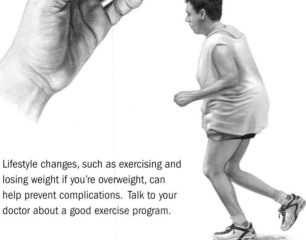

Lifestyle changes, such as exercising and losing weight if you're overweight, can help prevent complications. Talk to your doctor about a good exercise program.

How Is MVP Diagnosed?

The doctor diagnoses MVP on the basis of a physical examination. Blood moving against the valve in MVP produces a sound called a murmur. The doctor hears the murmur with a stethoscope. The timing and location of the murmur help the doctor tell which valve is affected.

The doctor may also order sonography of the heart (echocardiography) to confirm the diagnosis and estimate the degree of MVP.

How Is MVP Treated?

Treatment of MVP depends on how severe it is. People with no symptoms and no mitral regurgitation need no treatment.

If people have mitral regurgitation, attempts are made to prevent complications by using medicines and lifestyle changes.

DOs and DON'Ts in Managing Mitral Valve Prolapse:

✔ **DO** exercise on a regular basis.

✔ **DO** lose weight if you're overweight.

✔ **DO** call your doctor if you have new or worsening symptoms, especially chest pain, shortness of breath at rest, lightheadedness, palpitations, or new swelling in your feet or legs.

✔ **DO** call your doctor if you have side effects from your medicines.

⊘ **DON'T** use too much caffeine, because excess caffeine may worsen your symptoms.

FROM THE DESK OF

NOTES

FOR MORE INFORMATION

Contact the following sources:

* American College of Cardiology
  Tel: (800) 253-4636
  Website: http://www.acc.org
* American Heart Association
  Tel: (800) 242-8721
  Website: http://www.americanheart.org

Myocarditis is a rare condition in which the myocardium (heart muscle) is inflamed. It is sometimes difficult to diagnose because of lack of symptoms.

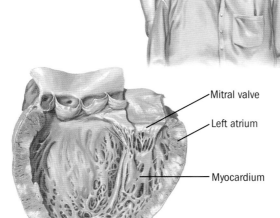

Mitral valve

Left atrium

Myocardium

Common symptoms of myocarditis

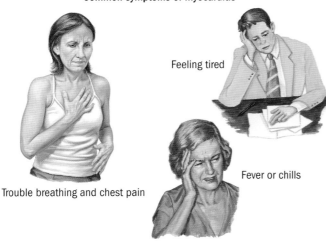

Feeling tired

Trouble breathing and chest pain

Fever or chills

Your doctor will do a physical examination and order electrocardiography (ECG) and laboratory tests to confirm myocarditis and find the cause.

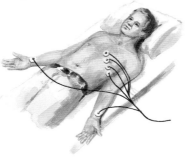

What Is Myocarditis?

Myocarditis is inflammation of heart muscle.

What Causes Myocarditis?

The many causes of the inflammatory response include injury, infections, radiation, and medicines. Most often, it is a virus, that causes myocarditis. Myocarditis is not contagious or hereditary.

What Are the Symptoms of Myocarditis?

Some people do not have any symptoms.

People who have early symptoms note chest pain, skipped heartbeats (palpitations), trouble breathing, fever or chills, inability to exercise, or feeling tired and run down much of the time. Irritation of the heart muscle may lead to abnormal heart rhythms (arrhythmias) and heart failure (when the heart doesn't pump blood well).

How Is Myocarditis Diagnosed?

Myocarditis is hard to diagnose because of the many causes and frequent lack of symptoms. The doctor diagnoses myocarditis by doing a physical examination, electrocardiography (ECG), and laboratory tests to look for damage to heart muscle. A biopsy of the heart muscle may also be done to confirm the diagnosis and help find the cause.

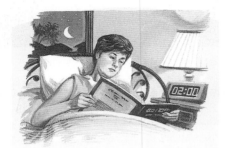

Symptoms usually disappear with rest and time.

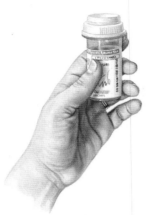

Your doctor may prescribe medicine to reduce inflammation and chest pain. Always tell your doctor about any drugs that you're taking, and read information provided on side effects.

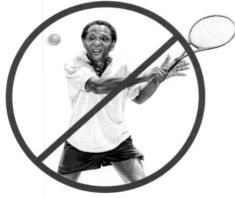

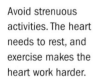

Avoid strenuous activities. The heart needs to rest, and exercise makes the heart work harder.

How Is Myocarditis Treated?

Treatment of chest pain and arrhythmias is most important. Heart failure must also be treated.

The doctor may prescribe nonsteroidal antiinflammatory drugs (NSAIDs) for inflammation and chest pain.

For more severe disease, steroid-containing medicines or immunosuppressive drugs may be used.

Medications may be given to control irregular heartbeat and improve heart function.

DOs and DON'Ts in Managing Myocarditis:

✔ **DO** take your medicines as prescribed for your symptoms.

✔ **DO** rest.

✔ **DO** call your doctor if you cannot tolerate your medicines or have a reaction to them.

✔ **DO** call your doctor if you have new or worsening chest pain, palpitations, shortness of breath, or fainting.

✔ **DO** call your doctor if you notice blood in your vomit or stools.

⊘ **DON'T** exercise until your doctor says that you can. Avoid strenuous exercise. Exercise increases the work of the heart, which may cause rapidly worsening inflammation and dangerous heart rhythm problems.

FROM THE DESK OF

NOTES

FOR MORE INFORMATION

Contact the following source:

• American Heart Association
  Tel: (800) 242-8721
  Website: http://www.americanheart.org

MANAGING YOUR
PERICARDITIS

The pericardium, a thin fibrous sac, covers the heart. This sac-like membrane helps hold the heart in place and lubricates it. Pericarditis is inflammation of the pericardium. More men than women are affected, often 20 to 50 years old. Early diagnosis and treatment may prevent complications.

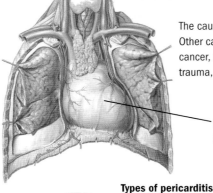

The cause is often a viral infection. Other causes are heart attacks, cancer, radiation, other infections, trauma, drugs, and allergy.

Pericardium of normal heart

Types of pericarditis

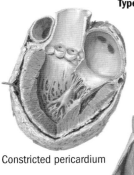

Constricted pericardium

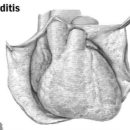

Mild pericarditis

Adhesive pericarditis

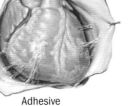

Symptoms include chest pain behind the breast bone that may go to the shoulder and neck, like pain of a heart attack. However, unlike the pain from a heart attack, it gets worse when taking a deep breath and is relieved by sitting up and leaning forward. Other symptoms are fever, palpitations, and cough. Constrictive pericarditis can cause legs and abdomen to swell and shortness of breath.

What Is Pericarditis?

The pericardium is the thin fibrous sac that covers the heart. This sac-like membrane helps hold the heart in position in the chest and lubricate the heart. Pericarditis is inflammation of the pericardium. It can be acute (sudden) or chronic (long-lasting). This inflammation may injure the membrane and cause complications. The pericardium can become scarred and thickened and the heart can be constricted (squeezed) (constrictive pericarditis). It may also cause another complication, reduced blood flow from the heart (cardiac tamponade). This occurs when too much fluid collects in the pericardium, so excess pressure on the heart doesn't let it fill correctly. Blood pressure and heart output can fall to dangerous levels. Untreated, cardiac tamponade can cause death.

More men than women are affected, often 20 to 50 years old. Most people recover in 2 weeks to 3 months. Early diagnosis and treatment may prevent complications.

What Causes Pericarditis?

The cause is often a viral infection. Other causes include myocardial infarctions (heart attacks), cancer, radiation, other infections (such as tuberculosis, fungal, and parasitic), trauma, medicines, and allergic reactions. It may have no known cause (idiopathic pericarditis).

What Are the Symptoms of Pericarditis?

Symptoms include sharp chest pain behind the sternum (breast bone) that may go to the shoulder and neck. Some people have dull, achy pain or pressure. Pain worsens with changes in position or with deep breathing. The pain is lessened by sitting forward. A fever may occur if infection is causing the pericarditis. Sometimes people feel palpitations (irregular or rapid heartbeats). Constrictive pericarditis can lead to severe swelling (edema) of the legs and abdomen (belly) and shortness of breath. Reduced blood flow from the heart causes symptoms of heart failure, including problems breathing and swelling in tissues of the legs, feet, or abdomen. The neck veins may also appear distended or very prominent.

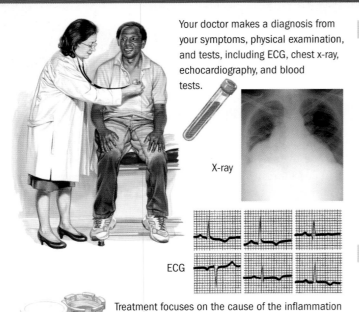

Your doctor makes a diagnosis from your symptoms, physical examination, and tests, including ECG, chest x-ray, echocardiography, and blood tests.

X-ray

ECG

Treatment focuses on the cause of the inflammation and pain. NSAIDs such as aspirin and ibuprofen are given for pain. In more severe cases, steroidal anti-inflammatory drugs may be used.

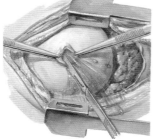

Surgery is rarely needed. The doctor cuts a window in the pericardium to let fluid drain out. For cardiac tamponade, the doctor must drain fluid from the sac (pericardiocentesis).

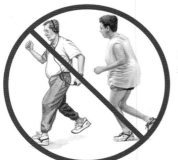

Don't exert yourself until after your symptoms have gone away.

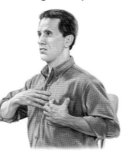

Call your doctor if you have new or worsening chest pain or pain with deep breaths or changes in position.

How Is Pericarditis Diagnosed?

The doctor makes a diagnosis from symptoms, a physical examination, and tests. Electrocardiography (ECG) may show signs of the inflammation. A chest x-ray may show an enlarged heart if fluid collects around the heart. Echocardiography may show fluid in the pericardial sac. Echocardiography is a type of ultrasound examination that uses sound waves to see the heart. The doctor may also order computed tomography (CT) or magnetic resonance imaging (MRI) if complications from pericarditis are suspected. Blood tests may be done to measure inflammation and look for infection.

How Is Pericarditis Treated?

Treatment focuses on the cause of the inflammation and pain. Nonsteroidal anti-inflammatory drugs (NSAIDs) such as aspirin and ibuprofen are given for pain. In more severe cases, steroidal antiinflammatory drugs such as prednisone may be used. If fluid in the pericardium affects how the heart works, an operation may be done to release the pressure. A window is cut in the membrane to let fluid drain out. For severe complications such as cardiac tamponade, the doctor must drain fluid from the sac (pericardiocentesis).

DOs and DON'Ts in Managing Pericarditis:

✔ **DO** take your medicines as prescribed.
✔ **DO** call your doctor if you have new or worsening chest pain or pain with deep breaths or changes in position.

🚫 **DON'T** exert yourself until after your symptoms have gone away.

FROM THE DESK OF

NOTES

FOR MORE INFORMATION
Contact the following sources:
• The American Heart Association
 Tel: (800) 242-8721
 Website: http://www.americanheart.org
• American College of Cardiology
 Tel: (800) 253-4636
 Website: http://www.acc.org

Peripheral arterial disease (PAD) refers to blockage of leg arteries by atherosclerosis, so legs have poor blood flow. In atherosclerosis, cholesterol plaques block arteries. PAD occurs in men and women equally.

Plaque formation in the walls of an artery

Locations of blockages

About half of people don't have symptoms, but the most common ones are pain, cramping, aching, and numbness. Others are heavy or tight feeling, cold skin, pale or bluish skin, and ulcers that don't heal.

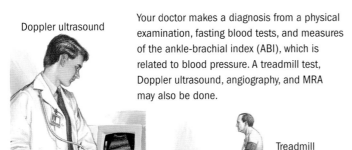

Doppler ultrasound

Your doctor makes a diagnosis from a physical examination, fasting blood tests, and measures of the ankle-brachial index (ABI), which is related to blood pressure. A treadmill test, Doppler ultrasound, angiography, and MRA may also be done.

Treadmill test

What Is Peripheral Arterial Disease (PAD)?

Peripheral arterial disease (PAD) refers to blockage of leg arteries by atherosclerosis (hardening of the arteries), so legs have poor blood flow. In atherosclerosis, cholesterol plaques block arteries. PAD occurs in men and women equally. It likely affects 8 to 10 million people in the United States.

What Causes PAD?

Fatty deposits build up inside arteries and make them narrower. Tobacco, diabetes, cholesterol, and high blood pressure make PAD likely. PAD isn't contagious or passed from parents to children.

What Are the Symptoms of PAD?

About half of people don't have symptoms. The most common symptoms are pain, cramping, aching, and numbness in the affected area. Others are heavy or tight feeling, cold skin, pale or bluish skin, pulse that's hard to feel, and sores or ulcers that don't heal. Aching or cramping leg pain often occurs during exercise and goes away during rest (intermittent claudication). If blood flow is completely blocked, the leg gets very painful and hard to move. In men, impotence can occur if vessels leading to the penis are affected.

How Is PAD Diagnosed?

The doctor makes a preliminary diagnosis from your symptoms, a physical examination, fasting blood tests, and by measuring the ankle-brachial index (ABI). The doctor gets the ABI by dividing the highest ankle blood pressure by the highest arm blood pressure. ABI values less than 1 are abnormal.

A treadmill test, Doppler ultrasound, angiography (a kind of x-ray with dye), and magnetic resonance angiography (MRA) may also be done to evaluate the extent of the disorder and areas of blockage.

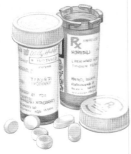

Treatment aims to reduce pain and prevent damage to the leg. Risks of getting a future heart attack or stroke must be lowered. Life-style changes are critical. Medicines can help blood flow, thin blood, dissolve clots, lower blood pressure, and lower cholesterol levels.

Angioplasty may be needed for a severely narrowed vessel. The doctor may put a small metal or mesh tube (stent) into the vessel to keep it open.

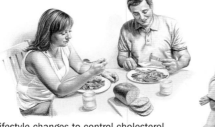

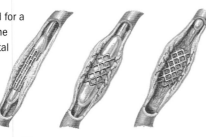

Lifestyle changes to control cholesterol, diabetes, and hypertension and to avoid tobacco are critical. Lose weight and get active. Walk for 20 to 30 minutes daily. Eat a heart-healthy diet.

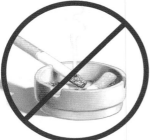

Stop smoking! Smoking is the biggest single risk factor for PAD and a major risk factor for heart attack and stroke.

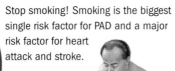

Take care of your feet. Examine them regularly, and avoid getting cuts or blisters. Call your doctor if you have a foot ulcer that doesn't heal.

How Is PAD Treated?

Treatment goals are to reduce pain and prevent damage to the affected area. Measures include avoiding tobacco, eating a healthy diet, and restricting salt. Diabetics should follow the American Diabetes Association (ADA) diet. Exercise such as walking 30 to 60 minutes per day helps walking distance and quality of life.

Medicines can help blood flow, thin blood, dissolve clots, lower blood pressure, and lower cholesterol levels.

The doctor may suggest angioplasty for a severely narrowed vessel. The doctor puts a wire (catheter) into the artery and inflates a tiny balloon to open the blocked artery. The doctor may put a small metal or mesh tube (stent) into the vessel to keep it open.

People sometimes need bypass surgery to get around the blockage.

DOs and DON'Ts in Managing PAD:

✔ **DO** understand that lifestyle changes for cholesterol, diabetes, hypertension, and tobacco are critical.

✔ **DO** eat a healthy diet, with less fat, especially saturated fat, and less salt. Eat plenty of fruits, vegetables, and whole-grain cereals.

✔ **DO** lose weight.

✔ **DO** get active. Walk for 20 to 30 minutes daily.

✔ **DO** take extra care with controlling your blood sugar if you have diabetes.

✔ **DO** take care of your feet. Examine them regularly, and avoid getting cuts or blisters. Call your doctor if you have a foot ulcer that doesn't heal.

🚫 **DON'T** smoke. Smoking is the biggest single risk factor for PAD and a major risk factor for heart attack and stroke.

FROM THE DESK OF

NOTES

FOR MORE INFORMATION

Contact the following sources:

• The National Heart, Lung, and Blood Institute
Tel: (301) 592-8573
Website: http://www.nhlbi.nih.gov

• American Heart Association
Tel: (800) 242-8721
Website: http://www.americanheart.org

Premature ventricular contractions (PVCs) are extra, abnormal heartbeats in the ventricles that occur too early. PVCs are very common and can happen in healthy people.

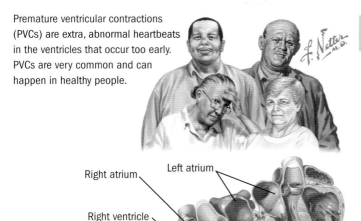

Right atrium

Left atrium

Right ventricle

Left ventricle

The heart has four pumping chambers, two upper (atria) and two lower (ventricles). Cells in the right atrium tell the ventricles to contract.

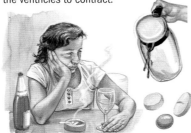

The most common causes are caffeine, nicotine, alcohol, and stress. Other causes are heart disease, high blood pressure, congestive heart failure, medicines, and illegal drugs.

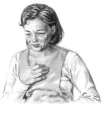

Most people don't have symptoms. Some have a feeling of the heart missing a beat followed by a stronger beat. Other symptoms are heart fluttering, palpitations, a sensation of heart pounding, and jumping.

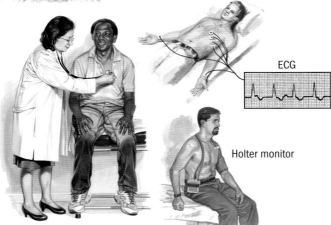

ECG

Holter monitor

Your doctor may find an irregular pulse during a physical examination. ECG, Holter monitoring, exercise stress testing, echocardiography, and an electrophysiology study may also be done.

What Are Premature Ventricular Contractions (PVCs)?

The heart has four pumping chambers, two upper ones (atria) and two lower ones (ventricles). Cells in the right atrium normally control heartbeats. Electrical impulses go from the atria to the ventricles and make them contract and pump blood from the heart to the body. Premature ventricular contractions (PVCs) are extra, abnormal heartbeats in the ventricles that occur too early in the rhythm sequence. These heartbeats don't work well in pumping blood through the body. This condition is known as an arrhythmia, a disorder of the heart's regular beating rhythm. The abnormal heartbeats will result in an irregular pulse.

PVCs are very common and occur in most people at some point. They can happen in otherwise healthy people and are usually harmless. Most people with PVCs don't need treatment.

What Causes PVCs?

The most common causes among healthy people are caffeine, nicotine, alcohol, and stress. Heart disease such as ischemia (reduced blood flow to the heart muscle), high blood pressure, congestive heart failure (reduced pumping of the heart), medicines, and illegal drugs are other causes.

What Are the Symptoms of PVCs?

Most people don't have symptoms. Some have a feeling of the heart missing a beat followed by a stronger beat. Other symptoms are fluttering, palpitations (irregular or rapid heartbeat), a sensation of heart pounding, and jumping.

How Are PVCs Diagnosed?

The doctor may find an irregular pulse during a physical examination. The doctor will diagnose PVCs by doing electrocardiography (ECG). The ECG records the heart's electrical activity. The test is best done while symptoms are occurring. Other tests include Holter monitoring. The Holter monitor records an ECG for 24 hours. Exercise stress testing may also be done. This test lets the doctor see effects of exercise on the heart's rhythms. Other tests are echocardiography (a type of ultrasound test that uses sound waves) and an electrophysiology study (checks the heart's electrical system). This test is done by a specialist in the hospital.

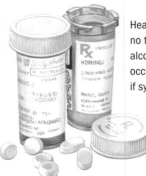

Healthy people with no symptoms need no treatment. Limiting or avoiding caffeine, alcohol, nicotine, and stress can make PVCs occur less often. Medicines can control PVCs if symptoms become severe.

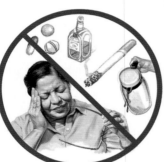

Exercise can help people who are inactive. An exercise stress test can be used to make sure that you can exercise safely.

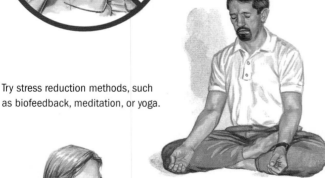

Reduce exposure to PVC triggers, such caffeine, alcohol, nicotine, drugs, and stress.

Try stress reduction methods, such as biofeedback, meditation, or yoga.

Call your doctor if you have palpitations, chest pain, shortness of breath, or fainting.

How Are PVCs Treated?

Healthy people with no symptoms need no treatment. The condition may go away on its own. Limiting or avoiding caffeine, alcohol, nicotine, and stress can make PVCs become less frequent. Medicines can control PVCs if symptoms become severe. These drugs include antiarrhythmic medicines, beta-blockers, and calcium channel blockers. Exercise can help people who are inactive.

DOs and DON'Ts in Managing PVCs:

✔ **DO** reduce exposure to PVC triggers, such caffeine, alcohol, nicotine, drugs, and stress.

✔ **DO** try stress reduction methods, such as biofeedback, meditation, or yoga.

✔ **DO** exercise. People with PVCs can usually exercise safely. PVCs may even stop during exercise. If PVCs increase in frequency with exercise, you may have heart disease. An exercise stress test can be used to make sure that you can exercise safely.

✔ **DO** call your doctor if you have palpitations, chest pain, shortness of breath, or fainting.

⊘ **DON'T** forget to take your prescribed medicines.

FROM THE DESK OF

NOTES

FOR MORE INFORMATION

Contact the following sources:

• American Heart Association
Tel: (800) 242-8721
Website: http://www.americanheart.org

• American College of Cardiology
Tel: (800) 253-4636
Website: http://www.acc.org

MANAGING YOUR
PULMONARY EMBOLISM

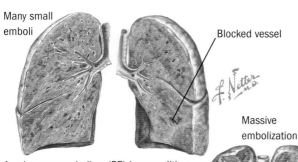

Many small emboli

Blocked vessel

Massive embolization

A pulmonary embolism (PE) is a condition that occurs in the lungs because of a blocked artery. The blockage results when a blood clot in a vein in another part of the body gets to the lungs. This clot that moves is called an embolus. It can be life-threatening and needs immediate treatment.

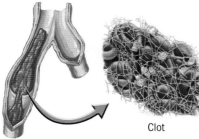

Clot

A clot is a clump of platelets, red blood cells, and protein. Clots usually form to help stop bleeding. Sometimes they occur for no reason. Clots can form during long periods of inactivity if blood moves too slowly through veins. Clots in lungs most often come from veins deep in the legs.

The most common symptoms are shortness of breath, chest pain, coughing up blood, and fast heartbeat.

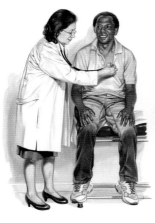

Angiogram showing blocked vessel

Your doctor makes a diagnosis from an examination, symptoms, and tests, including ECG, chest x-ray, blood tests, CT or lung scan. In rare cases when the tests are inconclusive and pulmonary embolus is still suspected, a special x-ray known as angiography may be done.

What Is a Pulmonary Embolism (PE)?

A pulmonary embolism (PE) is an emergency medical condition that occurs in the lungs as a result of a blocked artery. The blockage occurs when a blood clot dislodges from a vein (venous thrombus) in another part of the body (usually the legs) and reaches the lungs. It can be life-threatening and needs immediate treatment.

What Causes a PE?

A blood clot is a clump of platelets with red blood cells and the protein fibrin. Platelets are cells that help stop injured blood vessels from bleeding. Clots usually form to help stop bleeding, but sometimes they occur due to blood clotting abnormalities. A clot that stays in a vein is called a thrombus. One that moves to another part of the body is called an embolus. Clots can also form during long periods of inactivity if blood moves too slowly through the veins. The clot formed in another part of the body moves to the lungs through the bloodstream. Veins deep in the legs are the most common source of clots.

What Are the Symptoms of PE?

The most common symptoms are shortness of breath, chest pain, coughing up blood, and fast heartbeat. Nausea, fainting, sweating, wheezing, and clammy or bluish skin are others. The chest pain may last from minutes to hours.

How Is a PE Diagnosed?

The doctor makes a diagnosis from an examination and symptoms. Tests include electrocardiography (ECG), chest x-ray, blood tests, computed tomography (CT), or lung scan. Blood tests check for clotting problems (D-dimer) and lung gases such as oxygen. In rare cases when the tests are inconclusive and pulmonary embolus is still suspected, a special x-ray known as angiography may be done. Angiography requires injecting a dye in the veins before x-rays can be taken.

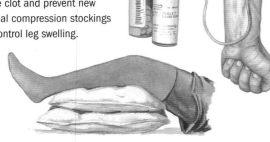

Treatment involves hospitalization and intravenous and oral medicines to dissolve the clot and prevent new ones. Special compression stockings may help control leg swelling.

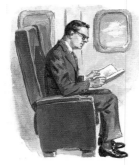

Move around when you're at work or traveling. If you can't get up, move your legs and bend your ankles and toes. Avoid long periods of bed rest or sitting or standing in one place.

Don't smoke! Smoking may increase blood clot formation. Don't be sedentary. Lose weight if you're overweight.

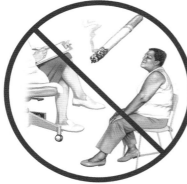

Call your doctor if you develop leg pain or swelling, have chest pain or are short of breath, or cough up blood.

How Is a PE Treated?

Treatment involves hospitalization and intravenous medicines (heparin) to dissolve the clot and stop new ones from forming. Anticoagulant drugs (warfarin) will also be given by mouth and continued for at least 6 months. Special compression stockings may help control swelling in the legs. The doctor will suggest that people who are overweight lose weight since obesity and sedentary lifestyle are major risk factors for pulmonary embolism.

In rare cases, a special (Greenfield) filter can be put in the main vein (vena cava) going from the legs and pelvis to the heart to stop clots from getting into the lungs.

DOs and DON'Ts in Managing PE:

✔ **DO** report bleeding or bruising easily to your doctor if you take medicine to prevent clots from forming.

✔ **DO** avoid activities that may cause injury.

✔ **DO** move around when you're at work or traveling. If you can't get up, move your legs and bend your ankles and toes. Avoid long periods of bed rest or sitting or standing in one place.

✔ **DO** call your doctor if you develop pain or swelling of your legs, have chest pain or are short of breath, or cough up blood.

✔ **DO** try to keep your feet higher than your hips when you're lying down or sitting.

⊘ **DON'T** smoke. Smoking may increase your risk of forming blood clots.

⊘ **DON'T** wear clothing that restricts blood flow in your legs.

⊘ **DON'T** forget that blood thinners such as warfarin require frequent monitoring with blood tests to ensure that you are receiving the correct dose.

FROM THE DESK OF

NOTES

FOR MORE INFORMATION

Contact the following sources:

• American College of Chest Physicians
Tel: (847) 498-1400, (800) 343-2227
Website: http://www.chestnet.org

• American Thoracic Society
Tel: (212) 315-8600
Website: http://www.thoracic.org/

Kidneys get blood through arteries that come from the aorta, connecting the heart. Renal artery stenosis is the narrowing or blocking of these arteries.

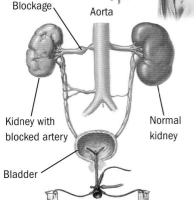

Blockage

Aorta

Kidney with blocked artery

Normal kidney

Bladder

Narrow arteries can lead to high blood pressure. Blockage of both arteries can cause serious problems including kidney failure.

Less urine

More urine

Causes include atherosclerosis and fibromuscular dysplasia, which block or narrow arteries.

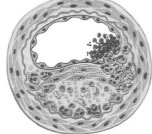

Plaque in atherosclerosis

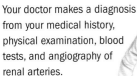

People usually have no symptoms. They don't know that they have renal artery stenosis until they develop high blood pressure or kidney failure.

Your doctor makes a diagnosis from your medical history, physical examination, blood tests, and angiography of renal arteries.

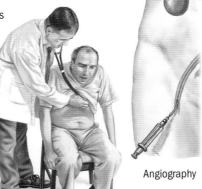

Angiography

What Is Renal Artery Stenosis?

Each kidney gets blood through an artery that comes from the aorta, the major blood vessel from the heart. Renal artery stenosis is the narrowing or complete blocking of arteries bringing blood to the kidneys. Narrow arteries can lead to high blood pressure (hypertension). When both arteries are blocked, serious problems, including kidney failure, can result. One or both kidneys can be blocked.

What Causes Renal Artery Stenosis?

In older people, the usual cause is atherosclerosis (hardening of the arteries). In atherosclerosis, fat, cholesterol, and other substances collect in artery walls. In younger adults, a condition known as fibromuscular dysplasia is the most common cause. In this illness, tissue grows in walls of renal arteries and narrows or blocks them.

What Are the Symptoms of Renal Artery Stenosis?

People usually have no symptoms. They don't know that they have it until they begin to have high blood pressure or kidney failure.

How Is Renal Artery Stenosis Diagnosed?

The doctor makes a diagnosis from a medical history and physical examination. Blood and urine tests and magnetic resonance angiography (MRA) of renal arteries may be done. MRA is a special x-ray of blood vessels bringing blood to kidneys.

How Is Renal Artery Stenosis Treated?

Treatment depends on the severity and cause of the stenosis and personal preference. Mild or moderate symptoms can sometimes be treated with medicine to control high blood pressure. A more severe condition may need the artery to be widened or reopened by surgery.

A treatment called angioplasty may be used instead of surgery. This treatment is more frequently performed when the cause is fibromuscular dysplasia but not atherosclerosis. A plastic balloon is used to open the narrowed artery. A metal or mesh tube called a stent may be put in to keep the artery open. The procedure may have to be repeated because narrowing may return. High blood pressure medicine may still be needed.

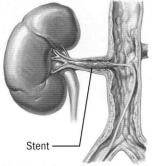
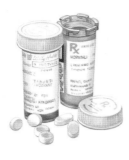

Stent

Treatment depends on the severity and cause of the stenosis and personal preference. Medicines to control high blood pressure are used for mild or moderate symptoms. More severe conditions may need the artery to be widened or reopened by surgery or angioplasty. A stent may be put in to keep the artery open.

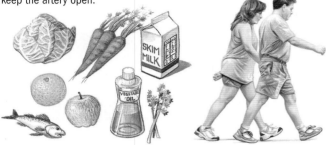

Keep your heart healthy. Exercise regularly to reduce complications, such as heart disease, caused by high blood pressure. Eat healthy foods. Lower your blood cholesterol levels, and follow a low-salt diet.

Stop smoking! Smoking worsens blood pressure control and may increase chances of getting heart disease.

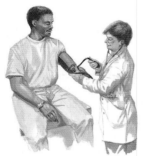

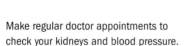

Make regular doctor appointments to check your kidneys and blood pressure.

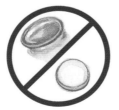

Don't take over-the-counter drugs, such as ibuprofen, or herbal preparations unless your doctor says you can. Some may not be safe to take with your condition.

DOs and DON'Ts in Managing Renal Artery Stenosis:

✔ **DO** take your medicine regularly and as directed. This is the most important thing you can do to delay or prevent worsening of kidney function.

✔ **DO** exercise regularly. Exercise will reduce the risk of complications, such as heart disease, caused by high blood pressure.

✔ **DO** eat healthy food. Follow your dietitian's advice to lower your blood cholesterol levels. High levels increase the risk of heart disease. A low-salt diet also helps lower blood pressure.

✔ **DO** call your doctor if your blood pressure stays high.

✔ **DO** call your doctor if you have side effects from medicines.

✔ **DO** make regular appointments with your doctor to check your kidneys and blood pressure.

⊘ **DON'T** smoke. Smoking can damage your arteries.

⊘ **DON'T** miss appointments to have your blood pressure checked. Do this at least every 6 months.

⊘ **DON'T** stop taking your medicine without asking your doctor.

⊘ **DON'T** take over-the-counter drugs, especially drugs similar to ibuprofen, unless your doctor says you can. Some may not be safe to take with your kidney condition and may make it worse.

⊘ **DON'T** take herbal preparations. Some may cause kidney disease.

FROM THE DESK OF

NOTES

FOR MORE INFORMATION

Contact the following sources:

• National Kidney Foundation
  Tel: (800) 622-9010
  Website: http://www.kidney.org

• National Kidney and Urologic Diseases
  Information Clearinghouse
  Tel: (800) 891-5390
  Website: http://kidney.niddk.nih.gov

MANAGING YOUR
RESTRICTIVE CARDIOMYOPATHY

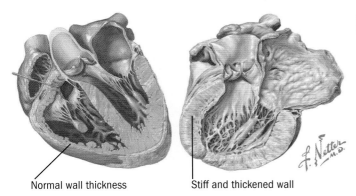

Normal wall thickness   Stiff and thickened wall

Restrictive cardiomyopathy is a heart muscle disease. Restrictive cardiomyopathy means that the heart is restricted in its ability to contract because the heart's inner lining becomes stiff. The heart can't expand correctly. The heart muscle thickens but is unable to function normally.

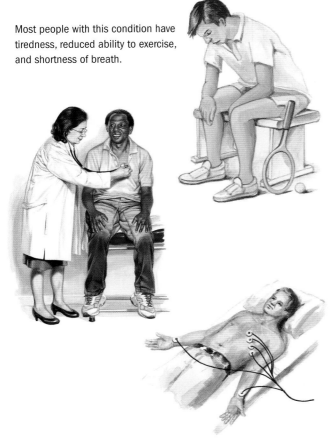

Most people with this condition have tiredness, reduced ability to exercise, and shortness of breath.

Your doctor will take a medical history and do physical examination for diagnosis. Your doctor may also order an ECG (shown here), chest x-rays, and echocardiography (ultrasound of the heart).

What Is Restrictive Cardiomyopathy?

Restrictive cardiomyopathy is a disease of heart muscle that prevents the muscle from contracting (squeezing) with normal force. The result is that the heart doesn't pump blood well. Restrictive cardiomyopathy means that the heart has a restricted ability to contract because the inner lining of the heart becomes stiff. The heart does not expand properly when it fills. The heart muscle thickens to make more muscle so it can increase its strength of contraction, but due to the abnormal filling of the heart is unable to function normally.

This type of heart disease is much less common than heart disease from coronary artery disease or heart valve problems.

What Causes Restrictive Cardiomyopathy?

Most of the time the cause is unknown. Amyloidosis, a condition in which abnormal deposits of protein in some body tissues occur, may be a cause. Sarcoidosis, a condition involving abnormal inflammation of lymph nodes and other tissues, may be another cause. It may also be caused by inflammatory or autoimmune conditions. Drinking alcohol in excess can make it worse.

What Are the Symptoms of Restrictive Cardiomyopathy?

Most people have tiredness, less ability to exercise, and shortness of breath. Swelling in the legs or feet, chest pain, or palpitations (feeling that the heart is skipping or beating too fast) may also occur. Cardiomyopathy can cause heart failure.

How Is Restrictive Cardiomyopathy Diagnosed?

The doctor may suspect the disorder on the basis of the medical history and physical examination. The doctor may also order electrocardiography (ECG) and chest x-rays. These tests usually show an enlarged heart. ECG may also show an irregular heartbeat (arrhythmia). Echocardiography (ultrasound examination of the heart) may be done to check the heart's pumping action. Blood tests may also be done to look for other causes.

In some cases, cardiac catheterization and biopsy of heart tissue may be done to confirm the diagnosis.

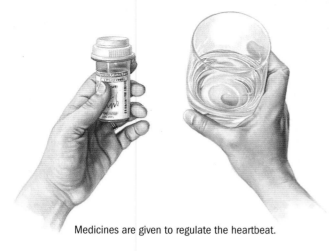

Medicines are given to regulate the heartbeat.

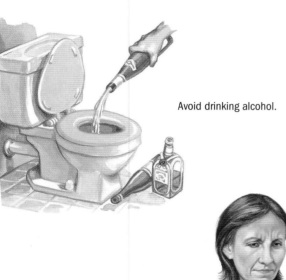

Avoid drinking alcohol.

Call your doctor if you have new or
worsening chest pain, shortness of
breath, swelling in the legs, or fainting.

How Is Restrictive Cardiomyopathy Treated?

Therapy is aimed at relieving symptoms of heart failure and correcting abnormal heart rhythms (arrhythmias).

Medications known as diuretics reduce fluid in the blood to decrease the work of the heart.

The doctor may prescribe drugs that regulate the heartbeat or drugs that suppress immune function (corticosteroids) to fight conditions causing the cardiomyopathy.

If the heart's pumping is very poor and symptoms of heart failure worsen, heart transplantation may be needed.

DOs and DON'Ts in Managing Restrictive Cardiomyopathy:

✔ **DO** eat a low-salt diet to reduce fluid accumulation.
✔ **DO** take all your prescribed medicines as directed.
✔ **DO** exercise when your doctor says that you can.
✔ **DO** call your doctor if you have new or worsening chest pain, shortness of breath, swelling in the legs, or fainting.

🚫 **DON'T** drink alcohol.

FROM THE DESK OF

NOTES

FOR MORE INFORMATION

Contact the following sources:

- American Heart Association
  Tel: (800) 242-8721
  Website: http://www.americanheart.org

- American College of Cardiology
  Tel: (800) 253-4636
  Website: http://www.acc.org

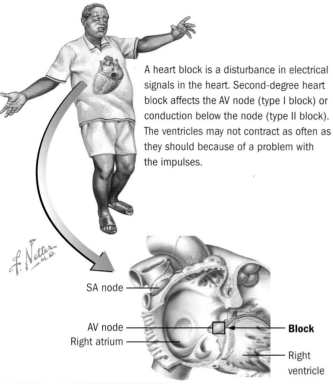

A heart block is a disturbance in electrical signals in the heart. Second-degree heart block affects the AV node (type I block) or conduction below the node (type II block). The ventricles may not contract as often as they should because of a problem with the impulses.

SA node

AV node
Right atrium

Block

Right ventricle

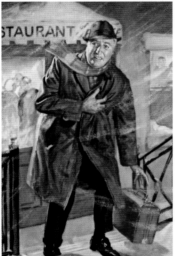

The cause is not always known. Heart conditions such as coronary artery disease and prior heart attacks can cause a heart block.

Half the people with second-degree heart block have no symptoms. Those with symptoms have fainting and feel tired and lightheaded.

What Is Second-Degree Heart Block?

The heart is a muscular pump with four chambers, two upper (left and right atria) and two lower (left and right ventricles). These contract and pump blood. Special tissue in the heart produces and sends electrical impulses to make the muscle contract. Normal electrical signals start from the sinoatrial (SA) node in the wall of the right atrium. From there the signal goes to the left atrium and reaches the atrioventricular (AV) node between the atria and ventricles. The signal then goes to the left and right bundle branches and finally the ventricles. There it stimulates ventricles to contract.

Heart block refers to a delay of electrical signals from the atria through the AV node. Second-degree heart block is one of three types of heart block; the others are first-degree and third-degree (or complete). It affects the AV node (type I block) or conduction below the node (type II block). The atria contract normally, but the ventricles may not contract as often as they should because of the delayed impulses.

People with type II block are at risk for complete heart block, cardiomyopathy (disease of heart muscle), or death from asystole (the heart stops beating).

What Causes Second-Degree Heart Block?

About half the time, the cause is unknown. Most other times, some type of heart disease exists, perhaps damage from a heart attack (myocardial infarction) or myocarditis (inflammation, or swelling, of heart muscle). Drugs, such as digoxin, or a congenital heart abnormality (present at birth) are other causes. Type II block usually results from heart disease.

What Are the Symptoms of Second-Degree Heart Block?

People may have no symptoms. When present, symptoms relate to not enough blood being pumped by the heart: feeling very tired, light-headed, or faint (syncope). Severe heart block can cause chest pain (angina) or stroke (not enough blood flow to the brain).

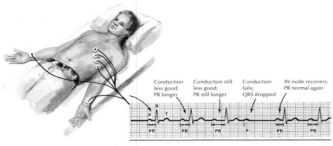

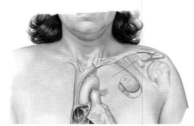

Your doctor will do electrocardiography (ECG) to see whether you have a heart block.

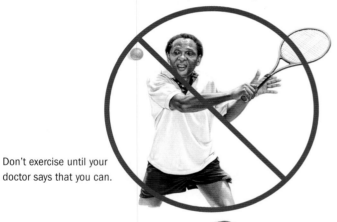

If you have symptoms, you will likely need a pacemaker to help your heart pump enough blood to meet your body's needs. A specialist who treats heart diseases (cardiologist) will determine the best type of pacemaker for you.

Don't exercise until your doctor says that you can.

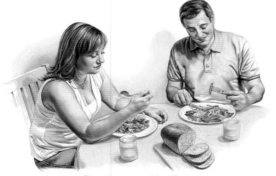

Eat a heart-healthy diet.

How Is Second-Degree Heart Block Diagnosed?

The doctor uses electrocardiography (ECG) for diagnosis. ECG measures the heart's electrical activity and will usually show some impulses from the atrium not reaching the ventricles.

How Is Second-Degree Heart Block Treated?

People without symptoms and no heart disease may not need any treatment.

Those with symptoms may need a pacemaker. Pacemakers are small electrical devices with a wire to the heart muscle that tells the ventricles to contract regularly (fixed-rate pacers) or to beat faster because of more activity (demand pacers). Pacemakers may be attached outside the body or implanted inside. New pacemakers are safer and better than old ones, but people should still be careful around strong magnetic or ultrasonic forces, such as those used in airport security screening.

DOs and DON'Ts in Managing Second-Degree Heart Block:

✔ **DO** eat a heart-healthy diet, low in fat and cholesterol.
✔ **DO** lose weight.
✔ **DO** stop smoking.
✔ **DO** call your doctor if you have dizziness, fainting, chest pain, or shortness of breath.

⊘ **DON'T** exercise until your doctor says that you can.

FROM THE DESK OF

NOTES

FOR MORE INFORMATION

Contact the following source:

• The American Heart Association
Tel: (800) 242-8721
Website: http://www.americanheart.org

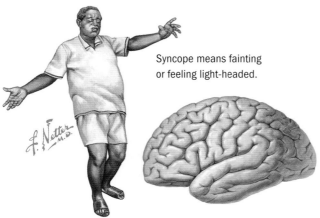

Syncope means fainting or feeling light-headed.

Blood carries oxygen to the brain. If blood (and thus oxygen) can't get to the brain, you can faint or feel light-headed. Anemia and dehydration are other causes of fainting.

ECG

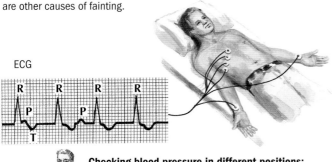

Checking blood pressure in different positions:

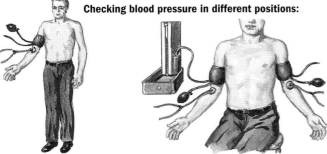

Standing

Right arm and left arm

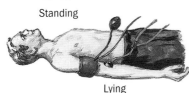

Lying

Your doctor will ask about your fainting, examine you, and order an ECG. Your doctor will also check your blood pressure with you in different positions (maybe with a tilt table) and before and after exercise.

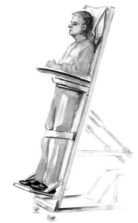

Tilt table testing

What Is Syncope?

Syncope means fainting or almost fainting or feeling light-headed.

What Causes Syncope?

People faint most often because they feel light-headed from hyperventilating or standing up too fast.

The usual cause is related to not enough blood flow to the brain, so not enough oxygen gets to the brain. Blood collecting in veins in the lower body because of gravity (venous pooling) or straining (Valsalva's maneuver) may prevent blood from reaching the brain. Damaged or stiff blood vessels and abnormal heart rhythms (arrhythmias) may also reduce blood flow.

Low blood pressure, ineffective pumping by the heart because of heart disease (heart failure), or heart valve abnormalities may cause fainting, as can anemia (low red blood cell count), drugs (especially those for high blood pressure), lung diseases, and too much water loss from the body (dehydration).

One type of fainting called vasovagal syncope refers to overstimulation of the vagus nerve, which lowers blood pressure and causes fainting. This type may occur with anxiety, pain, urination, or coughing.

What Are the Symptoms of Syncope?

Symptoms are sudden brief loss of consciousness, feeling dizzy or light-headed, and a heart rate that is too fast (palpitations) or too slow.

How Is Syncope Diagnosed?

The doctor will diagnose syncope on the basis of a history of fainting or feeling faint. Fainting once needs no medical care, but fainting often does. People with cardiovascular disease who faint should also see a doctor.

The doctor will do a physical examination and electrocardiography (ECG) and take blood pressure with the person in different positions (lying, sitting, standing, after exercise). Tilt table testing is a test done by specialists when the cause of syncope is unclear. It can check for symptoms with the body in different positions.

Blood sugar (glucose) level and blood count (hematocrit) may be checked.

If an irregular heartbeat is suspected, the doctor may use a Holter monitor, a device worn at home and work to monitor the heart rhythm.

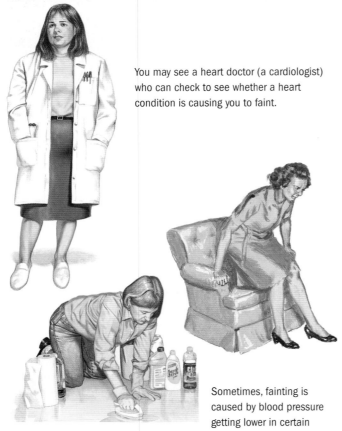

You may see a heart doctor (a cardiologist) who can check to see whether a heart condition is causing you to faint.

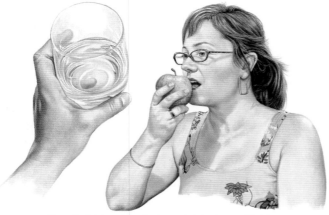

Sometimes, fainting is caused by blood pressure getting lower in certain positions, such as when standing from a sitting or kneeling position. This is called orthostatic hypotension. Keep a record of each fainting episode and what you were doing when it happened. Then, tell your doctor.

If you feel faint, sit or lie down. Drink plenty of fluids. If you have low blood sugar, eat something.

How Is Syncope Treated?

If not enough blood is pumped by the heart, the heart's condition must be checked. The doctor may suggest seeing a heart specialist (cardiologist).

For people with low blood pressure (hypotension) or heart disease, drugs that may be causing fainting are stopped on a trial basis.

DOs and DON'Ts in Managing Syncope:

✔ **DO** keep a record of fainting, for example, it happens when you suddenly stand from being seated.
✔ **DO** eat a proper diet and drink enough fluids. These are needed for avoiding fainting caused by low blood sugar and dehydration.
✔ **DO** sit or lie down if you feel faint, to help improve blood flow to the brain. Drink plenty of fluids once you are able to drink. If you have low blood sugar, eat something.
✔ **DO** call your doctor if you have fainting with chest pain, shortness of breath, or history of heart disease.

⊘ **DON'T** ignore any fainting episodes. Call your doctor.
⊘ **DON'T** put yourself in situations that make your fainting worse.

FROM THE DESK OF

NOTES

FOR MORE INFORMATION

Contact the following source:

• American Heart Association
Tel: (800) 242-8721
Website: http://www.americanheart.org

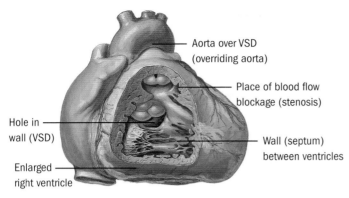

Tetralogy of Fallot, a heart abnormality present at birth, includes a ventricular septal defect (VSD), which is a hole in the wall (septum) between the right and left ventricles (lower chambers). This causes a mixing of oxygen-rich and oxygen-poor blood and increases pressure on the right ventricle. The right ventricle gets thick and blocks proper blood flow.

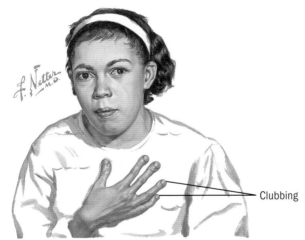

Children usually have a blue color (cyanosis) of the lips, nail beds, ears, and cheeks. They also have deformed fingers (clubbing).

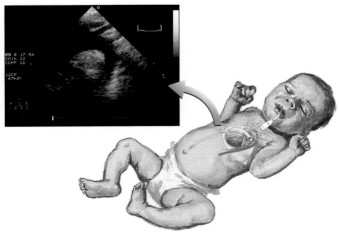

The doctor may suspect this disorder in an infant or child with cyanosis or heart murmur. For diagnosis, the doctor will order echocardiography. The doctor may also use blood tests, ECG, and x-rays.

What Is Tetralogy of Fallot?

Tetralogy of Fallot is a heart abnormality that is present at birth (congenital). The heart is a muscular pump with four chambers, two upper (left and right atria) and two lower (left and right ventricles). These contract and pump blood. A muscular wall (septum) separates the ventricles.

Tetralogy of Fallot has four features: (1) a hole between the ventricles called ventricular septal defect (VSD); (2) blocked flow of blood leaving the right ventricle (infundibular pulmonary stenosis); (3) an enlarged, thickened right ventricle; and (4) an aorta that gets mixed blood from both ventricles because it sits directly over the VSD (overriding aorta). The aorta is the main artery going from the heart to the body. The hole lets blood mix between ventricles, and pressure building in the right ventricle makes that ventricle larger. Blood without enough oxygen reaches body cells, causing a bluish tinge (cyanosis) of the lips, nails, and other body tissues.

What Causes Tetralogy of Fallot?

The cause is unknown.

What Are the Symptoms of Tetralogy of Fallot?

As a result of the blocking of blood flow from the right ventricle to the lungs, oxygen-poor blood is shunted (switched) from the right ventricle through the VSD to the left ventricle. The most common symptom is cyanosis, when lips, nail beds, ears, and cheeks turn blue. Some children squat after exercise, which reduces the amount of oxygen-poor blood shunting from the right ventricle to the left. Other symptoms include shortness of breath with exertion, weakness, fainting (syncope), clubbing of fingers, and heart murmurs. A heart murmur is a sound that the doctor hears with a stethoscope.

How Is Tetralogy of Fallot Diagnosed?

The doctor may suspect the diagnosis in any infant or child who has cyanosis and a heart murmur. The initial test is echocardiography, which uses sound waves to get pictures of the heart and its blood flow. The doctor will also order blood tests, electrocardiography (ECG), and chest x-rays. After the doctor makes the diagnosis, a heart catheterization may be done. In this test, a thin tube is put into a leg vein and passed up to the heart to measure pressure, oxygen levels, and degree of blood shunting among heart chambers.

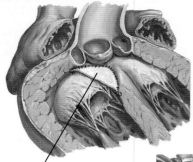

Almost all children with this disorder should have surgery. Surgery involves closing the VSD with a patch and relieving the blockage of blood flow from the right ventricle into the lungs.

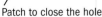
Patch to close the hole

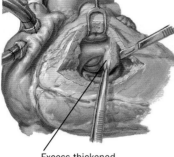

Excess thickened ventricle wall removed

Patches to relieve blockage

Your child will need to take antibiotics before dental work or operations.

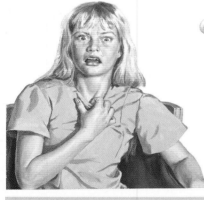

Call your doctor right away if your child has trouble breathing or turns blue.

How Is Tetralogy of Fallot Treated?

Surgery is the treatment of choice for almost all children with the abnormality. Surgery involves closing the VSD with a patch and relieving the blockage of blood flow from the right ventricle to the lungs.

DOs and DON'Ts in Managing Tetralogy of Fallot:

✔ **DO** realize that tetralogy of Fallot isn't very common.

✔ **DO** consult with a doctor specializing in heart diseases of children (pediatric cardiology).

✔ **DO** understand that children with tetralogy of Fallot need antibiotics before any dental work or surgery on the bowel or bladder to prevent heart infections.

✔ **DO** remember that fewer than 3% of people with this disorder reach age 40 without having surgery.

✔ **DO** call your doctor if your child has cyanosis or trouble breathing.

⊘ **DON'T** forget that nearly 40% of people with this tetralogy will have other heart abnormalities, such as atrial septal defect (a hole between the right and left atria) and lack of a pulmonary artery.

FROM THE DESK OF

NOTES

FOR MORE INFORMATION

Contact the following sources:

• American College of Cardiology
  Tel: (800) 575-9355
  Website: http://www.acc.org

• American Heart Association
  Tel: (800) 242-8721
  Website: http://www.americanheart.org

Angina occurs when the heart doesn't get enough oxygen. The usual cause is narrowed blood vessels (from atherosclerosis), but spasm of the coronary arteries can also cause it. Unstable angina has no pattern and doesn't go away (like stable angina). It's an emergency.

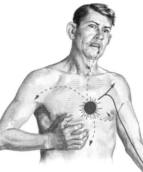

A blood clot partly blocking an artery will cause angina. If the clot grows and completely blocks the artery, a heart attack will occur.

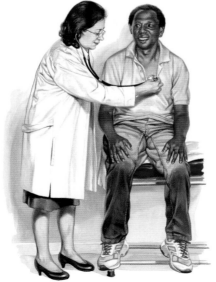

The usual symptom is a feeling of tightness, dull ache, or heaviness that begins in the chest and can spread to the neck, left shoulder, and down the arms, especially the left arm.

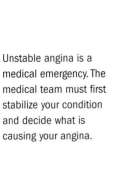

Unstable angina is a medical emergency. The medical team must first stabilize your condition and decide what is causing your angina.

What Is Unstable Angina?

Angina is chest pain resulting from reduced blood and oxygen to the heart. It can be a symptom of coronary artery disease, or atherosclerosis, when cholesterol and fats (plaque) build up inside arteries. Angina can also occur from a spasm of muscles in the coronary artery.

Unstable angina is less common than stable angina. Also, unstable angina pain doesn't follow a pattern, can happen without exertion, and doesn't go away by resting or taking medicine. Unstable angina is an emergency.

What Causes Unstable Angina?

Blood clots, which form plaques in the arteries, break open and block arteries. Clots may form, partly dissolve, and re-form. Unstable angina can occur whenever a clot blocks the coronary artery. Untreated clots may grow enough to block an artery completely and cause a heart attack.

What Are the Symptoms of Unstable Angina?

Symptoms include mild or severe discomfort or pain in the chest, felt as tightness, dull ache, or heaviness that may spread down the arms (especially left arm) or to the neck, shoulder, or jaw; shortness of breath; nausea; sweating; or weakness. Symptoms often occur at rest or with little physical exertion and are severe, long-lasting, and can't be predicted or helped by rest or medicine.

How Is Unstable Angina Diagnosed?

The doctor will take a medical history, do an examination, blood tests, electrocardiography (ECG), and chest x-rays. Emergency room doctors start treatment while they quickly find out how badly the heart is affected. Heart and breathing rates, blood pressure, and blood oxygen levels are measured.

If a blockage is suspected, the doctor may also look at heart arteries by a special x-ray test (coronary angiography). A specialist in heart diseases (cardiologist) passes a thin, flexible tube through an artery in the groin or arm to heart arteries.

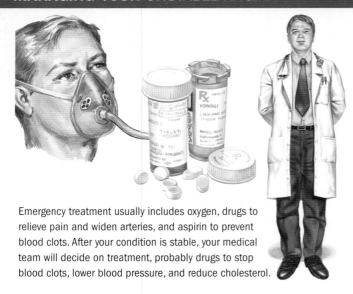

Emergency treatment usually includes oxygen, drugs to relieve pain and widen arteries, and aspirin to prevent blood clots. After your condition is stable, your medical team will decide on treatment, probably drugs to stop blood clots, lower blood pressure, and reduce cholesterol.

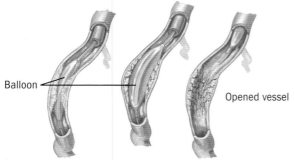

Balloon

Opened vessel

Severe angina that can't be treated with medicine may need angioplasty (opening clogged blood vessels with a balloon-like device).

Exercise under medical supervision to make the heart stronger and lose weight.

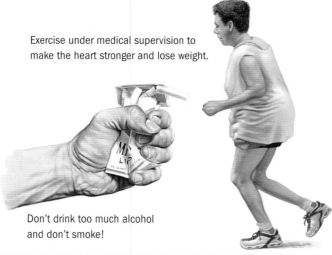

Don't drink too much alcohol and don't smoke!

FROM THE DESK OF

NOTES

How Is Unstable Angina Treated?

First, emergency room doctors stabilize a person's condition. Painkillers, aspirin (prevent blood clots), and oxygen (help breathing) may be given. A nitroglycerin capsule that dissolves inside the mouth widens the heart's blood vessels. Other drugs may be given to control blood pressure and open arteries.

Later treatments in the hospital (and after the hospital stay) include drugs (e.g., aspirin, clopidogrel, heparin) to stop clotting, medicines to lower blood pressure, and drugs (statins) to reduce blood cholesterol and fat levels.

Other treatments include operations called balloon angioplasty and stenting, and coronary artery bypass graft (CABG). For balloon angioplasty, blocked arteries are widened with a tiny balloon. A metal tube (stent) can be put in arteries to keep them open. In CABG, veins or arteries are transferred and sewn on (grafted) to blocked arteries so that blood flow can get past the blockage.

DOs and DON'Ts in Managing Unstable Angina:

✔ **DO** visit your doctor regularly and take all prescribed medicines.
✔ **DO** lose weight and eat healthy.
✔ **DO** always carry nitroglycerin with you and take it if needed.
✔ **DO** exercise only when approved to do so by your doctor.
✔ **DO** quit smoking.
✔ **DO** lower stress.
✔ **DO** know how and when to get medical care, because of heart attack risk.

⊘ **DON'T** delay getting medical care if symptoms worsen.
⊘ **DON'T** stop taking medicine without talking to your doctor.

FOR MORE INFORMATION

Contact the following sources:

• American Heart Association
 Tel: (800) 242-8721
 Website: http://www.americanheart.org

• American College of Cardiology
 Tel: (202) 375-6000
 Website: http://www.acc.org

• National Heart, Lung, and Blood Institute
 Tel: (301) 592-8573
 Website: http://www.nhlbi.nih.gov

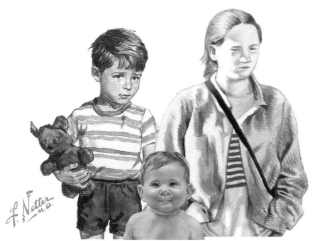

Ventricular septal defect (VSD) is a congenital defect (present at birth). It is more common in girls than in boys. The cause is unknown.

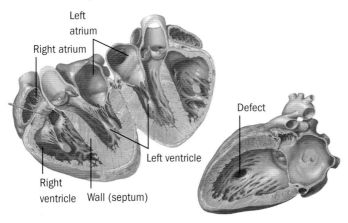

Left atrium

Right atrium

Defect

Left ventricle

Right ventricle   Wall (septum)

VSD is a hole in the wall (septum) in the heart muscle dividing the left and right ventricles (lower chambers). The hole lets blood from both sides of the heart mix, which reduces oxygen getting to the body.

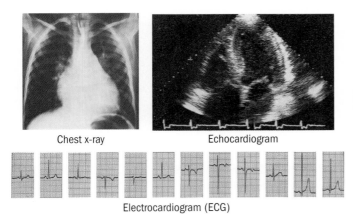

Chest x-ray   Echocardiogram

Electrocardiogram (ECG)

Diagnosis is based on symptoms, physical examination, and tests such as ECG, x-rays, and echocardiography (uses sound waves to get pictures of the heart).

What Is Ventricular Septal Defect?

The two ventricles are lower chambers of the heart and are divided by a wall (septum). Ventricular septal defect (VSD) is a hole in this septum. The left side of the heart normally pumps under higher pressure than the right side. The VSD produces a left-to-right switch (shunt) that allows blood from both sides of the heart to mix. The heart has trouble getting oxygen to the rest of the body because it pumps blood with less oxygen to the body. Circulation on the right side of the system can be overloaded, so increased pressure occurs in the lungs (pulmonary hypertension).

VSDs are the most common type of heart abnormality developing before birth (congenital). Defects usually close by themselves or are surgically closed in childhood, but they may last into adulthood. More girls than boys have VSDs.

A small defect may not cause a problem. Large defects can cause heart failure (the heart can't pump enough blood). The result is feeling tired, trouble breathing (especially with exertion), or chest pain. Sometimes the skin turns blue (cyanosis) because blood with less oxygen reaches the skin. Abnormal heart rhythms (arrhythmias) may develop. If a defect is near the aortic valve, damage to that valve may occur as children grow.

What Causes Ventricular Septal Defect?

The cause is unknown.

What Are the Symptoms of Ventricular Septal Defect?

The most common symptoms are a feeling of weakness, trouble breathing, chest pain, bluish color of the skin, and irregular heartbeat.

How Is Ventricular Septal Defect Diagnosed?

The doctor uses symptoms and a physical examination to make a diagnosis. Electrocardiography (ECG) may show abnormalities. A chest x-ray may also be abnormal and show enlargement of the heart and of lung vessels. Echocardiography (a test using sound waves to get pictures of the heart) can be used to study the heart's structure and pumping and measure how well the ventricles work, and examine blood flow.

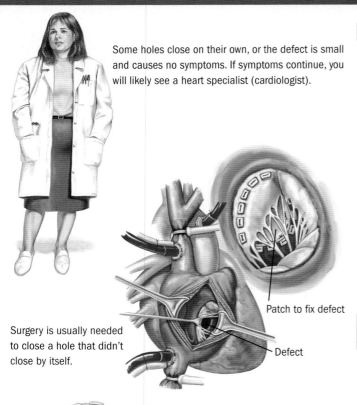

Some holes close on their own, or the defect is small and causes no symptoms. If symptoms continue, you will likely see a heart specialist (cardiologist).

Patch to fix defect

Defect

Surgery is usually needed to close a hole that didn't close by itself.

People with VSD (either open or surgically closed) need antibiotics before dental work and other surgeries to prevent bacterial infections of the lining of the heart.

Discuss exercise with your doctor. Many people can have a normal lifestyle, but each case is different so check with your doctor to be sure.

How Is Ventricular Septal Defect Treated?

People with a small defect or a defect that has closed may never have symptoms and usually need no treatment. If the defect lasts, treatment to correct the defect would likely be needed.

People with VSDs usually see a heart specialist (cardiologist). Treatment may involve surgery to correct the defect. Heart failure, if it occurs, can be treated with drugs to reduce the excess blood volume and help the heart contract better. Sometimes the aortic valve is replaced. If no other heart disease exists, correcting the defect usually allows a normal life span and lifestyle.

People with an open VSD or those who had surgery to close the VSD must take antibiotics before and after dental work or surgery. Antibiotics help prevent infection of the lining of the heart (bacterial endocarditis).

DOs and DON'Ts in Managing Ventricular Septal Defect:

✔ **DO** take your medicines as prescribed.
✔ **DO** call your doctor if you have VSD symptoms.

🚫 **DON'T** neglect worsening symptoms. See your doctor.

FROM THE DESK OF

NOTES

FOR MORE INFORMATION

Contact the following source:

• American Heart Association
 Tel: (800) 242-8721
 Website: http://www.americanheart.org

MANAGING YOUR
ACNE

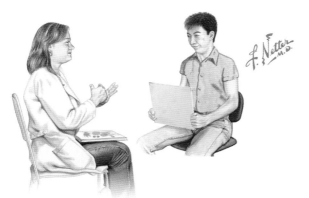

Acne is a very common condition, especially during adolescence. A number of things can help control it. Together, you and your doctor can find something that works for you.

Whitehead Skin pore **Blackhead**

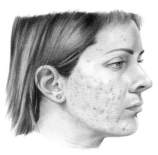

Oil gland

Oil glands become more active, and oil may become blocked at the skin pore and form a whitehead. A blackhead is a gland with an open pore.

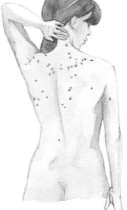

Pimples and cysts form when oil leaks into surrounding skin and causes redness (inflammation) and infection. Squeezing pimples can also cause scarring.

The upper back may also be involved.

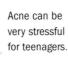

Acne can be very stressful for teenagers.

What Is Acne?

Acne vulgaris is called simply acne, pimples, or zits. Almost all teenagers have it. Acne usually gets better with age, but sometimes older people, especially women, can get acne.

What Causes Acne?

In the midteens, skin oil (sebaceous) glands begin to produce more oil. Oily skin usually results, but in some people this oil is blocked at skin pore openings. Bacteria, oil, and other materials block these pores. Blocked oil backs up and forms whiteheads; if pores are open to the air, blackheads form. Blocked oil in the skin causes redness (inflammation) and infection, and then pimples and cysts. Boys usually have more oily skin than girls and often worse acne. Foods do not affect acne. Acne is not an infection, so it cannot be caught from someone else.

What Are the Symptoms of Acne?

A rash usually occurs on the face, shoulders, and back. The small bumps can be whiteheads, blackheads, or pimples with pus.

How Is Acne Diagnosed?

Usually, the doctor just does a skin examination. Sometimes blood tests may be done to help pick the best medicine and to monitor side effects from treatment.

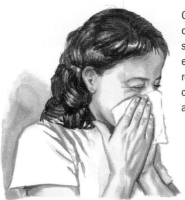

Gently wash your skin at least once a day. Products with salicylic acid may be very effective. Your doctor may also recommend special lotions or creams to apply to the acne-prone areas.

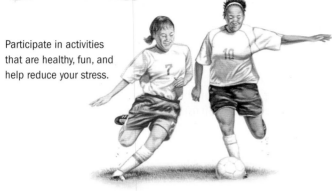

Participate in activities that are healthy, fun, and help reduce your stress.

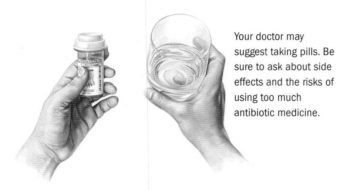

Your doctor may suggest taking pills. Be sure to ask about side effects and the risks of using too much antibiotic medicine.

Be patient. Prescription and over-the-counter creams and pills take time to work. Give treatment at least 8 to 10 weeks to start having an effect.

How Is Acne Treated?

Whatever the treatment, a few weeks may pass before acne improves. Sometimes, acne may worsen before improving.

A healthy diet, regular exercise, daily skin care with salicylic acid compounds and cleansing soaps, and gentle washing (no scrubbing) are important.

Treatment usually starts with lowest strength over-the-counter topical medicines (put on the skin). These drugs are usually antibiotics and peeling agents (comedolytics). Antibiotics include benzoyl peroxide, erythromycin, and clindamycin. The over-the-counter benzoyl peroxide has both peeling and antibiotic effects.

Additional prescription drugs include other peeling agents, antibiotics, and hormones.

Most people outgrow acne by their mid 20s. Rarely, severe cases may need special treatment, such as surgery.

DOs and DON'Ts in Managing Acne:

✔ **DO** eat a healthy diet, exercise regularly, and wash oily skin gently, at least twice daily, with medicated soap and water.
✔ **DO** use pills or creams according to your doctor's instruction.
✔ **DO** use oil-free cosmetics, suntan lotions, and shampoos.
✔ **DO** call your doctor if your acne gets worse despite treatment or if you have bad scarring.
✔ **DO** see a dermatologist if your doctor recommends it.
✔ **DO** call your doctor if you have emotional problems because of acne. Acne may cause embarrassment, anxiety, and social difficulties.

🚫 **DON'T** be impatient. Improvement usually takes a few weeks.
🚫 **DON'T** avoid specific foods unless you find that they make your acne worse.
🚫 **DON'T** pinch, squeeze, or pick your pimples. Infection and scarring can result.
🚫 **DON'T** sunbathe. It can make acne worse.
🚫 **DON'T** use over-the-counter acne drugs while you take prescription drugs, unless your doctor knows.

FROM THE DESK OF

NOTES

FOR MORE INFORMATION

Contact the following source:

• American Academy of Dermatology
930 North Meachum Road
Schaumburg, IL 60173
Tel: (866) 503-7546
Website: http://www.aad.org/

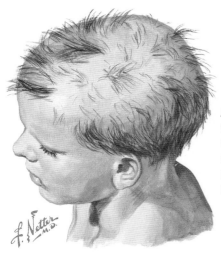

Alopecia means hair loss. People can lose hair because of infections, burns, severe illness, and even after having major surgery.

Some causes of alopecia

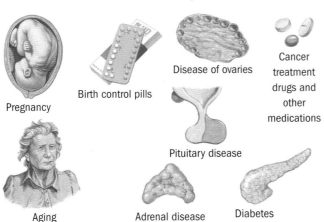

Pregnancy

Birth control pills

Disease of ovaries

Cancer treatment drugs and other medications

Pituitary disease

Aging

Adrenal disease

Diabetes

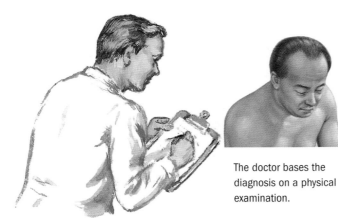

The doctor bases the diagnosis on a physical examination.

What Is Alopecia?

Alopecia means hair loss. Alopecia areata is hair loss in round patches on the scalp. Alopecia universalis refers to hair loss over the whole body.

What Causes Alopecia?

Heredity plays a major role in hair loss. Other contributing factors are the presence of male hormones, worry and stress, poor nutrition, low red blood cell count, thyroid problems, pregnancy, ringworm of the scalp, and medicines such as oral contraceptives, anticancer drugs, and statins.

Hair can also be lost because of hairstyles, pulling on hair, infections, burns, severe illness, and even after having major surgery.

Alopecia can be permanent or temporary (such as when caused by cancer treatment drugs).

What Are the Symptoms of Alopecia?

Hair can be lost from any part of the body, the scalp, eyebrows, underarms, genital area, arms, and legs. It can occur gradually or suddenly. Itching may occur, for example, when ringworm is the cause.

How Is Alopecia Diagnosed?

The doctor bases the diagnosis on the physical examination. Blood tests may be done to check for anemia, infection, arthritis, or hormone imbalances. Analysis of hair can also be performed.

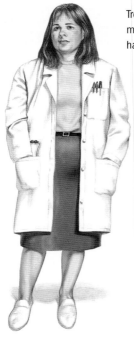

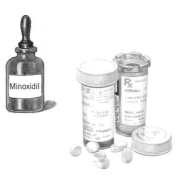

Treatments include using a topical solution and medicines. Follow your doctor's advice if you have anemia or thyroid problems.

Minoxidil

How Is Alopecia Treated?

Treatment doesn't always work. The doctor may suggest a solution (minoxidil) to put on areas with alopecia. It may help hair regrow but its effects vary greatly. The doctor may sometimes inject medicine (steroids) into small areas with alopecia.

Hair transplants can restore hair, and wigs and hair weaves may reduce the look of alopecia.

For alopecia on the scalp, the doctor can use scalp reduction therapy. In this therapy, the doctor removes a strip of scalp about every 4 weeks until edges of hair meet, or until scalp tissue becomes too thin.

Men with male pattern baldness can take finasteride (Propecia^R), a prescription drug taken by mouth, to minimize alopecia and promote regrowth of hair.

An illness causing alopecia, such as infection, ringworm, anemia, and hormone imbalance, will need treatment. Alopecia with reversible causes, such as pregnancy and stress, usually stops, and new hair grows, but this may take several months.

DOs and DON'Ts in Managing Alopecia:

✔ **DO** bathe and shampoo as usual.
✔ **DO** be sure to follow your doctor's advice if you have anemia or thyroid problems.
✔ **DO** avoid alkaline pH shampoos.
✔ **DO** pat your hair dry rather than rubbing it with a towel.
✔ **DO** use a comb rather than a brush, and avoid brushing your hair excessively when it is wet.
✔ **DO** use a conditioner for easier combing.
✔ **DO** call your doctor if signs of infection appear after treatment with steroid injections. These signs include redness, swelling, tenderness, and warmth at the site of injections.
✔ **DO** consider wearing a hairpiece or wig if you think this improves how you look.

⊘ **DON'T** tug on normal hair close to areas of alopecia.
⊘ **DON'T** damage your hair by bleaching, permanent waving, straightening, using hot combs or overly hot dryers, or excessive sun exposure.

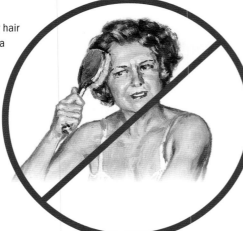

Don't brush your hair excessively. Use a comb.

FROM THE DESK OF

NOTES

FOR MORE INFORMATION

Contact the following source:

• The National Alopecia Areata Foundation
Tel: (415) 472-3780
Website: http://www.naaf.org/

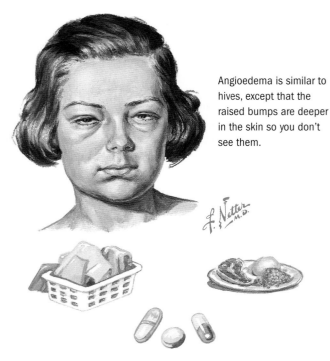

Angioedema is similar to hives, except that the raised bumps are deeper in the skin so you don't see them.

New foods, perfumes, drugs, soaps, and clothes are the usual causes of angioedema.

Areas commonly affected by angioedema:

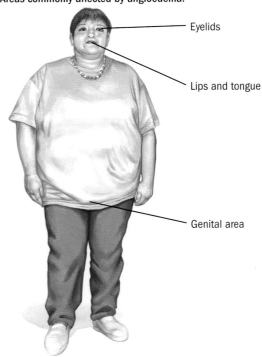

Eyelids

Lips and tongue

Genital area

What Is Angioedema?

Angioedema is an allergic reaction that is like the common skin condition of hives (urticaria). Hives are raised, red, itchy, irregular bumps on the skin. In angioedema, the same thing happens but it is deeper in the skin. The bumps cannot be seen but can be felt. Anyone can get angioedema. About 15% to 20% of all people will have at least one episode of hives or angioedema in their lifetime.

What Causes Angioedema?

Usual causes are taking new drugs, eating new foods, and wearing new perfumes. But even foods or drugs used in the past without problems can cause an allergic reaction later. Angioedema cannot be caught and is not an infection, although infections can cause it. Certain types are hereditary (may occur in family members).

What Are the Symptoms of Angioedema?

The main symptom is swollen skin that can be tender and painful. Swelling at one spot is usually present for only a day or two, but swelling will move from one spot to another and last for several days or may become chronic. Chronic angioedema, although uncomfortable and irritating, usually won't become more serious.

Angioedema can occur anywhere on the body but more often involves eyelids, lips, tongue, and genitals. Outside the body it is usually not dangerous. It can also occur inside the body, in intestines and lungs (airways), where it can potentially cause breathing difficulty, which can be serious and even fatal.

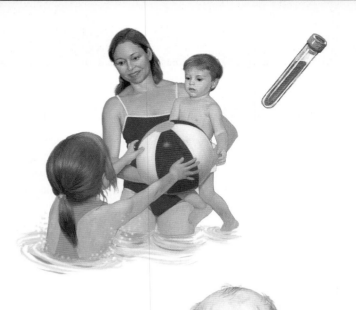

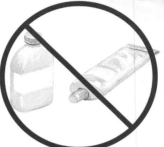

Diagnosis is usually made by finding swollen areas under the skin, reviewing family history, and blood tests.

Lotions and creams do not provide relief, because the angioedema is too deep for them to reach.

The best treatment is stopping exposure to the cause. Cold compresses may help you feel more comfortable. Your doctor may prescribe oral antihistamines or stronger medicine, such as steroids.

How Is Angioedema Diagnosed?

The doctor examines the swollen skin and the tendency of swelling to come and go for diagnosis. Blood tests can be done but don't always help or affect treatment. A family history is very important, so the doctor will ask family members about any episodes of angioedema.

How Is Angioedema Treated?

No cure exists, but symptoms can be controlled.

The best treatment is to remove the cause. However, the exact cause is often unknown or impossible to remove. Therefore the main approach to management is control of symptoms.

Application of cold compresses may provide comfort. Lotions and creams don't usually help because they don't get deep enough when they're applied to the skin.

Oral antihistamines work well, but the right dose must be taken regularly, or the angioedema may return. Antihistamines also may have side effects (drowsiness, dry mouth), but newer antihistamines have fewer of these effects. Stronger drugs (prednisone or other steroids) may help if antihistamines don't control the angioedema.

DOs and DON'Ts in Managing Angioedema:

✔ **DO** call your doctor immediately if you have trouble breathing, are wheezing, or have chest or abdominal pain. Angioedema may require long-term treatment.
✔ **DO** use cold compresses on swollen areas.
✔ **DO** take antihistamines in proper doses.
✔ **DO** note any possible causes (new foods, drugs, soaps, perfumes, clothes). Avoid those items that trigger the reaction. Ask your doctor about your drugs.
✔ **DO** call your doctor if your angioedema doesn't respond to 2 or 3 days of continuous antihistamines.
✔ **DO** call your doctor if you have repeated attacks of angioedema.

🚫 **DON'T** treat swelling with heat, creams, ointments, or lotions.

FROM THE DESK OF

NOTES

FOR MORE INFORMATION

Contact the following source:

• American Academy of Dermatology
930 North Meachum Road
Schaumburg, IL 60173
Tel: (866) 503-7546
Website: http://www.aad.org/

MANAGING YOUR
BALANITIS

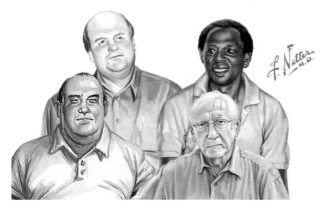

Balanitis is swelling and soreness or irritation of the head (tip) of your penis. It tends to occur more often in men who are not circumcised.

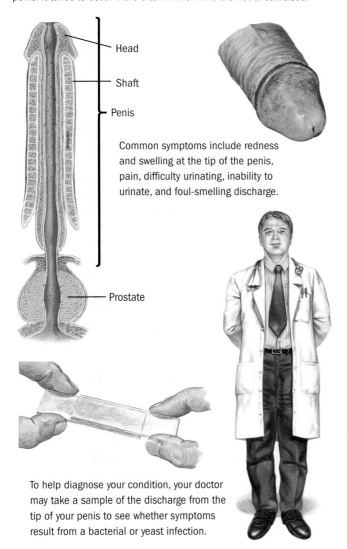

Head

Shaft

Penis

Common symptoms include redness and swelling at the tip of the penis, pain, difficulty urinating, inability to urinate, and foul-smelling discharge.

Prostate

To help diagnose your condition, your doctor may take a sample of the discharge from the tip of your penis to see whether symptoms result from a bacterial or yeast infection.

What Is Balanitis?

Balanitis is swelling (inflammation) and soreness or irritation of the head (tip, or glans) of the penis. It tends to occur more often in men who are not circumcised. It usually occurs with posthitis (inflammation of the foreskin, the thin sheath of skin that covers the head of the penis). Together the two types of inflammation are called balanoposthitis. Circumcised men never have balanoposthitis because they have no foreskin. These common disorders affect men and boys of all ages.

What Causes Balanitis?

Causes include bacterial or yeast infections, urinary tract infection, sexually transmitted disease, poor hygiene, contraceptive foams or creams, injury or trauma, sexual intercourse, and allergies. Also, a tight foreskin can trap urine, bacteria, and other microorganisms, which can cause balanitis.

What Are the Symptoms of Balanitis?

Common symptoms include redness and swelling at the tip of the penis or foreskin, pain, difficulty urinating, inability to urinate, and bad-smelling discharge. The foreskin can become red, swollen, and tender. In untreated balanitis, the shaft of the penis may become involved, and blisters and ulcers can form.

How Is Balanitis Diagnosed?

The doctor takes a medical history and does a physical examination. A sample of the discharge may be taken to see whether bacteria or yeast are causing symptoms.

The doctor may also do a blood test if a more serious disease, such as diabetes or syphilis, could be present.

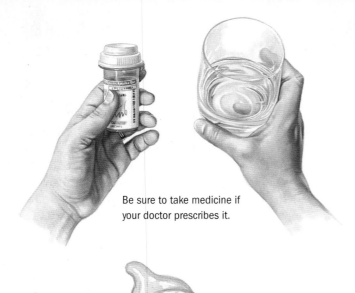

Be sure to take medicine if your doctor prescribes it.

If your balanitis is caused by an infection, be sure to wear a condom during sex, so that your partner does not become infected.

Call your doctor if, after treatment, you have trouble urinating or if your urine has blood or pus in it.

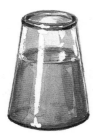

Use creams as recommended by your doctor.

How Is Balanitis Treated?

Balanitis and posthitis usually respond well to treatment. Treatment depends on age, cause, and whether the person is sexually active and circumcised. Treatment involves retracting the foreskin and soaking the area in lukewarm water. Mild cases need an antibiotic cream for the area. Men with more severe cases or with diabetes may take antibiotics by mouth. If the cause is a yeast or fungal infection, a topical antifungal cream is usually applied to the area. Sometimes corticosteroid creams are given to reduce swelling. Surgery is rarely required. Recovery time depends on the cause and whether the person follows the doctor's instructions. In simple cases, symptoms may improve or even disappear in 5 to 10 days. In complex cases, full recovery may take longer.

DOs and DON'Ts in Managing Balanitis:

✔ **DO** use good hygiene, including pushing back your foreskin and cleaning the tip of your penis.

✔ **DO** wear condoms during sex.

✔ **DO** use creams or antibiotic pills as directed by your doctor.

✔ **DO** try a milder soap to see if it helps relieve symptoms.

✔ **DO** call your doctor if swelling worsens even with treatment.

✔ **DO** call your doctor if your condition hasn't improved in 3 or 4 days.

✔ **DO** call your doctor if you have trouble producing urine or if you see blood or pus in your urine.

✔ **DO** call your doctor if balanitis returns, and consider circumcision if you get balanitis or posthitis over and over.

🚫 **DON'T** stop treatment early, especially if you take antibiotics. Even if symptoms are getting better or are gone, you need to finish taking the antibiotic. Otherwise, your symptoms can return.

🚫 **DON'T** have unprotected sex while getting treatment.

FOR MORE INFORMATION

Contact the following sources:

- American Urological Association
  Tel: (866) RING AUA (746-4282)
  Website: http://www.auanet.org/

- American Academy of Dermatology
  930 North Meachum Road
  Schaumburg, IL 60173
  Tel: (866) 503-7546
  Website: http://www.aad.org/

FROM THE DESK OF

NOTES

MANAGING YOUR
BASAL CELL SKIN CANCER

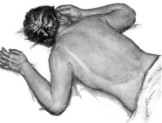

Exposure to ultraviolet light from the sun or tanning booth increases the risk of basal cell carcinoma (BCC), the most common type of skin cancer. It usually develops after age 40, but you most likely increased your risk of getting it when you were younger.

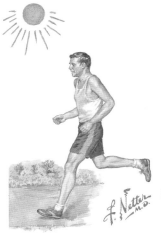

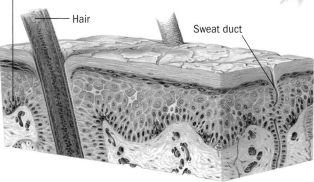

Basal cell layer

Hair

Sweat duct

Basal cells are at the bottom of the epidermis—the outermost layer of the skin.

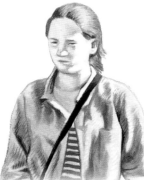

Risk factors
· Fair skin
· Freckles
· Burn more than tan in the sun
· Work outdoors
· Have HIV
· Family history of basal cell cancer

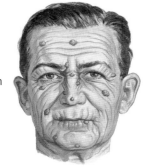

The doctor will suspect BCC based on the appearance of the skin but will need to do a biopsy for diagnosis.

What Is Basal Cell Skin Cancer?

The most common type of skin cancer is basal cell carcinoma (BCC). It grows very slowly and almost never spreads to other parts of the body. It usually grows on parts of the head and neck that had a lot of sun exposure. It occurs more commonly after age 40.

What Causes BCC?

Exposure to ultraviolet light (both UVA and UVB) from the sun or light in tanning salons increases the risk of BCC.

Risk of getting BCC is also greater for people who have fair skin and tend to freckle or burn instead of tan. Repeated sunburns or excessive childhood sun exposures, an outdoor job, HIV, medicine that suppresses the body's infection-fighting system, personal or family history of BCC, and radiation treatment can also increase risk.

What Are the Symptoms of BCC?

BCC usually does not cause any symptoms; however, it can sometimes bleed or scab. It may also be itchy, but it usually doesn't hurt.

Doctors classify the different types of BCC according to shape, appearance, and color. The most common have a raised, white or pink border and a central depression.

How Is BCC Diagnosed?

The doctor will suspect BCC based on the appearance of the skin but will need a biopsy to confirm the diagnosis. In a biopsy, a small piece of the skin area is removed and sent to the laboratory for study under a microscope.

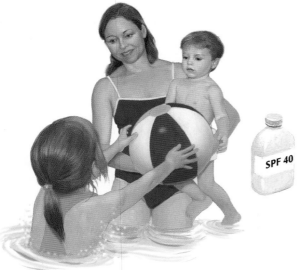

If your biopsy results show BCC, your doctor will remove it completely. Several methods are available depending on its location and your medical history.

Always wear sunscreen with SPF 15 or higher whenever you're in the sun. Teach your children the importance of sunscreen to reduce their risk of getting BCC.

Get a yearly skin examination. Your doctor may suggest an examination more than once a year.

How Is BCC Treated?

Treatment usually consists of doing a biopsy and later removing the skin lesion. Sometimes, the doctor will remove the abnormal area completely without doing a biopsy if the area is small.

BCC may in rare cases recur after treatment, especially on the ears, eyelids, scalp, and nose.

Other treatment methods are electrosurgery (using an electric needle), cryosurgery (freezing), radiation therapy, and Mohs' surgery. Mohs' surgery is a special method for removing BCCs on the nose or eyelid or large BCCs, or for recurrent BCC.

DOs and DON'Ts in Managing BCC:

✔ **DO** follow all your doctor's instructions after treatment.

✔ **DO** resume usual activities after you go home.

✔ **DO** avoid sunburns (especially small children).

✔ **DO** have a skin examination yearly, or more often if your doctor recommends it.

✔ **DO** call your doctor if you have a new mole or abnormal skin area, an area that doesn't heal or that bleeds often, a raised skin mole with a central depressed area, a mole that changes shape or color or that has irregular or unclear borders, or a mole that is asymmetric (one side looks different from the other).

✔ **DO** wear sunscreen with a sun protection factor (SPF) of 15 or higher, protective clothing, and hats.

✔ **DO** call your doctor if the incision becomes red and swollen or has drainage or if you have a temperature higher than 100° F.

🚫 **DON'T** go in the sun when it's hottest, especially from 11 am to 3 pm during summer days.

🚫 **DON'T** delay seeing your doctor if you have any warning signs of skin cancer.

FROM THE DESK OF

NOTES

FOR MORE INFORMATION

Contact the following sources:

• American Academy of Dermatology
  Tel: (866) 503-SKIN (503-7546)
  Website: http://www.aad.org

• American Cancer Society
  Tel: (800) ACS-2345 (227-2345)
  Website: http://www.cancer.org/

MANAGING YOUR
BEHÇET'S SYNDROME

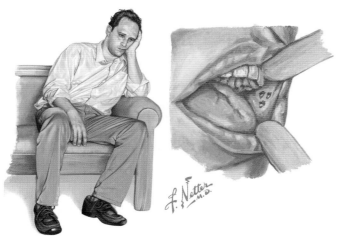

Behçet's syndrome occurs in men twice as often as in women. Most people have painful mouth sores, and more than 70% have skin blisters. Symptoms can include feeling tired, sluggish, or "down."

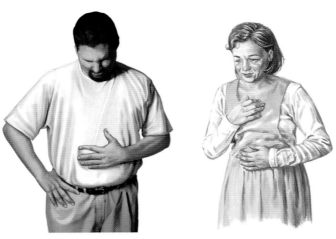

Symptoms also can include stomach pains, diarrhea, chest pain, and trouble breathing.

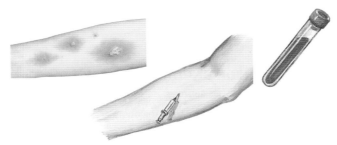

A pathergy (skin) test and blood tests are used for diagnosis.

What Is Behçet's Syndrome?

Behçet's syndrome is a lifelong illness that causes irritation (inflammation) and sores in blood vessels, mouth, genitals, eyes, joints, skin, brain, and nerves. This illness occurs when the immune system becomes too active and attacks parts of the body (autoimmune disease).

Behçet's syndrome occurs in men twice as often as in women and usually starts in early adulthood.

What Causes Behçet's Syndrome?

The cause of this rare syndrome is unknown. It is more common in people of Mediterranean, Middle Eastern, or Japanese descent.

What Are the Symptoms of Behçet's Syndrome?

Symptoms tend to come and go, with remissions sometimes lasting months or years. Most people have painful mouth sores; more than 70% have skin blisters that often occur after minor injuries to the skin. The many other possible symptoms include feeling tired, sluggish, or confused; fever; muscle and joint pain; feeling unwell or uncomfortable; eye pain and redness; trouble seeing; stomach pain or diarrhea; blood or mucus (thick slippery liquid) in bowel movements (stools); chest pain or trouble breathing; feeling tingling, numbness; feeling weak; having trouble with balance and walking; poor hearing; and headache or stiff neck.

How Is Behçet's Syndrome Diagnosed?

The doctor makes the diagnosis on the basis of a physical examination and possibly blood tests to rule out other diseases and check general health. Some tests will show inflammation. However, there are no specific tests to prove that Behçet's syndrome is present.

The doctor may also order a pathergy test. In this test, the skin of the forearm is poked with a needle and then checked later for a reaction (redness).

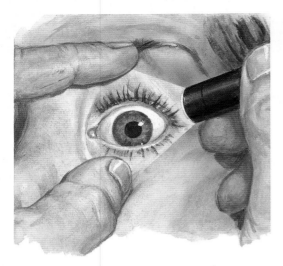

If your eyes are affected, your doctor will refer you to an eye doctor (ophthalmologist) for treatment.

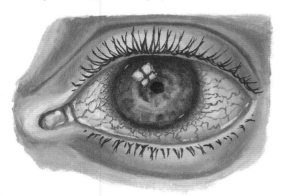

Your eyes may be inflamed (red), and you may have trouble seeing. Call your doctor immediately if your eyesight is affected.

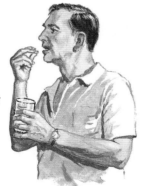

Take your medicine as your doctor instructs you to.

How Is Behçet's Syndrome Treated?

Treatment is effective in helping most symptoms. The doctor can prescribe medicine to reduce inflammation and help symptoms go away. Many types of drugs can be used, such as medicine to slow the immune system reaction, antibiotic mouthwashes for mouth sores, nonsteroidal antiinflammatory drugs (NSAIDs) for joint pain, and blood thinners to stop clots from forming.

The doctor will suggest an eye doctor (ophthalmologist) for treatment of eye problems.

DOs and DON'Ts in Managing Behçet's Syndrome:

✔ **DO** take your medicine as instructed. It can prevent serious complications, such as vision problems.
✔ **DO** call your doctor if you have symptoms that worry you.
✔ **DO** talk to your doctor before taking herbal remedies. Some don't go well with prescribed medicine.
✔ **DO** call your doctor immediately if your eyesight is affected.
✔ **DO** call your doctor if you have problems with your medicines. These side effects can include stomach pain, feeling sick, being sick, thrush, high blood pressure, trouble sleeping, feeling either very down or very high, convulsions, acne, sores that heal very slowly, stretch marks, or blurred vision.

⊘ **DON'T** forget to take your medicines.
⊘ **DON'T** forget doctor's appointments.

FROM THE DESK OF

NOTES

FOR MORE INFORMATION

Contact the following sources:
- American Behçet's Disease Association
  Tel: (800) 7BEHCET (723-4238)
  Website: http://www.behcets.com/
- **Website: www.nlm.nih.gov/medlineplus/ behcetssyndrome.html**

MANAGING YOUR
CANDIDIASIS

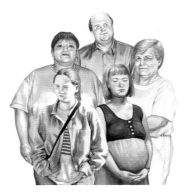

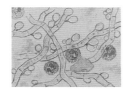

Candida under the microscope

Anyone can develop candidiasis, or infection with the yeast *Candida*, a fungus. *Candida* fungi normally live on the skin and are harmless, but they can overgrow and cause an infection.

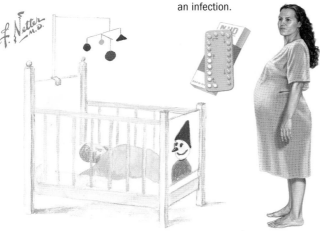

Pregnancy, diabetes, a weak immune system, certain medicines, and HIV infection can increase your risk of candidiasis. Diaper rash in babies is also usually due to candidiasis.

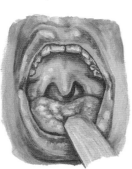

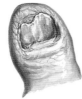

Candidiasis usually occurs in the genital area, mouth, skin folds, or nails.

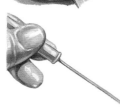

The doctor will use a swab to take samples from the mouth or genital area or will take scrapings from the nail and send them to a laboratory for diagnosis.

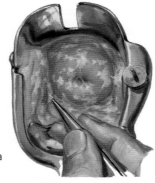

Genital area (cervix)

What Is Candidiasis?

Candidiasis is infection with a type of fungus, a yeast called *Candida*. Candidiasis can occur in genital areas, mouth, skin folds, or nails. In the vagina, candidiasis is called yeast vaginitis. In the mouth, candidiasis is called thrush. Diaper rash in babies is often due to candidiasis.

What Causes Candidiasis?

Anyone can get candidiasis. *Candida* fungi normally live on the skin and are harmless. Too much moisture favors overgrowth of the fungus and can lead to infection. Pregnancy, diabetes mellitus, weak immune system, and certain medicines such as antibiotics and corticosteroids can increase chances of infection.

What Are the Symptoms of Candidiasis?

Women with vaginal candidiasis have intense itching in the vagina. Burning during urination, white patches on the vagina surface, and an odorless cottage cheese–like liquid coming from the vagina may occur.

Mouth candidiasis causes raised white patches inside the mouth or on the tongue, splitting or cracking on the side of the mouth, and swollen gums or red and white sores on the gums.

Nail candidiasis causes swelling around nails and separation between nails and cuticles, pain around the nail base, and yellow or blackish-brown nails.

Skin with candidiasis may itch, look moist, and appear irritated.

How Is Candidiasis Diagnosed?

The doctor will use a swab to take samples from the affected area, such as the genitals or mouth, or will take scrapings from the nail and send them to a laboratory for diagnosis.

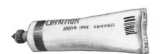
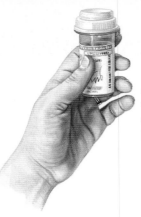

Antifungal medicine—pills, ointment, vaginal cream, suppositories, powder, or spray—usually clears up the infection in 1 to 2 weeks.

The fungus *Candida* needs moisture to live, so wear loose cotton clothing to keep your skin cool and dry and reduce infection risk.

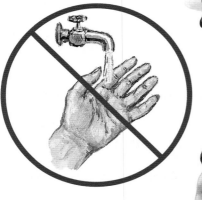

Don't keep your hands in water too long.

Keep your skin cool and dry.

How Is Candidiasis Treated?

The doctor will prescribe antifungal medicine (pills, ointment, vaginal cream, suppositories, powder, or spray). The doctor may want to treat partners with genital candidiasis to avoid spreading the infection. Wear loose cotton clothing to keep your skin cool and dry.

Genital candidiasis will clear up in 4 to 7 days. Mouth and skin candidiasis will clear up in 1 or 2 weeks. Nail candidiasis often needs longer treatment.

DOs and DON'Ts in Managing Candidiasis:

✔ **DO** keep your genital area clean and wear cotton, loose-fitting underpants if you have genital candidiasis. Lose weight if needed, and don't use harsh chemicals such as douches. Practice safe sex (use condoms).

✔ **DO** avoid oral sex if you have mouth candidiasis.

✔ **DO** dry your hands well after washing if you have nail candidiasis. Don't soak your hands in water.

✔ **DO** change the baby's diaper often and keep the area dry for diaper rash.

✔ **DO** keep your skin clean and dry.

✔ **DO** make sure that your diabetes is controlled.

✔ **DO** take antibiotics only when prescribed by your doctor.

✔ **DO** call your doctor if the infection continues despite treatment.

⊘ **DON'T** wear tight panty hose or have intercourse until the infection clears up if you have genital candidiasis.

⊘ **DON'T** put rubber pants on your baby. It will increase the risk of diaper rash.

FOR MORE INFORMATION

Contact the following sources:

• The American College of Obstetricians and Gynecologists
Website: http://www.acog.org

• Obgyn.net
Website: http://www.obgyn.net

• American Academy of Dermatology
Tel: (866) 503-SKIN (503-7546)
Website: http://www.aad.org

FROM THE DESK OF

NOTES

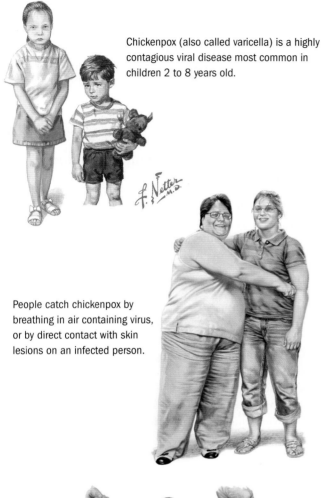

Chickenpox (also called varicella) is a highly contagious viral disease most common in children 2 to 8 years old.

People catch chickenpox by breathing in air containing virus, or by direct contact with skin lesions on an infected person.

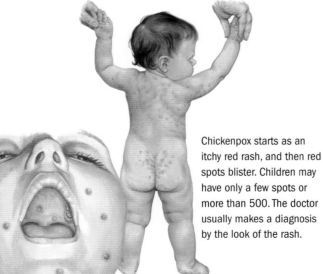

Chickenpox starts as an itchy red rash, and then red spots blister. Children may have only a few spots or more than 500. The doctor usually makes a diagnosis by the look of the rash.

What Is Chickenpox?

Chickenpox (also called varicella) is a highly contagious viral disease that affects skin and mucous membranes. Most cases occur in young people, often children 2 to 8 years old. Adults usually have a more severe illness that lasts longer.

People develop immunity or resistance to chickenpox when they get it the first time and are unlikely to get it again. Some people may later develop shingles (herpes zoster), a reactivation of chickenpox virus, if their immunity weekens.

Immunizations with varicella-zoster vaccine can prevent chickenpox and shingles.

What Causes Chickenpox?

The cause is varicella-zoster herpesvirus. People catch chickenpox, when they are around someone who has it, by breathing in droplets containing virus. People also catch it by direct contact with skin lesions on infected people.

What Are the Symptoms of Chickenpox?

Symptoms develop 7 to 21 days after exposure. They include slight fever, runny nose, slight cough, headache, tiredness, and no appetite.

Red spots that appear on the body 2 to 3 days later are an itchy rash that forms blisters, which dry and become scabs in 4 to 5 days. People may have only a few blisters, or more than 500 may appear. Chickenpox is usually contagious 1 to 2 days before the rash and up to 6 days after blisters form. The mouth, ears, and eyes can also have ulcers.

How Is Chickenpox Diagnosed?

The doctor will make a diagnosis by the medical history and by looking at the rash.

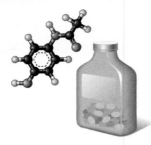

Nonaspirin products such as acetaminophen can reduce fever. DO NOT give aspirin to a child with chickenpox. Aspirin can cause Reye's syndrome. Recovery usually takes 7 to 10 days.

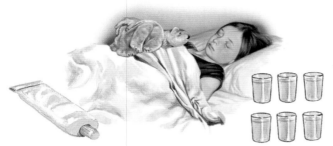

Encourage resting and drinking plenty of fluids. Lotions, such as calamine, and oatmeal baths may help the itching.

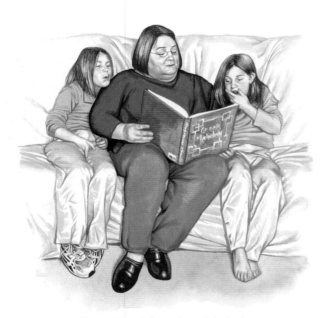

Be sure to rest, but quiet activity is ok.

How Is Chickenpox Treated?

Healthy children need no specific medicine but can get symptom relief. Nonaspirin products such as acetaminophen can reduce fever. DON'T give aspirin to children with chickenpox. Antihistamines, lotions such as calamine, and oatmeal baths can reduce itching. Drinking liquids and resting are recommended. To prevent spreading chickenpox, keep children away from others until blisters have crusted.

People at high risk for severe infection and people with impaired immune systems (e.g., those with bone marrow transplants or leukemia) may get antiviral drugs.

DOs and DON'Ts in Managing Chickenpox:

✔ **DO** call your doctor at once if you're pregnant and think that you were exposed to chickenpox.

✔ **DO** wash your hands regularly and wash bed linens and recently worn clothes with hot, soapy water.

✔ **DO** keep fingernails short to prevent scratching and avoid infection.

✔ **DO** rest, but allow quiet activity.

✔ **DO** use nonaspirin drugs for fever.

✔ **DO** notify school nurses and parents of playmates who may have been exposed.

✔ **DO** use antihistamines and cool sponge baths to reduce itching.

✔ **DO** call your doctor if your temperature is higher than 101°F or if weakness, headache, or sensitivity to light develop.

✔ **DO** call your doctor if vomiting, restlessness, and irritability occur, with decreased consciousness.

✔ **DO** know that a vaccine for chicken pox is available for those who have not yet had the disease.

⊘ **DON'T** scratch blisters or scabs.

⊘ **DON'T** expose pregnant women, newborns, elderly people, or those with low resistance to infection to chickenpox.

⊘ **DON'T** let infected children go to school or day care for at least 6 days after the first blisters appear. Dried, crusted scabs are not infectious.

⊘ **DON'T** give aspirin to children younger than 16 years because of the risk of Reye's syndrome.

FROM THE DESK OF

NOTES

FOR MORE INFORMATION

Contact the following sources:

• National Institute of Allergy and Infectious Diseases
  Tel: (866) 284-4107
  Website: http://www3.niaid.nih.gov

• The American Academy of Pediatrics
  Website: http://www.aap.org/topics.html

• U.S. Department of Health & Human Services
  Website: http://www.healthfinder.gov

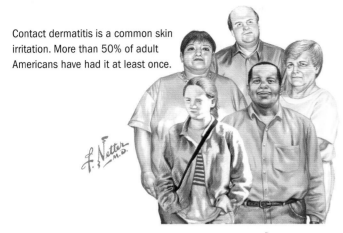

Contact dermatitis is a common skin irritation. More than 50% of adult Americans have had it at least once.

A substance produced by poison ivy, poison oak, and poison sumac is one common cause of contact dermatitis. Others include

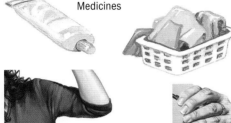

Medicines

Household cleaners and fragrances (e.g., in laundry soaps)

Clothing (wool)

The metal nickel (in jewelry)

Contact dermatitis looks like dry, red, or blistered areas on the skin.

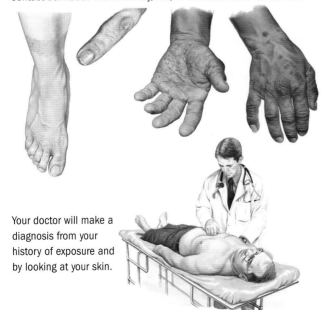

Your doctor will make a diagnosis from your history of exposure and by looking at your skin.

What Is Contact Dermatitis?

Contact dermatitis is a common skin irritation due to exposure to a skin irritant. Contact dermatitis is not infectious.

More than 50% of adult Americans have had it at least once.

What Causes Contact Dermatitis?

Causes include substances that come into direct contact with the skin and irritate it or cause skin allergies. The resin urushiol, produced by poison ivy, poison oak, and poison sumac plants, is a common cause. Contact with the substance may occur not only by touching the plants but also clothing or pets carrying the substance.

Other causes include clothing (wool), household cleaners, fragrances (e.g., in soaps, shampoos), the metal nickel, dyes, medicines, pesticides, and other chemicals.

What Are the Symptoms of Contact Dermatitis?

Symptoms include dry, red, or blistered skin; itching; and mild discomfort. Intense itching and burning of the skin develop 24 to 36 hours after exposure, followed by weeping blisters and crusting and swelling of the skin. The liquid in the blisters is not infectious to others.

Breathing in or swallowing the substance can cause wheezing or nausea. Scratching the skin may lead to infection.

How Is Contact Dermatitis Diagnosed?

The doctor will diagnose dermatitis from the history of exposure and by looking at the skin.

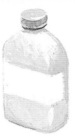

The best treatment is avoiding exposure. Lotions and oatmeal baths can be soothing.

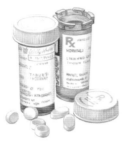

Other treatments include steroids and antihistamines.

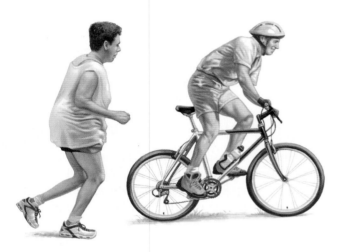

Although exercise is important, hot, sweaty skin will itch more. Wash and cool the skin soon after exercise.

How Is Contact Dermatitis Treated?

The best treatment is avoiding exposure. For example, avoid buying wool clothes and blankets if you are sensitive to wool products, and learn to recognize poison ivy. Wear gloves, long sleeves, and long pants to avoid contact with the plants and anything that has touched them.

Other treatments include topical or oral antiinflammatory drugs (steroids), antihistamines (for itching), and immunotherapy (desensitization) to minimize the reaction.

Steroids (such as prednisone) can be given in pill form, injection, or as creams and ointments.

Lotions, such as calamine, and oatmeal baths soothe oozing, blistery rashes and may be used as needed.

DOs and DON'Ts in Managing Contact Dermatitis:

✔ **DO** use your oral steroids as directed. Oral antihistamines can be used as needed and stopped if itching improves.
✔ **DO** use anti-itch lotions as needed, but avoid using them during the first hour after applying steroids, creams, or ointments. (Give the steroid time to soak in first!)
✔ **DO** eat a good diet.
✔ **DO** exercise, but realize that hot, sweaty skin will itch more. Wash and cool the skin soon after exercise.
✔ **DO** use a mild soap or cleanser to clean skin. Avoid extra irritation that might be caused by deodorants or fragrances in soaps.
✔ **DO** wash your skin immediately with soap and water if you're exposed to a substance that caused previous contact dermatitis.
✔ **DO** call your doctor if you have a fever, coughing, wheezing, vomiting, or diarrhea; if the rash worsens despite treatment; or if a new or different rash occurs.

⊘ **DON'T** skip doses of steroid medicines. Your dermatitis may worsen.
⊘ **DON'T** use antihistamine lotions or creams without your doctor's advice. These can cause rashes themselves!

FROM THE DESK OF

NOTES

FOR MORE INFORMATION

Contact the following sources:

• Asthma and Allergy Foundation of American
Tel: (800) 727-8462
Website: http://www.aafa.org

• American Academy of Dermatology
Tel: (866) 503-SKIN (503-7546)
Website: http://www.aad.org

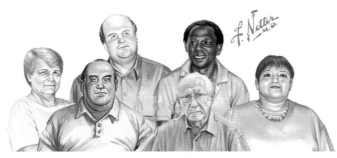

Dermatitis herpetiformis is an uncommon, hereditary, and chronic skin disorder. It usually affects adults between 20 and 60, males slightly more often than females.

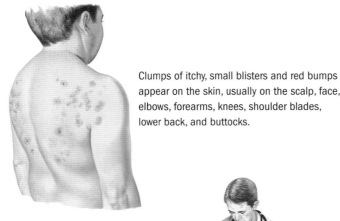

Clumps of itchy, small blisters and red bumps appear on the skin, usually on the scalp, face, elbows, forearms, knees, shoulder blades, lower back, and buttocks.

Your doctor will diagnose dermatitis herpetiformis from a history of exposure and by examining your skin.

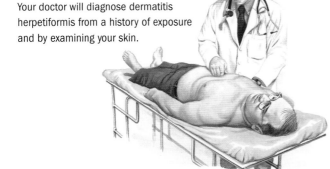

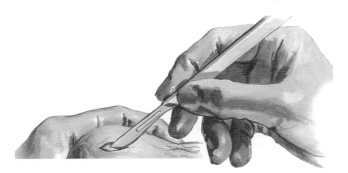

Your doctor may also do a skin biopsy, or remove a small piece of skin, for study to help make the diagnosis.

What Is Dermatitis Herpetiformis?

Dermatitis herpetiformis is a hereditary, chronic, recurrent skin disorder manifesting with clumps of small blisters (vesicles) and red bumps (papules). Outbreaks may last for days, weeks, months, or even years.

Dermatitis herpetiformis is uncommon. It usually affects adults between 20 and 60, but children may also have it. It occurs in males slightly more often.

Other family members may have a history of this condition. This disorder is not contagious and cannot be prevented.

What Causes Dermatitis Herpetiformis?

The cause is unknown, but the disorder is probably autoimmune (i.e., a condition in which the body's own immune system attacks itself, causing injury or disease).

Some people also have celiac disease (disorders in which people cannot digest gluten, a protein in grains such as wheat).

What Are the Symptoms of Dermatitis Herpetiformis?

Lesions are very itchy and may cause burning or stinging. The clumps of blisters are symmetric (i.e., similar on both halves of the body). Lesions usually involve the scalp, face, elbows, forearms, knees, shoulder blades, lower back, and buttocks.

Scratching may cause abrasions, crusting, and infections.

How Is Dermatitis Herpetiformis Diagnosed?

The doctor makes a diagnosis usually from the look of the skin. The doctor may also do a skin biopsy (i.e., removing a small piece of skin for study) or blood tests.

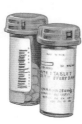
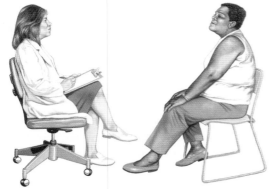

Treatment includes using medicines (e.g., steroids, calamine lotion) and cool-water soaks to improve symptoms, and avoiding triggers of the disorder, such as foods containing gluten.

Tell your doctor about all medicines that you take, including over-the-counter drugs, and talk to your doctor about concerns about your condition and drug side effects.

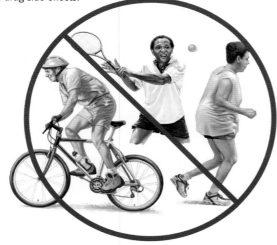

Avoid activities that can cause overheating or sweating or make the affected area too moist, because this can trigger or worsen your condition.

FROM THE DESK OF

NOTES

How Is Dermatitis Herpetiformis Treated?

Treatment depends on its location and how severe it is, its impact on quality of life, and response to therapy. The condition can be controlled but cannot be cured. Treatment includes avoiding triggers, general measures, and medicines. General measures involve soaking the area in cool water to soothe irritation and reduce itching and avoiding gluten in the diet.

Medicines (such as steroids, calamine lotion, antihistamines, and dapsone or sulfapyridine) can reduce inflammation (swelling, redness), improve symptoms, and reduce the severity and duration of the outbreak.

DOs and DON'Ts in Managing Dermatitis Herpetiformis:

✔ **DO** take medicines prescribed by your doctor.
✔ **DO** tell your doctor about all medicines, including over-the-counter drugs, that you take.
✔ **DO** read medicine labels and follow instructions.
✔ **DO** avoid gluten in your diet, which may improve the condition.
✔ **DO** avoid activities that cause overheating and too much sweating. Shower and clean skin lesions immediately if you sweat too much.
✔ **DO** use good skin hygiene to reduce risks of bacterial infection.
✔ **DO** keep follow-up doctor appointments.
✔ **DO** watch your skin for healing and signs of infection, including redness around skin lesions, pus, increased pain or swelling of the lesions or lymph nodes, and fever.
✔ **DO** wash clothing, towels, and linens often if skin lesions ooze, crust, or may be infected.
✔ **DO** call your doctor if lesions become worse or new lesions appear despite therapy.

⊘ **DON'T** stop taking your medicine or change the dose without asking your doctor.
⊘ **DON'T** do activities that can cause overheating or sweating.

FOR MORE INFORMATION

Contact the following source:

• American Academy of Dermatology
Tel: (866) 503-SKIN (503-7546)
Website: http://www.aad.org

CARING FOR YOUR BABY WITH
DIAPER RASH

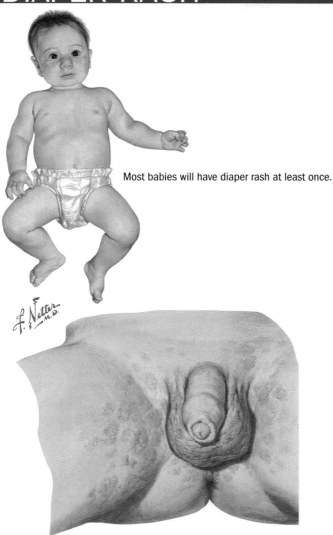

Most babies will have diaper rash at least once.

The cause can be irritating substances, yeast, or bacteria trapped against the baby's skin by the diaper. Synthetic absorbent materials in disposable diapers or germ-killing rinses can also cause irritation. The rash can be uncomfortable or painful.

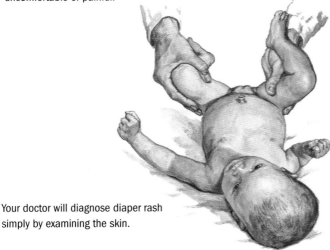

Your doctor will diagnose diaper rash simply by examining the skin.

What Is Diaper Rash?

Diaper rash, or diaper dermatitis, is a skin irritation underneath the area covered by a diaper. It affects most babies at least once.

What Causes Diaper Rash?

The cause can be irritating substances, yeast, or bacteria trapped against the baby's skin by the diaper. Materials such as synthetic absorbents in disposable diapers and germ-killing rinses can also cause irritation. Commercial diaper wipes are another source of irritation.

What Are the Symptoms of Diaper Rash?

Redness and irritation in the diaper area often begin with faint, raised, pink spots, which seem to get larger and soon cover the diaper area if untreated. In the worst cases, skin may look red and begin to peel. Skin folds may become raw. Babies are usually fretful and fussy and cry, especially after urinating or moving the bowels. Diaper rash doesn't usually cause a fever.

How Is Diaper Rash Diagnosed?

The doctor will make a diagnosis by examining the skin.

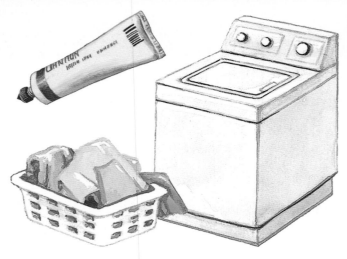

Topical creams and frequent diaper changes usually cure and prevent diaper rash. Also, switching disposable diaper brands or rinsing cloth diapers twice to remove an irritating rinse may solve the problem.

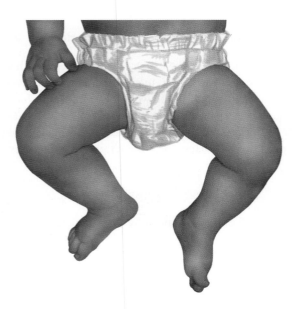

Sometimes a baby's skin is extra sensitive to one brand of diaper or wipes. Use warm water instead of wipes at least until the rash clears. Switch brands if cream and frequent changes don't help.

FROM THE DESK OF

NOTES

How Is Diaper Rash Treated?

Treatment includes use of creams and ointments on the skin (topical) and frequent diaper changes. If irritation from urine is the main problem, a simple ointment containing zinc oxide will often give relief. It should be applied at each diaper change, after the diaper area is gently cleaned with lukewarm water and patted dry.

If the rash lasts even with these treatments, changing the type of diaper may help. Some babies are sensitive to chemicals in cloth diaper rinses, and others are irritated by synthetic materials in disposable diapers. Switching disposable brands or rinsing cloth diapers twice may solve the problem.

If yeast (*Candida*) caused the rash, the doctor may prescribe an ointment containing nystatin or clotrimazole. This kind of rash, perhaps with yeast infection in the mouth (thrush), often occurs after antibiotic treatment for ear infections. The doctor may also prescribe nystatin drops for the thrush.

DOs and DON'Ts in Managing Diaper Rash:

✔ **DO** your best to prevent diaper rash by keeping your baby's diaper area as dry as possible.
✔ **DO** leave the skin open to fresh air as much as possible.
✔ **DO** diaper loosely, and change baby frequently.
✔ **DO** use lukewarm water with a soft washcloth for cleaning the diaper area after the baby urinates. A small amount of baby bath can be used on the washcloth for cleaning after bowel movements.
✔ **DO** apply zinc oxide or antiyeast ointment at each diaper change.
✔ **DO** call your doctor if the baby develops a fever.
✔ **DO** call your doctor if the rash worsens despite home treatment or if it goes beyond the diaper area.
✔ **DO** call your doctor if your baby refuses breast or bottle or if vomiting or diarrhea occurs.

⊘ **DON'T** wait for a doctor visit to begin treating diaper rash. If the diaper area looks red, begin frequent (hourly) diaper checks right away, and change the diaper if you note dampness.
⊘ **DON'T** use commercial diaper wipes because they'll worsen the rash.
⊘ **DON'T** use over-the-counter antibacterial ointments unless your doctor recommends them. These can cause irritation and rash themselves and are rarely needed.

FOR MORE INFORMATION

Contact the following source:
• American Academy of Dermatology
Tel: (866) 503-SKIN (7546)
Website: http://www.aad.org

MANAGING YOUR
DISCOID LUPUS ERYTHEMATOSUS

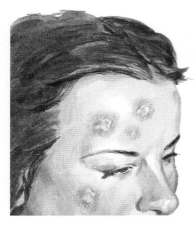

Discoid lupus erythematosus (DLE) is a chronic skin disorder with red, raised plaques (scales) having sharp edges. The cause is unknown, but DLE may be an autoimmune disorder, affecting women more than men. Other family members may have DLE, but it is not contagious.

What Is Discoid Lupus Erythematosus?

Discoid lupus erythematosus (DLE) is a chronic skin disorder with red, raised plaques (scales) having sharp edges. The lesions usually occur on sun-exposed areas, especially the face, scalp, and neck.

DLE can be more frequent and more severe in African Americans. It affects women more often than men, usually adults between ages 20 and 50. Remissions occur between episodes.

Other family members may have DLE, but it is not contagious.

Some people with DLE develop systemic lupus erythematosus (SLE), a more serious disease involving many body organs.

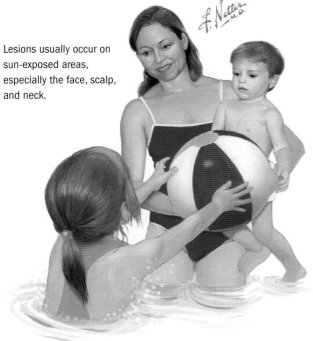

Lesions usually occur on sun-exposed areas, especially the face, scalp, and neck.

What Causes DLE?

The cause is unknown, but DLE is likely an autoimmune condition (i.e., one in which the body's immune system attacks itself, causing injury or disease). Exposure to sunlight may increase the risk of getting DLE.

What Are the Symptoms of DLE?

Lesions are red, raised bumps (papules; smaller than 1 centimeter) and scales (plaques; larger than 1 centimeter) with clear borders. Lesions may also have scaling and thinning (atrophy) of the skin. Scarring is common.

In African Americans, lesions may be darker than normal skin. Lesions tend to be round or oval with irregular borders. They involve the face, scalp, neck, nose, forearms, hands, fingers, and toes. Sometimes, the trunk and mucous membranes are involved. Scalp lesions are often related to hair loss.

Later lesions tend to be flat and faint pink or white. They tend to show atrophy and depression in the center, with slightly raised borders.

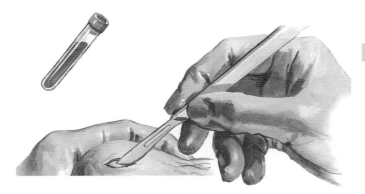

Your doctor will make a diagnosis by looking at your skin, as well as doing a skin biopsy and blood tests.

How Is DLE Diagnosed?

The doctor makes a diagnosis from the look of the skin. The doctor may do blood tests and a skin biopsy (removing a small piece of skin for study).

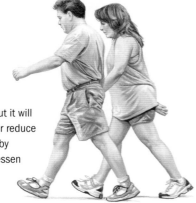

Treatment does not cure DLE, but it will make life easier for you. Avoid or reduce your exposure to sunlight (e.g., by wearing protective clothes) to lessen disease severity.

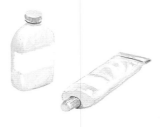

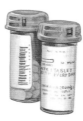

Your doctor may prescribe drugs, lotions, and ointments to help relieve symptoms.

Tell your doctor about all medicines that you take, including over-the-counter drugs, and talk to your doctor about concerns about your condition and drug side effects.

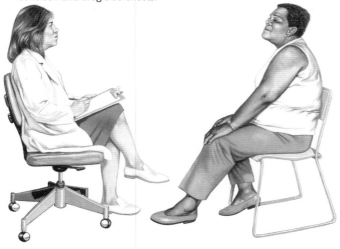

How Is DLE Treated?

Treatment depends on its location and how severe, its impact on quality of life, and response to therapy. DLE can be controlled but cannot be cured. Treatment lessens the severity of the condition and reduces scarring. Treatment includes avoiding triggers (sunlight and fluorescent lights), general measures, and medicines. Use maximum protection sunscreens and wear protective clothing.

Sunscreens with a sun protection factor (SPF) of 30, steroids, and drugs to inhibit the immune system can reduce inflammation (redness, swelling), scarring, and lessen the severity of DLE.

DOs and DON'Ts in Managing DLE:

✔ **DO** take medicines as prescribed.
✔ **DO** tell your doctor about all medicines, including over-the-counter drugs, that you take.
✔ **DO** read medicine labels and follow instructions.
✔ **DO** avoid exposure to sunlight and fluorescent lights to reduce the severity of DLE.
✔ **DO** keep follow-up doctor appointments.
✔ **DO** call your doctor if lesions become worse or new lesions appear despite therapy.
✔ **DO** call your doctor if you have new or unexplained symptoms.

🚫 **DON'T** stop taking your medicine or change the dose without asking your doctor.
🚫 **DON'T** suddenly stop using steroids or immunosuppressive therapy without asking your doctor.

FROM THE DESK OF

NOTES

FOR MORE INFORMATION

Contact the following sources:

• Lupus Foundation of America
Tel: (800) 558-0121
Website: http://www.lupus.org/newsite/index.html

• American Academy of Dermatology
Tel: (847) 330-0230
Website: http://www.aad.org

MANAGING YOUR
ECZEMA

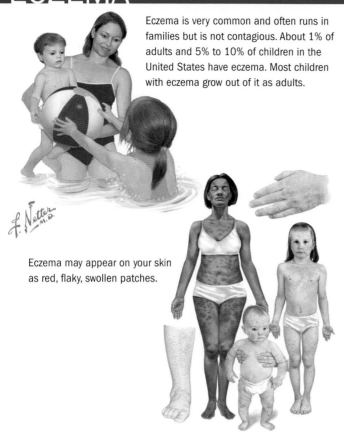

Eczema is very common and often runs in families but is not contagious. About 1% of adults and 5% to 10% of children in the United States have eczema. Most children with eczema grow out of it as adults.

Eczema may appear on your skin as red, flaky, swollen patches.

Things causing eczema or making it worse:

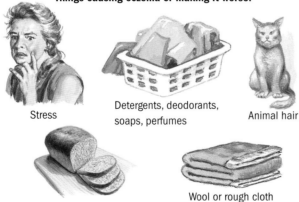

Stress

Detergents, deodorants, soaps, perfumes

Animal hair

Certain foods (e.g., wheat)

Wool or rough cloth

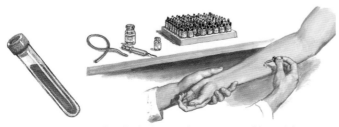

Your doctor can usually tell whether you have eczema without doing tests but may check your blood and skin to be sure.

What Is Eczema?

Eczema, or atopic dermatitis, is a skin disease caused by increased sensitivity to the environment. It often runs in families and may occur with hay fever, asthma, and nasal allergies. It cannot be caught. Eczema is very common, affecting 1% of adults and 5% to 10% of children in the United States. In most people, eczema goes away completely by adulthood.

This sensitivity causes inflammation (redness), itching, and scratching. Scratching, however, often makes itching worse and can cause breaks in the skin, increasing risks of infection.

What Causes Eczema?

Causes of eczema or things that make it worse include stress; very hot or cold air; foods including wheat, milk, eggs, and pod vegetables such as beans, peas, and lentils; certain types of cloth; perfumes; dust mites; and animal hair.

What Are the Symptoms of Eczema?

Eczema produces a rash that is red, swollen, itchy, dry, flaky, hard, thick, oozing, and crusty.

How Is Eczema Diagnosed?

The doctor can usually diagnose eczema without doing tests but may order general blood tests and skin testing when the diagnosis is unclear or when trying to determine the cause of the eczema.

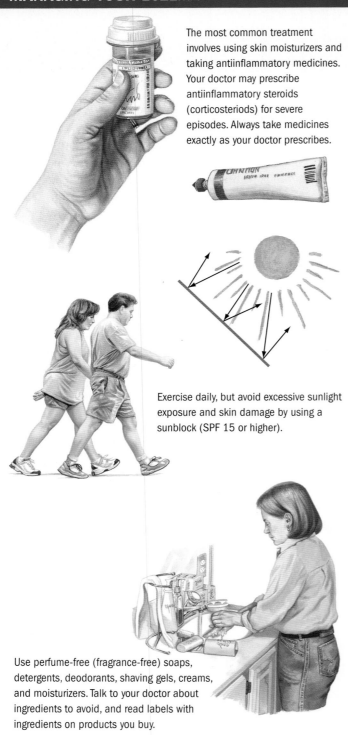

The most common treatment involves using skin moisturizers and taking antiinflammatory medicines. Your doctor may prescribe antiinflammatory steroids (corticosteriods) for severe episodes. Always take medicines exactly as your doctor prescribes.

Exercise daily, but avoid excessive sunlight exposure and skin damage by using a sunblock (SPF 15 or higher).

Use perfume-free (fragrance-free) soaps, detergents, deodorants, shaving gels, creams, and moisturizers. Talk to your doctor about ingredients to avoid, and read labels with ingredients on products you buy.

FROM THE DESK OF

NOTES

How Is Eczema Treated?

Four main ways of treating eczema involve avoiding triggers that cause or worsen it; keeping skin moist with special lotions, soaps, and bath products; treating redness and swelling with antiinflammatory medicines (corticosteroid creams and pills), tar, and light therapy; and helping stop itching with antihistamines, creams, and pills.

Simple, nonmedicated moisturizing cream may be used daily. Steroid creams are for severe itching.

Medicines taken by mouth (pills) to relieve itching include antihistamines, which calm nerve endings in skin. Corticosteroids given as pills can stop inflammation and itching and reduce redness, but they do have side effects (e.g., stomach ulcers, weight gain) when taken long term.

Covering the rash with bandages helps by keeping creams and lotions on the skin and protecting skin from being scratched.

DOs and DON'Ts in Managing Eczema:

✔ **DO** avoid triggers of the rash, including stress.

✔ **DO** moisturize your skin daily, even when you have no symptoms. Use an odor-free oil-based cream or ointment (not lotion), best applied just after bathing while skin is still damp. Use hypoallergenic products when possible. For severe itching, also use a very mild over-the-counter steroid cream (1% hydrocortisone). Bathe with warm, not hot, water and mild soap.

✔ **DO** take all pills prescribed by your doctor. Don't stop taking the medicines unless your doctor approves.

✔ **DO** avoid foods that cause your eczema to worsen.

✔ **DO** exercise daily, but avoid excessive sunlight exposure and skin damage with a sunblock (SPF 15 or greater).

✔ **DO** wash clothing and linens in fragrance-free soap; double rinse when possible.

✔ **DO** call your doctor if you have signs of infection (worsening redness, pus); wheezing or trouble breathing; or a severe stomachache or bone pain when taking steroid pills.

🚫 **DON'T** let your skin or home become too dry. A home humidifier may help.

🚫 **DON'T** forget your daily skin regimen even if you feel well. Plan ahead for trips by saving some of your usual products.

🚫 **DON'T** drive, cook, or operate machinery while using antihistamines if they make you sleepy.

FOR MORE INFORMATION

Contact the following sources:

• American Academy of Dermatology
Tel: (866) 503-SKIN (7546)
Website: http://www.aad.org

• Asthma and Allergy Foundation of America
Tel: (800) 727-8462
Website: http://www.aafa.org

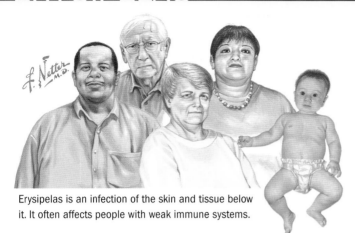

Erysipelas is an infection of the skin and tissue below it. It often affects people with weak immune systems.

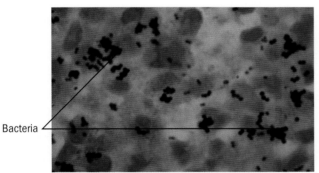

Bacteria

The infection is caused by a kind of bacteria called group A streptococci.

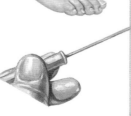

The leg is usually affected. The skin becomes red and swollen, feels tender and hot, and can have blisters. Other symptoms are fever, chills, headache, tiredness, loss of appetite, abdominal pain, and swollen glands.

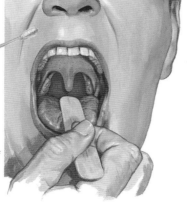

Your doctor may order cultures of your throat and nose, and blood tests to confirm the diagnosis.

What Is Erysipelas?

Erysipelas is an infection of the skin and tissue below it.

What Causes Erysipelas?

The cause is a type of bacteria called group A streptococci.

The infection may occur in people without medical problems but most often occurs in very young or elderly people and those who are infected with human immunodeficiency virus (HIV) or who have acquired immunodeficiency syndrome (AIDS). Diabetics and alcoholics are also more prone to it. It may also occur in wounds after surgery.

What Are the Symptoms of Erysipelas?

The skin becomes painful and then gets red and swollen, with a very distinct edge. The area is tender and hot. Small or large blisters may develop in the red area.

This infection may develop on the face, but is more common on the legs, after heart bypass surgery, often near the vein that was used in coronary artery bypass surgery.

Other symptoms are fever, chills, headache, tiredness, loss of appetite, belly (abdominal) pain, and swollen glands (lymph nodes).

How Is Erysipelas Diagnosed?

The doctor will make the diagnosis by obtaining a medical history and doing a physical examination. Nose and throat cultures for the streptococcus bacteria and blood tests (e.g., white blood cell count) may also be done to see whether an infection is present.

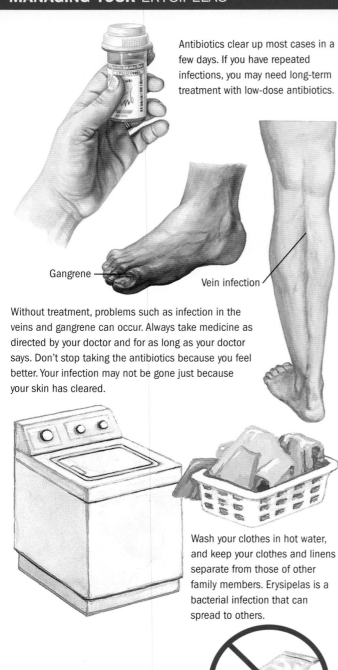

Antibiotics clear up most cases in a few days. If you have repeated infections, you may need long-term treatment with low-dose antibiotics.

Gangrene

Vein infection

Without treatment, problems such as infection in the veins and gangrene can occur. Always take medicine as directed by your doctor and for as long as your doctor says. Don't stop taking the antibiotics because you feel better. Your infection may not be gone just because your skin has cleared.

Wash your clothes in hot water, and keep your clothes and linens separate from those of other family members. Erysipelas is a bacterial infection that can spread to others.

Don't use creams, salves, or lotions on infected areas.

How Is Erysipelas Treated?

Antibiotics are the best treatment. For frequent or very severe infections, long-term treatment with low-dose antibiotics may be needed.

With proper treatment, most infections go away after few days. Without treatment, abscesses, infections in veins, and gangrene can develop. These problems are also more likely to occur in people with weakened immune systems, such as in diabetes, alcoholism, HIV infection, and those with previous blood clots in legs.

DOs and DON'Ts in Managing Erysipelas:

✔ **DO** elevate your leg to help with swelling.
✔ **DO** separate your towels, washcloths, and bedding from laundry of other household members. Use very hot water for washing.
✔ **DO** take all of your antibiotics, even after the skin clears.
✔ **DO** call your doctor if you have a reaction to your antibiotic, or if the rash and redness continue to spread.
✔ **DO** call your doctor if you have fever, chills, dizziness when you stand up, or rapid heart rate.

🚫 **DON'T** stop your antibiotic, even if the infection has greatly improved. Erysipelas is a serious infection. You must finish all the antibiotic that your doctor gave you.
🚫 **DON'T** put any salves, creams, or lotions on the infected part. If the area "weeps" a little, dress it with plain gauze.
🚫 **DON'T** let other family members use your towels. If the skin weeps, the substance may contain bacteria, and you can give the infection to others.

FROM THE DESK OF

NOTES

FOR MORE INFORMATION

Contact the following source:

- American College of Dermatology
  Tel: (866) 503-SKIN (7546)
  Website: http://www.aad.org

MANAGING YOUR
ERYTHEMA MULTIFORME

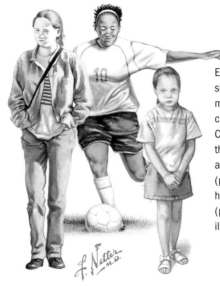

Erythema multiforme is a skin condition that in the mild form usually affects children and young adults. Causes, found in only half the cases, include infections, allergic reactions to drugs (penicillin, vaccines), hormone changes (pregnancy), and other illnesses (such as cancer).

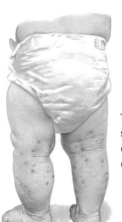

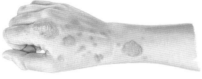

The skin shows redness, swelling, and sometimes blistering. The milder form usually doesn't cause complications and clears up on its own in 2 to 4 weeks.

Erythema multiforme major, also called Stevens-Johnson syndrome, is the more serious form that needs prompt medical care. Large blisters and ulcers form in the mouth and on the nose, eyes, genital area, arms, and skin.

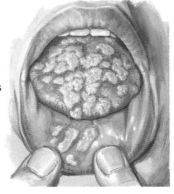

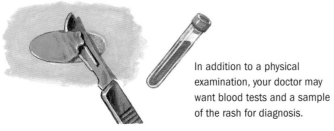

In addition to a physical examination, your doctor may want blood tests and a sample of the rash for diagnosis.

What Is Erythema Multiforme?

Erythema multiforme is a reddening, swelling, and sometimes blistering of the skin. A milder form, called erythema multiforme minor, usually doesn't cause complications and clears up on its own. The mild form usually affects children and young adults, lasts from 2 to 4 weeks, and can recur during the first few years. The more severe form, called Stevens-Johnson syndrome or erythema multiforme major, can cause serious symptoms that need prompt treatment and maybe hospitalization.

What Causes Erythema Multiforme?

The cause is unknown in half the cases. Most of these skin irritations result from infections, allergic reactions to drugs such as penicillin or vaccines, physical conditions such as pregnancy and other hormone changes, and illnesses such as cancer.

What Are the Symptoms of Erythema Multiforme?

Skin in the minor form has round red bumps and blisters on the face, lips, arms, and legs on both sides of the body. These bumps can look like red or pink targets; they can become large blisters. Fever and muscle and joint aches may be present.

In the serious form, people have high fever, large blisters, severe itching, and ulcers on membranes of the mouth, nose, eyes, genital area, arms, and skin. Without complications, symptoms go away in 4 weeks, but mouth sores can last for months. Untreated eye involvement can lead to blindness.

How Is Erythema Multiforme Diagnosed?

The doctor will examine the rash and take a medical history to make a diagnosis.

Blood tests may be done to check for an infection. A skin biopsy may also be done to rule out another medical condition. In a biopsy, a small sample of skin with the rash will be removed and studied with a microscope.

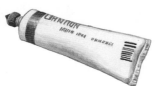

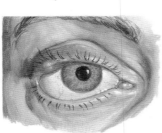

Most rashes will clear up in a few weeks. Your doctor may prescribe pills and steroid cream to reduce itching and swelling.

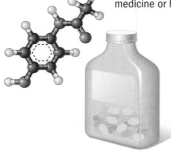

Your doctor may refer you to an eye specialist if the rash is in the eye area. If the rash near the eye goes untreated, it can cause blindness.

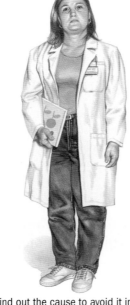

You'll want to find out the cause to avoid it in the future, if you can. Talk with your doctor to change medicine or hormones to avoid more episodes.

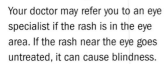

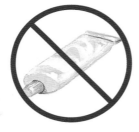

Don't apply skin creams or ointments to broken or bleeding skin. Take acetaminophen for pain unless your doctor says not to.

How Is Erythema Multiforme Treated?

Treatment focuses on controlling the cause and symptoms. For a drug reaction, the drug needs to be stopped. If a bacterial infection is the cause, antibiotics are given. Symptoms are relieved by using moist compresses (for itching), soothing lukewarm or cool baths, drugs such as steroid (prednisone) creams (for itching and swelling), mouthwashes and rinses (for mouth blisters), and eyewash and other topical medicine (for a rash near the eyes). Eye involvement may mean a visit to an eye specialist.

The severe disorder can cause major skin damage. In that case, hospitalization in a burn unit may be needed.

DOs and DON'Ts in Managing Erythema Multiforme:

✔ **DO** promptly treat any illness or condition that may lead to erythema multiforme. Avoid suspected causes as much as possible, such as drugs you are allergic to.

✔ **DO** eat a soft or liquid diet if you have mouth sores.

✔ **DO** apply cool wet Burow's solution compresses or just a cool wet cloth to blisters.

✔ **DO** call your doctor immediately if you have vision changes, eye pain, vomiting, or diarrhea.

✔ **DO** take acetaminophen for pain unless otherwise directed by your doctor.

✔ **DO** call your doctor if new symptoms occur during treatment, or if symptoms get much worse.

⊘ **DON'T** apply skin creams or ointments to broken or bleeding skin.

⊘ **DON'T** take hot baths or hot showers.

FROM THE DESK OF

NOTES

FOR MORE INFORMATION

Contact the following source:
• American Academy of Dermatology
  Tel: (866) 503-SKIN (7546)
  Website: http://www.aad.org

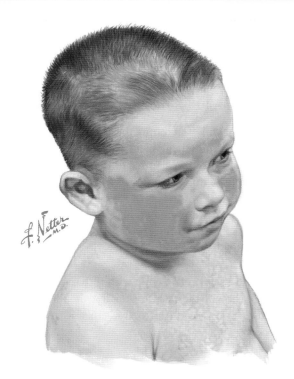

The rash of fifth disease looks as if a cheek was slapped or wind-burned. The rash sometimes spreads to other parts of the body.

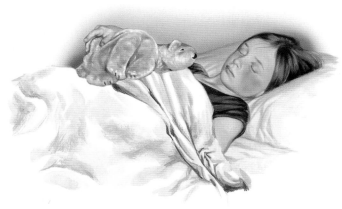

Rest is usually all it takes to feel better from this viral infection. The rash and any aches and pains will go away after 5 to 10 days.

What Is Fifth Disease?

Fifth disease is a mild, infectious viral illness that occurs in outbreaks, often during the winter and spring. The face has a characteristic rash. The name of the illness relates to its place in a list of childhood diseases developed in the early 1980s. It affects mostly children 5 to 14 years old.

Fifth disease can't be prevented, and children aren't contagious after the rash appears. People usually won't get fifth disease a second time, because immunity to the virus develops.

Healthy people rarely have complications, but children with sickle cell anemia have an increased risk of complications. A pregnant woman has a small risk of miscarriage if infection occurs during the first trimester.

What Causes Fifth Disease?

The cause is a virus called human parvovirus B19. It spreads by means of particles in the air.

What Are the Symptoms of Fifth Disease?

Symptoms usually appear 4 to 14 days after a child is exposed to someone with the disease. Symptoms, which usually last 5 to 10 days, include a fiery red rash on the cheeks that makes the cheek look like it was slapped. The rash then spreads to the rest of the body and has a lacy look to it. Slight tiredness, headache, and itching may occur. Some people have a fever. Adults may have mild pain and swelling in the joints. Many people have no symptoms.

How Is Fifth Disease Diagnosed?

The doctor will diagnose fifth disease on the basis of the physical examination and history. Blood tests aren't usually needed.

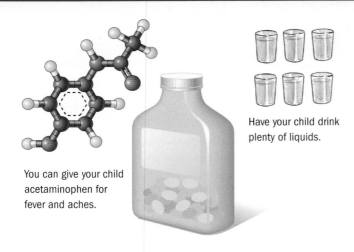

You can give your child acetaminophen for fever and aches.

Have your child drink plenty of liquids.

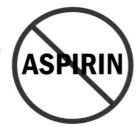

Don't give your child aspirin! It can cause dangerous complications, such as Reye's syndrome.

ASPIRIN

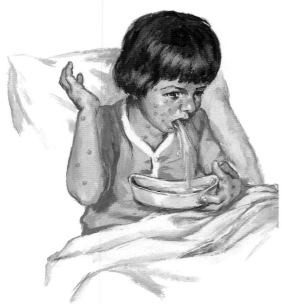

Symptoms of Reye's syndrome include vomiting, restlessness, irritability, and decreased level of consciousness.

How Is Fifth Disease Treated?

No specific treatment is needed, but symptoms can be controlled. Nonaspirin products (e.g., acetaminophen) can be given for fever and aches. Don't give aspirin to a child with fifth disease. Aspirin can lead to a serious complication called Reye's syndrome.

DOs and DON'Ts in Managing Fifth Disease:

✔ **DO** have your child rest during the early days of the illness.
✔ **DO** have your child drink plenty of liquids.
✔ **DO** use cool cloths or calamine lotion if the rash itches.
✔ **DO** call your doctor if symptoms get worse with normal treatment.
✔ **DO** call your doctor if your child gets symptoms of Reye's syndrome, such as vomiting, restlessness, irritability, and a decrease in the level of consciousness.

⊘ **DON'T** give aspirin to a child with fifth disease.
⊘ **DON'T** worry if the rash recurs after the illness is over, especially during exposure to the sun and temperature changes.

FROM THE DESK OF

NOTES

FOR MORE INFORMATION

Contact the following sources:

• National Institute of Allergy and Infectious Diseases
Tel: (301) 496-5717
Website: http://www3.niaid.nih.gov

• The American Academy of Pediatrics
Tel: (847) 434-4000
Website: http://www.aap.org

• National Institute of Child Health and Human Development
Tel: (800) 370-2943
Website: http://www.nichd.nih.gov

MANAGING YOUR
FOLLICULITIS

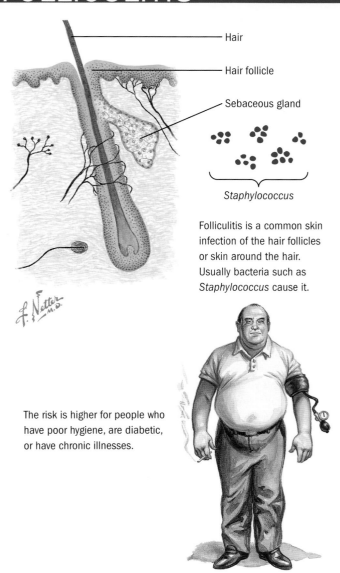

Hair

Hair follicle

Sebaceous gland

Staphylococcus

Folliculitis is a common skin infection of the hair follicles or skin around the hair. Usually bacteria such as *Staphylococcus* cause it.

The risk is higher for people who have poor hygiene, are diabetic, or have chronic illnesses.

Your doctor can usually diagnose folliculitis by looking at the skin. Small pustules or pimples around hair follicles can be seen.

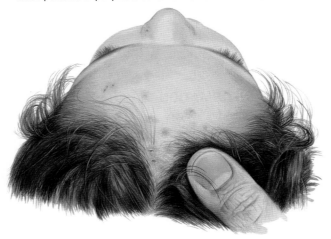

What Is Folliculitis?

Folliculitis is a common skin infection of hair follicles or skin around the hair. When follicles become damaged, they get infected and small, white, pus-filled bumps (pustules) appear on the skin's surface. The skin usually looks inflamed (red). It can affect people of any age and race.

What Causes Folliculitis?

Bacteria, usually ones called *Staphylococcus* or *Pseudomonas*, cause folliculitis. Anyone can get the infection, but people who have poor hygiene, are diabetic, or have chronic illnesses have a higher chance of getting it. Using public hot tubs or saunas in hotels is a major risk factor.

What Are the Symptoms of Folliculitis?

The most common symptom is a small pustule or pimple around a hair follicle. Pustules can appear anywhere on the body. They may be painful to touch. Skin around them may be red and itchy. Pimples can crust over.

How Is Folliculitis Diagnosed?

The doctor usually diagnoses folliculitis by looking at the skin. Sometimes, the doctor may want to take a sample of a pustule for study in a laboratory when the diagnosis is unclear or when suspecting folliculitis due to a bacteria resistant to common antibiotics.

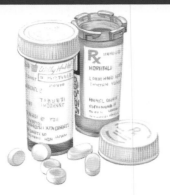

Mild cases may get better on their own, without treatment. People with more severe infection may need to take antibiotics by mouth.

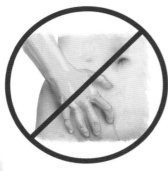

Don't scratch the pustules. Bathe at least once daily to keep your skin clean.

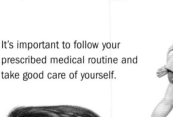

It's important to follow your prescribed medical routine and take good care of yourself.

Try to avoid shaving the area with pustules, such as your face and neck.

How Is Folliculitis Treated?

Mild cases may get better on their own, without treatment. They usually start to clear up in 2 to 3 days. The affected area should be washed with an antibacterial soap and kept very clean. Sometimes, over-the-counter antibiotic ointment can help healing. Folliculitis can come back, however.

People with more severe cases may need to take antibiotics by mouth. The doctor will prescribe these. Antibiotics usually heal folliculitis in 1 to 2 weeks.

DOs and DON'Ts in Managing Folliculitis:

✔ **DO** bathe at least once daily to keep your skin clean. Your doctor may prescribe a special soap to use.

✔ **DO** follow your prescribed medical treatment and take good care of yourself if you have diabetes or another chronic condition. You are more likely to get folliculitis.

✔ **DO** avoid using public hot tubs or saunas.

✔ **DO** use cool compresses for itching and irritation.

✔ **DO** try to keep clothing from rubbing against the pustules.

✔ **DO** try to avoid shaving the area with pustules, such as your face and neck. If that's not possible, use a clean new razor or an electric razor each time you shave.

✔ **DO** call your doctor if you have folliculitis that recurs.

✔ **DO** call your doctor if you develop signs of spreading infection.

🚫 **DON'T** scratch the affected area. That can cause the infection to spread.

🚫 **DON'T** share towels, face cloths, and clothing. Using personal items of others can spread the infection.

FROM THE DESK OF

NOTES

FOR MORE INFORMATION

Contact the following source:

• American Academy of Dermatology
Tel: (866) 503-SKIN (503-7546)
Website: http://www.aad.org

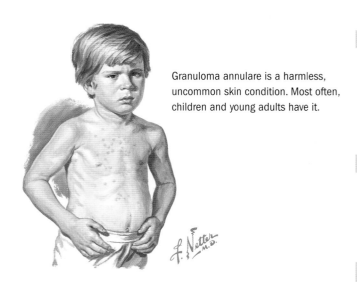

Granuloma annulare is a harmless, uncommon skin condition. Most often, children and young adults have it.

What Is Granuloma Annulare?

Granuloma annulare is a rather uncommon, harmless skin condition. Most often, children and young adults have it. It usually disappears on its own but often comes back. Treatment with medicine applied to the skin may help speed healing.

What Causes Granuloma Annulare?

The cause is unknown, but it cannot be caught and isn't passed from parents to children. Granuloma annulare does tend to return, but it isn't cancerous or life-threatening.

What Are the Symptoms of Granuloma Annulare?

Granuloma annulare may start as a small, red bump and develop into a ring of bumps or even many bumps. It appears evenly on both sides of the body. The bumps are red to tan, and the rings can grow up to a few inches but are usually smaller. The bumps are smooth and may have a shallow indented area in the center. Some bumps may go away in a few months, but others may last for years. The bumps may be tender or itchy. Granuloma annulare usually appears on the hands, feet, arms, and legs, and over joints (elbows and knees).

The disorder may start as a small, red bump and develop into a ring of bumps or many bumps. It usually appears on hands, feet, arms, and legs and over joints (elbows and knees).

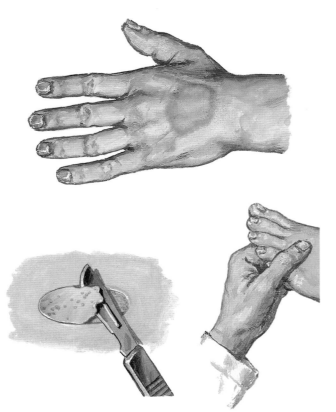

How Is Granuloma Annulare Diagnosed?

The doctor usually makes a diagnosis by looking at the skin. The doctor may do a minor skin biopsy to confirm the diagnosis. In a biopsy, a small piece of skin with the lesion is removed and studied under a microscope. A skin biopsy is generally not necessary and only done when the diagnosis is unclear.

Your doctor will look at your skin to make a diagnosis. A biopsy may also be done. In a biopsy, a small piece of skin with the lesion is removed and studied with a microscope.

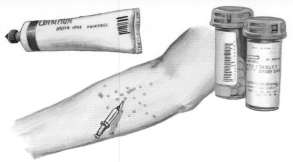

Treatment isn't usually needed, but your doctor may prescribe pills or steroid creams to put on the skin. Your doctor may also inject steroids directly into the affected area.

Don't put over-the-counter creams or ointments on the bumps without talking to your doctor first.

Call your doctor if you have itching or scaling or signs of infection, such as fever, swelling, or pus drainage.

How Is Granuloma Annulare Treated?

Treatment is usually not needed. Diet and exercise don't affect the condition. Most cases improve within months. People with this disorder have no restrictions.

The doctor may prescribe steroid creams to put on the skin. A small amount of cream or lotion is applied to the affected area. It is best to do this just before bedtime.

For severe or extensive cases of granuloma annulare, the doctor may prescribe medicine to be taken by mouth. The doctor may also inject steroids directly into the affected area. A special treatment combining a cream put on the skin and a special ultraviolet light therapy (called PUVA, for psoralen plus ultraviolet A) may also be used.

DOs and DON'Ts in Managing Granuloma Annulare:

✔ **DO** be patient. Granuloma annulare is not life-threatening.
✔ **DO** call your doctor if you have itching or scaling.
✔ **DO** call your doctor if you have signs of infection, such as fever, swelling, or pus drainage.

⊘ **DON'T** apply over-the-counter creams or ointments to the bumps without checking with your doctor first.
⊘ **DON'T** expect immediate improvement. It may take weeks or months for the skin lesions to resolve.

FROM THE DESK OF

NOTES

FOR MORE INFORMATION

Contact the following source:

• American Academy of Dermatology
Tel: (866) 503-SKIN (7546)
Website: http://www.aad.org

CARING FOR YOUR CHILD WITH
HAND, FOOT, AND MOUTH DISEASE

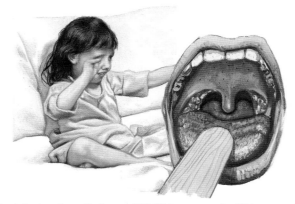

Hand, foot, and mouth disease (HFMD) is common in children younger than 10 and usually starts with a sore throat.

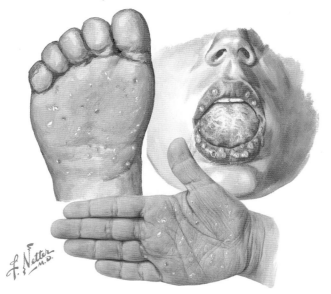

Small red blisters may develop on the palms, soles of the feet, and mouth.

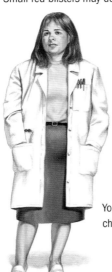

Your doctor makes a diagnosis by checking your child's symptoms and looking at the rash and sores.

What Is Hand, Foot, and Mouth Disease?

Hand, foot, and mouth disease (HFMD) is a common viral illness that starts in the throat and affects mainly children younger than age 10. The disease isn't serious, needs no specific treatment, and usually goes away within 2 weeks.

What Causes HFMD?

The cause is coxsackievirus A16. This virus can be found in bowel movements (stool) and body fluids of the nose and throat. It spreads from person to person by touching the body fluids of someone who is infected.

What Are the Symptoms of HFMD?

Symptoms usually start within a week after an exposure and include feeling sick, low-grade fever, sore throat, loss of appetite, headache, and a rash on the palms of the hands, soles of the feet, and buttocks. Sores may begin in the mouth—on the tongue, gums, and insides of the cheeks—several days after fever starts. They start as small red spots that blister.

How Is HFMD Diagnosed?

The doctor makes a diagnosis by checking symptoms and looking at the rash and sores. The doctor may take samples of stool or of fluid from the throat for testing.

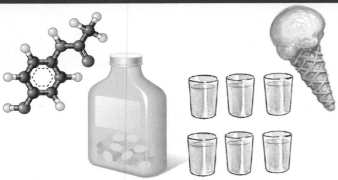

No specific treatment is needed, but medicine, such as acetaminophen, may reduce fever and help control pain. Encourage your child to drink liquids and eat soft foods, such as ice cream, custard, and Jell-O to keep your child hydrated.

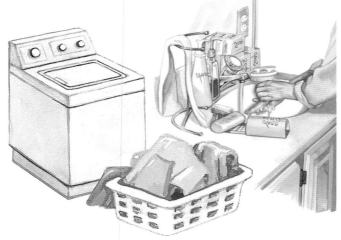

Avoid spreading the virus by washing your hands regularly, cleaning items and clothing that your child uses.

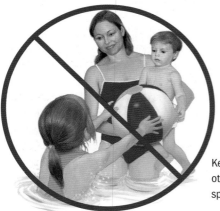

Keep your child away from other children to avoid spreading the virus.

How Is HFMD Treated?

No specific treatment is needed. Medicine such as acetaminophen may reduce fever and help control pain. Rinsing the mouth or gargling with warm salt water, taking antacids, and using topical anesthetic gels can relieve pain from mouth sores.

Children should rest until the fever is gone. Encourage drinking fluids and offer ice cream, custard, and Jell-O, because solid foods may not be tolerated.

To avoid spreading the disease, use separate eating utensils and boil them, or use disposable utensils. Boil pacifiers and bottle nipples separately from bottles. Keep the child away from other children.

DOs and DON'Ts in Managing HFMD:

✔ **DO** wash your hands, especially after changing diapers.
✔ **DO** wash contaminated surfaces.
✔ **DO** wash dirty clothing.
✔ **DO** call your doctor if symptoms get worse and don't improve within 2 weeks.
✔ **DO** keep your child away from others.
✔ **DO** use acetaminophen or tepid sponge baths for fever. Don't give aspirin.
✔ **DO** boil bottle nipples, pacifiers, and eating utensils after use.
✔ **DO** have your child use a mild saltwater solution to rinse the mouth.
✔ **DO** have your child rest until the fever is gone.
✔ **DO** have your child drink liquids and eat soft foods.
✔ **DO** call your doctor if your child gets a high fever that doesn't respond to acetaminophen or sponge baths.
✔ **DO** call your doctor if your child has trouble swallowing and can't take fluids.

⊘ **DON'T** let your child become dehydrated.
⊘ **DON'T** send your child to preschool or day care until the rash resolves and the child feels better.
⊘ **DON'T** share drinking cups or eating utensils.

FROM THE DESK OF

NOTES

FOR MORE INFORMATION

Contact the following sources:

• Centers for Disease Control and Prevention
  Division of Viral and Rickettsial Diseases
  Tel: (800) 311-3435
  Website: http://www.cdc.gov

• The American Academy of Pediatrics
  Tel: (847) 434-4000
  Website: http://www.aap.org

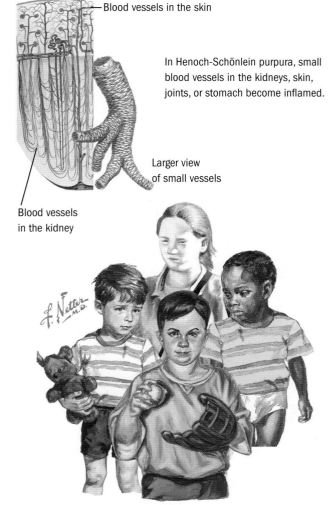

Blood vessels in the skin

In Henoch-Schönlein purpura, small blood vessels in the kidneys, skin, joints, or stomach become inflamed.

Larger view of small vessels

Blood vessels in the kidney

The disease affects mostly younger children, usually boys, but older children and adults can get it.

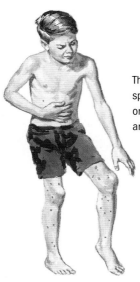

The first symptom may be small purplish spots (purpura), usually on the buttocks or legs. Joints, usually knees and ankles, are painfully swollen.

What Is Henoch-Schönlein Purpura?

Henoch-Schönlein purpura is a disease in which small blood vessels throughout the body become inflamed (swollen, red). These blood vessels may be in the skin, joints, stomach, or kidneys.

This disease is also called allergic purpura or anaphylactoid purpura. It affects mostly younger children (usually boys), but older children and adults may also get it.

Most people recover completely, but recovery may take several months. Also, because of possible kidney problems, regular follow-up blood pressure checks and urine tests will be needed for several months.

What Causes Henoch-Schönlein Purpura?

The cause isn't fully known. It usually occurs a few weeks after a strep throat infection or after a cold or other viral infections. Substances (antibodies) produced by the body's immune system to fight the initial infection may contribute to its development.

What Are the Symptoms of Henoch-Schönlein Purpura?

The first symptom may be small purplish spots (purpura), usually on the buttocks and legs. The ankles are always affected. The rash may first look like hives but usually changes to purplish or brownish bruises in 1 to 2 days.

Joints, usually knees and ankles, are painfully swollen. The pain may be so severe that walking is hard.

Other symptoms are pain in the belly (abdomen), nausea, vomiting, diarrhea, and blood in the stool or urine. Adolescent girls and women may have painful periods.

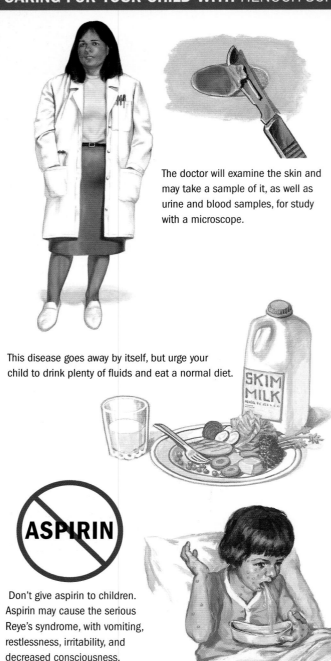

The doctor will examine the skin and may take a sample of it, as well as urine and blood samples, for study with a microscope.

This disease goes away by itself, but urge your child to drink plenty of fluids and eat a normal diet.

Don't give aspirin to children. Aspirin may cause the serious Reye's syndrome, with vomiting, restlessness, irritability, and decreased consciousness.

Over-the-counter medicine (such as acetaminophen) or prescription drugs may help control pain and fever.

How Is Henoch-Schönlein Purpura Diagnosed?

The doctor will examine the skin and may take a sample of it for study with a microscope. Urine and blood samples may also be taken.

If the doctor thinks that there may be a kidney problem, a kidney biopsy will be done. This biopsy involves using a hollow needle to remove a tiny bit of tissue from the kidney and sending it to a laboratory for study.

How Is Henoch-Schönlein Purpura Treated?

This disease goes away by itself. Symptoms may flare up and disappear several times. The doctor may prescribe medicine for the pain. Over-the-counter medicine, such as ibuprofen, naproxen, or acetaminophen, may also be used to control pain and fever.

DOs and DON'Ts in Managing Henoch-Schönlein Purpura:

✔ **DO** encourage your child to drink plenty of fluids and eat a normal diet as much as possible.

✔ **DO** call your doctor immediately if the abdominal pain gets worse or the bowel movements (stool) or urine contain blood; if there is puffiness, especially around the face or eyes; or if your child hasn't urinated in more than 12 hours.

✔ **DO** call your doctor immediately if your child appears very sick.

⊘ **DON'T** give aspirin to children, because it may cause a serious illness called Reye's syndrome and may cause increased bleeding from the blood vessels.

FROM THE DESK OF

NOTES

FOR MORE INFORMATION

Contact the following sources:

• American College of Rheumatology
  Tel: (404) 633-3777
  Website: http://www.rheumatology.org

• American Academy of Dermatology
  Tel: (866) 503-SKIN (7546)
  Website: http://www.aad.org

MANAGING
IMPETIGO

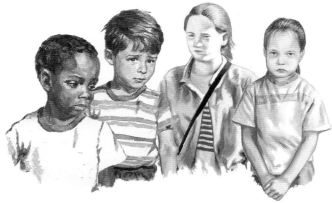

Impetigo is a mild skin infection. It occurs most often in babies and children. It spreads easily among them, especially when they're crowded together.

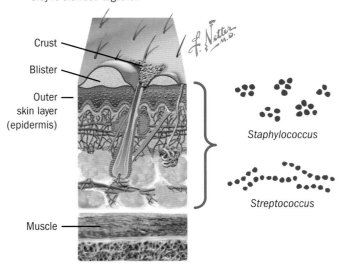

Crust

Blister

Outer
skin layer
(epidermis)

Staphylococcus

Streptococcus

Muscle

Bacteria called *Staphylococcus* (staph) and *Streptococcus* (strep) cause impetigo. They normally live on the skin surface but can go deeper and cause infection.

Impetigo starts with painless blisters, usually on the face, especially near the nose and mouth. Blisters fill with clear or yellow fluid and crust over.

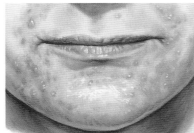

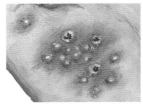

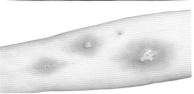

Your doctor makes a diagnosis from the look of the blisters and sores.

What Is Impetigo?

Impetigo is a very common, mild skin infection. It occurs most often in babies and children. It spreads easily from one person to another, especially when they're crowded together. Brothers and sisters and people who play contact sports can often get it.

What Causes Impetigo?

Two kinds of bacteria called *Staphylococcus* (staph) and *Streptococcus* (strep) cause impetigo, separately or together. These bacteria normally live on the skin surface, but they can get into top layers of the skin and cause infection. Impetigo is more likely when skin is hurt, such as with scratches, scrapes, or insect bites.

Young children can spread it because hands carry bacteria and the children touch each other a lot and don't wash their hands.

What Are the Symptoms of Impetigo?

Impetigo starts with painless blisters, usually on the face, especially around the nose and mouth. Blisters fill with clear or yellow fluid, eventually burst open, and leave a gold crust. Blisters may itch or burn. They don't usually leave scars.

Rarely, impetigo can lead to kidney inflammation, with blood or protein in the urine.

How Is Impetigo Diagnosed?

The doctor will make a diagnosis from the look of the skin blisters and sores. Tests may be done to find out which bacteria are causing the infection. A swab may be used to take a sample of fluid inside a blister. Blood or urine tests may also be done to be sure that bacteria haven't caused a complication.

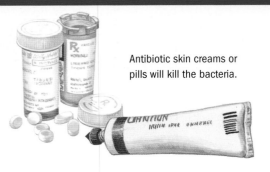

Antibiotic skin creams or pills will kill the bacteria.

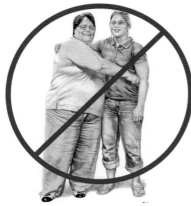

Avoid close contact with others so that you don't spread impetigo.

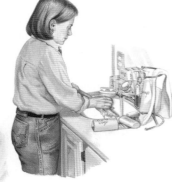

Call your doctor if your urine is discolored or has blood in it.

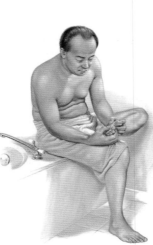

Keep your skin clean by hand washing. Bathe or shower at least once daily.

How Is Impetigo Treated?

Impetigo should be treated quickly to keep it from spreading under the skin and preventing additional damage. If left untreated, impetigo can continue for weeks, and the bacteria may, in rare cases, damage the kidneys.

Impetigo responds rapidly to medicine plus soaking and washing. Most cases go away within 7 to 10 days. Antibiotics, given as skin creams or pills, will kill the bacteria. Crusts that remain after blisters burst should be removed. Blisters are first soaked with a wet cloth. Then the area is washed with antibacterial soap.

DOs and DON'Ts in Managing Impetigo:

✔ **DO** keep your skin clean by hand washing. Maintain good hygiene. Bathe or shower at least once daily. Wash your whole body with an antibacterial soap.

✔ **DO** thoroughly wash skin scrapes and cuts and insect bites.

✔ **DO** keep toys and other objects that children play with clean.

✔ **DO** tell your doctor if you don't feel well while taking medicine.

✔ **DO** trim children's nails if scratching is a problem.

✔ **DO** call your doctor if you're not better in 7 to 10 days, you have persistent fever even with treatment, family members become infected, or your urine has blood in it.

⊘ **DON'T** scrape or scratch blisters.

⊘ **DON'T** have close contact with other people while you still have blisters.

⊘ **DON'T** shave infected areas or anywhere that is red and inflamed.

⊘ **DON'T** share washcloths, towels, or beds while you have impetigo.

FROM THE DESK OF

NOTES

FOR MORE INFORMATION

Contact the following source:

• American Academy of Dermatology
 Tel: (866) 503-SKIN (503-7546)
 Website: http://www.aad.org

MANAGING YOUR
KELOIDS

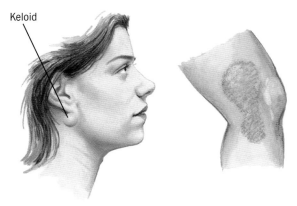

Keloid

Keloids and abnormally large (hypertrophic) scars are an overgrowth of scar tissue on the skin. They can appear anywhere, usually in a place that was injured, such as after ear piercing or severe acne.

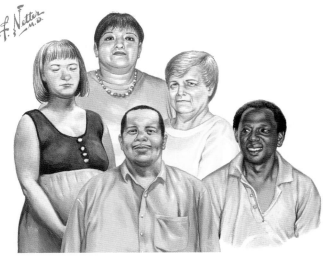

They can affect people of all skin types, but are more common in people with dark skin.

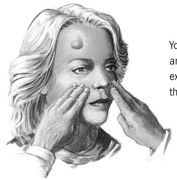

Your doctor can diagnose keloids and hypertrophic scars by examining you and noting how they look.

What Are Keloids?

Keloids and scars that are hypertrophic (meaning growing abnormally large) are an overgrowth of scar tissue on the skin. They can appear anywhere, usually in a place that was injured, such as after a burn, severe acne, or a scratch.

What Causes Keloids?

Keloids result from too much scar tissue forming as a wound heals. No one knows why they form. They cannot be caught from someone else and aren't skin cancer, but the tendency to get keloids often runs in families. Keloids affect people of all skin types but are more common in people with dark skin.

What Are the Symptoms of Keloids?

Keloids are raised lumps of pink, red, or dark scar tissue that go beyond the original wound. They sometimes start after very small wounds, such as ear piercing. They may grow large and don't get smaller with time, but they may become paler. Keloids are different from hypertrophic scars. A hypertrophic scar is raised, red and lumpy, or uneven. It doesn't spread beyond the original wound. It often gets smaller and paler over time.

Both hypertrophic scars and keloids are usually painless but can itch. If they form over a joint they may make it harder to move.

How Are Keloids Diagnosed?

The doctor makes a diagnosis from the look of the scar. Tests are usually not needed.

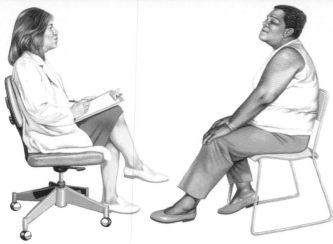

No one treatment works for everyone, but surgery, injections, dressings, freezing, and lasers have been used. If possible, the best thing may be to leave keloids alone. Talk to your doctor.

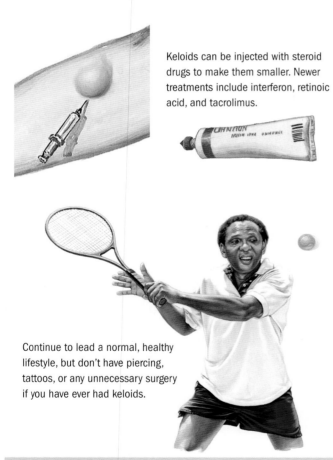

Keloids can be injected with steroid drugs to make them smaller. Newer treatments include interferon, retinoic acid, and tacrolimus.

Continue to lead a normal, healthy lifestyle, but don't have piercing, tattoos, or any unnecessary surgery if you have ever had keloids.

How Are Keloids Treated?

No one treatment is effective. With keloids, prevention is better than cure. Avoid body piercing, tattoos, or any kind of unnecessary surgery. If possible, the best thing may be to leave them alone.

Different treatments have had success but don't work for everyone. Keloids may come back in the same areas despite treatment. The various treatments include surgery, steroid injections, dressings, freezing, and lasers.

Surgery usually doesn't work because keloids often come back, sometimes larger than before. Injecting a steroid drug into the keloid may make it smaller. Dressings include pressure bandages or special dressing sheets placed over the area for several weeks or months. Freezing (cryosurgery) can make keloids flatter, and lasers can make the color paler and make the scar flatter.

Certain newer treatments, including chemotherapy drugs, interferon, imiquimod cream, retinoic acid, and tacrolimus, are sometimes successful.

DOs and DON'Ts in Managing Keloids:

✔ **DO** use makeup to help cover your scar if it bothers you. Special products are available.

✔ **DO** continue to lead a normal, healthy lifestyle. There are no restrictions for keloids.

✔ **DO** call your doctor when you see signs of keloids forming.

⊘ **DON'T** have piercings, tattoos, or any unnecessary surgery if you have ever had keloids.

FROM THE DESK OF

NOTES

FOR MORE INFORMATION

Contact the following source:

• American Academy of Dermatology
Tel: (866) 503-SKIN (7546)
Website: http://www.aad.org

LEPROSY

World incidence
(rate/1000)

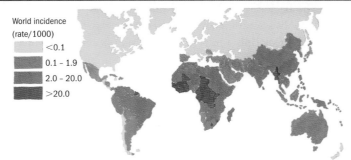

	<0.1
	0.1 - 1.9
	2.0 - 20.0
	>20.0

Leprosy is an infection that involves mainly the skin and nerves. About 650,000 new cases occur each year worldwide, about 150 in the United States. Today, leprosy found early can be treated and has no major lasting effects.

What Is Leprosy?

Also called Hansen's disease, leprosy is an infection that involves mainly the skin and nerves. The number of cases worldwide has fallen, so now 650,000 new cases are diagnosed yearly. Nearly three fourths of leprosy cases occur in India, Brazil, Bangladesh, Indonesia, and Myanmar. About 150 new cases occur yearly in the United States, more than 85% in immigrants.

There are two types: paucibacillary and multibacillary. In paucibacillary leprosy, people have fewer than five skin lesions and skin smears show no bacteria. In multibacillary leprosy, people have six or more skin lesions and bacteria are found.

Leprosy is more common in women than men. People of any age can get it, but it usually occurs in young children. Leprosy isn't cancer and can't be passed on. It can spread from person to person (through the respiratory tract or broken skin), but the risk of catching it is low. Found early, leprosy can be cured without major lasting effects.

What Causes Leprosy?

The cause is a kind of bacteria called *Mycobacterium leprae.*

What Are the Symptoms of Leprosy?

Skin and nerves that control muscle movement and feeling in the arms and legs are affected. A rash or lumps called nodules are usually noted first. Skin lesions may look darker or lighter than usual. Nodules have a clear center, with loss of feeling; the affected area can't sweat. Many people complain of feeling pins and needles in hands or feet and lumps along the nerve, especially on arms and legs.

Nerve involvement can lead to muscle weakness and wasting (atrophy), especially in hands and feet. Hands and feet contract and can't be used well, and foot drop and clawed hands and toes result. Leprosy involving facial nerves may cause the bridge of the nose to collapse, trouble closing upper eyelids, and loss of eyebrows.

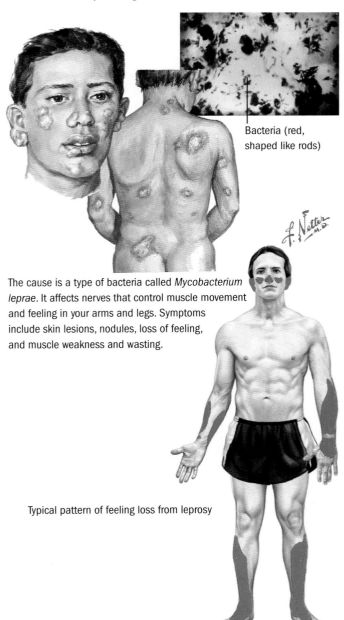

Bacteria (red, shaped like rods)

The cause is a type of bacteria called *Mycobacterium leprae*. It affects nerves that control muscle movement and feeling in your arms and legs. Symptoms include skin lesions, nodules, loss of feeling, and muscle weakness and wasting.

Typical pattern of feeling loss from leprosy

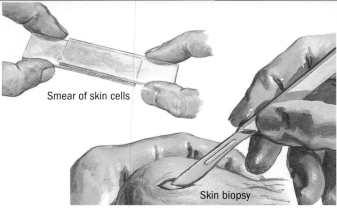

Smear of skin cells

Skin biopsy

For diagnosis, your doctor will study your skin cells (from a smear or biopsy) under a microscope, take a medical history, and do a physical examination.

Your doctor will prescribe an antibiotic or a combination of antibiotics, depending on the type of leprosy you have.

If nerves in your feet have been affected, ask your doctor about what shoes to wear to reduce or prevent skin problems and ulcers.

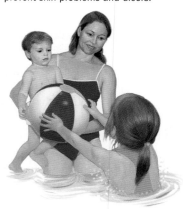

Although the risk of infecting others is low, it is possible. Your family members and close contacts should be examined often for signs of infection.

How Is Leprosy Diagnosed?

The doctor relies on a medical history and physical examination. The bacteria will be found on skin smears or biopsy. A smear involves scraping skin, smearing the sample on a slide, and looking at cells under a microscope. A biopsy involves removing a piece of skin (or nerve) for study under a microscope.

How Is Leprosy Treated?

Antibiotics (rifampin, dapsone) are usually given for pauci-bacillary leprosy. People with multibacillary leprosy take a combination of antibiotics. A doctor who specializes in infections should be involved in care.

DOs and DON'Ts in Managing Leprosy:

✔ **DO** take medicines as prescribed.
✔ **DO** get proper foot care and shoes if leprosy involves leg nerves, to prevent skin breakdown and ulcers.
✔ **DO** see an infectious disease expert. Call your doctor if you need a referral.
✔ **DO** call your doctor if you have a rash, tender lumps on your skin, muscle weakness, or a feeling of pins and needles going down your arms or legs.
✔ **DO** call your doctor if you have medicine side effects.

⊘ **DON'T** miss follow-up appointments.
⊘ **DON'T** forget that, although the risk of giving leprosy to someone else is low, your family members and close contacts should be examined often.

FROM THE DESK OF

NOTES

FOR MORE INFORMATION

Contact the following sources:

• American Leprosy Missions
  Tel: (800) 543-3135
  E-mail: amlep@leprosy.org

• International Federation of Anti-Leprosy Associations
  Website: http://www.ilep.org.uk/

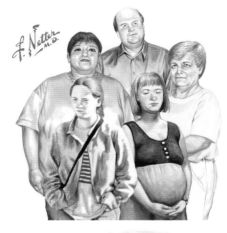

Lichen planus (LP) is a condition that affects your skin and mouth. It occurs at any age but is more common in people older than 40.

What Is Lichen Planus?

Lichen planus (LP) is an illness that affects the skin and mouth. It occurs at any age but is more common in people older than 40. It develops slowly and can spread for several months. No cure exists, but LP tends to disappear after 6 to 18 months. Some people have it more than once.

What Causes LP?

The cause is unknown. LP cannot spread to others by contact or germs. It doesn't run in families and isn't passed on from parents to children. Some medicines, including antimalarial drugs, penicillamine, tetracycline, water pills (diuretics), quinine, propranolol, and captopril, tend to cause LP-like reactions. LP isn't skin cancer.

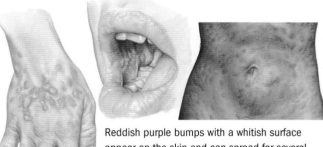

Reddish purple bumps with a whitish surface appear on the skin and can spread for several months. The bumps are raised, with flat tops and maybe white scales or flakes. Most often, they occur on wrists, forearms, and ankles.

What Are the Symptoms of LP?

LP can occur anywhere but is most common on inner wrists, forearms, and ankles. Small, very itchy bumps that are reddish-purple with a whitish surface appear. The bumps are raised, with flat tops and maybe white scales or flakes.

An irregular whitish line inside the mouth or vagina may also occur. Mouth sores may hurt. Patches of hair on the head may be lost.

The exact cause is unknown, but some medicines such as tetracycline, water pills (diuretics), quinine, propranolol, and captopril cause reactions.

How Is LP Diagnosed?

The doctor can diagnose LP by looking at the skin and mouth. The doctor may suggest seeing a specialist who treats skin problems (dermatologist). This doctor may remove a small piece of tissue (biopsy sample) for study, to help with diagnosis.

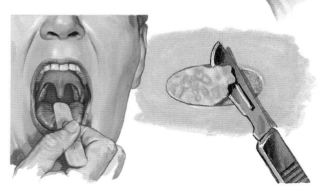

Your doctor will look at your skin and mouth. Your doctor may also do a biopsy (remove a small sample of the area, to study it under a microscope.

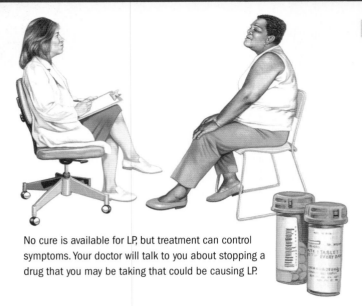

No cure is available for LP, but treatment can control symptoms. Your doctor will talk to you about stopping a drug that you may be taking that could be causing LP.

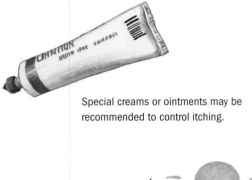

Special creams or ointments may be recommended to control itching.

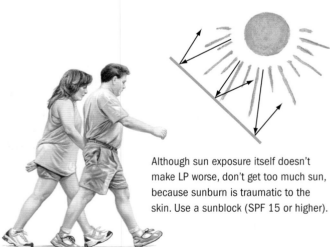

Although sun exposure itself doesn't make LP worse, don't get too much sun, because sunburn is traumatic to the skin. Use a sunblock (SPF 15 or higher).

How Is LP Treated?

If LP isn't itchy or painful, no treatment is needed. After about 4 months, the rash doesn't get worse.

For symptoms, LP has many treatments. Some treatments control symptoms (in days to weeks), and some may reduce the number of lesions. Because the cause is unknown, no specific treatment is effective in all people. Treatment can make your skin look better. Creams and ointments help control itching, as do antihistamines. Medicines should be applied just after bathing. Cortisone-like medicines are used most often.

For severe LP, there are medicines that can be taken by mouth. The affected area can be soaked in cool water to relieve itching.

Reducing stress, by using relaxation techniques or getting counseling, can help LP.

The doctor may suggest stopping a medicine that is related to LP. A substitute drug may be needed for chronic conditions such as high blood pressure.

DOs and DON'Ts in Managing LP:

✔ **DO** see your doctor regularly for oral cancer screening. LP in your mouth means that you may have a greater risk of getting oral cancer.

✔ **DO** treat your skin gently, because LP is caused by inflammation, and trauma can cause further lesions. No specific diet, exercise, or other medicines will cure LP.

✔ **DO** see your doctor if the lesions are scratched and become infected and drain pus.

✔ **DO** see an eye doctor (ophthalmologist) if irritation of the eye develops when you have this condition.

✔ **DO** call your doctor if your mouth lesions become so painful that you cannot eat.

⊘ **DON'T** scratch, to avoid starting new lesions.

⊘ **DON'T** use over-the-counter medicines, creams or lotions containing perfumes, or anything that can irritate the skin.

⊘ **DON'T** get too much sun, because sunburn is traumatic to the skin. Sun exposure itself doesn't make LP worse.

FROM THE DESK OF

NOTES

FOR MORE INFORMATION

Contact the following source:

• American Academy of Dermatology
Tel: (866) 503-SKIN (7546)
Website: http://www.aad.org/

MANAGING YOUR
MEASLES

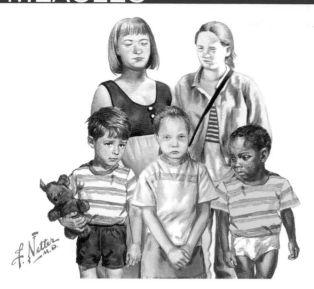

Measles is a highly contagious infection caused by a virus. Outbreaks are not as common today as before because of now-routine vaccinations. Most cases occur in preschool children and adolescents who didn't get immunized. Pregnant women should avoid getting measles because it can affect their unborn babies.

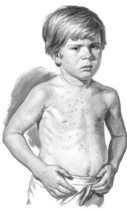

People generally catch measles by breathing in air droplets that contain virus. Symptoms start 1 to 2 weeks after exposure. Flulike symptoms are followed by tiny white-gray spots in the mouth and throat, and then a red-brown rash that starts on the forehead and around the ears and spreads to the body.

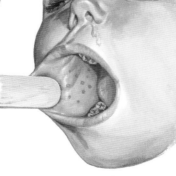

Your doctor will do a physical examination and ask your medical history. Blood tests may also be needed for diagnosis.

What Is Measles?

Measles is a highly contagious infection caused by a virus. The disease usually starts 7 to 14 days after exposure and lasts 4 to 10 days.

What Causes Measles?

Measles is caused by a virus that easily spreads among people. People breathe in droplets in the air that contain the virus when they are near someone who has it, or they touch things that are contaminated with the virus, such as drinking glasses, and then put their fingers in their mouths.

People don't get measles more than once.

The best way to stop measles is to get vaccinated. Most cases occur in preschool children, adolescents, young adults, and people who haven't had vaccinations. Adults may get measles if they only had one vaccine dose many years ago and may need a booster shot for travel to countries where measles is still common.

Complications include ear infections, pneumonia, strep throat, and meningitis.

What Are the Symptoms of Measles?

The first symptom is fever, followed by feeling tired, loss of appetite, and later, a runny nose, sneezing, dry hacking cough, and light sensitivity. Then, tiny white-gray spots appear in the mouth and throat, followed by a red-brown rash that starts on the forehead and around the ears and spreads to the body. The fever starts to go down on the second or third day of the rash. When the rash reaches the feet, it starts to fade. The rash can leave a brownish color that disappears in 7 to 10 days.

How Is Measles Diagnosed?

The doctor makes a diagnosis from the medical history and physical examination. No specific tests are needed, but a blood test may confirm the diagnosis.

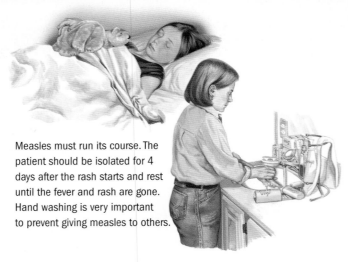

Measles must run its course. The patient should be isolated for 4 days after the rash starts and rest until the fever and rash are gone. Hand washing is very important to prevent giving measles to others.

Only use nonaspirin products, such as acetaminophen. Never give aspirin to a child younger than 16 who has a viral infection to avoid the serious Reye's syndrome.

All children should have measles vaccination as part of routine childhood immunizations. Some adults need a booster shot for travel to a country where measles is still common.

How Is Measles Treated?

People should be isolated for 4 days after the rash starts and rest until the fever and rash are gone. Saline eye drops can help eye irritation, and sunglasses help severe light sensitivity. Non-aspirin products (e.g., acetaminophen) should be given for fever. Never give aspirin to a child younger than 16 with a viral infection because of the risk of Reye's syndrome. Antibiotics aren't needed because the infection is due to a virus. Fluid intake should be increased.

DOs and DON'Ts in Managing Measles:

✔ **DO** tell your doctor if you're pregnant. Measles during pregnancy can affect your baby.

✔ **DO** cover your mouth when coughing.

✔ **DO** wash hands regularly and encourage others to do so.

✔ **DO** use a cool-mist vaporizer to soothe coughing.

✔ **DO** use saline eye drops for irritation and sunglasses for light sensitivity.

✔ **DO** call your doctor if a sore throat and high temperature develop during the illness, or if you have a severe headache, trouble breathing, chest pain, earache, increased drowsiness or weakness, and a cough with thick yellow sputum.

⊘ **DON'T** send a child with measles to school for about 10 days. They can give measles to others from 5 days before the first spots appear until at least 5 days after the rash develops.

⊘ **DON'T** give aspirin to a child younger than 16 during a viral infection to avoid Reye's syndrome.

FROM THE DESK OF

NOTES

FOR MORE INFORMATION

Contact the following sources:

• American Academy of Pediatrics
 Tel: (847) 434-4000
 Website: http://www.aap.org

• Pediatric Infectious Disease Society
 Tel: (703) 299-6764
 Website: http://www.pids.org

MANAGING YOUR
MELANOMA

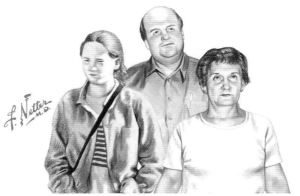

Melanoma is the most serious type of skin cancer. It usually is seen after adolescence. In the United States, the number of new cases increased greatly in the past 25 years. If found early, about 85% of melanomas are curable.

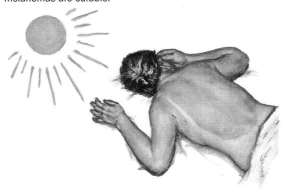

The cause of melanoma is usually too much sun. Risk factors include fair skin, blue eyes, freckles, having family members with melanoma, and going to tanning salons. People with dark skin can also get melanoma.

New moles or changes in moles that you already have can mean melanoma. The ABCD rule can help you remember symptoms to watch for:

Asymmetric shape
Border—irregular
Color—varied
Diameter—increasing (larger than 6 mm)

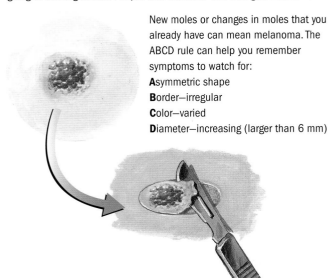

A biopsy of the mole is done to see whether it's cancerous. For the biopsy, a piece of the mole is removed for study with a microscope.

What Is Melanoma?

Melanoma is a skin cancer that begins in melanocytes. Melanocytes are skin cells that make pigment. Most melanomas appear as new moles; some start from a mole already present. Melanoma starts in the mole, spreads nearby and then deeper into the skin, into veins and lymph nodes, and finally into the liver, brain, lungs, and bones.

The number of new cases in the United States increased greatly in the last 25 years. If found early, about 85% of melanomas are curable.

What Causes Melanoma?

The cause is too much ultraviolet radiation from the sun, which hurts the skin. Higher risk is related to severe sunburns, light-colored skin, blue eyes, blond hair, getting freckles, using tanning salons, and having many abnormal moles or family members with melanoma. People with dark skin can also get melanoma.

What Are the Symptoms of Melanoma?

Initially there are no symptoms. When the melanoma spreads, symptoms include ABCD changes in a mole, swollen glands (lymph nodes), shortness of breath, bone pain (when melanoma spreads to bones), and headache, seizures, and visual problems (when melanoma spreads to brain). Skin signs of melanoma are *a*symmetry (the shape of one half doesn't match the other), irregular *b*order, uneven *c*olor, and increasing *d*iameter (change in size). These are known as ABCD changes.

How Is Melanoma Diagnosed?

The doctor makes a diagnosis by doing a biopsy (removing a piece of the mole and studying it with a microscope). The biopsy must be done for staging the cancer (how thick it is and how deep it goes in the skin). Also, to see whether the cancer spread (metastasized), the doctor looks for swollen lymph nodes during an examination and orders blood tests, chest x-rays, computed tomography (CT) of the head, and a bone scan.

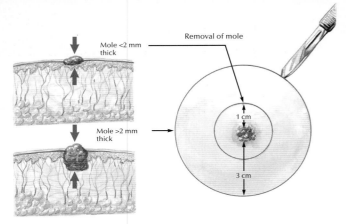

Mole <2 mm thick

Removal of mole

Mole >2 mm thick

1 cm

3 cm

All stages of melanoma need surgery. For early stages, when the cancer hasn't spread, the mole and skin around it will be removed. If the cancer spread, lymph nodes may also be removed. Advanced melanoma may also need radiation and chemotherapy.

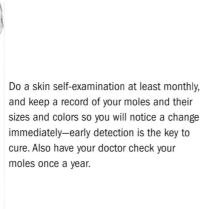

Don't go to tanning salons, and limit your time in the sun. Always wear sun block, at least SPF 30, and protective clothing. Avoid being in the sun between 10 AM and 4 PM, when the sun is strongest.

SPF 30

Do a skin self-examination at least monthly, and keep a record of your moles and their sizes and colors so you will notice a change immediately—early detection is the key to cure. Also have your doctor check your moles once a year.

How Is Melanoma Treated?

Treatment depends on the stage of the cancer and whether it spread to other organs. Early detection is critical for a cure, because advanced melanoma cannot be cured.

Surgery is done for all stages. For early stages, a surgeon cuts a wide margin of skin to make sure that all cancer is removed. If the melanoma has spread to other organs, surgery, radiation, chemotherapy, and immunotherapy help symptoms but usually don't cure it.

DOs and DON'Ts in Managing Melanoma:

✔ **DO** check your skin regularly for odd-looking new moles or changes in old moles. Call your doctor if you find any.

✔ **DO** have your doctor do a complete check of your skin at least yearly.

✔ **DO** avoid tanning booths.

✔ **DO** a skin self-examination at least once monthly. Look at all moles on your body or any new moles that have developed.

✔ **DO** use sunscreen with a sun protection factor (SPF) more than 30, which provides the best protection.

✔ **DO** remember that treating malignant melanoma requires a team effort, involving a primary care doctor, dermatologist (skin specialist), oncologist (cancer specialist), and surgeon.

✔ **DO** call your doctor if you feel swollen glands or you have pain, fever, or drainage after surgery.

🚫 **DON'T** stay out in the sun for long periods, especially if you burn easily.

🚫 **DON'T** delay calling your doctor if you see a mole that has changed or one that looks different.

FROM THE DESK OF

NOTES

FOR MORE INFORMATION

Contact the following sources:

• National Cancer Institute
Tel: (800) 422-6237
Website: http://www.cancer.gov

• American Academy of Dermatology
Tel: (866) 503-SKIN (7546)
Website: http://www.aad.org

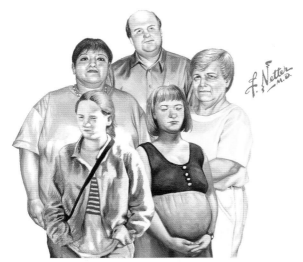

Molluscum contagiosum is an infection of the skin caused by a virus. It is fairly common in children (more often boys) and young adults. When it affects the genital area, it's called a sexually transmitted disease (STD).

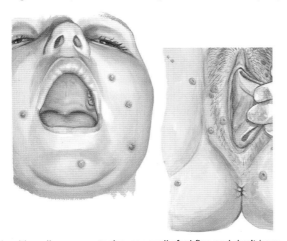

People with molluscum contagiosum usually feel fine and don't have itching, pain, or tenderness. Small bumps occur on the skin, often the face, eyelids, underarms, and thighs (groin).

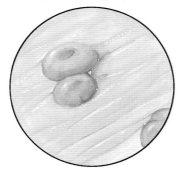

Your doctor will make a diagnosis just by looking at the bumps. These bumps are domed, with a pit and white curdlike material in the center. Your doctor may want to take a scraping of the bumps and look at the white material under a microscope.

What Is Molluscum Contagiosum?

Molluscum contagiosum is an infection of the top layers of the skin caused by a virus. It spreads easily and so is fairly common in children (more often boys) and young adults. When it affects the genital area, it's said to be a sexually transmitted disease (STD).

What Causes Molluscum Contagiosum?

The cause is a poxvirus (the same virus family that causes warts). The virus spreads by direct contact, touching either the infected skin of someone else or infected items such as clothes.

What Are the Symptoms of Molluscum Contagiosum?

Usually, people with molluscum contagiosum feel fine and don't have itching, pain, or tender spots. It takes from 2 to 7 weeks after exposure to see the rash. Small bumps occur on the skin in the affected part of the body, often in the face, eyelids, underarms, and thighs (groin). Usually, bumps don't appear on the palms of the hands, soles of the feet, and mouth.

The bumps are domed with a central pit and contain white curdlike (cheeselike) material. This material contains the virus.

The bumps usually go away on their own over several weeks, but some may last for months. They don't usually leave scars.

How Is Molluscum Contagiosum Diagnosed?

Tests are usually not needed. The doctor will usually diagnose the infection just by looking at the bumps on the skin. In some cases, the doctor may want to take a scraping of the bumps and look at it under a microscope.

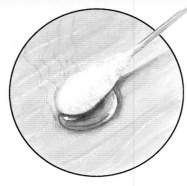

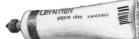

The bumps usually go away on their own, but people often have treatment to keep the virus from infecting someone else. Medicated creams, lasers, freezing, and scraping are ways to treat the bumps.

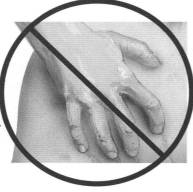

Don't scratch or pick at your bumps and then touch other parts of your body. You'll spread the virus and may get another infection with bacteria.

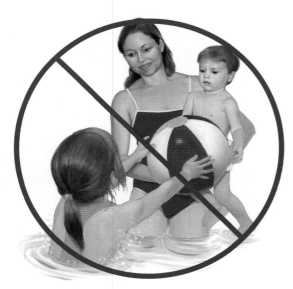

Don't use public swimming pools, saunas, and showers until the bumps are gone.

How Is Molluscum Contagiosum Treated?

The bumps usually go away on their own, but people often have treatment to keep the virus from infecting someone else or to keep the rash from spreading to other body parts. Treatments include removing the bumps by using lasers, freezing, or scraping. Sometimes these treatments leave scars. Special medicated skin creams can also help bumps go away.

Treatment may have to be repeated as new bumps appear. Also, people can get this infection more than once. Sharing contaminated hand towels or other personal items and having close contact with someone who has the infection should be avoided.

DOs and DON'Ts in Managing Molluscum Contagiosum:

✔ **DO** avoid sexual contact if the bumps involve the genital area.

✔ **DO** keep the affected area clean and covered with clothing or a bandage, to avoid spreading the virus.

✔ **DO** call your doctor if the bumps get worse.

🚫 **DON'T** share hand towels with another person until the bumps are gone.

🚫 **DON'T** scratch the bumps on your skin and then touch other parts of your body. You will spread the virus this way and may get another (bacterial) infection.

🚫 **DON'T** use public swimming pools, saunas, and showers until the bumps are gone, to avoid passing the infection to others.

FROM THE DESK OF

NOTES

FOR MORE INFORMATION

Contact the following source:

• American Academy of Dermatology
Tel: (866) 503-SKIN (7546)
Website: http://www.aad.org

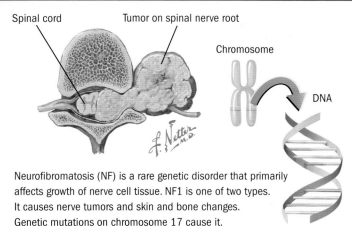

Spinal cord   Tumor on spinal nerve root

Chromosome

DNA

Neurofibromatosis (NF) is a rare genetic disorder that primarily affects growth of nerve cell tissue. NF1 is one of two types. It causes nerve tumors and skin and bone changes. Genetic mutations on chromosome 17 cause it.

Symptoms

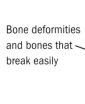

Usually present at birth and almost always show up before a child is 10 years old

Curved spine (scoliosis)

Small brown patches (café-au-lait spots), mostly on the chest, back, and tummy

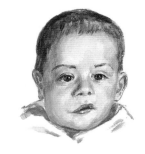

Bone deformities and bones that break easily

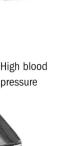

High blood pressure

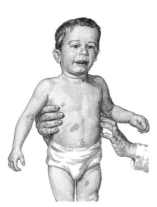

Your doctor will ask about family medical history and will do physical and eye examinations.

What Is Neurofibromatosis Type 1?

Neurofibromatosis (NF) is a genetic disorder that primarily affects growth of nerve cell tissue. It causes nerve tumors and skin and bone changes. Two types occur, type 1 (NF1) and type 2 (NF2). NF1 is also called von Recklinghausen's disease. NF1 isn't common, occurring in 1 of every 4000 people. It affects men and women equally and has been related to tumors of the brain, eye, and spinal cord and certain types of leukemia. There is no cure for it yet.

What Causes NF1?

NF1 is inherited, but more than half of people have no family history of NF1. It happens because of genetic mutations on chromosome 17. Each child born to a parent with NF1 has a 50% chance of getting it.

What Are the Symptoms of NF1?

Symptoms include small brown patches (café-au-lait spots), mostly on the chest, back, and tummy. Present from birth, they vary in size.

Several types of growths develop in and under the skin. They often appear in late childhood or early adolescence. They also vary from smaller than 1 inch to many inches. Larger ones can be disfiguring.

Other symptoms are freckling in body parts that normally don't get sun (such as armpits and groin), learning problems (e.g., learning disabilities and low IQ, in about half of children), curved spine, bones that break easily, and high blood pressure.

Growths in different places in the body cause symptoms. Growths inside the head or on the spine can lead to seizures, loss of vision, and leg weakness (paralysis).

How Is NF1 Diagnosed?

The doctor will ask about family medical history and will do physical and eye examinations. Electroencephalography (EEG), which records brain waves, is done for seizures. Children have their IQ tested.

A biopsy is done if cancer is possible. In a biopsy, a sample of the growth is removed and studied.

No general treatment is available, but certain treatments may control symptoms. Your doctor will watch for and treat complications.

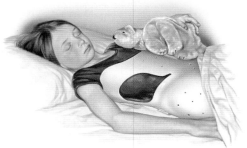

A back brace and bone surgery may be suggested for scoliosis.

Surgery to remove painful or disfiguring tumors may be an option, but tumors may grow back and in greater numbers.

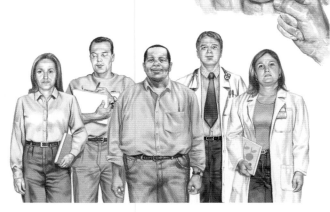

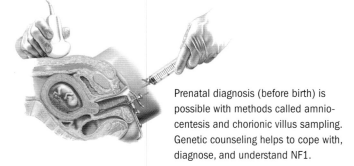

Find doctors and hospitals with experience treating NF1. A team approach is needed for management. Don't be afraid to get a second opinion.

Prenatal diagnosis (before birth) is possible with methods called amniocentesis and chorionic villus sampling. Genetic counseling helps to cope with, diagnose, and understand NF1.

How Is NF1 Treated?

No general treatment is available, but specific treatments may control symptoms. The doctor will watch for and treat complications. Children with learning disabilities need special schooling. Physical and occupational therapy can help. Physical therapy benefits people with a curved spine and broken bones. Occupational therapy teaches people how to manage normal activities.

Surgery can help with bone abnormalities. Scoliosis may need surgery plus back braces. Painful or disfiguring tumors can be removed but may grow back. For rare cancerous tumors, surgery, radiation, or chemotherapy can be used.

DOs and DON'Ts in Managing NF1:

✔ **DO** find doctors and hospitals that have experience with NF1.

✔ **DO** realize that NF1 diagnosis before birth is possible with methods called amniocentesis and chorionic villus sampling.

✔ **DO** call your doctor if you see café-au-lait spots or freckles in your groin or armpit.

✔ **DO** call your doctor if you have new nervous system problems (hearing loss, muscle weakness, or difficulty with walking or balance).

⊘ **DON'T** be afraid to ask for a second opinion.
⊘ **DON'T** forget that NF1 is rare and will need a team approach for management.

FROM THE DESK OF

NOTES

FOR MORE INFORMATION

Contact the following sources:

• Neurofibromatosis, Inc.
 Tel: (800) 942-6825
 Website: http://www.nfinc.org

• National Neurofibromatosis Foundation, Inc.
 Tel: (800) 323-7938
 Website: http://www.neurofibromatosis.org

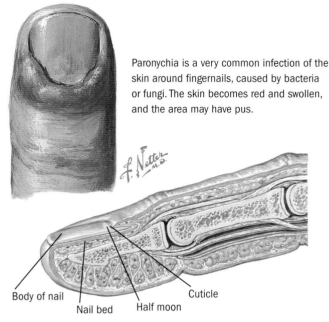

Paronychia is a very common infection of the skin around fingernails, caused by bacteria or fungi. The skin becomes red and swollen, and the area may have pus.

Body of nail   Cuticle
Nail bed   Half moon

The nail body lies on top of the nail bed. An infection can happen when the seal between the body and bed is broken.

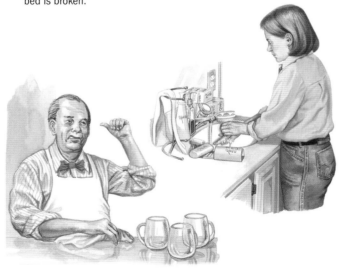

You may be more prone to developing the infection if your hands are often wet (such as dishwashers and bartenders). Biting nails or hangnails, thumb sucking, penetrating injuries (e.g., from splinters), and exposure to harsh chemicals, acrylic nails, or nail glue can lead to infection.

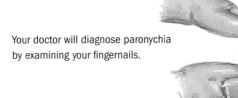

Your doctor will diagnose paronychia by examining your fingernails.

What Is Paronychia?

Paronychia is a common infection under the skin around the fingernails. It can be acute (come on suddenly) or chronic (last a long time). It occurs more in females than males. An abscess, or pus, can form if the infection is not treated.

What Causes Paronychia?

Bacteria (usually the ones called *Staphylococcus* and *Streptococcus*) or fungi cause paronychia by getting into the skin through a wound. These wounds can come from biting nails or hangnails; thumb sucking; penetrating injuries; foreign bodies such as splinters; and exposure to harsh chemicals, acrylic nails, or nail glue. People who often have wet hands that aren't dried well (such as dishwashers, bartenders, and housekeepers) and people who have diabetes have a higher risk of getting paronychia.

What Are the Symptoms of Paronychia?

Redness and swelling of the skin near the fingernail occur first. Then, fluid or pus may be seen under the nail. The area is usually very tender and feels puffy or fluid filled. As paronychia continues, throbbing pain often occurs.

How Is Paronychia Diagnosed?

The doctor will diagnose paronychia by doing an examination of the fingernails.

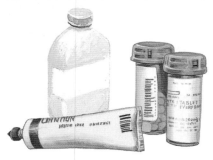

Treatment can be simply soaking in water with liquid antibacterial soap. Your doctor may prescribe a topical antibiotic cream or lotion (if bacteria are the cause) or an antifungal medicine given by mouth (if a fungus is the cause).

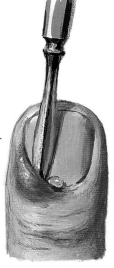

Your doctor may need to drain the pus.

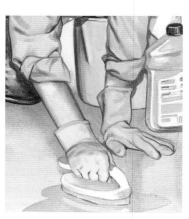

Wear vinyl gloves to prevent contact with irritating substances, such as water, soap, detergent, scouring pads, and chemicals.

How Is Paronychia Treated?

Antibiotics are used if paronychia is due to a bacterial infection, or antifungal medications are used if it is due to a fungus. The doctor may also drain the area of pus. Draining the pus usually provides a complete cure. Draining may involve making a small cut over the area or separating a small part of the nail from the skin. In advanced cases, a small piece of nail may be removed, but the nail almost always grows back.

DOs and DON'Ts in Managing Paronychia:

✔ **DO** protect your hands from water. Keep them clean and dry. Wash with soap and water after doing dirty work.

✔ **DO** wear vinyl gloves to prevent contact with irritating substances, such as water, soap, detergent, metal scrubbing pads, scouring pads, and chemicals, such as paint, paint thinner, turpentine, and polishes for cars, floors, shoes, metal, and furniture. Also wear gloves when you peel or squeeze lemons, oranges, sour fruits, tomatoes, or potatoes.

✔ **DO** wear leather or heavy-duty fabric gloves for housework or gardening.

✔ **DO** keep your bandage clean and dry. Change it at least twice daily.

✔ **DO** leave hangnails alone and avoid injuring your fingertips.

✔ **DO** take prescribed antibiotics as directed.

✔ **DO** call your doctor if the pad of your finger becomes swollen or painful, or your finger or knuckle becomes swollen or hurts to bend.

✔ **DO** call your doctor if you have red streaks from the infected area, fever, or chills.

✔ **DO** call your doctor if your pain lasts for more than 24 hours after treatment.

✔ **DO** call your doctor if you have a reaction to your medicine.

⊘ **DON'T** try to drain paronychia yourself with pins or knives.

⊘ **DON'T** bite your nails.

⊘ **DON'T** allow the wound to become dirty.

FROM THE DESK OF

NOTES

FOR MORE INFORMATION

Contact the following source:

• American Academy of Dermatology
  Tel: (866) 503-SKIN (7546)
  Website: http://www.aad.org

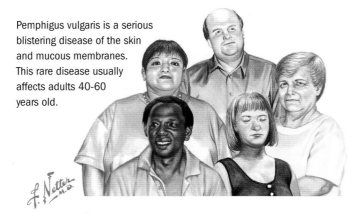

Pemphigus vulgaris is a serious blistering disease of the skin and mucous membranes. This rare disease usually affects adults 40-60 years old.

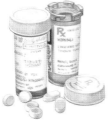

Certain drugs can trigger pemphigus vulgaris.

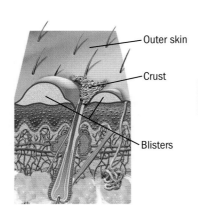

- Outer skin
- Crust
- Blisters

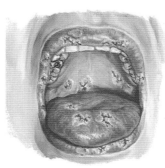

Painful sores in the mouth, nose, throat, vagina, and anus occur first. The skin shows small blisters and large ones that break easily, weep, and form crusts. These lesions can get serious bacterial infections.

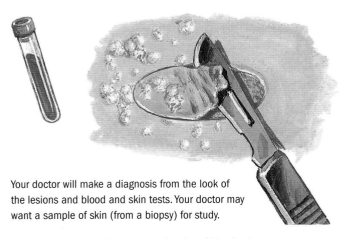

Your doctor will make a diagnosis from the look of the lesions and blood and skin tests. Your doctor may want a sample of skin (from a biopsy) for study.

What Is Pemphigus Vulgaris?

Pemphigus vulgaris is a serious blistering disease of the skin and mucous membranes. It has large blisters (bullae) that break down and form crusts.

Pemphigus vulgaris is rare. It affects men and women equally, usually adults 40 to 60 years old.

What Causes Pemphigus Vulgaris?

Pemphigus vulgaris is likely an autoimmune illness. Autoimmune means that the body's own immune system attacks the body and causes disease. Certain drugs can trigger it. It's not an infection or cancer.

What Are the Symptoms of Pemphigus Vulgaris?

Painful ulcers of the mucous linings of the mouth, nose, throat, vagina, and anus are the first symptoms. Many people cannot eat, become weak and tired, and lose weight. Dehydration and malnutrition can result.

The skin may not be affected for months. Skin lesions are usually small blisters (vesicles) and larger ones (bullae) that are flabby, easily broken, and weeping. As bullae burst, they weep fluid, bleed easily, and crust. These lesions can get bacterial infections. Scarring can also occur. Irritated mucous membranes can cause trouble swallowing, painful swallowing, and bleeding.

How Is Pemphigus Vulgaris Diagnosed?

The doctor makes a diagnosis from the look of the lesions and blood and skin tests. The doctor may do a skin biopsy (remove a small piece of skin) for study in the laboratory.

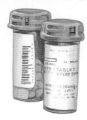

Pemphigus vulgaris can be fatal in rare cases if not treated aggressively. Immunosuppressants lessen effects of the immune attack and reduce blisters, inflammation, and pain. Powder and creams can also reduce symptoms.

If you have this disease, listen to your doctor to help reduce complications. Your doctor may prescribe a combination of drugs. Severe illness needs other measures, including intravenous fluids, surgical removal of dead tissue, and intensive wound care. You may need to stay in the hospital.

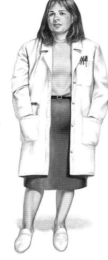

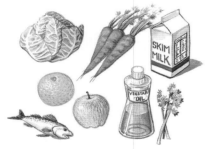

Eat a well-balanced diet. You may be malnourished because of the pain with eating and swallowing.

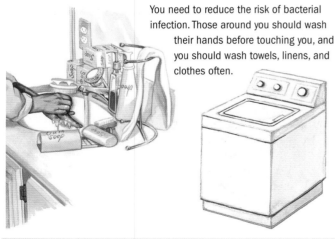

You need to reduce the risk of bacterial infection. Those around you should wash their hands before touching you, and you should wash towels, linens, and clothes often.

FROM THE DESK OF

NOTES

How Is Pemphigus Vulgaris Treated?

Pemphigus vulgaris can be fatal in rare cases if not treated aggressively. Immunosuppressive medicines lessen effects of the immune attack; reduce blisters, inflammation, and pain; and promote healing. These medicines include corticosteroids, intravenous immune globulins, and immunosuppressants such as methotrexate and cyclophosphamide. Talc or powder for wounds and bed linens (plus antibiotic ointments put on the skin) can reduce symptoms.

Severe illness needs other measures, including intravenous fluids, surgical removal of dead tissue (débridement), antibiotics for serious bacterial infections, and intensive wound care. Plasmapheresis is also used with medicines. In plasmapheresis, blood is taken from the body and put into a machine to remove antibodies causing pemphigus vulgaris. Healthier blood is then put back into the body. These measures often mean hospitalization.

Eating a healthy diet is important. Cleaning and watching wounds can prevent infections.

DOs and DON'Ts in Managing Pemphigus Vulgaris:

✔ **DO** take medicines as prescribed. Follow all instructions. Tell your doctor about all your medicines (including over-the-counter).

✔ **DO** eat a well-balanced diet. Follow a liquid or soft diet if needed.

✔ **DO** keep follow-up doctor appointments.

✔ **DO** use cleaning baths, wound care, and dressings as directed.

✔ **DO** check your lesions carefully. Call your doctor if you have signs of bacterial infection, such as redness, pus, pain or swelling, and fever.

✔ **DO** clean towels, linens, and clothing often.

✔ **DO** call your doctor if you have symptoms of another illness (fever, confusion, weakness).

🚫 **DON'T** stop your medicines or change the dose unless your doctor says you can.

🚫 **DON'T** stop taking steroids or immunosuppressants suddenly, to avoid a rebound worsening of your condition.

🚫 **DON'T** share towels, linens, or clothing with other people.

🚫 **DON'T** swim or use a Jacuzzi until your doctor says you can.

🚫 **DON'T** do activities that may contaminate skin wounds.

FOR MORE INFORMATION

Contact the following source:

• American Academy of Dermatology
Tel: (866) 503-SKIN (503-7546)
Website: http://www.aad.org

MANAGING
SUN POISONING

Sun poisoning (photodermatitis) is an itchy, scaly, blistery reddening of the skin. The skin is abnormally sensitive to sunlight or ultraviolet rays A (UVA) or B (UVB).

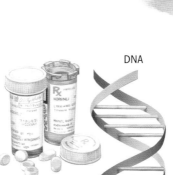

DNA

Sensitivity to sun exposure can be genetic, but often the cause can be traced to chemicals in medicines, cosmetics, and food (e.g., limes). Certain diseases can also make skin sensitive to light.

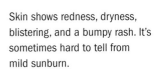

Skin shows redness, dryness, blistering, and a bumpy rash. It's sometimes hard to tell from mild sunburn.

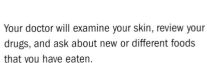

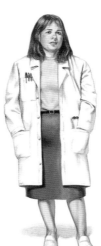

Your doctor will examine your skin, review your drugs, and ask about new or different foods that you have eaten.

What Is Sun Poisoning?

Sun poisoning, also known medically as photodermatitis, is an itchy, scaly, blistery reddening of the skin. The skin is abnormally sensitive to effects of sunlight or ultraviolet rays A (UVA) or B (UVB). It can begin suddenly (acute) or be ongoing (chronic). How much exposure to sunlight or ultraviolet light (e.g., from a tanning bed) will cause problems is different for each person.

More than 10% of people in the United States have had sun poisoning.

What Causes Sun Poisoning?

Sensitivity to sun exposure can run in families (be genetic). Often, the cause can be traced to chemicals in medicines, cosmetics, and foods. Certain diseases, such as lupus and eczema, can also make skin sensitive to light.

What Are the Symptoms of Sun Poisoning?

Symptoms include skin that is red and dry. It may have blisters and a bumpy rash. The rash may feel painful or itchy. It's sometimes hard to tell from mild sunburn.

Long-term effects include skin thickening and scarring and an increased risk of skin cancer.

How Is Sun Poisoning Diagnosed?

The doctor will make a diagnosis from the history of exposure and a skin examination. The doctor will review the medicines you are taking and ask about new or different foods you have eaten.

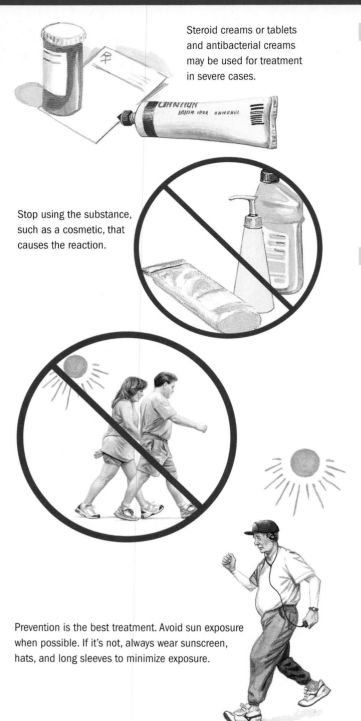

Steroid creams or tablets and antibacterial creams may be used for treatment in severe cases.

Stop using the substance, such as a cosmetic, that causes the reaction.

Prevention is the best treatment. Avoid sun exposure when possible. If it's not, always wear sunscreen, hats, and long sleeves to minimize exposure.

How Is Sun Poisoning Treated?

Prevention is the best treatment for this disorder. However, if that's impossible, therapy is aimed at minimizing inflammation (swelling, redness) of damaged skin and relieving pain. Steroid creams or tablets may be prescribed. Antibacterial creams may be prescribed for burn-like reactions and suspected infection.

Avoiding the sun and the substance causing attacks are critical. If being outside in the sun cannot be avoided, a sunblock for both UVA and UVB light with an SPF of 15 or greater should be applied. Be sure to ask the doctor and pharmacist about avoiding sun exposure while taking any drugs.

DOs and DON'Ts in Managing Sun Poisoning:

✔ **DO** take medicines only as prescribed. Avoid ultraviolet light exposure as much as possible while taking drugs such as tetracycline antibiotics, sulfa drugs, and thiazide diuretics. These drugs cause greater sensitivity to light.

✔ **DO** use sunscreen, hats, and long sleeves to minimize effects of unavoidable exposure.

✔ **DO** avoid "natural" fruit-based skin lotions and cosmetics, because they may contain sensitizers as well.

✔ **DO** check with your doctor before using any tanning device.

✔ **DO** call your doctor if you develop fever or if your symptoms don't improve with treatment.

⊘ **DON'T** take sun exposure for granted. Once you've had sun poisoning, your skin will always be sensitive to the combination of the sun and the chemical you're sensitized to.

⊘ **DON'T** rely on sun lotions and lightweight clothing to provide protection for long periods.

⊘ **DON'T** rely on clouds for sunblock. They don't block ultraviolet light.

FROM THE DESK OF

NOTES

FOR MORE INFORMATION

Contact the following source:

• American Academy of Dermatology
  Tel: (866) 503-SKIN (503-7546)
  Website: http://www.aad.org

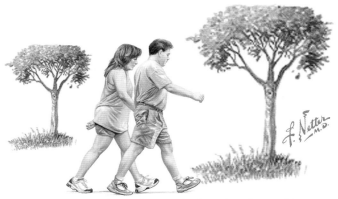

Pityriasis rosea is a rash, usually on the back, trunk, and arms. It's more common in spring and fall and usually affects men and women, 10 to 35 years old. It's not contagious. The cause is unknown.

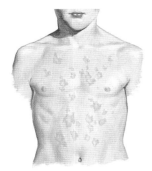

The rash starts as a single small round or oval spot, 1 to 2 inches across, usually on the trunk. Then, more spots form: oval, smaller, usually less than ¼ inch across. They are pink, red, or tan (or lighter) and may have a scale around the borders.

With the rash, other symptoms may include:

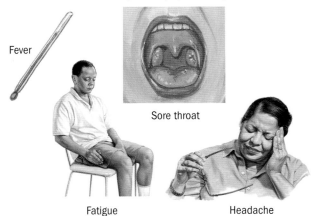

Fever

Sore throat

Fatigue

Headache

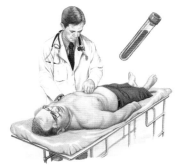

Diagnosis can usually be made from a medical history and physical examination. Blood tests and a biopsy are rarely needed but may be done to check for other causes of the rash.

What Is Pityriasis Rosea?

Pityriasis rosea is a rash that is usually on the trunk. The rash starts as a single, small, round or oval spot that measures 1 to 2 inches across. This first spot is called a herald patch. Then, more spots start to form, from a few spots to over 100, following the lines of the trunk, in a Christmas tree pattern over the back, trunk, and chest. The neck, arms, legs, and face may also be involved. These oval spots are smaller than the first, usually less than ¼ inch across. They are pink, red, or tan (or lighter) and may have a scale around their borders. The rash should heal in 2 to 8 weeks without scars. Sometimes, the rash can last longer. Dark-skinned people may have some long-lasting lighter brown spots.

The rash most often affects men and women, 10 to 35 years old.

What Causes Pityriasis Rosea?

The cause isn't known, but it's believed that a viral infection is the most likely cause. It's more common in the spring and fall than other seasons. It's not contagious.

What Are the Symptoms of Pityriasis Rosea?

Most people don't have symptoms. Some have mild itching with the rash. Other symptoms may include fatigue, fever, headache, and sore throat. Symptoms are usually gone by the time the rash appears.

How Is Pityriasis Rosea Diagnosed?

The doctor will make a diagnosis from a medical history and physical examination. Other tests are generally not necessary, but in some cases the doctor may order blood tests to make sure that another condition isn't causing the rash. Rarely, the doctor may also scrape the rash to collect some skin or cut out (biopsy) a small piece of skin that will be checked with a microscope.

The treatment goal is to reduce itching. It doesn't shorten the course of the disorder. Over-the-counter medicines such as calamine lotion and Benadryl can help itching.

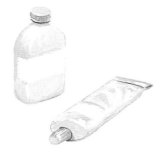

Exposure to sunlight may help, but sunburns should be avoided. Ask your doctor for guidelines.

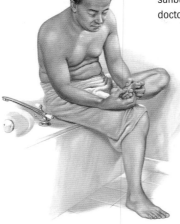

Aveeno® oatmeal baths can help itching. Heat will worsen the itching, so don't take a hot bath or use the sauna.

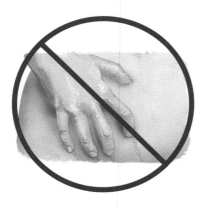

Don't scratch at your rash. It will make it worse and take longer to heal.

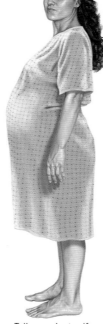

Tell your doctor if you're pregnant.

How Is Pityriasis Rosea Treated?

Treatment is aimed at reducing itching. It doesn't shorten the course of the disorder. Over-the-counter medicines such as calamine lotion, Benadryl, and Aveeno oatmeal baths can help itching. Ultraviolet light treatments may also be prescribed in some cases. Exposure to sunlight may help, but sunburns should be avoided. Prednisone may be prescribed by your physician if the itching is severe.

The doctor may want to make sure that the rash is going away during an office visit in 2 to 3 weeks.

DOs and DON'Ts in Managing Pityriasis Rosea:

✔ **DO** tell your doctor about your medicines, including prescription and over-the-counter ones.

✔ **DO** tell your doctor if you're pregnant.

✔ **DO** call your doctor if your symptoms get worse, you have a fever, or the rash has pus coming from it.

✔ **DO** call your doctor if medicines don't help the itching after a few days of using them.

✔ **DO** call your doctor if you're not better in 6 to 8 weeks.

✔ **DO** call your doctor if you have symptoms of another infection, such as high temperature, pus drainage, or swelling.

⊘ **DON'T** take a hot bath or sauna. Heat will worsen the itching.

⊘ **DON'T** use lotion too often, maybe once per day or every other day, if your skin gets too dry.

FROM THE DESK OF

NOTES

FOR MORE INFORMATION

Contact the following source:

• American Academy of Dermatology
Tel: (847) 330-0230, (866) 503-7546
Website: http://www.aad.org

Psoriasis is a common chronic skin disorder that often comes and goes. It can be mild to severe. It's a lifelong disorder that usually starts in adolescence or early adulthood.

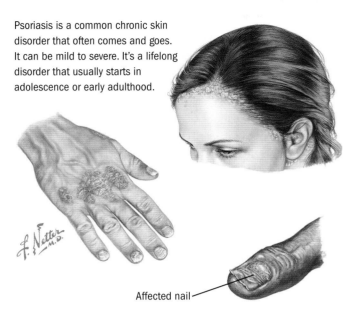

Affected nail

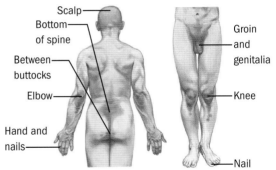

Scalp
Bottom of spine
Between buttocks
Elbow
Hand and nails
Groin and genitalia
Knee
Nail

Lesions are slightly raised, silvery white scales with red or pink margins. Lesions may be single, in certain body parts, or all over the body.

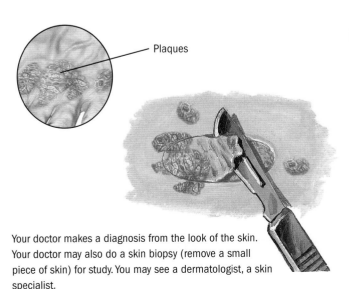

Plaques

Your doctor makes a diagnosis from the look of the skin. Your doctor may also do a skin biopsy (remove a small piece of skin) for study. You may see a dermatologist, a skin specialist.

What Is Psoriasis?

Psoriasis is a chronic skin disorder that often comes and goes. It can be mild to severe. Psoriasis is common but occurs less in African, Asian, and Native American people. It affects men and women equally. It is a lifelong disorder that usually starts in adolescence or early adulthood.

Outbreaks can start with minor injury, stress, infections, exposure to cold and dry climates, obesity, and other auto-immune conditions. They can also occur without an obvious reason.

What Causes Psoriasis?

The cause is unknown but psoriasis is likely autoimmune. Autoimmune means that the body's immune system attacks normal parts of the body and causes injury or disease. Psoriasis is not infectious or cancerous.

What Are the Symptoms of Psoriasis?

Skin lesions are slightly raised, silvery white scales with red or pink margins. Painful cracks can appear. Lesions may be single, in certain body parts, or all over the body.

Skin of the scalp, face, elbows, hands, knees, feet, chest, lower back, and folds between buttocks is usually affected. Fingernails and toenails are often involved.

Itching may be present, and joint pain sometimes occurs. Scratching can cause bacterial infections. The skin's appearance can lead to feeling embarrassed.

How Is Psoriasis Diagnosed?

The doctor makes a diagnosis from the look of the skin. The doctor may do a skin biopsy (i.e., remove a small piece of skin) for study when the diagnosis is unclear.

Psoriasis isn't curable. Treatment of mild-to-moderate psoriasis is aimed at controlling symptoms by using topical creams, ointments, shampoos, and lotions. These help reduce inflammation, scaling, and itching.

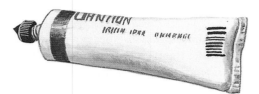

Other treatments may include immunosuppressant drugs such as methotrexate and isotretinoin, antihistamines, and antibiotics.

Take time to have good skin hygiene. Oatmeal baths to loosen scales can improve the appearance of your skin and make topical medicines work better.

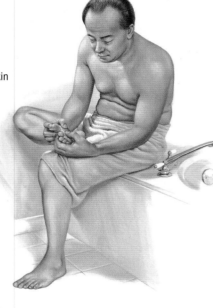

Moderate exposure to sunlight may help your rash, but ask your doctor first before you use exposure to sunlight as a treatment.

How Is Psoriasis Treated?

Psoriasis is treatable but not curable. A doctor who treats skin problems (dermatologist) may be involved in care. Avoiding things that trigger psoriasis and using prescribed medications can control and lessen symptoms. General measures include good skin hygiene, avoiding skin injury and dryness, exposing skin to moderate sunlight, and oatmeal baths. Treatment of mild to moderate psoriasis includes topical creams, lotions, shampoos, and ointments containing coal tar. These will reduce inflammation (redness), scaling, and itching. Steroids and other antiinflammatory drugs applied to skin (topical) are for mild to moderate cases and as combination therapy for more severe cases. Other treatments include salicylic acid in mineral oil (removes plaques), PUVA (psoralen and exposure to ultraviolet light A [UVA]), immunosuppressant drugs (e.g., methotrexate, isotretinoin), antihistamines (for itching), and antibiotics (for secondary bacterial infections).

DOs and DON'Ts in Managing Psoriasis:

✔ **DO** take medicines as prescribed by your doctor.
✔ **DO** tell your doctor about all of your medicines, including over-the-counter.
✔ **DO** expose your skin to some sunlight.
✔ **DO** maintain good skin hygiene.
✔ **DO** keep follow-up doctor appointments.
✔ **DO** watch your skin for healing and for bacterial infections. Redness around skin lesions, pus, pain or swelling of lesions or lymph glands, and fever are signs.
✔ **DO** avoid skin injuries and dry skin. These can trigger outbreaks.
✔ **DO** call your doctor if signs of infection appear, lesions become worse, or new lesions start even with therapy.
✔ **DO** call your doctor if you see pustules on the skin, especially with fever, fatigue, muscle aches, or joint pain or swelling.

⊘ **DON'T** stop your medicine or change the dose without asking your doctor.
⊘ **DON'T** exceed recommended medicine doses.
⊘ **DON'T** use over-the-counter topical steroids on the face or genitals without checking with your doctor.
⊘ **DON'T** stop steroids or immunosuppressants suddenly, to avoid rebound worsening of psoriasis.

FOR MORE INFORMATION

Contact the following sources:

• American Academy of Dermatology
Tel: (866) 503-SKIN (503-7546)
Website: http://www.aad.org

• National Psoriasis Foundation
Tel: (503) 244-7404, (800) 723-9166
Website: http://www.psoriasis.org

FROM THE DESK OF

NOTES

MANAGING YOUR RINGWORM

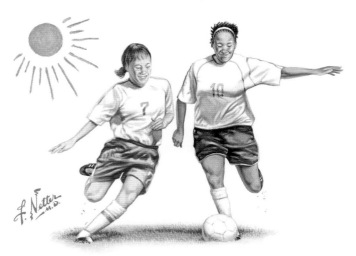

Ringworm (tinea corporis) is a very common skin infection caused by a fungus, not a worm. People of all ages can get ringworm, but it's seen more often in children. It usually occurs in hot, humid weather. Ringworm can be passed to other people.

Ringworm can occur anywhere on the body. The first symptom is usually itching. The skin shows ring-shaped, raised, red-to-brown patches.

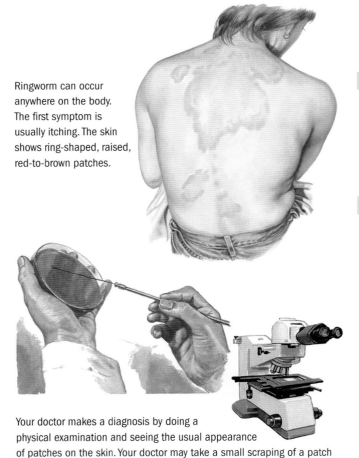

Your doctor makes a diagnosis by doing a physical examination and seeing the usual appearance of patches on the skin. Your doctor may take a small scraping of a patch for study with a microscope, because the fungus that causes the infection is so small that it can be seen only with a microscope.

What Is Ringworm?

Ringworm is a general name for a very common skin infection. The name ringworm comes from the appearance (ring-shaped or oval patches), not the cause, of the infection. The cause is not a worm at all but is actually a fungus. These fungal infections are named according to where they occur, such as ringworm of the body (tinea corporis), ringworm of the scalp (tinea capitis), athlete's foot (tinea pedis, ringworm of the feet), and jock itch (tinea cruris, ringworm of the groin).

People of all ages can get ringworm, but it's seen more often in children, diabetics and, athletes. Ringworm commonly occurs during hot, humid weather.

What Causes Ringworm?

Fungi that cause ringworm are very small and can be seen only with a microscope. They are passed among other people or animals. They can also be found in towels, carpet, bedding, showers, and baths.

What Are the Symptoms of Ringworm?

The most common symptom is itching. Ringworm on the body or face starts as slightly raised, ring-shaped or oval, red-to-brown, round, itchy patches on the skin. Sometimes, scaling or flaking of the skin occurs.

How Is Ringworm Diagnosed?

The doctor makes a diagnosis by doing a physical examination and seeing the typical appearance of patches on the skin. Sometimes, a small scraping of an affected area can be studied under a microscope to confirm the diagnosis.

Over-the-counter antifungal creams, ointments, and powders applied to the infected area usually clear up the infection. Treatment continues for 7 days after the rash is gone.

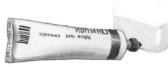

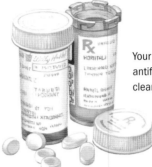

Your doctor may prescribe pills or stronger antifungal cream if your infection doesn't clear up with other treatments.

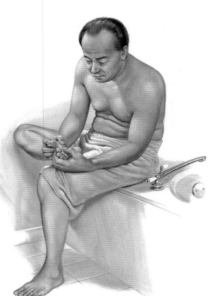

Keep your body clean and dry to prevent spreading the infection and getting another infection. Don't share towels with others, and when possible, don't use public showers, such as those at a gym.

How Is Ringworm Treated?

Over-the-counter medicines can treat mild cases. A small amount of antifungal cream, ointment, or powder is applied to affected areas twice daily, for 7 days after areas have healed. Calamine lotion twice daily can help reduce severe itching. Diphenhydramine (Benadryl®) and other antihistamines can also help itching.

The doctor can prescribe a stronger skin cream if over-the-counter medicines don't work. Treatment continues for 7 days after the infection seems to be over to prevent another infection.

For severe cases, when medicines applied to the skin don't work, medicine taken by mouth can be used.

DOs and DON'Ts in Managing Ringworm:

✔ **DO** use good general hygiene and keep the skin clean and dry.

✔ **DO** apply medicines as directed.

✔ **DO** bathe or shower daily. Gently wash affected areas with a cloth, dry off, then apply cream or ointment.

✔ **DO** wear clean, dry clothes. Cotton or other absorbent cloth is best. Avoid nylon.

✔ **DO** wear loose-fitting underwear and clothes.

✔ **DO** wash your hands after touching soil, plants, and animals, including pets (such as cats).

✔ **DO** avoid touching ringworm patches on other people or contaminated items, such as clothes, combs, showers, and pools.

✔ **DO** call your doctor if you get symptoms of another infection, such as fever, pus drainage, oozing, crusting, or swelling.

✔ **DO** call your doctor if you see skin changes, such as scarring or bleeding.

🚫 **DON'T** scratch or rub infected areas to avoid spreading the infection or causing another infection.

🚫 **DON'T** let anyone else come into contact with your clothing or other items (such as a hairbrush) that may have touched the infection.

FROM THE DESK OF

NOTES

FOR MORE INFORMATION

Contact the following sources:

• National Institute of Allergic and Infectious Diseases
Tel: (301) 496-5717
Website: http://www.niaid.nih.gov

• American Academy of Dermatology
Tel: (866) 503-SKIN (7546)
Website: http://www.aad.org

MANAGING YOUR
ROSACEA

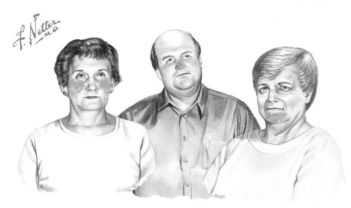

Rosacea is a skin disease that usually affects the middle of the face. Rosacea is most common during or after middle age and is often called adult acne. People of northern European descent and those with fair complexions are more likely to have rosacea.

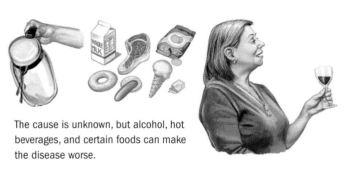

The cause is unknown, but alcohol, hot beverages, and certain foods can make the disease worse.

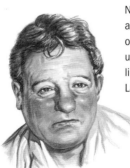

Nose, cheeks, and forehead skin is affected. Redness, swelling, and pimples or pustules appear. Small blood vessels under the skin can get bigger. They look like thin red lines. Skin can become oily. Larger bumps on the nose may occur.

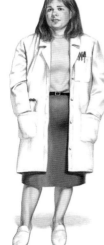
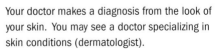

Your doctor makes a diagnosis from the look of your skin. You may see a doctor specializing in skin conditions (dermatologist).

What Is Rosacea?

Rosacea is a skin disease that usually affects the middle of the face. Women are more likely to show symptoms on the chin and cheeks, whereas in men the nose is commonly involved. Rosacea is most common during or after middle age and is often called adult acne. People of northern European descent and those with fair complexions are more likely to have rosacea. It's treatable but usually not curable.

What Causes Rosacea?

The cause is unknown. Alcohol, hot beverages, and certain foods do not cause it but can make it worse.

What Are the Symptoms of Rosacea?

The skin of the nose, cheeks, chin, and forehead is affected. Redness, swelling, and pimples or pustules appear on the skin. Small blood vessels under the skin can get bigger and noticeable. They look like thin red lines on the face or nose. Skin can become oily. In more severe cases, larger bumps on the nose occur. Rarely, eyes and eyelids are affected, with swelling, redness, dry eyes, and burning.

Rosacea has three stages, each with different symptoms. Early symptoms include flushing or redness that comes and goes. Spicy food, sunlight, or alcohol can trigger these. Middle stage symptoms are the same but last longer. Skin may burn or sting, and eyes feel itchy or gritty. In the advanced stage, redness becomes permanent, small and sometimes painful pimples may appear, skin may burn or sting, eyes may be watery and irritated, and the nose can become red and swollen.

Because their skin looks similar to that of chronic alcohol abusers, people with rosacea are often thought of as being closet alcoholics. This isn't true.

How Is Rosacea Diagnosed?

The doctor makes a diagnosis from the physical examination.

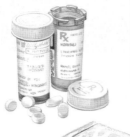

Mild cases can sometimes be treated with a topical antibiotic cream (metronidazole, clindamycin, erythromycin) or oral antibiotics. Rosacea often returns and may need a regular smaller dose of medicine to control it. Early treatment may slow disease progress.

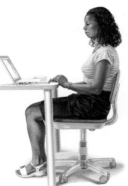

Take an active role in your treatment, because outbreaks can be triggered by something you ate, drank, or used on your face. Keep a diary of your activities, foods eaten, and personal care items used when a flare-up occurs to see whether you can find a pattern.

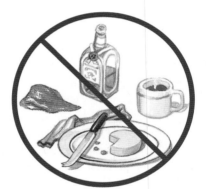

Don't eat foods that make rosacea worse. These may include hot liquids and spicy foods, chocolates, cheeses, nuts, iodized salt, and seafood. Don't drink alcohol.

Wash your face twice a day with a washcloth and mild soap.

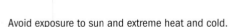

Avoid exposure to sun and extreme heat and cold.

How Is Rosacea Treated?

Mild cases can sometimes be treated with a topical antibiotic cream (metronidazole, clindamycin, erythromycin) or antibiotics taken by mouth. Rosacea often returns and may need a smaller dose of medicine taken regularly to control symptoms. Early treatment may slow disease progress. In more severe cases, a combination of medicines may be needed. Severe nose swelling in rare cases needs surgery, but laser treatment may help. A laser is sometimes used for large veins and redness. The doctor will usually suggest seeing a dermatologist (specialist in skin diseases).

DOs and DON'Ts in Managing Rosacea:

✔ **DO** wash your face twice a day with a washcloth and mild soap.

✔ **DO** follow your doctor's instructions about soaps, sunscreens, and medicines. Early treatment may prevent some long-term effects.

✔ **DO** keep a diary of activities performed, kinds of foods eaten, and personal care items used when a flare-up occurs to see whether you can find a pattern. For example, if your skin becomes irritated and red when you eat chili peppers, they probably trigger symptoms.

✔ **DO** change to milder soap or skin creams that don't contain perfumes, alcohol, or harsh additives, to minimize skin irritation.

✔ **DO** call your doctor if you have symptoms involving your eyes or eyelids.

✔ **DO** call your doctor if treatment isn't helping after 3 or 4 weeks.

⊘ **DON'T** eat foods that make rosacea worse. These may include hot liquids and spicy foods, chocolates, cheeses, nuts, iodized salt, and seafood.

⊘ **DON'T** drink alcohol.

⊘ **DON'T** get exposed to sun without sunscreen and avoid extreme heat and cold.

FROM THE DESK OF

NOTES

FOR MORE INFORMATION

Contact the following sources:

- National Rosacea Society
  Tel: (888) NO-BLUSH (662-5874)
  Website: http://www.rosacea.org
- American Academy of Dermatology
  Tel: (847) 330-0230, (866) 503-7546
  Website: http://aad.org

MANAGING
SCABIES

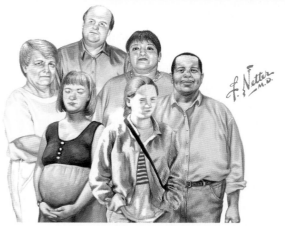

Scabies is a very common skin infection that causes an extremely itchy rash. Anyone can catch scabies, but it occurs much more in young children. It doesn't depend on your hygiene.

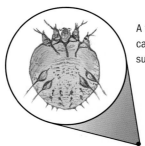

A tiny mite, about the size of a pin head, causes scabies. Mites burrow into the surface of the skin, but not very far.

Severe itching, especially at night, is common. Tiny pimples, tiny blisters, or bumps that break easily when scratched and tiny, very itchy burrows on the skin are symptoms.

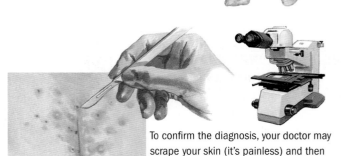

To confirm the diagnosis, your doctor may scrape your skin (it's painless) and then use a microscope to look for the mites in the skin sample.

What Is Scabies?

Scabies is a very common skin infection that causes an extremely itchy rash. It's not dangerous and doesn't usually lead to lasting damage, but excessive scratching can result in a skin bacterial infection. Anyone can catch scabies, but it occurs much more in young children. Children often get scabies from their classmates and bring the infection home and spread it to their family. It's also common in people who live together, such as those in nursing homes.

What Causes Scabies?

The cause is a tiny mite that burrows into the skin. The mite is only slightly larger than the head of a pin and doesn't burrow very far. The infection spreads easily from person to person by skin-to-skin contact, such as sharing a bed with an infected person. It doesn't depend on personal cleanliness.

What Are the Symptoms of Scabies?

Severe itching, especially at night, is common. Tiny pimples, tiny blisters, or bumps that break easily when scratched and tiny, very itchy burrows on the skin are manifestations of scabies. Blisters usually form a thin line between fingers and on skin folds of the wrist, elbows, knees, breasts, shoulder blades, or penis. Children and babies often have the rash on the head, neck, face, palms (hands), and soles (feet).

Scratching can cause hives, skin scaling, sores, blisters, and small blisters around the nose and mouth.

How Is Scabies Diagnosed?

The doctor makes the diagnosis by looking closely at the skin. No other tests are generally needed. The doctor may painlessly scrape the skin to get a sample containing mites and put it on a slide for study with a microscope.

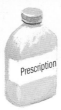

The most common treatment is to apply a prescription lotion on the skin which kills the mites. Lotions must be put on the whole body below the face and be left on for a specific time before being washed off.

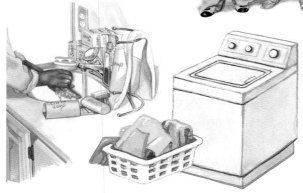

All people who were in close contact should be treated at the same time.

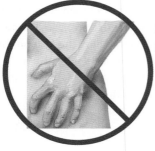

Wash your hands often to avoid spreading the mites. Wash all clothes, bedding, and toys with hot, soapy water.

Don't scratch, to avoid getting a bacterial infection.

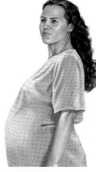

Tell your doctor if you're pregnant or if you have a young child. Some medicines may not be safe for your child.

FROM THE DESK OF

NOTES

How Is Scabies Treated?

The standard treatment is a topical prescription lotion, such as permethrin or lindane, which kills the mites. These lotions are put on the whole body, left on for a specific time, and then washed off. These medicines are usually safe, but caution is especially important with infants younger than 2 years and with pregnant women. In these situations permethrin is preferred over lindane. All close family contacts should be treated at the same time.

All clothes, bedding, and toys must be washed with hot, soapy water.

Severe itching may need antihistamines or topical salves and corticosteroids. Elderly people and those with weak immune (infection-fighting) systems can get more serious infections and need stronger treatment. In resistant cases an oral medication (ivermectin) can be prescribed by your doctor.

DOs and DON'Ts in Managing Scabies:

✔ **DO** use medications or lotions as instructed by your doctor.

✔ **DO** wash all clothing, bedding, and towels that you've used in the past 2 days in hot water. Keep your bedding and clothing separate.

✔ **DO** put items that can't be washed into plastic bags, and keep them there for 14 days to kill the mites.

✔ **DO** clean chairs, mattresses, and other items with a special solution (called antiseptic scabicide) that kills mites.

✔ **DO** use good personal hygiene.

✔ **DO** wash your hands often.

✔ **DO** call your doctor if you show redness, pus, swelling, or pain after treatment.

✔ **DO** call your doctor if itching or pain lasts for 1 to 2 weeks after treatment.

⊘ **DON'T** share bedding.

⊘ **DON'T** wash off prescribed cream before 8 to 12 hours.

⊘ **DON'T** use home remedies such as detergents, scrubbing, or kerosene.

⊘ **DON'T** use steroid creams unless your doctor prescribes them.

FOR MORE INFORMATION

Contact the following sources:

• Centers for Disease Control and Prevention
Tel: (800) 311-3435
Website: http://www.cdc.gov

• American Academy of Dermatology
Tel: (866) 503-7546
Website: http://www.aad.org

CARING FOR YOUR CHILD WITH
SCARLET FEVER

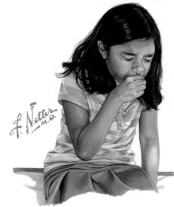

Scarlet fever is a contagious infection in children that is caused by bacteria. It starts as a reaction to certain kinds of strep infections.

Swollen glands

Coated tongue

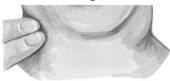

The first symptoms will usually be a sore throat, fever, swollen glands in the neck, loss of appetite, headache, and coughing. The tongue, tonsils, and the back of the throat may have a whitish coating. After 4 to 5 days, the tongue becomes red (strawberry or raspberry tongue).

A bright red rash develops a few days after the sore throat. It looks like sunburn on the face and neck and then moves down the body.

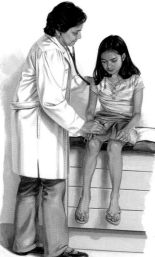

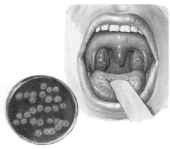

Bacterial culture

The doctor will examine your child and take a small scraping from the throat and send it for culture, to see which bacteria grow.

What Is Scarlet Fever?

Scarlet fever is a common illness in children. It starts as a bacterial infection in the throat. A reaction to a toxin (poison) produced by a specific kind of bacteria causes a bright red rash. Not everyone who has this type of infection will have scarlet fever.

What Causes Scarlet Fever?

The kind of bacteria named *Streptococcus* (strep) is the cause. The infection is contagious and spread by direct contact, from the day the sore throat starts until 24 to 48 hours after starting antibiotics.

What Are the Symptoms of Scarlet Fever?

First symptoms are usually a bad sore throat, fever (higher than 101° F), swollen glands in the neck, cough, headaches, and loss of appetite. Tonsils and the back of the throat may have a whitish coating or look red and swollen. The tongue may be coated.

A bright red rash is the most striking symptom. It usually starts several days after the sore throat, first on the neck and face and then the chest and back. The tongue becomes red (strawberry or raspberry tongue). Areas with the rash turn white when they're pressed on. By the sixth day, the rash starts to fade and the skin begins to peel. The skin peeling may last 1 to 2 weeks before returning to normal.

How Is Scarlet Fever Diagnosed?

The doctor will make a diagnosis from the medical history and physical examination. A small scraping from the child's throat will be taken and sent for culture, to show which bacteria are in the throat.

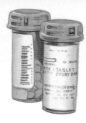

Your child will need to take antibiotics, such as penicillin or erythromycin. Be sure that your child takes all the medicine, for as long as your doctor prescribes.

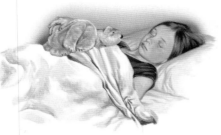

Your child should get plenty of rest and be kept away from others to prevent spreading the infection.

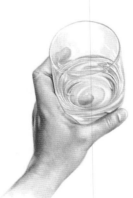

Have your child drink plenty of fluids to keep hydrated.

Wash your hands often while caring for your sick child. Keep drinking glasses and eating utensils separate, and wash them in very hot soapy water.

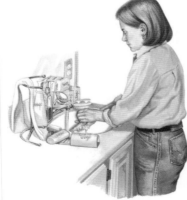

How Is Scarlet Fever Treated?

Treatment includes antibiotics, such as penicillin or erythromycin, and bed rest. Children should be kept away from others to prevent disease spread. No special diet is needed, but fluid intake should be increased. Using a cool mist vaporizer and gargling with warm salt water can help the sore throat.

DOs and DON'Ts in Managing Scarlet Fever:

✔ **DO** give the medicine on schedule and for as many days as your doctor directs.

✔ **DO** make your child comfortable. Give soft foods and liquids and make sure your child drinks plenty of fluids. Use a humidifier to add moisture to the air.

✔ **DO** keep your child away from other family members from the day he or she develops a sore throat until 2 days after antibiotics are started. Your child can usually return to school within 2 weeks.

✔ **DO** keep drinking glasses and eating utensils separate, and wash them in very hot soapy water.

✔ **DO** wash your own hands often.

✔ **DO** trim your child's fingernails to prevent scratches if the rash itches.

✔ **DO** call your child's doctor if fever (temperature higher than 101° F) returns after it went away for a few days.

✔ **DO** call your child's doctor if nausea or vomiting, severe headache or earache, or chest pain and a cough that produces thick sputum develop.

✔ **DO** call your child's doctor if areas of peeling skin show signs of infection.

⊘ **DON'T** let your sick child play with other children.

⊘ **DON'T** let your sick child skip doses or stop antibiotics before they are finished.

⊘ **DON'T** send your child to school until the infection is over.

FOR MORE INFORMATION

Contact the following sources:

• National Institute of Allergy and Infectious Diseases
Tel: (301) 496-5717
Website: http://www3.niaid.nih.gov

• The American Academy of Pediatrics
Tel: (847) 434-4000
Website: http://www.aap.org

• National Institute of Child Health and Human Development
Tel: (800) 370-2943, (301) 496-5133
Website: http://www.nichd.nih.gov

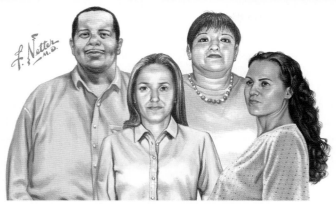

Scleroderma is a disorder that causes the body to make too much collagen. Women are affected more often than men, usually starting at age 30 to 50. Collagen is the main protein in connective tissue, and too much collagen causes skin and organs to get thick and stiff. The cause isn't known, but scleroderma is an autoimmune disorder.

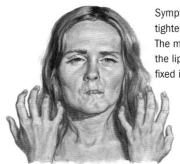

Symptoms include thickening and tightening of facial skin, which gets rigid. The mouth looks small and constricted, the lips thin. Fingers become partly fixed in a flexed position.

Complications of scleroderma

Kidney failure

Heart failure

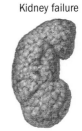
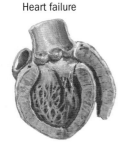

Organs can be affected, slowly losing function as they become thick and stiff.

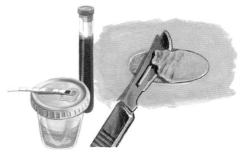

For diagnosis, your doctor will take a medical history and examine you and may order blood and urine tests, ECG, x-rays, and biopsy.

What Is Scleroderma?

Scleroderma is a disorder that causes the body to make too much collagen, the result being inflammation (swelling) and stiffness. Collagen is the main protein in connective tissue, which supports the organs and skin. Too much collagen causes skin and organs to get thick and stiff. Scleroderma can affect the heart, esophagus (tube connecting the mouth and stomach), kidneys, lungs, blood vessels, and skin.

Scleroderma affects women four times more often than men, usually starting at age 30 to 50.

What Causes Scleroderma?

The cause is unknown, but scleroderma is an autoimmune disorder. In autoimmune disorders, the body's own immune system mistakenly attacks normal parts of the body and causes disease.

What Are the Symptoms of Scleroderma?

People can have many symptoms. Mild to severe symptoms depend on the organs affected. Most common symptoms are dry eyes and mouth, joint stiffness and pain, heartburn, muscle pain, numbness, poor circulation, poor wound healing, swallowing problems, weakness, and weight loss. Skin becomes thick, hard, and tight and loses flexibility. The face looks mask-like, with thin lips and furrowing around the mouth. Fingers become thick, stiff, painful, and less moveable.

Complications include kidney failure (most common cause of death), heart failure, abnormal heart rhythms, high blood pressure, poor lung function, heartburn, and constipation.

How Is Scleroderma Diagnosed?

The doctor will take a medical history, do an examination, order blood and urine tests, do electrocardiography (ECG), and x-rays. The ECG measures the heart's electrical activity. A small piece of skin may be taken and looked at with a microscope. Since scleroderma affects many organs, your primary care doctor may refer you to a rheumatologist (specialist of muscle joint diseases), a nephrologist (kidney specialist), a dermatologist (skin specialist), a cardiologist (heart specialist), a pulmonologist (lung specialist), or a gastroenterologist (specialist of digestive tract).

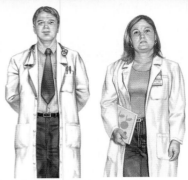

No cure exists, but your medical team can help you control symptoms, reduce the severity of the illness, treat and prevent complications, and help you stay in a healthy state of mind.

Don't smoke!

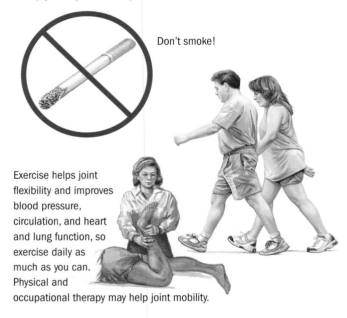

Exercise helps joint flexibility and improves blood pressure, circulation, and heart and lung function, so exercise daily as much as you can. Physical and occupational therapy may help joint mobility.

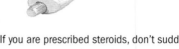
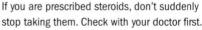

Take care of your skin. Use sunscreen and moisturizers, and avoid drying soaps, getting cut or burned, and cold weather.

SPF 30

If you are prescribed steroids, don't suddenly stop taking them. Check with your doctor first.

How Is Scleroderma Treated?

Scleroderma isn't curable. Treatment is aimed at controlling symptoms, relieving symptoms, and treating or preventing complications. Treatment consists of general measures and medicines. General measures include medications for heartburn or gastroesophageal reflux; avoiding smoking, alcohol, and caffeine; and not eating close to bedtime or lying down. For joint pain and stiffness, use mild heat. Avoid very cold temperatures and skin injuries and burns such as from hot water. Psychological counseling and biofeedback may help depression. Physical therapy and occupational therapy improve joint mobility.

Helpful medicines include steroids, over-the-counter antacids or prescription drugs (gastroesophageal reflux), blood pressure drugs, aspirin or anti-inflammatory drugs (arthritis), and immunomodulators (which help the immune system). Lotions, moisturizers, and bath oils soften the skin.

DOs and DON'Ts in Managing Scleroderma:

✔ **DO** raise the head of your bed with blocks to prevent acid reflux and heartburn while sleeping. Eat small meals. Avoid alcohol, tobacco, caffeine, and fatty and spicy foods.
✔ **DO** wear warm clothing. Avoid cold weather.
✔ **DO** use sunscreen, and avoid skin-drying hot baths or showers and harsh soaps.
✔ **DO** exercise regularly.
✔ **DO** stop smoking.
✔ **DO** call your doctor if you have worse or new symptoms.

⊘ **DON'T** stop taking your medicine or change your dosage because you feel better unless your doctor says to.
⊘ **DON'T** smoke.
⊘ **DON'T** stop steroids suddenly.

FROM THE DESK OF

NOTES

FOR MORE INFORMATION
Contact the following sources:
• Scleroderma Foundation
  Tel: (877) 722-4673
  Website: http://www.scleroderma.org
• American Academy of Dermatology
  Phone: (866) 503-7546
  Website: http://www.aad.org

MANAGING YOUR
SHINGLES

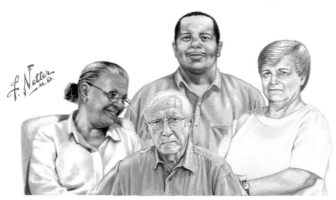

Herpes zoster, or shingles, is caused by the same virus that causes chickenpox. After chickenpox, the virus stays inactive and can become active again if the immune system weakens. People older than 50 are more prone to shingles.

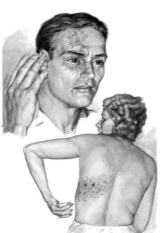

The virus lives in nerves near your spine. Activated virus moves along the nerves to the skin and causes a rash in groups or bands at nerve endings. The rash can occur anywhere. Blisters usually go away in a few weeks. Severe pain (called postherpetic neuralgia) can last more than 30 days.

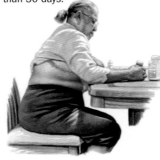

Your doctor will diagnose shingles by examining your skin. Blood tests may be done, and blister fluid may be studied if the diagnosis is unclear.

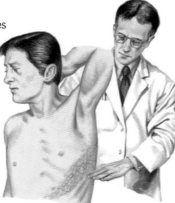

What Is Shingles?

Herpes zoster, also called shingles, is an uncomfortable and often very painful outbreak of skin blisters and sores. One of every 10 people who had chickenpox as children can have shingles later.

There isn't any cure, but some medicines can help relieve symptoms and prevent complications. Also, a vaccine (Zostavax) is now available for prevention in people 60 years and older.

What Causes Shingles?

The cause is varicella-zoster virus, the same virus that causes chickenpox. After people have chickenpox, the virus usually stays inactive. But if antibodies to this virus get low decades later, the virus can become active and cause shingles.

People who have not been vaccinated for chickenpox can catch it from someone with active shingles.

What Are the Symptoms of Shingles?

The virus lives in nerves near the spine. Activated virus travels along the nerves to the skin. It then causes a rash on the skin in groups or bands at the nerve endings. The rash usually stays as a band going across part of the body on one side. The rash can occur anywhere.

Early vague symptoms are mild itching, tingling, pain, headache, fever, or flulike syndrome. The rash that follows consists of many small, fluid-filled blisters in groups that dry, scab over, and heal (like chickenpox) in a few weeks. Healing is usually complete. Scars may persist in the area of the blisters.

The amount of pain and discomfort of shingles varies from person to person.

A significant number of people, especially those older than 50, can have pain (called postherpetic neuralgia) for more than 30 days. It can be very severe and interfere with daily activity.

People who scratch the rash can also get a bacterial infection.

Shingles on the face can involve the eyes, which is serious and can cause scarring and blindness.

How Is Shingles Diagnosed?

The doctor will diagnose shingles by examining the skin. Blood tests are rarely needed. Blister fluid may be studied if the diagnosis is unclear.

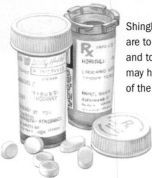

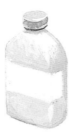

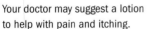

Shingles has no cure, so the goals of treatment are to reduce the pain and duration of infection and to prevent complications. Antiviral drugs may help but must be given within 2 or 3 days of the start of symptoms.

Your doctor may suggest a lotion to help with pain and itching.

Avoid contact with anyone who never had chickenpox or didn't get immunized, pregnant women, children, or people with weak immune systems such as those with cancer or AIDS.

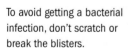

To avoid getting a bacterial infection, don't scratch or break the blisters.

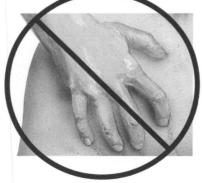

How Is Shingles Treated?

The main goals are to shorten the infection, reduce discomfort, and prevent complications. Antiviral medicine, started early (within 2 or 3 days), can help the rash and pain. These drugs include acyclovir, valacyclovir, and famciclovir. Other drugs and lotions can help with pain and itching.

DOs and DON'Ts in Managing Shingles:

✔ **DO** tell your doctor about your medical problems and prescriptions and over-the-counter medicines.

✔ **DO** tell your doctor if you're pregnant or breast-feeding.

✔ **DO** keep blisters clean. Don't bandage the blisters.

✔ **DO** avoid anyone who never had chickenpox or didn't get immunized, pregnant women, or people with cancer.

✔ **DO** get medical care as soon as you think that you may have shingles.

✔ **DO** call your doctor if the rash is on your face or nose, the pain doesn't get better after the rash heals, or the rash looks infected.

⊘ **DON'T** stop taking your medicine or change your dose because you feel better unless your doctor tells you.

⊘ **DON'T** shave the area with the rash.

⊘ **DON'T** scratch, contaminate, or break the blisters.

FROM THE DESK OF

NOTES

FOR MORE INFORMATION

Contact the following source:

• American Academy of Dermatology
Tel: (866) 503-SKIN (7546)
Website: http://www.aad.org

MANAGING YOUR
SQUAMOUS CELL CARCINOMA

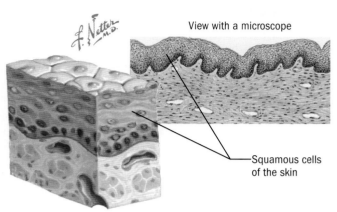

View with a microscope

Squamous cells of the skin

Squamous cells are in the part of the skin called the epidermis. These cells, near the skin surface, are often exposed to UV sunlight. They can become abnormal and grow into a common skin cancer called squamous cell carcinoma.

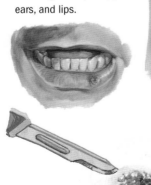

Long-term sun exposure is the main cause of squamous cell carcinoma. Other risk factors are radiation exposure and having light-colored skin, blue or green eyes, and blond or red hair.

Squamous cell carcinoma usually starts as a red crusty patch and may grow to look like a wart or sore. It can grow anywhere, including hands, scalp, ears, and lips.

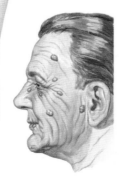

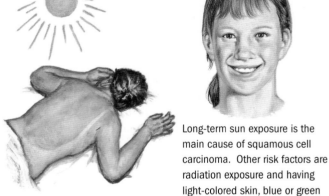

Your doctor will examine your skin, but a biopsy is needed for diagnosis. For a biopsy, a tiny piece of skin is shaved off and sent to a laboratory for study.

What Is Squamous Cell Carcinoma?

Squamous cells form the part of the skin called the epidermis. Cutaneous squamous cell carcinoma is a common kind of skin cancer that involves these cells. It occurs most often in people older than age 50.

What Causes Squamous Cell Carcinoma?

The cause is usually longtime sun exposure. Exposure to many x-rays and having light-colored skin, blue or green eyes, and blond or red hair can also give people greater risks of having this cancer.

What Are the Symptoms of Squamous Cell Carcinoma?

This cancer usually starts as a reddish skin patch with a crusty surface. It may grow and look like a wart or sore. It can grow anywhere, including hands, scalp, ears, and lips. It can form a sore that bleeds on and off. A sore that doesn't heal may mean squamous cell carcinoma.

How Is Squamous Cell Carcinoma Diagnosed?

The doctor will examine the skin, but a skin biopsy is needed for diagnosis. For a biopsy, a tiny piece of skin is shaved off and sent to a laboratory for study. A dermatologist (specialist in skin diseases) may do this.

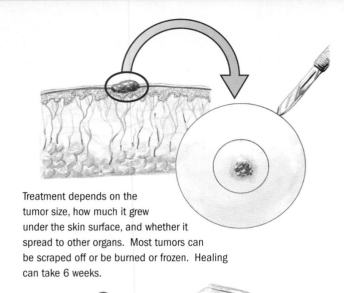

Treatment depends on the tumor size, how much it grew under the skin surface, and whether it spread to other organs. Most tumors can be scraped off or be burned or frozen. Healing can take 6 weeks.

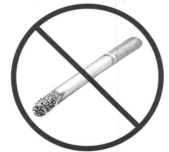

Wear protective clothing and sunscreens with high SPF values. Use a lot of sunscreen. Don't forget your face, backs of your hands, and ears. Avoid too much sun, especially the strongest midday sun—10 AM to 2 PM.

Watch for changes in the look, color, size, or texture of a lesion on your skin. Call your doctor if you see these changes.

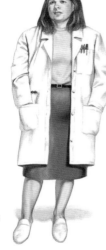

Don't smoke. Cigarette, cigar, and pipe smoking can cause squamous cell carcinoma of the lips and mouth.

How Is Squamous Cell Carcinoma Treated?

Squamous cell carcinoma can most often be cured by taking off the cancer. The way to do this depends on the size of the tumor growing below the skin surface.

Small tumors can be burned with an electric needle and scraped out. Some can be removed by freezing. These procedures are usually done in the doctor's office.

Larger tumors need to be cut out. The doctor may use a special type of surgery called Mohs micrographic surgery. This operation involves slowly removing layers of skin until the whole cancer is gone. The wound may take up to 6 weeks to heal. The doctor must be told about any signs of infection during this time.

Rarely, the tumor spreads. If it has spread to other areas, a doctor specializing in treating cancer can treat this tumor with radiation or cancer drugs.

Squamous cell carcinoma can come back, so regular follow-up appointments are a must to find new squamous cell carcinomas early.

DOs and DON'Ts in Managing Squamous Cell Carcinoma:

✔ **DO** avoid too much sun, especially the strongest sun during the middle of the day (between 10 AM and 2 PM).

✔ **DO** wear sunscreens with high sun protection factors and protective clothing when you're in the sun.

✔ **DO** use a lot of sunscreen. Don't forget your face, the backs of your hands, and your ears.

✔ **DO** stay out of tanning parlors.

✔ **DO** watch for changes in the look, color, size, or texture of a lesion on your skin. Call your doctor if you see these changes. Also call if you have pain, inflammation, bleeding, or itching of a skin lesion.

✔ **DO** call your doctor if you see new growth in the area of the skin where the cancer was removed.

🚫 **DON'T** smoke. Cigarette, cigar, and pipe smoking can cause squamous cell carcinoma of the lips and mouth.

🚫 **DON'T** miss follow-up doctor appointments for early detection of possible cancers.

FROM THE DESK OF

NOTES

FOR MORE INFORMATION

Contact the following source:

• American Cancer Society
Tel: (800) ACS-2345 (227-2345)
Website: http://www.cancer.org

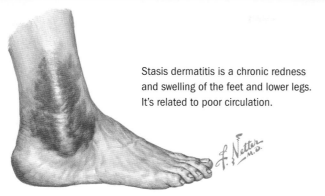

Stasis dermatitis is a chronic redness and swelling of the feet and lower legs. It's related to poor circulation.

What Is Stasis Dermatitis?

Stasis dermatitis is chronic inflammation (redness, swelling) and irritation of the skin, usually in the lower legs. It's related to poor circulation of blood and lymphatic fluids, with fluids moving slowly up from the feet to the heart. It's very common, affecting 50% of Americans with certain risk factors. It usually occurs in middle-aged and elderly people.

What Causes Stasis Dermatitis?

Contributing factors include prolonged standing, varicose veins, inactivity, obesity, and congestive heart failure. These factors lead to leg swelling (edema).

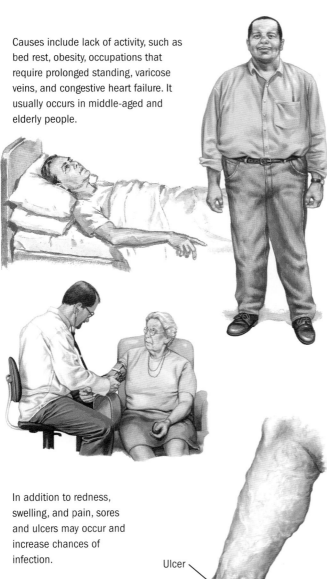

Causes include lack of activity, such as bed rest, obesity, occupations that require prolonged standing, varicose veins, and congestive heart failure. It usually occurs in middle-aged and elderly people.

What Are the Symptoms of Stasis Dermatitis?

Symptoms include reddened, swollen feet and lower legs and often shiny skin and painful feet. Small sores or ulcers may appear on feet or lower legs and may not heal well. Swelling and skin breakdown lead to infection, which may be one ulcer or become severe and involve deeper tissues (muscle or bone). Severe pain and swelling limit activity, as walking becomes more painful. This decreased movement makes the condition even worse.

How Is Stasis Dermatitis Diagnosed?

The doctor will make a diagnosis by examining the feet and legs. If the doctor suspects heart failure or other disorders, more tests will be done.

How Is Stasis Dermatitis Treated?

Fluid trapped in feet and lower legs must be reduced. If the leg swelling is severe, mechanical devices such as hospital-grade support hose or leg compression pumps move fluid from legs if used correctly. Diuretics (water pills) may also help some, but not all, people, and can cause dehydration and low potassium levels.

Steroid and zinc oxide creams and paste may be used for small ulcers. Antibiotics may be prescribed for skin infection. In severe cases, a special wrap filled with gelatin and containing zinc (called Unna's boot) may protect and heal skin and stop more swelling.

In addition to redness, swelling, and pain, sores and ulcers may occur and increase chances of infection.

Ulcer

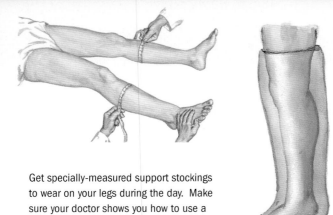

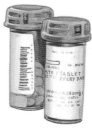

Get specially-measured support stockings to wear on your legs during the day. Make sure your doctor shows you how to use a compression pump if you need one.

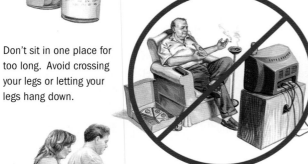

Take medicines such as diuretics (to remove fluids) and antibiotics (for infections) exactly as prescribed.

Don't sit in one place for too long. Avoid crossing your legs or letting your legs hang down.

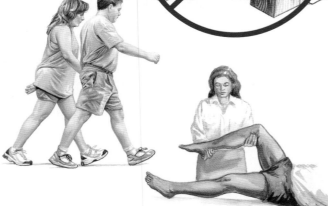

If your doctor approves, exercise daily. Walking can improve circulation. If walking is too hard, physical therapy may help your strength and range of motion.

DOs and DON'Ts in Managing Stasis Dermatitis:

✔ **DO** take diuretics exactly as prescribed.

✔ **DO** use prescribed mechanical devices such as support hose or compression pumps every day. The hose should be ordered specifically for you, with your exact leg measurements. Put the hose on in the morning after bandaging ulcers or sores. Remove them at night for sleeping.

✔ **DO** learn to use your compression pump properly, for several sessions each day.

✔ **DO** eat a low-fat, low-cholesterol diet and avoid too much salt. Ask your doctor about the amount of salt you may have. Usually, more than 4 grams of sodium will increase foot swelling.

✔ **DO** ask your doctor about drinking water. You may need less than the usual 8 glasses daily.

✔ **DO** exercise daily. Mild to moderate exercise (walking) can improve circulation. If walking is too hard for you, physical therapy may improve strength and range of motion. Raising your legs when you sit or lie down may help.

✔ **DO** call your doctor if you notice new sores, ulcers, or redness in your feet or legs.

✔ **DO** call your doctor if you have more leg swelling even after using support hose or compression pumps.

✔ **DO** call your doctor if you have fever, chills, or shortness of breath.

⊘ **DON'T** miss blood tests for potassium and kidney function tests.

⊘ **DON'T** exercise without your doctor's OK.

⊘ **DON'T** sit for long periods with your legs crossed or your feet hanging down.

FROM THE DESK OF

NOTES

FOR MORE INFORMATION

Contact the following sources:

• American Heart Association
  Tel: (800) 242-8721
  Website: http://www.americanheart.org

• American Academy of Dermatology
  Tel: (866) 503-SKIN (503-7546)
  Website: http://www.aad.org

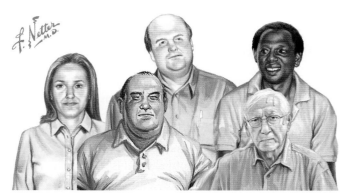

Stevens-Johnson syndrome is a very serious allergic skin disorder that requires emergency care. More men than women get it.

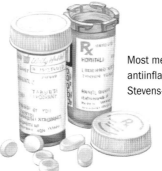

Most medicines, including antibiotics and antiinflammatory drugs, can cause Stevens-Johnson syndrome.

Flulike symptoms with fever are usually the first signs of the syndrome.

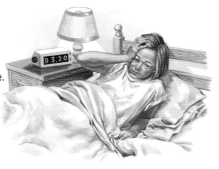

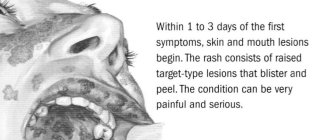

Within 1 to 3 days of the first symptoms, skin and mouth lesions begin. The rash consists of raised target-type lesions that blister and peel. The condition can be very painful and serious.

What Is Stevens-Johnson Syndrome?

Stevens-Johnson syndrome is an acute allergic inflammatory skin disease. It isn't very common and cannot be caught. More men than women get it. Most cases have a strong relation to exposure to specific medicines, starting 1 to 3 weeks after the first drug exposure. The disease can cause serious symptoms that need prompt treatment and maybe treatment in the intensive care unit of a hospital.

What Causes Stevens-Johnson Syndrome?

Stevens-Johnson syndrome is usually due to a reaction to a medicine. Most drugs can cause Stevens-Johnson syndrome, but the more common ones are sulfa antibiotics, nonsteroidal antiinflammatory drugs (NSAIDs), anticonvulsants, and allopurinol (used for gout). In rare cases, an infection (e.g., with bacteria or virus) or cancer may cause Stevens-Johnson syndrome. Sometimes the cause is unknown.

What Are the Symptoms of Stevens-Johnson Syndrome?

The syndrome begins with a high fever and flulike symptoms. After 1 to 3 days, skin lesions appear. The rash consists of raised target-type lesions, which look like blisters. The lesions will peel off and leave red, oozing skin. Mild to moderate skin tenderness and burning or itching of the eyes occur. People may have painful mouth lesions that make it hard to swallow and ulcers on membranes of the nose, eyes, and genital area. Mouth sores can last for months.

Other possible symptoms are sensitivity to light, anxiety, and painful urination. Fingernails may also be shed.

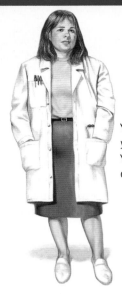

Your doctor will diagnose your condition from your medical history and a physical examination. You may need to be hospitalized in a specialized center such as a burn unit for intensive care.

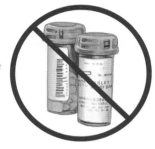

Any medicines thought to be causing the syndrome must be stopped right away.

You must be especially careful not to get an infection. Be sure that people treating you have washed their hands.

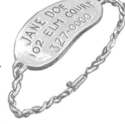

Wear a medical ID bracelet naming the medicine thought to cause the syndrome.

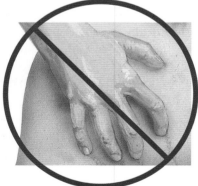

Don't scratch the rash!

FROM THE DESK OF

NOTES

How Is Stevens-Johnson Syndrome Diagnosed?

A doctor will diagnose Stevens-Johnson syndrome on the basis of a medical history of exposure to medicines and the physical examination.

How Is Stevens-Johnson Syndrome Treated?

Any medicine that may be the cause must be stopped immediately. If blistering and peeling are severe, a hospital stay may be needed. People are often placed in special burn units where damaged skin can get the best care. Topical ointments will be applied to the rash, and intravenous fluids will be given to prevent dehydration. Prevention of infection is the main concern. Medicated rinses can treat mouth lesions.

DOs and DON'Ts in Managing Stevens-Johnson Syndrome:

✔ **DO** wash hands carefully. Anyone caring for the lesions should do this to prevent infection.
✔ **DO** maintain good nutrition. A liquid diet may help if pain occurs with swallowing.
✔ **DO** drink enough fluids to prevent dehydration.
✔ **DO** wear a medical ID bracelet naming the medicine suspected of causing the syndrome.
✔ **DO** call your doctor if you get a high fever.
✔ **DO** call your doctor if you cannot drink enough fluids or have good nutrition because of mouth lesions.
✔ **DO** call your doctor if symptoms worsen.

⊘ **DON'T** scratch the lesions or peel the loose skin.
⊘ **DON'T** use the medicine suspected of causing the syndrome.

FOR MORE INFORMATION

Contact the following sources:

- National Institute of Arthritis and Musculoskeletal and Skin Diseases of the NIH
  Tel: (877) 226-4267
  Website: http://www.niams.nih.gov
- American Academy of Allergy, Asthma & Immunology
  Tel: (800) 822-2762
  Website: http://www.aaaai.org
- American Academy of Dermatology
  Tel: (866) 503-SKIN (7546)
  Website: http://www.aad.org

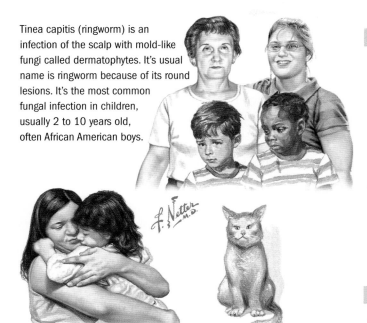

Tinea capitis (ringworm) is an infection of the scalp with mold-like fungi called dermatophytes. It's usual name is ringworm because of its round lesions. It's the most common fungal infection in children, usually 2 to 10 years old, often African American boys.

The cause is the common fungus named *Trichophyton*. People get it by direct contact with infected people or infected animals, especially cats and dogs.

Symptoms may be mild and first include redness and swelling of the scalp, followed by hair loss. Infected hairs become brittle and broken. Pus-filled blister-like lesions called kerions may occur.

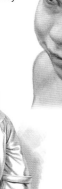

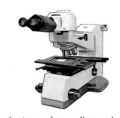

Your doctor makes a diagnosis by a skin examination. The doctor may take small samples of hair or infected skin with fungi for culture, to see whether fungi grow. A microscope is used to study them.

What Is Tinea Capitis?

Tinea capitis (ringworm) is an infection of the scalp (and sometimes eyebrows and eyelashes) with mold-like fungi called dermatophytes. It's widely known as ringworm because of its round lesions. It is a common childhood disease that is often confused with other scalp conditions, and is the most common fungal infection in children. Ages usually affected are 2 to 10 years. Tinea capitis is slightly more common in African American children. In adults, more women than men are infected. Because symptoms are often mild, it can go untreated for long periods. Tinea capitis is easily cured but usually requires weeks to months of treatment. If left untreated, it can cause hair loss.

What Causes Tinea Capitis?

The cause is a very common fungus named *Trichophyton*. People get it by direct contact with infected people or infected animals, especially cats and dogs.

What Are the Symptoms of Tinea Capitis?

Symptoms may be mild and first include redness and swelling (inflammation) of the scalp, followed by hair loss. Infected hairs become brittle and broken. Pustules called kerions, or small, pus-filled, blister-like lesions, may be present. Some people may have a tender, swollen area with drainage. Severe ringworm can also cause fever and enlarged lymph nodes (glands).

How Is Tinea Capitis Diagnosed?

The doctor makes a diagnosis by a skin examination. The doctor may take small samples of hair or infected skin with fungi for culture, to see whether fungi grow. A microscope is used to study them. Culture results are usually available after several days.

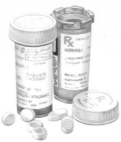

Oral medicines (such as griseofulvin or terbinafine) can cure tinea capitis, but treatment usually takes weeks to months. It's very important to finish the full course of treatment and follow the doctor's instructions. Otherwise, the infection can return.

The doctor may also prescribe special creams or shampoos (such as selenium sulfide) if needed.

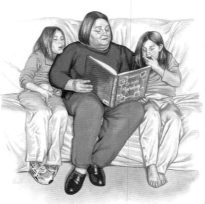

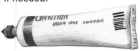

Avoid contact with infected people. Check family members for the disorder. Don't share combs, brushes, or hats with other people.

Check pets (such as cats, dogs, hamsters, and guinea pigs) for skin infections or irritations, and take your pet to your veterinarian if infections are present.

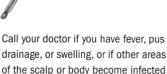

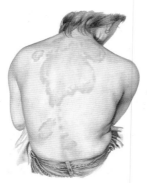

Call your doctor if you have fever, pus drainage, or swelling, or if other areas of the scalp or body become infected even with treatment.

How Is Tinea Capitis Treated?

Medicines taken by mouth (such as griseofulvin or terbinafine) can cure tinea capitis, but treatment usually takes weeks to months. Rarely, these drugs cause changes in liver function tests, and the doctor may order laboratory tests to make sure that the liver is working properly. It's very important to finish the full course of treatment and follow the doctor's instructions. Otherwise, the disorder can return.

The doctor may also prescribe special creams or shampoos (such as selenium sulfide) if needed.

DOs and DON'Ts in Managing Tinea Capitis:

✔ **DO** avoid contact with infected people.
✔ **DO** wash your hair after every haircut.
✔ **DO** continue treatment until your doctor tells you to stop.
✔ **DO** check pets (such as cats, dogs, hamsters, and guinea pigs) for skin infections or irritations, and if they're present, have your veterinarian treat your pets.
✔ **DO** check brothers and sisters for ringworm of the scalp.
✔ **DO** call your doctor if you have fever, pus drainage, or swelling.
✔ **DO** call your doctor if other areas of the scalp or body become infected even with treatment.
✔ **DO** call your doctor if tinea capitis comes back after you have finished the treatment.

⊘ **DON'T** share combs, brushes, or hats with other people.
⊘ **DON'T** get close haircuts, shave your head, or wear caps as long as you're taking your medicine.

FROM THE DESK OF

NOTES

FOR MORE INFORMATION

Contact the following source:

• American Academy of Dermatology
  Tel: (847) 330-0230, (866) 503-7546
  Website: http://www.aad.org

MANAGING YOUR
TINEA CRURIS

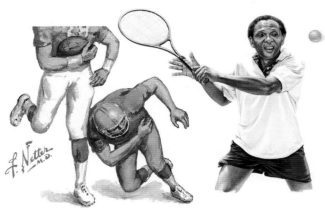

Tinea cruris is commonly called jock itch. It is a fungal infection of the groin and upper thighs and usually affects males. Females and non-athletes can also get it.

Male   Female

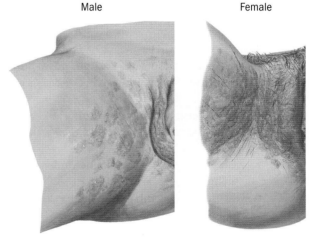

The skin in the groin and upper thighs becomes slightly raised, red to brown, and itches. Both sides of the groin may show patches, scaling with sharp edges, or small blisters. The rash is contagious as long as you have redness and scaling.

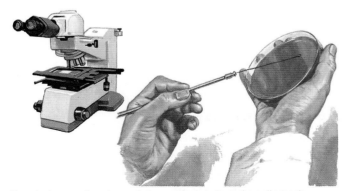

Your doctor usually only needs to examine you to make a diagnosis. Sometimes, your doctor may take a small sample of the infected skin and culture it (put it in a dish and let it grow). The culture is then studied under a microscope to see whether a fungus is present and what kind it is.

What Is Tinea Cruris?

Tinea cruris is a very common fungal infection of the skin in the groin and upper thighs. It occurs most often in men and adolescent boys. Tinea cruris can be cured in 2 to 3 weeks with the right treatment.

Tinea cruris is also called ringworm of the groin and is related to other similar fungal infections that are named according to where they occur, such as ringworm of the body (tinea corporis), ringworm of the scalp (tinea capitis), and athlete's foot (tinea pedis, ringworm of the feet).

What Causes Tinea Cruris?

The cause is a very common fungus that can be seen only with a microscope. Factors that increase the risk for infection include excessive sweating, athlete's foot, obesity, hot humid weather, and use of public baths or showers.

What Are the Symptoms of Tinea Cruris?

Symptoms include usually slightly raised, red-to-brown skin that itches. The skin may show patches, scaling with sharp edges, or small blisters. Both sides of the groin are usually affected, and pain in the groin may occur.

As long as redness and scaling are present, the infection can be passed to other people.

Scratching can cause oozing, swelling, and infections caused by other organisms.

How Is Tinea Cruris Diagnosed?

The doctor makes a diagnosis by doing an examination of the skin. The doctor may take small samples of infected skin if the diagnosis is unclear. These samples are cultured and studied under a microscope. Culture results are usually available after several days.

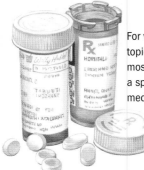

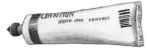

For very mild cases, only over-the-counter topical antifungal cream may be needed. In most cases, however, your doctor will prescribe a special antifungal cream or, for severe cases, medicine taken by mouth.

Wear loose-fitting, clean cotton underwear, especially when participating in physical activities. Boxer shorts are preferred.

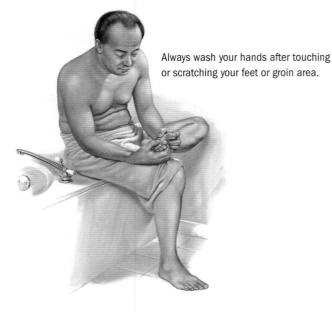

Always wash your hands after touching or scratching your feet or groin area.

How Is Tinea Cruris Treated?

In very mild cases, topical antifungal cream or ointment available without a prescription may be used. Treatment with the cream continues for 7 days after the area has cleared.

Most people, however, may need prescription antifungal creams ordered by the doctor.

The doctor may also prescribe medicines to be taken by mouth for severe or resistant infections. When such medicine is prescribed, the full course of therapy must be finished as prescribed.

DOs and DON'Ts in Managing Tinea Cruris:

✔ **DO** dry the groin with a separate towel after bathing or showering to prevent the infection from spreading to other areas.

✔ **DO** wear loose-fitting, clean cotton underwear. Boxer shorts are preferred. Change underwear daily or more often to keep the groin dry.

✔ **DO** call your doctor if the rash doesn't improve after 2 weeks of treatment.

✔ **DO** call your doctor if you have signs of another infection, such as fever, pus drainage, oozing, crusting, or swelling.

✔ **DO** call your doctor if you have scarring or bleeding.

🚫 **DON'T** share towels.

🚫 **DON'T** touch or scratch your feet and then touch your groin area.

🚫 **DON'T** wear nylon or other synthetic underwear that keeps moisture in the groin area.

🚫 **DON'T** wear clothes that rub or irritate the skin.

FROM THE DESK OF

NOTES

FOR MORE INFORMATION

Contact the following source:

• American Academy of Dermatology
Tel: (866) 503-SKIN (7546)
Website: http://www.aad.org

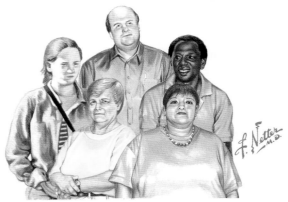

Tinea infections (ringworm) are very common skin disorders caused by fungi called dermatophytes—not worms. The infections are named for where they occur, such as ringworm of the body (tinea corporis), ringworm of the scalp (tinea capitis), athlete's foot (tinea pedis, ringworm of the feet), jock itch (tinea cruris, ringworm of the groin), and nail ringworm (tinea unguium).

Ringworm of the body causes a ring-shaped rash, usually on the legs or trunk of the body.

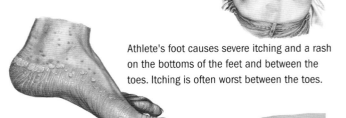

Athlete's foot causes severe itching and a rash on the bottoms of the feet and between the toes. Itching is often worst between the toes.

Jock itch affects the inner thighs and groin. It causes pain and severe itching and usually a rash of red, ring-like patches that grow outward in the crease of the thighs. The patches usually have bumps and a different color than nearby skin.

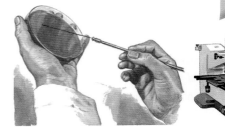

Your doctor makes a diagnosis by examining you and seeing the usual appearance of patches on the skin. Your doctor may take a small scraping of a patch for study with a microscope, because the fungi that cause the infection are so small that they can be seen only with a microscope.

What Are Tinea Infections?

Tinea infections (or ringworm) are caused by different fungi. The name ringworm comes from the appearance (ring-shaped or oval patches), not the cause, of the infection. Different fungi affect different parts of the body. These infections are named according to where they occur, such as ringworm of the body (tinea corporis), ringworm of the scalp (tinea capitis), athlete's foot (tinea pedis, ringworm of the feet), jock itch (tinea cruris, ringworm of the groin), and nail ringworm (tinea unguium).

What Causes Tinea Infections?

These infections aren't caused by worms but by fungi (microscopic plants) called dermatophytes. The more common ones are named *Trichophyton*, *Microsporum*, and *Epidermophyton*. Fungi that cause ringworm are very small, can be seen only with a microscope, and thrive in warm, moist areas.

What Are the Symptoms of Tinea Infections?

The most common symptom is itching. Sometimes scaling or flaking of the skin occurs.

On the body, ringworm starts as slightly raised, ring-shaped or oval, red-to-brown patches on the skin that itch. It usually develops on the legs or on the trunk of the body.

Jock itch is a tinea infection on the inner thighs. It causes pain and severe itching and usually produces a rash of red, ring-like patches that grow outward in the crease of the thighs. The rash usually has bumps and a different color than the skin around it.

Athlete's foot is another tinea infection affecting areas between the toes and bottoms of the feet. It causes severe itching, a rash, scaling, dead skin, burning, small blisters, and a musty or unpleasant odor. Dry skin may flake, peel, or crack. Itching is often worst between the toes.

How Are Tinea Infections Diagnosed?

The doctor makes a diagnosis by doing a physical examination and seeing the typical appearance of patches on the skin. The doctor may also take a sample of the skin for study under a microscope to confirm the diagnosis.

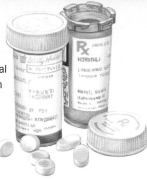

You can use over-the-counter antifungal cream, or your doctor can prescribe an antifungal cream to rub on the rash. For serious infections, your doctor can prescribe medicines taken by mouth.

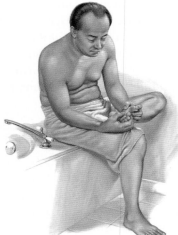

Use good general hygiene, including keeping the skin clean and dry. Take extra care if you use public showers, such as those at the gym.

If you have athlete's foot, wear cotton socks, not synthetic ones that don't allow your feet to breathe. Sneakers should also be well ventilated.

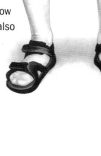

For jock itch, wear loose-fitting, clean cotton underwear, especially when participating in physical activities. Boxer shorts are preferred.

How Are Tinea Infections Treated?

Over-the-counter medicines (antifungal cream, ointment, or powder) can treat mild cases.

The doctor can prescribe antifungal cream to rub on the infected area or antifungal medicines to be taken by mouth for worse cases.

Jock itch usually improves in 2 to 8 weeks. Body ringworm usually gets better in 4 weeks, and athlete's foot may take longer.

DOs and DON'Ts in Managing Tinea Infections:

✔ **DO** use good general hygiene. Bathe or shower daily.
✔ **DO** keep infected skin clean and dry.
✔ **DO** wear loose-fitting underwear (for prevention of jock itch).
✔ **DO** wear cotton socks and well-ventilated sneakers with small holes to keep your feet dry (for prevention of athlete's foot).
✔ **DO** apply medicines exactly as directed.
✔ **DO** wear clean, dry clothes. Cotton or other absorbent cloth is best. Avoid nylon.

⊘ **DON'T** scratch or rub the infected area.
⊘ **DON'T** let anyone come in contact with your clothing or other items (such as a hairbrush) that may touch the infection. Don't touch ringworm patches on other people or contaminated items, such as clothes or combs.
⊘ **DON'T** shower in public places.
⊘ **DON'T** scratch or rub infected areas to avoid spreading the infection or causing another infection.

FROM THE DESK OF

NOTES

FOR MORE INFORMATION

Contact the following source:

• American Academy of Dermatology
  Tel: (866) 503-SKIN (7546)
  Website: http://www.aad.org

MANAGING YOUR ATHLETE'S FOOT

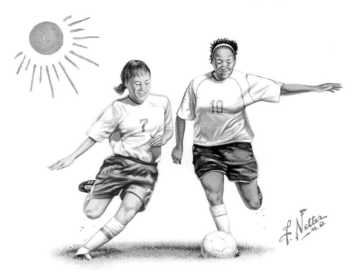

Tinea pedis is an infection of the foot and is one of the most common infections in people. It's also called athlete's foot or ringworm of the feet. It can occur anytime in adolescents and adults, but usually happens in warmer weather, when moist, sweaty feet and socks are more common.

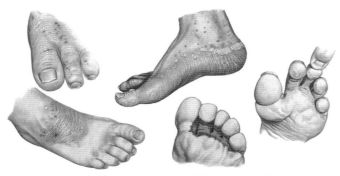

The cause is usually a fungus, ones named *Trichophyton* or *Epidermophyton*. These fungi are very small and can be seen only with a microscope. The most common symptoms are cracked skin between the toes and on the bottoms of the feet, plus itching.

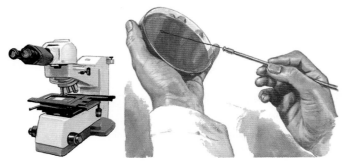

Your doctor makes a diagnosis by examining you and seeing the usual appearance of the skin. Your doctor may take a small scraping of a patch for study with a microscope, because the fungus that causes the infection is so small that it can be seen only with a microscope.

What Is Tinea Pedis?

Tinea pedis is an infection of the foot caused by a fungus. It is one of the most common infections that people get. It's also called athlete's foot or ringworm of the feet. Ringworm is a general name for these common skin infections. The name comes from the appearance (ring-shaped or oval patches), not the cause, of the infection. These infections are named according to where they occur, such as ringworm of the body (tinea corporis), ringworm of the scalp (tinea capitis), athlete's foot (tinea pedis), and jock itch (tinea cruris, ringworm of the groin).

Tinea pedis is most often seen in adolescents and adults during warm weather, but it can occur at any time.

Tinea pedis can be cured in 2 to 3 weeks, but it reappears often if things aren't done to prevent it.

What Causes Tinea Pedis?

The cause is usually a fungus, ones named *Trichophyton* or *Epidermophyton.* These fungi are very small and can be seen only with a microscope. Moist, sweaty feet and socks, hot humid weather, and use of public showers increase the chance of getting this infection.

What Are the Symptoms of Tinea Pedis?

The most common symptoms are cracked and boggy skin between the toes, plus itching. Tinea pedis also affects the bottoms of the feet. Scaling, dead skin, burning, and small blisters sometimes occur, as well as a musty or unpleasant odor. Dry skin may flake, peel, or crack. Itching is often worst between the toes. Scratching it can cause a red (inflamed) or weeping rash.

How Is Tinea Pedis Diagnosed?

The doctor makes a diagnosis by doing a physical examination and seeing the typical appearance of the skin. Sometimes, a small scraping of an affected area can be studied under a microscope to confirm the diagnosis.

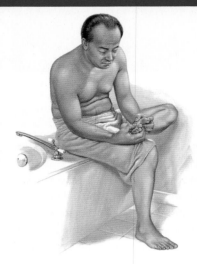

Wash your feet and then you can take off scales and dead skin. Wash and dry your feet at least once per day during and after treatment.

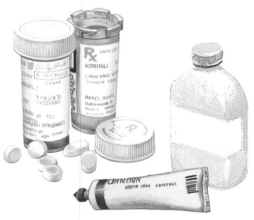

You can apply an over-the-counter antifungal powder, cream, or ointment to affected areas. Your doctor can also prescribe stronger topical medicines, or for serious infections, medicines that you take by mouth.

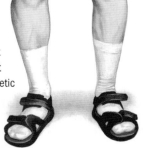

Wear sandals without socks to keep feet dry. When wearing socks, make sure that they are clean and dry. Don't wear synthetic socks—buy only cotton or wool.

How Is Tinea Pedis Treated?

It is important to keep the feet dry. Wear sandals if possible.

Feet should be washed, and then scales and dead skin can be removed.

An antifungal powder, cream, or ointment that is available without a prescription can be applied to affected areas. The doctor can also prescribe topical antifungal medicines.

To prevent the infection from returning, the medicine should be continued for 1 week after the symptoms and rash disappear.

DOs and DON'Ts in Managing Tinea Pedis:

✔ **DO** wash and dry your feet at least once per day during and after treatment, to make sure that the infection doesn't return.

✔ **DO** wear clean, dry socks made of cotton or wool.

✔ **DO** change socks daily or more often if necessary to keep your feet dry.

✔ **DO** wear sandals instead of going barefoot when in public places, such as locker rooms or showers. Also wear well-ventilated sneakers to keep your feet dry.

✔ **DO** wash and dry your feet immediately after exercising.

✔ **DO** call your doctor if your rash doesn't get better after 1 week of treatment.

✔ **DO** call your doctor if you see signs of another infection, such as fever, pus drainage, or red streaks on your feet.

⊘ **DON'T** scratch your feet.

⊘ **DON'T** wear synthetic socks. These keep moisture around the feet.

FROM THE DESK OF

NOTES

FOR MORE INFORMATION

Contact the following source:

• American Academy of Dermatology
Tel: (866) 503-SKIN (7546)
Website: http://www.aad.org

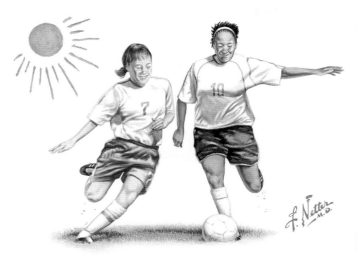

Tinea versicolor is a rash caused by fungus that usually lives on the skin. Teenagers and young adults can get it, more often in warmer weather, because fungus grows easily in heat and humidity. Unlike similar infections, tinea versicolor won't be passed among people.

What Is Tinea Versicolor?

Tinea versicolor is a rash caused by a fungus that normally lives on the skin. The infection affects the top layer of the skin and causes many irregular spots that are pale brown, pink, or white. Sometimes scales are seen on the rash. The rash usually appears on the upper body of both dark- and light-skinned people.

 The rash is more common in the summer. It usually affects teenagers and young adults and rarely affects elderly people and children, except in tropical areas where people of any age can have it.

What Causes Tinea Versicolor?

Tinea versicolor is caused by the fungus *Malassezia furfur*, which is a kind of yeast. Heat and humidity increase the risk of having tinea versicolor, as can too much sweating, oily skin, hormone changes, and a weak immune system. It cannot be caught from someone else.

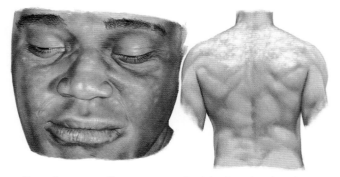

The rash occurs on the upper arms, chest, back, and neck and sometimes the face. The rash can be various colors and has small, white-to-pink or tan-to-dark spots with sharp edges and scales.

What Are the Symptoms of Tinea Versicolor?

Most people who have this rash don't have symptoms, but some have mild itching and increased sweating. The rash can be various colors and has small, white to pink or tan to dark spots with sharp edges and scales. It occurs on the upper arms, chest, back, and neck and sometimes the face. Light skin may show faint or tan to pink spots, but dark skin may show light or dark spots. The affected skin doesn't tan normally.

How Is Tinea Versicolor Diagnosed?

The doctor can usually make a diagnosis by the look of the skin. Ultraviolet light may be used to see the rash more clearly. Also, the doctor may gently scrape the rash to get some skin to look at under a microscope if is the diagnosis is unclear.

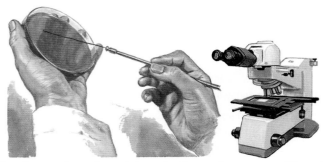

Your doctor makes a diagnosis by seeing the usual appearance of the rash on the skin. Your doctor may take a small scraping of a patch for study with a microscope if the diagnosis isn't clear.

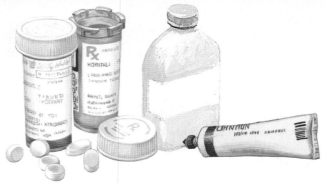

Your doctor may prescribe a cream, lotion, or pills to treat the rash. Treatment may last up to 1 month, but your skin may take several months to return to normal. So don't be discouraged if it doesn't look normal after a few weeks.

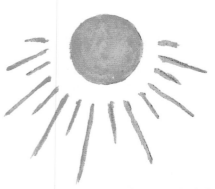

Sunlight may help your rash, but ask your doctor whether being in the sun is good for you, and if so, how long you should stay in the sun. Using sunscreen is also important.

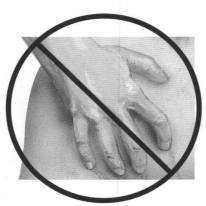

Don't scratch at the rash. If the itching really bothers you, talk to your doctor about medicine to help relieve it.

How Is Tinea Versicolor Treated?

The usual treatment is medicated skin cream, lotion, or gel. If the rash is severe or doesn't get better with over-the-counter products, the doctor can prescribe stronger medicine, either topical (applied to the skin) or given by mouth as pills. Sunlight may help the skin get better. Medicine is also given for itching.

Treatment usually lasts 1 to 2 weeks, but may take up to 1 month. The skin should return to normal after several months, without scars.

The rash can come back and will need treatment again.

DOs and DON'Ts in Managing Tinea Versicolor:

✔ **DO** tell your doctor about medicines you take, including prescription drugs and ones you buy over the counter.

✔ **DO** tell your doctor if you're pregnant.

✔ **DO** call your doctor if your symptoms get worse or you have a fever.

🚫 **DON'T** stop taking your medicine or change your dosage because you feel better.

FROM THE DESK OF

NOTES

FOR MORE INFORMATION

Contact the following source:

• American Academy of Dermatology
Tel: (866) 503-SKIN (7546)
Website: http://www.aad.org

MANAGING
HIVES

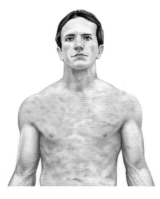

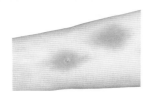

The medical term for hives is urticaria, also called wheals (bumps). Swollen, small, pale red bumps or larger patches suddenly appear on the skin. Other symptoms are itching and, less often, burning or stinging.

f. Netter M.D.

Some common causes of allergic urticaria

Drugs such
as penicillin

Insect stings
and bites

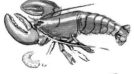

Foods such as
shellfish and nuts

Causes of nonallergic urticaria

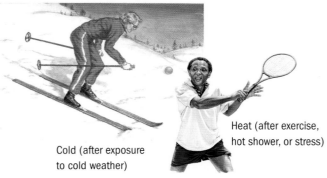

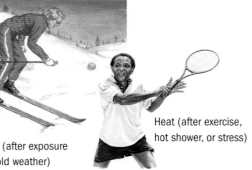

Cold (after exposure
to cold weather)

Heat (after exercise,
hot shower, or stress)

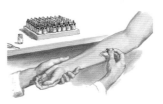

To find the cause, your doctor will ask questions about when you get the hives, what you eat, where you work, how long the hives lasted, and what things may have triggered them. Tests of blood, urine, and skin may be done.

What Are Hives?

The medical term for hives is urticaria, also called wheals (bumps). Swollen, small, pale red bumps or larger patches suddenly appear on the skin. Severe itching usually follows. Each bump tends to go away in 24 hours without leaving marks, but then others appear. They can be very small to large. Scratching can cause the affected skin area to get larger, leading to big, fiery red patches. Hives usually don't last long. When they last more than 6 weeks, they're called chronic; when they last less than 6 weeks, they're called acute.

What Causes Hives?

Hives can be allergic or nonallergic, but often the cause remains unknown. Allergic hives, the least common, are triggered by an overreaction of the immune system to certain things, most commonly foods (nuts, shellfish), insect stings and bites, and drugs (e.g., penicillin).

Causes of nonallergic hives include cold (after exposure to cold weather) and heat (after exercise, hot shower, or stress).

What Are the Symptoms of Hives?

Symptoms include itching, or less often burning or stinging; raised, often red, swellings; and separate swellings that usually go away in 24 hours, but new ones often appear as the old ones disappear.

How Are Hives Diagnosed?

The doctor will ask about symptoms: when they appeared, how long they lasted, what things may have triggered them. If the doctor thinks that an allergy is the cause, seeing a specialist in allergies may be suggested. A diary of foods eaten, drugs taken, illnesses, work and home life, and when symptoms appear should be kept.

No specific tests are used for these conditions, so the choice of tests depends on answers to questions about symptoms and a full physical examination. Sometimes, blood and urine tests and skin testing may be done.

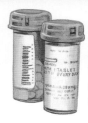

Antihistamines (like those taken for hay fever) are the most common treatment. For complicated or severe hives, your doctor may prescribe drugs called corticosteroids (prednisone) for a short time.

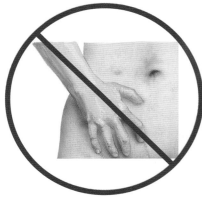

Avoid anything your doctor says will trigger your hives. Stress can make your symptoms worse. Don't scratch; it may make the hives worse.

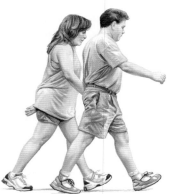

Wear looser fitting clothes that don't rub against your skin.

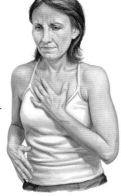

Call your doctor if you have shortness of breath or wheezing. Also call your doctor if you develop a swollen tongue, lips, or face.

How Are Hives Treated?

Antihistamines (like those taken for hay fever) are the most common treatment. In complicated or severe cases, drugs called corticosteroids (prednisone) may be prescribed for a short time.

DOs and DON'Ts in Managing Hives:

✔ **DO** avoid anything your doctor says will trigger your condition.

✔ **DO** take your prescribed drugs and follow directions for their use.

✔ **DO** avoid stress. This can make your symptoms worse.

✔ **DO** call your doctor if you have shortness of breath or wheezing.

✔ **DO** call your doctor if you develop a swollen tongue, lips, or face.

⊘ **DON'T** wear tight-fitting clothes that can rub your skin.

⊘ **DON'T** towel yourself vigorously after a bath or shower, because this can increase the area of skin affected.

⊘ **DON'T** scratch, because this can make the hives worse.

⊘ **DON'T** drink alcohol or eat spicy foods. These can make your condition worse.

⊘ **DON'T** use harsh soaps or wash too much. Dry skin can cause more itching.

FROM THE DESK OF

NOTES

FOR MORE INFORMATION

Contact the following sources:

• American Academy of Allergy, Asthma & Immunology
Tel: (800) 822-2762
Website: http://www.aaaai.org/

• American Academy of Dermatology
Tel: (866) 503-7546
Website: http://www.aad.org

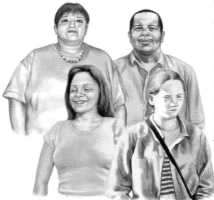

Vitiligo is a fairly common skin condition involving loss of pigmentation (color) in the skin. Vitiligo affects people of all races and ethnic groups. It can occur at any age, but half of the cases occur in people younger than 20. The cause isn't known.

What Is Vitiligo?

Vitiligo is a fairly common skin condition involving loss of pigmentation (color) in the skin. Color is lost in patches, often on the back of the hands, face, and armpits. Vitiligo affects people of all races and ethnic groups. It can occur at any age, but half of the cases occur in people younger than 20. Vitiligo can cause serious cosmetic changes in the skin. It's not life threatening or curable, but some skin pigment may return on the face and neck. It's sometimes related to other illnesses such as thyroid diseases.

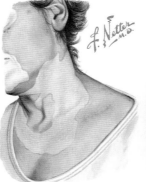

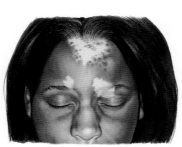

What Causes Vitiligo?

The cause is unknown. Vitiligo isn't cancerous and is not contagious. It can run in families.

What Are the Symptoms of Vitiligo?

Small areas of skin lose pigment and color and become flat and white. Patches can't be felt with the fingers. They don't hurt or itch. They vary in size and may be up to an inch across. Patches spread to form larger areas with irregular shapes. They often occur on both sides of the body in about the same place. Sometimes hair in the area also loses pigment.

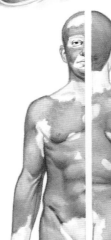

The skin develops small areas that lose pigment and therefore color. These patches are flat and white. Patches spread to form larger irregular areas. They usually occur on both sides of the body in about the same place.

How Is Vitiligo Diagnosed?

The doctor will examine the skin to make a diagnosis and may suggest seeing a doctor who specializes in skin diseases (dermatologist). The doctor may take a small sample of skin (biopsy sample) for closer study with a microscope.

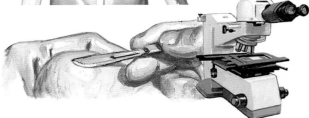

Your doctor will examine your skin to make a diagnosis and may suggest seeing a skin doctor (dermatologist). A small sample of skin may be taken (biopsy). The sample will be checked with a microscope.

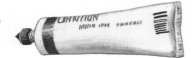

For limited patches, a steroid cream applied to the skin can help. Best results may take 3 to 4 months.

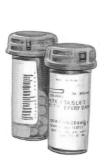

Specialized light therapy, or PUVA, involves applying medicines called psoralens, followed by exposure to ultraviolet light. Psoralens can also be taken as pills.

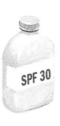

Use sunscreen on areas with vitiligo.

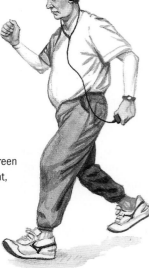

If you can't avoid the sun, use a sunscreen with an SPF of 15 or higher. Wear a hat, long-sleeved shirt, and long pants.

How Is Vitiligo Treated?

Treatment involves a combination of cosmetics, prescription creams, and specialized light therapy.

Mild vitiligo may not need treatment. People with small patches can do well with cosmetic stains and makeup. Fair-skinned people may benefit from avoiding tanning by using sunscreens with an SPF of 15 or higher and keeping away from direct sunlight.

For limited patches, a steroid cream applied to the skin can help. Best results may take 3 or 4 months. Steroid creams should not be put on eyelids, armpits, or groin areas.

Specialized light therapy, or PUVA, consists of applying a solution of medicines called psoralens, followed by ultraviolet light. Psoralens can also be taken as pills. This treatment is best for the face, neck, trunk, upper arms, and upper legs. Results begin after 25 to 50 treatments depending on areas involved. Major side effects are severe sunburn and blistering.

DOs and DON'Ts in Managing Vitiligo:

✔ **DO** use sunscreen in areas with vitiligo.
✔ **DO** contact your doctor if new symptoms develop. Drugs for vitiligo may have side effects.
✔ **DO** use a sunscreen with an SPF of 15 or higher and wear a hat, long-sleeved shirt, and long pants.
✔ **DO** call your doctor if you get severe reddening or blistering during treatment.

⊘ **DON'T** expose yourself to direct sunlight, especially between 11 AM and 3 PM during summer.
⊘ **DON'T** get sunburns or tan. When skin not affected by vitiligo tans, affected areas will become more obvious.

FROM THE DESK OF

NOTES

FOR MORE INFORMATION

Contact the following sources:

• National Vitiligo Foundation
Tel: (614) 261-8145
Website: http://www.nvfi.org

• American Academy of Dermatology
Tel: (866) 503-SKIN (503-7546)
Website: http://www.aad.org

MANAGING YOUR
WARTS

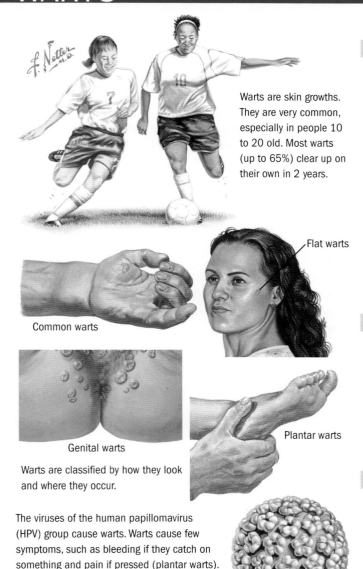

Warts are skin growths. They are very common, especially in people 10 to 20 old. Most warts (up to 65%) clear up on their own in 2 years.

Common warts

Flat warts

Genital warts

Plantar warts

Warts are classified by how they look and where they occur.

The viruses of the human papillomavirus (HPV) group cause warts. Warts cause few symptoms, such as bleeding if they catch on something and pain if pressed (plantar warts).

HPV cell

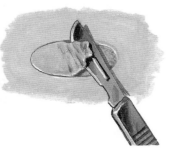

Your doctor will diagnose warts by examining your skin. If the diagnosis is unclear, your doctor may take a small piece of the wart (biopsy) to look at with a microscope.

What Are Warts?

Warts are skin growths. They are classified by how they look and where they occur. Common warts occur on hands, arms, and legs. These warts often look like little rough cauliflowers. Periungual warts occur around fingernails. Flat warts, on the face, knees, and elbows of children and young women, are slightly raised and flesh colored. Genital warts on genital and rectal areas are often sexually transmitted. Plantar warts on bottoms of feet are often passed along by bare feet. Filiform warts are small with hairlike pieces.

Warts are very common, especially in people 10 to 20 years old. Most warts (up to 65%) disappear on their own without treatment in 2 years. They often come back, even when treated.

What Causes Warts?

The viruses of the human papillomavirus (HPV) group cause warts. Different types of viruses tend to infect different body parts. Warts can be passed from one person to another. Scratching and picking warts also spreads the infection. Skin that is moist from soaking or that has cuts or scratches is more likely to become infected by virus and form warts.

What Are the Symptoms of Warts?

Most warts are little more than unpleasant growths on skin. They sometimes catch and bleed if they're on the face and head. Plantar warts may cause pain and tenderness when stepping on the foot.

How Are Warts Diagnosed?

The doctor will diagnose warts by examining the skin. If the diagnosis is unclear, the doctor may remove a small piece of wart (biopsy) for study with a microscope.

No treatment may be needed for painless warts. You should avoid spreading the virus by making sure your wart is covered when using community swimming pools, locker rooms, or showers.

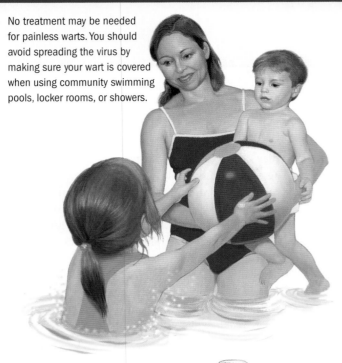

Common warts on arms, hands, and legs can be treated by salicylic and lactic acids in solution. Other treatments include freezing, drugs to stimulate the immune system, surgery, and burning with lasers or electricity.

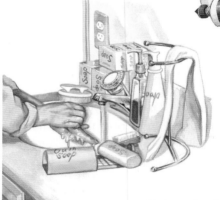

Wash your hands well after touching the wart to avoid spreading the virus.

How Are Warts Treated?

Treatment is usually but not always successful, and not all warts need treatment. Treatment itself can often cause problems, such as pain, infection, and scarring.

Warts causing no pain may need no treatment. Spreading the virus should be avoided, for example, by making sure the wart is covered when using community swimming pools, locker rooms, or showers.

Treatment depends somewhat on the wart location. Common warts on arms, hands, and legs can be treated with salicylic acid in solution. The solution is put on warts each night and each morning dead skin is peeled off.

Plantar warts can be treated with 40% salicylic acid plasters. Flat warts are often treated by skin peeling using tretinoin cream or 5-fluorouracil. Genital warts almost always need a doctor's visit for both partners. Treatment is usually with a blistering agent. If these treatments don't work, your doctor may prescribe stronger medicine, such as imiquimod cream or trichloroacetic acid.

Other treatments include freezing, injecting warts with drugs that stimulate the immune (infection-fighting) system, surgically cutting them, and burning them with a laser or electricity.

DOs and DON'Ts in Managing Warts:

✔ **DO** wash your hands well after touching warts to avoid spreading them.

✔ **DO** call your doctor if you have warts that cannot be treated by over-the-counter salicylic acid solutions.

✔ **DO** call your doctor if your warts aren't better after several weeks of treatment.

⊘ **DON'T** scratch, pick, or cut warts.

⊘ **DON'T** shave or cut hair over warts.

FROM THE DESK OF

NOTES

FOR MORE INFORMATION

Contact the following sources:

• American Academy of Dermatology
Tel: (888) 462-3376
Website: http://www.aad.org

• American Podiatric Medical Association
Tel: (800) 366-8227
Website: http://www.apma.org

MANAGING YOUR
ACROMEGALY

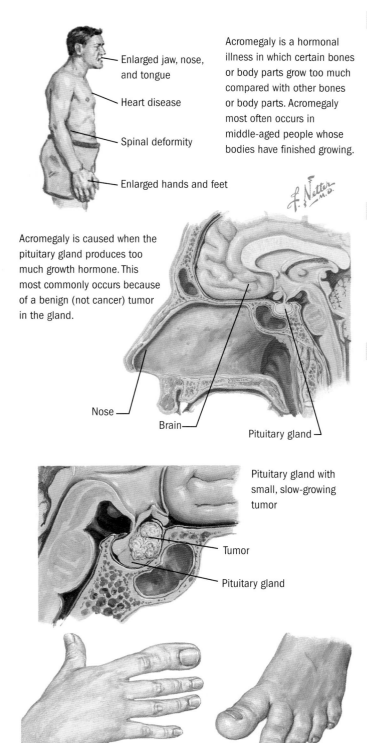

Acromegaly is a hormonal illness in which certain bones or body parts grow too much compared with other bones or body parts. Acromegaly most often occurs in middle-aged people whose bodies have finished growing.

Enlarged jaw, nose, and tongue

Heart disease

Spinal deformity

Enlarged hands and feet

Acromegaly is caused when the pituitary gland produces too much growth hormone. This most commonly occurs because of a benign (not cancer) tumor in the gland.

Nose

Brain

Pituitary gland

Pituitary gland with small, slow-growing tumor

Tumor

Pituitary gland

The most common symptom of acromegaly is enlargement of the feet, hands (so gloves, rings, and shoes are too tight), head, or face.

What Is Acromegaly?

Acromegaly is an illness in which some soft skin and bones of the head, face, hands, and feet can grow out of proportion to the rest of your body. Acromegaly is rare; only about 750 people per year are diagnosed with it in the U.S. However, 10 to 20 times as many people currently live with it.

Acromegaly usually occurs in middle-aged adults who finished growing in height but then other body parts start growing. Children can also have acromegaly.

What Causes Acromegaly?

This illness is caused by production of too much growth hormone made by the body's pituitary gland. This gland makes too much growth hormone because of a benign (not cancer) tumor, or growth. This tumor usually occurs in the same part of the brain as the pituitary gland.

What Are the Symptoms of Acromegaly?

Enlargement of bones of the hands, feet, head, or face is a common symptom. Others include headaches, blurred vision, joint pain, numbness and tingling of the fingers, high blood pressure, carpal tunnel syndrome (numbness of fingers), high blood sugar (glucose) level, changes in a woman's periods (menstrual cycle), impotence in men, and excess growth of skin on the forehead, jaw, lips, and tongue. Snoring and space between the teeth may increase, and the voice may get deeper. Acromegaly may also cause arthritis, heart disease, and sleep apnea.

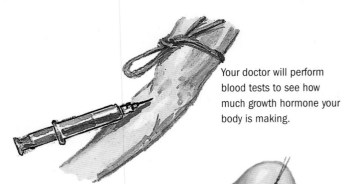

Your doctor will perform blood tests to see how much growth hormone your body is making.

Surgery through the nose to reach the pituitary and remove the tumor.

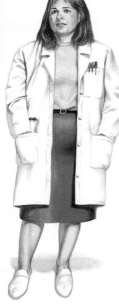

Be sure to have your eyes checked frequently, and contact your doctor if you have severe headaches that become worse over time.

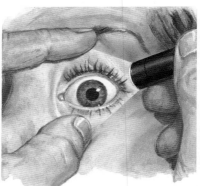

Follow your doctor's recommendations. Remember that it is not typical for all symptoms to go away immediately, so don't get discouraged.

How Is Acromegaly Diagnosed?

The doctor will perform a physical examination and do blood tests to measure the amount of growth hormone.

An MRI (magnetic resonance imaging) or CT (computed tomography) scan of the pituitary gland will be done to find the tumor.

How Is Acromegaly Treated?

Early diagnosis and treatment of overproduction of growth hormone are needed to prevent acromegaly.

Surgery may be done to remove the tumor. Surgery is done through the nose or above the lip, so no scarring occurs.

Radiation to the pituitary gland and medicine are other treatments. Often, a combination of all these methods is used.

The doctor may suggest seeing an endocrinologist, a doctor who treats hormone problems.

Acromegaly requires lifelong treatment. Surgery often succeeds, but hormone levels may not return to normal, and medicines may be needed even after surgery.

DOs and DON'Ts in Managing Acromegaly:

✔ **DO** follow your doctor's recommendations about medicines.

✔ **DO** see your doctor regularly. Your doctor will check your blood pressure, blood sugar level, and heart to monitor for complications of this disease. Your eyes should also be checked regularly.

✔ **DO** contact your doctor if you have vision changes, worsening headaches, or get new nerve pains or numbness, or pain or pressure in the chest.

✔ **DO** call your doctor if you have side effects from your medicines, including nausea, dizziness, or lightheadedness.

⊘ **DON'T** expect all your symptoms to go away immediately.

⊘ **DON'T** be afraid to try a combination of treatments.

⊘ **DON'T** forget to have your eyes examined.

FROM THE DESK OF

NOTES

FOR MORE INFORMATION

Contact the following source:

• Pituitary Network Association
  Post Office Box 1958
  Thousand Oaks, CA 91358
  Tel: (805) 499-9973
  Website: http://www.pituitary.com

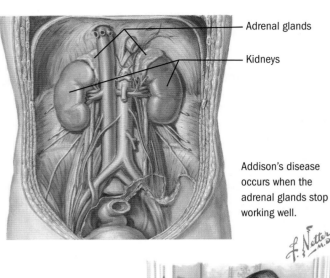

Adrenal glands

Kidneys

Addison's disease occurs when the adrenal glands stop working well.

What Is Addison's Disease?

Addison's disease is a condition in which the adrenal glands don't work well. The two small adrenal glands sit atop the kidneys. They usually produce hormones called cortisol and aldosterone. Without these hormones, salt and water in the body is lost in urine, which makes blood pressure fall too low. Also, potassium builds up to a dangerous level. There is no effective way to prevent Addison's disease.

What Causes Addison's Disease?

Addison's disease develops because the immune system (infection-fighting system) doesn't work well. In an auto-immune disease, the body makes substances (antibodies) that damage adrenal glands. Other causes include infections (e.g., tuberculosis, AIDS), cancer, bleeding, and blocked blood vessels. Adrenal glands may also develop poorly from birth. Surgery, medicines with harmful side effects, and x-ray treatments can also cause the disorder.

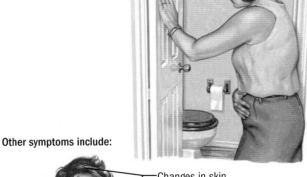

Symptoms of Addison's disease include fatigue and feeling sick to the stomach.

What Are the Symptoms of Addison's Disease?

Some people may have no symptoms. Others may feel weak, tired, or sick to the stomach; there may also be weight loss, decreased appetite, low blood pressure, depression, or skin and hair changes. Darkening of the skin over knuckles, knees, elbows, toes, or lips, creases of palms, and mucous membranes may be present.

People with addisonian crisis have a more serious illness that is a medical emergency. The sudden crisis usually results from stress, such as surgery, trauma, or illness. Symptoms may include severe nausea and vomiting, diarrhea, very low blood pressure, leg and stomach pain, and coma.

Other symptoms include:

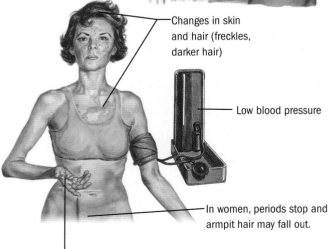

Changes in skin and hair (freckles, darker hair)

Low blood pressure

In women, periods stop and armpit hair may fall out.

Darkening of skin over knuckles, knees, elbows, toes, palm creases, and lips

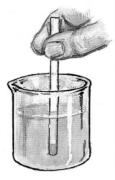

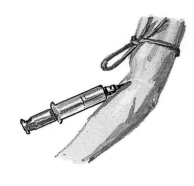

Testing of blood and urine samples will help diagnose what is wrong.

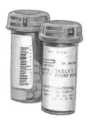

Treatment of both Addison's disease and addisonian crisis involves medicines such as hydrocortisone, fludrocortisone, and prednisone.

Be sure to visit your doctor regularly, and take any medicine prescribed.

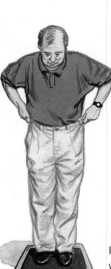

If you have sudden weight loss, are vomiting, or have a fever, call your doctor right away!

FROM THE DESK OF

NOTES

How Is Addison's Disease Diagnosed?

The doctor will order blood and urine laboratory tests and measurements of adrenal hormones.

The doctor may also want x-rays and CT (computed tomography) scans to show the size of the heart (which may be smaller) and adrenal glands.

How Is Addison's Disease Treated?

Medicine to replace adrenal hormones includes hydrocortisone, fludrocortisone, and prednisone. These medications work well for this lifelong illness.

DOs and DON'Ts in Managing Addison's Disease:

✔ **DO** see your doctor regularly.
✔ **DO** take medicine as recommended by your doctor.
✔ **DO** talk to your doctor before you have surgery (to adjust your dose) and before using other prescription drugs.
✔ **DO** wear a medical alert bracelet.
✔ **DO** carry an emergency pack with medicine. Be sure that you and your family know how to give this medicine. Always be prepared for addisonian crisis.
✔ **DO** avoid stress.
✔ **DO** watch your lifestyle. Drink alcohol only in moderation. Eat a well-balanced diet with enough regular table salt.
✔ **DO** exercise, but don't overdo it.
✔ **DO** call your doctor when you feel poorly (nausea, vomiting, fever) or feel weak and tired and have weight loss.
✔ **DO** slowly decrease your medicine if your doctor recommends it. You'll avoid complications, such as weight gain, diabetes, and high blood pressure, from too much medicine.

⊘ **DON'T** eat too much potassium (foods like oranges and salt substitutes).
⊘ **DON'T** skip doses of medicine.

FOR MORE INFORMATION

Contact the following sources:

- National Adrenal Disease Foundation
  505 Northern Boulevard, Suite 200
  Great Neck, NY 11021
  Tel: (516) 487-4992

- National Institute of Diabetes and Digestive and Kidney Diseases
  Website: http://www.niddk.nih.gov/index.htm

- Medic Alert Foundation International
  Tel: (209) 668-3333

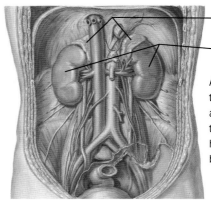

Aldosteronism occurs when the adrenal glands, which lie above the kidneys, produce too much aldosterone, a hormone that helps regulate blood pressure.

— Adrenal glands

— Kidneys

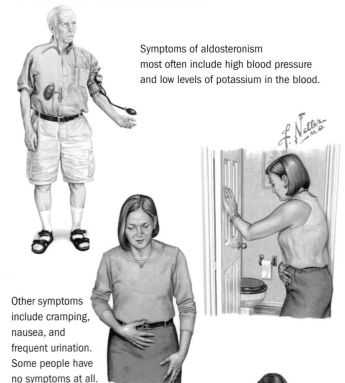

Symptoms of aldosteronism most often include high blood pressure and low levels of potassium in the blood.

Other symptoms include cramping, nausea, and frequent urination. Some people have no symptoms at all.

Testing of urine or blood samples can confirm the diagnosis. The plasma renin activity (PRA) blood test can tell whether primary (low PRA) or secondary (high PRA) aldosteronism is present.

What Is Aldosteronism?

Aldosteronism is an illness caused by too much aldosterone, a hormone produced by adrenal glands. These two small glands sit atop the kidneys. Aldosteronism leads to high blood pressure and low blood potassium levels.

What Causes Aldosteronism?

Aldosterone is a hormone that regulates blood pressure by increasing sodium and fluid levels in the blood and increasing removal of potassium by kidneys. The two main types of aldosteronism are primary and secondary. Primary aldosteronism means that extra aldosterone comes from adrenal glands themselves, usually because of a growth (or tumor). This usually benign (not cancerous) tumor is called an adenoma. This disorder is also called Conn's syndrome. Bilateral adrenal hyperplasia, an illness in which both glands are enlarged and overproduce aldosterone, may also cause this condition.

Secondary aldosteronism means that the illness results from other conditions, such as congestive heart failure, liver failure, kidney disease, and dehydration, or certain medicines, such as diuretics or fludrocortisone.

Aldosteronism accounts for less than 1% of cases of high blood pressure in the United States.

What Are the Symptoms of Aldosteronism?

High blood pressure, weakness, cramping, nausea, constipation, muscle spasm, and frequent urination may occur. Some people have no symptoms.

How Is Aldosteronism Diagnosed?

High blood pressure and low blood potassium levels may indicate aldosteronism.

High aldosterone levels can be measured in blood or urine. A special blood test called plasma renin activity (PRA) can tell whether primary or secondary aldosteronism is present. A specialist called an endocrinologist will use special tests for primary aldosteronism.

An MRI (magnetic resonance imaging) or CT (computed tomography) scan of the belly (abdomen) may be done to help identify the cause of aldosteronism.

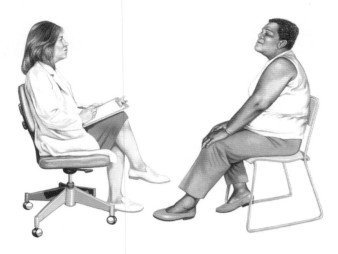

Talk to the doctor about all your symptoms. Be sure to take salt tablets and specific medicines, if the doctor prescribes them, according to the doctor's instructions.

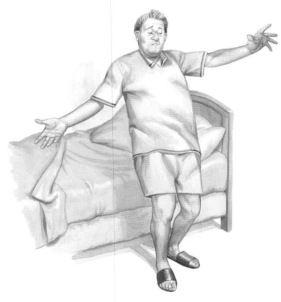

If you feel weak and tired or dizzy when you stand up, call your doctor right away. You might need extra or different treatment.

How Is Aldosteronism Treated?

Untreated aldosteronism can cause uncontrolled high blood pressure, which can be a risk factor for stroke or heart disease. People with very low potassium levels may also have an abnormal heart beat. Treatment for Conn's syndrome involves tumor removal by surgery.

Bilateral adrenal hyperplasia can't be cured unless both adrenal glands are removed. This removal may cause more side effects than wanted. Therefore people with this illness take spironolactone, a diuretic. This drug helps keep blood potassium levels normal. Side effects may include gynecomastia (breast development in men), impotence, and feeling tired and drowsy.

For aldosteronism resulting from other illnesses, treatment of the condition causing higher aldosterone levels will help.

DOs and DON'Ts in Managing Aldosteronism:

✔ **DO** follow your doctor's instruction to add salt to each meal or take salt tablets for special tests.

✔ **DO** tell your doctor if you have a history of congestive heart failure before beginning this high-salt diet.

✔ **DO** find an experienced surgeon to remove the tumor if present.

✔ **DO** call your doctor if you have male breast development, impotence, nausea, drowsiness, or lethargy while taking spironolactone.

✔ **DO** call your doctor for cramps or rapid heart beats. Your potassium level may be dangerously low.

✔ **DO** call your doctor if you feel extremely weak and tired or dizzy when you stand up. You may need extra hormone replacement after surgery.

🚫 **DON'T** let your potassium level fall below normal, especially if you're taking diuretics. Follow dietary instructions from your doctor and have frequent blood tests to check potassium levels.

FROM THE DESK OF

NOTES

FOR MORE INFORMATION

Contact the following sources:

- National Adrenal Disease Foundation
  505 Northern Boulevard, Suite 200
  Great Neck, NY 11021
  Tel: (516) 487-4992

- The Endocrine Society
  435 East West Highway, Suite 500
  Bethesda, MD 20814-4410
  Tel: (888) 363-6274

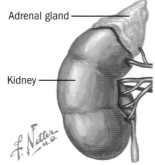

Adrenal gland

Kidney

Cushing's syndrome is a disorder caused by high levels of the hormone cortisol. Cortisol controls blood pressure (especially during stress), but too much cortisol causes body changes. Adrenal glands, which are found on top of the kidneys, produce cortisol.

What Is Cushing's Syndrome?

Cushing's syndrome is a rare endocrine illness caused by exposure of body tissues to too much cortisol in the bloodstream. Produced by the adrenal glands, cortisol is a substance (hormone) that helps the body control blood pressure and respond to stress. Extra cortisol, however, produces abnormal body changes.

Cushing's syndrome occurs most often in women 25 to 45 years old. It may increase the risk of getting diabetes, hypertension, osteoporosis, and obesity.

What Causes Cushing's Syndrome?

Extra cortisol may come from medicines prescribed by doctors for other conditions (e.g., asthma, bronchitis, arthritis). Certain tumors may produce excess cortisol. These tumors may be in the pituitary gland, adrenal gland, or other places.

Symptoms include:

Red cheeks

Fat pads (buffalo hump)

Thin skin

High B.P.

Thin arms and legs

Moon face

Excess hair growth in women (face, neck, chest, stomach)

Bruises easily

Stretch marks

Loosely hanging abdomen

Poor wound healing

What Are the Symptoms of Cushing's Syndrome?

Symptoms are weight gain, rounded face, fat around the neck, and thin arms and legs. Children are obese and grow slowly. The stomach, legs, arms, and breasts may show purplish-pink stretch marks. Thin, delicate skin bruises easily and heals poorly. Bones are weak and brittle and may break. Hormonal changes in women mean that they usually have too much hair growth on the face, neck, chest, stomach, and thighs. Periods may be irregular or stop. Men may be impotent. Other symptoms are urinating often, severe tiredness, weak muscles, high blood pressure, personality changes, and feeling irritable, anxious, and depressed.

How Is Cushing's Syndrome Diagnosed?

The doctor will make a diagnosis by doing a physical examination and testing blood and urine.

If cortisol levels are high, another doctor (an endocrinologist, a specialist who treats diseases of glands and hormones) will order other tests. These tests usually involve taking medicine and providing blood and urine samples. Computed tomography (CT) or magnetic resonance imaging (MRI) of the belly (abdomen) to look for tumors of adrenal glands (located above the kidneys) or of the brain to look for pituitary gland tumors may be done.

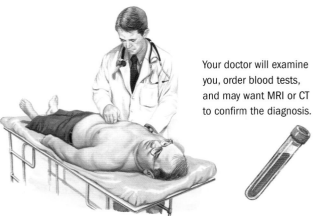

Your doctor will examine you, order blood tests, and may want MRI or CT to confirm the diagnosis.

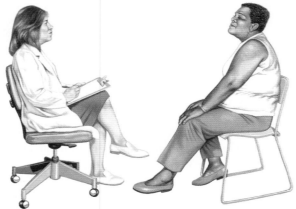

Your doctor will develop a treatment plan based on possible causes of Cushing's and your cortisol levels. Get regular checkups to control symptoms. Heavy drinking and a history of depression can cause false-positive results on tests, so truthful answers to questions about drinking and depression will help diagnosis and treatment.

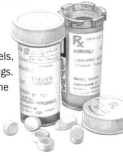

Certain medicines can increase cortisol levels, so your doctor may change your current drugs. Your doctor may also prescribe new medicine to block effects of cortisol on your body.

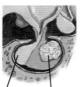

An abnormal growth, such as a pituitary tumor, may cause the increased cortisol level. In these cases, treatment of the growth may involve surgery, radiation, and drugs (chemotherapy).

Pituitary Tumor
gland

Don't become discouraged. You may become frustrated during the recovery period. Look for a support group in your community for people with Cushing's syndrome. If you can't find a group, try starting one.

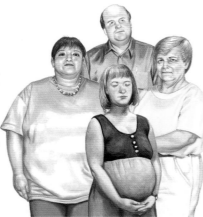

FROM THE DESK OF

NOTES

How Is Cushing's Syndrome Treated?

If medicine is the cause, the doctor can change the dose to lower the cortisol levels or give medicine that blocks effects of cortisol on the body.

For an abnormal growth (tumor), treatment may include surgery to remove the growth, radiation, and drugs (chemotherapy).

If no cause is found, rarely adrenal glands are removed to prevent extra cortisol from being made. Medicine to replace missing cortisol is then needed.

Recovery time depends on duration of the illness, cortisol levels, and basic health.

DOs and DON'Ts in Managing Cushing's Syndrome:

✔ **DO** minimize using corticosteroid hormones.
✔ **DO** see your doctor regularly. Have regular checkups for blood sugar level, blood pressure, and bone density.
✔ **DO** look for a nearby support group.
✔ **DO** tell your doctor if you have had depression or drink alcohol daily.
✔ **DO** find an experienced surgeon if you need surgery.
✔ **DO** eat less fat and calories.
✔ **DO** call your doctor if you have a fever, infection, or increased bruising or you gain too much weight.
✔ **DO** call your doctor for weakness or dizziness after surgery.

⊘ **DON'T** become discouraged.
⊘ **DON'T** begin exercise until your doctor checks blood pressure, blood sugar, and bones.
⊘ **DON'T** overeat.

FOR MORE INFORMATION

Contact the following sources:

• American Association of Clinical Endocrinologists
Tel: (904) 353-7878
Website: http://www.aace.com

• Cushing's Support and Research Foundation
Tel: (617) 723-3824

• National Institute of Diabetes and Digestive and Kidney Diseases
Tel: (301) 496-3583
Website: http://www.endocrine.niddk.nih.gov/pubs/cushings/cushings.htm

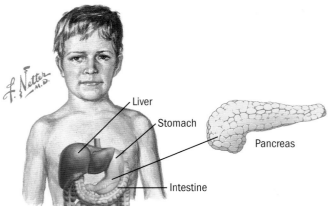

In diabetes mellitus type 1, the pancreas doesn't make enough insulin, so people have too much sugar (glucose) in the blood, and not enough glucose gets into the body cells.

Diabetes is a lifelong condition. Your child will need your help in developing good habits to control diabetes.

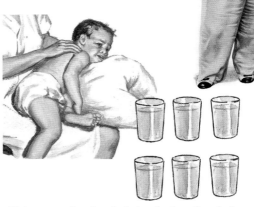

Diabetes warning signs include urinating often, feeling very thirsty and hungry, and feeling tired and weak.

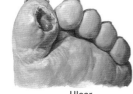

Ulcer

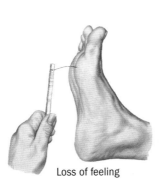

Loss of feeling

Uncontrolled diabetes can cause eye disease, reduce blood circulation in feet, and cause ulcers, infections, and loss of feeling. It may also lead to kidney failure that could mean your child would need dialysis.

What Is Diabetes Mellitus Type 1?

Diabetes mellitus type 1 (or just diabetes) is a lifelong disorder that prevents your child's body from getting energy from food. Most cases start in children 12 to 15 years old.

In diabetes, the body doesn't produce enough insulin, a hormone produced by special beta cells in the pancreas. Insulin is vital because it controls the amount of sugar (glucose) absorbed by body cells from the blood. The body needs sugar for energy. People with diabetes have too much sugar in the blood, and not enough glucose gets into body cells.

What Causes Diabetes?

Not enough insulin is the cause. In most diabetic people, the body's own defense, the immune system, destroys beta cells in the pancreas, but the reason for this isn't known.

Other causes are some diseases, such as cystic fibrosis, and surgical removal or severe inflammation (swelling, irritation) of the pancreas.

What Are the Symptoms of Diabetes?

Diabetes warning signs include urinating frequently, feeling very thirsty and hungry, getting infections, losing weight quickly, and feeling tired and weak. Symptoms of uncontrolled diabetes also include blurred vision or blindness, slow-healing skin sores, numbness in hands or feet, and kidney failure (needing dialysis).

In diabetic ketoacidosis, another complication of diabetes, substances (ketones) form when fats break down faster than kidneys can remove them. Ketones in blood make the blood dangerously acidic, which affects organs including the brain.

How Is Diabetes Diagnosed?

For diagnosis, the doctor uses a medical history, physical examination, and different measures of blood sugar (fasting level, average levels during 2 to 3 months [hemoglobin A1c test], glucose tolerance test).

The doctor may test the kidney function (serum creatinine level test), and check the urine (urine microalbumin level).

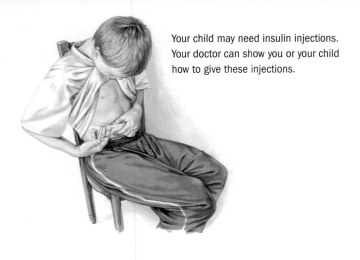

Your child may need insulin injections. Your doctor can show you or your child how to give these injections.

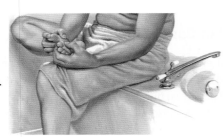

Help your child do regular foot check-ups.

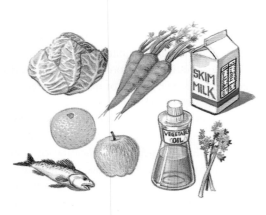

A healthy diet of lean protein and high fiber is essential. Ask your doctor for nutrition plans for your child.

How Is Diabetes Treated?

A special diet will help control blood sugar. A nutritionist can help manage this diet. A glucometer can be used to check blood sugar levels.

The doctor will explain how to give insulin injections at home. Children 7 to 10 years old can often check their own blood sugar levels. Children can also learn how to watch for signs of low blood sugar. Children 10 to 12 years old can often give themselves insulin.

The doctor will suggest exercises, because exercise affects blood sugar levels.

Regular foot care and eye checkups are needed to prevent complications.

DOs and DON'Ts in Managing Diabetes Mellitus:

✔ **DO** prepare the special diet and have your child eat snacks at the same time every day, as instructed by your doctor.

✔ **DO** make sure that your child gets enough exercise and sleep.

✔ **DO** check your sick child's blood sugar level. Call your doctor if your child has fever, nausea, or vomiting and can't keep down solids or liquids.

✔ **DO** call your doctor right away if your child's blood sugar level is too high.

✔ **DO** take your child to the hospital right away if he or she has a seizure, can't wake up, or loses consciousness.

✔ **DO** follow your doctor's orders about insulin exactly.

✔ **DO** give your child a sugar snack or glass of orange juice if the sugar level is too low and call the doctor to adjust future insulin doses.

🚫 **DON'T** let your child eat too much sugar.

🚫 **DON'T** give your child too much insulin.

🚫 **DON'T** let your child become dehydrated.

🚫 **DON'T** serve foods that are not suggested by your doctor.

FROM THE DESK OF

NOTES

FOR MORE INFORMATION

Contact the following sources:

• National Diabetes Information Clearinghouse
Tel: (800) 860-8747
Website: http://www.niddk.nih.gov/health/diabetes/diabetes.htm

• American Diabetes Association (ADA)
Tel: (800) DIABETES (342-2383)
Website: http://www.diabetes.org

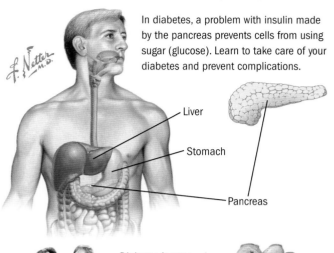

In diabetes, a problem with insulin made by the pancreas prevents cells from using sugar (glucose). Learn to take care of your diabetes and prevent complications.

Liver

Stomach

Pancreas

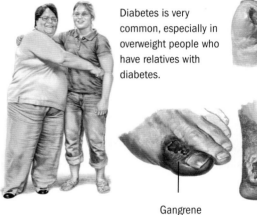

Diabetes is very common, especially in overweight people who have relatives with diabetes.

Ulcers

Gangrene

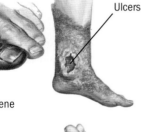

Uncontrolled diabetes can cause eye disease.

Loss of feeling

Diabetes may reduce circulation in your feet and cause ulcers, infections, and other problems.

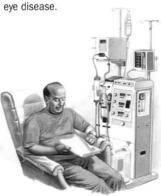

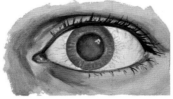

Untreated diabetes may lead to kidney failure that could require dialysis.

What Is Diabetes Mellitus Type 2?

Diabetes mellitus type 2, or type 2 diabetes (abbreviated DM), is one type of diabetes. In DM, a problem with insulin prevents body cells from using sugar (glucose) in food. Insulin is a chemical made by the pancreas. Insulin helps sugar enter body cells, which use the sugar for energy. DM involves poor responses of cells to insulin (insulin resistance) in type 2 DM, lack of insulin in type 1 DM, and too much sugar in the blood (hyperglycemia) in both types of DM.

People of any age can have DM. Type 2 DM occurs more often in overweight adults, especially those with diabetic relatives. DM is a lifelong illness.

Another name for type 2 DM is adult-onset diabetes.

What Causes Type 2 Diabetes?

In DM, when cells don't have or don't respond to insulin, they can't get the sugar. Sugar stays in the blood until some extra sugar goes into urine and is removed. Too much blood sugar damages blood vessels, which can cause serious diseases.

What Are the Symptoms of Type 2 Diabetes?

Symptoms start slowly but get worse, although some people have no symptoms. Some people complain of often being thirsty and hungry and may need to urinate often.

More symptoms are tiredness, blurred vision, chest pain or other heart trouble, weight gain or loss, foot ulcers, numbness or tingling in hands or feet, sores that don't heal, infections, and impotence (in men).

Serious complications of long-term DM include blindness, kidney failure, nerve damage, coronary heart disease, and peripheral vascular disease.

How Is Type 2 Diabetes Diagnosed?

The doctor uses a medical history, physical examination, and blood sugar levels for diagnosis.

Other laboratory tests include average sugar levels during 2 to 3 months (hemoglobin A1C [HbA1c] test) and glucose tolerance test. The doctor will also test the kidneys with blood and urine tests and the blood fat (lipid) level.

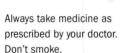

All diabetics should check blood glucose levels at home. You can learn the signs that tell you that your sugar level is too low.

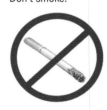

Always take medicine as prescribed by your doctor. Don't smoke.

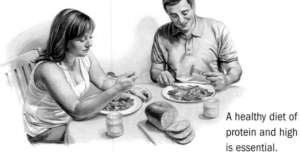

Take good care of your feet. Check them regularly.

A healthy diet of lean protein and high fiber is essential.

How Is Type 2 Diabetes Treated?

Many people control DM through just diet and exercise. New diet rules allow many food choices, but avoiding high-sugar and high-fat foods is important. Exercise helps control weight and keep blood sugar level down, and the body uses insulin better.

Some people need medicine, however. Medicine for type 2 DM usually consists of pills to help the body use sugar. If the pills don't work, insulin is given by injection.

Blood sugar levels must be tested often (usually at least daily). Being under the care of specialists (endocrinologist, podiatrist, eye doctor) in addition to your primary care doctor can also help prevent complications from diabetes.

DOs and DON'Ts in Managing Diabetes Mellitus Type 2:

✔ **DO** keep your blood sugar level near normal.
✔ **DO** exercise regularly.
✔ **DO** keep to a normal body weight.
✔ **DO** eat regular meals.
✔ **DO** eat healthy: whole-grain foods, fruit, vegetables, and high-quality proteins. Avoid high-sugar, high-fat, and white flour foods.
✔ **DO** keep alcohol intake low.
✔ **DO** have your eyes checked yearly and visit the dentist twice yearly.
✔ **DO** quit smoking.
✔ **DO** take good care of your feet. Visit your podiatrist at least twice per year.
✔ **DO** call your doctor if you have a fever or vomiting and cannot eat or drink.
✔ **DO** call your doctor if you have high or low blood sugar levels that you cannot explain.

🚫 **DON'T** smoke.
🚫 **DON'T** drink liquor or high-sugar liquids.

FOR MORE INFORMATION

Contact the following sources:
• National Diabetes Information Clearinghouse
  Tel: 1-800-860-8747
  Website: http://www.niddk.nih.gov/health/diabetes/diabetes.htm
• American Diabetes Association
  Tel: 1-800-DIABETES (1-800-342-2383)
  Website: http://www.diabetes.org

FROM THE DESK OF

NOTES

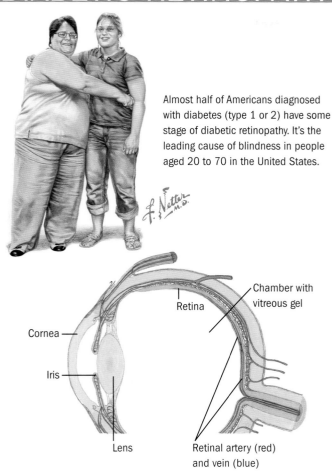

Almost half of Americans diagnosed with diabetes (type 1 or 2) have some stage of diabetic retinopathy. It's the leading cause of blindness in people aged 20 to 70 in the United States.

Cornea

Iris

Lens

Retina

Chamber with vitreous gel

Retinal artery (red) and vein (blue)

The retina is the part of the eye that lets us see. In diabetic retinopathy, blood vessels swell and leak fluid or blood, which causes blurred vision, or abnormal blood vessels form on the retina.

Normal retinal blood vessels

Macula

Nonproliferative retinopathy

Proliferative retinopathy

Bleeding (hemorrhages)

Small areas of balloonlike swelling in tiny blood vessels

New abnormal, fragile retinal blood vessels grow

What Is Diabetic Retinopathy?

Diabetic retinopathy is an eye disease caused by diabetes mellitus. It affects the retina, the part of the eye that lets us see. Diabetes hurts the retina's tiny blood vessels and can cause swelling and leaking of fluid into the eye. Extra retinal blood vessels can grow, which damages eyesight. Diabetic retinopathy is the leading cause of blindness in people 20 to 70 years old. All people with diabetes—type 1 or 2—are at risk. Almost half of Americans with diabetes have some stage of diabetic retinopathy. There are four stages of diabetic retinopathy. The first is early mild nonproliferative retinopathy, with small balloon-like swollen areas in tiny retinal blood vessels. Then moderate nonproliferative retinopathy occurs, with blocked blood vessels. Severe nonproliferative retinopathy follows (more blood vessels are blocked, and new vessels grow). In the advanced stage (proliferative retinopathy), new abnormal, fragile blood vessels grow along the retina and watery soft gel (vitreous gel) inside the eye.

What Causes Diabetic Retinopathy?

Damaged blood vessels can cause vision loss when fragile, abnormal blood vessels grow and leak blood into the center of the eye. This advanced stage is called proliferative retinopathy. Also, fluid can leak into the center of the macula of the eye, where sharp, straight-ahead vision occurs. The macula swells (macular edema) and vision becomes blurry.

What Are the Symptoms of Diabetic Retinopathy?

Symptoms include seeing a few specks of blood or floating spots. Bleeding (hemorrhages) in the vitreous can occur, without pain, and lead to blurred vision or blindness. Diabetic retinopathy often has no warning signs.

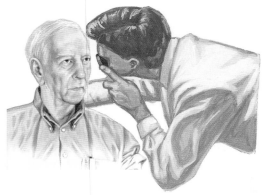

Your doctor will examine your eyes if you could have diabetic retinopathy. Your doctor will look for leaking blood vessels, retinal swelling (macular edema), damaged nerve tissue, and pale fatty deposits on the retina.

Two treatments for the disease are laser surgery and vitrectomy.

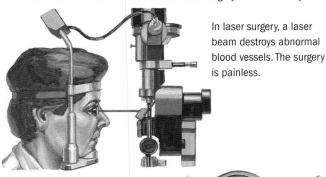

In laser surgery, a laser beam destroys abnormal blood vessels. The surgery is painless.

In vitrectomy, the watery substance (vitreous gel) that has blood in it is removed from the middle of the eye.

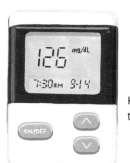

Keep your blood sugar levels under control to prevent the disease from getting worse.

FROM THE DESK OF

NOTES

How Is Diabetic Retinopathy Diagnosed?

The doctor makes a diagnosis by doing an examination to look for leaking blood vessels, retinal swelling, damaged nerve tissue, and pale fatty deposits on the retina. The doctor may order fluorescein angiography (using a special dye to see leaking vessels).

How Is Diabetic Retinopathy Treated?

For early disease, no treatment may be needed.

Two treatments can help people with advanced disease: laser surgery and vitrectomy (another operation). In the first procedure, which is painless, a laser beam is used to destroy abnormal blood vessels. Focal laser surgery is used for macular edema; a small laser burns slow leakage from vessels. A similar scatter laser treatment helps shrink abnormal blood vessels in proliferative retinopathy. In vitrectomy, blood that leaked from vessels is removed.

Control of blood sugar (glucose) levels and other risk factors (blood pressure and cholesterol) is important to prevent worsening disease.

DOs and DON'Ts in Managing Diabetic Retinopathy:

✔ **DO** watch your diet to control blood sugar levels.

✔ **DO** exercise.

✔ **DO** remember that untreated diabetic retinopathy can cause severe vision loss and blindness.

✔ **DO** remember that macular edema may need focal laser treatment more than once.

✔ **DO** call your doctor if you have symptoms of uncontrolled diabetes (e.g., increased thirst, increased urination, increased appetite with weight loss).

✔ **DO** call your doctor if you notice vision changes.

⊘ **DON'T** smoke or drink alcohol.

⊘ **DON'T** wait until you have symptoms. Get yearly eye examinations.

⊘ **DON'T** forget that proliferative retinopathy and macular edema can develop without symptoms.

FOR MORE INFORMATION

Contact the following sources:

• American Academy of Ophthalmology
Tel: (415) 561-8500
Website: http://www.aao.org

• American Diabetes Association
Tel: (800) DIABETES (342-2383)
Website: http://www.diabetes.org

• National Eye Institute
Tel: (301) 496-5248
Website: http://www.nei.nih.gov

MANAGING YOUR
ERECTILE DYSFUNCTION

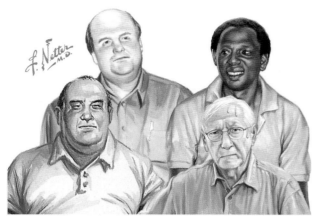

Erectile dysfunction (ED) is the inability to get or keep an erection. It becomes more common with age and affects 30% of men in their 70s.

Causes of ED

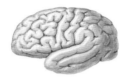

Psychological factors:
Depression, anxiety, stress

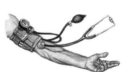

Vascular (blood vessel) factors: Diabetes, high blood pressure, drugs, atherosclerosis, high cholesterol, cigarette smoking

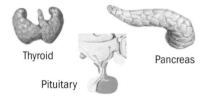

Thyroid

Pituitary

Pancreas

Hormonal factors:
Thyroid, pituitary, and pancreas (diabetes) disorders

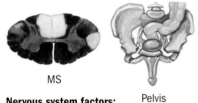

MS

Pelvis

Nervous system factors:
Multiple sclerosis (MS), pelvic fractures, radiation or surgery of pelvic organs, spinal cord injury

Cross section of penis

Flaccid state

Erect state

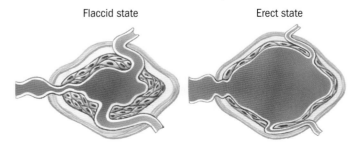

The main symptom is loss of the erection, because blood flow to the penis (which causes the erection) is lost or doesn't occur.

What Is Erectile Dysfunction?

Erectile dysfunction (ED), or male impotence, is a man's inability to get or keep an erection long enough to finish sexual activity. ED causes great distress and problems with relationships.

The percentage of men affected with ED increases with age. About 10% of men in their 60s and 30% in their 70s have ED.

What Causes Erectile Dysfunction?

Causes are both physical and psychological (psychogenic). Most older men with ED have heart and blood vessel disease. Other causes are medicines, nervous system problems, hormone deficiency, diabetes, hypertension, and smoking. Psychogenic ED, a result of emotional problems, is much more common and harder to diagnose.

What Are the Symptoms of Erectile Dysfunction?

The main symptom is inability to get or keep an erection until the end of sexual activity.

If the cause is psychological, men may have associated anxiety, mood swings, depression, insomnia, and concerns about sexual performance.

If the cause is physical, symptoms of medical illness may include poor circulation in the legs, chest pains, or shortness of breath with exercise (possible heart disease). Diabetes is frequently associated with ED.

How Is Erectile Dysfunction Diagnosed?

The doctor will ask about the firmness and duration of erections at different times (e.g., sex with partners, erections after sleep). Discussing sexual dysfunction with a doctor is very important because many conditions causing it can be successfully treated. If a man has no diseases that cause ED and can have an erection with masturbation or early morning awakening, he likely has ED due to psychological causes.

Your doctor will ask about the firmness and duration of erections at different times (e.g., sex with partners, in early morning). Talking with your doctor is very important because many causes of ED can be treated. Your doctor may give you medicine to increase blood flow to the penis (e.g., Viagra®, Levitra®, Cialis®).

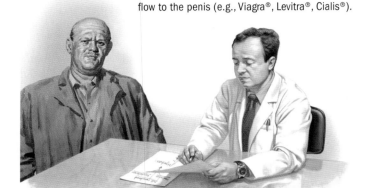

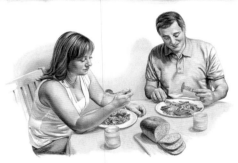

One of the most important things you can do is to relax with your partner. You and your partner can enjoy many sexual activities without intercourse. Focusing on pleasing your partner may help.

Exercise regularly, communicate with your partner, and eat a healthy diet.

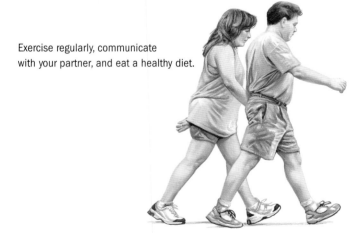

How Is Erectile Dysfunction Treated?

The basic treatment for performance anxiety is to ask the man to make love with his partner without trying intercourse, to show him how lovemaking can feel without a concern with failure. This method (called sensate focus) lets the man have a different focus: pleasing his partner and himself.

Men with physical causes of ED have options, including such medicines as sildenafil (Viagra®), vardenafil (Levitra®), or tadalafil (Cialis®). Men who use nitroglycerin products and those who should avoid sexual activity because of cardiovascular disease shouldn't take these drugs. Other treatment modalities include use of a vacuum pump or injection of a substance (papaverine) into the penis to increase blood flow to the penis. Men can also have surgery to put a prosthesis into the penis.

DOs and DON'Ts in Managing Erectile Dysfunction:

✔ **DO** discuss ED with your doctor.
✔ **DO** make sure that you tell your doctor all the medicines that you take because many, including antidepressants, can cause ED.
✔ **DO** talk with your partner. Keep lines of communication open.
✔ **DO** exercise regularly, eat a healthy diet, and relax.
✔ **DO** call your doctor if you see blood or discharge from your penis, sexual intercourse becomes painful, your erection lasts long after intercourse, or you have severe depression or suicidal thoughts.

⊘ **DON'T** expect to have normal sex during times of stress, grieving, or depression.
⊘ **DON'T** take Viagra®, Levitra®, or Cialis® if you use nitroglycerin products. These medicines may also interfere with vision and shouldn't be used within several hours of operating an airplane.

FROM THE DESK OF

NOTES

FOR MORE INFORMATION

Contact the following sources:

• WebMD
  Erectile Dysfunction Health Center
  Website: http://www.webmd.com/erectile-dysfunction/ default.htm

• American Academy of Family Physicians
  Tel: (800) 274-2237
  Website: http://www.aafp.org

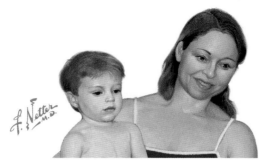

Galactorrhea is a condition in which an abnormal discharge comes from the nipple. It's fairly common in women who have had children and women who were recently pregnant or stopped breast-feeding.

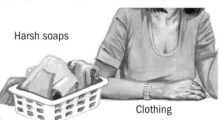

Harsh soaps

The cause is usually breast irritation, which can happen with injuries, surgery, squeezing the nipples, soaps, creams, and scratchy clothing. In women it's most likely to occur when estrogen (female hormone) levels change (such as when starting or stopping birth control pills).

Clothing

Birth control pills

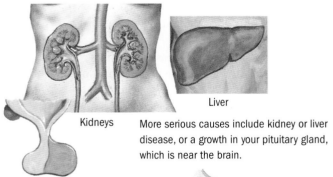

Liver

Kidneys

More serious causes include kidney or liver disease, or a growth in your pituitary gland, which is near the brain.

Pituitary gland

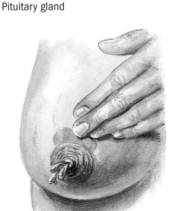

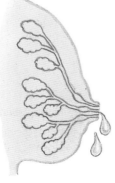

The main symptom is a milky fluid that seeps from the nipples of your breast.

What Is Galactorrhea?

Galactorrhea is a condition in which an abnormal discharge comes from the breast. A milky fluid seeps from the nipples of women who are not breast-feeding. It's fairly common in women who have had children and in women who were recently pregnant or stopped breast-feeding. It also occurs somewhat often in newborn infants (this used to be called witch's milk). In most women, it usually stops without treatment. It is a rare condition in men.

What Causes Galactorrhea?

The cause is usually irritation or stimulation of the breast, which can happen with an injury, surgery, or just squeezing the nipples. Soaps, creams, and scratchy clothing can also cause it.

In most women, galactorrhea is most likely when the level of female hormone (estrogen) changes, such as when starting or stopping birth control pills, after surgery to remove the ovaries, or after an abortion.

In women who never had a baby or in men, it can be due to a more serious problem. Such causes include medicines, kidney or liver disease, or a growth in the pituitary gland (an endocrine gland near the brain). This growth can be very serious because it may be cancerous, and this gland controls many body functions.

What Are the Symptoms of Galactorrhea?

The main symptom is a milky fluid seeping from the nipples. It may seep on its own or only if the nipples are squeezed.

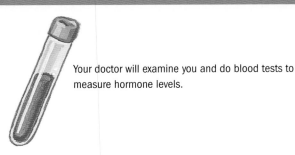
Your doctor will examine you and do blood tests to measure hormone levels.

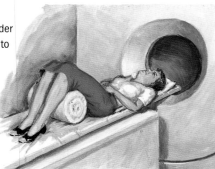
Your doctor may also order MRI or CT of your head, to see whether you have a growth on the pituitary gland. Surgery, medications, or radiation therapy will be used to treat a growth.

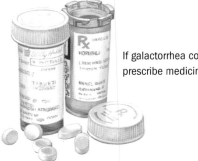
If galactorrhea continues, your doctor may prescribe medicine that will make it stop.

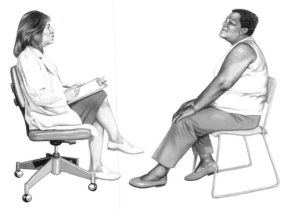
Keep all appointments with your doctor, and call your doctor if you have symptoms that worry you.

How Is Galactorrhea Diagnosed?

The doctor will do a physical examination and blood tests to measure hormone levels, such as prolactin.

Your doctor may also order magnetic resonance imaging (MRI) or computed tomography (CT) of the head. These tests take pictures of the inside of the head and may show whether there is a growth on the pituitary gland.

How Is Galactorrhea Treated?

If medicine is the cause, the doctor may say to stop taking it. If galactorrhea continues, the doctor may prescribe a medicine that will stop it.

Surgery, radiation therapy, or medications will be used to treat a growth on the pituitary gland. With surgery, the growth will be removed. With radiation therapy, a special x-ray machine is used and causes the growth to shrink. Radiation therapy works slowly, often taking several months to shrink the tumor. Medication will decrease the abnormal hormone levels produced by the pituitary.

DOs and DON'Ts in Managing Galactorrhea:

✔ **DO** wear a breast binder. A breast binder or firmly fitting bra can help prevent fabric from rubbing your nipples, which can cause stimulation or irritation and lead to galactorrhea.

✔ **DO** keep all doctor appointments.

✔ **DO** call your doctor about symptoms that worry you.

⊘ **DON'T** squeeze your breasts or nipples. This can stimulate your breasts and cause more milky fluid to seep from your nipples.

⊘ **DON'T** forget follow-up doctor appointments.

FROM THE DESK OF

NOTES

FOR MORE INFORMATION

Contact the following sources:

• Pituitary Network Association
Tel: (805) 499-9973
Website: http://www.pituitary.org

• American Academy of Family Physicians
Tel: (800) 274-2237
Website: http://www.aafp.org

MANAGING YOUR
GRAVES' DISEASE

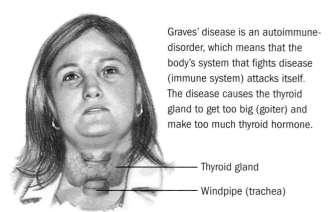

Graves' disease is an autoimmune-disorder, which means that the body's system that fights disease (immune system) attacks itself. The disease causes the thyroid gland to get too big (goiter) and make too much thyroid hormone.

— Thyroid gland
— Windpipe (trachea)

An overactive thyroid gland leads to abnormal heartbeats, high blood pressure, and nervousness.

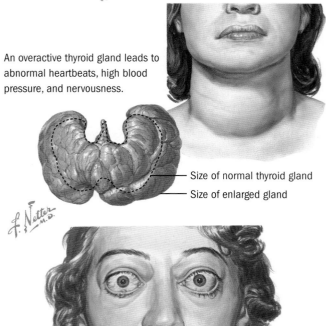

— Size of normal thyroid gland
— Size of enlarged gland

Graves' disease also causes eye problems, such as bulging of the eyeball, a staring look, blurred vision, and dryness.

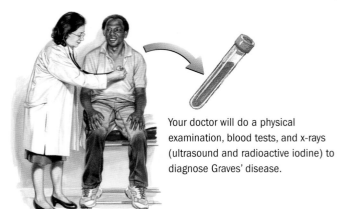

Your doctor will do a physical examination, blood tests, and x-rays (ultrasound and radioactive iodine) to diagnose Graves' disease.

What Is Graves' Disease?

The thyroid is an important endocrine gland found in the front of the neck. It produces substances (hormones) that act on metabolism and control mood, weight, and energy. Graves' disease is an autoimmune disease that is the most common cause of too much thyroid hormone (hyperthyroidism). It affects primarily women. An autoimmune disease is one in which the immune system of the body attacks itself and destroys healthy organs or tissues.

What Causes Graves' Disease?

The cause is substances called antibodies that stimulate the thyroid to get too big (goiter) and make too much hormone. Eye disease can result. It may run in families but cannot be caught from someone else.

What Are the Symptoms of Graves' Disease?

Symptoms include problems with the thyroid, eyes, and rarely the skin. Eye problems include blurred vision, dryness, bulging of the eyeball (exophthalmos), or a staring look. Double vision and blindness can occur if Graves' disease isn't treated.

An overactive thyroid gland results in fast or irregular heartbeat, high blood pressure, diarrhea, weight loss, increased sweating, and nervousness. Long-term complications include heart failure, bone loss (osteoporosis), and stroke.

How Is Graves' Disease Diagnosed?

The doctor will make a diagnosis from the medical history, physical examination, and blood tests for thyroid function and antibody levels.

X-rays (ultrasound of the gland and radioactive iodine study) may also be done.

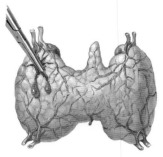

Before treatment—large thyroid that bleeds easily

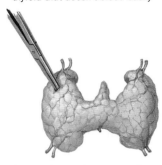

After drug treatment—smaller thyroid that doesn't bleed easily

Medicines, surgery, or radioactive iodine can be used to prevent the thyroid from making the hormone.

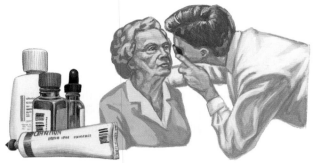

An eye doctor (ophthalmologist) must treat eye problems. Treatment includes eye drops, ointments, laser therapy, medications, and surgery. You should see your eye doctor at least once yearly.

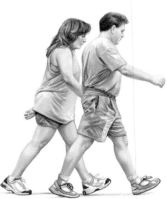

Exercise daily if your doctor says that you can. Regular exercise can improve your sense of well-being and overall health!

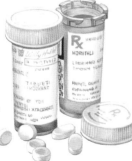

Thyroid medicines must be taken exactly as directed, because they leave the body very quickly.

How Is Graves' Disease Treated?

High thyroid hormone levels and eye problems can both be treated.

Medicine, surgery, and/or radioactive iodine are used for high hormone levels. Medicines such as propylthiouracil (PTU) and methimazole prevent the thyroid from producing hormone. Other medicines that may help are beta-blockers (such as propranolol), which reduce the hormone's damaging effect on the heart. These drugs have side effects and should be used with care.

Radioactive iodine usually has few side effects, gives permanent results, and is very effective, but it cannot be used during pregnancy. It can be done as an outpatient or with a short hospital stay. The long-term risk is an underactive thyroid (hypothyroidism), so thyroid supplements may be needed lifelong after radioactive iodine treatment.

People who cannot have radiation therapy or cannot use oral antithyroid medicines may have surgery. Surgery risks damage to vocal cord nerves and glands that regulate calcium.

An eye doctor (ophthalmologist) should check for eye problems at least once yearly. Treatments for eye disease include laser therapy, surgery, eye drops, medications, and ointments.

DOs and DON'Ts in Managing Graves' Disease:

✔ **DO** take your medicines exactly as prescribed. Skipping doses makes medicines useless.
✔ **DO** exercise daily if your doctor says you can. Daily exercise can improve your well-being and health.
✔ **DO** visit your eye doctor at least once yearly or more, if needed.
✔ **DO** call your doctor if you have palpitations, shortness of breath, chest pain, or sudden worsening of nervousness or jitters.
✔ **DO** call your doctor if you have eye pain or vision changes, sore throat, fever, chills, nausea, or vomiting.

⊘ **DON'T** skip medicine doses.
⊘ **DON'T** miss your laboratory test appointments.

FROM THE DESK OF

NOTES

FOR MORE INFORMATION

Contact the following source:

• Thyroid Foundation of America
Tel: (800) 832-8321
Website: http://www.allthyroid.org

MANAGING YOUR
GYNECOMASTIA

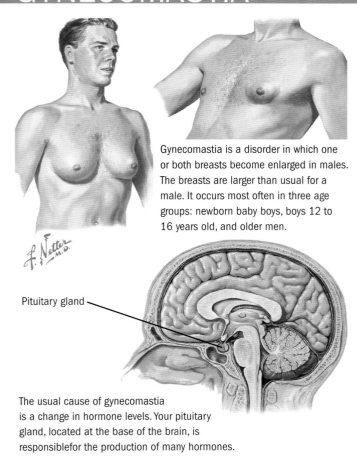

Gynecomastia is a disorder in which one or both breasts become enlarged in males. The breasts are larger than usual for a male. It occurs most often in three age groups: newborn baby boys, boys 12 to 16 years old, and older men.

Pituitary gland

The usual cause of gynecomastia is a change in hormone levels. Your pituitary gland, located at the base of the brain, is responsiblefor the production of many hormones.

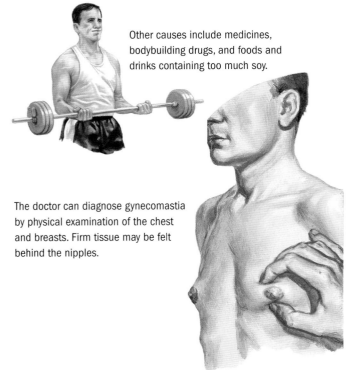

Other causes include medicines, bodybuilding drugs, and foods and drinks containing too much soy.

The doctor can diagnose gynecomastia by physical examination of the chest and breasts. Firm tissue may be felt behind the nipples.

What Is Gynecomastia?

Gynecomastia is a disorder in which one or both breasts become enlarged in males. It occurs most often in three age groups: newborn baby boys, boys 12 to 16 years old, and older men. In the boys, breasts may return to normal in 6 months to 3 years after puberty.

What Causes Gynecomastia?

The usual cause in boys is a change in hormone levels during puberty. Hormone changes can also occur in baby boys and older men.

Some medicines, illegal drugs, and drugs used for bodybuilding can cause gynecomastia, as can foods and drinks containing too much soy. Rare causes include tumors, birth defects, and liver disease.

What Are the Symptoms of Gynecomastia?

Breasts are larger than is typical for males. An area of firm tissue can be felt behind the nipples. Breasts may be tender but aren't usually painful.

How Is Gynecomastia Diagnosed?

The doctor can diagnose gynecomastia by physical examination of the chest and breasts. Blood tests may be done to check hormone levels and look for other causes. Sometimes other tests, such as mammography and a sonogram of the breast are needed to exclude breast tumors.

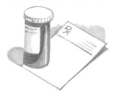

Treatment includes weight loss in overweight males, avoidance of medicines associated with gynecomastia, or surgery (breast reduction). Boys 12 to 16 years old and newborn babies aren't usually treated.

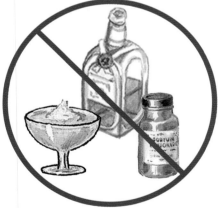

If you are overweight, talk to your doctor about an exercise and diet plan.

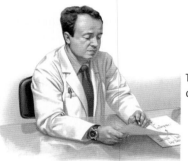

Talk to a counselor if you're distressed about your condition.

Don't take bodybuilding drugs, drink alcohol in excess, or eat or drink soy-containing products.

How Is Gynecomastia Treated?

Treatment includes lifestyle changes to promote weight loss, avoidance of medications associated with gynecomastia, or surgery. Many times, lifestyle changes alone are enough. Boys 12 to 16 years old and newborn babies aren't usually treated. If the condition has lasted less than 1 year, it usually responds well to treatment. It may not go away in someone who has finished puberty and has gynecomastia lasting for more than 1 year.

For hormone level problems, medicine may balance the levels and may help breast tissue return to normal. The doctor may suggest seeing a specialist called an endocrinologist, a doctor who is an expert in the study of hormones.

When other treatments fail, an operation called breast reduction surgery can remove breast tissue. This operation is generally thought of as cosmetic and may not be covered by medical insurance.

DOs and DON'Ts in Managing Gynecomastia:

✔ **DO** tell your doctor about medicines you take.
✔ **DO** tell your doctor about cosmetic products you use.
✔ **DO** tell your doctor if you don't feel well while taking medicine for gynecomastia.
✔ **DO** talk to a counselor if you're distressed about your condition.
✔ **DO** lose weight if you're overweight.
✔ **DO** call your doctor if your breasts become sore or red, because you may have an infection.

⊘ **DON'T** drink alcohol in excess.
⊘ **DON'T** use bodybuilding drugs.
⊘ **DON'T** include large amounts of soy products in your diet.
⊘ **DON'T** use cosmetics that include the female hormone estrogen.

FROM THE DESK OF

NOTES

FOR MORE INFORMATION

Contact the following source:

• American Society of Plastic Surgeons
  Tel: (888) 475-2784
  Website: http://www.plasticsurgery.org

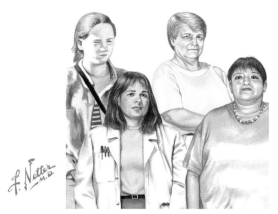

Hirsutism is the growth of too much hair on the face and body of women in places usually seen in men. It's very common, occurring in 5% to 10% of women, and isn't usually serious.

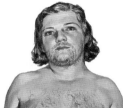

Dark, thick hair grows on the upper lip, chin, and sideburns. Hair also grows on the upper back, neck, chest, thighs, and belly.

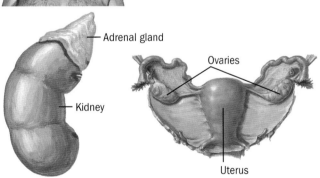

Women normally make small amounts of male sex hormones (androgens) in the ovaries and adrenal glands. Problems in these organs can lead to too much hormone being made. Serious causes of hirsutism may also cause menstrual problems, acne, and deepening of the voice.

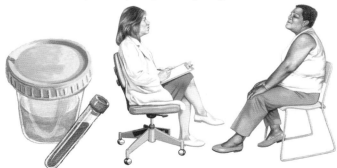

Your doctor will examine you and take blood and urine samples to test. Imaging, such as a CT or MRI, may also be done for diagnosis.

What Is Hirsutism?

Hirsutism refers to the growth of too much hair on the face and body in women. Thick, dark hair grows in areas where men have hair: upper lip, chin, and sideburns. Hirsutism is very common, occurring in 5% to 10% of women, and it's usually not serious. Increased body hair is also normal in Caucasian women of Mediterranean origin. Most women do not need medical care. Therapy may improve hirsutism, but it may take months to work. Hirsutism cannot be prevented.

What Causes Hirsutism?

The cause is production of too much male sex hormones (called androgens). Women normally make small amounts of androgens in their ovaries and adrenal glands. Problems in these organs can lead to too much hormone being made. Certain endocrine disorders (e.g., Cushing's syndrome, acromegaly) may cause hair to grow. Tumors in adrenal glands or ovaries may also cause high hormone levels. Other less serious disorders of these organs, including polycystic ovary syndrome (PCOS) and congenital adrenal hyperplasia (CAH), can also lead to hirsutism.

Other sources of androgens are medicines, including steroids, phenytoin, diazoxide, progestins, cyclosporine, and minoxidil.

Some women have idiopathic hirsutism, meaning that the cause is unknown.

What Are the Symptoms of Hirsutism?

Hair develops on the face (as a beard or mustache) and body, specifically the upper lip, chin, sideburns, upper back, neck, chest, thighs, belly, and around the nipples. Hair becomes thick and dark. Women may also have problems with periods, with fertility, and have acne.

Serious causes can mean rapid growth of hairs, balding, deepening of the voice, muscle development, change in sexual desire, or infertility.

How Is Hirsutism Diagnosed?

The doctor will do a physical examination and take blood and urine samples to measure levels of the androgens called testosterone and dehydroepiandrosterone sulfate (DHEAS). The doctor may order computed tomography (CT) or magnetic resonance imaging (MRI) to check organs that may be the cause.

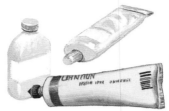

Mild cases need no treatment. Ways to remove unwanted hair include shaving, plucking, waxing, using creams (depilatories), electrolysis, and laser light (permanent removal).

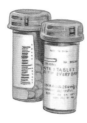

Medicine containing female sex hormone is usually prescribed for menstrual problems. It may take 6 months to see results, so be patient.

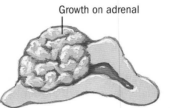

Growth on adrenal

If growths on the adrenal glands or ovaries are causing hirsutism, you'll need surgery to remove the growths.

Growth on ovary

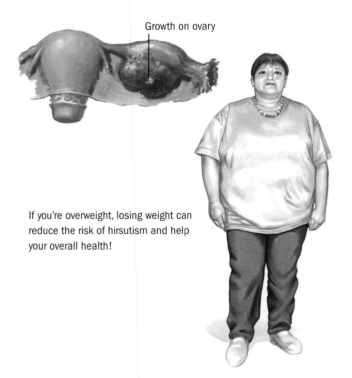

If you're overweight, losing weight can reduce the risk of hirsutism and help your overall health!

How Is Hirsutism Treated?

Treatment depends on the cause. No treatment may be needed for a mild case with no menstrual problems. Ways to remove unwanted hair include medicines, shaving, plucking, bleaching, waxing, using creams (depilatories), and electrolysis or laser light (for permanent removal).

For hirsutism related to menstrual problems, the doctor may prescribe medicine that contains female sex hormones. Other treatment may be needed to get pregnant.

Growths on ovaries or adrenal glands can be removed surgically.

DOs and DON'Ts in Managing Hirsutism:

✔ **DO** follow your doctor's advice. Contact your doctor if you had successful treatment and unwanted hair returns.

✔ **DO** lose weight if you're overweight. Weight loss reduces hirsutism.

✔ **DO** tell your doctor if you shaved, plucked, or bleached your hair or if you received electrolysis.

✔ **DO** tell your doctor if you want to become pregnant.

✔ **DO** consider bleaching, shaving, and electrolysis.

✔ **DO** call your doctor if you notice male pattern hair growth.

✔ **DO** call your doctor if you have side effects from your medicine.

○ **DON'T** use medicine that contains male sex hormones unless your doctor prescribes it.

○ **DON'T** expect hirsutism to go away completely or immediately. Successful drug treatment may take 3 to 6 months.

FROM THE DESK OF

NOTES

FOR MORE INFORMATION

Contact the following source:

• The Endocrine Society
Tel: (301) 941-0200
Website: http://www.endo-society.org

MANAGING YOUR
HOT FLASHES

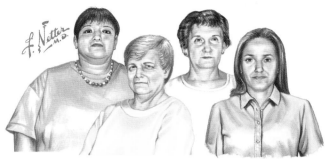

Hot flashes are sudden feelings of intense warmth that start in the neck, face, or chest. They affect 75% of women after menopause.

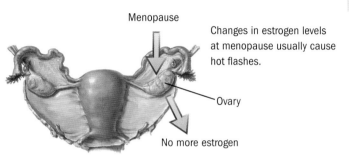

Menopause

Changes in estrogen levels at menopause usually cause hot flashes.

Ovary

No more estrogen

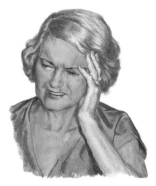

The face, neck, chest, back, and arms become red (flushed), followed by heavy sweating.

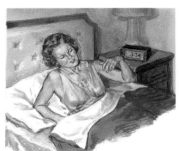

Flashes can be as mild as a light blush or bad enough to wake you from a sound sleep (night sweats).

Your doctor may order blood tests, such as thyroid function tests, and special hormone studies (e.g., follicle stimulating hormone, luteinizing hormone, serum estrogen) for diagnosis.

What Are Hot Flashes?

Hot flashes are sudden feelings of intense warmth that start in the neck, face, or chest and often occur with sweating and anxiety. Hot flashes occur most often in women at menopause (change of life, when periods stop). Most begin 1 to 2 years before menopause and stop after 2 years, but some women have hot flashes for more than 15 years! They affect 75% of women after menopause.

What Causes Hot Flashes?

Changes in the level of the female hormone estrogen at menopause usually cause hot flashes. Chemotherapy causing ovaries to stop working and use of tamoxifen, a drug treatment for breast cancer, are other causes.

Hormone therapy to block or inhibit the male hormone testosterone, used in men for prostate cancer, and the medication niacin can also cause flushing.

Hot flashes cannot be caught or passed on from parents to children (inherited).

What Are the Symptoms of Hot Flashes?

Symptoms include sudden feelings of heat in the upper or whole body. The face, neck, chest, back, and arms become red (flushed). Heavy sweating and cold shivering can follow. Flashes can be mild or bad enough to awaken people from sound sleep (called night sweats). Most flashes last between 30 seconds and 5 minutes and vary in frequency, with one third of women reporting more than 10 flashes per day.

Palpitations, brisk reflexes, and increases in temperature, heart rate, and blood flow to the hands and face also occur.

How Are Hot Flashes Diagnosed?

The doctor may order blood tests (such as thyroid function tests) and special hormone studies (e.g., follicle stimulating hormone, luteinizing hormone, estrogen level) to find out whether another condition may be causing hot flashes. Such other conditions include hyperthyroidism (overactive thyroid gland), anxiety, lymphoma, and carcinoid syndrome (rare tumor in the gastrointestinal system).

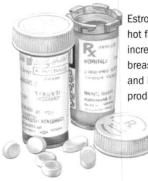

Estrogen replacement therapy can reduce hot flashes by 80% to 90% but may increase the risk of getting uterine cancer, breast cancer, heart attacks, strokes, and blood clots. Options such as herbal products have also been tried.

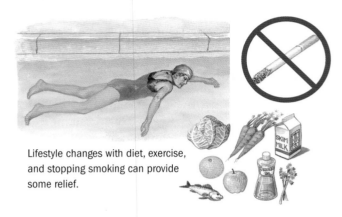

Lifestyle changes with diet, exercise, and stopping smoking can provide some relief.

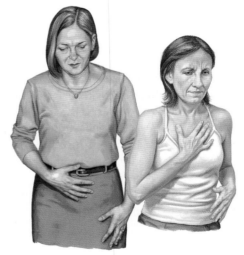

Call your doctor if you have hot flashes occurring with other symptoms, such as diarrhea, nausea, vomiting, fever, chills, palpitations, chest pains, or abdominal pains.

FROM THE DESK OF

NOTES

How Are Hot Flashes Treated?

The cause of the hot flashes must be treated. For example, giving estrogen to postmenopausal women to replace missing hormone, called estrogen replacement therapy (ERT), reduces hot flashes by 80% to 90%. Estrogen therapy may increase the risk of uterine cancer, breast cancer, heart attacks, strokes, and blood clots and can have side effects of abdominal bloating and breast tenderness. Options such as herbal products have also been tried but are generally ineffective.

Other drugs, including antidepressants called selective serotonin reuptake inhibitors (e.g., fluoxetine, paroxetine), anti-seizure medications (e.g., gabapentin), vitamin E, and soy protein (estrogens from plants), are often used with limited success.

DOs and DON'Ts in Managing Hot Flashes:

✔ **DO** realize that nonmedical treatments (e.g., air conditioners, fans, cold water) have been tried with different degrees of success. Lifestyle changes with diet, exercise, and stopping smoking can provide some relief.

✔ **DO** call your doctor if you also have other symptoms, such as diarrhea, nausea, vomiting, fever, chills, palpitations, chest pains, or pains in the abdomen (belly). These may suggest other conditions (e.g., infections, hyperthyroidism, carcinoid syndrome, myocardial infarction).

✔ **DO** call your doctor if you think that you're going through menopause and have concerns about using ERT.

🚫 **DON'T** use medicines for hot flashes unless hot flashes are severe and have a major impact on your life.

FOR MORE INFORMATION

Contact the following source:

• American College of Obstetricians and Gynecologists
Tel: (202) 638-5577
Website: http://www. acog.org

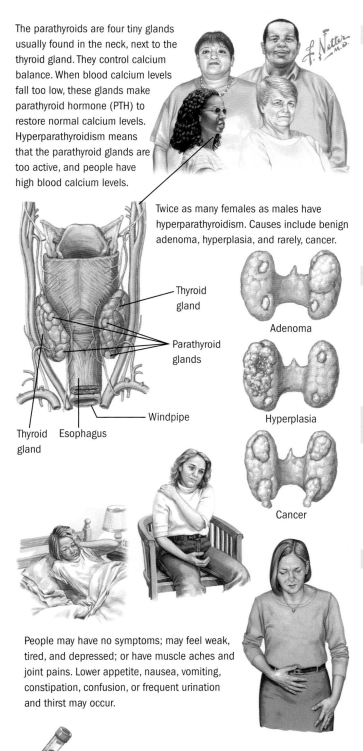

The parathyroids are four tiny glands usually found in the neck, next to the thyroid gland. They control calcium balance. When blood calcium levels fall too low, these glands make parathyroid hormone (PTH) to restore normal calcium levels. Hyperparathyroidism means that the parathyroid glands are too active, and people have high blood calcium levels.

Twice as many females as males have hyperparathyroidism. Causes include benign adenoma, hyperplasia, and rarely, cancer.

Thyroid gland

Parathyroid glands

Windpipe

Thyroid gland   Esophagus

Adenoma

Hyperplasia

Cancer

People may have no symptoms; may feel weak, tired, and depressed; or have muscle aches and joint pains. Lower appetite, nausea, vomiting, constipation, confusion, or frequent urination and thirst may occur.

Your doctor makes a diagnosis by measuring blood levels of calcium and PTH. High levels of both confirm the diagnosis.

What Is Hyperparathyroidism?

The parathyroids are four tiny glands usually found in the neck, next to the thyroid gland. They control calcium balance in the body. When blood calcium levels fall too low, these glands make a hormone to restore normal calcium levels. This hormone is named parathyroid hormone (PTH). Hyperparathyroidism means that the parathyroid glands are too active, and people have high blood calcium levels. Untreated hyperparathyroidism can lead to osteoporosis, kidney stones, high blood pressure, inflammation (swelling) of the pancreas, or stomach ulcers.

About 100,000 people per year are diagnosed with hyperparathyroidism, twice as many females as males.

What Causes Hyperparathyroidism?

Most people (85%) have a benign (not cancerous) parathyroid gland tumor (adenoma). Others may have enlarged parathyroid glands (hyperplasia). Rarely, the cause is cancer. Aging increases the risk. Some people have disorders related to other endocrine conditions.

What Are the Symptoms of Hyperparathyroidism?

People may have no symptoms. Some may feel weak, tired, and depressed or have muscle aches and joint pains. They may have less appetite, nausea, vomiting, constipation, confusion, or frequent urination and thirst.

How Is Hyperparathyroidism Diagnosed?

The doctor makes a diagnosis by measuring blood levels of calcium and PTH. High levels of both confirm the diagnosis.

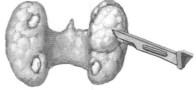
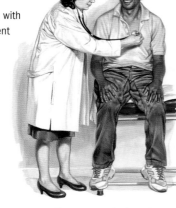

Only people with high calcium levels, bothersome symptoms, or possible cancer need surgery. Following surgery, a low calcium level, temporary or permanent, may occur. Calcium and vitamin D supplements may be taken to restore normal levels.

The doctor may just watch people with enlarged parathyroids, with frequent measurement of blood calcium levels. In an emergency (very high calcium levels), intravenous fluids and medicines may be given to lower the levels.

Don't let yourself become dehydrated. Dehydration will increase your calcium levels.

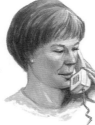

Call your doctor if you notice muscle spasms, face twitching, or numbness around the lips after surgery on the parathyroid glands. These symptoms of a very low blood calcium level are due to underactive parathyroids and need attention right away.

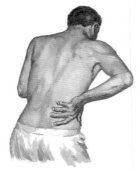

Call your doctor if you have symptoms of a kidney stone, including severe pain on your side or back and blood in your urine.

FROM THE DESK OF

NOTES

How Is Hyperparathyroidism Treated?

A parathyroid gland tumor is best removed surgically. Only people with high calcium levels, bothersome symptoms, or possible cancer need surgery. Surgery cures 95% of people. Complications of surgery include low calcium level, bleeding, and infection. The low calcium level that occurs may be temporary or permanent. Many doctors suggest taking calcium and vitamin D supplements.

The doctor may just watch people with enlarged parathyroids and monitor them with frequent measurement of blood calcium levels. In an emergency (a very high calcium level), intravenous fluids and medicines may be given to lower the levels.

DOs and DON'Ts in Managing Hyperparathyroidism:

✔ **DO** tell your doctor if you have a family history of parathyroid or other endocrine tumors. Make sure that your doctor has your old records of blood calcium measures.

✔ **DO** drink plenty of water to prevent high blood calcium levels.

✔ **DO** find an experienced surgeon for your operation.

✔ **DO** see your doctor regularly if no surgery is planned. Blood, urine, bone density, and kidney function tests should be done regularly.

✔ **DO** call your doctor if you become dehydrated or immobilized because of trauma or illness, as this may affect your calcium level.

✔ **DO** call your doctor if you have symptoms of a kidney stone, including severe pain on your side or back and blood in your urine.

✔ **DO** call your doctor if you notice muscle spasms, face twitching, or numbness around the lips after surgery on the parathyroid glands. These symptoms of a very low blood calcium level are due to a low level of parathyroid hormone and need attention right away.

⊘ **DON'T** let yourself become dehydrated. Dehydration will increase your calcium level.

⊘ **DON'T** take calcium supplements unless your doctor approves. They can lead to kidney stone formation and high blood calcium levels.

FOR MORE INFORMATION

Contact the following sources:

• American Association of Clinical Endocrinologists
  Tel: (904) 353-7878
  Website: http://www.aace.com

• National Health Information Center
  Tel: (800) 336-4797
  Website: http://www.health.gov/nhic/

Hyperthyroidism is an illness caused by a thyroid gland that's too active. Three times more women than men have it.

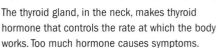

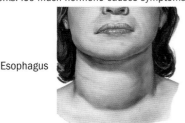

The thyroid gland, in the neck, makes thyroid hormone that controls the rate at which the body works. Too much hormone causes symptoms.

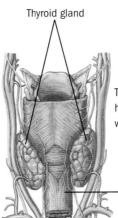

Thyroid gland

Esophagus

Windpipe

Goiter

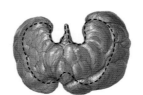

Dashed line shows normal gland size

Bulging eyes, eye irritation

The most common cause is Graves' disease. People with this disease have an enlarged thyroid gland (goiter) and may have bulging eyeballs (exophthalmos). Other causes are thyroiditis, toxic adenoma, and using too much thyroid medicine. Sometimes the cause isn't known.

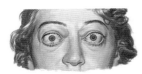

Symptoms include

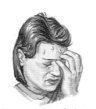

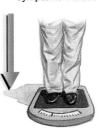

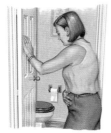

Nervousness, fatigue, sweating

Weight loss

Frequent bowel movements or diarrhea

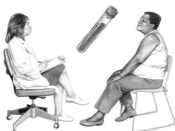

Your doctor makes a diagnosis from a medical history, physical examination, and blood tests. A thyroid scan or ultrasonography may be done. The doctor may also suggest seeing an endocrinologist.

What Is Hyperthyroidism?

Hyperthyroidism is an illness caused by a thyroid gland that's too active. The thyroid gland is located in the neck and makes thyroid hormone. This hormone controls the rate at which the body works. Too much hormone causes symptoms of hyperthyroidism. Three times more women than men have an overactive thyroid.

What Causes Hyperthyroidism?

The most common cause is a condition called Graves' disease. This disease causes 80% to 90% of cases. This disease is thought to be autoimmune. Autoimmune means that the body's own immune system attacks itself. In Graves' disease, the thyroid gland is attacked. Other less common causes include thyroiditis, toxic adenoma, and using too much thyroid medicine. Thyroiditis is inflammation of the thyroid. An adenoma is a thyroid tumor that makes thyroid hormone. Sometimes the cause isn't known. This illness can run in families, but it's not contagious.

What Are the Symptoms of Hyperthyroidism?

Symptoms include nervousness, sweating, fatigue, and fast or skipped heartbeats or other heart rhythm abnormalities such as atrial fibrulation. Others are eye irritation, weight loss, sensitivity to heat, and frequent bowel movements or diarrhea. People with Graves' disease have an enlarged thyroid gland (goiter) and may have bulging eyeballs (exophthalmos).

How Is Hyperthyroidism Diagnosed?

The doctor makes a diagnosis from the medical history, physical examination, and blood tests to measure blood thyroid hormone levels. The doctor may also order a thyroid scan or ultrasonography to get pictures of the thyroid gland.

The doctor may also suggest seeing a thyroid specialist (endocrinologist).

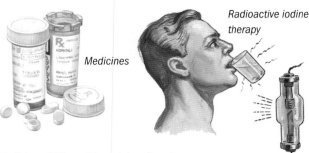

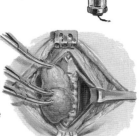
Medicines

Radioactive iodine therapy

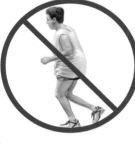
Surgery

Medicines (PTU, methimazole), radioactive therapy, and surgery lower thyroid hormone levels. Radioactive iodine is used to destroy the thyroid. Radiotherapy is best for people older than 21 and younger people who can't control the disease with medicines. Surgery is for people with large thyroids that interfere with neck structures, people who don't want radioactive iodine, and pregnant women, who shouldn't use radioactive iodine.

Don't exercise until your illness is controlled.

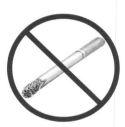

Don't smoke! Smoking may worsen eye problems from Graves' disease. Protect your eyes by wearing sunglasses and using artificial tears if you have exophthalmos.

Call your doctor if you have palpitations, serious weight loss, diarrhea, tremors, restlessness, anxiety, or mood swings.

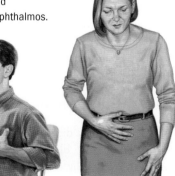

How Is Hyperthyroidism Treated?

Thyroid hormone levels are lowered with medicines, radiation therapy, or surgery. Medicines may be needed for a few months, a few years, or more. Ones that prevent thyroid hormone production include propylthiouracil (PTU) and methimazole. They can be used as the main therapy or to prepare for other treatments.

Radioactive iodine is used to destroy the thyroid. This therapy is best for people older than 21 and younger people who can't control their disease with medicines.

Surgery is for people with large thyroid glands that block or interfere with other structures in the neck. People who don't want to use radioactive iodine may have surgery. Pregnant women may also need surgery.

DOs and DON'Ts in Managing Hyperthyroidism:

✔ **DO** protect your eyes if you have eye complications of Graves' disease. Use sunglasses and artificial tears, and wear eye protection at night.

✔ **DO** remember that radioactive iodine shouldn't be used during pregnancy. It may cause an underactive thyroid condition in the baby.

✔ **DO** realize that successful treatment means that you need lifelong care. The doctor must check you for onset of an underactive thyroid gland (hypothyroidism) after treatment and for possible recurrence of hyperthyroidism.

✔ **DO** call your doctor if you have palpitations, serious weight loss, diarrhea, or tremors.

✔ **DO** call your doctor if you have restlessness, anxiety, or mood swings.

⊘ **DON'T** do physical exercise until your illness is controlled.

⊘ **DON'T** smoke. Smoking may worsen eye problems.

⊘ **DON'T** forget that complications of surgery may include paralysis of vocal cords, underactive thyroid (hypothyroidism), and calcium problems. Calcium problems can result if parathyroid glands are accidentally removed.

⊘ **DON'T** forget that hyperthyroidism may recur after surgery in 10% to 15% of people.

FROM THE DESK OF

NOTES

FOR MORE INFORMATION

Contact the following sources:

• American Association of Clinical Endocrinologists
  Tel: (904) 353-7878
  Website: http://www.aace.com

• Thyroid Foundation of America
  Tel: (800) 832-8321
  Website: http://www.allthyroid.org

Hypoglycemia means that your blood sugar (glucose) level is too low. It occurs when insulin and glucose aren't in balance. In diabetes, usually the blood sugar level is too high but sometimes it can be low after excessive doses of insulin or diabetic medications.

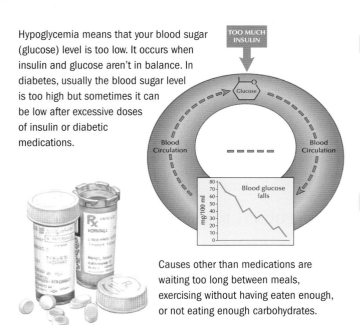

Causes other than medications are waiting too long between meals, exercising without having eaten enough, or not eating enough carbohydrates.

Symptoms include:

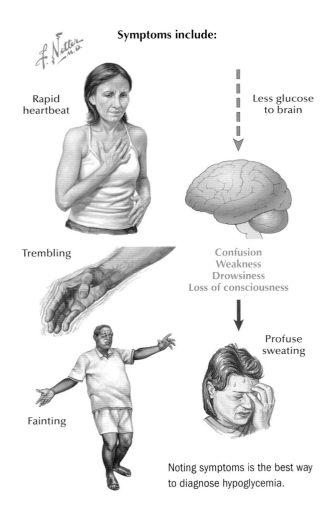

Rapid heartbeat

Less glucose to brain

Trembling

Confusion
Weakness
Drowsiness
Loss of consciousness

Profuse sweating

Fainting

Noting symptoms is the best way to diagnose hypoglycemia.

What Is Hypoglycemia?

Hypoglycemia means that a person's blood sugar (glucose) level is too low. In diabetes, the blood sugar level is usually too high (hyperglycemia), but sometimes blood sugar can be low after treatment. Because hypoglycemia can cause people to pass out (lose consciousness), symptoms must be recognized and treated right away.

What Causes Hypoglycemia?

Hypoglycemia occurs when insulin and glucose aren't in balance. This problem can occur after taking too much insulin or another diabetes medicine, not eating enough or waiting too long between meals (such as overnight), exercising without having eaten enough, or not eating enough carbohydrates. Foods rich in carbohydrates include pasta, rice, potatoes, bread, tortillas, cereal, milk, yogurt, fruit, and sweets.

What Are the Symptoms of Hypoglycemia?

Symptoms include shakiness; dizziness; sweating; hunger; headache; rapid heartbeats; pale skin color; sudden moodiness or behavior problems, such as crying for no reason; clumsy, jerky movements; confusion or trouble paying attention; tingling around the mouth; and seizures.

How Is Hypoglycemia Diagnosed?

Symptoms are the best way to tell whether hypoglycemia is occurring. People having any of the symptoms should immediately have a sugar snack and check their blood glucose level right away.

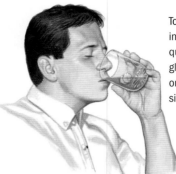

To get a normal balance between insulin and glucose, eat sugar quickly. This snack could be three glucose tablets (from a drugstore), one-half cup of fruit juice, or five or six pieces of hard candy.

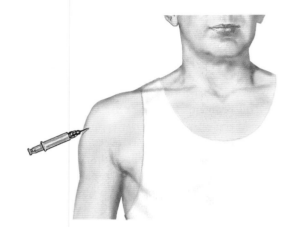

Be sure that people at work and at home know how to give you a shot of glucagon if you lose consciousness.

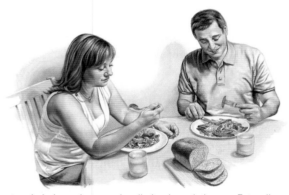

Prevent an imbalance between insulin levels and glucose. Eat well-balanced meals with the right amount of carbohydrates. Carbohydrate-rich foods include pasta, rice, potatoes, bread, tortillas, cereal, milk, yogurt, fruit, and sweets.

FROM THE DESK OF

NOTES

How Is Hypoglycemia Treated?

To return the balance between insulin and glucose to normal, sugar should be eaten quickly. Three glucose tablets (available at a drugstore), one-half cup of fruit juice, or five or six pieces of hard candy should help. This snack should help within 15 to 20 minutes, when the blood sugar level should be checked again. If the level isn't normal, another snack should be eaten and blood sugar level checked again 15 to 20 minutes later.

If these snacks don't help and loss of consciousness occurs, emergency treatment is needed. A doctor or someone trained to give shots (family members or co-workers) can give a shot of glucagon. If no one who knows about glucagon is available, someone should call 911 immediately.

DOs and DON'Ts in Managing Hypoglycemia:

✔ **DO** take steps to prevent an imbalance between insulin levels and glucose.
✔ **DO** eat regular, well-balanced meals with the amount of carbohydrates that your doctor or dietitian approved.
✔ **DO** take your insulin or other diabetic medicine as prescribed.
✔ **DO** check your blood sugar level according to the schedule that your doctor gave you.
✔ **DO** keep sugar pills, fruit juice, or hard candy handy.
✔ **DO** be aware of symptoms of hypoglycemia.
✔ **DO** eat enough carbohydrates before exercise and snack during exercise if needed.
✔ **DO** eat snacks as soon as your sugar level is too low or you get symptoms.
✔ **DO** explain to people with whom you live and work that you have diabetes and how to inject glucagon if you lose consciousness.
✔ **DO** call your doctor if you have hypoglycemic symptoms. Your medicine doses may need adjusting.

⊘ **DON'T** wait too long between meals.
⊘ **DON'T** exercise without eating enough carbohydrates.
⊘ **DON'T** ignore symptoms of hypoglycemia or put off treating hypoglycemia. Hypoglycemia can lead to coma and brain damage.
⊘ **DON'T** become discouraged if you have type 1 diabetes and it takes time to adjust your insulin dose to allow exercise.

FOR MORE INFORMATION

Contact the following source:

• American Diabetes Association
 Tel: (800) 342-2383
 Website: http://www.diabetes.org

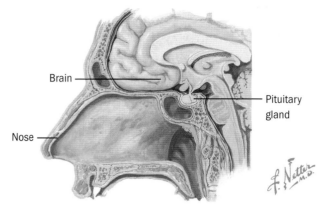

Hypopituitarism, or underactive pituitary gland, occurs when the pituitary gland doesn't produce enough hormones. The pituitary is important for controlling water balance, blood pressure, sexual function, stress responses, and metabolism.

Causes include pituitary tumors or other brain tumors, pituitary bleeding or surgery, trauma, brain infections, stroke, congenital abnormalities, and brain radiation.

Pituitary gland with small, slow-growing tumor

Trauma (skull fracture) causing bleeding

Stroke (bleeding in brain)

Symptoms include headache, blurred vision, and sensitivity to light. You can have other symptoms if other organs such as ovaries, testes, thyroid, or adrenal glands are affected.

What Is Hypopituitarism?

Hypopituitarism, or underactive pituitary gland, occurs when the pituitary gland doesn't produce enough hormones. It's a rare medical disorder. The pituitary, located below the brain, is called the master gland because it helps control other glands that also produce hormones. These other glands include the thyroid, adrenals, and sex organs. This disorder can affect just one other gland, a number of others, or all others, with effects that may be gradual or sudden and dramatic. The pituitary is important for regulating water balance, blood pressure, sexual function, stress responses, and basic metabolism. In hypopituitarism, these hormone systems don't work as well as they should.

What Causes Hypopituitarism?

The many causes include pituitary tumors or other brain tumors, brain infections, pituitary bleeding, trauma, pituitary surgery, stroke, congenital malformations, rare hereditary conditions, and radiation to the brain for tumors.

What Are the Symptoms of Hypopituitarism?

Some people have no symptoms until a stressful situation occurs. Others have symptoms that start suddenly. These symptoms include headache, blurred vision, and increased sensitivity to light with neck stiffness.

Symptoms depend on the organ system that is affected. An affected thyroid gland may cause you to feel weak and tired, become constipated, feel bloated, and gain weight. Affected ovaries may cause changes in periods, vaginal dryness, and painful intercourse. Affected testicles may cause problems in getting an erection. Affected adrenal glands may cause weakness, dizziness when standing, feeling sick to the stomach, and pain in the belly (abdomen). Children with hypopituitarism grow slowly.

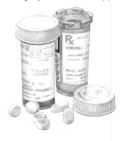

Your doctor will do a physical examination and test your blood and urine to measure hormone levels.

Your doctor will prescribe medicine to replace hormones that your body doesn't make. You may have to take medicine for the rest of your life. Medicine can stop the symptoms from happening again.

Surgery may be necessary if an abnormal growth in the pituitary or nearby tissues are causing your disorder. The growth might be removed by an operation through the nose.

Wear a medical alert bracelet showing that you have hypopituitarism.

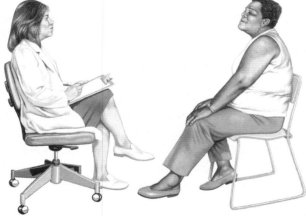

See your doctor regularly to make sure that your hormone levels are normal.

How Is Hypopituitarism Diagnosed?

The doctor will ask questions and do a physical examination. The doctor will take samples of blood and urine to measure hormone levels. The doctor may also prescribe medicine to see whether these hormone levels change after taking medicine. A special imaging test called magnetic resonance imaging (MRI) may be done of the pituitary to see if it has changed.

How Is Hypopituitarism Treated?

Treatment is based on the cause of the hypopituitarism. The doctor will prescribe medicine to replace each hormone that the body doesn't make. People with hypopituitarism may have to take medicine for the rest of their lives. Taking the medicine can stop the symptoms from happening again. Surgery may be necessary if abnormal growths in the pituitary gland or nearby tissues of the brain are causing hypopituitarism.

DOs and DON'Ts in Managing Hypopituitarism:

✔ **DO** take your medicine as prescribed.
✔ **DO** see your doctor regularly to make sure that your hormone levels are normal.
✔ **DO** make sure that you understand how to use the medicine.
✔ **DO** wear a medical alert bracelet showing that you have hypopituitarism.
✔ **DO** call your doctor if you have a fever, nausea, or vomiting or if you feel weak or dizzy.
✔ **DO** ask your doctor about purchasing a home emergency treatment kit.

⊘ **DON'T** stop taking your medicine without informing your doctor.
⊘ **DON'T** leave home without your emergency treatment kit, if you have one.

FROM THE DESK OF

NOTES

FOR MORE INFORMATION

Contact the following source:

• American Association of Clinical Endocrinologists
  Tel: (904) 353-7878
  Website: http://www.aace.com

MANAGING YOUR
HYPOTHYROIDISM

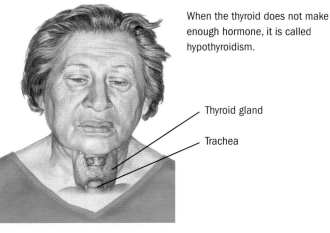

When the thyroid does not make enough hormone, it is called hypothyroidism.

Thyroid gland

Trachea

Symptoms may include tiredness, coldness, constipation, swollen face and eyelids, and changes in voice and hair texture.

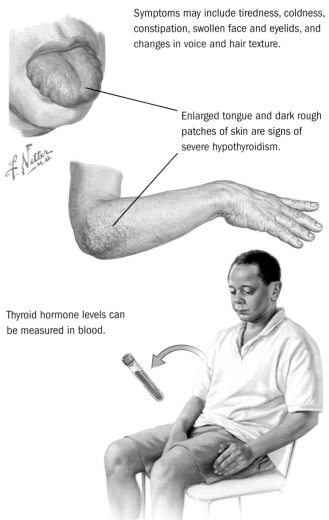

Enlarged tongue and dark rough patches of skin are signs of severe hypothyroidism.

Thyroid hormone levels can be measured in blood.

What Is Hypothyroidism?

Hypothyroidism is a disorder of the thyroid gland, which is an endocrine gland in your neck. The thyroid produces hormones (thyroxine or T_4 and triiodothyronine or T_3). These hormones affect how the body works (e.g., control metabolism). In hypothyroidism, the gland doesn't make enough thyroid hormone. Hypothyroidism affects both sexes. It can occur at any age but is more common in adult women.

What Causes Hypothyroidism?

Hypothyroidism is usually caused when the body makes antibodies (proteins that are part of the immune system) against its own thyroid gland. This form is called an autoimmune disease. It can also occur after treatment for hyperthyroidism (overactive thyroid) and as a side effect of some medicines.

What Are the Symptoms of Hypothyroidism?

Mild hypothyroidism may not cause symptoms. One person will probably not have all the symptoms but may have several of the following ones.

Poor appetite and difficulty with bowel movements (constipation) may lead to gaining or losing weight. Anemia may develop. Becoming pale, feeling cold and unable to sweat, and often feeling tired are possible.

Problems with mental abilities may include poor memory and feeling depressed. Trouble sleeping at night and numbness and tingling in hands and feet may occur.

Hair may become coarse, thin, or grow slowly. The voice may get deeper and hoarse. Some people may feel the effects in other parts of the body. They may have shortness of breath and changes in heart rate. Fluid may be retained, especially around the eyes. Women may have problems with periods. Both men and women may have less interest in sex. In severe hypothyroidism, the tongue may become enlarged (macroglossia) and the skin may look darkened and rough (hyperkeratosis).

How Is Hypothyroidism Diagnosed?

The doctor will do a complete physical examination and measure levels of thyroid hormones in the blood.

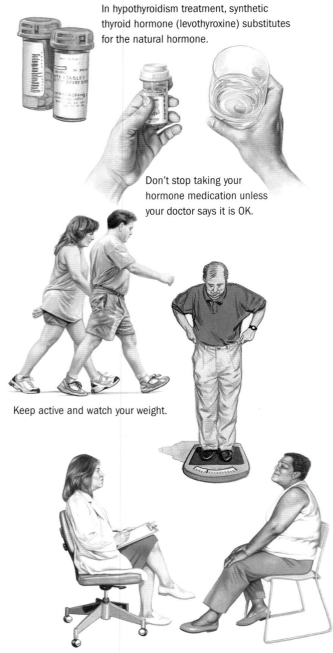

In hypothyroidism treatment, synthetic thyroid hormone (levothyroxine) substitutes for the natural hormone.

Don't stop taking your hormone medication unless your doctor says it is OK.

Keep active and watch your weight.

See your doctor regularly to monitor hormone levels.

How Is Hypothyroidism Treated?

Medicine can replace hormones that your body doesn't make. It is inexpensive, very effective, and available in many doses to properly treat each patient. The goal is to provide the body with enough hormone so that it works normally.

The medicine, called synthetic thyroid hormone or levothyroxine, should be taken daily because the body needs a new supply each day. Regular blood tests will ensure the right dose. The right dose of the synthetic hormone has no side effects. Doses that are too high may cause palpitations, nervousness, shakiness, bone loss, and increased bowel movements. These symptoms should prompt blood tests to check whether the dose should be changed.

Patients should start feeling better within a few weeks after starting thyroid medicine.

DOs and DON'Ts in Managing Hypothyroidism:

✔ **DO** follow your doctor's advice.
✔ **DO** see your doctor regularly to check hormone levels.
✔ **DO** contact your doctor if your condition changes or new problems develop.
✔ **DO** let your doctor know if you become pregnant or want to get pregnant.
✔ **DO** keep your weight within normal limits.
✔ **DO** stay as active as possible.

⊘ **DON'T** stop taking your medicine because you feel better, unless your doctor says it's ok. Hypothyroidism usually needs lifelong treatment.

FROM THE DESK OF

NOTES

FOR MORE INFORMATION

Contact the following sources:

• American Association of Clinical Endocrinologists
Tel: (904) 353-7878
Website: http://www.aace.com

• Thyroid Foundation of America
Tel: (800) 832-8321
Website: http://www.allthyroid.org

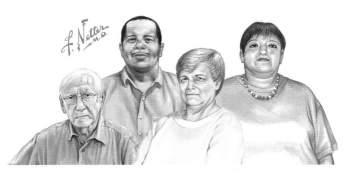

We have many hormones in our body, each with different functions. Antidiuretic hormone (ADH) is important for normal water balance. Too much ADH leads to the syndrome of inappropriate antidiuretic hormone secretion (SIADH). The body can't get rid of water and has low blood sodium levels.

Many different conditions and drugs can cause SIADH including

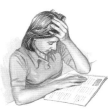

Antidepressants, anti-anxiety agents, anti-psychotic agents, and antiseizure drugs

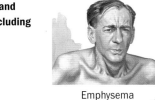

Emphysema

Brain tumor

Lung cancer (most common cause)

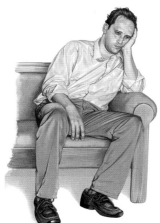

Early SIADH has no symptoms. Untreated SIADH may cause lethargy, weakness, seizures, and coma.

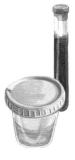

Your doctor will order blood and urine tests to check for SIADH.

What Is Syndrome of Inappropriate Secretion of Diuretic Hormone?

Antidiuretic hormone (ADH) is important for normal water balance in the body. Too much ADH leads to the syndrome of inappropriate antidiuretic hormone secretion (SIADH). The body can't get rid of water (water retention) and has lower blood sodium levels.

What Causes SIADH?

Causes include many different conditions and drugs. Certain tumors, such as lung cancer, and chronic lung diseases may produce ADH. Common drugs are antidepressants, antianxiety agents, antipsychotic agents, diuretics, and seizure medicines. More advanced cases with very low serum (blood) sodium levels usually occur in hospitalized people who are having surgery or are being treated for brain tumors, seizure disorders, lung cancers, or other chronic conditions.

What Are the Symptoms of SIADH?

Early SIADH has no symptoms. Untreated SIADH may cause lethargy, weakness, seizures, coma, and even death. People with quickly falling serum sodium levels have worse symptoms.

How Is SIADH Diagnosed?

The doctor makes a diagnosis with blood and urine tests that the body has too much water for the amount of sodium. Other causes of low sodium levels, such as an underactive thyroid (hypothyroidism) or adrenal insufficiency (Addison's disease), must be ruled out before SIADH can be diagnosed.

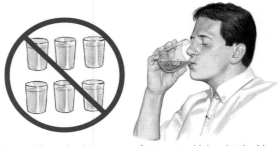

Your doctor will restrict the amount of water you drink to let the blood sodium levels return to normal. Water restriction is usually all that's needed.

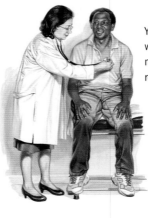

Your doctor will work with you to find out what may have caused SIADH. If it was medicine, your doctor may suggest replacing that drug.

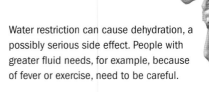

Water restriction can cause dehydration, a possibly serious side effect. People with greater fluid needs, for example, because of fever or exercise, need to be careful.

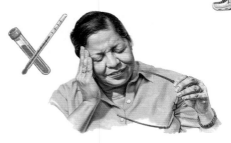

Get your serum sodium levels measured regularly, when your doctor suggests. Call your doctor if you feel weak or very tired, if you have an illness with a fever, and before you have elective surgery.

How Is SIADH Treated?

SIADH can be cured by removing the cause (drug or tumor) and by treating the underlying condition. Water restriction is the key to treatment. Less water intake allows serum sodium levels to rise normally. The maximum amount of water that people are allowed to drink is just slightly more than the amount of urine that they produce.

People need regular serum sodium measurements to make sure that water restriction has worked. Some people may need a medicine called demeclocycline. In emergency situations your physician may prescribe a strong diuretic such as furosemide.

DOs and DON'Ts in Managing SIADH:

✔ **DO** restrict the amount of water you drink. This may be the only treatment you need.

✔ **DO** understand the reason for your SIADH. If you treat the underlying cause, SIADH will go away.

✔ **DO** have regular follow-up serum sodium measurements.

✔ **DO** call your doctor if you feel weak or extremely tired, or if you have an illness with a fever.

✔ **DO** call your doctor if you are to have elective surgery.

⊘ **DON'T** assume that you have SIADH just because you have a low blood sodium level. Other disorders must be excluded.

FROM THE DESK OF

NOTES

FOR MORE INFORMATION

Contact the following source:

• American Association of Clinical Endocrinologists
Tel: (904) 353-7878
Website: http://www.aace.com

UNDERSTANDING
INFERTILITY

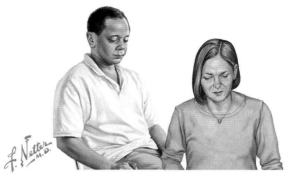

Infertility affects up to 18% of Americans. Infertility means being unable to get pregnant after 1 year of trying. The cause may be in the woman or man or both. Trying to find the cause can be hard. You and your partner should discuss what's involved in an infertility evaluation, including the cost.

Possible causes of male infertility:

Low sperm count: less than 20 million sperm per milliliter of semen (normal is 20-300 million)

Normal shape	Abnormal shapes

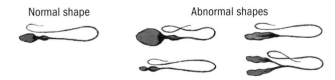

Sperm movement and shape: Sperm must travel, so if they can't move properly, abnormal movement may cause infertility. The sperm shape may also prevent it from reaching or entering the egg.

Possible causes of female infertility:

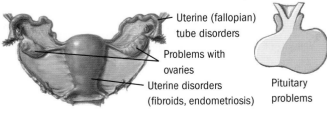

Uterine (fallopian) tube disorders

Problems with ovaries

Uterine disorders (fibroids, endometriosis)

Pituitary problems

What Is Infertility?

The inability to become pregnant and have children affects 8% to 18% of people in the United States. Usually, 80% to 90% of normal couples become pregnant during 1 year of attempting to do so. Infertility usually means being unable to get pregnant after 1 year of trying.

Infertility may be divided into primary and secondary on the basis of reproductive history. Women who were never pregnant are in the primary group. Women who were pregnant more than 1 year before are in the secondary group. Slightly more than half of people with infertility fall into the primary group. It's harder to become pregnant after the age of 30.

What Causes Infertility?

About 35% to 50% of infertility is due to a male factor such as low sperm count, abnormal sperm shape, or abnormal sperm motion (motility).

About 50% to 60% of infertility is related to female conditions. These conditions include fallopian tube disease, disorders related to ovaries (ovulation), and factors related to the uterus or cervix. The reason for infertility of the other 10% to 20% of couples isn't known (idiopathic).

What Are the Symptoms of Infertility?

The symptom is being unable to get pregnant after 1 year of regular intercourse without contraception.

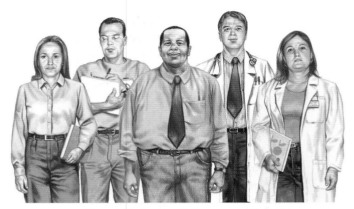

Initial testing to find a cause can be simple, such as getting a sperm count or blood tests to measure hormones. In up to 15% of couples, no cause is found.

Your medical team will discuss possible treatments with you and your partner.

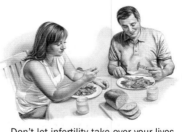

Don't let infertility take over your lives. Remember to continue nurturing your relationship by talking to one another and doing things that you enjoy together.

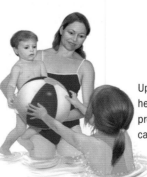

Up to 85% of infertile couples can be helped, so stay positive. If you can't get pregnant, alternatives such as adoption can provide you with the gift of parenting.

How Is Infertility Diagnosed?

Testing to find a cause ranges from simple things, such as getting a sperm count, to much more complicated testing. This testing includes blood tests (to measure female hormones, such as estrogen, progesterone, and follicle-stimulating hormone), ultrasound of the uterus and ovaries, and even laparascopic surgery to look at the reproductive organs. Before testing, it is important to understand what's involved in an infertility evaluation, including the methods, how long it will take, the limits, and the cost.

How Is Infertility Treated?

Treatment is based on finding out the reasons for infertility and overcoming them so that it's possible to get pregnant. Ways to do this include lifestyle changes (such as losing or gaining weight), medicines (for medical conditions), hormones, and drugs, such as clomiphene citrate, to make the ovaries start to release eggs. Surgery (such as to unblock fallopian tubes) and other methods, such as intrauterine insemination and in vitro fertilization, may also be tried.

DOs and DON'Ts in Managing Infertility:

✔ **DO** talk to your doctor if you're worried about getting pregnant.

✔ **DO** continue to have intercourse according to your usual schedule.

✔ **DO** eat a healthy diet and exercise in moderation. Excessive exercise and weight loss may cause fertility problems by interfering with ovulation and menses.

🚫 **DON'T** give up: up to 85% of infertile couples may be helped.

🚫 **DON'T** let the process of trying to get pregnant get in the way of the rest of your relationship.

🚫 **DON'T** smoke or drink alcohol if you are trying to get pregnant.

FOR MORE INFORMATION

Contact the following sources:

• American College of Obstetricians and Gynecologists
Tel: (202) 638-5577
Website: http://www.acog.org

• WebMD
Website: http://www.webmd.com

• U.S. Department of Health and Human Services
Websites: http://womenshealth.gov
http://www.4women.gov/faq/infertility.cfm

FROM THE DESK OF

NOTES

MANAGING YOUR
KLINEFELTER'S SYNDROME

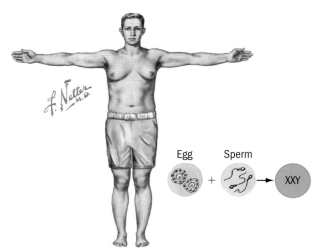

Klinefelter's syndrome is an inherited disorder of males. Males have an extra X chromosome and don't develop normal male sexual characteristics of puberty; however, most men with Klinefelter's syndrome can live normal lives.

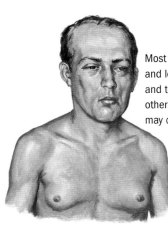

Most teenagers and men have long arms and legs compared with the body trunk, and teenagers may be less muscular than other boys. Men are infertile, and some may develop breasts (gynecomastia).

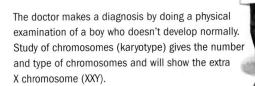

The doctor makes a diagnosis by doing a physical examination of a boy who doesn't develop normally. Study of chromosomes (karyotype) gives the number and type of chromosomes and will show the extra X chromosome (XXY).

What Is Klinefelter's Syndrome?

Klinefelter's syndrome is an inherited disorder of males. It can affect different stages of development—physical, language, and social. Normal male sexual characteristics of puberty don't develop.

Klinefelter's syndrome affects about 1 in 400 to 1 in 1000 males.

What Causes Klinefelter's Syndrome?

The cause is a defect in sex chromosomes. Normal females have a chromosome pattern of 46,XX. Normal males have a 46,XY pattern. In this syndrome, the pattern is 47,XXY. This extra X chromosome interferes with normal male sexual development in the womb and at puberty.

What Are the Symptoms of Klinefelter's Syndrome?

Most teenagers and men have long arms and legs compared with the body trunk. Teenagers may be less muscular than other boys, have problems expressing themselves, be shy, and have trouble being part of a social group. Men have a low sperm count or no sperm and therefore are infertile. The testicles are small and firm, and some men may have breasts (gynecomastia). Men may have problems with erections, small penis, poor beard growth, and little underarm or pubic hair. Symptoms vary greatly.

This syndrome leads to osteoporosis (low bone density), an increased risk for breast cancer, and sometimes personality disorders.

How Is Klinefelter's Syndrome Diagnosed?

The doctor makes a diagnosis by doing a physical examination of a boy who doesn't develop normally. Analysis of chromosomes (karyotype) done from obtaining a smear from cells inside your mouth (buccal smear) gives the number and type of chromosomes. Sometimes, a man sees a doctor because of impotence (cannot get an erection) or infertility (inability to father children). Blood tests show a low level of testosterone (male hormone) and high level of another hormone, follicle-stimulating hormone (FSH).

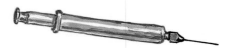

Infertility can't be treated, because testes can't make sperm. However, replacing testosterone, given as an injection or skin patch, can induce the development of male secondary sexual characteristics.

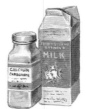

Calcium and vitamin D

Osteoporosis may be treated with testosterone plus enough calcium and vitamin D and regular weight-bearing exercises. These will prevent fractures.

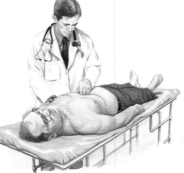

See an endocrinologist if you have concerns about male sexual development or function.

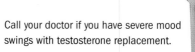

Call your doctor if you have severe mood swings with testosterone replacement.

How Is Klinefelter's Syndrome Treated?

No treatment for infertility is possible, because testes cannot make sperm. Replacing testosterone will help the male secondary sexual characteristics. Testosterone, given as an injection or skin patch, leads to normal male muscle development and hair growth (beard, underarms, and genitals). Excess testosterone may cause mood changes, aggressive behavior, abnormal prostate growth, or high blood pressure. Use of the testosterone patch may cause a local skin reaction.

Gynecomastia can be treated surgically (breast reduction). Lumps in the breast should be checked for breast cancer.

Osteoporosis may be treated with testosterone plus enough calcium and vitamin D and regular weight-bearing exercises.

DOs and DON'Ts in Managing Klinefelter's Syndrome:

✔ **DO** see an endocrinologist if you have concerns about male sexual development or function. An endocrinologist is a doctor who specializes in diseases of the endocrine system.

✔ **DO** see a surgeon if gynecomastia is troubling or you note a breast lump.

✔ **DO** call the doctor if you have severe mood swings with testosterone replacement.

✔ **DO** call the doctor if you notice sudden bone pain in the back, hip, wrist, or rib.

✔ **DO** call the doctor if you have a rash while using a testosterone patch.

✔ **DO** ask your doctor about support groups if you're interested in learning from others with Klinefelter's syndrome.

🚫 **DON'T** assume your child has Klinefelter's syndrome because he's behind his peers in pubertal development. See a pediatric endocrinologist.

🚫 **DON'T** forget that you can get help if you're having emotional problems with your diagnosis.

🚫 **DON'T** put the testosterone patch on the same spot of skin every time, to prevent skin irritation.

FROM THE DESK OF

NOTES

FOR MORE INFORMATION

Contact the following source:

• American Association of Clinical Endocrinologists
Tel: (904) 353-7878
Website: http://www.aace.com

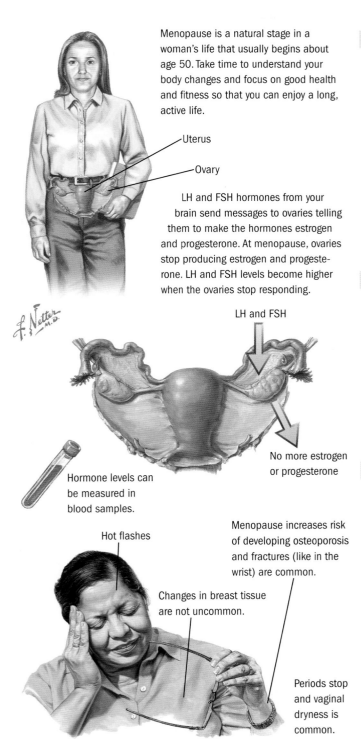

Menopause is a natural stage in a woman's life that usually begins about age 50. Take time to understand your body changes and focus on good health and fitness so that you can enjoy a long, active life.

Uterus

Ovary

LH and FSH hormones from your brain send messages to ovaries telling them to make the hormones estrogen and progesterone. At menopause, ovaries stop producing estrogen and progesterone. LH and FSH levels become higher when the ovaries stop responding.

LH and FSH

No more estrogen or progesterone

Hormone levels can be measured in blood samples.

Hot flashes

Menopause increases risk of developing osteoporosis and fractures (like in the wrist) are common.

Changes in breast tissue are not uncommon.

Periods stop and vaginal dryness is common.

Hormone alterations cause changes throughout the body. The major change is that periods stop.

What Is Menopause?

Menopause is the time in a woman's life when menstrual periods have stopped for at least 1 year. It is often called the change of life. Menopause is not an illness.

Periods become irregular and stop because ovaries stop producing hormones, and hormone levels change. Hormones are chemicals in the body that control certain body functions. The hormone estrogen in women helps control the menstrual cycle. As a woman ages, the amount of estrogen decreases.

Most women go through menopause at about age 50 or 51. Sometimes menopause happens earlier (at 40 years), and sometimes later (at 60 years).

What Are the Symptoms of Menopause?

The most common symptoms are hot flashes and end of periods. Hot flashes can be very mild (feeling a little warmth in the face) to very severe (becoming red in the face and sweating excessively). A hot flash only lasts a few minutes. Hot flashes can disturb sleep, so women may feel very tired during the day.

Other symptoms include vaginal dryness, vaginal sensitivity, pain during intercourse, bladder control problems, weight gain, loss of sex drive (libido), and mood swings.

How Is Menopause Diagnosed?

Hot flashes and the end of periods for about 6 months mean that menopause is occurring.

Blood tests for follicle-stimulating hormone (FSH) and luteinizing hormone (LH) levels can be done to find out whether ovaries are slowing down or no longer working.

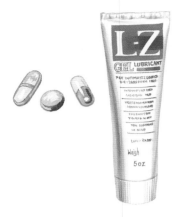

No special treatments are needed, because this process is natural. However some women with severe symptoms use HRT. Lubricants can help vaginal dryness.

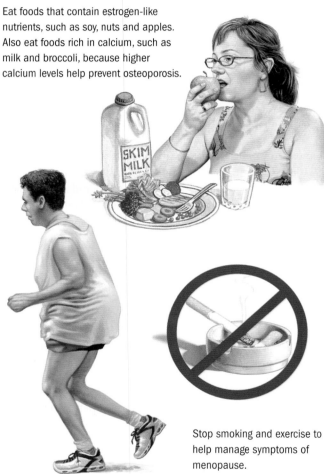

Eat foods that contain estrogen-like nutrients, such as soy, nuts and apples. Also eat foods rich in calcium, such as milk and broccoli, because higher calcium levels help prevent osteoporosis.

Stop smoking and exercise to help manage symptoms of menopause.

How Is Menopause Treated?

Treatment of mild symptoms with drugs is unnecessary.

The most effective treatment for severe symptoms is hormone replacement therapy (HRT). Women with a uterus need estrogen and progesterone. Estrogen relieves symptoms of menopause very well. Progesterone reduces the risk of developing uterine cancer while taking estrogen. Women without a uterus do not take progesterone. Because taking hormones may slightly increase the risk of developing breast cancer, HRT should be prescribed as needed for each woman and only at the lowest effective dose. Vaginal creams or lubricants may help dryness and pain during intercourse.

During menopause, metabolism slows down and muscle tends to turn into fat. It becomes more important to eat healthy, low-fat foods and to exercise. Exercise helps burn calories and keep up bone strength and muscle mass. Exercise also increases the body's metabolism for several hours, which helps weight loss.

DOs and DON'Ts in Managing Menopause:

✔ **DO** follow a healthy diet. Eating and drinking products that contain chemicals called plant estrogens may help. Such foods include fennel, soy, nuts, whole grains, and apples.

✔ **DO** take care of your health. Exercise. Women who have gone through menopause may be more likely to develop certain diseases, including heart disease and osteoporosis.

✔ **DO** get regular checkups.

✔ **DO** tell your doctor if you don't feel well while using HRT. Estrogen sometimes has side effects.

✔ **DO** use simple exercises called Kegel exercises to improve bladder control if you have problems with it.

⊘ **DON'T** drink beverages containing caffeine.

⊘ **DON'T** drink alcohol in excess.

⊘ **DON'T** eat hot spicy foods.

FROM THE DESK OF

NOTES

FOR MORE INFORMATION

Contact the following sources:

• National Women's Health Resource Center
  Tel: (877) 986-9472
  Website: http://www.healthywomen.org

• American College of Obstetricians and Gynecologists
  Tel: (202) 638-5577
  Website: http://www.acog.org

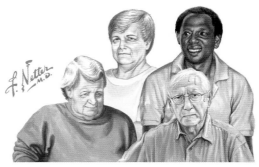

If you have metabolic syndrome, you may have a greater chance of getting cardiovascular disease (such as heart disease and stroke), kidney disease, and diabetes. More older people (70 or more) have it than younger people (20 to 29).

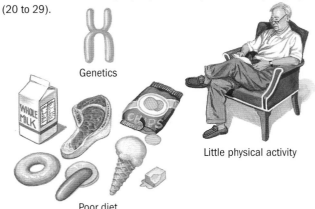

Genetics

Little physical activity

Poor diet

The exact cause isn't known, but genetics and lifestyle factors (e.g., diet, amount of food eaten, physical inactivity) are important.

The doctor may diagnose metabolic syndrome if you have three of these risk factors:

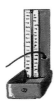

High blood pressure

High cholesterol (too much LDL), but low HDL levels

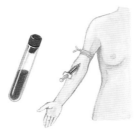
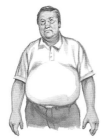

High fasting blood sugar (glucose) level

Too much fat around the waist (abdomen)

What Is Metabolic Syndrome?

Metabolic syndrome refers to the presence of several factors that increase your risk of getting cardiovascular disease (such as heart disease and stroke), kidney disease, and diabetes.

Nearly 47 million adults in the United States have the syndrome. It's more common in middle-aged and elderly people.

What Causes Metabolic Syndrome?

The exact cause is unknown, but genetics and lifestyle choices (e.g., diet, food intake, physical inactivity) both play a role. Metabolic syndrome can't be caught or passed from person to person.

What Are the Symptoms of Metabolic Syndrome?

Metabolic syndrome has no specific symptoms. Many people don't know that they have it and find out only after blood tests, measurements of the waist, and blood pressure readings show its presence.

How Is Metabolic Syndrome Diagnosed?

The doctor makes a diagnosis if the combination of certain risk factors is present: too much fat around the waist (abdomen), so that the waist measures more than 40 inches in men and 35 inches in women. A second factor is high blood triglyceride levels (higher than 150 mg/dl). Triglycerides are a kind of fat in the blood. Another factor is a high-density lipoprotein (HDL) level lower than 40 mg/dl in men and 50 mg/dl in women. HDL is good cholesterol, because it carries cholesterol including low-density lipoprotein (LDL, or bad cholesterol) away from the arteries and back to the liver for removal from the body. Other factors are high blood pressure (130/85 mmHg or higher), and a high fasting blood sugar (glucose) level (100 mg/dl or higher).

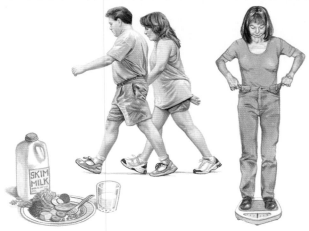

Changes in lifestyle—diet, weight, and exercise—are important. These changes, plus using less salt, can reduce blood pressure.

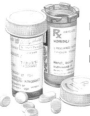

If these changes don't work, your doctor may prescribe medicines such as statins (e.g., lovastatin, pravastatin, atorvastatin).

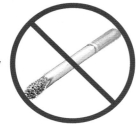

Don't smoke. Cigarette smoking is a major risk factor for coronary artery disease.

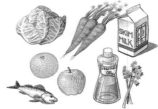

Eat a low-fat diet.

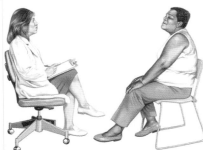

Talk to your doctor about high blood pressure, diet, and exercise, or if you have symptoms of diabetes (increased thirst, increased urination, blurred vision, and overeating).

FROM THE DESK OF

NOTES

How Is Metabolic Syndrome Treated?

First, changes in lifestyle, specifically diet, weight, and exercise, are important. A small weight loss can lead to a great decrease in blood pressure, blood fat levels, and blood glucose levels.

Diet changes to lower cholesterol include using unsaturated fats instead of saturated fats, reducing total fat intake to 30% of daily calories, and eating no more than 300 mg of cholesterol daily. Also, less salt should be used.

Moderate daily exercise, defined as 30 minutes of brisk walking or 15 minutes of running, can produce important health benefits.

Weight loss, exercise, and less salt can reduce blood pressure. If they don't, the doctor may prescribe medicines.

The doctor may prescribe cholesterol-lowering medicine, such as statins (e.g., lovastatin, pravastatin, simvastatin, atorvastatin, rosuvastatin), if lifestyle changes don't lower cholesterol levels.

DOs and DON'Ts in Managing Metabolic Syndrome:

✔ **DO** remember that fasting for at least 12 hours before testing is needed for accurate blood cholesterol, triglycerides, and glucose levels.

✔ **DO** call your doctor if you have high blood pressure, you need advice about diet or exercise, or you have symptoms of diabetes (increased thirst, increased urination, blurred vision, and overeating).

✔ **DO** call your doctor if you want to know your blood levels of total cholesterol, HDL (good) cholesterol, LDL (bad) cholesterol, and triglycerides.

⊘ **DON'T** smoke. Cigarette smoking is a major risk factor for coronary artery disease.

⊘ **DON'T** forget that reasonable lifestyle changes can have big benefits in reducing chances of getting metabolic syndrome and cardiovascular disease.

FOR MORE INFORMATION

Contact the following sources:

• American College of Cardiology
 Tel: (800) 253-4636
 Website: http://www.acc.org

• American Heart Association
 Tel: (800) 242-8721
 Website: http://www.americanheart.org

MANAGING YOUR
OSTEOPOROSIS

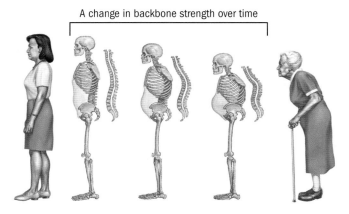

A change in backbone strength over time

Osteoporosis is the thinning of the bones. Bones become fragile and loss of height is common as the back bones begin to collapse.

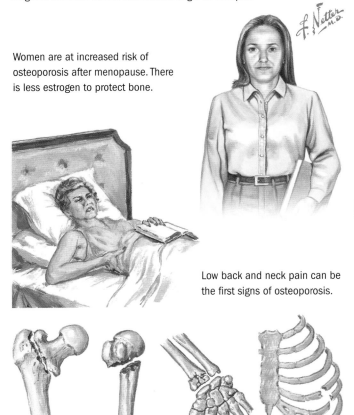

Women are at increased risk of osteoporosis after menopause. There is less estrogen to protect bone.

Low back and neck pain can be the first signs of osteoporosis.

Fractures of the hip, wrist, arm, and rib are common in people with osteoporosis.

What Is Osteoporosis?

Osteoporosis is the continuing thinning and loss of density in bones (bone mass), which makes bones more brittle, fragile, and likely to break after minor trauma. Loss of height and back pain are common. Women are at special risk for osteoporosis after their menstrual periods end (menopause), because quicker bone loss occurs after reduced production of the hormone estrogen. Estrogen blocks a protein that weakens bones.

Osteoporosis is a silent disease, and it may not be evident until a bone breaks.

What Causes Osteoporosis?

Normal bone formation needs the minerals calcium and phosphate. If the body does not get enough calcium from the diet, bone production and bone tissues may suffer.

The main causes of osteoporosis include aging, which leads to a drop in estrogen in women at menopause and a drop in testosterone (a male hormone) in men. Other causes are being underweight, lifestyle habits (being sedentary or inactive), alcohol use, cigarette smoking, eating disorders, taking certain drugs, some chronic diseases, and long-term bed rest or immobilization.

What Are the Symptoms of Osteoporosis?

No symptoms may be obvious early in the disease, but in time, low back and neck pain, stooped posture, and gradual loss of height may be seen. In other cases the first sign is a fracture (ribs, wrists, or hips). Bones (vertebrae) in the spine may collapse (become flattened or compressed) and break, which is the most common fracture. Hip fractures can cause the greatest disability.

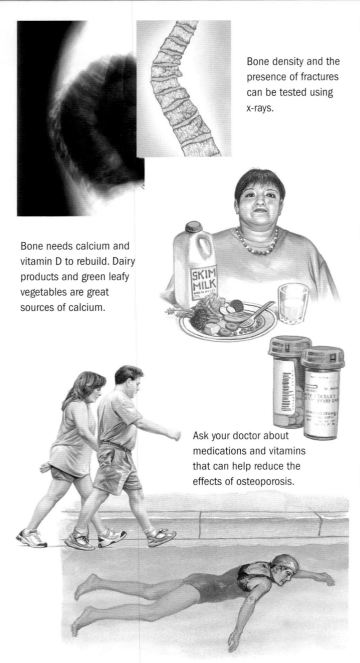

Bone density and the presence of fractures can be tested using x-rays.

Bone needs calcium and vitamin D to rebuild. Dairy products and green leafy vegetables are great sources of calcium.

Ask your doctor about medications and vitamins that can help reduce the effects of osteoporosis.

Regular weight-bearing and muscle strengthening exercises may help reduce fracture risk.

How Is Osteoporosis Diagnosed?

The physician will take a medical history and do a physical examination to look for age-related signs of a deformed spine. Laboratory tests can measure calcium and vitamin D levels. An x-ray examination called DEXA can measure bone density at important places, such as the spine and the hip. Screening for osteoporosis may be recommended for all women after menopause and for men with risk factors such as long-term use of corticosteroids such as prednisone, which predisposes to osteoporosis.

How Is Osteoporosis Treated?

Lifestyle changes may help reduce fracture risk. Such changes include doing regular weight-bearing and muscle-strengthening exercises, stopping smoking, limiting alcohol intake, and getting enough calcium and vitamin D in the diet. Calcium supplements may increase calcium intake, with vitamin D used to help the body absorb calcium. Treatments focus on slowing down or stopping bone loss and on preventing bone fractures by minimizing the risk of falls.

Different drugs, including bisphosphonates such as alendronate, and adequate supplementation of calcium and vitamin D are used as well.

DOs and DON'Ts in Managing Osteoporosis:

✔ **DO** regular weight-bearing and muscle-strengthening exercises as suggested by your doctor.
✔ **DO** make sure you get enough calcium and vitamin D. Eat a healthy diet that is rich in calcium-containing foods, such as dairy products, fish, beans, and green leafy vegetables.
✔ **DO** take your medicines as prescribed.
✔ **DO** discuss screening for osteoporosis with your doctor.

🚫 **DON'T** smoke.
🚫 **DON'T** drink alcohol in excess.

FROM THE DESK OF

NOTES

FOR MORE INFORMATION

Contact the following sources:

* NIH Osteoporosis and Related Bone Diseases
  Tel: (800) 624-BONE
  Website: http://www.osteo.org
* National Osteoporosis Foundation
  Tel: (800) 223-9994
  Website: http://www.nof.org

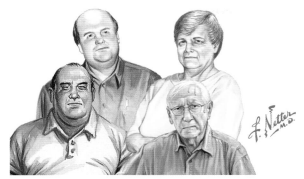

Paget's disease affects up to 4% of Caucasians of Northern European descent older than 40, in more males than females. It's much less common in other ethnic groups.

What Is Paget's Disease of Bone?

Paget's disease is a disorder with abnormal bone formation. Bone cells (osteoblasts) normally form new bone in smooth even layers, like a bricklayer building a brick wall. At the same time, other bone cells (osteoclasts) knock down older parts of this bony structure and take pieces away in the process called resorption. Formation and resorption are balanced, so bones grow straight and strong. In Paget's disease, the process is unbalanced, as if the wall had bricks facing in all directions, weakened by gaps and holes. These bones break easily.

Any bone can be affected, but the skull, spine, leg, pelvis, and collar bone are usually involved.

Up to 4% of Caucasians of Northern European descent older than 40, more males than females, have Paget's disease. It's much less common in other ethnic groups. Paget's disease can be mild to severe. Most people have the mild form that doesn't need treatment.

Paget's disease is a disorder with abnormal bone formation. Bone formation and bone resorption (breakdown) are out of balance.

Normal bone   Bone in Paget's disease

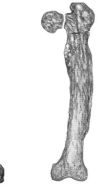

What Causes Paget's Disease of Bone?

The cause is unknown.

What Are the Symptoms of Paget's Disease of Bone?

Many people have no symptoms. The most common symptom is mild to severe bone pain that is worse at night. Other symptoms include warmth and swelling over the bone (especially skull or long leg bones), large skull, bone breaks, curved spine, deformed bones, headache, hearing loss, joint pain and stiffness, loose teeth, trouble moving, numbness and tingling in hands or feet, shortness of breath, and nerve problems.

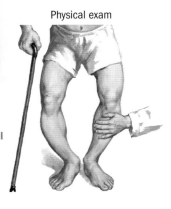

Many people have no symptoms, but the most common one is bone pain that is worse at night. Others are bone breaks, curved spine, and deformed bones. Hearing loss and headache can occur when the disease affects the skull.

Physical exam

How Is Paget's Disease of Bone Diagnosed?

The doctor will take a medical history, do a physical examination, and order bone x-rays. Blood and urine may be tested. Bone scan and hearing and vision tests may also be done.

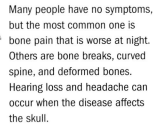

Blood and urine tests

X-rays

After taking your medical history and doing a physical exam, your doctor will x-ray your bones and order blood and urine tests. Bone scan may also be done.

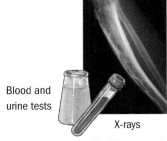

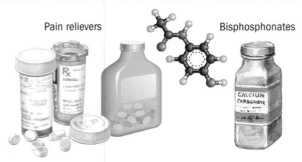

Pain relievers   Bisphosphonates

Treatment depends on the severity of symptoms. Mild pain relievers such as acetaminophen or ibuprofen may be enough. For moderate to severe disease, other medicines (bisphosphonates) are given.

Exercising is important, because being immobile may cause high calcium levels in blood and urine and lead to kidney stones.

Try to avoid injury. Accident-proof your home. Sleep on a firm bed to support your back.

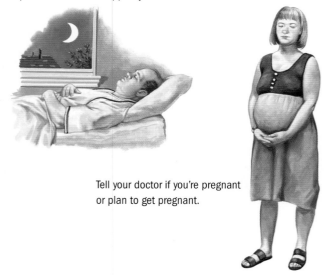

Tell your doctor if you're pregnant or plan to get pregnant.

How Is Paget's Disease of Bone Treated?

Treatment depends on the severity of symptoms. Mild pain relievers such as acetaminophen or ibuprofen may be enough. Moderate to severe disease is treated with other medicines (bisphosphonates) for pain and to slow new bone growth.

A cane may be helpful for balance and weight-bearing pain.

Exercising is important, because not moving may cause high calcium levels in blood and urine and lead to kidney stones. Surgery may be needed to fix a bone or when weight-bearing bones break.

DOs and DON'Ts in Managing Paget's Disease of Bone:

✔ **DO** tell your doctor about your other medical problems (especially kidney or liver).

✔ **DO** tell your doctor if you're pregnant or plan to get pregnant.

✔ **DO** sleep on a firm bed to support your back.

✔ **DO** exercise and stay slim. Ask your doctor which exercises are right for you.

✔ **DO** try to avoid injury. Accident-proof your home. For example, put hand rails next to your tub and toilet and don't use throw rugs.

✔ **DO** call your doctor if your bone pain or hearing worsens, your ankles swell, or you have shortness of breath on exertion.

⊘ **DON'T** stop taking your medicine or change your dosage because you feel better unless your doctor says to.

⊘ **DON'T** exercise, do heavy work, or play sports without your doctor's OK.

FROM THE DESK OF

NOTES

FOR MORE INFORMATION

Contact the following sources:

• The Paget Foundation
  Tel: (800) 23-PAGET (237-2438), (212) 509-5335
  Website: http://www.paget.org

• The Endocrine Society
  Tel: (888) 363-6274
  Website: http://www.endo-society.org

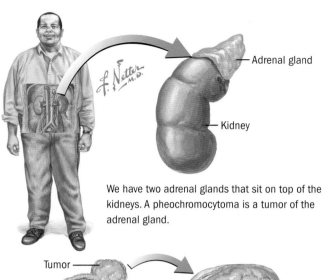

We have two adrenal glands that sit on top of the kidneys. A pheochromocytoma is a tumor of the adrenal gland.

Adrenal gland

Kidney

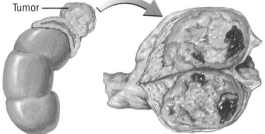

Tumor

The cause of adrenal gland tumors is unknown.

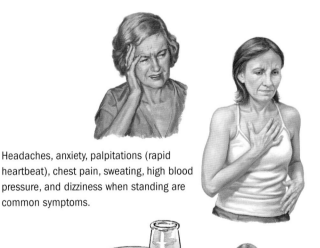

Headaches, anxiety, palpitations (rapid heartbeat), chest pain, sweating, high blood pressure, and dizziness when standing are common symptoms.

If your medical history and examination suggest a pheochromocytoma, your doctor will do urine and blood tests to measure hormone levels. CT or MRI may be done to look for the tumor.

What Is Pheochromocytoma?

Humans have two adrenal glands located above the kidneys. They make substances called hormones that regulate blood pressure, fluid metabolism, and other body functions. A pheochromocytoma is an uncommon tumor of the adrenal gland. Rarely, tumors develop outside the adrenal glands.

Pheochromocytomas secrete epinephrine or related compounds. High blood pressure, heart palpitations, headaches, and sweating are the result. Pheochromocytomas account for a very small number of hypertension cases.

What Causes Pheochromocytoma?

The cause is unknown. Most tumors aren't related to family history, but about 10% are part of familial endocrine tumor disorders.

What Are the Symptoms of Pheochromocytoma?

Common symptoms are headaches that come and go, anxiety, palpitations (abnormal, rapid heartbeats), sweating, high blood pressure, heat intolerance, and dizziness when standing. Some people have none.

Uncontrolled hypertension can cause vision loss, heart disease, kidney disease, and stroke.

How Is Pheochromocytoma Diagnosed?

Your doctor may suspects a pheochromocytoma because of your medical history and physical examination. Urine and blood tests will be done to measure hormone levels. One urine test, a 24-hour collection, measures substances called catecholamines. You should be in a nonstressful place when this test is done. You shouldn't drink alcohol or caffeine or take amphetamines, benzodiazepines, certain antidepressants, or lithium when doing the test. These substances may lead to false levels.

Magnetic resonance imaging (MRI) or CT scans may be done to look for the tumor. Tumors outside the adrenals may need whole-body imaging with special nuclear medicine tests.

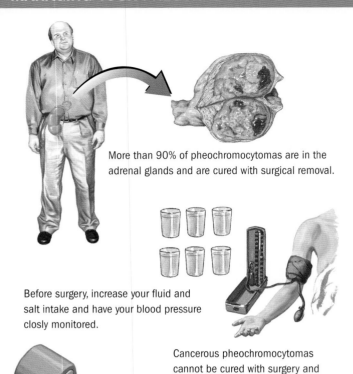

More than 90% of pheochromocytomas are in the adrenal glands and are cured with surgical removal.

Before surgery, increase your fluid and salt intake and have your blood pressure closly monitored.

Cancerous pheochromocytomas cannot be cured with surgery and need a combination of chemotherapy, radiation therapy, and other treatments.

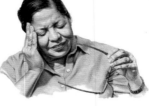

Don't exercise strenuously until your pheochromocytoma is removed.

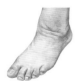

Call your doctor if you have a severe headache, chest pains, palpitations, ankle swelling, or other symptoms.

How Is Pheochromocytoma Treated?

More than 90% of pheochromocytomas are in the adrenal glands and can be cured with surgery. Medicines to control blood pressure should be given before surgery.

Complications from surgery include bleeding and infection. Temporary low and high blood pressure readings can occur while the tumor is being removed.

Pheochromocytomas that are malignant and have spread cannot be cured with surgery. A combination of chemotherapy, radiation therapy, and other treatments is used to help control the disease.

DOs and DON'Ts in Managing Pheochromocytoma:

✔ **DO** tell your doctor if you had pheochromocytomas before or family members have endocrine tumors. Your family may need screening blood or urine tests.

✔ **DO** call your doctor if you have vision changes, severe headache, weakness on one side of the body, chest pains, or increasing palpitations.

✔ **DO** call your doctor if you have ankle swelling, shortness of breath, or weakness or dizziness when standing.

✔ **DO** call your doctor if symptoms return after surgery.

⊘ **DON'T** do strenuous exercise until your pheochromocytoma has been removed.

⊘ **DON'T** expect that your high blood pressure will be completely normal after the operation. Some permanent changes may have already occurred in the kidneys and blood vessels.

FROM THE DESK OF

NOTES

FOR MORE INFORMATION

Contact the following sources:

• National Adrenal Diseases Foundation
Tel: (516) 487-4992
Website: http://www.nadf.us/

• The Endocrine Society
Tel: (888) 363-6274
Website: http://www.endo-society.org

MANAGING YOUR
PITUITARY ADENOMA

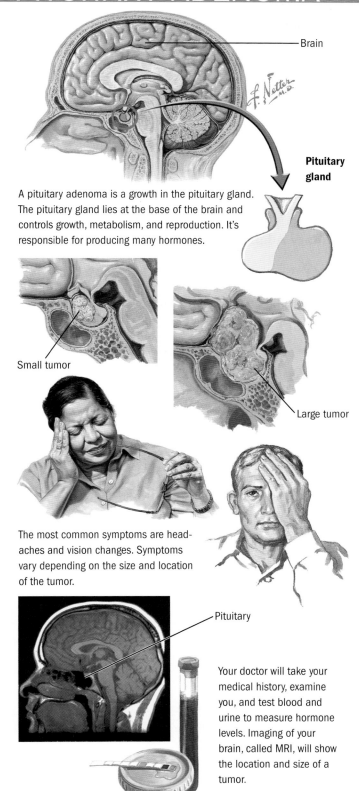

Brain

A pituitary adenoma is a growth in the pituitary gland. The pituitary gland lies at the base of the brain and controls growth, metabolism, and reproduction. It's responsible for producing many hormones.

Pituitary gland

Small tumor

Large tumor

The most common symptoms are headaches and vision changes. Symptoms vary depending on the size and location of the tumor.

Pituitary

Your doctor will take your medical history, examine you, and test blood and urine to measure hormone levels. Imaging of your brain, called MRI, will show the location and size of a tumor.

What Are Pituitary Adenomas?

A pituitary adenoma is a growth in the pituitary gland. The pituitary gland, or master gland, lies at the base of the brain and controls growth, metabolism, and reproduction. This gland makes a number of hormones including corticotropin (ACTH), which causes the adrenal gland to produce corticosteroids, and thyroid-stimulating hormone (TSH), which causes the thyroid gland to make thyroid hormone. The pituitary also makes growth hormone (GH), which controls body growth; prolactin, which is needed for breast development and milk production; follicle-stimulating hormone (FSH) and luteinizing hormone (LH), which work in sexual development and reproduction; antidiuretic hormone, which is needed for water balance and blood pressure; and oxytocin, which helps the uterus contract during childbirth.

Adenomas can cause the pituitary to make too much or too little of a hormone. A very large adenoma can press on the brain itself and cause headaches and other symptoms.

What Causes Pituitary Adenomas?

The cause is unknown.

What Are the Symptoms of Pituitary Adenomas?

Symptoms depend on the size of the growth and its effects in the body. The most common symptoms are headache and vision changes. There are many other possible symptoms, including acne, loss of menstrual periods, inability to get pregnant (women), nipple discharge, inability to have an erection, easy bruising, too much body hair, large jaw, joint pain, oily skin, round face, thin skin, and vaginal dryness.

How Are Pituitary Adenomas Diagnosed?

The doctor will take a medical history, do a physical examination, and test blood and urine to measure hormone levels. Magnetic resonance imaging (MRI) of the brain will be done to find the tumor and measure its size. Vision tests will be done to rule out damage to the visual areas near the pituitary.

The doctor may suggest seeing an endocrinologist and a neurosurgeon. An endocrinologist is a doctor who specializes in disorders of the endocrine system. A neurosurgeon is a doctor who specializes in brain surgery.

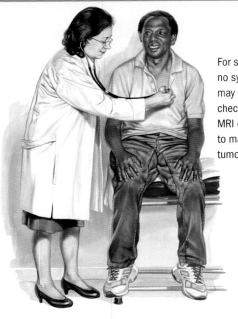

For small growths causing no symptoms, your doctor may suggest just getting a checkup, blood tests, and MRI every few months to make sure that the tumor isn't growing.

If the tumor is causing too much or too little hormone to be made, medicine can help get things back in balance.

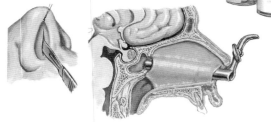

Surgery may be needed. The type of operation depends on the size and location of the tumor. In one type of operation, the surgeon goes through the inside of the nose to reach and remove the tumor.

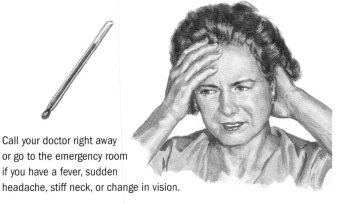

Call your doctor right away or go to the emergency room if you have a fever, sudden headache, stiff neck, or change in vision.

FROM THE DESK OF

NOTES

How Are Pituitary Adenomas Treated?

Treatment depends on the adenoma size and its effects. Treatment may involve surgery, radiation, and medicines.

People with very small growths and no symptoms usually don't need treatment. Every few months, blood tests and MRI will be done to make sure that it's not growing.

If an adenoma is making too much hormone, drugs will be given to prevent more hormone from being made and to control symptoms.

If an adenoma is causing a lack of a hormone, the missing hormone will be prescribed (hormone replacement therapy).

Surgery and radiation, if needed, will depend on the adenoma size and location.

DOs and DON'Ts in Managing Pituitary Adenomas:

✔ **DO** tell your doctor about your other medical problems.

✔ **DO** tell your doctor about medicines you take, including prescription and over-the-counter drugs.

✔ **DO** tell your doctor if you're pregnant or plan to get pregnant.

✔ **DO** call your doctor right away or go to the emergency room if you have a fever, stiff neck, sudden headache, or change in vision.

🚫 **DON'T** stop taking your medicine or change your dose, even if you feel better, unless your doctor says you can.

FOR MORE INFORMATION

Contact the following source:

• National Brain Tumor Society
Tel: (800) 934-2873
Website: http://www.braintumor.org

Polycystic ovarian syndrome (PCOS) usually starts in women younger than 30. It's a hormonal condition in which ovaries have many cysts (fluid-filled sacs).

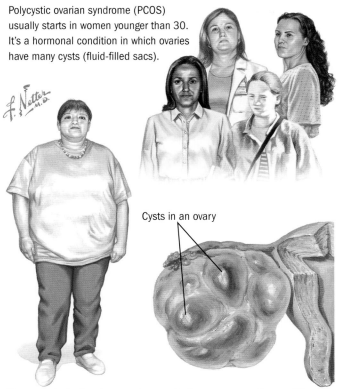

Cysts in an ovary

The cause isn't clear but may be genetic. In some cases, the condition seems to be linked to weight gain. The most common symptom is irregular periods.

Other symptoms

Too much hair on the face, chest, and stomach

Infertility

Depression

Acne

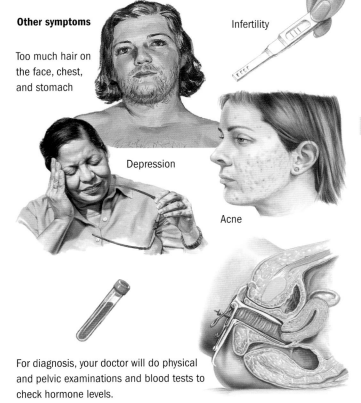

For diagnosis, your doctor will do physical and pelvic examinations and blood tests to check hormone levels.

What Is Polycystic Ovarian Syndrome?

Polycystic ovarian syndrome (PCOS) is a condition in which ovaries have many cysts (fluid-filled sacs). It's also called Stein-Leventhal syndrome. PCOS is a disorder related to the body's hormones. For example, the pituitary gland, which is at the base of the brain, makes hormones that tell the body how to work. One of these hormones tells the ovary when to release an egg. When the pituitary gland is overactive and makes too much hormone, ovaries get cysts.

PCOS usually starts in women younger than 30.

What Causes Polycystic Ovarian Syndrome?

The cause of changes in hormone levels isn't clear. One possibility is genetic reasons that cause PCOS in overweight or obese women. Also, it's related to type 2 diabetes.

What Are the Symptoms of Polycystic Ovarian Syndrome?

The most common symptom is irregular periods. They occur a few times a year, sometimes only once a year, and sometimes not at all. Bleeding can be very light or very heavy. Other symptoms include acne; hair loss on the head; too much hair on the face (can be thick and dark), chest, or stomach; high cholesterol levels; high blood pressure; deep voice; oily skin; dark rash on the neck, underarm, or groin; trouble getting pregnant (infertility); depression; and weight gain.

How Is Polycystic Ovarian Syndrome Diagnosed?

The doctor will take a medical history, do a physical and pelvic examination, and order blood tests to measure hormone levels and rule out other illnesses. Blood pressure and blood glucose and cholesterol levels will be measured. The doctor will also order ultrasonography of the ovaries to see how many cysts they have. The doctor may suggest a visit to a gynecologist (a doctor who specializes in female reproductive health) and to an endocrinologist (a specialist in hormone disorders).

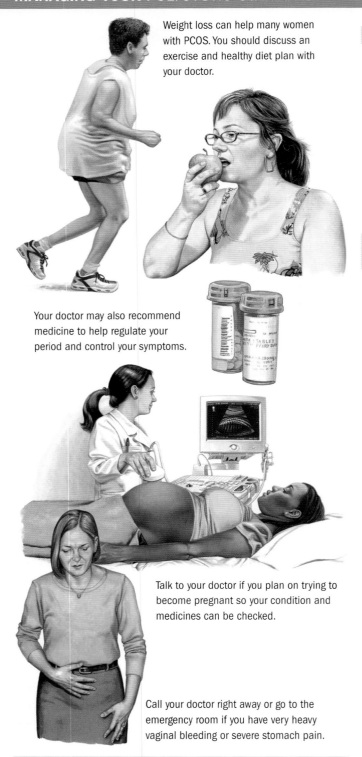

Weight loss can help many women with PCOS. You should discuss an exercise and healthy diet plan with your doctor.

Your doctor may also recommend medicine to help regulate your period and control your symptoms.

Talk to your doctor if you plan on trying to become pregnant so your condition and medicines can be checked.

Call your doctor right away or go to the emergency room if you have very heavy vaginal bleeding or severe stomach pain.

How Is Polycystic Ovarian Syndrome Treated?

Treatment depends on how severe symptoms are and if pregnancy is wanted. Overweight women will need to diet and exercise. Weight loss can help many women with PCOS.

Medicine can be given to make periods more regular, control other symptoms, and help in becoming pregnant. Surgery (laparoscopic ovarian wedge resection) is sometimes performed to decrease hormone release from the ovaries.

High blood pressure, diabetes, and high cholesterol should also be treated.

DOs and DON'Ts in Managing Polycystic Ovarian Syndrome:

✔ **DO** follow your doctor's directions and take your medicine.
✔ **DO** tell your doctor about your other medical problems.
✔ **DO** tell your doctor about your medicines, including prescription and nonprescription drugs.
✔ **DO** tell your doctor if you're pregnant or trying to have a baby.
✔ **DO** see your doctor regularly. Get a pelvic examination every year.
✔ **DO** try to lose weight by eating a healthy diet and exercising.
✔ **DO** call your doctor right away or go to the emergency room if you have very heavy vaginal bleeding or severe stomach pain.

🚫 **DON'T** stop taking your medicine just because you feel better.
🚫 **DON'T** abuse alcohol.
🚫 **DON'T** use any other medicines, including herbal supplements, without asking your doctor first.

FROM THE DESK OF

NOTES

FOR MORE INFORMATION

Contact the following source:

• Polycystic Ovarian Syndrome Association
Tel: (877) 755-7276
Website: http://www.pcosupport.org

MANAGING
PROLACTINOMA

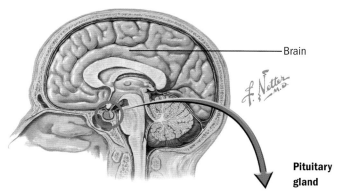

Brain

Pituitary gland

The pituitary gland lies at the bottom of the brain and controls growth, metabolism, and reproduction. It also secretes many hormones, including prolactin. Prolactin is the hormone that stimulates milk production after pregnancy.

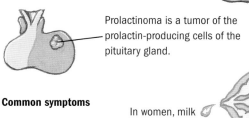

Prolactinoma is a tumor of the prolactin-producing cells of the pituitary gland.

Common symptoms

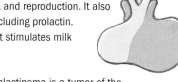

In women, milk production without pregnancy

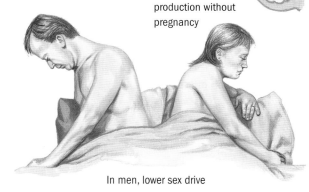

In men, lower sex drive

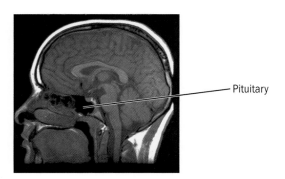

Pituitary

Prolactin levels can be checked by blood tests. High prolactin levels can also be caused by drugs or another condition, such as liver or kidney disease. To confirm the diagnosis, MRI of the pituitary gland is needed.

What Are Prolactinomas?

A prolactinoma is a tumor of the prolactin-producing cells of the pituitary gland. The pituitary gland, or master gland, lies at the bottom of the brain and controls growth, metabolism, and reproduction. One of the many hormones secreted by the pituitary is prolactin. Prolactin causes a woman's breasts to secrete milk after pregnancy. Tumors in prolactin-secreting cells of the pituitary cause too much prolactin to get into the bloodstream.

Prolactinomas are rare and occur in 1 or 2 people in 10,000. Most are curable.

What Causes Prolactinomas?

The cause is unknown.

What Are the Symptoms of Prolactinomas?

Women may have changes in menstruation (periods) or produce milk when they aren't pregnant. High prolactin levels may lower estrogen levels, which lead to vaginal dryness and painful intercourse.

Males may notice impotence or lower sex drive.

Untreated prolactinomas may lead to reduced amounts of mineral in bones (osteoporosis). Tumors may also press on nerves near the pituitary, such as optic nerves, which are important for vision. The result may be decreased peripheral vision.

How Are Prolactinomas Diagnosed?

The doctor diagnoses a prolactinoma by finding high blood prolactin levels. Breast stimulation will also increase prolactin levels, as will many drugs, especially antidepressants. People with hypothyroidism (low thyroid gland function) or advanced liver or kidney disease can also have high prolactin levels. The doctor will take into account medicines you are taking and other medical disorders when making the diagnosis.

Magnetic resonance imaging (MRI) of the brain will show a tumor in the pituitary gland.

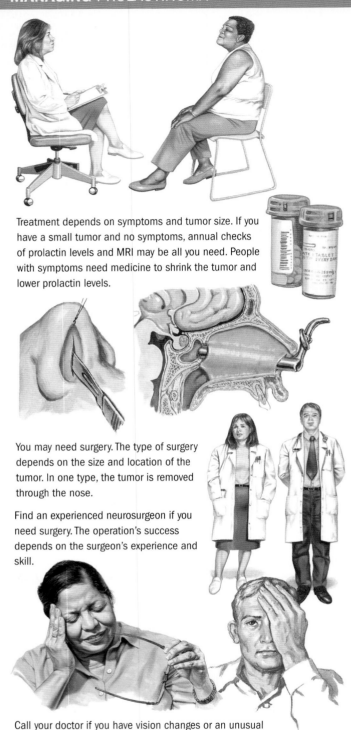

Treatment depends on symptoms and tumor size. If you have a small tumor and no symptoms, annual checks of prolactin levels and MRI may be all you need. People with symptoms need medicine to shrink the tumor and lower prolactin levels.

You may need surgery. The type of surgery depends on the size and location of the tumor. In one type, the tumor is removed through the nose.

Find an experienced neurosurgeon if you need surgery. The operation's success depends on the surgeon's experience and skill.

Call your doctor if you have vision changes or an unusual increase in headaches.

How Are Prolactinomas Treated?

The best treatment depends on symptoms and tumor size. The treatment goal is to have normal reproductive and pituitary function and minimize symptoms, such as production of breast milk and changes in periods.

Some people with very small tumors (called microadenomas), who have no symptoms may be followed up with annual MRI and prolactin level tests. Many of these small prolactinomas don't get larger.

People with symptoms need medicine (e.g., bromocriptine and cabergoline) to shrink the tumor and reduce prolactin levels.

If medicine isn't tolerated or doesn't control tumor growth, surgery is used and can be very successful. But tumors may come back after surgery. Larger tumors (macroadenomas) can be treated with surgery, irradiation of the pituitary, and medications. The tumor may also be destroyed with radiation delivered through multiple parts (stereotactic surgery, also called gamma knife surgery).

DOs and DON'Ts in Managing Prolactinomas:

✔ **DO** make sure that your prolactin level was measured after an 8-hour fast, and that there was no recent breast stimulation, to get an accurate prolactin level.

✔ **DO** find an experienced surgeon if you need surgery. A neurosurgeon (doctor who specializes in surgery for the nervous system) should do the operation. Success depends on the neurosurgeon's experience and skill.

✔ **DO** call your doctor if you have vision changes or an unusual increase in headaches.

✔ **DO** call your doctor if you have nausea or dizziness from the medicine.

✔ **DO** call your doctor if you feel extremely weak and tired or urinate often after surgery.

⊘ **DON'T** forget to use birth control if you're sexually active after starting treatment. With successful treatment, women will again have normal periods and men will have normal testosterone levels.

FROM THE DESK OF

NOTES

FOR MORE INFORMATION

Contact the following sources:

• National Brain Tumor Society
Tel: (800) 934-2873
Web: http://www.braintumor.org

• Pituitary Tumor Network Association
Tel: (805) 499-9973

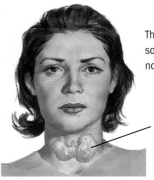

The butterfly-shaped thyroid sometimes develops a lump, or nodule.

Thyroid gland with nodule

Most nodules are benign with no noticeable symptoms, but because some can be problematic or cancerous, it is important to investigate the nature of the nodule(s).

Some nodules lead to an overactive thyroid and cause tremor, anxiety, and hunger.

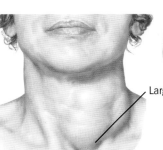

Large thyroid nodule

Other nodules might be visible as a swollen thyroid.

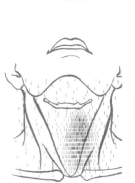

Thyroid scan showing overactive nodule

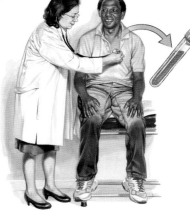

Blood tests and imaging (x-ray, sonogram, radioactive iodine scan) can show the thyroid nodule.

What Is a Thyroid Nodule?

The thyroid gland lies in the neck. It is part of the endocrine system and produces a substance (thyroid hormone) that helps control metabolism. A thyroid nodule is a lump on this gland. Nodules may be caused by an infection, cyst, benign tumor, or malignant tumor of the thyroid. Most nodules are benign tumors or cysts filled with fluid. Because some thyroid nodules are cancerous, all nodules should be examined.

What Are the Symptoms of a Thyroid Nodule?

Most people don't know that they have a nodule. Some people may have no symptoms. Others may feel or see a soft, painless swelling near the thyroid in the neck. Most nodules are benign, cold (inactive) nodules, with no effect on health. Hot (overactive) nodules cause anxiety, sweating, weight loss, hunger, and tremor by producing excess thyroid hormone (hyperthyroidism).

A rock-hard nodule that grows rapidly and causes a voice change (hoarseness) or swallowing difficulty suggests cancer and should be removed quickly.

How Is a Thyroid Nodule Diagnosed?

A sonogram (which uses sound waves to make pictures of body parts) can tell whether nodules are present and whether a nodule is solid. Solid nodules may be cancerous.

Specialists may also discover nodules on x-ray films of the chest or neck done for other reasons. After nodules are found, two important questions need answers:

- Is the thyroid working normally?
- Is the nodule benign or malignant?

Thyroid function blood tests answer the first question. Most people have normal thyroid function.

A special test (radioactive iodine scan) can tell whether an overactive nodule is producing too much hormone and must be treated.

A doctor will check a tissue sample (biopsy) of the nodule to see whether the nodule is benign. A fine-needle aspiration biopsy (FNAB) is used to get this sample.

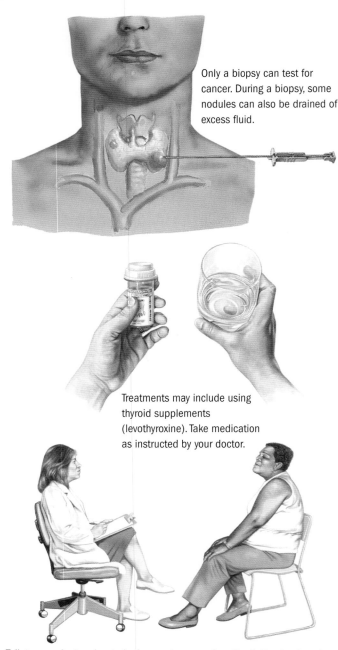

Only a biopsy can test for cancer. During a biopsy, some nodules can also be drained of excess fluid.

Treatments may include using thyroid supplements (levothyroxine). Take medication as instructed by your doctor.

Talk to your doctor about whether surgery or radioactive iodine treatments might be a better option for you.

How Is a Thyroid Nodule Treated?

Most nodules are benign. Benign solid nodules are easily treated with thyroid supplements (levothyroxine) that help prevent nodule growth. Nodules that contain only fluid are drained during the FNAB.

Surgery may be needed to remove large nodules if they could be cancerous or if they crush blood vessels or other tissues in the neck. If the whole tumor cannot be removed, radioactive iodine can destroy remaining cancer cells. This treatment also destroys normal thyroid cells, so after treatment most people develop an underactive thyroid (hypothyroidism) and need medicine to replace thyroid hormone.

Complications after surgery include bleeding, infection, low calcium levels from damage to the parathyroid glands near the thyroid during surgery, or damage to vocal cords. An experienced surgeon usually causes few complications, however. Hormone therapy for benign nodules can lead to an overactive thyroid (hyperthyroidism). Radioactive iodine therapy may cause other glands to swell and dry out.

DOs and DON'Ts in Managing a Thyroid Nodule:

✔ **DO** have an FNAB of any suspicious nodule.

✔ **DO** find an experienced thyroid specialist.

✔ **DO** examine your neck to find new nodules.

✔ **DO** tell your doctor if you had radiation therapy to the neck or a family history of thyroid cancer.

✔ **DO** call your doctor if you develop symptoms after treatment or surgery.

⊘ **DON'T** stop taking or changing your medicine because you feel better unless your doctor tells you to.

FROM THE DESK OF

NOTES

FOR MORE INFORMATION

Contact the following source:

- American Thyroid Association
  Tel: (703) 998-8890
  Website: http://www.thyroid.org

MANAGING YOUR
THYROIDITIS

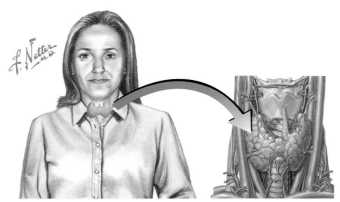

The thyroid is a small gland in the middle of the neck. It helps control metabolism. Thyroiditis is inflammation of this gland. It may cause an overactive thyroid (called hyperthyroidism) or underactive thyroid (called hypothyroidism).

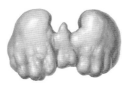

Thyroid gland showing Hashimoto's thyroiditis

The most common kind of thyroiditis is Hashimoto's thyroiditis. Many more women than men get it. The cause is the body's own immune system attacking thyroid cells. Another type of thyroiditis can occur in women who were recently pregnant.

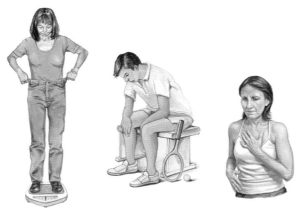

Common symptoms of an overactive gland are weight loss, diarrhea, irregular periods, racing heartbeat, and anxiety. An underactive gland causes weight gain, constipation, tiredness, and depression.

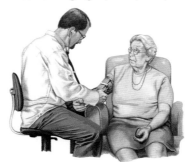

Your doctor will take a medical history, examine you, and order blood tests. A special x-ray called radioactive iodine uptake (RAIU) may also be done.

What Is Thyroiditis?

The thyroid is a small gland in the middle of the neck and is important for controlling metabolism. Thyroiditis is inflammation (swelling) of this gland. Inflammation may result in an overactive gland (called hyperthyroidism) or underactive gland (called hypothyroidism).

The most common type of thyroiditis is Hashimoto's thyroiditis. About 10 times more women than men get it, up to 2% of women in the United States. Other types called subacute and silent thyroiditis can also result in an overactive thyroid. Postpartum thyroiditis occurs in women who were recently pregnant. Thyroiditis can lead to both overactive and underactive thyroid symptoms depending on its stage.

What Causes Thyroiditis?

Many things can cause thyroiditis. In the most common type, the body's own immune (infection-fighting) system attacks thyroid cells. The result may be high hormone levels (hyperthyroidism) followed by low hormone levels (hypothyroidism).

What Are the Symptoms of Thyroiditis?

Symptoms depend on the type of thyroiditis and how severe it is. The most common symptoms of acute disease in early stages are enlarged thyroid, sometimes pain and tenderness in the thyroid, and sometimes dry eyes and dry mouth. One type, painless thyroiditis, causes no pain. Symptoms of hyperthyroidism occur in silent, subacute, or early postpartum thyroiditis. They include weight loss, greater appetite, diarrhea, irregular periods, racing heartbeat, anxiety, heat sensitivity, and shaking. Hypothyroidism may cause weight gain, less appetite, constipation, tiredness, depression, cold sensitivity, and weakness. In subacute thyroiditis, which occurs after a viral infection, an enlarged thyroid may cause neck pain and swelling. Postpartum thyroiditis may cause anxiety (hyperthyroid) and depression and fatigue (hypothyroid).

How Is Thyroiditis Diagnosed?

The doctor takes a medical history, does a physical examination, and orders blood tests. These tests measure thyroid-stimulating hormone (TSH) and antithyroid antibodies. A special x-ray called radioactive iodine uptake (RAIU) may also be done.

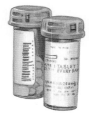

People treated with thyroid hormone usually need lifelong therapy. For Hashimoto's disease, levothyroxine will replace missing hormone. Antiinflammatory medicine may be needed if pain is present. It may be 4 to 6 weeks before you start to feel better, so don't get discouraged.

Pregnancy affects your condition, so tell your doctor if you are or are planning to become pregnant. You can then discuss the best treatment approach for you.

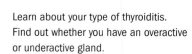

Physical activity is good for the body, but if you have hyperthyroid or hypothyroid symptoms, don't exercise too vigorously until your condition is treated.

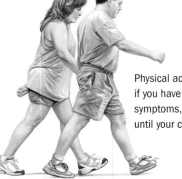

Learn about your type of thyroiditis. Find out whether you have an overactive or underactive gland.

How Is Thyroiditis Treated?

People treated with thyroid hormone will likely need lifelong therapy. People with Hashimoto's disease take levothyroxine (thyroid hormone) to replace missing hormone.

Silent and subacute thyroiditis may go away without treatment or may need antiinflammatory medicines. These drugs include a nonsteroidal antiinflammatory drug (NSAID) or prednisone for pain. A beta-blocker such as propranolol or atenolol may be given for rapid heartbeats.

DOs and DON'Ts in Managing Thyroiditis:

✔ **DO** follow-up with your doctor. Thyroiditis changes over time and you usually change from being hyperthyroid to hypothyroid.
✔ **DO** learn about your type of thyroiditis. Find out whether you have an overactive or underactive gland.
✔ **DO** take your medicine as prescribed.
✔ **DO** tell your doctor if you're pregnant or breastfeeding or want to become pregnant.
✔ **DO** call your doctor if you have chest pain, chest pressure, or palpitations after starting thyroid hormone therapy.
✔ **DO** call your doctor if you have a high fever or severe illness.
✔ **DO** call your doctor if you have a reaction to medicine.
✔ **DO** call your doctor if you feel sick even with treatment for several weeks.

⊘ **DON'T** expect an overnight response to treatment. You'll need 4 to 6 weeks before you begin to feel better.
⊘ **DON'T** exercise too hard if you have symptoms.

FROM THE DESK OF

NOTES

FOR MORE INFORMATION

Contact the following sources:

• American Association of Clinical Endocrinologists
Tel: (904) 353-7878
Website: http://www.aace.com

• American Thyroid Association
Tel: (718) 882-6047
Website: http://www.thyroid.org/patients/patients.html

CARING FOR YOUR CHILD WITH TURNER'S SYNDROME

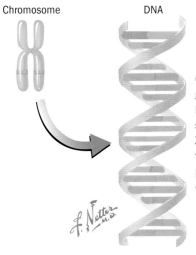

Chromosome   DNA

Chromosomes consist of genes that are made of DNA. Normal females have two XX sex chromosomes (boys have XY). A girl born without one of the X chromosomes will have physical abnormalities. This disorder is Turner's syndrome.

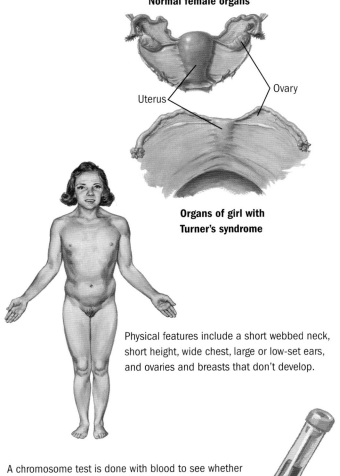

Normal female organs

Uterus   Ovary

Organs of girl with Turner's syndrome

Physical features include a short webbed neck, short height, wide chest, large or low-set ears, and ovaries and breasts that don't develop.

A chromosome test is done with blood to see whether an X chromosome is missing. This confirms the diagnosis.

What Is Turner's Syndrome?

Turner's syndrome is a genetic disorder related to a defect in chromosomes. Chromosomes consist of genes that are made up of DNA. Chromosomes inside cells contain a unique blueprint for each person's development. Turner's syndrome affects only girls, who are missing a chromosome that females normally have. This defect leads to physical symptoms that vary and can be mild or severe.

What Causes Turner's Syndrome?

The cause is one of the X chromosomes in females being partly or completely missing. The reason why this chromosome is missing is unknown.

What Are the Symptoms of Turner's Syndrome?

Babies with Turner's syndrome grow slowly and often have feeding problems.

Common physical features include a short webbed neck, short height, wide chest, large or low-set ears, and low hairline at the back of the neck.

Ovaries often don't develop, so neither do breasts. Older girls will be late having their first period or may not have periods. Almost all girls are unable to become pregnant.

Heart and kidney problems, hearing loss, and clumsiness may be present. Usually, girls and women have normal intelligence but rarely may have slight learning problems.

How Is Turner's Syndrome Diagnosed?

A doctor may suspect Turner's syndrome because of a baby's appearance. A chromosome test is done to see whether an X chromosome is missing and confirm the diagnosis. For this test, a small sample of blood is collected. Chromosomes from blood cells are counted, and their size and shape are studied. This arrangement of chromosomes is called a karyotype.

Other tests may be needed to check for other problems, such as heart or kidney disorders, caused by Turner's syndrome.

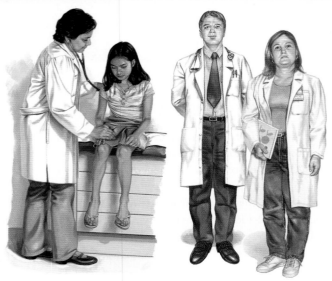

In addition to a primary care doctor, specialists can help provide the best treatment. A geneticist specializes in chromosome problems, and an endocrinologist specializes in hormone treatments.

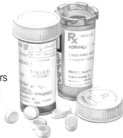

Hormones can help improve some abnormalities. Growth hormones can increase a girl's height by a few inches. Female hormones given in early teen years can help breast development and getting menstrual periods.

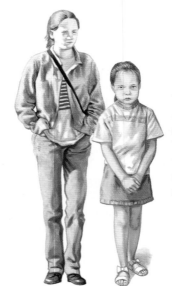

Teenage years can be hard for anyone and may be more so for someone with Turner's syndrome. Talk to your doctor if your child needs help with school, is feeling depressed, or wants to find a support group.

How Is Turner's Syndrome Treated?

Treatment with hormones can help correct some abnormalities. Hormones are chemicals in the body that control growth and other body functions.

Growth can improve by giving growth hormones. This treatment can increase height by several inches.

In early teen years, female hormones may be given. They will help physical development, such as breast growth and starting periods.

Other medicines are used as needed, such as for heart or kidney problems.

Specialists will help the doctor choose the best treatment. These specialists include a geneticist for chromosome problems and an endocrinologist for hormone treatment.

DOs and DON'Ts in Managing Turner's Syndrome:

✔ **DO** use medicines as directed.
✔ **DO** follow up with an endocrinologist in addition to your primary care doctor.
✔ **DO** help your daughter exercise, eat healthy, and keep to a normal body weight.
✔ **DO** call the doctor if she needs special help with school.
✔ **DO** call the doctor if she feels depressed.
✔ **DO** look for and join a support group. Ask your doctor for help finding one or for more information.

🚫 **DON'T** stop using medicines without asking your doctor first.

FROM THE DESK OF

NOTES

FOR MORE INFORMATION

Contact the following source:

• Turner Syndrome Society
  Tel: (800) 365-9944
  Website: http://www.turnersyndrome.org

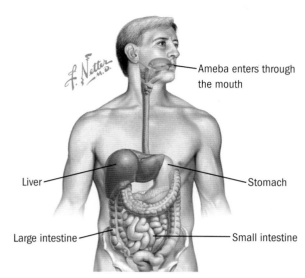

Ameba enters through the mouth

Liver

Stomach

Large intestine

Small intestine

Amebiasis is an infection of the intestine and sometimes the liver. It is caused by the ameba *Entamoeba histolytica*, a parasite.

The parasite infects and damages the stomach and intestine.

Ulcers in the intestine

People usually get the infection by drinking dirty water or eating contaminated food. Rarely, the ameba spreads through the blood to the lung, liver, brain, and other organs.

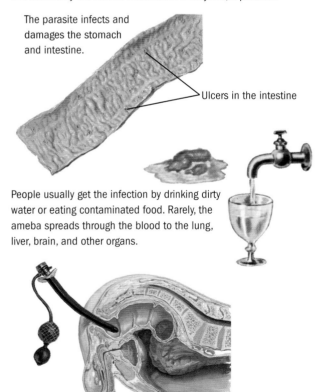

Your doctor may ask you for stool sample to be examined under a microscope to see if parasites or cysts are there. If needed, a scope with a light at the end (called a sigmoidoscope or colonoscope) may be inserted into the anus where small pieces of tissue can be taken and then studied to check for the parasite.

What Is Amebiasis?

Amebiasis is an infection of the large intestine and sometimes the liver.

What Causes Amebiasis?

Amebiasis is caused by an ameba, the parasite *Entamoeba histolytica*. It is common in subtropical locations, especially in crowded or unsanitary living conditions. Amebic dysentery (or gastrointestinal amebiasis) is diarrhea caused by the parasite, which damages the stomach and intestine. People usually get the parasite by drinking dirty water or eating contaminated food. Flies or other insects also spread the infection. Amebic dysentery can also be caught from a sexual partner during anal sex.

What Are the Symptoms of Amebiasis?

Symptoms usually begin 2 to 4 weeks after infection, or months later. Some people have no symptoms (but may be carriers). The most common symptoms are diarrhea (10 to 12 small bowel movements daily), bloody diarrhea, stomach cramps, stomach tenderness (soreness), mucus (slippery, thick liquid) in the stool (feces or diarrhea), and gas. Other symptoms include fever, back pain, and tiredness.

How Is Amebiasis Diagnosed?

The doctor will take a medical history and do an examination. Three or more samples of stool are studied under a microscope to find parasites or cysts. The doctor may recommend sigmoidoscopy or colonoscopy (using a small tube, or scope, with a lighted tip) to get small samples from the intestine to examine.

In most cases, your doctor will give you medicine that kills the parasites. The medicine should be taken according to your doctor's instructions. Take all the medicine prescribed.

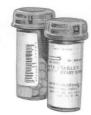
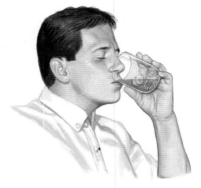
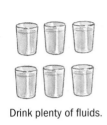

Drink plenty of fluids.

Always wash your hands with soap and warm water after using the bathroom.

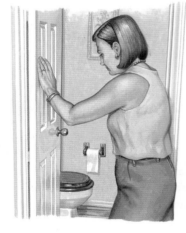

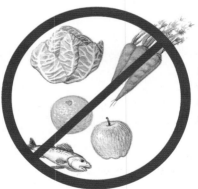

Prevent reinfection: Don't eat raw vegetables, unpeeled fruit, or raw fish in questionable areas.

How Is Amebiasis Treated?

With treatment, most people get better in 10 to 20 days. In most cases, medicine kills the ameba. It is critical to take all the medicine prescribed by the doctor. The doctor will recheck the stool after treatment to make sure all parasites are gone.

Medicines include metronidazole and iodoquinol. Side effects include nausea, headache, dry mouth or metallic taste, and darkened urine. Don't drink alcohol when taking these drugs.

Bed rest may be needed in severe cases, with normal activities then resumed gradually. Fluids must be increased to prevent dehydration. In serious cases, intravenous fluids may be given.

DOs and DON'Ts in Managing Amebiasis:

✔ **DO** take your medicine as prescribed.
✔ **DO** increase fluid (water) intake.
✔ **DO** wash hands often with soap and warm water.
✔ **DO** drink bottled or boiled water or soda if traveling in developing countries.
✔ **DO** make sure all food is well cooked.
✔ **DO** call your doctor right away if you have a high fever, bloody diarrhea, stomach pain, pain in the right upper side of your stomach, or yellowing of the skin.
✔ **DO** practice safe sex (use a latex condom).
✔ **DO** call your doctor if you cannot take the fluids or medicines prescribed.

⊘ **DON'T** drink alcohol during treatment.
⊘ **DON'T** swim in fresh water outside the United States or Western Europe, or in dirty pools.
⊘ **DON'T** eat raw vegetables, unpeeled fruit, raw fish, or shellfish in questionable areas. Don't have ice in your drinks or eat ice cream.
⊘ **DON'T** stop taking your medicine or change your dose because you feel better unless your doctor tells you to.

FROM THE DESK OF

NOTES

FOR MORE INFORMATION

Contact the following sources:

* National Institute of Allergy and Infectious Diseases
  Tel: (866) 284-4107
  Website: http://www.healthfinder.gov

* Centers for Disease Control and Prevention
  Tel: (800) 311-3435
  Website: http://www.cdc.gov

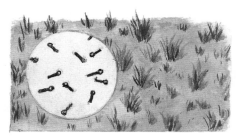

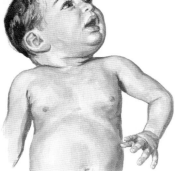

Bacteria occur widely in nature and form spores that resist heat.

A common cause of botulism is eating improperly preserved home-processed foods.

Infant botulism occurs when a child eats the spores (like in contaminated honey), which then grow in the intestines and produce toxin.

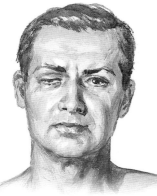

One symptom is drooping eyelids. Others include difficulty swallowing and muscle weakness.

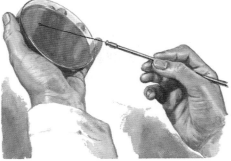

Laboratory tests to diagnose botulism can take up to 4 days to complete.

What Is Botulism?

Botulism is a disease caused by toxins (poisons) that are produced by a bacteria named *Clostridium botulinum*. These bacteria occur widely in soils and grow from spores (the resting stage) only in the right conditions. The three types of botulism are food related, wound related, and infant botulism. In the United States, an average of 110 cases are reported yearly. Of these, about 25% are related to the food type, 72% to the infant type, and 3% to the wound type.

These toxins also have value in medical treatments, such as relieving muscle spasms (twitching) and removing wrinkles (cosmetic use).

What Causes Botulism?

The bacteria produce seven toxins (labeled A through G). Types A, B, E, and F cause disease in humans, in people of all ages. Botulism cannot be transmitted from person to person.

People get food-borne botulism from eating food containing the toxin. A common cause is improperly preserved home-processed foods.

Wound botulism is most often related to illegal drug use and to crush injuries. Spores contaminate a wound and produce toxin that gets into the bloodstream.

Infants can eat spores, which then grow in the intestines and produce toxin.

What Are the Symptoms of Botulism?

First symptoms are drooping eyelids, blurred vision, double vision, slurred speech, difficulty swallowing, dry mouth, and muscle weakness. Most symptoms start 12 to 36 hours after eating tainted foods. If the disease isn't diagnosed and treated early, it may lead to paralysis of arms, legs, trunk, and breathing muscles. People may need a mechanical ventilator to help their breathing.

About 5% to 10% of people with food-borne botulism die.

How Is Botulism Diagnosed?

Botulism has symptoms similar to those of other neurological diseases, so diagnosis is difficult and it is often misdiagnosed. Laboratory tests to prove it can take up to 4 days to complete, and only certain laboratories can do them.

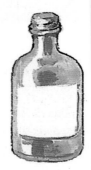

Botulism can be treated with an antitoxin.

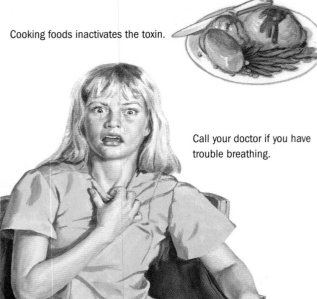

Cooking foods inactivates the toxin.

Call your doctor if you have trouble breathing.

How Is Botulism Treated?

The doctor treats botulism by checking and observing symptoms, providing supportive care, and giving an antitoxin (a chemical to counteract the toxin). The antitoxin slows the paralysis and may also make the symptoms less severe and stop them sooner.

DOs and DON'Ts in Managing Botulism:

✔ **DO** realize that most outbreaks are related to eating home-canned foods, especially vegetables. Avoid eating contaminated food. You can get instructions on safe home canning from the U.S. Department of Agriculture.

✔ **DO** understand that the toxin is destroyed by high temperatures. Boil foods for at least 10 minutes.

✔ **DO** realize that infant botulism occurs when an infant eats spores of the bacteria. Many cases have occurred after eating contaminated honey.

✔ **DO** keep all wounds clean. Proper wound care and avoiding illegal drug use reduces your risk of getting wound botulism.

✔ **DO** call your doctor if you have trouble breathing or swallowing or note muscle weakness, double vision, or slurred speech.

✔ **DO** call your doctor if you have a contaminated wound.

⊘ **DON'T** do drugs!

⊘ **DON'T** forget that botulism is not spread from one person to another.

FROM THE DESK OF

NOTES

FOR MORE INFORMATION

Contact the following source:

• Centers for Disease Control and Prevention
  Tel: (800) 232-4636
  Website: http://www.bt.cdc.gov

MANAGING YOUR BURNS

The seriousness of a burn depends on how deep the injury goes.

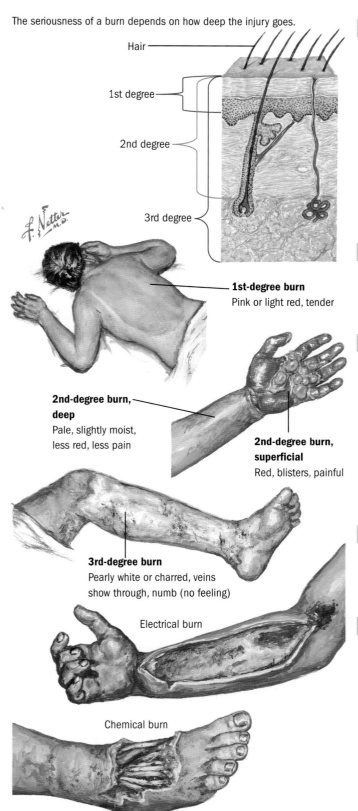

Hair

1st degree

2nd degree

3rd degree

1st-degree burn
Pink or light red, tender

2nd-degree burn, deep
Pale, slightly moist, less red, less pain

2nd-degree burn, superficial
Red, blisters, painful

3rd-degree burn
Pearly white or charred, veins show through, numb (no feeling)

Electrical burn

Chemical burn

What Are Burns?

Thermal burns are injuries to the skin (and deeper structures) caused by too much heat or certain types of light. Intense heat for a short time (e.g., hot grease) and low heat or light over long times (e.g., heating pads or sun) produce burns. The depth of tissue injury determines burn severity. Thermal burns are usually classified as first, second, and third degree. Electricity and chemicals such as acids and alkali may also cause burns. Chemical burns are more complicated and hard to classify. Electrical burns may be deep enough to reach muscles and bones and are sometimes called fourth-degree (black or char) burns.

What Causes Burns?

Burns can be caused by fire, steam, electricity, sun, chemicals, and hot liquids or objects.

What Are the Symptoms of Burns?

Symptoms vary with the degree of damage to body tissues. First-degree burns produce painful, red areas in the surface (superficial) skin, but no blisters. Second-degree burns affect deeper skin, with blisters and light charring, and are very painful. Third-degree burns damage the whole skin depth, so the skin looks pale, charred, and leathery. These burns aren't painful because the nerves in the burned area have been damaged.

How Are Burns Diagnosed?

The diagnosis is made by examining the skin. Symptoms will help determine the degree of burn.

How Are Burns Treated?

Small first-degree burns may not require any treatment. Putting the burned area in cold water (not ice) or using wet compresses can reduce pain and swelling of minor burns. Breaking blisters can cause infection, so this should be avoided. Using aloe vera and acetaminophen or ibuprofen can help pain. Protection with dressings and antibiotic ointment may prevent infection.

Treatment for first-degree burns includes putting the burned area in cold water or using wet compresses (not ice directly on the burn), using aloe vera and taking medicine for pain.

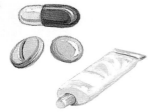

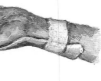

Your doctor should see second-degree burns larger than the size of your palm. All third-degree burns and worse need a doctor's immediate care. Call 911 for emergency help.

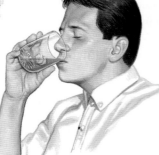

Drink plenty of fluids, because burns cause you to lose water.

Avoid sun on your burns while healing—it increases scarring. Do not put butter on burns.

Practice fire safety: wear protection, fireproof your home and business, and teach children safety rules.

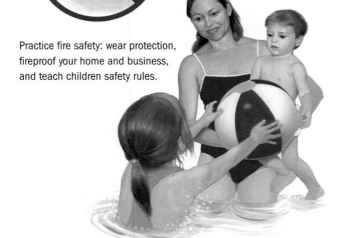

Medical evaluation and treatment is needed for: (1) second-degree burns larger than the person's palm; (2) any second-degree burns of hands, feet, face, or genitals; and (3) second-degree burns anywhere on infants. All third- and fourth-degree burns (which are life-threatening) need a doctor's immediate care. A doctor should always see chemical burns.

The doctor will gently remove dead skin layers (débridement), change dressings, and watch for infections. Some severe burns need specialized treatment, including surgical grafting of skin and use of special pressure garments, at special centers.

For severe burns, call 911 for help.

DOs and DON'Ts in Managing Burns:

✔ **DO** change your dressing and apply fresh antibiotic ointment at prescribed times.

✔ **DO** use pain medicines as directed.

✔ **DO** drink extra fluids and eat a healthy diet.

✔ **DO** keep follow-up doctor appointments.

✔ **DO** call your doctor if you have fever; chills; increasing pain; or pus, foul odor, or red streaking from your wound.

✔ **DO** call your doctor if you have a reaction to medicine.

✔ **DO** practice fire safety: wear protection, fireproof your home and business, and teach children safety rules.

⊘ **DON'T** ignore second-degree burns.

⊘ **DON'T** put butter on burns.

⊘ **DON'T** let bandages become dirty or wet.

⊘ **DON'T** exercise or return to work until your doctor says to.

⊘ **DON'T** expose healing burns to sunlight (increases scarring).

⊘ **DON'T** try to peel dead skin layers.

FROM THE DESK OF

NOTES

FOR MORE INFORMATION

Contact the following source:

• Burn Survivor Resource Center
Tel: (800) 669-7700
Wesite: http://burnsurvivor.com/survivorlinks.html

MANAGING YOUR
CARBON MONOXIDE POISONING

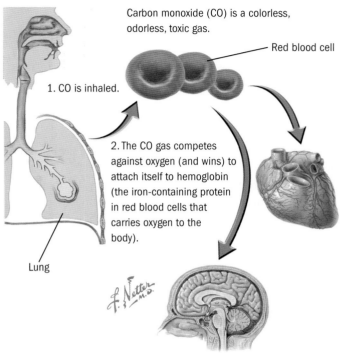

Carbon monoxide (CO) is a colorless, odorless, toxic gas.

Red blood cell

1. CO is inhaled.

2. The CO gas competes against oxygen (and wins) to attach itself to hemoglobin (the iron-containing protein in red blood cells that carries oxygen to the body).

Lung

3. Less oxygen gets to tissues, especially organs that need the most, such as the brain and heart.

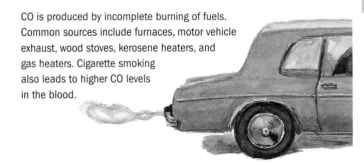

CO is produced by incomplete burning of fuels. Common sources include furnaces, motor vehicle exhaust, wood stoves, kerosene heaters, and gas heaters. Cigarette smoking also leads to higher CO levels in the blood.

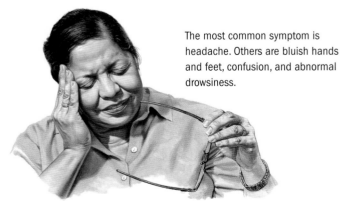

The most common symptom is headache. Others are bluish hands and feet, confusion, and abnormal drowsiness.

What Is Carbon Monoxide Poisoning?

Carbon monoxide (abbreviated as CO) is a colorless, odorless, toxic gas that doesn't irritate the skin or eyes. CO in air is breathed in and easily absorbed through lungs. It is better than oxygen in binding with hemoglobin in red blood cells. Hemoglobin is the iron-containing protein in these cells that carries oxygen to body tissues. This means that when too much carbon monoxide is in the environment, less oxygen gets to tissues, especially organs needing the most oxygen, such as the brain and heart.

CO poisoning accounts for almost 4000 deaths yearly in the United States. Exposures may be accidental (less often) or on purpose (suicide attempts).

What Causes Carbon Monoxide Poisoning?

CO is produced by incomplete burning of fuels. Sources include furnaces, motor vehicle exhaust fumes, wood stoves, kerosene heaters, and gas heaters. Even cigarette smoking causes a higher CO level in the bloodstream.

What Are the Symptoms of Carbon Monoxide Poisoning?

The most common symptom is headache. Others include nausea, weakness, dizziness, difficulty concentrating, chest pain, shortness of breath, and visual problems. Most common physical problems include cherry-red lips, bluish hands and feet, bleeding in the back of the eye (retina), and mental changes including confusion, lethargy, and coma.

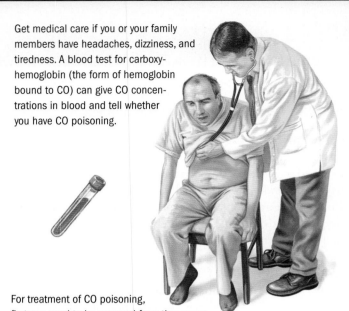

Get medical care if you or your family members have headaches, dizziness, and tiredness. A blood test for carboxyhemoglobin (the form of hemoglobin bound to CO) can give CO concentrations in blood and tell whether you have CO poisoning.

For treatment of CO poisoning, first you need to be removed from the source of the CO. Then, you will be given 100% oxygen to improve your oxygen level.

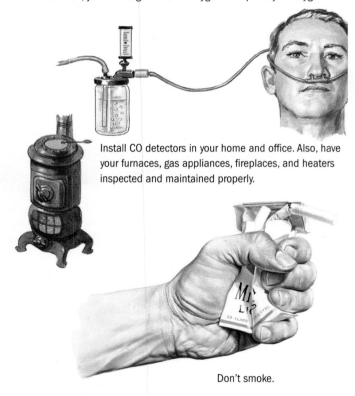

Install CO detectors in your home and office. Also, have your furnaces, gas appliances, fireplaces, and heaters inspected and maintained properly.

Don't smoke.

How Is Carbon Monoxide Poisoning Diagnosed?

Symptoms can mimic other diseases. A blood test for carboxyhemoglobin (the form of hemoglobin bound to CO) can give CO concentrations in blood. The doctor can order other tests.

How Is Carbon Monoxide Poisoning Treated?

First, people must be removed from the source of CO (e.g., defective appliances, house fire). Then, 100% oxygen is immediately given to compete for binding sites in hemoglobin and to improve oxygen delivery to the oxygen-deprived tissues. Oxygen is given until the level of carboxyhemoglobin in blood is zero. In severe cases, a mechanical ventilator may be used to deliver oxygen.

Another treatment is hyperbaric oxygen therapy. It increases the amount of oxygen dissolved in blood. Hyperbaric oxygen chambers are for certain people, such as those with a carboxyhemoglobin level higher than 40%, those in a coma or unconscious, and pregnant women with a CO level higher than 15%.

DOs and DON'Ts in Managing Carbon Monoxide Poisoning:

✔ **DO** remember that the best treatment is prevention. Avoid enclosed garages with running vehicles. Have furnaces, gas appliances, fireplaces, and heaters inspected and maintained properly.
✔ **DO** install CO alarms in your home and office.
✔ **DO** call your doctor if you think that you or someone else had exposure to CO or if you have symptoms of CO poisoning.

⊘ **DON'T** smoke. Smoking only increases the CO level in your system and leads to other medical problems.
⊘ **DON'T** use outdoor gas grills inside buildings.
⊘ **DON'T** work in a closed garage on a vehicle that is running. It only takes 10 minutes before life-threatening concentrations of CO build up in your body.

FROM THE DESK OF

NOTES

FOR MORE INFORMATION

Contact the following sources:

• Consumer Product Safety Commission
Tel: (800) 638-2772

• Medline Plus
Website: http://www.nlm.nih.gov/medlineplus/carbonmonoxidepoisoning.html

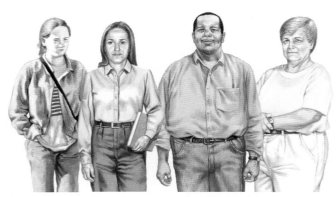

Bacterial food poisoning is a common illness resulting from eating contaminated food. Similar symptoms often occur in a group of people who ate the same foods.

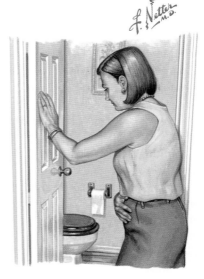

Bacteria named *Escherichia coli (E. coli), Salmonella,* and *Campylobacter* are common causes. Symptoms usually start 24 to 48 hours after eating the food. They include nausea, vomiting, abdominal cramps, diarrhea, fever, and blood in the stool.

Your doctor makes a diagnosis from your medical history, physical examination, and symptoms. Your doctor may order blood tests and stool cultures for more severe illness.

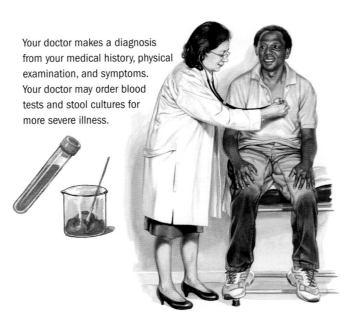

What Is Bacterial Food Poisoning?

Bacterial food poisoning is a common illness resulting from eating contaminated food.

What Causes Bacterial Food Poisoning?

Various bacteria cause this condition. Bacteria named *Escherichia coli* (*E. coli*), *Salmonella*, and *Campylobacter* are common causes. Rarely, bacteria named *Clostridium* will cause the illness called botulism.

What Are the Symptoms of Bacterial Food Poisoning?

Symptoms usually start 24 to 48 hours after eating the food. Nausea and vomiting develop, with cramps in the abdomen (belly). Diarrhea is common. Certain bacteria may produce blood in the bowel movements (stool). Fever may also be present. In severe illness, diarrhea and vomiting can lead to severe dehydration and to abnormalities in chemicals called electrolytes.

How Is Bacterial Food Poisoning Diagnosed?

The doctor makes a diagnosis from the medical history, physical examination, symptoms, and the occurrence of similar symptoms in a group of people who ate the same foods. The doctor may order blood tests and stool cultures for more severe cases.

How Is Bacterial Food Poisoning Treated?

This self-limited disease will usually go away in a few days, but one rare form, botulism, is life-threatening. The key to treatment is to replace fluids and electrolytes. Fluids such as clear broth or special oral glucose-electrolyte preparations can be taken by mouth in small, frequent sips, even if vomiting continues. Sucking ice chips, if possible, will help. Special rehydration fluids can be used. Avoid dairy products until symptoms go away.

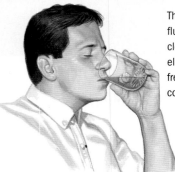

The key to treatment is replacing fluids and electrolytes. You can drink clear broth or special oral glucose-electrolyte preparations. Take small frequent sips, even if vomiting continues.

Rest in bed, but stay near the bathroom.

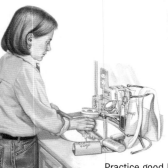

Practice good hygiene when preparing food. Wash hands between handling different foods.

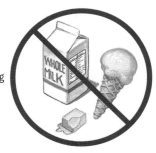

Eat a soft, bland diet if you can. Avoid dairy products and antacids containing magnesium if you have diarrhea.

Severe symptoms may mean a hospital stay and intravenous fluids. Antibiotics may help treat certain bacteria.

Medicines to stop vomiting (antiemetics) and others to control diarrhea are usually given for only severe illness.

DOs and DON'Ts in Managing Bacterial Food Poisoning:

✔ **DO** rest in bed, but stay near the bathroom or bedpan.

✔ **DO** try to drink fluids even when vomiting.

✔ **DO** eat a soft, bland diet if you can. Slowly (over 1 or 2 days) return to a normal diet.

✔ **DO** avoid dairy products and antacids containing magnesium if you have diarrhea.

✔ **DO** contact the local health department if many people who ate the same food are ill.

✔ **DO** use good hygiene when preparing foods. Wash hands between handling different foods. Keep cooking areas and utensils clean.

✔ **DO** cook and store foods properly. Throw out foods that don't smell right or are in bulging cans.

✔ **DO** wash your hands after using the bathroom.

✔ **DO** call your doctor if young children or older adults have symptoms.

✔ **DO** call your doctor if symptoms worsen after treatment begins.

✔ **DO** call your doctor if vomiting is so severe that you cannot keep liquids down.

✔ **DO** drink only bottled water when traveling (especially in foreign countries). Don't use ice cubes in drinks because these may be made with contaminated water.

🚫 **DON'T** eat raw seafood or meat or unpasteurized foods.

🚫 **DON'T** eat fresh vegetables that weren't properly washed.

🚫 **DON'T** drink tap water or eat raw foods when traveling in foreign countries. Fruits that you can peel before eating are usually safe.

FROM THE DESK OF

NOTES

FOR MORE INFORMATION

Contact the following sources:

• U.S. Department of Agriculture, Food Safety and Inspection Service
Tel: (888) 674-6854
Website: http://www.usda.gov/

• International Association for Medical Assistance to Travelers
Tel: (716) 754-4883
Website: http://www.iamat.org

MANAGING YOUR
FROSTBITE

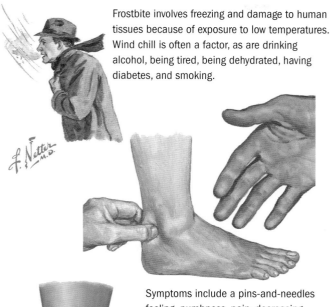

Frostbite involves freezing and damage to human tissues because of exposure to low temperatures. Wind chill is often a factor, as are drinking alcohol, being tired, being dehydrated, having diabetes, and smoking.

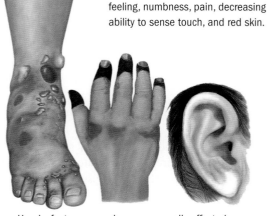

Symptoms include a pins-and-needles feeling, numbness, pain, decreasing ability to sense touch, and red skin.

Hands, feet, nose, and ears are usually affected.

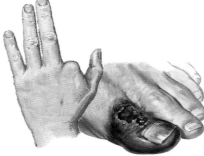

Recovery of nearby tissues can take weeks, and loss of skin, fingers, and toes, as well as deformity and discoloration (gangrene), can occur.

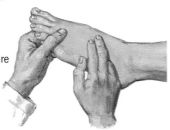

Your doctor will diagnose frostbite on the basis of a history of exposure to freezing temperatures and a physical examination.

What Is Frostbite?

Frostbite is the condition in which living human tissues freeze and are damaged because of exposure to low temperatures. Frostbite will most likely affect the hands, feet, nose, and ears.

Frostbite can be a very serious injury. Recovery of nearby tissues can take weeks. People can lose skin, fingers, and toes as well as have deformities and discoloration. People who have frostbite may also suffer from low body temperature (hypothermia).

Children and the elderly are at greater risk than adults.

What Causes Frostbite?

Exposure of bare or poorly protected skin, hands, and feet to freezing temperatures will cause frostbite. Increased wind speed, known as wind chill, is often a factor. Drinking alcohol, being tired, being dehydrated, taking beta-blockers (medicine for heart disease), smoking, and having diabetes, peripheral vascular disease (of arteries), peripheral neuropathy (nervous system disorder), and Raynaud's syndrome increase the risk of frostbite.

What Are the Symptoms of Frostbite?

Symptoms include a pins-and-needles feeling, numbness, pain, decreasing ability to sense touch, and red skin. If the problem is recognized and treated at this stage, mild swelling and peeling of the skin may be the only effects. As the process gets worse, the affected area becomes pale and firm. As the area is rewarmed, large blisters, blood blisters, and dead tissue that looks black, blue, or dark gray (from gangrene) can occur.

How Is Frostbite Diagnosed?

The doctor will diagnose frostbite on the basis of the history of exposure to freezing temperatures and a physical examination.

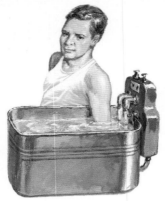

The best treatment is prevention! If frostbite occurs, it's best to put the injured area in warm water (104°F). Don't use hot water, which may cause more injury.

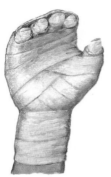

If blisters occur, don't break them. Wrap the area in dry, clean bandages and get emergency care.

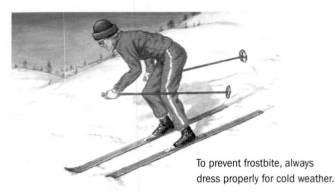

To prevent frostbite, always dress properly for cold weather.

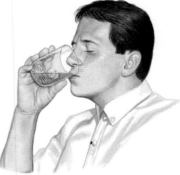

Drink plenty of nonalcoholic liquids.

How Is Frostbite Treated?

The best treatment is prevention! Dress properly for the weather and make sure children are protected and watched closely.

Drink plenty of nonalcoholic and noncaffeinated liquids. Plan ahead and limit exposure to cold when possible.

If frostbite is possible, get to shelter and warmth immediately. Immersing the injured area in warm water (104° F) is best. Don't use hot water because it may cause more injury.

If possible, rewarm the entire body, encourage fluid intake, and raise the affected area after rewarming.

If blisters occur, don't burst them. Wrap the area in dry, clean bandages and get emergency care.

DOs and DON'Ts in Managing Frostbite:

✔ **DO** watch weather conditions and dress properly.
✔ **DO** drink plenty of nonalcoholic liquids.
✔ **DO** get indoors at the first sign of symptoms.
✔ **DO** protect and watch small children closely in freezing weather.
✔ **DO** raise the injured area after rewarming.
✔ **DO** warm the entire body if possible.
✔ **DO** remove all wet clothing as soon as possible.
✔ **DO** get emergency care immediately if blisters or dead tissue appear.
✔ **DO** call your doctor if you think that you have frostbite.

⊘ **DON'T** rub the injured area with snow! This makes the injury worse.
⊘ **DON'T** drink alcohol before going out in freezing cold.
⊘ **DON'T** become tired or dehydrated in freezing weather.
⊘ **DON'T** ignore frostbite's early symptoms: pain, numbness, and redness.
⊘ **DON'T** burst blisters that form.
⊘ **DON'T** let frostbitten parts freeze again.

FROM THE DESK OF

NOTES

FOR MORE INFORMATION

Contact the following source:

• American Red Cross
Tel: (800) REDCROSS (733-2767)
Website: http://www.redcross.org

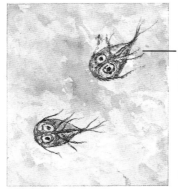

A tiny parasite so small that you can't see it, named *Giardia*, causes giardiasis, an intestinal infection.

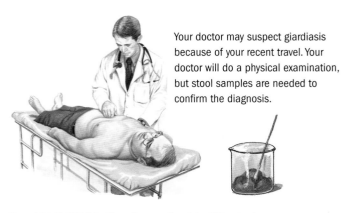

Drinking water or eating food that is contaminated with the parasite leads to giardiasis. People who travel to countries with poor water supply and sanitation systems are at risk of getting giardiasis.

Life cycle of *Giardia*

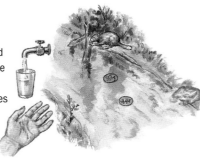

Stomach

Bowel (small intestine)

Parasites leave the body in stool.

Parasite

Parasites multiply in your body.

Parasites attach to the bowel and cause pain and diarrhea.

Your doctor may suspect giardiasis because of your recent travel. Your doctor will do a physical examination, but stool samples are needed to confirm the diagnosis.

What Is Giardiasis?

Giardiasis is an intestinal illness caused by a parasite. It's one of the main causes of diarrhea in the United States. Giardiasis isn't usually serious, but complications, such as absorption problems, weight loss, and fluid loss, can occur.

What Causes Giardiasis?

The cause is a tiny parasite you can't see named *Giardia*. Drinking water or eating food that contains *Giardia* can result in giardiasis. It's very easy to get it when traveling to countries with infected water supplies.

Giardiasis also spreads easily in crowded or unclean places or in areas with a poor water supply or sanitation system. Children in day care centers and preschools are at risk. Drinking stream water while camping or hiking, or swimming in a pool contaminated with *Giardia* can lead to giardiasis.

People who had stomach surgery have a higher risk for infection because stomach acid usually protects against infection. The risk is also greater for oral-anal and oral-genital sexual practices.

What Are the Symptoms of Giardiasis?

Up to half of people with giardiasis have no symptoms.

When symptoms occur, they'll start in 1 to 3 weeks after entry of *Giardia* into the body. Diarrhea starts suddenly. Bowel movements (stools) will be very watery and foul smelling. Stomach cramping, indigestion, discomfort at the top of the stomach, belching, gas, slight fever, and weight loss are other symptoms. Sometimes, symptoms keep returning for several months.

How Is Giardiasis Diagnosed?

The doctor may suspect giardiasis on the basis of travel history, symptoms, and physical examination. Diagnosis is made by studying samples of stool in the laboratory.

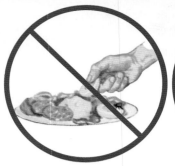
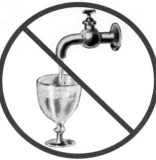

Prevention is the best treatment—be careful about drinking water or eating food that may not be safe. Don't drink from rivers and ponds when hiking or camping. Drink bottled water when in countries with questionable water supplies, and don't use ice cubes (possibly made with contaminated water).

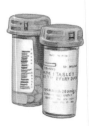

Your doctor will prescribe antiparasitic medicine, which works very well.

Drink at least eight glasses of water a day if you have giardiasis. You must replace body fluids lost because of diarrhea.

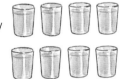

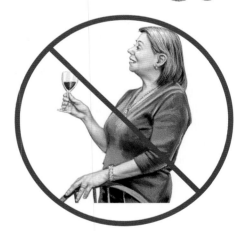

Don't drink alcohol when taking your medicine. It interacts with the medicine and causes stomach cramps.

How Is Giardiasis Treated?

Oral antiparasitic medicines such as metronidazole are taken to get rid of the parasite.

A hospital stay and intravenous fluids may be needed for severe diarrhea and loss of too much body fluid.

Prevention is the best treatment. Be careful about drinking water or eating food that may not be safe. Don't drink from surface water (rivers and ponds) when hiking or camping. If in doubt, boil the water, drink bottled water, or treat water with chemical purifiers available in camping supply stores.

Also, frequent hand washing is important, especially before meals, for people who have diarrhea or are around others with diarrhea, and after handling soiled diapers. Keep children with giardiasis home from day care and away from other children until symptoms improve.

DOs and DON'Ts in Managing Giardiasis:

✔ **DO** drink only bottled water when traveling, and don't use ice cubes (they may be made with contaminated water).

✔ **DO** drink plenty of fluids (at least eight glasses of water or liquid daily) if you have giardiasis.

✔ **DO** wash your hands often, especially after handling soiled diapers, to prevent the infection from spreading.

✔ **DO** keep children with giardiasis home until symptoms are better, to prevent spread of infection to others.

✔ **DO** call your doctor if you have new, unexplained symptoms. Sometimes the medicine causes side effects.

⊘ **DON'T** drink alcohol. It interacts with medicines and causes stomach cramps and nausea.

⊘ **DON'T** use nonprescription drugs for stomach problems. They can mask symptoms.

FROM THE DESK OF

NOTES

FOR MORE INFORMATION

Contact the following source:

• Centers for Disease Control and Prevention
Tel: (404) 639-3534, (800) 311-3435
Website: http://www.cdc.gov

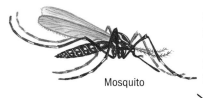
Mosquito

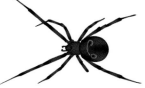

Biting insects include ants, fleas, flies, no-see-ums, and mosquitoes. Stinging insects include bees, wasps, and hornets.

Black widow

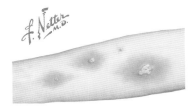
Spiders, scorpions, ticks, and mites are arachnids. The main poisonous spiders include the brown recluse and black widow.

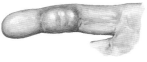

Most insect bites cause local pain or itching and then redness and swelling. Stings cause local pain and swelling.

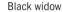

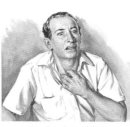
Bites can become infected.

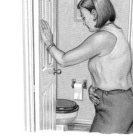
Trouble breathing   Diarrhea

People who get many stings or who have allergies to stings can have swelling, weakness, confusion, trouble breathing, fainting, vomiting, and diarrhea.

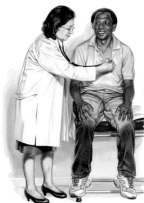

Diagnosis is based on your medical history and physical examination.

What Are Bites and Stings?

Biting insects include ants, fleas, flies, no-see-ums (flies called midges), and mosquitoes. Stinging insects include bees, wasps, and hornets. These insects are usually a nuisance, but some people are may have allergic responses to bites or stings. Some insects pass diseases to people.

The group called arthropods that includes insects also includes arachnids—spiders, scorpions, ticks, and mites. The main poisonous spiders in the United States are the brown recluse, black widow, tarantula, and hobo. Most spider bites are uncomfortable but heal without problems.

What Are the Symptoms of Bites and Stings?

Local pain or itching occur first, then redness and swelling. Bites can become infected. Stings cause local pain and swelling. Many stings can cause swelling, weakness, confusion, trouble breathing, fainting, vomiting, and diarrhea. Kidney failure, cardiac arrest, and death can occur with severe allergies. Disorders such as Lyme disease are spread by ticks, and encephalitis is spread by mosquitoes.

Brown recluse spider bites can cause stinging, redness, and swelling and blood-filled blisters, ulcers, and infection. Hobo spider bites cause similar problems plus headaches and muscle aches. Black widow spider bites usually cause intense burning, sometimes followed by spasms of the abdomen (belly), limbs, and back, with high blood pressure, sweating, and vomiting. Tarantula bites are like wasp stings with severe pain, redness, and swelling.

How Are Bites and Stings Diagnosed?

Diagnosis is based on a medical history and physical examination. Blood tests are needed for only Lyme disease or Rocky Mountain fever or if fever, rash, headache, or joint pains are present.

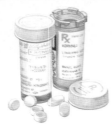

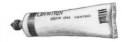

For most bites and stings, applying ice cold or cold packs will help itching and swelling, as will steroid creams and antihistamines.

You may need a tetanus shot for black widow or tarantula bites.

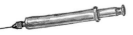

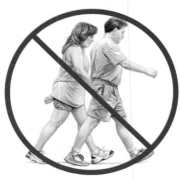

Wear long sleeves and pants and a hat when you are outdoors in mosquito- and tick-infested areas and use repellents. Put screens in the doors and windows in your home.

Don't scratch the bite area. It will make the skin reaction worse.

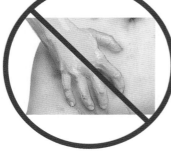

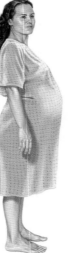

Call your doctor if an ulcer from a bite gets larger or becomes infected, you're pregnant, or you have new painful muscle spasms or trouble breathing.

How Are Bites and Stings Treated?

It's best to avoid getting bitten or stung. Use repellents, wear long sleeves and pants and a hat, and put screens in doors and windows. For most bites and stings, ice or cold packs, steroid creams, and antihistamines help itching and swelling. Oral steroids are used to treat severe reactions or many bites or stings. Antibiotics are given for tick fevers such as Lyme disease.

Hives or more severe allergic reactions need quick medical care. Some people with severe allergy must use epinephrine self-injectors.

Most spiders try to avoid humans and bite only when trapped. Bites usually heal on their own, but applying cold packs (ice) and elevating the limb if the bite is on a leg or arm will help. A tetanus shot, pain medicines, and muscle relaxants may be needed. Black widow antivenin is given for very severe cases (trouble breathing) or for pregnant women with black widow bites. Steroids and antihistamines may help relieve itching from tarantula bites.

DOs and DON'Ts in Managing Bites and Stings:

✔ **DO** carry epinephrine if you're sensitive to stings.
✔ **DO** remove ticks (especially the head) as soon as possible.
✔ **DO** rest an area bitten by a spider, keep it elevated, and consider applying ice. Take pain medicines as prescribed.
✔ **DO** call your doctor if you have an infected bite or allergic reactions (hives, itching, and trouble breathing, swallowing, or talking).
✔ **DO** call your doctor if a bite ulcer gets larger or becomes infected, you're pregnant, or you have new painful muscle spasms, trouble breathing, or chronic health problems.

⊘ **DON'T** go in wooded areas without wearing protective clothing.
⊘ **DON'T** scratch bite areas.

FOR MORE INFORMATION

Contact the following sources:

- American Academy of Dermatology
  Tel: (847) 330-0230
  Website: http://www.aad.org
- National Institute of Allergy and Infectious Diseases
  Tel: (866) 284-4107
  Website: http://www.niaid.nih.gov
- National Institute of Environmental Health Sciences
  Tel: (919) 541-3345
  Website: http://www.niehs.nih.gov

FROM THE DESK OF

NOTES

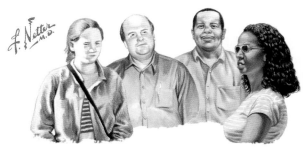

Lyme disease is an infection that affects many parts of the body, including skin, joints, and nervous system. This illness was first seen in 1975. More than 150,000 cases have been reported in the United States since 1980.

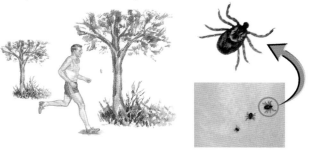

A bacteria named *Borrelia burgdorferi* causes it. A tick bite passes the bacteria to people. Deer living in heavily wooded areas often carry these ticks.

Flu-like symptoms, including headache, fever, fatigue, rash, and joint pain, are usually the first symptoms.

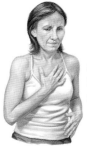

As the infection progresses, chest pain, shortness of breath, dizziness, arthritis-like symptoms in joints, and neurological problems may occur.

Tick bites often may leave a large, bull's-eye type of rash that lasts a few days.

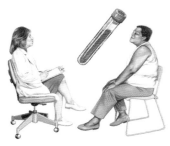

Tell your doctor if you've been in a wooded area where ticks may live. This information will help with your diagnosis. Your doctor will examine you and do blood tests.

What Is Lyme Disease?

Lyme disease is an infection that affects many parts of the body, including the skin, joints, and nervous system. This illness was first recognized in 1975. More than 150,000 cases have been reported in the United States since 1980. It's named for the Connecticut town where the first case was found. Most cases occur in the Northeast US, but cases have also been reported in several other states including California, Wisconsin, and Minnesota.

What Causes Lyme Disease?

A bacteria named *Borrelia burgdorferi* causes it. A tick bite passes bacteria to people. Deer often carry these ticks.

What Are the Symptoms of Lyme Disease?

People may only have one or a few symptoms before the disease is diagnosed and treated. Early symptoms are flu-like ones: headache, joint and muscle pain, fever, chills, fatigue, and enlarged lymph glands. A rash may appear on the site of the tick bite, often on the armpit, groin, or thigh. It's raised or flat, and red with a white area in the middle. Tick bites usually leave a large, bull's-eye type of rash that lasts for a few days.

Untreated flu-like symptoms may get worse. Neck stiffness, shortness of breath, chest pain, and dizziness may occur. Then, without treatment, people may develop arthritis-like symptoms in joints, rash, continued fatigue and heart problems, and neurological symptoms, such as confusion, weakness in the face, arm, and legs; or even paralysis in the face.

How Is Lyme Disease Diagnosed?

The doctor will do a physical examination and take a medical history. Living or recent travel in areas of high prevalence, such as New England, makes the diagnosis more likely. The doctor must know about recent tick bites or outings to wooded areas or fields where deer ticks live. Deer ticks are so small, you may not even know you were bitten. Most people with Lyme disease do not remember getting bitten by a tick or having a bull's-eye type of rash. The doctor will do a blood test for bacteria that cause Lyme disease. The doctor may do other tests to rule out illnesses with similar symptoms.

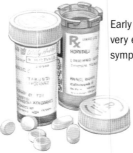

Early treatment with antibiotics is usually very effective. If the illness is very advanced, symptoms may not go away completely.

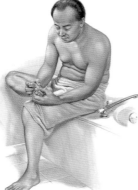

Young children and pregnant women need different medicine, so tell your doctor if you may be pregnant.

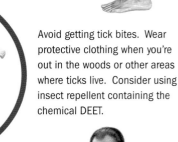

Avoid getting tick bites. Wear protective clothing when you're out in the woods or other areas where ticks live. Consider using insect repellent containing the chemical DEET.

Check your body for tick bites after any possible exposure to ticks.

How Is Lyme Disease Treated?

Early treatment with antibiotics is usually very effective. If the illness is very advanced, symptoms may not completely go away. The duration of therapy and type of antibiotic used depend on the stage of the disease. Different medicine is used for young children and pregnant women. During antibiotic treatment, acetaminophen or nonsteroidal antiinflammatory drugs (NSAIDs) can be used for pain. Other types of treatment may also be necessary, for example, for heart or neurological problems.

DOs and DON'Ts in Managing Lyme Disease:

✔ **DO** take antibiotics as directed.

✔ **DO** tell your doctor if your symptoms don't improve or you have side effects from medicine.

✔ **DO** avoid getting bitten by a tick. Avoid areas where ticks live, especially in spring and summer when they are most numerous. Wear protective clothing when you're out in the woods or other areas where deer ticks live. Use insect repellent containing the chemical called DEET.

✔ **DO** check your body for tick bites after any possible exposure to ticks.

✔ **DO** call your doctor if treatment doesn't help your symptoms in a reasonable amount of time.

✔ **DO** call your doctor if you have new or unexplained symptoms.

⊘ **DON'T** wait to see whether side effects from medicines go away.

FROM THE DESK OF

NOTES

FOR MORE INFORMATION

Contact the following sources:

• Lyme Disease Foundation, Inc.
Tel: 800-886-LYME (886-5963)
Website: http://www.lyme.org

• Arthritis Foundation
Tel: (800) 283-7800
Website: http://www.arthritis.org

• U.S. Department of Health and Human Services
Websites: http://womenshealth.gov

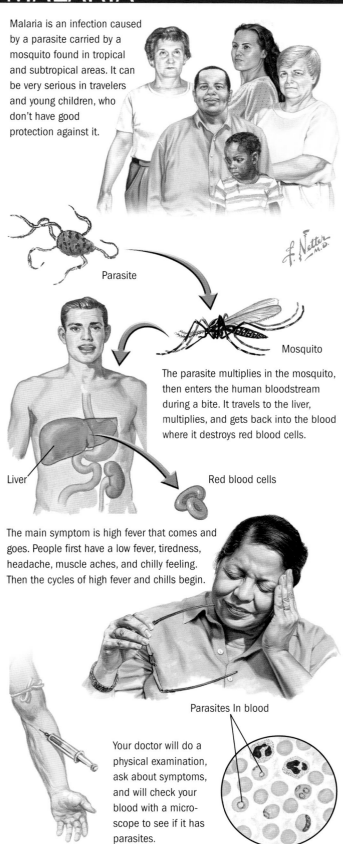

Malaria is an infection caused by a parasite carried by a mosquito found in tropical and subtropical areas. It can be very serious in travelers and young children, who don't have good protection against it.

Parasite

Mosquito

The parasite multiplies in the mosquito, then enters the human bloodstream during a bite. It travels to the liver, multiplies, and gets back into the blood where it destroys red blood cells.

Liver

Red blood cells

The main symptom is high fever that comes and goes. People first have a low fever, tiredness, headache, muscle aches, and chilly feeling. Then the cycles of high fever and chills begin.

Parasites In blood

Your doctor will do a physical examination, ask about symptoms, and will check your blood with a microscope to see if it has parasites.

What Is Malaria?

Malaria is an infection caused by a parasite carried by a mosquito found in tropical and subtropical areas. It involves the blood cells, liver, and nervous system.

About 300 to 500 million cases of malaria occur worldwide every year, but only about 1200 in the United States. It occurs mainly in immigrants or travelers returning from areas with malaria.

What Causes Malaria?

The parasite named *Plasmodium* is the cause. Four types (species) infect humans: *P. falciparum, P. vivax, P. malariae,* and *P. ovale*. The parasite is passed along by bites of a female mosquito of the genus *Anopheles*. The parasite enters the human bloodstream during a bite. It travels to the liver, multiplies, and then reenters the bloodstream where it destroys red blood cells. Some parasites stay in the liver and are released later, which causes attacks off and on.

What Are the Symptoms of Malaria?

The main symptom is high fever. Symptoms can start 10 to 35 days after the mosquito bite. During the first 2 or 3 days, people have a low-grade fever, tiredness, headache, muscle aches, and chilly feeling. Then a cold stage (hard shaking chills for 1or 2 hours) is followed by a hot stage (high fever for 12 to 24 hours with rapid breathing and heavy sweating). These attacks come and go every 2 or 3 days. Untreated, they can continue for years.

How Is Malaria Diagnosed?

The doctor will do a physical examination, ask about symptoms, and examine blood with a microscope. The diagnosis is confirmed if parasites are seen inside red blood cells with the microscope on a specially stained blood smear. Newer blood tests such as polymerase chain reaction (PCR) can also be used for diagnosing malaria.

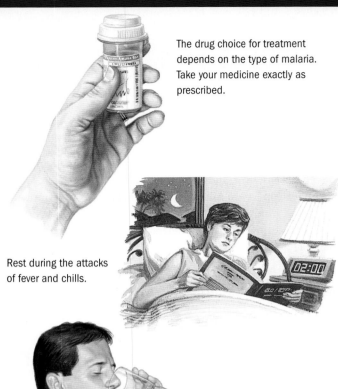

The drug choice for treatment depends on the type of malaria. Take your medicine exactly as prescribed.

Rest during the attacks of fever and chills.

Drink more fluids during attacks.

Before traveling to a country with malaria, visit your doctor to talk about prevention medicine available.

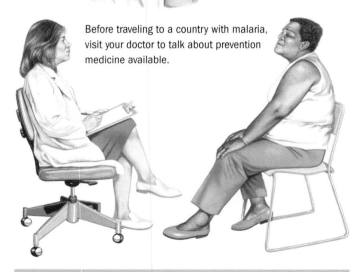

How Is Malaria Treated?

The treatment is medicine. The drug choice depends on the type of malaria. Most people with mild malaria start to feel better within 48 hours after treatment begins. However, parasites can be resistant to drugs. If symptoms don't get better, different treatment is needed. People with severe malaria take longer to recover.

DOs and DON'Ts in Managing Malaria:

✔ **DO** take preventive medicine when traveling in a country with malaria. To find out which countries have malaria, call the International Travelers' Hotline at (404) 332-4559.

✔ **DO** take your medicine exactly as directed by your doctor. Take it at the same time every day.

✔ **DO** finish all the medicine, to treat malaria effectively and prevent the parasite from becoming resistant to the drug.

✔ **DO** protect others by making your environment mosquito free.

✔ **DO** rest during fevers and chills. Begin normal activities slowly.

✔ **DO** drink more fluids during the attacks.

✔ **DO** call your doctor if you can't drink fluids.

✔ **DO** call your doctor if you still have symptoms, such as fever and chills, after treatment or if you get new symptoms.

✔ **DO** call your doctor if you have severe side effects from medicines.

⊘ **DON'T** skip doses of medicine or stop taking it because symptoms have gone.

⊘ **DON'T** donate blood until your doctor says you can.

FROM THE DESK OF

NOTES

FOR MORE INFORMATION

Contact the following sources:

• National Center for Preparedness, Detection, and Control of Infectious Diseases
Tel: (800) 311-3435
Website: http://www.cdc.gov/ncpdcid

• CDC Travelers' Health webpage
Tel: (800) 232-4636
Website: http://wwwn.cdc.gov/travel/default.aspx

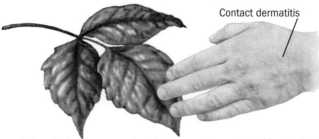

Contact dermatitis

Poison ivy is a common plant that can cause a severe skin reaction (contact dermatitis) in sensitive people. Contact with any part of the poison ivy plant or oils from the plant on clothing or pets can cause an allergic reaction.

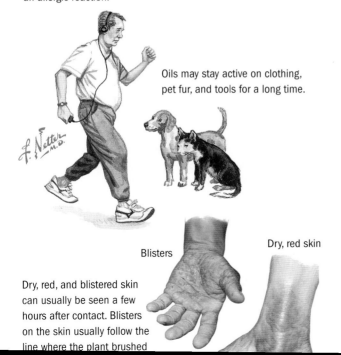

Oils may stay active on clothing, pet fur, and tools for a long time.

Blisters

Dry, red skin

Dry, red, and blistered skin can usually be seen a few hours after contact. Blisters on the skin usually follow the line where the plant brushed

What Is Poison Ivy?

Poison ivy is a common plant that can cause a severe skin reaction (contact dermatitis) in sensitive people. Affected skin may be dry and red and can blister. This dermatitis isn't contagious, but contact with resin on the skin of affected people can cause a reaction.

What Causes Poison Ivy?

Contact with any part of the plant or with the oily substance (resin) that the plant makes can cause the reaction. Contact can occur directly, by touching the plant, or indirectly, by touching something carrying the oils, such as pets. Oils on clothing, pet fur, and tools may stay active for a long time and can be the source of the rash.

What Are the Symptoms of Poison Ivy?

The main symptom is skin that looks dry, red, or blistered, usually within few hours of contact. Blisters on the skin usually follow the line where the plant brushed the skin. Other symptoms include itching and mild pain, but not fever. Because the skin is fragile, scratching may in some cases lead to infection, which may need antibiotic treatment.

How Is Poison Ivy Diagnosed?

The doctor will diagnose poison ivy dermatitis by a skin examination.

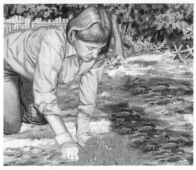

The best treatment is avoidance. Learn to recognize the plant and avoid contact. Wearing gloves, long sleeves, and long pants when outdoors or gardening will prevent exposure.

Other treatments include anti-inflammatory drugs (steroids) used orally or topically, antihistamines for itching, and immunotherapy (desensitization) to minimize reactions.

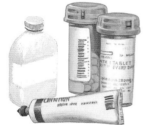

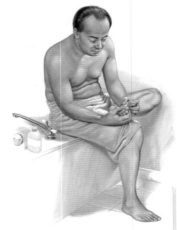

Use steroid ointments and creams on clean, dry skin. Repeat two or three times per day as directed.

When to call your doctor...

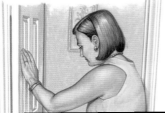

How Is Poison Ivy Treated?

The best treatment is avoidance. Learn how to recognize the plant, and avoid contact as much as possible. Wearing gloves, long sleeves, and long pants when outdoors or gardening will prevent exposure.

Other treatments include oral (by mouth) or topical (put on the skin) antiinflammatory drugs (steroids). Also, antihistamines can reduce itching, and immunotherapy (desensitization) can minimize reactions. Steroids are powerful drugs and quickly reduce swelling and irritation but also may have serious side effects. For these reasons, steroids are usually prescribed for short periods. Antihistamines can cause sleepiness, so being careful is important when driving, cooking, or using machinery when taking them. Anti-itch lotions, such as calamine, and oatmeal baths are soothing for oozing, blistery rashes and may be used as needed.

DOs and DON'Ts in Managing Poison Ivy:

✔ **DO** use oral steroids each day as prescribed. Oral antihistamines can be used as needed and may be skipped if itching improves.

✔ **DO** use steroid ointments and creams on clean, dry skin. Repeat two or three times per day as directed.

✔ **DO** use anti-itch lotions as needed, but avoid using them during the first hour after applying steroid creams or ointments. Give the steroid time to soak in first!

✔ **DO** call your doctor if you have a fever, vomiting, or diarrhea.

✔ **DO** call your doctor if your rash worsens despite treatment, or you get a new or different rash.

⊘ **DON'T** skip doses of steroid medicines. Your dermatitis may worsen.

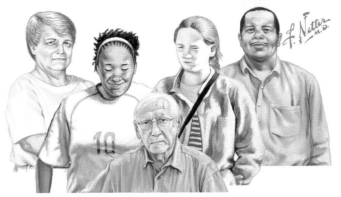

Rabies occurs most often in teens younger than 16 and adults older than 55. It is an infection caused by an animal with the rabies virus.

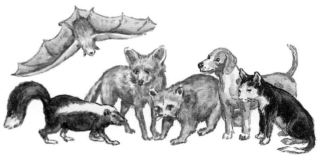

Rabies exists mainly in skunks, raccoons, bats, and foxes, but pets such as cats and dogs can get it. A virus named rhabdovirus is the cause.

First symptoms may be general, such as fever, headache, and feeling down. Later, nervous system symptoms occur, such as being agitated and restless. Fear of water occurs during this stage. If untreated, rabies can lead to death.

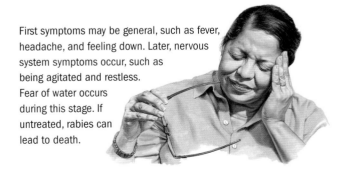

What Is Rabies?

Rabies is an infection caused by the rabies virus. People get the virus after being bitten by an infected animal. Rabies exists mainly in wildlife, most frequently in skunks, raccoons, bats, and foxes. Pets including cats and dogs can also get it.

Only about two cases occur yearly in the United States, most caused by wild animal bites. Rabies is more common in developing countries.

What Causes Rabies?

The cause is the virus named rhabdovirus in saliva of infected animals.

What Are the Symptoms of Rabies?

The time from infection with the virus to first symptoms averages 35 to 65 days. First symptoms may be general, such as fever, headache, and feeling down. Also, loss of appetite, nausea, and pain or numbness at the bite site may last for the first 3 to 4 days.

Later, nervous system symptoms occur, including being agitated and restless with extreme hyperactivity, with bizarre behavior and calm periods. Hallucinations, muscle spasms, and paralysis may also occur. The fear of water (hydrophobia) occurs during this stage.

Unfortunately, if rabies isn't treated soon after exposure, it almost always leads to coma, convulsions, and death, usually by the 4th to 7th day after onset of symptoms.

How Is Rabies Diagnosed?

A doctor will examine the wound and do blood tests. The animal may be captured and killed so that its brain can be checked for the presence of rabies virus.

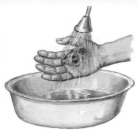

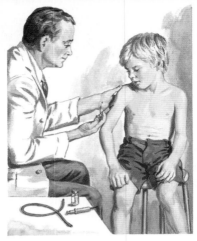

Treatment is first washing the wound and then HRIG and HDCV. HRIG is given once with half the dose near the wound and half given as a shot into a muscle. HDCV is given as five shots.

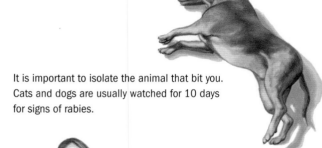

It is important to isolate the animal that bit you. Cats and dogs are usually watched for 10 days for signs of rabies.

Call your doctor if you have a reaction (such as pain or swelling) to rabies vaccine.

How Is Rabies Treated?

All bite wounds should be cleaned immediately with soap and water and in the emergency room with povidone-iodine or something similar. Then, treatment depends on the risk of rabies. For simple dog or cat bites, the animal is observed for 10 days and, if it's healthy and not showing rabid behaviors, no treatment is needed. For an animal with rabid behavior, the doctor will start treatment with human rabies immune globulin (HRIG) and human diploid cell rabies vaccine (HDCV).

HRIG is given once with half the dose usually injected near the wound and the other half given as a shot into a muscle. HDCV is given in five doses on days 0, 3, 7, 14, and 28. Treatment should continue even if local reactions to the vaccine occur.

A tetanus booster may also be given.

DOs and DON'Ts in Managing Rabies:

✔ **DO** ask your doctor or emergency room staff to tell state and local health department and animal control agencies about your animal bite.

✔ **DO** realize that the animal that bit you should be isolated. Cats and dogs are usually watched for 10 days for signs of rabies.

✔ **DO** remember that animal bites occurring outside the United States should be considered high risk for rabies. Get prompt medical care.

✔ **DO** realize that most rabid animals are weak, agitated, and dangerous.

✔ **DO** go to the closest emergency department if you have an animal bite.

✔ **DO** call your doctor if you have a reaction (e.g., pain, swelling) to rabies vaccine.

⊘ **DON'T** forget that most rabid animals have odd behavior. They may approach people, drool from the mouth, and seem weak. They may attack anything that moves.

MANAGING
SALMONELLOSIS

Salmonella

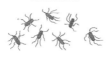

Salmonellosis is an infection of the stomach and intestines that's caused by *Salmonella*, a kind of bacteria. It's similar to stomach flu.

Eating contaminated foods (eggs, beef, poultry, fruit) or drinking contaminated water or milk can lead to infection. Food handlers who don't wash their hands after going to the bathroom can also spread it.

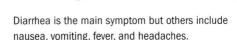
Diarrhea is the main symptom but others include nausea, vomiting, fever, and headaches.

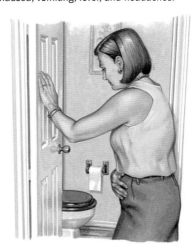

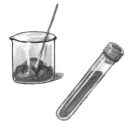
Your doctor makes a diagnosis by testing a stool sample. Blood tests are sometimes done to rule out other diseases.

What Is Salmonellosis?

Salmonella is the name of a kind of bacteria. Salmonellosis is an infection of the stomach and intestines that's caused by *Salmonella*. It's similar to stomach flu. Most people with mild infection get better in 4 to 7 days without treatment. An epidemic can occur when many people eat the same contaminated foods, such as at a restaurant. Some people have such severe diarrhea that they may need a hospital stay for intravenous fluids and antibiotics.

What Causes Salmonellosis?

People get *Salmonella* infection by eating contaminated foods, especially eggs, beef, poultry, or fruit, or by drinking contaminated water or milk. Cooking helps reduce but does not eliminate chances of getting infected. *Salmonella* can spread among people when they don't wash their hands after going to the bathroom. *Salmonella* can also spread from pets, such as turtles and iguanas, to people.

What Are the Symptoms of Salmonellosis?

Diarrhea is the main symptom. It may be mild, with two or three loose bowel movements (stools) daily. It may be severe, with watery diarrhea every 10 or 15 minutes. Other symptoms are blood in stool, stomach cramps, vomiting, fever, and headaches.

How Is Salmonellosis Diagnosed?

The doctor makes a diagnosis by testing stool, blood, and urine samples. Blood tests are also done to rule out other diseases.

How Is Salmonellosis Treated?

Mild infections (gastroenteritis) don't usually need medicine. Most go away in 24 to 48 hours.

If possible, infected people should be isolated or at least use a separate bathroom. Good hand washing is essential to avoid spreading the infection.

People who have fever and more severe infection (typhoid fever) will need antibiotics. Drinking more fluids helps prevent dehydration. A liquid diet including Gatorade® or Pedialyte® should be followed until diarrhea stops. Then, eating regular foods can slowly begin again. Dairy products can make the diarrhea worse and should be avoided for several days.

People with severe diarrhea may need intravenous fluids.

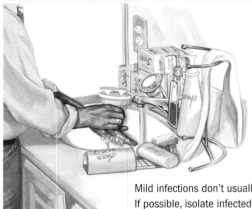

Mild infections don't usually need medicine. If possible, isolate infected people. Wash your hands well after using the bathroom to avoid spreading the infection.

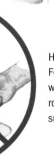

Drink more fluids to prevent dehydration.

Handle and store food correctly. For example, don't let a salad with mayonnaise sit for hours at room temperature or in the hot sun.

If possible, have the infected person use a separate bathroom. If it's not possible, don't let others use the same bathroom unless it was well cleaned.

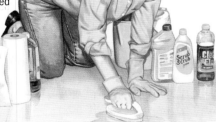

FROM THE DESK OF

NOTES

DOs and DON'Ts in Managing Salmonellosis:

✔ **DO** thoroughly cook food such as meat and poultry.

✔ **DO** handle and store food correctly. For example, don't let a salad with mayonnaise sit for hours at room temperature.

✔ **DO** drink only pasteurized milk.

✔ **DO** use only bottled water when traveling. Ask your doctor about how to prepare if you're traveling to a developing country.

✔ **DO** avoid contact with anyone who has a *Salmonella* infection.

✔ **DO** avoid animals, such as pet turtles, that could be infected.

✔ **DO** wash your hands well after using the bathroom to avoid spreading the infection.

✔ **DO** drink watered-down electrolyte solutions, such as sports drinks, until diarrhea stops.

✔ **DO** eat a bland, high-calorie, well-balanced diet after diarrhea stops.

✔ **DO** call your doctor if you're dehydrated (have dry wrinkled skin and dark or less urine).

✔ **DO** call your doctor if you have symptoms longer than 48 hours, high fever, worse diarrhea, or yellow skin or eyes.

⊘ **DON'T** let others use the same bathroom unless it was thoroughly cleaned.

⊘ **DON'T** eat raw or undercooked poultry or eggs or drink unpasteurized milk.

FOR MORE INFORMATION

Contact the following sources:

• Centers for Disease Control and Prevention
Tel: (800) 232-4636
Website: http://www.cdc.gov/salmonella

• Intestinal Disease Foundation
Tel: (412) 261-5888
Website: http://www.intestinalfoundation.org

• National Institute of Allergy and Infectious Diseases
Tel: (866) 284-4107
Website: http://www3.niaid.nih.gov/topics/salmonellosis/default.htm

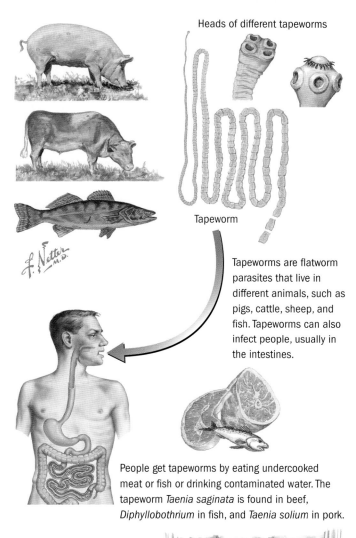

Heads of different tapeworms

Tapeworm

Tapeworms are flatworm parasites that live in different animals, such as pigs, cattle, sheep, and fish. Tapeworms can also infect people, usually in the intestines.

People get tapeworms by eating undercooked meat or fish or drinking contaminated water. The tapeworm *Taenia saginata* is found in beef, *Diphyllobothrium* in fish, and *Taenia solium* in pork.

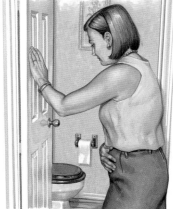

Symptoms of intestinal infection, when present, include diarrhea, nausea, pain in the upper abdomen, weight loss, loss of appetite, and weakness.

The doctor can find a tapeworm infection with stool samples. Samples are checked for worm eggs and body parts in a laboratory.

What Is Tapeworm Infection?

Tapeworms are flatworm parasites that live in different animals such as pigs, cattle, sheep, and fish. Tapeworms can also infect people and live in the intestines. People can eat eggs or baby worms (larvae) in contaminated food or water. Eggs and larvae can pass out of the body with bowel movements (stools). Eggs can also hatch into larvae that move out of the intestines, form cysts in other organs (lungs and liver), and cause serious illness.

People usually get it when traveling to developing countries such as those in Asia, Latin America, or Africa. It isn't common in the United States.

What Causes Tapeworm Infection?

The tapeworm named *Taenia saginata* is found in beef, *Diphyllobothrium* occurs in fish, and *Taenia solium* is found in pork. Eating undercooked meat or fish or drinking contaminated water can lead to infection.

What Are the Symptoms of Tapeworm Infection?

Many times people don't have symptoms. Parts of worms might appear in stools. Symptoms of intestinal infection, when present, include diarrhea, nausea, pain in the upper abdomen (belly), unexplained weight loss, loss of appetite, weakness, and anemia (low blood count).

Symptoms of damage from cysts in other organs include fever and nervous system symptoms (such as seizures if larvae get to the brain).

How Is Tapeworm Infection Diagnosed?

The doctor can find a tapeworm infection through a stool sample. The sample is checked in a laboratory for worm eggs and body parts.

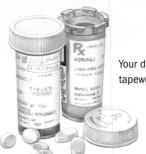

Your doctor will prescribe a drug to kill the tapeworm. Usually, only one dose is needed.

How Is Tapeworm Infection Treated?

Drugs can kill the tapeworm. One dose is usually all that's needed. When more than just intestines are affected, treatment is more difficult.

After treatment, another stool specimen should be checked in 3 to 6 weeks to make sure that the infection is gone. Activities and diet can remain normal.

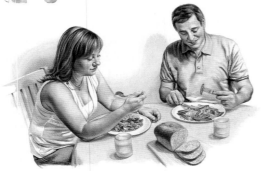

Stomach upset can be lessened by taking the medicine with food.

DOs and DON'Ts in Managing Tapeworm Infection:

✔ **DO** take your medicine as directed.

✔ **DO** have a follow-up doctor's examination in 3 to 6 weeks.

✔ **DO** have all family members checked for the infection.

✔ **DO** buy only meats that have been inspected.

✔ **DO** cook your beef, pork, and fish so that it's well done (to at least 150° F).

✔ **DO** call your doctor if you have symptoms after treatment.

✔ **DO** use good hygiene. Washing your hands after going to the bathroom will prevent infections.

⊘ **DON'T** miss your follow-up examination.

⊘ **DON'T** eat raw or undercooked meats or fish, especially when traveling in a foreign country. When traveling, don't eat fruits and vegetables until they're washed and cooked with safe water.

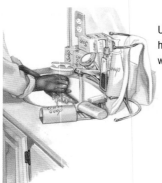

Use good hygiene. Washing your hands after going to the bathroom will prevent infections.

Have a follow-up doctor's examination in 3 to 6 weeks.

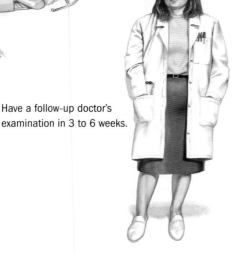

FROM THE DESK OF

NOTES

FOR MORE INFORMATION

Contact the following source:

• Centers for Disease Control and Prevention
Tel: (800) 311-3435
Website: http://www.cdc.gov

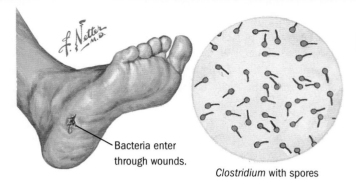

Bacteria enter through wounds.

Clostridium with spores

Tetanus is a disease caused by a type of bacteria named *Clostridium tetani*. The bacteria can be found primarily in the soil. Spores of bacteria usually get into people through a puncture wound.

What Is Tetanus?

Tetanus is a disease caused by a type of bacteria named *Clostridium tetani*. These bacteria occur worldwide and are found primarily in the soil. The bacteria produce poison that damages nerves. Muscles controlled by these nerves become stiff or locked in place. Locked muscles in the face is why tetanus is also called lockjaw. If not treated quickly, the disease can be fatal, such as when muscles used for breathing stop working. Types of tetanus include generalized, localized, and neonatal (in newborns).

Tetanus isn't contagious, and vaccination can prevent it.

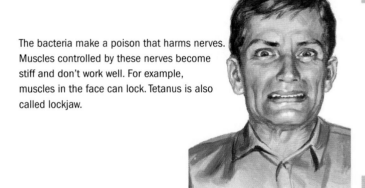

The bacteria make a poison that harms nerves. Muscles controlled by these nerves become stiff and don't work well. For example, muscles in the face can lock. Tetanus is also called lockjaw.

What Causes Tetanus?

Contamination of a wound, usually following a puncture wound, with bacterial spores causes the disease. Spores enter the wound, multiply, and make a toxin (poison) that binds to nerve endings. The toxin reaches the spinal cord and base of the brain. The toxin blocks chemical signals from the brain and spinal cord to muscles. Muscles have severe spasms, breathing can stop, and death can occur. Neonatal tetanus usually results from infection of the umbilical cord stump.

What Are the Symptoms of Tetanus?

Generalized tetanus is most common. Muscles get rigid and painful spasms occur about 7 days after the injury. Affected muscles are most often in the jaw, neck, shoulder, back, abdomen (belly), arm, and thigh. Muscles of the face contract, so the face has a grimace. Some people get violent, painful, generalized muscle spasms. The illness may be mild (rigid muscles with few spasms), moderate (lockjaw and trouble swallowing), or severe (violent spasms and breathing cessation).

Localized tetanus is not common. Symptoms occur in muscles near the wound.

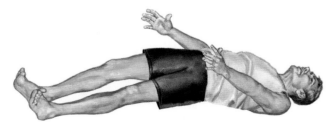

Symptoms of generalized tetanus, the most common type, are rigid muscles and painful muscle spasms.

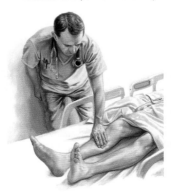

Your doctor diagnoses tetanus by a physical examination, especially of muscles and nerves. Your doctor may rub a swab on the wound and have it checked for tetanus bacteria.

How Is Tetanus Diagnosed?

The doctor diagnoses tetanus by doing a physical examination, especially of muscles and nerves. The doctor may rub a swab on the wound and send it to a laboratory. It will be checked for tetanus bacteria. Blood tests may also be done.

Diagnosis of neonatal tetanus is based on symptoms in a newborn.

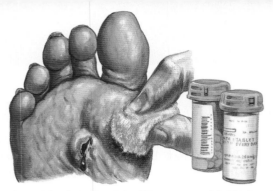

All wounds must be cleaned and dead tissue removed. Antibiotics will be prescribed. Human tetanus immunoglobulin is given to make the tetanus toxin harmless.

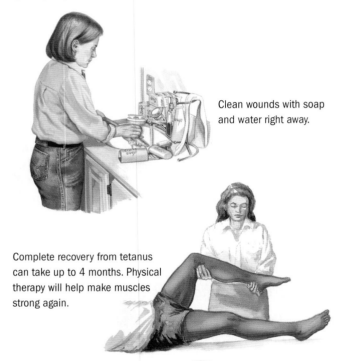

Clean wounds with soap and water right away.

Complete recovery from tetanus can take up to 4 months. Physical therapy will help make muscles strong again.

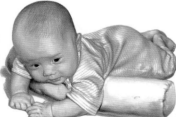

The best treatment is prevention by vaccination. Babies should get their first tetanus vaccine at 2 months of age.

How Is Tetanus Treated?

The doctor treats tetanus by removing the toxin source, making toxin harmless, preventing and treating muscle spasms, and providing support.

All wounds must be cleaned and dead tissue removed. Antibiotics will be given to kill bacteria.

Antitoxin called human tetanus immunoglobulin is injected, to make the toxin harmless.

Drugs such as diazepam and lorazepam will control spasms.

A breathing machine may be needed by people with lockjaw, those who have trouble swallowing, and those with muscle spasms.

Tetanus may last for a 2 to 3 months. Complete recovery can take up to 4 months. Physical therapy will help make muscles strong again.

DOs and DON'Ts in Managing Tetanus:

✔ **DO** clean wounds with soap and water right away.
✔ **DO** call your doctor if you have a wound and don't know if you need tetanus vaccine.
✔ **DO** call your doctor if you have muscle spasms, trouble swallowing, or trouble breathing.
✔ **DO** vaccinate your children; start vaccination in babies at 2 months. Stay up-to-date with tetanus vaccines. Adults should have booster shots every 10 years.
✔ **DO** call your doctor if you need a tetanus booster.

⊘ **DON'T** ignore any wounds.
⊘ **DON'T** forget that the best treatment is prevention by vaccination.

FROM THE DESK OF

NOTES

FOR MORE INFORMATION

Contact the following source:

• Centers for Disease Control and Prevention
Tel: (800) 311-3435
Website: http://www.cdc.gov

In achalasia, the muscle between the esophagus and stomach, called the lower esophageal sphincter, does not relax after swallowing, which interrupts the flow of liquids and food into the stomach.

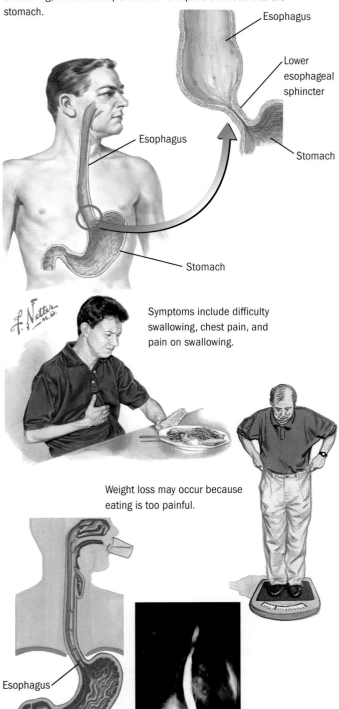

Esophagus

Lower esophageal sphincter

Esophagus

Stomach

Stomach

Symptoms include difficulty swallowing, chest pain, and pain on swallowing.

Weight loss may occur because eating is too painful.

Esophagus

Your doctor may order a barium esophagography. This is an x-ray taken after you drink barium to show your esophagus.

What Is Achalasia?

Achalasia is a disorder of the esophagus, the tube connecting the mouth and stomach. With achalasia, the esophagus has trouble moving liquid and solids down to the stomach. This movement is called peristalsis. Also, the muscle between the esophagus and stomach (the lower esophageal sphincter) does not relax after swallowing. Achalasia may occur at any age but is more common in older people. It cannot be prevented.

What Causes Achalasia?

The causes are usually unknown but may include damage to nerves of the esophagus, infections, and heredity.

What Are the Symptoms of Achalasia?

The main symptom is difficulty swallowing. Problems with liquids usually occur first, followed by problems with solid foods. Weight loss can occur because eating is too difficult or painful.

Other symptoms include chest pain, painful swallowing, coughing, wheezing, heartburn, belching, and vomiting. In advanced cases, halitosis (bad breath) can occur.

How Is Achalasia Diagnosed?

The doctor will order a barium swallow x-ray, or esophagography. This study will show narrowing of the lower part of the esophagus and widening of the upper part.

Pressure measurements (manometry) may be done to prove an absence of peristalsis and increased pressure at the lower esophageal sphincter.

Endoscopy (using a small lighted tube with a tiny video camera at the tip) can confirm a tight sphincter or obtain a piece of tissue to make sure that other diseases aren't causing symptoms.

Endoscopy

In endoscopy, a small tube with a tiny video camera (a scope) is inserted down into your esophagus to confirm the diagnosis or to get a tissue sample for study.

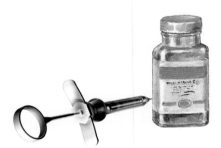

Medicine can lower the pressure at the lower esophageal sphincter and help your symptoms.

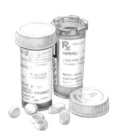

Before considering surgery, your doctor may try Botox® injections into your lower esophageal sphincter.

How Is Achalasia Treated?

There is no cure, but treatment can improve symptoms and help prevent complications.

The treatment goal is to reduce pressure at the lower esophageal sphincter. This is done by dilating the sphincter with special instruments or balloons. Even after dilation, the esophagus will not have normal movement. The dilation may have to be repeated if symptoms come back.

Medicines such as long-acting nitrates or calcium channel blockers can lower the pressure at the sphincter. The drugs are usually used in people who can't have the dilation.

Injection of Botox® (botulinum toxin) in the sphincter is a newer treatment that the doctor may try before considering surgery. If other treatments fail, the doctor may operate to reduce pressure in the sphincter (called esophagomyotomy). Surgery can be done laparoscopically (by using a very small incision instead the usual large one).

Without treatment, complications can arise. These include tearing (perforation) of the esophagus, return of acid or food from the stomach into the esophagus (gastroesophageal reflux disease, or GERD), and aspiration pneumonia. Some people may develop esophageal cancer.

DOs and DON'Ts in Managing Achalasia:

✔ **DO** eat and chew slowly.
✔ **DO** call your doctor if you have persistent difficulty swallowing, if painful swallowing develops, or if symptoms remain after treatment.
✔ **DO** call your doctor if you vomit blood or you have other new symptoms.

⃠ **DON'T** eat or drink while lying down.
⃠ **DON'T** drink hot or cold liquids, because they may make the condition worse.

FROM THE DESK OF

NOTES

FOR MORE INFORMATION

Contact the following source:

• National Digestive Diseases Information Clearinghouse
E-mail: nddic@aerie.com
Website: http://www.niddk.nih.gov/health/digest/ nddic.htm

MANAGING YOUR
ALCOHOLIC HEPATITIS

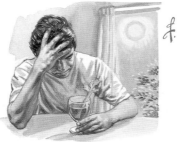

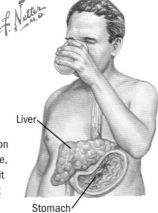

Liver

Stomach

Alcoholic hepatitis, or liver inflammation caused by drinking alcohol, is treatable, so take steps now to control it before it becomes cirrhosis, a liver disease that can't be cured.

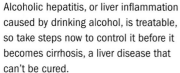

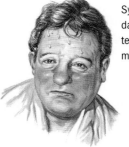

Symptoms may include a flu-like feeling, dark urine, general itching, high body temperature, and possible coma. Symptoms may not appear until the disease is severe.

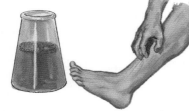

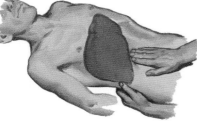

Your doctor may suspect alcoholic hepatitis because you have a long history of heavy alcohol use, and your liver seems enlarged (hepatomegaly) during a physical examination.

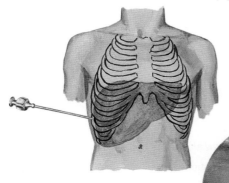

To confirm the diagnosis, the doctor may perform a liver biopsy. A needle is inserted through the skin to take out a tiny piece of the liver for study.

What Is Alcoholic Hepatitis?

Alcoholic hepatitis is inflammation (swelling) of the liver. It is treatable, but for any treatment to work, drinking alcohol must stop. With continued drinking, alcoholic hepatitis can progress to cirrhosis of the liver. Cirrhosis is an illness that can't be cured. In cirrhosis, normal liver tissue is destroyed and replaced by scar tissue. In time, the liver stops working.

The disease usually affects people older than 30.

What Causes Alcoholic Hepatitis?

Alcoholic hepatitis is caused by drinking too much alcohol for a long time.

What Are the Symptoms of Alcoholic Hepatitis?

Symptoms may not appear until damage to the liver is severe.

Symptoms are similar to those of viral hepatitis. The first symptoms are rashes, pain in the joints, and a flu-like feeling. People who drink alcohol may also be malnourished.

As the disease progresses, later symptoms include yellowish skin and whites of the eyes (jaundice); pale or clay-colored stools; dark urine; general itching; high temperature; swelling of the abdomen (belly) caused by fluid; painful, tender, and enlarged liver; mental confusion; and possible coma.

How Is Alcoholic Hepatitis Diagnosed?

The doctor may suspect the disease because of a history of drinking too much alcohol, abnormal blood tests suggesting inflammation of the liver, and an abnormal physical examination that shows an enlarged liver. To confirm the diagnosis, the doctor may recommend a liver biopsy. For a biopsy, the doctor inserts a hollow needle through the skin and takes out a tiny piece of liver tissue for study in the laboratory.

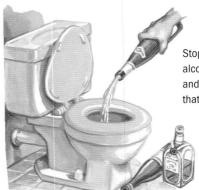

Stop drinking. If you don't, alcoholic hepatitis will progress and damage the liver so much that it can't be treated.

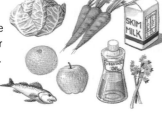

Many people with this disease are not well nourished. Work with your doctor to create a nutritional diet.

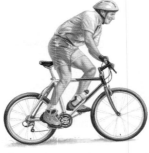
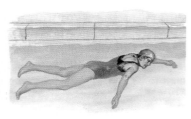

Start a good exercise program. This will help your body and state of mind.

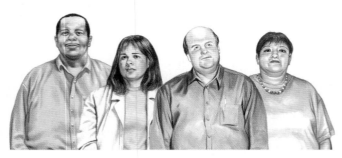

It's estimated that more than 15 million adults in the U.S. are alcoholics or have alcohol-related problems. Rehabilitation programs are available to help you stop drinking. Reach out to these programs. Your doctor can also help by explaining what to expect from your body when you stop drinking and by treating any medical issues.

FROM THE DESK OF

NOTES

How Is Alcoholic Hepatitis Treated?

Treatment of hepatitis is supportive, meaning that the goal is to improve the person's overall health and increase strength. The key is to stop drinking alcohol. An alcohol rehabilitation program can offer important help with this. Malnourishment is improved by following a good diet, one that is high in carbohydrates and calories. Intravenous feedings may be needed in people with extremely poor nutritional status. Eating less salt (sodium) may also be important to prevent abdominal swelling. Vitamin supplements are also needed, especially vitamin B and folic acid. It may take the liver weeks to months to heal.

DOs and DON'Ts in Managing Alcoholic Hepatitis:

✔ **DO** stop drinking.
✔ **DO** seek treatment for your alcohol problem.
✔ **DO** eat a well-balanced, high-calorie diet. People who drink too much alcohol are often malnourished.
✔ **DO** take vitamins, especially vitamin B and folic acid.
✔ **DO** change your activity according to your symptoms. A good fitness program may help with fatigue.
✔ **DO** call your doctor if you develop symptoms suggesting alcoholic hepatitis.
✔ **DO** call your doctor if you develop symptoms after prolonged or heavy drinking.

⊘ **DON'T** drink alcohol. You could get cirrhosis of the liver.
⊘ **DON'T** salt your food. Eating salt can make swelling of the abdomen worse.
⊘ **DON'T** use drugs, including acetaminophen, sedatives, and tranquilizers, that can harm the liver.

FOR MORE INFORMATION

Contact the following sources:
- Alcoholics Anonymous
  Tel: (212) 870-3400
  Website: http://www.alcoholics-anonymous.org
- American Liver Foundation
  Tel: (800) GOLIVER (465-4837)
  E-mail: webmail@liverfoundation.org
  Website: http://www.liverfoundation.org
- National Institute of Alcohol Abuse and Alcoholism
  Tel: (301) 443-3860
  Website: http://www.niaaa.nih.gov

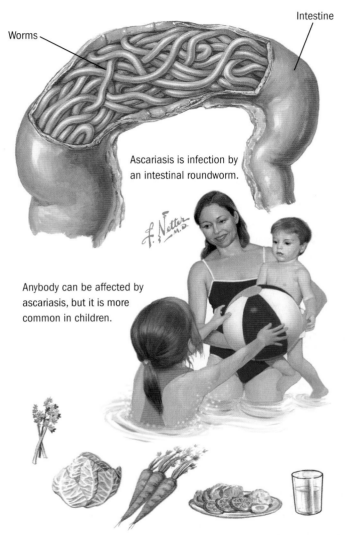

Worms

Intestine

Ascariasis is infection by an intestinal roundworm.

Anybody can be affected by ascariasis, but it is more common in children.

The infection is spread by contact with contaminated water, food, or hands, such as by eating poorly washed raw vegetables grown in contaminated soil.

What Is Ascariasis?

Ascariasis is infection by the worm *Ascaris lumbricoides*. It is the most common intestinal worm. This large roundworm can easily be seen without a microscope.

Ascariasis affects only humans. Anybody can get it, but it is more common in children.

What Causes Ascariasis?

The parasite is never passed from person to person. Worm eggs are spread by contact with contaminated water, food, or hands (e.g., by eating poorly washed raw vegetables grown in contaminated soil). Untreated young worms (larvae) travel from the intestine to other parts of the body, such as the lungs. They then return to the intestine where they become adults and lay eggs.

What Are the Symptoms of Ascariasis?

Symptoms include restlessness at night, being irritable, tiredness, poor appetite, weight loss, pain in the abdomen (belly), and sometimes diarrhea and fever. Worms may sometimes be seen in bowel movements. In lungs, larvae can cause wheezing.

How Is Ascariasis Diagnosed?

Study of stool samples to find worms or eggs confirms the diagnosis.

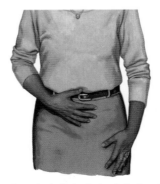

Symptoms include having pain in the abdomen (belly) and being restless at night.

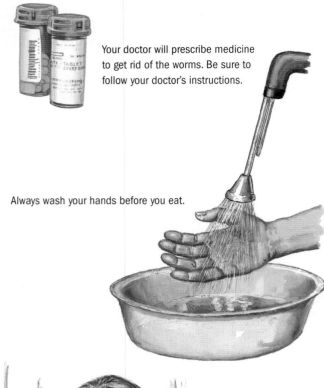

Your doctor will prescribe medicine to get rid of the worms. Be sure to follow your doctor's instructions.

Always wash your hands before you eat.

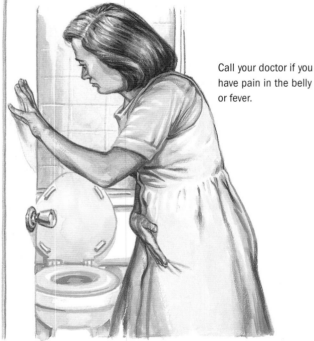

Call your doctor if you have pain in the belly or fever.

How Is Ascariasis Treated?

Medicine is used to kill the worms. These drugs cannot be used in pregnant women.

Management includes attention to habits: wash hands carefully after using the toilet and always before eating. Shower daily and clean the anal area. Boil or soak linens, nightclothes, towels, and washcloths used by someone with roundworms in an ammonia solution (1 cup of ammonia to 5 gallons of water).

After treatment, bathroom floors and fixtures should be scrubbed. Toys should be sterilized or scrubbed with ammonia solution and then rinsed with clear water.

DOs and DON'Ts in Managing Ascariasis:

✔ **DO** avoid contaminated food and drink.
✔ **DO** take medicine as directed by your doctor.
✔ **DO** tell your doctor if you think you're pregnant.
✔ **DO** wash your hands thoroughly before eating and after using the toilet.
✔ **DO** shower instead of taking tub baths.
✔ **DO** boil soiled linens if possible, or soak them in an ammonia solution before washing.
✔ **DO** sterilize toys or scrub with ammonia solution, then rinse with clear water.
✔ **DO** have pets treated for worms.
✔ **DO** clean bathroom fixtures thoroughly after treatment.
✔ **DO** have all family members checked for infection.
✔ **DO** drink only bottled water when traveling in underdeveloped countries.
✔ **DO** call your doctor if you have a fever, severe abdominal pain, chest pain, or shortness of breath.
✔ **DO** call your doctor if you continue to have symptoms after treatment.

⊘ **DON'T** eat unwashed vegetables.
⊘ **DON'T** drink tap water when traveling in underdeveloped countries.
⊘ **DON'T** share towels or washcloths.

FROM THE DESK OF

NOTES

FOR MORE INFORMATION

Contact the following sources:

• Intestinal Disease Foundation
Tel: (412) 261-5888, Monday through Friday from 9:30 am to 3:30 pm (EST)

• National Institute of Allergy and Infectious Disease
Tel: (866) 284-4107, (301) 496-5717
Website: http://www3.niaid.nih.gov/

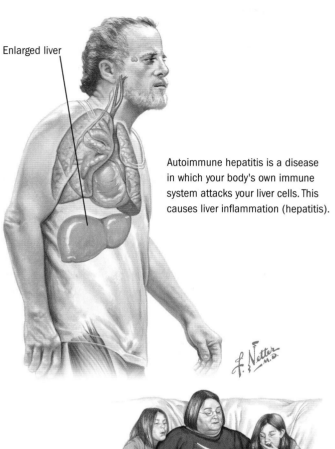

Enlarged liver

Autoimmune hepatitis is a disease in which your body's own immune system attacks your liver cells. This causes liver inflammation (hepatitis).

What Is Autoimmune Hepatitis?

Autoimmune hepatitis is a disease in which the body's own immune system attacks its liver cells. This causes hepatitis, or liver inflammation (swelling). Autoimmune hepatitis is not contagious and cannot be prevented.

About 70% of people with autoimmune hepatitis are women, most between 15 and 40. Untreated, this serious disease gets worse. It can last for years and can lead to liver cirrhosis (scarring and hardening) and liver failure.

What Causes Autoimmune Hepatitis?

The cause is unknown. A substance (antigen) may cause the immune system to attack liver cells. Most experts think that genetics may make some people more likely to have autoimmune diseases.

What Are the Signs and Symptoms of Autoimmune Hepatitis?

Fatigue is common. Other signs are enlarged liver (hepatomegaly), jaundice (yellowish skin), itching, rashes, joint pain, and discomfort in the abdomen (belly). Symptoms range from mild to severe.

People with advanced disease are more likely to have such symptoms as fluid in the abdomen (ascites) and mental confusion.

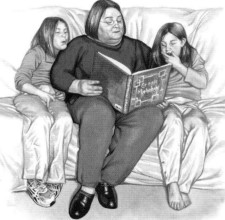

Most experts think that genetics may make some people more likely to get autoimmune diseases, such as autoimmune hepatitis.

How Is Autoimmune Hepatitis Diagnosed

The doctor makes a diagnosis on the basis of symptoms, blood test results, x-rays (ultrasound or computed tomography [CT] of the liver to rule out other causes), and liver biopsy.

Blood tests for liver enzymes and autoantibodies are needed. The tests also help tell autoimmune hepatitis from viral hepatitis (e.g., hepatitis A, B, or C) or metabolic diseases. Antibodies are proteins made by the immune system. In autoimmune hepatitis, antibodies attack and destroy liver cells. The pattern and level of these antibodies can tell the type of disease (type I, usually in women, or II, more common in girls).

For a liver biopsy, a tiny liver sample is removed with a hollow needle and examined under a microscope.

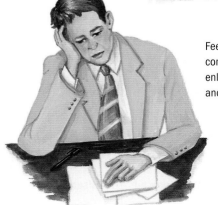

Feeling tired is the most common symptom. An enlarged liver, jaundice, and itching are other signs.

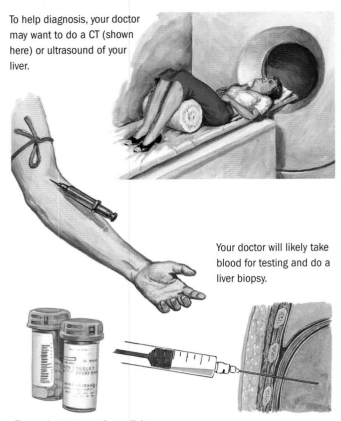

To help diagnosis, your doctor may want to do a CT (shown here) or ultrasound of your liver.

Your doctor will likely take blood for testing and do a liver biopsy.

The main treatment is medicine to slow down the overactive immune system.

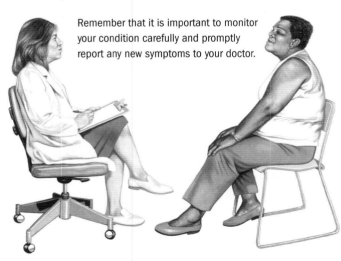

Remember that it is important to monitor your condition carefully and promptly report any new symptoms to your doctor.

How Is Autoimmune Hepatitis Treated?

The main treatment for both types is medicine (corticosteroid called prednisone) to slow an overactive immune system.

In most people, the disease goes into remission with proper treatment, but may recur. Lifelong treatment may be needed.

People who don't respond to standard therapy or who have severe side effects may be helped by other immunosuppressive drugs.

People who develop liver failure may need a liver transplant, a promising treatment, with a 5-year survival rate of 70% to 80%.

DOs and DON'Ts in Managing Autoimmune Hepatitis:

✔ **DO** remember that monitoring of your condition is important. Report any new symptoms to your doctor promptly.

✔ **DO** call your doctor if you notice skin color changes, side effects from medicines, joint pains, or abdominal swelling.

🚫 **DON'T** ignore drug side effects, such as weight gain, anxiety, confusion, thinning of bones (called osteoporosis), thinning of the hair and skin, diabetes, high blood pressure, and cataracts.

🚫 **DON'T** use alcohol. It may further damage your liver.

FROM THE DESK OF

NOTES

FOR MORE INFORMATION

Contact the following source:

• National Institute of Diabetes and Digestive and Kidney Disease (NIDDK)
2 Information Way
Bethesda, MD 20892-3570
E-mail: nddic@info.nddk.nih.gov
Tel: (800) 891-5389
Website: http://digestive.niddk.nih.gov/ddiseases/pubs/ autoimmunehep/

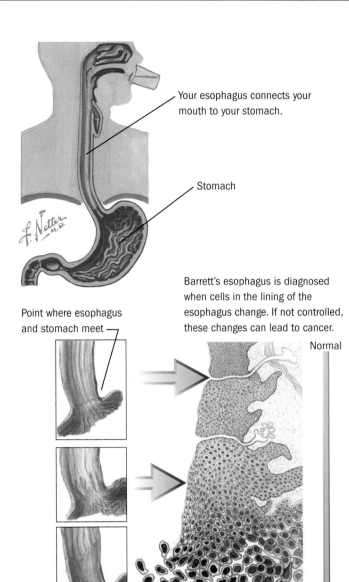

Your esophagus connects your mouth to your stomach.

Stomach

Point where esophagus and stomach meet

Barrett's esophagus is diagnosed when cells in the lining of the esophagus change. If not controlled, these changes can lead to cancer.

Normal

Precancer

Symptoms are similar to those of gastroesophageal reflux disease (GERD). Barrett's esophagus may actually be caused by GERD.

What Is Barrett's Esophagus?

Barrett's esophagus is condition in which cells lining the esophagus are abnormal. The esophagus is a long muscular tube that moves food down from the mouth to the stomach. At its lower end is a small band of muscle (sphincter) that prevents stomach acid from moving back up into the esophagus (reflux). Cells called squamous (flat) cells line the esophagus. In Barrett's esophagus, these cells become another type, called columnar (cells that look like columns). About 5% to 10% of people with this disorder develop cancer of the esophagus.

What Causes Barrett's Esophagus?

The cause is unknown, but it is thought to start from acid reflux disease. It can occur in 10% to 15% of people with acid reflux. It is not hereditary and is not spread from person to person.

What Are the Symptoms of Barrett's Esophagus?

Most symptoms are similar to those in people with acid reflux or acid indigestion. Heartburn is characteristic and usually occurs at night, often waking people from sleep.

Other symptoms include chest pain, difficulty swallowing, food getting stuck or having to vomit food, shortness of breath, wheezing, laryngitis, and hoarseness.

How Is Barrett's Esophagus Diagnosed?

The doctor usually diagnoses the disorder by using endoscopy (placing a lighted tube into the mouth and down into the esophagus). The doctor examines the esophagus and can take samples of any possible problem areas (by a biopsy, or removing a small piece of tissue for study under a microscope).

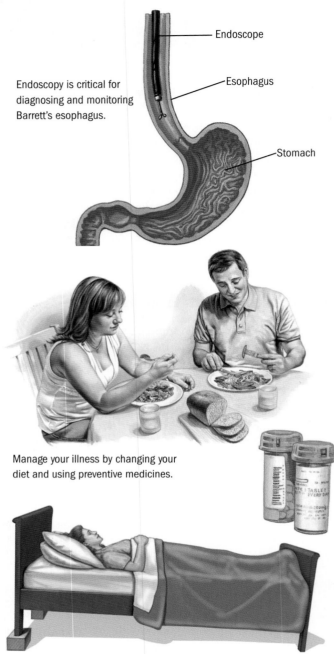

Endoscope

Esophagus

Stomach

Endoscopy is critical for diagnosing and monitoring Barrett's esophagus.

Manage your illness by changing your diet and using preventive medicines.

Elevating the head of the bed is especially good for minimizing nighttime GERD.

How Is Barrett's Esophagus Treated?

The goal is to prevent acid from refluxing into the esophagus. This protects the esophageal lining and may prevent development of Barrett's esophagus. Drugs can limit the amount of acid reaching the lining. These drugs including antacids, H_2-antagonists (e.g., ranitidine, cimetidine), proton pump inhibitors (e.g., omeprazole, lansoprazole), and medicines that improve gastrointestinal motion (e.g., metoclopramide). Proton pump inhibitors are most effective and preferred.

The major complication is development of esophageal cancer, but the doctor can monitor the esophagus by frequent endoscopy to check for cancer. Other complications include bleeding from ulcers and narrowing (stricture) of the esophagus.

DOs and DON'Ts in Managing Barrett's Esophagus:

✔ **DO** remember that the only way to diagnose the disorder is by tissue biopsy via endoscopy. A gastroenterologist (a specialist who treats diseases of the stomach and bowel) will do this.

✔ **DO** remember that acid reflux tends to occur more frequently at night when you lie flat. Elevating the head of the bed will help.

✔ **DO** lose weight.

✔ **DO** make lifestyle changes and take medicines to lower your risk of getting Barrett's esophagus.

✔ **DO** call your doctor if you have heartburn that medicine doesn't help, food gets stuck in your throat and you throw up, or you have trouble swallowing and lose weight.

✔ **DO** call your doctor if you vomit blood.

⊘ **DON'T** drink. Alcohol increases acid reflux.

⊘ **DON'T** eat large meals before going to bed.

⊘ **DON'T** drink coffee or eat chocolate and fats; they can increase acid reflux. Calcium channel blockers can also trigger reflux.

FOR MORE INFORMATION

Contact the following sources:

• American College of Gastroenterology
  Tel: (703) 820-7400
  Website: http://www.acg.gi.org

• Gastro-Intestinal Research Foundation
  Tel: (312) 332-1350
  Website: http://www.girf.org

FROM THE DESK OF

NOTES

MANAGING
CELIAC DISEASE

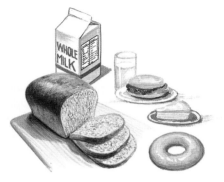

Celiac disease is a food allergy. The allergy is to a substance called gluten. Many grains such as wheat, rye, and barley contain gluten.

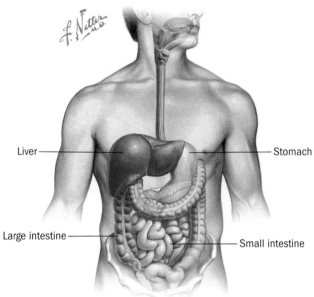

Liver

Stomach

Large intestine

Small intestine

The allergy mostly affects the small intestine and prevents the body from using nutrients. It usually first appears in babies when they start eating food containing gluten.

Symptoms include diarrhea, swollen belly or pain in the belly, light tan or gray stools that may be watery, mouth ulcers, weight loss, and failure to grow.

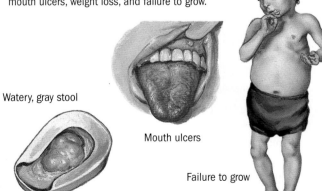

Watery, gray stool

Mouth ulcers

Failure to grow

What Is Celiac Disease?

Celiac disease is a food allergy that prevents the body from using certain nutrients. The allergy is to a substance (protein) called gluten. Gluten is found in many grains, such as wheat, rye, oats, and barley. The allergy mostly affects the small intestine, which is where the food travels after it leaves the stomach.

It usually first appears in babies when they start eating food containing gluten. Celiac disease is more common in those of Western European descent. It often runs in families.

Celiac disease is not curable but can be controlled with a gluten-free diet.

What Causes Celiac Disease?

An allergic reaction to gluten causes celiac disease, which is also called nontropical sprue and gluten enteropathy. The small intestine cannot absorb some nutrients.

What Are the Symptoms of Celiac Disease?

Symptoms include diarrhea, with light tan or gray stools that may be watery or part solid, often smell bad, and look oily or frothy; weight loss; failure to grow and develop (babies and children); frequent gas; swollen abdomen (belly) or abdominal pain; mouth ulcers; tiredness, or weakness; paleness; rash; and muscle cramps.

Diagnosis is by testing blood and stools to check for antibodies and a lack of nutrients. A stool sample may also be checked to test for the presence of parasites and other diseases that have signs and symptoms similar to celiac disease.

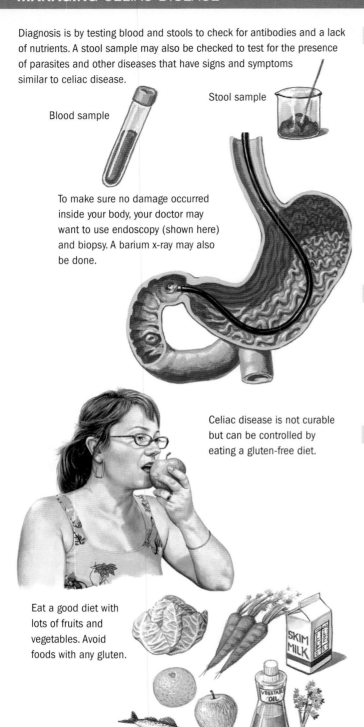

Blood sample

Stool sample

To make sure no damage occurred inside your body, your doctor may want to use endoscopy (shown here) and biopsy. A barium x-ray may also be done.

Celiac disease is not curable but can be controlled by eating a gluten-free diet.

Eat a good diet with lots of fruits and vegetables. Avoid foods with any gluten.

SKIM MILK

VEGETABLE OIL

How Is Celiac Disease Diagnosed?

The doctor tests blood to check for lack of nutrients and antibodies produced in response to gluten.

The doctor may do other tests (such as endoscopy) to look for damage inside the digestive tract caused by the allergy. In endoscopy, a thin, flexible tube with a camera on one end is put into the throat and then down through the stomach into the small intestine. Then the doctor removes a piece of tissue for study under a microscope (biopsy). In a newer test, capsule endoscopy, a small camera in a swallowed pill can look inside the bowels.

The doctor may also do x-rays (small bowel series), which are taken after drinking a white chalky liquid (barium).

How Is Celiac Disease Treated?

The main treatment is eating a special diet that avoids anything containing gluten, which includes grains, particularly wheat, barley, and rye.

Food supplements to help boost low nutrient levels and medicine to help control the allergy may also be required.

DOs and DON'Ts in Managing Celiac Disease:

✔ **DO** get the help of a dietitian or nutritionist to plan your diet.

✔ **DO** follow the gluten-free diet every day. Stay on your diet, even when you feel good.

✔ **DO** take recommended or prescribed food supplements.

✔ **DO** find a support group if you are interested in learning from others with celiac disease.

✔ **DO** call your doctor if symptoms don't improve after 3 weeks of new diet.

✔ **DO** call your doctor if fever develops.

⊘ **DON'T** eat anything that has even a small amount of gluten.

⊘ **DON'T** eat or drink dairy products until your doctor or dietitian approves them.

FROM THE DESK OF

NOTES

FOR MORE INFORMATION

Contact the following sources:

• Celiac Disease Foundation
Tel: (818) 990-2354
Website: http://www.celiac.org

• Celiac Sprue Association (CSA)/USA
Tel: (877) CSA-4-CSA (272-4272)
Website: http://www.csaceliacs.org

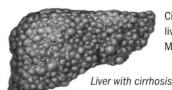

Liver with cirrhosis

Cirrhosis is long-term scarring of the liver, so the liver stops working normally. More men than women have it.

Of the many causes, chronic alcohol abuse is the most common. Other causes include prescription and illegal drugs, fatty liver, and liver infections.

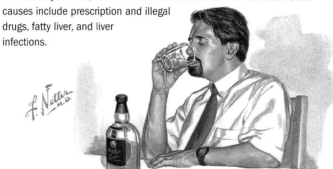

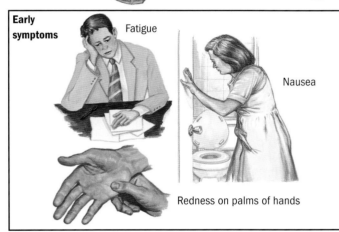

Early symptoms

Fatigue

Nausea

Redness on palms of hands

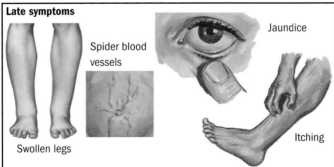

Late symptoms

Spider blood vessels

Swollen legs

Jaundice

Itching

Your doctor will take a medical history, examine you, and do blood and urine tests to see whether your liver is working well. A liver biopsy is the best way to tell that you have cirrhosis.

Liver biopsy

What Is Cirrhosis?

Cirrhosis is a long-term illness involving scarring of the liver. Scarring stops the liver from working normally, which causes problems in the whole body.

Cirrhosis is one of the top 10 causes of death in the United States. Prognosis depends on how much the liver is damaged.

What Causes Cirrhosis?

Of the many causes, the usual one is chronic alcohol abuse. Others include prescription and illegal drugs, fatty liver, liver infections, inherited diseases (such as hemochromatosis and cystic fibrosis), chronic viral hepatitis, toxic substances, and primary biliary cirrhosis (which causes bile duct blockage).

What Are the Symptoms of Cirrhosis?

The most common symptoms of early stages are tiredness (fatigue), weakness, little or no appetite, nausea, weight loss, enlarged liver, and red palms of hands. The symptoms of late stages are yellowing of eyes and skin (jaundice), brown or dark yellow urine, hair loss, changes in blood vessels in skin and around the belly button (spider blood vessels), breast growth in men, easy bruising and bleeding, diarrhea, mental confusion, swollen belly from fluid accumulation (ascites) and swollen legs (edema), large spleen, hemorrhoids, and coma.

How Is Cirrhosis Diagnosed?

The doctor uses a medical history and physical examination for diagnosis. Blood tests, x-rays, computed tomography (CT), and liver biopsy may be done to make the diagnosis. In a biopsy, the best test for diagnosis, the doctor takes a small piece of liver tissue for study.

Medicines can be given for fluid accumulation (edema), mental confusion, and to decrease pressure in the blood vessels in the belly (portal hypertension).

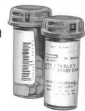

The key to treatment is removing the cause. If you drink alcohol, stop immediately.

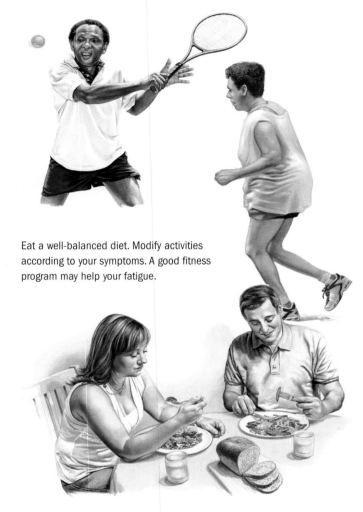

Eat a well-balanced diet. Modify activities according to your symptoms. A good fitness program may help your fatigue.

How Is Cirrhosis Treated?

The key to treatment is removing the cause. The main treatment is then supportive and includes a high-calorie diet and salt (sodium) and fluid restriction (to control fluid accumulation). For severe fluid accumulation in the belly (ascites) or edema, diuretic medicines can be given. Other drugs are given for mental confusion and coma.

Treatment of the complication of increased pressure in the blood vessels in the belly (portal hypertension) depends on its severity. Medicines, endoscopy (a lighted flexible tube used to look at the esophagus, stomach, and small intestine) with treatment of bleeding, surgery, shunting of the blood vessels (portacaval shunt), and liver transplantation are treatment options.

DOs and DON'Ts in Managing Cirrhosis:

✔ **DO** stop drinking alcohol. An alcohol rehabilitation program can help.
✔ **DO** eat a well-balanced diet. You may need to limit protein because the liver may be unable to use it.
✔ **DO** change activities according to your symptoms. A good fitness program may help fatigue.
✔ **DO** get hepatitis B vaccine if you're in a high-risk group (e.g., health care worker, homosexual), and get treated promptly for hepatitis.
✔ **DO** have family members checked for cirrhosis if your family has a history of cirrhosis or inherited diseases that cause it.
✔ **DO** call your doctor if during treatment you vomit blood or have black stool (bowel movements), bright red blood in your stool, increase in fluid accumulation in your belly or feet, or fever.

⊘ **DON'T** use alcohol.
⊘ **DON'T** use medicines, such as acetaminophen, sedatives, and tranquilizers, that can harm the liver.

FOR MORE INFORMATION

Contact the following sources:

• American Liver Foundation
  Tel: (800) GO-LIVER (465-4837)
  Website: http://www.liverfoundation.org

• American College of Gastroenterology
  Phone: (703) 820-7400
  Website: http://www.acg.gi.org

• Alcoholics Anonymous
  Phone: (212) 870-3400
  Website: http://www.aa.org

FROM THE DESK OF

NOTES

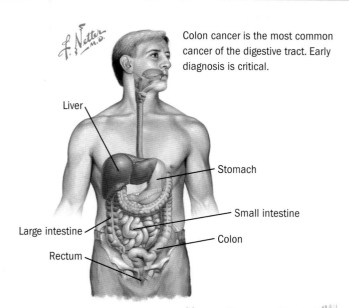

Colon cancer is the most common cancer of the digestive tract. Early diagnosis is critical.

Liver

Stomach

Small intestine

Large intestine

Colon

Rectum

Change in bowel habits, stool appearance, or pain may be the first symptoms of colon cancer, but sometimes there are no symptoms.

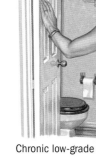

Polyp

The cancer usually starts as a polyp, but some polyps are harmless.

Chronic low-grade bleeding may lead to anemia (low blood).

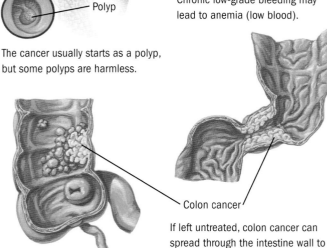

Colon cancer

If left untreated, colon cancer can spread through the intestine wall to the liver and other areas of the body.

What Is the Colon?

The colon is part of the digestive system. Food moves from the mouth to the stomach. Several hours later, it moves into the intestines, first the small intestine and then the large intestine. After digestion of food is finished, what's left leaves the body as waste (stool) through the rectum. The colon is the last part of the large intestine, just before the rectum.

What Is Colon Cancer?

Colon cancer is a tumor in the colon. It is the most common cancer of the digestive tract. Other names are adenocarcinoma of the colon and colorectal cancer (often the lower rectum and sigmoid part of the colon are involved). The cancer can also be found in the first part of the colon (cecum). Colon cancer can also spread (metastasize) to other parts of the body.

Colon cancer usually starts as a small growth (polyp) on the surface of the colon. Some polyps are harmless, but some can turn into cancer.

What Are Symptoms of Colon Cancer?

Symptoms to be aware of are a change in bowel habits, such as constipation or diarrhea, a change in stool size (e.g., pencil-thin) or stool appearance (e.g., black and tarry), rectal bleeding, and abdominal pain.

Sometimes no symptoms are present, but iron deficiency anemia from long-term blood loss may occur.

Early diagnosis is critical because undetected or untreated cancer usually spreads through the intestine wall into neighboring areas and into the liver. Sometimes it can also spread to lungs and bones.

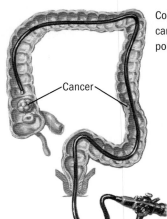

Colonoscopy is used to detect cancer as well as precancerous polyps.

Cancer

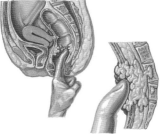

Tumors near the rectum can be found with a rectal exam.

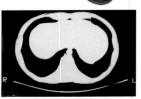

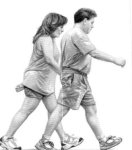

CT imaging can sometimes reveal polyps. CT is also used to see if cancer has spread beyond the colon.

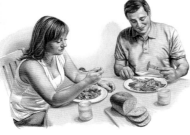

To reduce the risk of developing colon cancer, eat a high-fiber diet and exercise.

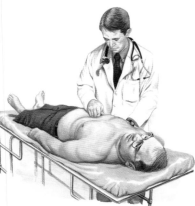

Get an annual physical including a rectal exam if you are over 50 or in a higher risk group. Discuss screening colonoscopy with your doctor.

How Is Colon Cancer Diagnosed?

The doctor will do a complete physical examination, including a digital rectal examination (DRE), and take one or more stool samples. These samples are analyzed for any occult (hidden) blood. This testing can find bleeding in the intestine, but results can be inaccurate because certain medicines or red meat may produce positive results that are really normal (false-positive results).

The doctor also looks inside the colon with a flexible tube called a colonoscope. This scope is passed through the rectum to see the whole colon. The doctor can see problem areas and biopsy (take samples of) these areas and remove any polyps. The samples are studied under a microscope to look for cancerous cells. Other tests, such as computed tomography (CT), of the abdomen and pelvis may be done to see whether cancer has moved to other parts of the body.

A newer screening test involves using CT only for the intestine (CT colonography). This test is also called virtual colonoscopy. Any possible problem areas found by CT colonography will need a follow-up colonoscopy to see whether they are cancerous.

DOs and DON'Ts in Diagnosing and Preventing Colon Cancer:

✔ **DO** realize the importance of colon screening for everyone, starting at age 50 or earlier for people who have family members with colon cancer.
✔ **DO** follow your doctor's advice.
✔ **DO** eat a high-fiber diet.
✔ **DO** watch your weight.
✔ **DO** exercise. Exercising can improve your overall health.

🚫 **DON'T** forget the importance of screening.
🚫 **DON'T** smoke.

FROM THE DESK OF

NOTES

FOR MORE INFORMATION

Contact the following sources:

• Colon Cancer Alliance
  Tel: (877) 422-2030
  Website: http://www.ccalliance.org

• American Cancer Society
  Tel: (800) ACS-2345
  Website: http://www.cancer.org

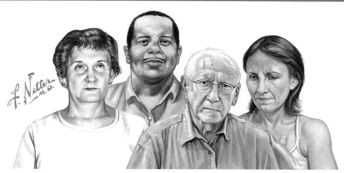

Constipation is having bowel movements less frequently than usual. There is no one normal number of bowel movements per week for everyone.

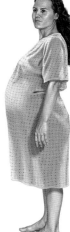

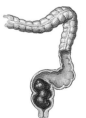

There are many causes, including not enough fluid and fiber intake, stress, inactivity, age, and pregnancy.

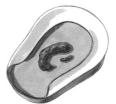

Hard stool   Blood in stool

Symptoms include straining to move bowels, dry or hard stools, bloating of the abdomen (belly), and pain or bleeding from the rectum.

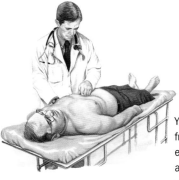

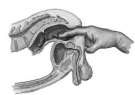

Digital rectal exam

Your doctor makes a diagnosis from your medical history, physical examination (especially of the abdomen), and maybe a digital rectal examination and other tests.

What Is Constipation?

Constipation is having bowel movements less frequently than usual. There is no normal number of bowel movements per week for everyone. Some people move their bowels three times daily and others do it once every 3 days.

What Causes Constipation?

Constipation is due to slow movement of stools (feces) through the colon. The many causes include benign conditions, such as not enough fluid and fiber intake, inactivity, pregnancy, recent travel, and stress, to more serious conditions, such as bowel obstruction because of colon cancer. Constipation is usually harmless and due to lifestyle changes. Medicines such as pain relievers containing narcotics, antihistamines, and some antidepressants are other common causes.

What Are the Symptoms of Constipation?

Symptoms include straining to move bowels, dry or hard stools, bloating of the abdomen (belly), pain or bleeding from the rectum during or after a bowel movement, and feeling that the bowel movement wasn't enough, with a need to go again.

How Is Constipation Diagnosed?

The doctor makes a diagnosis from the medical history, including recent lifestyle changes (stress, travel, fluid intake) and medicines. The doctor will also do a physical examination, especially of the abdomen. The doctor may also do a digital rectal examination to check for problems such as hemorrhoids and rectal fissures, to look for stool in the rectum and its consistency, and to test for blood in the stool.

If the stool contains blood, a colonoscopy and blood tests may be done. In a colonoscopy, a specialist uses a small tube attached to a lighted instrument to look at the colon. Blood tests will check for anemia.

If a lump or mass in the abdomen is found, additional tests such as computed tomography of the abdomen and pelvis may be needed.

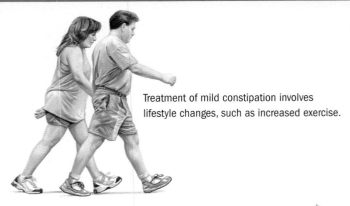

Treatment of mild constipation involves lifestyle changes, such as increased exercise.

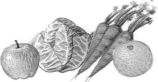

Include lots of fiber in your diet, such as with fruits, vegetables, and whole grains.

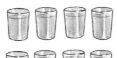

Drink enough fluids (six to eight glasses daily).

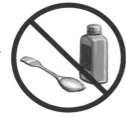

Don't use laxatives on a daily basis.

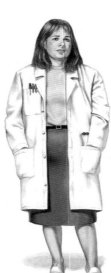

Don't ignore continuing constipation—talk to your doctor. It could be a sign of something serious.

How Is Constipation Treated?

Treatment of mild constipation involves lifestyle changes, with increased exercise and intake of fluids (six to eight glasses daily) and fiber. Laxatives are best avoided because people can become dependent on them. If needed, use natural laxatives such as prune juice. Set a regular time each day for bowel movements. Take enough time, and don't rush. Hot water or coffee a few minutes before may help stimulate the movement.

For moderate to severe constipation, stool softeners, over-the-counter laxatives, and enemas may be needed. Avoid harsh laxatives.

DOs and DON'Ts in Managing Constipation:

✔ **DO** tell your doctor about laxatives you use regularly.
✔ **DO** include lots of fiber in your diet, such as with fruits, vegetables, and whole grains.
✔ **DO** drink enough fluids, especially in warm weather.
✔ **DO** avoid over-the-counter products such as antihistamines that may cause constipation.
✔ **DO** call your doctor if constipation lasts even with lifestyle changes.
✔ **DO** call your doctor if you have rectal pain or bleeding with your bowel movements.
✔ **DO** call your doctor if you have a fever or abdominal pain.

🚫 **DON'T** use laxatives daily.
🚫 **DON'T** rush your bowel movements.
🚫 **DON'T** ignore continuing constipation. It could be a sign of something serious.

FROM THE DESK OF

NOTES

FOR MORE INFORMATION

Contact the following source:

• American College of Gastroenterology
Tel: (703) 820-7400
Website: http://www.acg.gi.org

Crohn's disease affects women slightly more than men. The cause isn't known, but it may be an autoimmune disorder and seems to run in families.

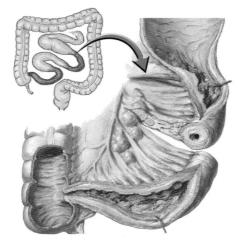

Crohn's disease is a disorder that causes inflammation of the bowel wall. The lower digestive tract gets sore and swollen.

Common symptoms include

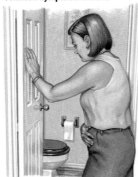

Middle or lower abdominal pain (may be worse after eating), diarrhea, vomiting

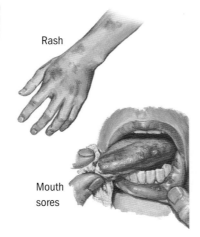

Rash

Mouth sores

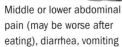

For diagnosis, your doctor uses symptoms and testing such as blood, abdominal CT, and colonoscopy.

What Is Crohn's Disease?

Crohn's disease is a disorder that causes inflammation (swelling, redness) of the wall of the bowel (intestines). Nutrients and vitamins in food may not be easily absorbed.

Most people have this disorder throughout life, but with treatment most people can often live a normal life. It affects women slightly more than men, usually between 15 and 25 years old. It is not contagious and cannot be prevented.

What Causes Crohn's Disease?

The cause is unknown. It's thought to be an autoimmune disease, which means that the body's immune system reacts against its own tissues. It seems to run in families.

What Are the Symptoms of Crohn's Disease?

Common symptoms include middle or lower abdominal (belly) pain (may be worse after eating), and diarrhea (sometimes bloody). Other possible symptoms are joint pain, eyelid redness and swelling, skin lesions, mouth sores, weight loss, tiredness, and fever.

Many complications, such as bowel blockages, can occur. Fistulas (abnormal passages) and fissures (cracks in the skin) in and around the anus and rectum can form and lead to infections.

How Is Crohn's Disease Diagnosed?

The doctor uses symptoms, blood tests, and abdominal CT to make a diagnosis and exclude other causes. The doctor may suggest seeing a digestive disease specialist (gastroenterologist).

Colonoscopy is used to examine the inside of the large intestine (colon). In colonoscopy, the gastroenterologist inserts a flexible tube (which holds a scope and camera) into the rectum and then up into the intestine. During this test, the doctor takes a sample of tissue (biopsy) for study with a microscope.

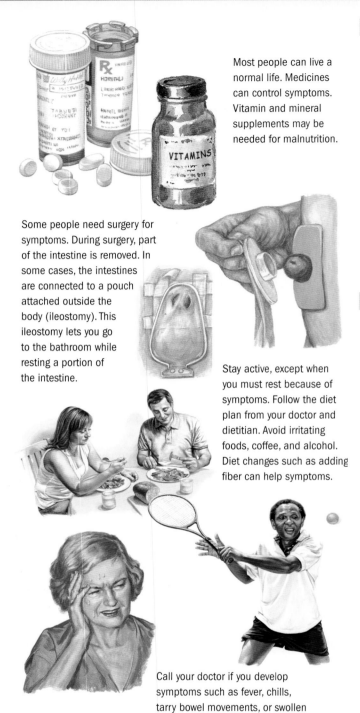

Most people can live a normal life. Medicines can control symptoms. Vitamin and mineral supplements may be needed for malnutrition.

Some people need surgery for symptoms. During surgery, part of the intestine is removed. In some cases, the intestines are connected to a pouch attached outside the body (ileostomy). This ileostomy lets you go to the bathroom while resting a portion of the intestine.

Stay active, except when you must rest because of symptoms. Follow the diet plan from your doctor and dietitian. Avoid irritating foods, coffee, and alcohol. Diet changes such as adding fiber can help symptoms.

Call your doctor if you develop symptoms such as fever, chills, tarry bowel movements, or swollen abdomen.

How Is Crohn's Disease Treated?

The goals of treatment are to relieve symptoms, control inflammation, and prevent complications. People without symptoms need no treatment. Mild diarrhea is controlled with medicine and dietary fiber. Severe symptoms need antiinflammatory drugs. Antibiotics may help infections. Pain relievers are given for abdominal pain and cramping; vitamin and mineral supplements, for malnutrition. Diet changes such as adding some fiber also help. High-nutrition liquid formulas may be used during severe symptoms to rest the intestines.

About 70% of people need surgery for symptoms. During surgery, part of the intestine is removed. In very bad cases, intestines are connected to a pouch attached outside the body (ileostomy pouch), which allows going to the bathroom.

DOs and DON'Ts in Managing Crohn's Disease:

✔ **DO** stay active, except when you must rest because of symptoms.

✔ **DO** take medicines as advised by your doctor.

✔ **DO** follow the diet plan from your doctor and dietitian.

✔ **DO** see your doctor regularly.

✔ **DO** tell your doctor if you have medicine side effects.

✔ **DO** call your doctor if you have a fistula and leak stool through the skin or vagina, have increased number of bowel movements, start bleeding, or have tarry-looking stool.

✔ **DO** call your doctor if you get fever or chills or a swollen abdomen.

⊘ **DON'T** eat a fatty diet.

⊘ **DON'T** eat foods that irritate your bowels or drink coffee and alcohol.

FROM THE DESK OF

NOTES

FOR MORE INFORMATION

Contact the following sources:

• Crohn's and Colitis Foundation of America
Tel: (800) 343-3637
Website: http://www.ccfa.org

• National Digestive Diseases Information Clearinghouse
Tel: (800) 891-5389
Website: http://www.niddk.nih.gov/health/digest/nddic.htm

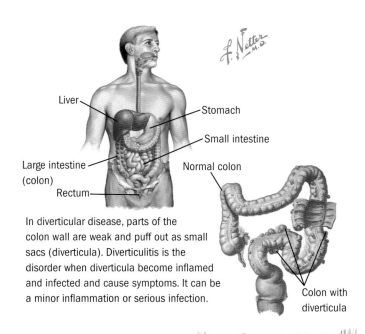

In diverticular disease, parts of the colon wall are weak and puff out as small sacs (diverticula). Diverticulitis is the disorder when diverticula become inflamed and infected and cause symptoms. It can be a minor inflammation or serious infection.

What Is Diverticulitis?

The large intestine (colon) is the last part of the digestive tract. Food passes through it just before waste leaves the body as a bowel movement (stool). In diverticular disease, parts of the colon wall are weak. These weak places can puff out like small sacs (diverticula). Each sac is called a diverticulum. These parts can become red and swollen (inflamed) and infected. Diverticulitis is the disorder when diverticula become inflamed and infected. Diverticulitis can be a minor inflammation or a serious infection.

Diverticulitis occurs in about half of people who have diverticuli. About 3 cases per 100 people occur each year. With treatment the prognosis is good, but relapses do occur. Complications include hemorrhage (bleeding), perforation (rupture), bowel blockage, and abscesses.

What Causes Diverticulitis?

Diverticuli become inflamed and infected, and small abscesses form and then burst, which causes symptoms. This disorder can occur if food moves too slowly through the colon. Pressure in the colon from this food causes weak spots and sacs. Diverticulitis is not contagious or cancerous.

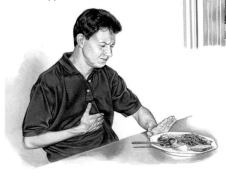

Symptoms are cramping and pain in the abdomen, usually in the left lower part. Pain is usually severe and starts suddenly. Other symptoms are fever, chills, constipation or diarrhea, and loss of appetite and nausea.

What Are the Symptoms of Diverticulitis?

Symptoms are cramping and pain in the abdomen (belly) that stops and starts but then becomes constant. The pain is usually in the left lower abdomen. It's usually severe and starts suddenly. Other symptoms are fever, chills, constipation or diarrhea, and loss of appetite and nausea.

How Is Diverticulitis Diagnosed?

The doctor will make a diagnosis from a medical history, physical examination, blood tests, x-rays, and computed tomography (CT). Blood tests will check for infection. CT will show the inflammation and infection. Certain tests such as colonoscopy and barium enema shouldn't be done during acute diverticulitis because they may cause the colon to burst at the place of diverticulitis.

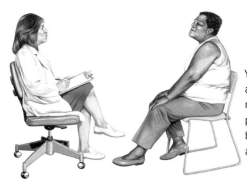

Your doctor will make a diagnosis from your medical history, physical examination, blood tests, x-rays, and CT.

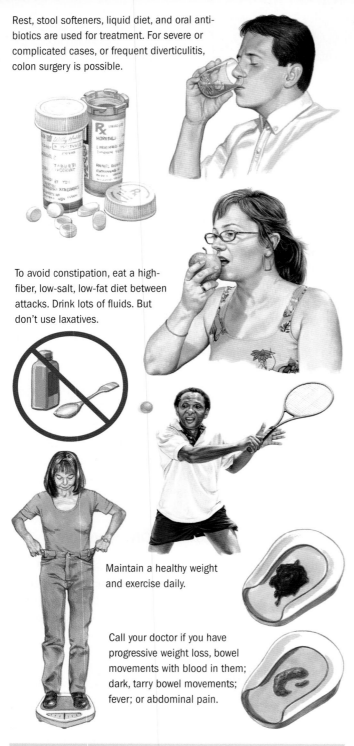

Rest, stool softeners, liquid diet, and oral antibiotics are used for treatment. For severe or complicated cases, or frequent diverticulitis, colon surgery is possible.

To avoid constipation, eat a high-fiber, low-salt, low-fat diet between attacks. Drink lots of fluids. But don't use laxatives.

Maintain a healthy weight and exercise daily.

Call your doctor if you have progressive weight loss, bowel movements with blood in them; dark, tarry bowel movements; fever; or abdominal pain.

How Is Diverticulitis Treated?

Outpatient treatment is usual, unless symptoms are severe and widespread infection or complications occur. Rest, stool softeners, liquid diet, and oral antibiotics are used. If a hospital stay is needed, treatment is similar, but intravenous fluids and antibiotics are given, together with pain medicine. At first, eating may not be allowed. Then, high-fiber, low-fat foods are slowly returned to the diet.

For severe or complicated cases, surgical removal of the affected part of the colon is possible. Surgery is also used for frequent diverticulitis.

DOs and DON'Ts in Managing Diverticulitis:

✔ **DO** take medicines as prescribed.
✔ **DO** eat a high-fiber, low-salt, low-fat diet between attacks to avoid constipation. This will reduce your chances of getting diverticulitis.
✔ **DO** drink plenty of fluids between attacks.
✔ **DO** keep physically active between attacks.
✔ **DO** maintain your correct weight. Try to lose weight if you're overweight.
✔ **DO** maintain good bowel habits by trying to have a bowel movement daily.
✔ **DO** call your doctor if you have blood in your stool or dark, tarry bowel movements or unexplained weight loss.
✔ **DO** call your doctor if abdominal pain develops or becomes worse.
✔ **DO** call your doctor if you get a fever.

⊘ **DON'T** strain with bowel movements.
⊘ **DON'T** use laxatives.

FROM THE DESK OF

NOTES

FOR MORE INFORMATION

Contact the following source:

• National Digestive Diseases Information Clearinghouse
Tel: (800) 891-5389
Website: http://www.niddk.nih.gov/health/digest/nddic.htm

MANAGING YOUR
DIVERTICULOSIS

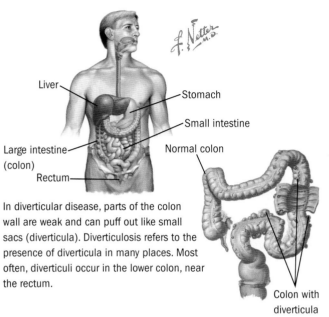

Liver
Stomach
Small intestine
Large intestine (colon)
Normal colon
Rectum

In diverticular disease, parts of the colon wall are weak and can puff out like small sacs (diverticula). Diverticulosis refers to the presence of diverticula in many places. Most often, diverticuli occur in the lower colon, near the rectum.

Colon with diverticula (diverticulosis)

The cause isn't known. Diverticulosis can occur if food moves too slowly through the colon, so people who eat a high-fat diet without much fiber are more likely to have diverticula.

Most people have no symptoms. Some have mild cramping in the left side of the abdomen, often relieved by a bowel movement or passing gas. Constipation may sometimes occur.

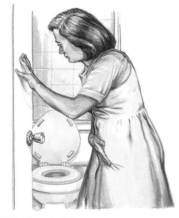

Your doctor will do a colonoscopy or rarely a barium enema x-ray examination for diagnosis.

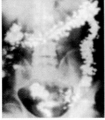

Barium enema x-ray showing diverticulosis

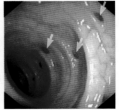

Diverticula seen during colonoscopy

What Is Diverticulosis?

The large intestine (colon) is the last part of the digestive tract. Food passes through it just before waste leaves the body as a bowel movement (stool). In diverticular disease, parts of the colon wall are weak. These weak places can puff out like small sacs (diverticula). Each sac is called a diverticulum. These parts can become red and swollen (inflamed) and infected. Diverticulosis refers to the presence of diverticula in many places. Most often, diverticuli occur in the lower part of the colon (sigmoid and distal colon) near the rectum.

The condition is a lifelong problem. Up to 20% of the general population has diverticulosis. Older people tend to have diverticuli more often than younger people. Up to 50% of people at age 50 will have them. Complications include infection (diverticulitis) and bleeding.

What Causes Diverticulosis?

The cause is the bulging (herniation) of the colon wall (mucosa) through the muscular layer of the colon. The reason for the herniation is unknown. Diverticulosis can occur if food moves too slowly through the colon. People who eat a low-fiber diet are much more likely to form diverticula. It's not contagious or cancerous.

What Are the Symptoms of Diverticulosis?

Most people don't have any symptoms. About 10% to 20% of people have mild cramping in the left side of the abdomen (belly). A bowel movement or passing gas often relieves the cramping. Constipation may be an occasional problem.

How Is Diverticulosis Diagnosed?

The doctor will make a diagnosis by a colonoscopy. In a colonoscopy, the doctor looks at the whole colon using a lighted flexible tube put through the rectum. The tube has a tiny camera that lets the doctor look for problem spots and take pictures. Before this test, a laxative must be taken to empty all food from the colon. Rarely a barium enema may be done in place of colonoscopy. For the barium enema x-ray examination, a liquid containing the substance barium is placed in the rectum. The liquid makes it easier to see inside the colon. Diverticulosis is often found when tests are done for another disorder.

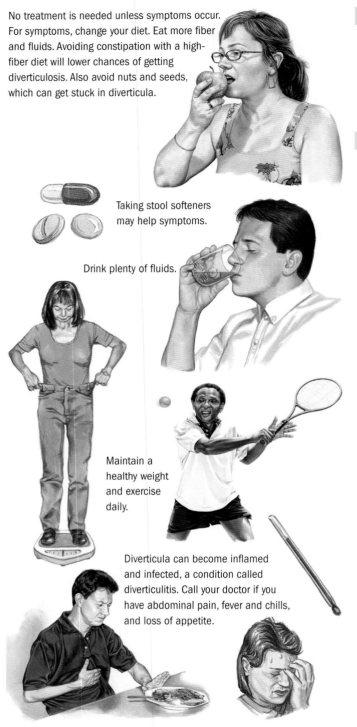

No treatment is needed unless symptoms occur. For symptoms, change your diet. Eat more fiber and fluids. Avoiding constipation with a high-fiber diet will lower chances of getting diverticulosis. Also avoid nuts and seeds, which can get stuck in diverticula.

Taking stool softeners may help symptoms.

Drink plenty of fluids.

Maintain a healthy weight and exercise daily.

Diverticula can become inflamed and infected, a condition called diverticulitis. Call your doctor if you have abdominal pain, fever and chills, and loss of appetite.

How Is Diverticulosis Treated?

No treatment is needed unless symptoms occur. For symptoms, a change in diet, with more fiber and fluids, and use of stool softeners will help. Avoid nuts and seeds, which can get stuck in diverticula.

DOs and DON'Ts in Managing Diverticulosis:

✔ **DO** eat a high-fiber, low-salt, low-fat diet. Avoiding constipation with a high-fiber diet will lower chances of getting diverticulosis.

✔ **DO** drink plenty of fluids.

✔ **DO** keep physically active.

✔ **DO** maintain your correct weight. Try to lose weight if you're overweight.

✔ **DO** maintain good bowel habits by trying to have a bowel movement daily.

✔ **DO** call your doctor if you have blood in your stool or dark, tarry bowel movements.

✔ **DO** watch for signs of diverticulitis and complications, such as abdominal pain and fever.

✔ **DO** call your doctor if you have a fever or abdominal pain or your pain becomes worse.

⊘ **DON'T** strain with bowel movements.

⊘ **DON'T** use laxatives.

FROM THE DESK OF

NOTES

FOR MORE INFORMATION

Contact the following source:

• National Digestive Diseases Information Clearinghouse
Tel: (800) 891-5389
Website: http://www.niddk.nih.gov/health/digest/nddic.htm

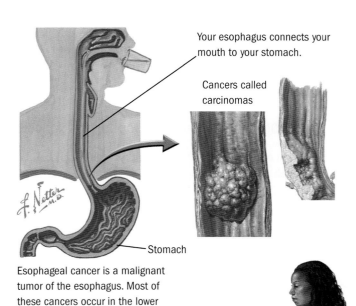

Your esophagus connects your mouth to your stomach.

Cancers called carcinomas

Stomach

Esophageal cancer is a malignant tumor of the esophagus. Most of these cancers occur in the lower esophagus.

The cause isn't known, but risk factors include heavy alcohol and tobacco use.

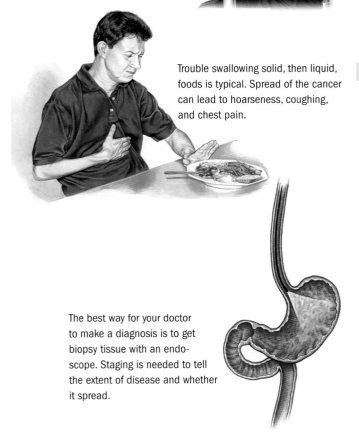

Trouble swallowing solid, then liquid, foods is typical. Spread of the cancer can lead to hoarseness, coughing, and chest pain.

The best way for your doctor to make a diagnosis is to get biopsy tissue with an endo-scope. Staging is needed to tell the extent of disease and whether it spread.

What Is Esophageal Cancer?

The esophagus is the part of the digestive tract that connects the mouth with the stomach. Esophageal cancer is a cancerous (malignant) tumor of this tube. Most of these cancers occur in the lower part of the esophagus. More than 10,000 new cases are diagnosed in the United States every year.

What Causes Esophageal Cancer?

The cause is unknown. Certain risk factors, such as heavy alcohol and tobacco use, increase the chances of getting this cancer. It isn't contagious. Acid reflux from the stomach that occurs for a long time can lead to changes in the lining of the esophagus (Barrett's esophagus), which can lead to esophageal cancer.

What Are the Symptoms of Esophageal Cancer?

Trouble swallowing solid foods is the usual symptom. As the tumor grows, liquids become hard to swallow, and pain with swallowing can occur. Cancer usually spreads nearby, to lungs, windpipe, lymph glands, and liver. Hoarseness, coughing, coughing up or vomiting blood, and chest pain can result.

How Is Esophageal Cancer Diagnosed?

The best way for the doctor to make a diagnosis is with an endoscope and biopsy. With this lighted tube, passed through the mouth into the esophagus, the doctor can get tissue to study with a microscope. X-ray studies, a barium swallow examination or esophagography, can also be done.

After diagnosis, staging is needed to tell the extent of disease and whether it spread. A physical examination, blood tests, and computed tomography (CT) of the chest and abdomen are used. Spread to the voice box (larynx) is checked with laryngoscopy. Spread to the lungs may be checked with bronchoscopy. These examinations use lighted tubes passed into the larynx or lungs.

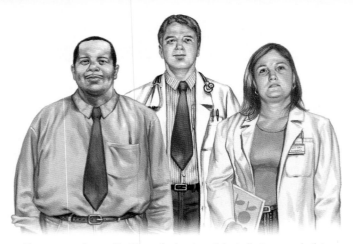

You may need a medical team for treatment, including an oncologist, surgeon, and nutritionist. Don't be afraid to seek second opinions.

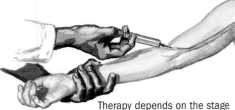

Therapy depends on the stage of disease and its spread. It can include surgery, radiation, and chemotherapy.

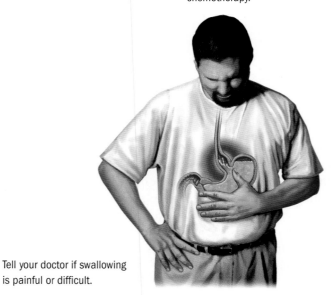

Tell your doctor if swallowing is painful or difficult.

How Is Esophageal Cancer Treated?

Therapy depends on the stage of disease and its spread. It can include surgery, radiation, and chemotherapy (cancer-fighting drugs). In an operation called esophagectomy, the surgeon removes the cancerous part of the esophagus and lymph glands. Radiation is used instead of surgery when the tumor is too large to remove or the person cannot undergo an operation. Chemotherapy can be used with radiation and surgery.

DOs and DON'Ts in Managing Esophageal Cancer:

✔ **DO** treat chronic acid reflux to avoid precancerous conditions such as Barrett's esophagus.

✔ **DO** ask about your prognosis. This cancer is hard to cure.

✔ **DO** understand that nutrition is important before and after the operation. Eat high-calorie foods and nutritional supplements. A nutritionist (diet specialist) can help.

✔ **DO** ask for help from support groups.

✔ **DO** call your doctor if you have pain with swallowing, trouble swallowing, or food getting stuck when eating.

✔ **DO** call your doctor if you cough up or vomit blood.

✔ **DO** call your doctor if you have shortness of breath and fever.

✔ **DO** call your doctor if you cannot eat and continue to lose weight.

⊘ **DON'T** smoke.

⊘ **DON'T** drink alcohol in excess.

⊘ **DON'T** miss follow-up appointments, such as with your primary care doctor, surgeon, and oncologist (cancer specialist).

FROM THE DESK OF

NOTES

FOR MORE INFORMATION

Contact the following sources:

• National Cancer Institute
Tel: (800) 422-6237
Website: http://www.cancer.gov

• American Cancer Society
Tel: (800) 227-2345
Website: http://www.cancer.org

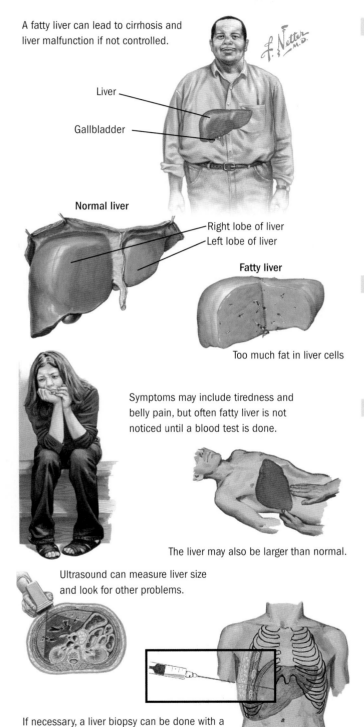

A fatty liver can lead to cirrhosis and liver malfunction if not controlled.

Liver

Gallbladder

Normal liver

Right lobe of liver
Left lobe of liver

Fatty liver

Too much fat in liver cells

Symptoms may include tiredness and belly pain, but often fatty liver is not noticed until a blood test is done.

The liver may also be larger than normal.

Ultrasound can measure liver size and look for other problems.

If necessary, a liver biopsy can be done with a special needle to take out a piece of the liver.

What Is Fatty Liver?

A fatty liver refers to a collection of too much fat in liver cells that often occurs in patients with diabetes or obesity or patients who drink too much alcohol. A fatty liver by itself is not harmful, but prolonged swelling (inflammation) of a fatty liver can lead to scarring (cirrhosis) and poor functioning of the liver.

Nonalcoholic fatty liver disease (nonalcoholic steatohepatitis, or NASH) is inflammation of a fatty liver that is not caused by alcohol or hepatitis. It is more common in overweight people, but the specific cause is unknown. NASH is not transmitted from person to person or from generation to generation. NASH is the most common liver disease in teenagers and the third leading cause of liver disease in adults.

What Are the Symptoms of Fatty Liver?

Most patients with fatty liver or NASH do not know they have it because they usually have no symptoms. Some patients may feel tired, have pain in the abdomen (belly), or just not feel right.

How Is Fatty Liver Diagnosed?

The doctor may make this diagnosis by accident when testing for another complaint. Often, liver function blood test results are not normal. In this case, the doctor will take a detailed history and do a physical examination and other studies to rule out common causes of these results (such as hepatitis, alcohol, or too much iron in the liver). At an examination, the doctor may feel for a liver or spleen that is too large but in most cases this will not be evident on physical examination.

The doctor may also want special x-ray studies and scans to take pictures of organs in the body: ultrasound scan, computed tomography (CT), or magnetic resonance imaging (MRI).

A diagnosis of NASH is proved by a liver biopsy. In a biopsy, a large needle is inserted into the liver. Then, a small piece of the liver is removed and examined under a microscope.

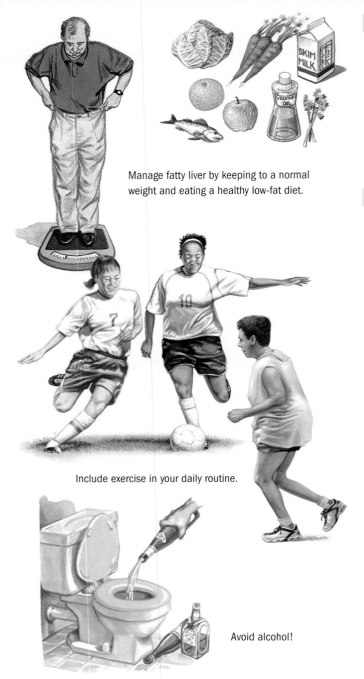

Manage fatty liver by keeping to a normal weight and eating a healthy low-fat diet.

Include exercise in your daily routine.

Avoid alcohol!

How Is Fatty Liver Treated?

Weight loss and avoiding alcohol are the best ways to treat fatty liver.

If you have NASH and are obese or diabetic or have high cholesterol, you should lose weight and control your blood sugar and lipid levels by eating a good diet and exercising.

Your doctor may try drugs to reduce the liver's fats and inflammation.

DOs and DON'Ts in Managing Fatty Liver:

✔ **DO** realize that often a liver biopsy is not done and fatty liver or NASH is diagnosed by ruling out other causes such as alcohol or virus (called a diagnosis of exclusion).

✔ **DO** ask your doctor about drugs that can hurt the liver, such as acetaminophen and some used for diabetes and high cholesterol.

✔ **DO** lose weight if you are obese.

⊘ **DON'T** drink alcohol. Avoiding alcohol may help get rid of the fat stored in liver cells.

⊘ **DON'T** forget that a few patients with NASH can get liver cirrhosis and have complications from liver failure, for example, yellow skin color (jaundice), fluid in and swelling of the belly (ascites), and swelling (edema) of the legs.

FROM THE DESK OF

NOTES

FOR MORE INFORMATION

Contact the following source:

• National Digestive Diseases Information Clearinghouse
Tel: (800) 860-8747
Website: http://www.niddk.nih.gov/health/diabetes/diabetes.htm

CARING FOR YOUR CHILD WITH
ENCOPRESIS

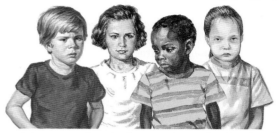

Encopresis is passage of stool or feces on places other than the toilet by children past toilet training age. To make a diagnosis of encopresis, the child must be at least 4 years old, and encopresis must occur at the rate of at least one episode a month for 3 months or more.

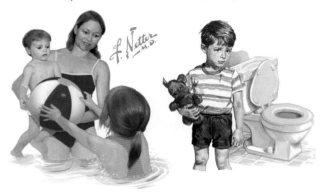

The cause is unknown, but encopresis may occur after constipation, illness, or change in diet. Stressful events such as birth of a sibling, starting a new school, and moving can be involved, as can too much stress during toilet training.

In some families in which punishment is too strict or abusive, a child may put feces in places to cause anger or irritation, even smeared on furniture or walls.

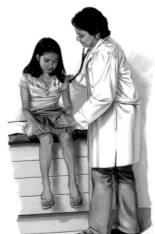

Your child's doctor will do a medical examination and laboratory and x-ray studies to rule out other diseases. Psychiatric, psychosocial, and family interviews may be needed.

What Is Encopresis?

Encopresis is passage of stools (bowel movements) or feces on places other than the toilet by children past the toilet training age (4 years old). These places can be clothing or floors. More boys than girls are affected. It can be involuntary or voluntary. To make a diagnosis of encopresis, it must occur at the rate of at least one episode a month for 3 months or more. It cannot be due only to a substance (for example, a laxative) or other medical conditions. It most commonly occurs in children with constipation. "Primary encopresis" means that the child never mastered toilet training. In "secondary encopresis" the child was toilet trained for at least 1 year or more before the development of encopresis.

What Causes Encopresis?

The cause is unknown, but encopresis may occur after constipation, illness, or change in diet. Stressful events such as birth of a sibling, starting a new school, and moving can be involved. Too much stress during toilet training can lead to anxiety, so-called pot phobia, and encopresis.

The three types of encopresis (which can overlap) include voluntary control (children choose inappropriate places), true failure to control bowels, and soiling caused by liquid feces (from constipation and overflow or from anxiety). In the first type, encopresis tends to be temporary. Children may put feces in places (such as furniture or walls) to cause anger. In the second group, medical illness may stop children from learning to control their bowels. In the third group, children may have a medical condition that causes diarrhea.

How Is Encopresis Diagnosed?

The doctor will do a medical examination and laboratory and x-ray studies to rule out other diseases. Psychiatric, psychosocial, and family interviews will get information about the child's development, behaviors, and stressful events.

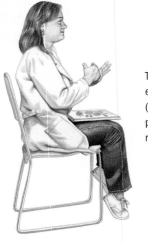

Treatment includes assessment; education; focus on toilet training (possibly laxatives and enemas), proper diet, and, in cases of relapse, biofeedback.

Avoid constipation by feeding a high-fiber diet and having your child drink plenty of water.

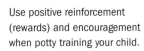

Use positive reinforcement (rewards) and encouragement when potty training your child.

Call your doctor if your child has symptoms such as fever, nausea, vomiting, hard stools, diarrhea with dehydration, or blood in the stool or around the rectum.

How Is Encopresis Treated?

Treatment involves four stages: the first (assessment) will find out whether encopresis is primary or secondary and rule out physical conditions.

The second involves advice, with education about diet, toileting, and parental punishment.

The third stage focuses on toilet training, eating a high-fiber diet, and toileting after meals for a maximum of 15 minutes. Laxatives and enemas (bisacodyl) may be used. The fourth stage consists of biofeedback, but only for children who relapse after training.

Other treatments include behavior therapy such as positive reinforcement and family therapy to shift the family's focus away from encopresis. Behavior therapy plus laxatives works well, in about 75% of cases, in reducing encopretic episodes. Biofeedback for control of the external sphincter muscle also works relatively well.

A healthy, high-fiber diet is often suggested, with bran added to cereals, fruit, and milkshakes.

DOs and DON'Ts in Managing Encopresis:

✔ **DO** avoid constipation by feeding a high-fiber diet and having your child drink plenty of water.

✔ **DO** understand that relapses are normal, so don't get discouraged and be patient.

✔ **DO** call your doctor if your child has a fever, begins to have nausea or vomiting, or has especially hard stools.

✔ **DO** call your doctor if your child has diarrhea and becomes really dehydrated.

✔ **DO** call your doctor right away if you see blood in your child's stool or blood around the rectum.

⊘ **DON'T** start toilet training too early, and don't be too forceful. Use positive reinforcement (rewards) and encouragement.

FROM THE DESK OF

NOTES

FOR MORE INFORMATION

Contact the following sources:

• American Academy of Pediatrics
Tel: (847) 434-4000
Website: http://www.aap.org

• American Psychiatric Association
Tel: (888) 357-7924
Website: http://www.psych.org

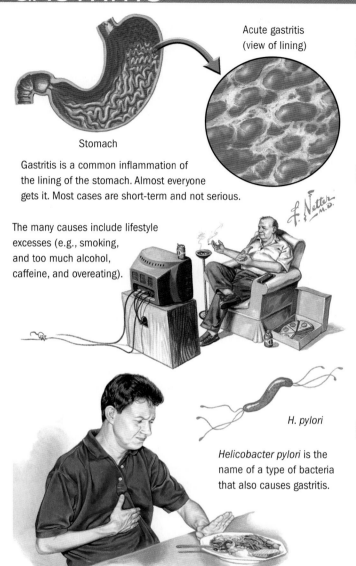

Acute gastritis
(view of lining)

Stomach

Gastritis is a common inflammation of the lining of the stomach. Almost everyone gets it. Most cases are short-term and not serious.

The many causes include lifestyle excesses (e.g., smoking, and too much alcohol, caffeine, and overeating).

H. pylori

Helicobacter pylori is the name of a type of bacteria that also causes gastritis.

The main symptoms are discomfort in the upper abdomen and cramps. Eating often makes the discomfort worse.

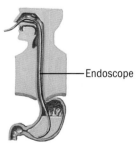

Endoscope

Your doctor will diagnose gastritis by using your medical history and physical examination. Sometimes your doctor may use upper endoscopy to rule out more serious conditions.

What Is Gastritis?

Gastritis is an inflammation (swelling, redness) of the lining of the stomach. This common condition affects almost everyone at some point in life. Most cases are short-term and have no lasting effects.

What Causes Gastritis?

The many causes include lifestyle excesses (e.g., smoking, alcohol, caffeine, and overeating). Gastritis is also a side effect of many medicines, such as aspirin and nonsteroidal anti-inflammatory drugs (NSAIDs). Other causes are bacterial and viral infections, stress from surgery, kidney failure, severe burns, and trauma. These things may increase acid production in the stomach or weaken the lining of the stomach. The bacterium named *Helicobacter pylori* is one of the more common causes of gastritis.

One type of gastritis that doesn't involve increased acid is atrophic gastritis. In this type, the stomach lining becomes damaged and shrunken.

What Are the Symptoms of Gastritis?

The main symptoms are discomfort in the upper abdomen (belly) and cramps. Eating often makes the pain worse. Many people have less appetite. Pain may radiate to the chest, so people think that it's related to the heart. Other symptoms may be bad breath, a burning acid taste in the mouth, and sometimes nausea, vomiting, and bleeding.

How Is Gastritis Diagnosed?

The doctor will diagnose gastritis by using the medical history. A physical examination is usually normal or may show slight pain in the stomach area.

The doctor sometimes schedules upper endoscopy (looking at the stomach through a lighted, flexible tube) to rule out more serious conditions such as stomach ulcers or cancer. During endoscopy, the doctor can take a sample of stomach tissue (biopsy). This tissue can be checked for bacteria (*H. pylori*).

If endoscopy isn't done and symptoms continue, other tests may be done. These tests will also look for *H. pylori* by checking blood, stools (bowel movements), or breath.

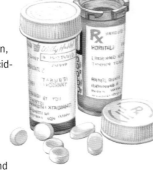

Treatment focuses on symptoms and the cause. For *H. pylori* infection, a combination of antibiotics and acid-reducing medicines will cure it.

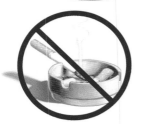

Eat regularly and not in excess.

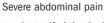

Stop smoking.

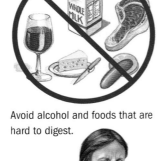

Avoid alcohol and foods that are hard to digest.

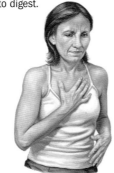

Severe abdominal pain

Call your doctor if abdominal pain is severe; you get severe chest pain that moves to the neck, jaw, or arm and occurs with sweating or shortness of breath; you have dark tarry stools; or you vomit blood.

Radiating chest pain with shortness of breath

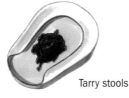

Tarry stools

FROM THE DESK OF

NOTES

How Is Gastritis Treated?

Treatment focuses on symptoms and avoiding the cause. For *H. pylori* infection, a combination of antibiotics and acid-reducing medicines will cure it. Medications such as ibuprofen, naproxen, or aspirin and alcoholic beverages should be avoided.

Mild symptoms are controlled with antacids, over-the-counter histamine-2 (H_2) blockers, or proton pump inhibitors (PPIs). H_2 blockers include famotidine and ranitidine. PPIs include omeprazole and pantoprazole. H_2 blockers and PPIs block stomach acid production. Antacids neutralize stomach acid. Some of these medicines are also available in prescription strength.

For severe gastritis with bleeding, a hospital stay may be needed. Intravenous fluids and medicines are given to control symptoms, reduce stomach acid, and protect the stomach lining.

DOs and DON'Ts in Managing Gastritis:

✔ **DO** eat regularly and not in excess.
✔ **DO** use antacids and over-the-counter H_2 blockers or PPIs for mild symptoms.
✔ **DO** call your doctor if abdominal pain becomes severe or you vomit blood.
✔ **DO** call your doctor if symptoms don't get better after 3 to 5 days of treatment.
✔ **DO** call your doctor if you get severe chest pain that radiates to your neck, jaw, or arm and is associated with sweating or shortness of breath.
✔ **DO** call your doctor if you have blood with bowel movements or dark tarry stools.

⊘ **DON'T** smoke.
⊘ **DON'T** drink alcohol.
⊘ **DON'T** eat foods that are hard to digest.
⊘ **DON'T** use medicines that can irritate your stomach, such as aspirin and NSAIDs.

FOR MORE INFORMATION

Contact the following sources:

• National Digestive Diseases Information Clearinghouse
Tel: (800) 891-5389
Website: http://www.niddk.nih.gov/health/digest/nddic.htm

• American Gastroenterological Association
Tel: (301) 654-2055
Website: http://www.gastro.org

• American College of Gastroenterology
Tel: (703) 820-7400
Website: http://www.acg.gi.org

MANAGING YOUR
GASTROENTERITIS

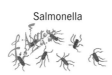

Salmonella

Salmonellosis is an infection of the stomach and intestines that's caused by *Salmonella*, a kind of bacteria. It's similar to stomach flu.

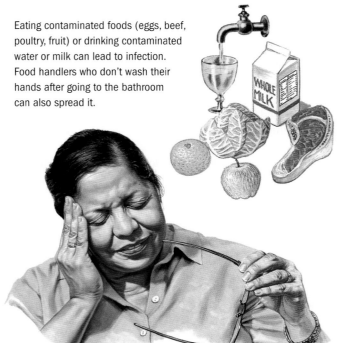

Eating contaminated foods (eggs, beef, poultry, fruit) or drinking contaminated water or milk can lead to infection. Food handlers who don't wash their hands after going to the bathroom can also spread it.

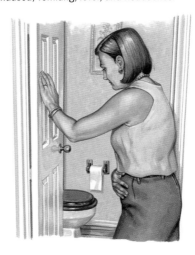

Diarrhea is the main symptom but others include nausea, vomiting, fever, and headaches.

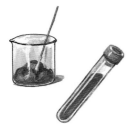

Your doctor makes a diagnosis by testing a stool sample. Blood tests are sometimes done to rule out other diseases.

What Is Gastroenteritis?

Gastroenteritis is inflammation (redness, swelling) of the stomach and intestines. Viral gastroenteritis, often called stomach flu, is an infection caused by a virus that affects the stomach and small intestine.

What Causes Gastroenteritis?

Many viruses can cause gastroenteritis. These viruses include rotaviruses and noroviruses. People get the virus by eating or drinking contaminated food or water, or by directly contacting someone infected by the virus, such as by shaking hands, kissing, or sharing a drink, food, or utensils. Often, someone with the virus handles food without washing hands after using the bathroom, so the virus is passed on by eating the food.

What Are the Symptoms of Gastroenteritis?

The most common symptoms are vomiting and diarrhea. Others include headache, fever, abdominal cramping, loss of appetite, feeling tired and weak, nausea, chills, and aching muscles.

How Is Gastroenteritis Diagnosed?

The doctor will do a physical examination and review the symptoms. The doctor may also order tests to rule out certain conditions, such as appendicitis, dehydration, or a serious infection.

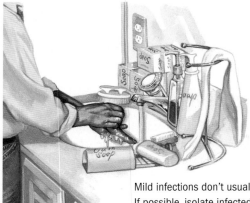

Mild infections don't usually need medicine. If possible, isolate infected people. Wash your hands well after using the bathroom to avoid spreading the infection.

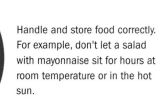

Drink more fluids to prevent dehydration.

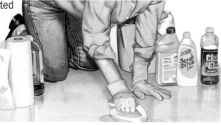

Handle and store food correctly. For example, don't let a salad with mayonnaise sit for hours at room temperature or in the hot sun.

If possible, have the infected person use a separate bathroom. If it's not possible, don't let others use the same bathroom unless it was well cleaned.

How Is Gastroenteritis Treated?

Medicines such as antibiotics aren't used for viral gastro-enteritis. Antibiotics don't work on viruses, and overusing them can result in growth of antibiotic-resistant bacteria.

The most important thing to do is avoid dehydration (loss of too much body fluid).

Drinking clear fluids allows the stomach and intestines to rest and get better. Fluids should be drunk slowly. Fluid loss from diarrhea and vomiting can affect babies and children more than adults, so they may need oral rehydration solutions (such as Pedialyte®). Drinking fluids should start slowly.

If the stomach can keep fluids down, soft, bland foods can be tried slowly. Such foods include toast, broth, apples, bananas, and rice. Avoid dairy products, caffeine, and alcohol.

Medicine may be used to treat symptoms such as nausea, vomiting, fever, and body aches.

People usually get better in a few days, but if not, another visit to the doctor may be needed.

DOs and DON'Ts in Managing Gastroenteritis:

✔ **DO** clean surfaces that have been touched by infected people.
✔ **DO** drink clear fluids, then add food gradually.
✔ **DO** wash your hands often, especially after using the bathroom.
✔ **DO** call your doctor if you have persistent vomiting or diarrhea.

⊘ **DON'T** have close contact (for example, by shaking hands) with others until symptoms have resolved.
⊘ **DON'T** give your child medicine without asking your doctor.

FROM THE DESK OF

NOTES

FOR MORE INFORMATION

Contact the following sources:

• American Gastroenterological Association
Tel: (301) 654-2055
Website: http://www.gastro.org

• American College of Gastroenterology
Tel: (301) 263-9000
Website: http://www.acg.gi.org

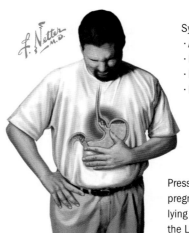

Symptoms of GERD include:
· Acid, sour taste in mouth
· Bloated stomach and belching
· Pain in throat and chest
· Hoarseness, coughing

Pressure from being overweight, pregnant, having a hiatal hernia, or lying down after a meal can cause the LES muscle to open.

Food passing normally from esophagus to stomach

LES muscles functioning properly; food remains in stomach

LES muscles not working properly; food refluxes into esophagus

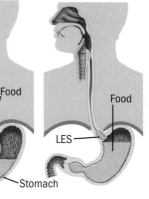
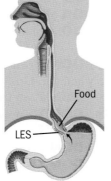

Esophagus
Food
Food
Food
LES
LES
LES
Stomach

If the LES does not function properly, the contents of the stomach may return upward into the esophagus. The stomach contents contain acid, and they irritate the sensitive lining of the esophagus.

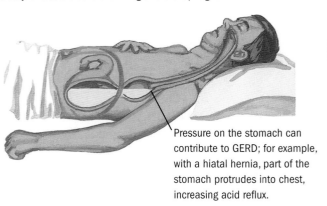

Pressure on the stomach can contribute to GERD; for example, with a hiatal hernia, part of the stomach protrudes into chest, increasing acid reflux.

What Is Gastroesophageal Reflux Disease (GERD)?

GERD (acid reflux disease) occurs when stomach acid flows up into the esophagus (the tube connecting the mouth with the stomach). The stomach can handle stomach acid, but the throat and esophagus can't. As a result, stomach acid in these areas may cause damage. To some extent, everyone has acid reflux. Normal reflux usually happens after meals, is brief and without symptoms, and rarely happens during sleep. Normal reflux becomes GERD when symptoms occur frequently (generally at least two or three times a week) or the esophagus becomes damaged.

What Are the Causes of GERD?

Abnormalities of the lower esophageal sphincter (LES), a muscle at the bottom of the esophagus, cause GERD. Other causes include hiatal hernias and other pressures on the stomach, such as pregnancy. A hiatal hernia is the bulging of the upper part of the stomach into the chest through an enlarged opening in the diaphragm (the sheet of muscle separating the bottom of the ribcage from the abdomen).

What Are the Symptoms of GERD?

The most common symptom is heartburn, a burning feeling in the middle of the chest. It sometimes spreads to the throat. An acid taste may occur. Heartburn affects about 10 million adults in the United States daily. Other symptoms include chronic cough, hoarseness, upset stomach, stomach bloating, and wheezing. More serious symptoms are bleeding, weight loss, and difficulty swallowing.

How Is GERD Diagnosed?

The doctor relies on symptoms and the response to treatment for diagnosis. Life-threatening diseases, such as heart disease, that can cause symptoms similar to those of GERD must be ruled out. Specific tests are needed for an unclear diagnosis or more serious symptoms. These tests may include upper GI (gastrointestinal) x-ray series, endoscopy (using a scope to look at your esophagus and stomach directly), 24-hour esophageal pH study (measurement of acidity), and esophageal manometry (measures esophageal muscle pressure).

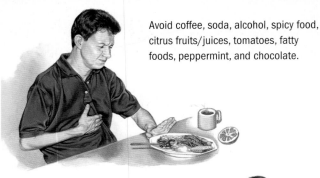

Avoid coffee, soda, alcohol, spicy food, citrus fruits/juices, tomatoes, fatty foods, peppermint, and chocolate.

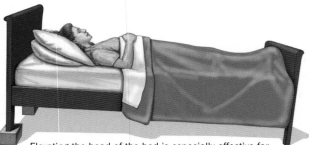

Eating smaller portions, avoiding late meals, and maintaining a healthy weight can help in GERD management.

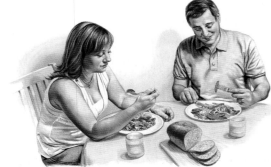

Elevating the head of the bed is especially effective for those with nighttime symptoms of GERD.

Take medication if recommended by your doctor.

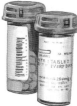

How Is GERD Treated?

First options for mild reflux include eating smaller portions and changing the diet. Certain foods, such as tomatoes and fatty foods, and medicines, such as aspirin, can make symptoms worse. Over-the-counter drugs, including antacids and acid-blocking medicines called H2-blockers, may help. Antacids neutralize stomach acid. H2-blockers (e.g., ranitidine or famotidine) prevent or block production of stomach acid. These drugs can be taken before eating to prevent heartburn. Omeprazole is another over-the-counter drug now available, which blocks the action of stomach cells responsible for making acid. It is generally more effective than antacids and H2-blockers.

People with severe or frequent symptoms may need prescription drugs. The doctor may perform an operation called fundoplication to strengthen the LES.

DOs and DON'Ts in Managing GERD:

✔ **DO** eat a healthy diet, rich in fruits, vegetables, and low-fat dairy products. Lower your intake of saturated and total fats.

✔ **DO** raise the head of your bed 6 to 8 inches.

✔ **DO** maintain a healthy body weight.

✔ **DO** take medicines recommended by your doctor.

🚫 **DON'T** eat reflux-inducing foods, such as citrus fruits and juices, coffee, peppermint, chocolate, and spicy foods.

🚫 **DON'T** eat large meals.

🚫 **DON'T** eat meals late in the day.

🚫 **DON'T** lie down just after eating.

🚫 **DON'T** wear tight-fitting clothing.

🚫 **DON'T** smoke or use tobacco products.

FROM THE DESK OF

NOTES

FOR MORE INFORMATION

Contact the following sources:

• American Gastroenterological Association
Tel: (301) 654-2055
Website: http://www.gastro.org

• American College of Gastroenterology
Tel: (703) 820-7400
Website: http://www.acg.gi.org

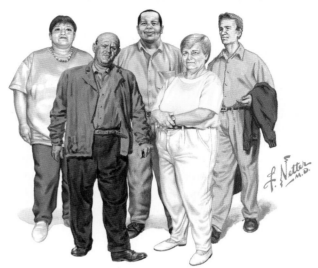

Glossitis is inflammation of the tongue. This common condition affects people of all ages, but more men than women.

The many causes include infections (e.g., syphilis and HIV) and irritants, such as tobacco, alcohol, and hot or spicy foods. Other causes include diet (e.g., lack of iron or B vitamins) and skin diseases (e.g., lichen planus).

Types of glossitis

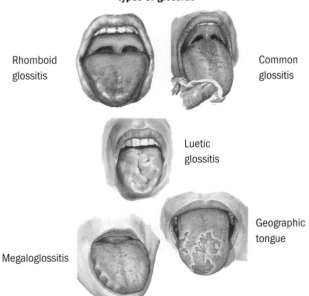

Rhomboid glossitis

Common glossitis

Luetic glossitis

Geographic tongue

Megaloglossitis

The tongue usually changes color, gets swollen, and hurts. White patches or little ulcers may also appear.

What Is Glossitis?

Glossitis is inflammation (redness, swelling) of the tongue. This common condition may come and go quickly or last several weeks. It may appear alone or be part of another illness. It affects people of all ages and seems to occur more often in men than women.

What Causes Glossitis?

The many causes include bacterial and viral infections; trauma or mechanical irritation from hot beverages, teeth, and dental appliances; local irritants, such as tobacco, alcohol, and hot or spicy foods; aphthous ulcers; and allergic reactions to toothpaste, mouthwash, or other substances put in the mouth.

Other causes affecting the whole body include diet (e.g., lack of iron or B vitamins), skin diseases (e.g., lichen planus), and infections (e.g., syphilis and human immunodeficiency virus, or HIV).

What Are the Symptoms of Glossitis?

Symptoms depend on the cause. The tongue usually changes color, gets swollen, and hurts. The color changes from a dark beefy red to fiery red to pale to white, and the tongue looks inflamed or irritated. Pain may be bad enough to make chewing, swallowing, or talking hard to do. Sometimes, the tongue gets white patches or little ulcers. Symptoms usually go away in about 2 weeks, depending on the cause.

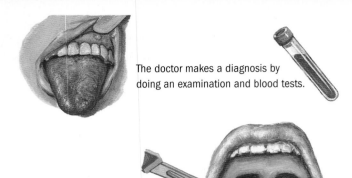

The doctor makes a diagnosis by doing an examination and blood tests.

If glossitis doesn't go away, your doctor may do a biopsy. A very tiny piece of tongue tissue is removed and studied with a microscope.

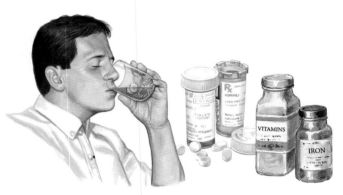

Treatment depends on the cause. The doctor may prescribe medicine, iron, or B vitamins. You may also use mouth rinses to help symptoms.

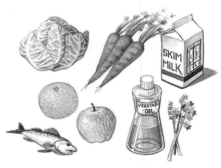
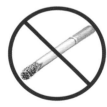
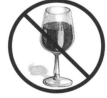

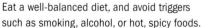

Eat a well-balanced diet, and avoid triggers such as smoking, alcohol, or hot, spicy foods.

How Is Glossitis Diagnosed?

Glossitis is diagnosed by your doctor with a physical examination. Blood tests may be done to help find the cause. The doctor may also test the tongue for infection.

If glossitis doesn't go away, the doctor may do a biopsy. A very tiny piece of tongue tissue is removed and studied with a microscope.

How Is Glossitis Treated?

The treatment depends on the cause. The doctor may prescribe medicine, especially if an infection occurs. People with poor nutrition may need to take vitamins or iron pills. Other pills may help stop the swelling. Sometimes, medicines are placed on the tongue for swelling and pain. Medicated mouth rinses may also give relief.

DOs and DON'Ts in Managing Glossitis:

✔ **DO** eat a well-balanced diet, or follow a bland or liquid diet if your doctor tells you to.

✔ **DO** keep your mouth clean. Brush and floss your teeth and clean your tongue after each meal.

✔ **DO** see your dentist regularly. If you wear dentures, have your dentist check the fit.

✔ **DO** keep heartburn under control, as stomach acid can irritate your esophagus and mouth.

✔ **DO** rinse your mouth if you use inhaled steroids for a lung condition after each time you breathe in the steroids.

✔ **DO** avoid things that you know will trigger your condition. Triggers include hot or spicy foods, alcohol, smoking and tobacco in all forms, tartar-control toothpaste or toothpaste containing peroxide, and mouthwash.

✔ **DO** call your doctor if you have breathing, speaking, chewing, or swallowing problems. These may mean that a swollen tongue is blocking your airways. This emergency needs immediate medical care.

✔ **DO** call your doctor if symptoms of glossitis last for more than 10 days.

⊘ **DON'T** smoke, and avoid all forms of tobacco.

⊘ **DON'T** drink alcohol or use spicy foods..

FROM THE DESK OF

NOTES

FOR MORE INFORMATION

Contact the following source:

• American Dental Association
  Tel: (312) 440-2500
  Website: http://www.ada.org

More than 25 million Americans have halitosis, or foul- or unpleasant-smelling breath.

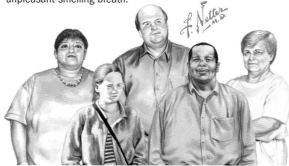

The most common causes are breakdown of food in the mouth by bacteria and other mouth-related problems. Other causes include various medical disorders.

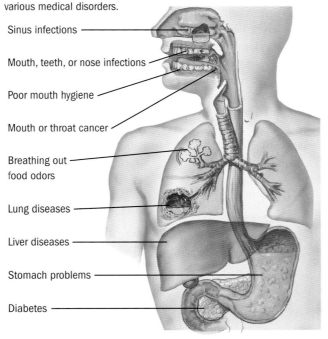

Sinus infections

Mouth, teeth, or nose infections

Poor mouth hygiene

Mouth or throat cancer

Breathing out food odors

Lung diseases

Liver diseases

Stomach problems

Diabetes

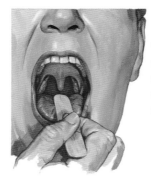

Your doctor makes a diagnosis by taking a medical history, doing an examination (especially of the mouth and nose), and maybe ordering other tests (for a possible medical condition).

What Is Halitosis?

Halitosis is the medical word for bad breath. More than 25 million Americans have foul- or unpleasant-smelling breath.

What Causes Halitosis?

The most common cause is the breakdown of food in the mouth by bacteria that live there. Certain foods may make it worse.

Medical conditions causing bad breath include infected teeth, gums, or oral tissues; cancer of the mouth; the common cold; lung and sinus infections; postnasal drip; infections such as tonsillitis, strep throat, and mononucleosis; untreated nasal polyps; diabetes; and other diseases of the stomach, lungs, liver, and kidneys.

Medicines such as antihistamines may cause halitosis because they dry the mouth. A dry mouth can also occur because of stress or nervous tension. Saliva is the mouth's natural mouthwash. It has antibiotic substances that get rid of mouth bacteria, so less saliva can mean bad breath. Tobacco and alcoholic beverages can also cause halitosis.

What Are the Symptoms of Halitosis?

People usually don't notice their own mouth odor, even after breathing out into their hand or licking the hand to smell the odor. They usually become aware of halitosis only when they see others avoiding them or when someone tells them. Bad breath tends to get worse and occur more often with aging. The odor intensity varies.

How Is Halitosis Diagnosed?

The doctor makes a diagnosis by taking a medical history and doing a physical examination, especially of the mouth and nose. The doctor may also do a sniff test (the doctor smells air that the person breathes out through just the nose and then just the mouth) and a throat culture if a sore throat or mouth sores are present. More tests may be done if other medical conditions may be the cause.

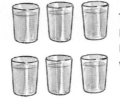

The key to treatment is good oral hygiene. Daily brushing and flossing are essential. Keep your mouth moist by drinking enough water.

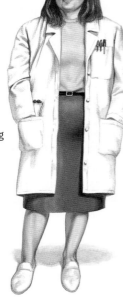

Get treatment for medical diseases that may be causing bad breath. Call your doctor or dentist if bad breath lasts a long time and simple treatments don't work.

Snack on carrots, celery, or other vegetables to help prevent plaque.

Avoiding certain foods and tobacco can help eliminate halitosis. These foods include garlic, onions, cheese, spices, cabbage, horseradish, eggs, broccoli, fish, red meat, peppers, alcohol, and coffee.

How Is Halitosis Treated?

The key to treatment is good oral hygiene. Daily brushing and flossing are essential. Using an over-the-counter mouthwash helps remove food particles and odors. Regular dental checkups are a must to prevent, identify, and treat problems.

Avoiding certain foods and tobacco can also help. These foods include garlic, onions, cheese, spices, orange juice, and soda. If a medical condition is the cause, that condition should be treated.

DOs and DON'Ts in Managing Halitosis:

✔ **DO** brush with baking soda toothpaste, floss between the teeth, and clean the tongue after each meal.

✔ **DO** make sure that your mouth is moist by drinking adequate water. Hold water in the mouth for as long as possible, swishing it hard to remove food particles.

✔ **DO** increase saliva production by chewing sugarless gum or sugarless candy mints.

✔ **DO** snack on carrots, celery, or other vegetables to help prevent plaque.

✔ **DO** use an oral irrigation device to clean the teeth.

✔ **DO** avoid foods and beverages that can cause bad breath, such as garlic, raw onions, cabbage, horseradish, eggs, broccoli, brussels sprouts, fish, red meat, peppers, alcohol, and coffee.

✔ **DO** call your doctor or dentist if bad breath becomes chronic and simple treatments don't work.

⊘ **DON'T** smoke cigarettes or use tobacco.

FROM THE DESK OF

NOTES

FOR MORE INFORMATION

Contact the following source:

• American Dental Association
Tel: (312) 440-2500
Website: http://www.ada.org

MANAGING YOUR
HELICOBACTER PYLORI INFECTION

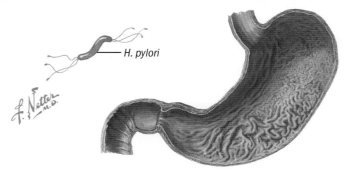

— H. pylori

The type of bacteria called *Helicobacter pylori* (or *H. pylori*) causes a stomach infection. It's the most common cause of gastritis.

What Is a *Helicobacter pylori* Infection?

Gastritis is inflammation (swelling) of the lining of the stomach because of a stomach infection. The bacteria called *Helicobacter pylori* (also called *H. pylori*) causes this infection. It's the most common cause of gastritis worldwide. No way to prevent it is known.

What Causes an *H. pylori* Infection?

How people get this infection is unclear. Possible sources of bacteria may be contaminated water or utensils. *H. pylori* can grow in the stomach lining covered by a layer of mucus that protects it from stomach acid.

What Are the Symptoms of an *H. pylori* Infection?

The main symptom is chronic stomach upset. Pain in the upper abdomen (belly) and cramps may be present and are often made worse by eating. Many people will have less appetite. Bad breath (halitosis) may also be present. A burning acid taste in the mouth, nausea, vomiting, and bleeding may occur.

Many people may have no symptoms, and the infection is found when a stomach biopsy is done during upper endoscopy.

Main symptoms are pain in the upper abdomen and cramps. Eating often makes pain worse. Your doctor makes a diagnosis from a history of these symptoms and breath, stool, and blood tests.

How Is an *H. pylori* Infection Diagnosed?

The doctor makes a diagnosis from a history of stomach upset, pain, and cramps. Sometimes, upper endoscopy (looking at the stomach through a lighted, flexible tube) is done to confirm the diagnosis and rule out other causes. A stomach biopsy (removing a small piece of tissue) may be done to test for bacteria in the stomach and to exclude other stomach diseases.

A breath test (testing with a substance called urea) or stool test may also be used for diagnosis. Blood tests can also measure antibodies to *H. pylori*, but these won't tell whether the infection is new or old because antibodies to the bacteria can last for several years after treatment.

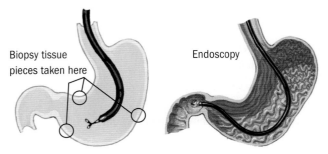

Biopsy tissue pieces taken here

Endoscopy

Your doctor can do upper endoscopy (looking at the stomach through a lighted, flexible tube) to confirm the diagnosis. A stomach biopsy (removing a small piece of tissue) may also be done.

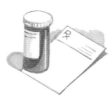

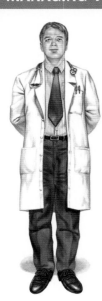

Your doctor may prescribe one of three or four drugs to be taken for several days. These include antibiotics and acid-suppressing medicines.

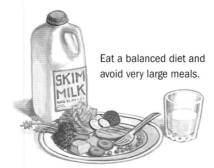

Eat a balanced diet and avoid very large meals.

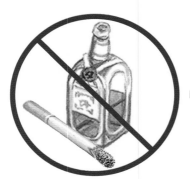

Don't smoke or drink alcohol.

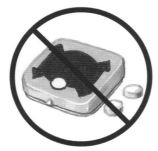

Don't take medicines that can irritate your stomach, such as aspirin and NSAIDs.

How Is an *H. pylori* Infection Treated?

Three or four drugs may be taken for several days. These usually include the following types of medicines: (1) antibiotics (e.g., clarithromycin, amoxicillin, tetracycline, metronidazole, or some combination); (2) acid-suppressing drugs (e.g., omeprazole, lansoprazole, and pantoprazole); and (3) bismuth subsalicylate (Pepto-Bismol™).

Complications, such as stomach ulcers, bleeding, and increased risk of stomach cancer, can occur in people with long-lasting infection left untreated.

DOs and DON'Ts in Managing *H. pylori* Infection:

✔ **DO** eat regularly and in moderation.

✔ **DO** take medicines as directed by your doctor.

✔ **DO** call your doctor if abdominal pain becomes severe or if symptoms don't improve 2 to 3 days after treatment.

✔ **DO** call your doctor if you have side effects from the medicines.

✔ **DO** call your doctor if you vomit blood or you have blood with bowel movements or dark tarry stools.

⊘ **DON'T** smoke.

⊘ **DON'T** drink alcohol.

⊘ **DON'T** take medicines that can irritate your stomach, such as aspirin and nonsteroidal antiinflammatory drugs (NSAIDs).

FROM THE DESK OF

NOTES

FOR MORE INFORMATION

Contact the following sources:

• National Digestive Diseases Information Clearinghouse
Tel: (800) 891-5389
Website: http://www.niddk.nih.gov/health/digest/nddic.htm

• American College of Gastroenterology
Tel: (703) 820-7400
Website: http://www.acg.gi.org

MANAGING YOUR
HEMOCHROMATOSIS

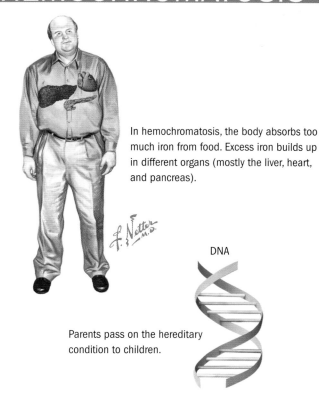

In hemochromatosis, the body absorbs too much iron from food. Excess iron builds up in different organs (mostly the liver, heart, and pancreas).

DNA

Parents pass on the hereditary condition to children.

Common symptoms include:

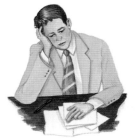 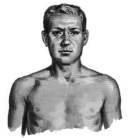 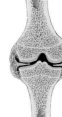

Fatigue   Darkening of the skin   Joint pain

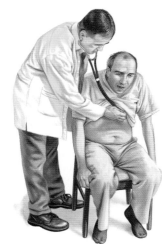 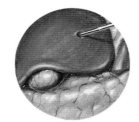

Biopsy

Your doctor makes a diagnosis from your medical history, physical examination, and blood tests. A liver biopsy may be done to confirm it.

What Is Hemochromatosis?

Hemochromatosis is a condition in which the body stores too much iron. The excess iron builds up in different organs (mostly the liver, heart, and pancreas) and damages them. Hemochromatosis is more common in caucasians.

Hemochromatosis is not contagious. It's not curable, but treatment can sometimes reverse symptoms. Men have symptoms more often and at an earlier age than women, because women lose iron during menstrual periods.

What Causes Hemochromatosis?

The most common form in the United States is called primary, or hereditary (passed on from parents to children), hemochromatosis. People who inherit a copy of the gene from both parents (2 or 3 per 1000 people) are at risk.

What Are the Symptoms of Hemochromatosis?

The abnormal gene is present at birth, but symptoms usually don't show up until adulthood. The most common symptoms are fatigue, joint pain, darkening of the skin and other organs, arthritis, weakness, erectile dysfunction in men or loss of interest in sex, and pain in the abdomen (belly).

Diabetes, liver disease, heart disease, thyroid disease, or reproductive system problems can occur.

How Is Hemochromatosis Diagnosed?

The doctor makes a diagnosis from the medical history, physical examination, and additional tests. Blood tests called transferrin saturation and ferritin level that measure the amount of iron in blood are done. Computed tomography (CT) or magnetic resonance imaging (MRI) of the liver may be done.

A biopsy of the liver is usually needed to confirm the diagnosis. In a biopsy, a long hollow needle is put into the liver, a piece of liver tissue is removed for study with a microscope. The iron level in the tissue will also be measured.

Special genetic tests can now check for the gene for hemochromatosis.

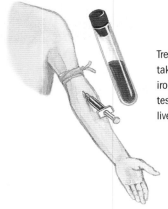

Treatment involves removing iron by taking blood until you have a normal iron level. You'll have regular blood tests to measure iron levels and liver function.

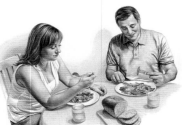 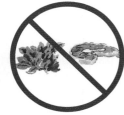

Eat a balanced diet, but avoid foods with a lot of iron.

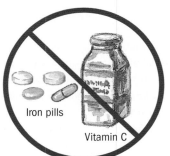

Don't take iron pills or vitamin C. They can increase the harmful effects of iron.

Iron pills

Vitamin C

Don't drink alcohol, because it increases your risk for liver disease.

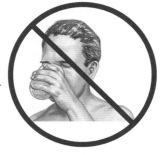

How Is Hemochromatosis Treated?

The best therapy is removal of iron by taking blood (phlebotomy) once or twice weekly until the iron level is at or near normal.

Regular blood tests to measure iron levels and liver function will also be needed.

When phlebotomy is not possible or is insufficient and the disease is advanced, a medication called deferoxamine may also be given. It is known as an iron chelating agent and helps to remove iron from the body.

DOs and DON'Ts in Managing Hemochromatosis:

✔ **DO** eat a balanced diet, but avoid red meat and eat more fruits and vegetables.

✔ **DO** restrict exercise if you have heart disease caused by hemochromatosis. Otherwise exercise as tolerated.

✔ **DO** ask other family members to be tested for hereditary hemochromatosis. If diagnosed, they should begin treatment before heart or liver disease develops.

✔ **DO** call your doctor if you have fever, chest pain, shortness of breath, or abdominal pain.

⊘ **DON'T** take iron pills or vitamin C. They can increase the harmful effects of iron.

⊘ **DON'T** drink alcohol. It increases your risk for liver disease.

FROM THE DESK OF

NOTES

FOR MORE INFORMATION

Contact the following sources:

• National Heart, Lung, and Blood Institute
Tel: (301) 592-8573
Website: http://www.nhlbi.nih.gov

• American College of Gastroenterology
Tel: (703) 820-7400
Website: http://www.acg.gi.org

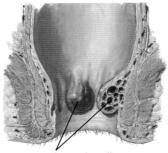

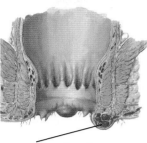

Internal swollen
blood vessels

External swollen
blood vessels

Hemorrhoids, which are inflamed blood vessels, can be inside the anus
(internal) or under the skin around it (external).

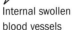

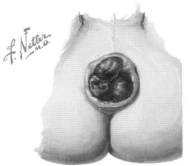

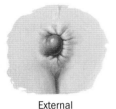

External

Internal

Hemorrhoids are very common. Increased pressure and straining to move
the bowels, as well as other conditions, can cause them.

Symptoms include pain during bowel
movements and blood covering stools,
on toilet paper, or in the toilet.

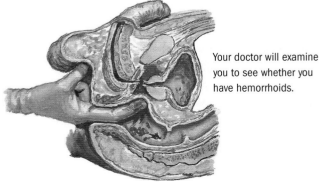

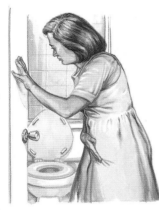

Your doctor will examine
you to see whether you
have hemorrhoids.

What Are Hemorrhoids?

Hemorrhoids (also called piles) are inflamed, swollen blood vessels located in and around the anus and lower rectum. These vessels can stretch under pressure, like varicose veins in the legs. Hemorrhoids are either inside the anus (internal) or under the skin around the anus (external). About 50% of the adult population of the United States, both men and women, have hemorrhoids.

Hemorrhoids aren't usually dangerous or life-threatening. They aren't contagious.

What Causes Hemorrhoids?

Causes include increased pressure and swelling from straining to move the bowel and conditions such as pregnancy and chronic constipation or diarrhea. Heredity and aging are other factors.

What Are the Symptoms of Hemorrhoids?

Many people have hemorrhoids but not all have symptoms. Pain or tenderness can occur during bowel movements. The most common symptom of internal hemorrhoids is bright red blood covering stools (bowel movements), on toilet paper, or in the toilet. Internal hemorrhoids may poke through to outside the body and become irritated and painful. These are protruding hemorrhoids. Symptoms of external hemorrhoids include painful swelling or hard lump near the anus. Straining, rubbing, or cleaning around the anus may cause irritation with bleeding and itching. Draining mucus may cause itching.

How Are Hemorrhoids Diagnosed?

The doctor may suspect hemorrhoids from the symptoms and will make a diagnosis by doing a physical examination. Hemorrhoids can be painless, and the doctor may find them on routine physical examinations.

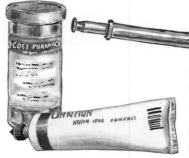

Creams, suppositories, and stool softeners are used for treatment. For serious cases, surgery can remove or reduce hemorrhoid size. Another method is sclerotherapy (injection of a chemical) to shrink hemorrhoids.

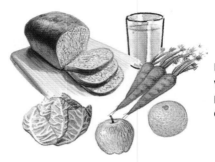

Eat more grains, fruits, and vegetables, and drink plenty of fluids, especially water.

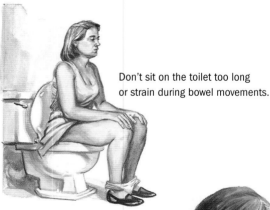

Don't sit on the toilet too long or strain during bowel movements.

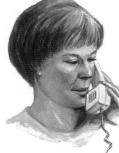

Call your doctor if you see blood in your stool or on toilet paper. You should also call your doctor if you have anal pain, burning, or itching.

FROM THE DESK OF

NOTES

How Are Hemorrhoids Treated?

Soft bowel movements are important for preventing and treating hemorrhoids. Eating a high-fiber diet and drinking plenty of fluids are important. Measures to reduce symptoms include warm tub or sitz baths several times a day. Ice packs can help reduce swelling. Cream or suppositories can be applied to the affected area. If hemorrhoids are very inflamed, the doctor may prescribe cortisone cream. Daily use of stool softeners such as docusate during flare-ups helps. Most people get better in about 2 weeks if they follow the doctor's suggestions.

Some hemorrhoids are treated surgically to remove or reduce the size of hemorrhoids. These methods include rubber band ligation, sclerotherapy, electric or laser heat (laser coagulation) or infrared light (infrared photocoagulation), and hemorrhoidectomy. For ligation, a rubber band around the bottom of the hemorrhoid cuts off circulation, and the hemorrhoid goes away. Sclerotherapy uses a chemical to shrink hemorrhoids. For heat and light methods, special tools are used to burn hemorrhoids. Hemorrhoidectomy is surgery to remove hemorrhoids permanently.

DOs and DON'Ts in Managing Hemorrhoids:

✔ **DO** eat more grains, fruits, and vegetables.
✔ **DO** drink more liquid, especially water.
✔ **DO** remember that many problems in your rectal area have similar symptoms and are incorrectly said to be hemorrhoids. Call your doctor for an examination.
✔ **DO** avoid anything that will cause constipation.
✔ **DO** remember that straining can make hemorrhoids worse.
✔ **DO** call your doctor if you see blood on your stool or toilet paper or in the toilet.
✔ **DO** call your doctor if you have anal pain, burning, or itching or if you have fever or drainage after surgery.

⊘ **DON'T** strain during bowel movements.

FOR MORE INFORMATION

Contact the following sources:

• American Gastroenterological Association
Tel: (301) 654-2055
Website: http://www.gastro.org

• National Digestive Diseases Information Clearinghouse
Tel: (800) 891-5389
Website: http://www.niddk.nih.gov/health/digest/nddic.htm

• American College of Surgeons
Tel: (312) 202-5000, (800) 621-4111
Website: http://www.facs.org

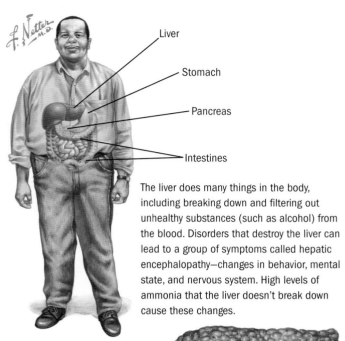

The liver does many things in the body, including breaking down and filtering out unhealthy substances (such as alcohol) from the blood. Disorders that destroy the liver can lead to a group of symptoms called hepatic encephalopathy—changes in behavior, mental state, and nervous system. High levels of ammonia that the liver doesn't break down cause these changes.

Cirrhosis is long-term scarring of the liver, so the liver stops working well. More than 50% of people with cirrhosis have hepatic encephalopathy.

Liver with cirrhosis

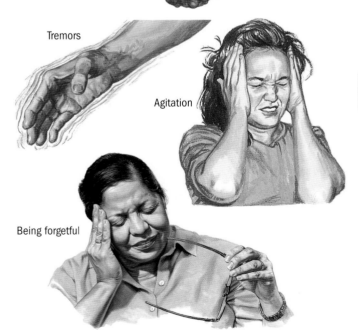

Tremors

Agitation

Being forgetful

Symptoms include being disoriented, forgetful, and confused. Jaundice, problems speaking, tremors, being agitated, and uncoordinated movements are others, as are sleepiness, mood changes, memory loss, being less responsive, and coma.

What Is Hepatic Encephalopathy?

Hepatic encephalopathy refers to changes in behavior, mental state, and nervous system in people with liver failure. It's not a disease but a group of symptoms seen in people whose livers don't work well. High levels of ammonia in the bloodstream and brain are thought to cause these changes. Bacteria in the stomach and intestines make ammonia. Usually, the liver makes ammonia harmless. However, people with liver disease have more ammonia because their liver doesn't work. Ammonia enters the blood, gets to the brain, hurts the brain, and causes symptoms.

This encephalopathy occurs in more than 50% of all people with liver cirrhosis. Untreated, it can lead to coma and death. It's not contagious and cannot be passed from parents to children.

What Causes Hepatic Encephalopathy?

Disorders that destroy the liver and cause liver failure can lead to hepatic encephalopathy. Some of these disorders are viral hepatitis (such as hepatitis B and hepatitis C), severe infections, autoimmune diseases, cancer, and Reye's syndrome. Medicines such as nonsteroidal antiinflammatory drugs and toxins such as alcohol are other causes. People with cirrhosis can get encephalopathy from using sedatives and analgesics. Gastrointestinal bleeding can also increase the risk of hepatic encephalopathy.

What Are the Symptoms of Hepatic Encephalopathy?

Symptoms include being disoriented, forgetful, and confused. People feel sleepy and have mood changes, lethargy, and memory loss. Coma can occur. Others include jaundice, problems speaking, tremors, being agitated, and uncoordinated movements. People usually have signs of liver disease such as jaundice, enlarged breasts and small testicles (men), fluid in the abdomen (belly), and swelling in the legs.

Hepatic encephalopathy is divided into grades 1 to 4. Grade 1 involves mild confusion, poor attention, being irritable, and decreased ability to do mental tasks. In grade 2, people have lethargy, drowsiness, personality changes, and great trouble doing mental tasks. In grade 3, people are sleepy (but can be aroused), cannot do mental tasks, and are disoriented (place and time). In grade 4, coma occurs.

Symptoms are similar to those of many other disorders, so a physical exam, blood tests, and x-rays may be needed to rule out other causes.

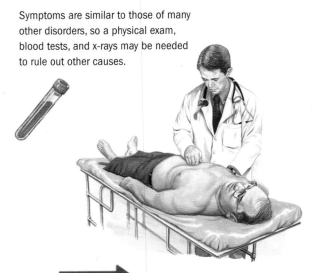

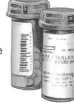

The treatment goals are to find and treat the causes, such as drugs and metabolic problems. Almost all people need hospitalization.

Antibiotics such as neomycin are used to kill bacteria in the intestine. A drug called lactulose acts as a laxative and helps empty the bowel. These treatments lead to lower ammonia levels in the body.

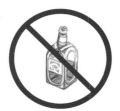

Don't drink alcohol, especially if you already have cirrhosis.

How Is Hepatic Encephalopathy Diagnosed?

The doctor will do a complete physical examination. The doctor may order blood tests and x-rays to rule out other problems, because hepatic encephalopathy mimics symptoms of other disorders. These disorders include alcohol withdrawal, sedative overdose, meningitis, low blood sugar, brain cancer, and blood clots in the brain.

How Is Hepatic Encephalopathy Treated?

Treatment goals are to find and treat causes, such as drugs, GI bleeding, and metabolic problems. Almost all people need hospitalization. Gastrointestinal bleeding must be stopped and other causes must be eliminated. A drug called lactulose acts as a laxative and helps empty the intestines, so bacteria cannot make ammonia. Sometimes, an antibiotic called neomycin is used. This drug kills bacteria in the intestine so that there is less ammonia.

DOs and DON'Ts in Managing Hepatic Encephalopathy:

✔ **DO** remember that this encephalopathy may be reversible. However, the chance of death is high if coma occurs.

✔ **DO** call your doctor if a family member with liver disease has behavior, personality, or mental changes.

⊘ **DON'T** drink alcohol, especially if you have cirrhosis.

⊘ **DON'T** forget that common over-the-counter and prescription sleeping drugs can cause the disorder in people with liver disease.

FROM THE DESK OF

NOTES

FOR MORE INFORMATION

Contact the following sources:

• American Gastroenterological Association
Tel: (301) 654-2055
Website: http://www.gastro.org

• National Digestive Diseases Information Clearinghouse
Tel: (800) 891-5389
Website: http://www.niddk.nih.gov/health/digest/nddic.htm

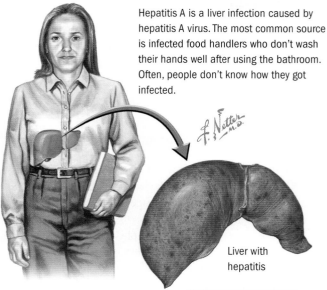

Hepatitis A is a liver infection caused by hepatitis A virus. The most common source is infected food handlers who don't wash their hands well after using the bathroom. Often, people don't know how they got infected.

Liver with hepatitis

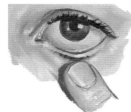

The main symptom is jaundice (yellow skin and whites of the eyes).

Others symptoms

Pale or clay-colored stools, dark urine

Abdominal pain

Flu-like symptoms

Itching

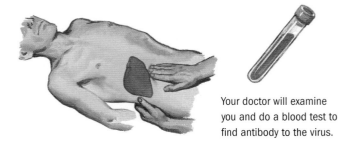

Your doctor will examine you and do a blood test to find antibody to the virus.

What Is Hepatitis A?

Hepatitis A is infection of the liver with the hepatitis A virus. About 150,000 people are infected every year in the United States. Most people recover in 2 to 6 months without serious health problems.

People with hepatitis A very rarely develop liver failure.

What Causes Hepatitis A?

The cause is the hepatitis A virus. Food (such as shellfish from polluted water) or water contaminated with infected stools (bowel movements) can spread the virus. The most common source of spread is infected food handlers who don't wash their hands well after using the bathroom. Direct contact with infected people will pass the infection to others. Outbreaks occur most often in day care centers, military bases, and institutions for disabled. In more than 40% of cases, it isn't known how people get infected.

What Are the Symptoms of Hepatitis A?

Not all people have symptoms. Symptoms may occur, usually during the first month following infection. The main symptom is jaundice (yellow skin and whites of the eyes), plus pale or clay-colored stools, dark urine, and itching all over the body. Flu-like symptoms of fatigue, loss of appetite, nausea and vomiting, low-grade fever, and pain in the abdomen (belly) in the liver area may occur before jaundice.

How Is Hepatitis A Diagnosed?

The doctor will do a physical examination and a blood test to show antibody to the virus. The antibody is a substance made by the immune, or infection-fighting, system. Liver function tests will also be much higher than normal.

No specific treatment exists. Most people can be cared for at home. Proper rest for several days after diagnosis is important. Eat a well-balanced, high-protein diet.

How Is Hepatitis A Treated?

No specific treatment exists. Most people can be cared for at home. Proper rest for several days after diagnosis is important. During this time, intimate contact with other people should be avoided. The diet should be balanced and include high-calorie foods. People who come in close contact with the infected person and who have not been previously vaccinated should be given immune serum globulin within 2 weeks of exposure by their physician.

DOs and DON'Ts in Managing Hepatitis A:

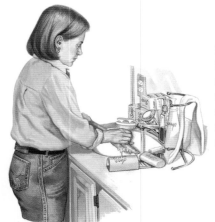

Make sure you wash your hands if you have hepatitis or care for someone who does, if you're a restaurant worker, or if you work in a day care center and change diapers.

✔ **DO** get plenty of rest and eat a well-balanced diet.

✔ **DO** make sure to wash your hands if you have hepatitis or care for someone who does, especially if you contact fecal material.

✔ **DO** use separate or disposable eating and drinking utensils.

✔ **DO** wash your hands properly after changing a diaper and before doing anything else if you work in a day care center. Restaurant workers should always wash their hands properly.

✔ **DO** use proper protection, such as gloves and eyeglasses, if you're exposed to fecal material and other body fluids on the job.

✔ **DO** call your doctor if you were exposed to someone with hepatitis A or you have symptoms of the disease.

✔ **DO** call your doctor if your hepatitis symptoms don't go away within 4 weeks.

⊘ **DON'T** drink alcohol. Avoid substances that may hurt the liver.

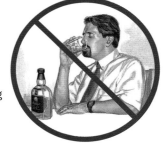

Don't drink alcohol or anything that may harm the liver.

FROM THE DESK OF

NOTES

FOR MORE INFORMATION

Contact the following sources:

• Hepatitis Foundation International
Tel: (800) 891-0707
Website: http://www.hepfi.org/

• American Gastroenterological Association
Tel: (301) 654-2055
Website: http://www.gastro.org

• National Digestive Diseases Information Clearinghouse
Tel: (800) 891-5389
Website: http://www.niddk.nih.gov/health/digest/nddic.htm

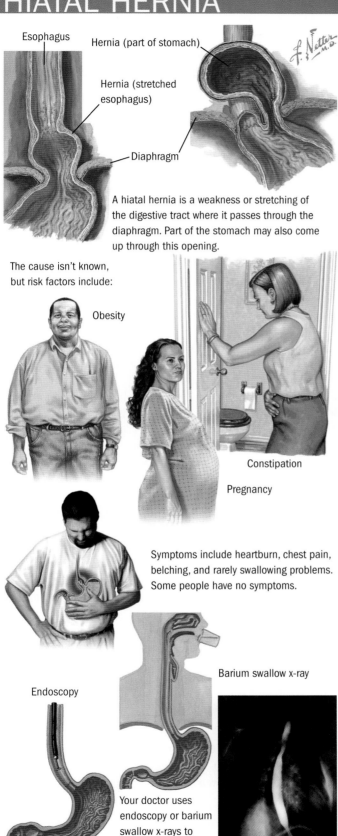

Esophagus   Hernia (part of stomach)

Hernia (stretched esophagus)

Diaphragm

A hiatal hernia is a weakness or stretching of the digestive tract where it passes through the diaphragm. Part of the stomach may also come up through this opening.

The cause isn't known, but risk factors include:

Obesity

Constipation

Pregnancy

Symptoms include heartburn, chest pain, belching, and rarely swallowing problems. Some people have no symptoms.

Barium swallow x-ray

Endoscopy

Your doctor uses endoscopy or barium swallow x-rays to detect a hiatal hernia.

What Are Hiatal Hernias?

A hiatal hernia is a weakness or stretching of the digestive tract where it passes through the diaphragm. The diaphragm is the muscle separating the chest from the abdomen (belly). Because of this stretching, acid from the stomach may flow back into the esophagus (the tube that connects the mouth and stomach). This acid causes irritation. Part of the stomach may also come up through the opening into the lower chest. Hiatal hernias can affect people of all ages, but they are more common in people older than 50.

What Causes Hiatal Hernias?

The cause is unknown, but many factors increase the chance of getting hiatal hernias. These factors may include obesity, pregnancy, straining or lifting with tightened abdominal muscles, coughing, abdominal trauma, and long-lasting constipation or straining with bowel movements.

What Are the Symptoms of Hiatal Hernias?

People often have no symptoms, but when they do occur, they are usually about an hour after meals. They include heartburn, chest pain, belching, and rarely swallowing problems. Bending over or lying down can make heartburn worse. A complication is bleeding, caused by irritation of the esophagus.

How Are Hiatal Hernias Diagnosed?

The doctor uses endoscopy or barium swallow x-rays to diagnose hiatal hernias. In endoscopy, a small lighted tube with a tiny camera on the end is passed into the esophagus to see the hernia. Pressure measurements (manometry) may be done to prove that there is lower pressure where the esophagus and stomach meet.

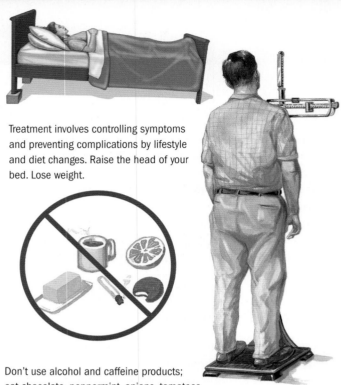

Treatment involves controlling symptoms and preventing complications by lifestyle and diet changes. Raise the head of your bed. Lose weight.

Don't use alcohol and caffeine products; eat chocolate, peppermint, onions, tomatoes, spicy, or fatty foods; or drink citrus juices, which make symptoms worse. Eat small meals instead of large ones. Don't smoke.

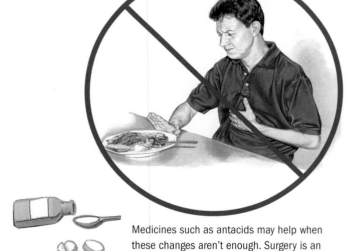

Medicines such as antacids may help when these changes aren't enough. Surgery is an option for serious cases.

How Are Hiatal Hernias Treated?

The goals of treatment are to control symptoms and prevent complications. The main approach is changing lifestyle and diet. Raising the head of the bed 4 to 6 inches (with wooden blocks or bricks, not pillows) will keep stomach acid from backing up and reaching the esophagus during sleep. Avoid foods and drinks that make symptoms worse.

Medicines can be used when these changes aren't enough. Antacids neutralize stomach acid, and drugs to reduce stomach acid include ranitidine, famotidine, and proton pump inhibitors such as omeprazole.

If symptoms cannot be controlled or complications such as scarring, ulceration, or bleeding occur, surgery may be needed to correct the hernia.

DOs and DON'Ts in Managing Hiatal Hernias:

✔ **DO** lose weight if you're overweight.

✔ **DO** eat slowly. Eat four or five small daily meals instead of one or two large meals.

✔ **DO** call your doctor if you feel that food stops beneath the breastbone.

✔ **DO** call your doctor if you have pain with shortness of breath, sweating, or nausea.

✔ **DO** call your doctor if you vomit blood or vomit often.

✔ **DO** call your doctor if symptoms don't improve after 1 month of treatment.

⊘ **DON'T** drink alcohol and caffeine products (coffee, tea, cocoa, cola).

⊘ **DON'T** eat fried, spicy, and fatty foods; citrus juices; peppermint; and spices that may irritate the hernia.

⊘ **DON'T** eat large meals.

⊘ **DON'T** eat anything for at least 2 hours before bedtime.

⊘ **DON'T** bend over or lie down right after eating.

⊘ **DON'T** smoke.

⊘ **DON'T** wear tight-fitting pants, belts, and undergarments.

FROM THE DESK OF

NOTES

FOR MORE INFORMATION

Contact the following source:

• American College of Gastroenterology
Tel: (703) 820-7400
Website: http://www.acg.gi.org

MANAGING YOUR
HOOKWORM INFECTION

Hookworms are parasitic worms that affect more than 1 billion people worldwide.

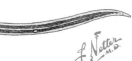

Infections are common in tropical and subtropical areas with poor sanitation. People can get infected by eating or drinking contaminated food or water. Often, worms get into people through the skin as shown here:

1. Eggs pass from infected people in the stool and get into soil.

2. Immature worms (larvae) develop in eggs.

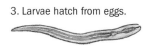

3. Larvae hatch from eggs.

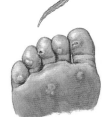

4. Larvae enter through skin (foot).

Symptoms include itching and redness of the skin where larvae entered the body (often the feet).

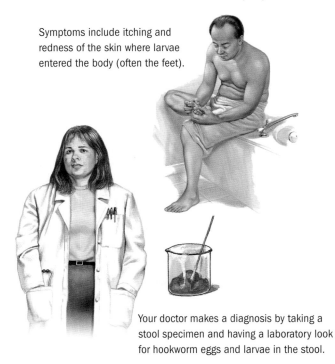

Your doctor makes a diagnosis by taking a stool specimen and having a laboratory look for hookworm eggs and larvae in the stool.

What Are Hookworm Infections?

Hookworms, also known as roundworms, are parasitic worms. They cause common infections in tropical and subtropical areas with poor sanitation. Hookworms affect more than 1 billion people worldwide. In the United States, hookworm infections are more common in southern states. Hookworms can cause serious problems, such as anemia and protein deficiency, for newborns, children, pregnant women, and malnourished people. Skin, lungs, and intestines are involved. Other complications include tiredness, breathing problems, enlarged heart, and irregular heartbeat.

What Causes Hookworm Infections?

Two kinds of roundworms infect people. Their names are *Ancylostoma duodenale* and *Necator americanus*. Infected people pass worm eggs in their stools (bowel movements). The eggs can hatch in moist soil and incubate for 2 days before they become larvae (young, immature forms). Then, larvae can get inside people through their skin (often bare feet) and travel through the bloodstream to the lungs and intestines. People can also get hookworms by eating contaminated food and drinking contaminated water.

What Are the Symptoms of Hookworm Infection?

Symptoms include itching and redness of the skin where larvae entered the body (commonly the feet). A skin infection caused by scratching may also be present.

When larvae travel through the lungs, a dry cough, bloody sputum, wheezing, and low-grade fever may occur. After 2 weeks, larvae make their way to the upper small intestine (bowel) where the adult worms attach to the intestinal lining and suck blood. At this point, loss of appetite, diarrhea, abdominal pain, and anemia can occur. Or people may have no symptoms.

How Are Hookworm Infections Diagnosed?

The doctor makes a diagnosis by taking a stool specimen and sending it to a laboratory to look for hookworm eggs and larvae in the stool. A chest x-ray may be done to look for infection in the lungs. Blood tests may also be done to check for low blood (anemia) and malnutrition.

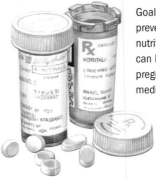

Goals of treatment are to cure the infection, prevent and treat complications, and improve nutrition. Medicines can kill the worms but can hurt a fetus, so tell your doctor if you're pregnant. Don't skip doses or stop your medicine before you finish taking all of it.

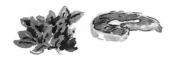

Many people develop anemia, so increased intake of iron through diet and supplements may be needed for up to 3 months.

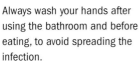

Always wash your hands after using the bathroom and before eating, to avoid spreading the infection.

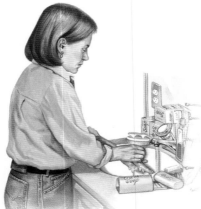

When walking in public areas, always wear shoes to reduce the chance of hookworms entering through the skin on your feet.

How Are Hookworm Infections Treated?

Treatment goals are to cure the infection, prevent and treat complications, and improve nutrition. The doctor will prescribe medicine, such as albendazole or mebendazole, to kill the worms. These drugs cannot be taken during pregnancy because they may harm the fetus.

If anemia is present, the doctor will prescribe iron pills. After anemia is corrected, a high-protein diet and vitamin supplements may be needed for about 3 months.

DOs and DON'Ts in Managing Hookworm Infections:

✔ **DO** take medicines as prescribed.
✔ **DO** eat a high-protein diet for 3 months.
✔ **DO** take vitamin supplements and iron as directed by your doctor.
✔ **DO** tell your doctor if you're pregnant.
✔ **DO** wash your hands well after using the bathroom and before eating.
✔ **DO** call your doctor if skin at the point of worm entry appears infected, red, swollen, and warm.
✔ **DO** call your doctor if you get a fever, chest pain, or shortness of breath.
✔ **DO** call your doctor if you cannot keep foods or fluids down.

🚫 **DON'T** skip doses or stop your medicine before you finish taking all of it.
🚫 **DON'T** walk barefoot in public areas, especially when visiting tropical regions.

FOR MORE INFORMATION

Contact the following sources:
- National Institute of Allergy and Infectious Diseases
  Tel: (866) 284-4107
  Website: http://www3.niaid.nih.gov/topics/hookworm/
- American College of Gastroenterology
  Tel: (703) 820-7400
  Website: http://www.acg.gi.org
- Centers for Disease Control and Prevention
  Tel: (800) 311-3435
  Website: http://www.cdc.gov

FROM THE DESK OF

NOTES

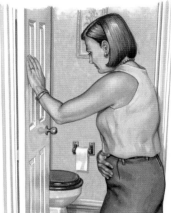

In IBS, colon contractions are abnormal and can cause abdominal pain and discomfort, diarrhea, or constipation at different times.

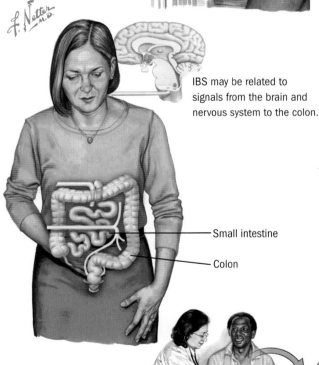

IBS may be related to signals from the brain and nervous system to the colon.

Small intestine

Colon

Your doctor may want to do blood and imaging tests to rule out other diseases.

What Is Irritable Bowel Syndrome (IBS)?

IBS is a common digestive disorder that affects about 20% of people in the United States, mostly women. It affects how the large intestine (colon) works.

Food moving through the digestive tract passes from the small intestine to the colon. The main function of the colon is to absorb water. Muscles in the colon usually contract in a way that pushes stool (waste products) through. In IBS, these muscle contractions may be abnormal. Too many contractions may cause diarrhea. Slowed or fewer contractions may cause constipation. Irregular or intermittent (spasmodic) muscle contractions may cause pain or a feeling of urgent need to move the bowels (go to the bathroom).

What Causes IBS?

The cause is unknown but appears to be related to the nervous system. People with IBS have a colon that reacts very strongly to signals from the brain. Many people find that stress, anxiety, and emotional upset trigger symptoms. Certain foods or eating too much or too little may also cause the colon to overreact.

What Are the Symptoms of IBS?

The most common symptoms are pain in the abdomen (belly), bloating, and constipation or diarrhea or both. Other symptoms include an urgent need to move the bowels and feeling of incomplete evacuation. These symptoms come and go over days, weeks, or months.

How Is IBS Diagnosed?

Not everyone who has gastrointestinal symptoms has IBS. The doctor diagnoses IBS by taking a careful medical history to detail the symptoms. No test can prove that someone has IBS. The doctor may use blood tests, x-rays, and looking at the colon through a thin, flexible tube (special instrument called an endoscope) to rule out other disorders.

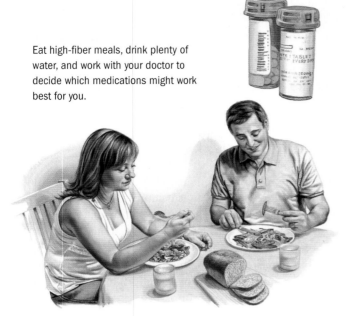

Eat high-fiber meals, drink plenty of water, and work with your doctor to decide which medications might work best for you.

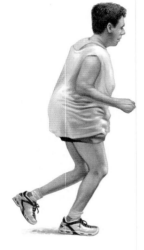

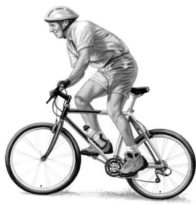

Getting regular exercise and reducing stress can also help relieve symptoms of IBS.

How Is IBS Treated?

Lifestyle changes may help relieve IBS symptoms. These changes include eating a high-fiber diet, avoiding foods that make symptoms worse, eating regular meals that are not too big, drinking enough water, getting regular exercise, and reducing stress.

Several medicines are available for IBS. The doctor can help decide which are best. Over-the-counter laxatives should be taken only under a doctor's direction, because overuse of laxatives may be harmful. Tranquilizers and antidepressants may also help people with IBS.

DOs and DON'Ts in Managing IBS:

✔ **DO** learn what foods worsen your symptoms and avoid them.
✔ **DO** eat a good diet with high-fiber foods, including whole grains, fruits, and vegetables. Fiber supplements may help if your diet does not have enough fiber.
✔ **DO** eat regular, balanced meals.
✔ **DO** drink plenty of water to help the colon work correctly.
✔ **DO** take medicines as instructed by your doctor.
✔ **DO** exercise. Try to do 30 minutes of moderate physical activity daily.
✔ **DO** try to lower stress. Don't take on more work or obligations than you can handle.

🚫 **DON'T** take over-the-counter laxatives without a doctor telling you to do so.
🚫 **DON'T** skip meals, and don't eat extra-large meals.

FROM THE DESK OF

NOTES

FOR MORE INFORMATION

Contact the following sources:

• American Academy of Family Physicians
  Tel: (913) 906-6000
  Website: http://www.aafp.org

• American Gastroenterological Association
  Tel: (301) 654-2055
  Website: http://www.gastro.org

• American College of Gastroenterologists
  Tel: (703) 820-7400
  Website: http://www.acg.gi.org

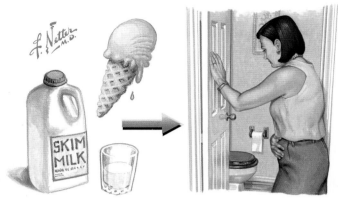

Lactose intolerance is common and means that your body has trouble digesting milk and other dairy products. Symptoms start 30 minutes to 2 hours after eating dairy foods and include stomach pain and cramps, bloating, nausea, diarrhea, gas, feeling sick, and rumbling sounds in the abdomen.

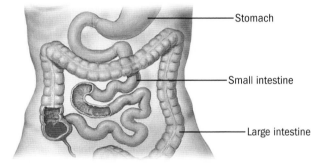

Stomach

Small intestine

Large intestine

Cells in the small intestine produces lactase, an enzyme that breaks down the sugar, lactose, that is found in milk products. If the cells are damaged by injury or disease, lactase production is low and a person becomes "lactose intolerant" because this sugar remains undigested.

Almost half of all babies with persistent diarrhea have it. It's more common in African Americans, Asians, and Mexican Americans.

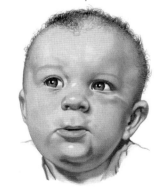

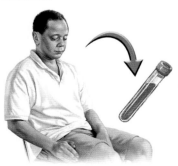

Your doctor will take your medical history and examine you. Tests are done to measure absorption of lactose in the digestive tract and to exclude other causes of your symptoms.

What Is Lactose Intolerance?

Lactose is a sugar in dairy products such as cheese and milk. Lactase, an enzyme in the intestines, digests lactose. Without enough lactase, lactose intolerance can occur.

Lactose intolerance is common. It affects almost 50 million Americans. Almost half of all babies with persistent diarrhea have it. Anyone can have it, but it's more common in African Americans, Asians, and Mexican Americans.

What Causes Lactose Intolerance?

Cells that make lactase enzyme can be damaged by injury or diseases, and then don't make enough lactase. Rarely, children are born with a lactase enzyme deficiency and cannot make lactase.

What Are the Symptoms of Lactose Intolerance?

Most symptoms occur within 30 minutes to 2 hours after eating milk products. They include stomach pain and cramps, bloating, nausea, diarrhea, gas, feeling sick, and rumbling sounds in the abdomen (belly). Children have slightly different symptoms: foamy diarrhea, diaper rash, slowed growth and development, and sometimes vomiting.

How Is Lactose Intolerance Diagnosed?

The doctor will take a medical history and do a physical examination. Tests are done to measure absorption of lactose in the digestive tract. These tests are the lactose tolerance test, hydrogen lactose breath test (most accurate test), and stool acidity test (for children). Rarely, a small tissue sample (biopsy) may need to be taken from the intestine for study when the diagnosis is unclear.

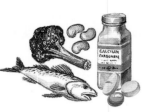

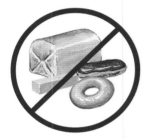

Babies and young children should not have foods containing lactose. Older children and adults usually can have some lactose but should figure out how much they can have. Get enough calcium and vitamin D from diet or supplements. Instead of calcium pills, you can eat more foods such as broccoli, greens, and fish with soft bones (salmon, sardines).

Don't eat foods that may contain hidden lactose. These foods include bread and baked goods, processed breakfast cereals, instant potatoes, soups, breakfast drinks, margarine, lunch meats, salad dressings, candies, and mixes for pancakes, biscuits, and cookies.

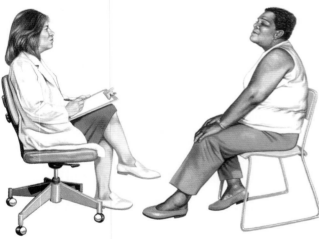

Talk to your doctor about over-the-counter lactase enzymes (drops or chewable). Drops can be put into milk. Chewable tablets help people digest solid foods with lactose.

How Is Lactose Intolerance Treated?

Babies and young children shouldn't have foods containing lactose. Older children and adults usually don't have to avoid lactose completely but should figure out the amount that they can have, based on symptoms after ingestion of lactose. Calcium and vitamin D pills may be needed to replace what would normally be obtained from milk. Calcium is very important for children, teenagers, and pregnant, breastfeeding, and postmenopausal women. Instead of calcium pills, eating more calcium-rich foods, such as shrimp, broccoli, and leafy green vegetables, is possible. Over-the-counter lactase enzymes (drops or chewable) are available. Drops can be put into milk. Chewable tablets help people digest solid foods.

Symptoms take about 3 weeks to go away once eating dairy products stops.

DOs and DON'Ts in Managing Lactose Intolerance:

✔ **DO** get enough calcium and vitamin D, from diet or supplements. Read food labels to see whether food contains lactose or has too much vitamin D and calcium. High-calcium foods include broccoli, kale, greens, oysters, and fish with soft bones (salmon, sardines).

✔ **DO** tell your doctor about all your medicines. Some contain lactose.

✔ **DO** consider breastfeeding your baby if you have a family history of lactose intolerance.

✔ **DO** give babies soy-based formula, not milk.

✔ **DO** call your doctor if a milk-free diet doesn't help symptoms.

✔ **DO** call your doctor if your child doesn't gain weight or refuses food or formula.

⊘ **DON'T** eat foods that may contain hidden lactose. These foods include bread and baked goods, processed breakfast cereals, instant potatoes, soups, breakfast drinks, margarine, lunch meats, salad dressings, candies, and mixes for pancakes, biscuits, and cookies.

⊘ **DON'T** take medicines that contain lactose as a base.

FOR MORE INFORMATION

Contact the following sources:

• American College of Gastroenterology
Tel: (703) 820-7400
Website: http://www.acg.gi.org

• National Digestive Diseases Information Clearinghouse
Tel: (800) 891-5389
Website: http://www.niddk.nih.gov/health/digest/nddic.htm

FROM THE DESK OF

NOTES

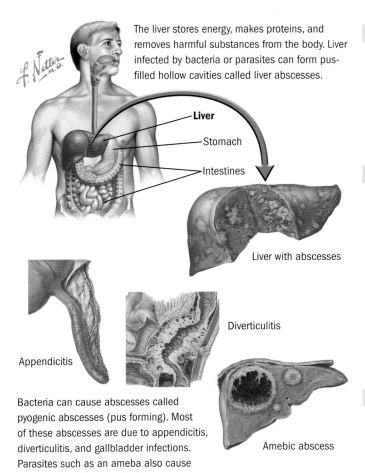

The liver stores energy, makes proteins, and removes harmful substances from the body. Liver infected by bacteria or parasites can form pus-filled hollow cavities called liver abscesses.

Liver

Stomach

Intestines

Liver with abscesses

Diverticulitis

Appendicitis

Bacteria can cause abscesses called pyogenic abscesses (pus forming). Most of these abscesses are due to appendicitis, diverticulitis, and gallbladder infections. Parasites such as an ameba also cause abscesses (called amebic abscesses).

Amebic abscess

What Are Liver Abscesses?

The liver is an important organ with many functions: it stores energy, makes proteins, and removes harmful substances from the body. When infected by bacteria or parasites, the liver can form small holes that fill with pus. Any pus-filled hollow pockets or cavities in the liver are called liver abscesses.

What Causes Liver Abscesses?

Bacteria can cause abscesses that are called pyogenic abscesses (meaning forming pus). Infections spread from appendicitis, diverticulitis, and gallbladder cause most pyogenic abscesses. Parasites such as the ameba *Entamoeba histolytica* also cause abscesses (called amebic abscesses). Most of these occur because of poor sanitation. People get these parasites by eating food contaminated by stools (bowel movements) of infected people. Drinking and eating contaminated water and food can also transfer parasites to people. Worldwide, amebic abscesses are more common than pyogenic abscesses.

What Are the Symptoms of Liver Abscesses?

Symptoms may not appear right away. Symptoms include fever, chills, sweats, nausea, vomiting, and diarrhea. Pain over the right upper part of the abdomen (belly) usually occurs.

Other less common symptoms are chest pain, loss of appetite, and jaundice (yellow color of skin and eyes).

How Are Liver Abscesses Diagnosed?

The doctor usually finds liver abscesses by ultrasonography, which uses sound waves to make pictures of the liver. Computed tomography (CT) of the abdomen is better for

Most people need two or three different drugs to treat the abscess. Usually, antibiotics are given intravenously until fever and infection are gone. You may need to be hospitalized for severe infections.

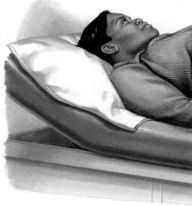

Similar to a liver biopsy to diagnose your condition, a needle may need to be passed into your abscess to drain pus if you have pyogenic abscesses.

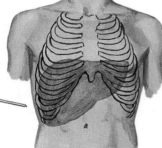

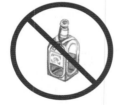

Don't drink alcohol when taking medicines for liver abscesses.

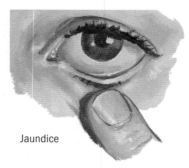

Jaundice

Call your doctor if your skin or eyes turn yellow (jaundice),

How Are Liver Abscesses Treated?

The best treatment is draining pus and using antibiotics. Most people need two or three different antibiotics. Usually, antibiotics are given intravenously until fever and infection are gone.

People with pyogenic abscesses have pus drained from the abscesses. This is done by passing a needle through into the abscesses and draining the pus. Drainage of an amebic abscess isn't needed, unless antibiotic treatment doesn't work or a pyogenic cause is suspected.

DOs and DON'Ts in Managing a Liver Abscess:

✔ **DO** remember that most people with pyogenic liver abscesses improve within 2 weeks of antibiotic treatment and drainage. The fever usually resolves in most people with amebic abscesses in 4 to 5 days of treatment.

✔ **DO** take your antibiotics as instructed. Finish taking all the medicine, even if you feel better.

✔ **DO** wash your hands before eating.

✔ **DO** call your doctor if you have severe abdominal pain, vomiting, diarrhea, fever, chills, and sweats.

✔ **DO** call your doctor if your skin turns yellow.

⊘ **DON'T** drink alcohol when taking medicines prescribed for liver abscesses.

⊘ **DON'T** drink tap water in countries where water may be contaminated.

⊘ **DON'T** ignore symptoms.

⊘ **DON'T** forget that untreated pyogenic liver abscess is fatal in nearly 100% of cases!

MANAGING YOUR
LIVER CANCER

Hepatoma is the most common cancer of the liver. In the United States, about 6000 new cases are diagnosed each year. Hepatomas are more common in men than women, usually occurring in people 50 to 70 years old.

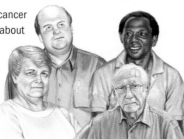

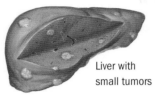

Liver with small tumors

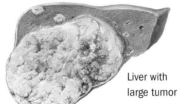

Liver with large tumor

Symptoms include:

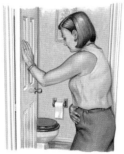

Abdominal pain

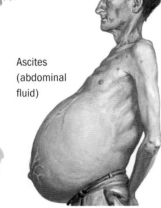

Ascites (abdominal fluid)

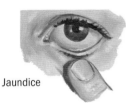

Jaundice

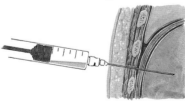

Diagnosis is hard because hepatomas don't have many early symptoms. To help diagnosis, your doctor can do blood tests, ultrasound, CT, MRI, and liver biopsy.

Liver biopsy

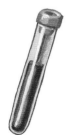

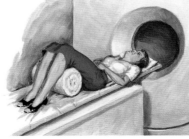

Blood test

CAT scan

What Is Liver Cancer?

Hepatoma (also called hepatocellular carcinoma) is the most common cancer of the liver. It's a primary tumor, meaning the tumor started growing in the liver and did not spread from someplace else in the body.

In the United States, about 6000 new cases occur each year. Hepatomas are more common in men than women, usually occurring in people 50 to 70 years old. Unfortunately, many hepatomas are found late. Early diagnosis gives the best hope for cure.

What Causes Liver Cancer?

Hepatoma occurs most often in people with cirrhosis (liver scarring), chronic hepatitis B, or chronic hepatitis C or after severe liver damage from chronic alcohol abuse. Hepatomas aren't contagious or passed from parents to children.

What Are the Symptoms of Liver Cancer?

One third of people do not have any symptoms. Symptoms may include pain in the abdomen (belly), an abdominal mass, abdominal fluid (ascites), and jaundice (yellow skin color). Later, weakness, loss of appetite, weight loss, and fatigue can occur.

How Is Liver Cancer Diagnosed?

Diagnosis is difficult because hepatomas often don't have many early symptoms. To help diagnosis, the doctor may initially do blood tests called alpha-fetoprotein and liver function tests for people with cirrhosis or hepatitis B or C. However, these tests are not diagnostic because not everyone with a hepatoma has abnormal blood tests, so the doctor may want imaging studies called ultrasound, computed tomography (CT), or magnetic resonance imaging (MRI). If these imaging studies show a probable tumor, a liver biopsy will be done. In a biopsy, liver tissue is taken with a needle and looked at with a microscope.

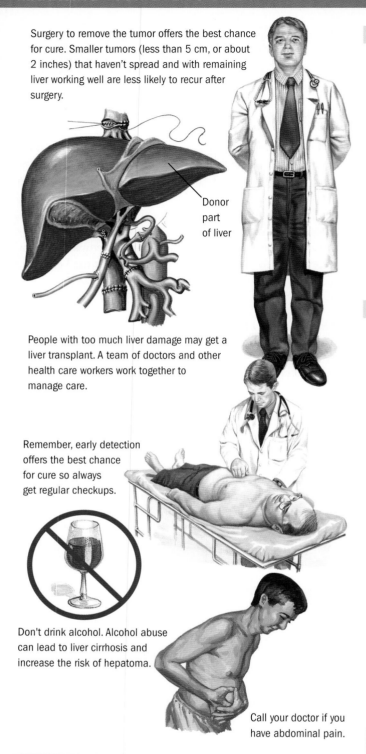

Surgery to remove the tumor offers the best chance for cure. Smaller tumors (less than 5 cm, or about 2 inches) that haven't spread and with remaining liver working well are less likely to recur after surgery.

Donor part of liver

People with too much liver damage may get a liver transplant. A team of doctors and other health care workers work together to manage care.

Remember, early detection offers the best chance for cure so always get regular checkups.

Don't drink alcohol. Alcohol abuse can lead to liver cirrhosis and increase the risk of hepatoma.

Call your doctor if you have abdominal pain.

How Is Liver Cancer Treated?

Untreated people have a rapid downhill course. Surgery offers the best chance for cure, but most people cannot have surgery because of cirrhosis or tumor spread. Smaller tumors (less than 5 cm, or about 2 inches) that haven't spread and with remaining liver working well are less likely to recur after surgery.

People who cannot have surgery may have other treatments, including injecting chemotherapy drugs into the artery that feeds the tumor or injecting ethanol (alcohol) directly into the tumor to destroy it.

People with very large tumors or with too much liver damage may be candidates for liver transplantation. A team of doctors and other health care workers must work together to manage care.

DOs and DON'Ts in Managing Liver Cancer:

✔ **DO** call your doctor if you have abdominal pain or vomit blood.

✔ **DO** tell your doctor if you have a drinking problem.

✔ **DO** tell your doctor if you feel a mass or large lump in the right upper part of your abdomen (belly).

🚫 **DON'T** drink alcohol. Alcohol abuse can lead to cirrhosis and increase the risk of hepatoma.

🚫 **DON'T** miss follow-up doctor appointments.

FROM THE DESK OF

NOTES

FOR MORE INFORMATION

Contact the following sources:

- American Liver Foundation
  Tel: (800) 223-0179
  Website: http://www.liverfoundation.org

- American Cancer Society
  Tel: (800) 227-2345
  Website: http://www.cancer.org

- National Cancer Institute Cancer Information Service
  Tel: (800) 422-6237
  Website: http://www.cancer.gov

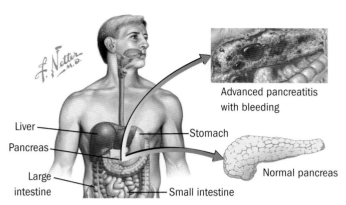

The pancreas is in the abdomen, surrounded by the stomach, intestines, and other organs. Pancreatitis is inflammation (swelling) of the pancreas.

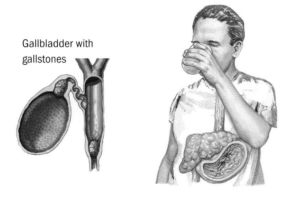

The most common causes are gallstones and alcohol use.

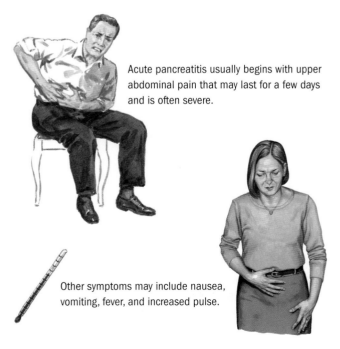

Acute pancreatitis usually begins with upper abdominal pain that may last for a few days and is often severe.

Other symptoms may include nausea, vomiting, fever, and increased pulse.

What Is Acute Pancreatitis?

The pancreas is a gland in the abdomen, surrounded by the stomach, intestines, and other organs. It makes substances called pancreatic juices (containing digestive enzymes) and hormones including insulin. These digestive enzymes are then sent to the small intestine.

Pancreatitis is inflammation (swelling) of the pancreas. It occurs when these digestive enzymes begin attacking the pancreas.

Pancreatitis can be acute, which occurs suddenly and may be life-threatening with many complications. Continuing injury to the pancreas may lead to a long-lasting (chronic) form. Pancreatitis cannot be caught.

About 50,000 to 80,000 cases of acute pancreatitis occur in the United States yearly. About 20% of cases are severe. In very severe cases, shock and sometimes death can occur.

What Causes Acute Pancreatitis?

The most common causes are gallstones and alcohol use. Others include prescribed drugs, surgery to the abdomen (belly), pancreatic or intestinal abnormalities, and rarely infection (e.g., mumps), blockage or scarring of the pancreas, cancer, and pancreatic infection. Sometimes, the cause is unknown.

What Are the Symptoms of Acute Pancreatitis?

The first symptom is usually upper abdominal pain that may last for a few days and is often severe. It may also reach the back and the chest. Pain may be sudden, intense or mild, and get worse with eating. A swollen, very tender abdomen may occur. Other symptoms may include nausea, vomiting, fever, and increased pulse.

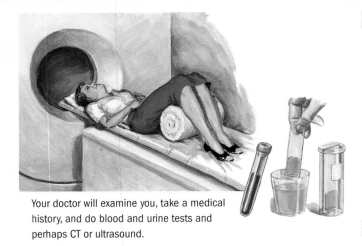

Your doctor will examine you, take a medical history, and do blood and urine tests and perhaps CT or ultrasound.

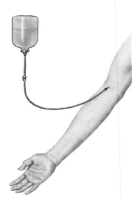

Treatment is usually supportive and in the hospital. You may be unable to eat for a few days but will get intravenous fluids and pain relievers.

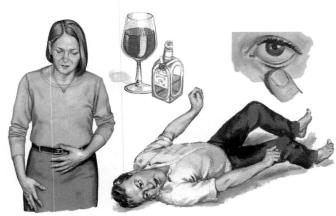

Call your doctor if you have abdominal pain, fever, jaundice, or alcohol-related seizures or an alcohol problem.

How Is Acute Pancreatitis Diagnosed?

To make a diagnosis, the doctor uses a medical history and physical examination, plus blood and urine tests and maybe computed tomography (CT) or ultrasound of the stomach.

The blood test checks the level of amylase or lipase (digestive enzymes made in the pancreas), which get high when the pancreas is inflamed. Blood levels of calcium, magnesium, sodium, potassium, and bicarbonate may also change. Sugar and lipid (fat) levels in blood may also increase. After the pancreas recovers, these levels usually go back to their baseline.

How Is Acute Pancreatitis Treated?

Treatment is usually supportive and in the hospital. Intravenous fluids increase blood volume and replace electrolytes such as potassium and calcium. If someone cannot control vomiting, a tube is temporarily passed through the nose to the stomach to remove fluid and air.

People with mild pancreatitis may be unable to eat for 3 or 4 days but are given intravenous fluids and pain relievers. People with severe pancreatitis may get intravenous feeding for longer periods. Surgery may be needed for infections, cysts, or bleeding. Attacks caused by gallstones may be treated with gallbladder removal or bile duct surgery when the pancreatitis subsides.

DOs and DON'Ts in Managing Acute Pancreatitis:

✔ **DO** remember that pancreatitis can be life-threatening and needs emergency treatment.

✔ **DO** call your doctor if you have abdominal pain, vomit blood, or have a problem with alcohol, jaundice (yellow skin and eyes), fever (101° F or higher), weight loss, muscle cramps, or seizures from alcohol withdrawal.

🚫 **DON'T** drink alcohol. Heavy drinking can cause pancreatitis. Don't be afraid to ask for help if you cannot stop drinking alcohol.

FROM THE DESK OF

NOTES

FOR MORE INFORMATION

Contact the following sources:

• American Gastroenterological Association
Tel: (301) 654-2055
Website: http://www.gastro.org

• National Digestive Diseases Information Clearinghouse
Tel: (800) 891-5389
Website: http://www.niddk.nih.gov/health/digest/nddic.htm

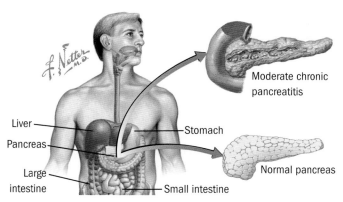

The pancreas is in the abdomen, surrounded by the stomach, intestines, and other organs. Pancreatitis is inflammation (swelling) of the pancreas.

Liver

Pancreas

Large intestine

Stomach

Small intestine

Moderate chronic pancreatitis

Normal pancreas

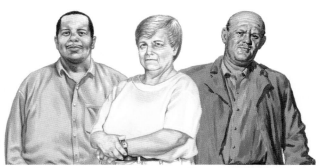

Chronic pancreatitis isn't common. Men are affected more often than women.

Alcohol abuse is the major cause.

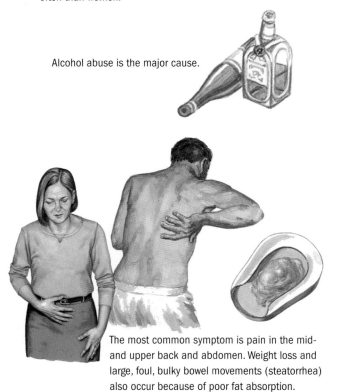

The most common symptom is pain in the mid- and upper back and abdomen. Weight loss and large, foul, bulky bowel movements (steatorrhea) also occur because of poor fat absorption.

What Is Chronic Pancreatitis?

The pancreas is a gland in the abdomen (belly), surrounded by the stomach, intestines, and other organs. It makes substances called pancreatic juices (containing digestive enzymes) and the hormones insulin and glucagon.

Pancreatitis is inflammation (swelling) of the pancreas. It occurs when these digestive enzymes begin attacking the pancreas. Pancreatitis can be acute (occurs suddenly). Continuing injury to the pancreas may lead to a long-lasting (chronic) form. The pancreas doesn't make its enzymes, causing an inability to digest and absorb fat in the diet. Insulin production also decreases.

Chronic pancreatitis isn't common. More men than women are affected. Pancreatitis cannot be caught.

What Causes Chronic Pancreatitis?

Alcohol abuse is the major cause. Other causes are hemochromatosis (too much iron in the blood) and cystic fibrosis. Sometimes the cause is unknown.

What Are the Symptoms of Chronic Pancreatitis?

The most common symptom is pain in the mid- and upper back and abdomen that varies in intensity. It may be a low-grade, lasting pain with repeated acute attacks. The pain may be constant and severe.

Another symptom is weight loss, which occurs because the body cannot absorb fat properly (malabsorption). Large, foul, bulky bowel movements, or stools (called steatorrhea) occur because of this problem with fat absorption. People can also have a distended abdomen and fever.

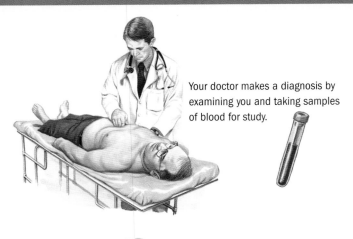

Your doctor makes a diagnosis by examining you and taking samples of blood for study.

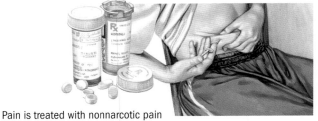

Pain is treated with nonnarcotic pain relievers. Insulin injections are used to control blood sugar levels.

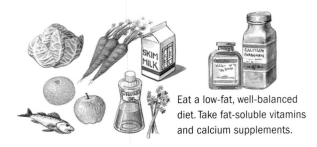

Eat a low-fat, well-balanced diet. Take fat-soluble vitamins and calcium supplements.

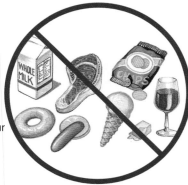

Avoid fatty foods, alcohol, and caffeinated beverages. Call your doctor if you can't control pain or you get a fever.

How Is Chronic Pancreatitis Diagnosed?

The doctor diagnoses chronic pancreatitis by reviewing the medical history and doing a physical examination. Samples of blood are studied for signs of this disease.

How Is Chronic Pancreatitis Treated?

The first treatment goal is to manage pain, usually by using nonnarcotic pain relievers. Referral to a pain specialist may help. In rare cases, if pain cannot be controlled, surgery is a possibility. Surgery involves draining the pancreatic duct (tube connecting the pancreas and bile duct). In advanced cases, all or part of the pancreas can be removed.

The second goal is replacing digestive enzymes and insulin that the pancreas normally makes. In severe cases, insulin replacement may also be necessary. Pancreatic enzymes, as tablets, are taken with meals and snacks. Insulin injections are used to control the blood sugar (glucose) level. Supplements of vitamins A, D, and K may be needed because of poor absorption.

DOs and DON'Ts in Managing Chronic Pancreatitis:

✔ **DO** eat a low-fat, well-balanced diet.
✔ **DO** take oral fat-soluble vitamin supplements and calcium supplements.
✔ **DO** take pancreatic enzyme supplements as prescribed.
✔ **DO** call your doctor if you cannot control pain with prescribed drugs. See a pain specialist if pain control is difficult.
✔ **DO** call your doctor if you get symptoms of pancreatitis or symptoms worsen or don't improve with treatment.
✔ **DO** call your doctor if you get a fever.

⊘ **DON'T** eat fatty foods.
⊘ **DON'T** drink alcohol or caffeinated beverages.
⊘ **DON'T** use narcotics for pain control for long periods.

FROM THE DESK OF

NOTES

FOR MORE INFORMATION

Contact the following sources:

• American Gastroenterological Association
Tel: (301) 654-2055
Website: http://www.gastro.org

• National Digestive Diseases Information Clearinghouse
Tel: (800) 891-5389
Website: http://www.niddk.nih.gov/health/digest/nddic.htm

MANAGING YOUR
PEPTIC ULCER

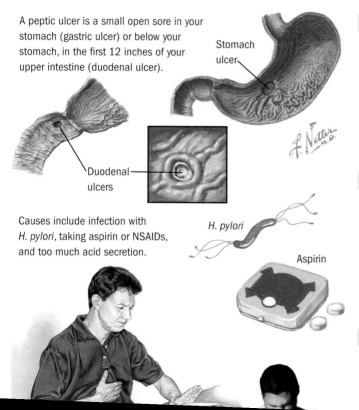

A peptic ulcer is a small open sore in your stomach (gastric ulcer) or below your stomach, in the first 12 inches of your upper intestine (duodenal ulcer).

Stomach ulcer

Duodenal ulcers

Causes include infection with H. pylori, taking aspirin or NSAIDs, and too much acid secretion.

H. pylori

Aspirin

What Are Peptic Ulcers?

Peptic ulcers are small open sores in the stomach or upper intestine. Sores occur when the lining of the stomach or intestine breaks down and exposes tissue underneath. Ulcers may be gastric (stomach) or duodenal (first 12 inches of the small intestine). Duodenal ulcers occur four times more often than gastric ulcers. Peptic ulcer disease (PUD) is common.

What Causes Peptic Ulcers?

Three things cause most peptic ulcers: infection with the kind of bacteria named *Helicobacter pylori* (*H. pylori*), taking aspirin or similar medicines (nonsteroidal antiinflammatory drugs, or NSAIDs, such as ibuprofen), and too much acid secretion. Ulcers aren't contagious but may run in families. Smoking increases the risk of stomach ulcers.

What Are the Symptoms of Peptic Ulcers?

The main symptom is stomach pain that feels like heartburn, indigestion, or hunger. A burning, boring, or gnawing feeling can last from 30 minutes to 3 hours. It's usually felt in the upper _____ sometimes occurs below the breastbone.

Medicines reduce acid production in the stomach and treat *H. pylori* infection if you have one.

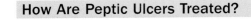

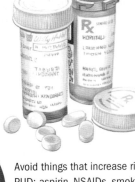

Avoid things that increase risk of PUD: aspirin, NSAIDs, smoking, and alcohol.

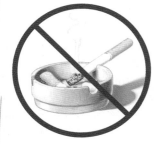

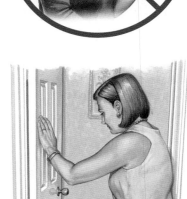

Call your doctor if you have diarrhea. Also call your doctor if you have blood in your stools or vomit or if stools are dark and tarry.

How Are Peptic Ulcers Treated?

Treatment heals the ulcer, helps symptoms, stops relapses, and avoids complications. With treatment, people usually start to feel better in about 2 weeks. Relapses can occur if the risk factors persist.

Two treatment options are drugs and surgery. Medicines to reduce stomach acid include antacids, histamine-2 blockers such as ranitidine or famotidine, and proton pump inhibitors such as omeprazole. Sucralfate is another medication that can form a protective coating on the ulcer to help it heal. Antibiotics, proton pump inhibitors, and bismuth can be used for *H. pylori* infection.

Surgery is used when drugs don't work or serious complications occur. Today, surgery is rarely needed.

DOs and DON'Ts in Managing Peptic Ulcers:

✔ **DO** avoid things that increase the risk of PUD: aspirin, NSAIDs, smoking, and drinking alcohol.

✔ **DO** call your doctor if you have diarrhea.

✔ **DO** call your doctor if your vomit is bloody or looks like coffee grounds.

✔ **DO** call your doctor if blood is in your stools or stools are dark and tarry.

✔ **DO** call your doctor if you are unusually weak or pale.

✔ **DO** call your doctor if pain doesn't get better with treatment.

Primary biliary cirrhosis refers to scarring of the liver caused by blockage of the tiny bile tubules (ducts) inside the liver. It accounts for 10% of liver cirrhosis cases. Most cases occur in women 30 to 60 years old.

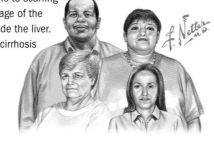

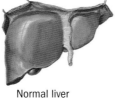

Normal liver

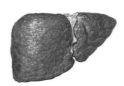

Diseased liver

An early symptom is itching on the whole body or just palms and feet. Other symptoms include:

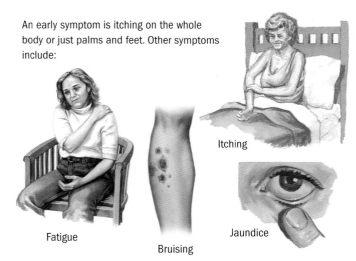

Fatigue

Bruising

Itching

Jaundice

Your doctor makes a preliminary diagnosis from symptoms, a physical examination, and blood tests. A liver biopsy is the best way to confirm the diagnosis.

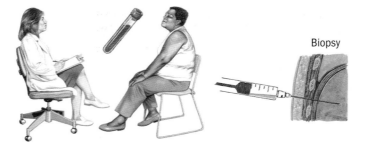

Biopsy

What Is Primary Biliary Cirrhosis?

Primary biliary cirrhosis refers to scarring of the liver caused by blockage of the tiny bile tubules (ducts) inside and outside the liver. This disorder accounts for 10% of all cases of liver cirrhosis. About 90% of all cases occur in women 30 to 60 years old.

What Causes Primary Biliary Cirrhosis?

The exact cause is unknown, but it's thought to be an autoimmune disorder. Autoimmune means that the body's immune system attacks the body's own tissues.

What Are the Symptoms of Primary Biliary Cirrhosis?

An early symptom is itchiness of the whole body or just palms and feet. Jaundice (yellow skin) follows. Fatigue and easy bruising are other symptoms. As the liver becomes more scarred, it fails, so fluid in the belly (ascites), leg swelling, confusion, and lethargy occur. Other complications are bleeding from the esophagus from enlarged veins known as varices that develop in people with cirrhosis and vitamin deficiencies, osteoporosis, and joint pains.

How Is Primary Biliary Cirrhosis Diagnosed?

The doctor makes a preliminary diagnosis from symptoms, physical examination, and blood tests. The blood tests are liver function tests and a specific test for antimitochondrial antibody. Almost 90% of people have this antibody. A liver biopsy is the best way to confirm the diagnosis. In a biopsy, the doctor puts a needle into the liver to get a small sample for study with a microscope.

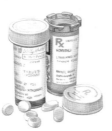

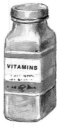

No specific treatment is available. The drugs ursodiol and colchicines are used to relieve symptoms and improve blood tests. Cholestyramine helps itchiness. Vitamins and minerals are used to prevent osteoporosis and night blindness.

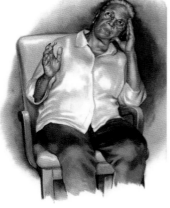

For confusion or lethargy from advanced liver failure, lactulose can be used.

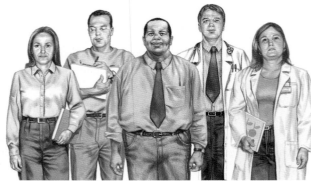

In the most advanced cases, liver transplantation can be an option. A team made up of your primary doctor, gastroenterologist, surgeon, and transplant surgical group will help make the decision about transplantation. Don't be afraid to ask for second opinions.

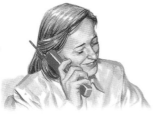

Call your doctor if you have yellow skin, itching, easy bruising, leg swelling, or bleeding.

How Is Primary Biliary Cirrhosis Treated?

No specific treatment is available. Treatment is for relief of symptoms. Treatment includes the drugs ursodiol and colchicine to help symptoms and decrease liver damage. Cholestyramine helps itchiness.

For confusion or lethargy from advanced liver failure, a medicine called lactulose can be used. The lactulose syrup acts as a laxative and may cause diarrhea. By causing diarrhea, lactulose gets rid of metabolic wastes such as ammonia. High ammonia levels cause confusion and lethargy. Confusion and thought processes get better after the lactulose syrup lowers the ammonia levels.

In the most advanced cases, liver transplantation is an option for better survival. A team made up of the primary doctor, gastroenterologist (specialist in digestive system diseases), surgeon, and transplant surgical team will help make the decision about transplantation.

DOs and DON'Ts in Managing Primary Biliary Cirrhosis:

✔ **DO** get the opinion of a gastroenterologist if you may have this disorder.
✔ **DO** call your doctor if you have yellow skin or persistent itchiness.
✔ **DO** call your doctor if you have easy bruising, leg swelling, or bleeding.

⊘ **DON'T** ignore jaundice, especially with itchiness.
⊘ **DON'T** be afraid to ask for second opinions about diagnosis or treatment.

FROM THE DESK OF

NOTES

FOR MORE INFORMATION

Contact the following sources:

• National Digestive Diseases Information Clearinghouse
Tel: (800) 891-5389
Website: http://digestive.niddk.nih.gov

• American College of Gastroenterology
Tel: (703) 820-7400
Website: http://www.acg.gi.org

MANAGING YOUR
ANAL ITCHING

Anal itching, or pruritus ani, is a burning or itching of the anus and skin around it. It's common and affects both sexes and people of all ages. People with diabetes may have more risk of getting this condition.

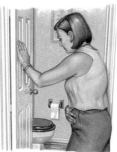

Possible causes include

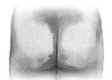

Psoriasis

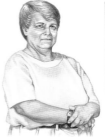

Menopausal women

Diarrhea

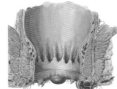

Hemorrhoids

Symptoms include itching (worse at night), redness of skin around the anus, and skin abrasions caused by scratching. Skin thickening and chronic inflammation can occur.

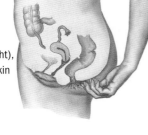

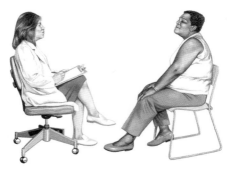

Your doctor makes a diagnosis from symptoms and an examination of the rectum and the skin surrounding it. Laboratory and microscopic studies are sometimes needed to identify fungi, eggs, or mites.

What Is Anal Itching?

Anal itching has the medical name pruritus ani. It's a burning or itching of the anus and skin around it. It's common and affects both sexes and people of all ages. People with diabetes may have more risk of getting this condition. Treatment can control symptoms, but the problem can come back.

What Causes Anal Itching?

Often, the cause is unknown. The many causes include infections with yeast, herpesvirus, human papillomavirus (HPV, which causes genital warts), pinworms, mites (which cause scabies), and lice. Skin conditions, such as contact dermatitis, psoriasis, and seborrheic dermatitis, may start as anal itching. Soaps, contraceptive jellies and foams, scented toilet paper, deodorant sprays, and douches can cause contact dermatitis. People with chronic diarrhea may have itching. Diseases of the rectum, such as hemorrhoids, fissures (tears), fistulas, and rectal prolapse, may cause itching. Women near or after menopause (change of life) may have itching caused by vaginal discharge or low estrogen levels.

What Are the Symptoms of Anal Itching?

Symptoms include itching, redness of skin around the anus, and skin abrasions caused by scratching. Itching is often intense and worse at night. Skin thickening and chronic inflammation (swelling, redness) can occur. Damaged skin can get a bacterial infection.

How Is Anal Itching Diagnosed?

The doctor makes a diagnosis from symptoms and an examination of the rectum and the skin surrounding it. Laboratory studies are sometimes needed to identify fungi. Examinations with a microscope may be needed to look for pinworm eggs or mites in skin.

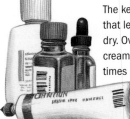

The key to treatment is self-care and avoiding things that lead to itching. Keep the area clean, cool, and dry. Over-the-counter hydrocortisone ointment or cream can control mild itching. It's applied three times a day, but not for more than 5 days. If these medicines don't help, the doctor may prescribe stronger drugs.

Lose weight if you're overweight.

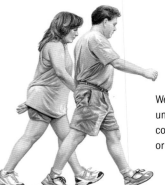

Wear loose-fitting clothing and cotton underwear. Don't overdo activities that could cause the area to get too wet or sweaty.

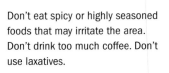

Don't eat spicy or highly seasoned foods that may irritate the area. Don't drink too much coffee. Don't use laxatives.

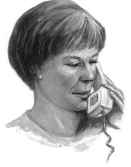

Call your doctor if you have a fever if symptoms continue even with self-care.

How Is Anal Itching Treated?

The key to treatment is self-care and avoiding the things that lead to itching. Keep the area clean, cool, and dry. Over-the-counter hydrocortisone ointment or cream can control itching. It's applied three times a day, rubbed in gently until it disappears. Hydrocortisone shouldn't be used for longer than 5 days because it may cause more irritation and damage the skin.

If over-the-counter medicine doesn't help, the doctor may prescribe a stronger topical cortisone or other drugs. Yeast, herpes, genital warts, scabies, and infections with pinworms and lice must be treated with the right medicines. Rectal diseases may need other treatments.

DOs and DON'Ts in Managing Anal Itching:

✔ **DO** keep the area clean, cool, and dry.
✔ **DO** use plain, unscented soaps.
✔ **DO** clean the area with moistened unscented tissue or tufts of cotton after bowel movements.
✔ **DO** lose weight if you're overweight.
✔ **DO** wear loose clothing and cotton underwear.
✔ **DO** use tampons for your periods. They may be more comfortable than sanitary napkins.
✔ **DO** call your doctor if the area seems to be infected.
✔ **DO** call your doctor if you have a fever or if symptoms continue even with self-care.

⊘ **DON'T** have contact with irritating substances that can cause itching.
⊘ **DON'T** wear tight-fitting underwear made from synthetic materials.
⊘ **DON'T** overdo activities that could cause the area to get too wet or sweaty.
⊘ **DON'T** eat spicy or highly seasoned foods that may irritate the area.
⊘ **DON'T** drink too much coffee.
⊘ **DON'T** use laxatives.

FROM THE DESK OF

NOTES

FOR MORE INFORMATION

Contact the following source:

• American Academy of Dermatology
  Tel: (847) 330-0230, (866) 503-7546
  Website: http://www.aad.org

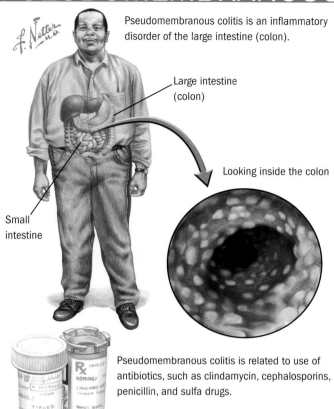

Pseudomembranous colitis is an inflammatory disorder of the large intestine (colon).

Large intestine (colon)

Looking inside the colon

Small intestine

Pseudomembranous colitis is related to use of antibiotics, such as clindamycin, cephalosporins, penicillin, and sulfa drugs.

Symptoms are diarrhea that is watery and yellow-green, smells bad, and may be bloody. Cramps, abdominal pain, and fever are other symptoms.

Your doctor makes a diagnosis by doing stool cultures that grow the bacteria. Sigmoidoscopy or colonoscopy may also be done if there is no improvement with treatment. In these procedures, a lighted flexible tube (colonoscope) is put into the rectum to look at the bowel and to get pieces of colon tissue for study with a microscope.

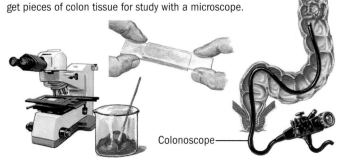

Colonoscope

What Is Pseudomembranous Colitis?

Pseudomembranous colitis is a disorder involving inflammation (swelling, redness) of the large intestine (colon, or bowel). It's related to use of antibiotics. Antibiotics given to treat an infection can make bacteria, such as the one named *Clostridium difficile*, that normally live in the bowel grow excessively. The colon becomes inflamed and severe diarrhea occurs.

This disorder affects 6 of 100,000 people treated with antibiotics. It occurs more often in adults than in children and in people in hospitals and nursing homes. Patients who had recent surgery or are having cancer treatments have a slightly greater chance of getting it.

Most people respond to treatment and have no lasting effects. Untreated, the condition can lead to severe dehydration from the diarrhea, and in rare cases can be fatal.

What Causes Pseudomembranous Colitis?

The antibiotics most frequently responsible for this colitis are penicillins, cephalosporins, clindamycin, and sulfa drugs. However, any antibiotic may cause the disease.

What Are the Symptoms of Pseudomembranous Colitis?

Symptoms are diarrhea that is watery and yellow-green, smells foul, and may be bloody. Cramps and pain in the abdomen (belly) and fever also occur.

Symptoms usually start 4 to 10 days after beginning antibiotics. However, some people may not have symptoms until after stopping the antibiotics.

Severe colitis may have symptoms of shock, low blood pressure, weak pulse, and increased heart rate.

How Is Pseudomembranous Colitis Diagnosed?

The doctor diagnoses the condition by doing cultures of stools (bowel movements) that grow the bacteria. Blood tests may also be done to check for signs of infection and dehydration. If the diagnosis isn't clear or therapy isn't helping, sigmoidoscopy or colonoscopy can be done. In these procedures, a lighted flexible tube is inserted into the rectum to look at the bowel and to get tissue samples for study with a microscope.

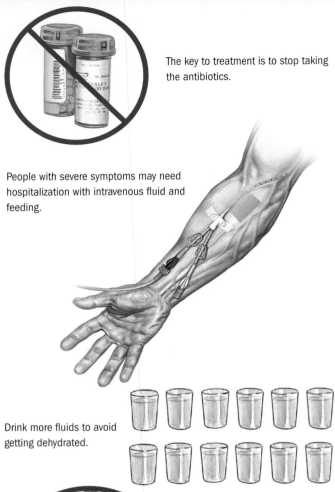

The key to treatment is to stop taking the antibiotics.

People with severe symptoms may need hospitalization with intravenous fluid and feeding.

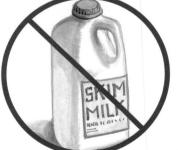

Drink more fluids to avoid getting dehydrated.

Avoid dairy products, which may make diarrhea worse.

Don't take antidiarrhea medicine without talking to your doctor about it first.

How Is Pseudomembranous Colitis Treated?

The key to treatment is to stop taking the antibiotics. People with severe symptoms may need hospitalization with intravenous fluid. The diet is then slowly returned to normal. Antibiotics such as metronidazole and vancomycin are prescribed for severe colitis.

DOs and DON'Ts in Managing Pseudomembranous Colitis:

✔ **DO** stop taking all antibiotics.
✔ **DO** increase drinking fluids to avoid dehydration.
✔ **DO** avoid dairy products, which may make diarrhea worse.
✔ **DO** call your doctor if you have symptoms of pseudomembranous colitis, such as diarrhea, bloody stool, and abdominal pain, especially when taking or just finishing antibiotics.
✔ **DO** call your doctor if your symptoms don't get better with treatment.
✔ **DO** call your doctor if new symptoms appear during treatment.
✔ **DO** call your doctor if you see signs of dehydration, such as dry skin and mouth, rapid pulse, confusion, and tiredness.

⃠ **DON'T** use antidiarrheal agents unless your doctor says that you should.

FROM THE DESK OF

NOTES

FOR MORE INFORMATION

Contact the following source:

• National Digestive Diseases Information Clearinghouse
Tel: (800) 891-5389
Website: http://www.niddk.nih.gov/health/digest/nddic.htm

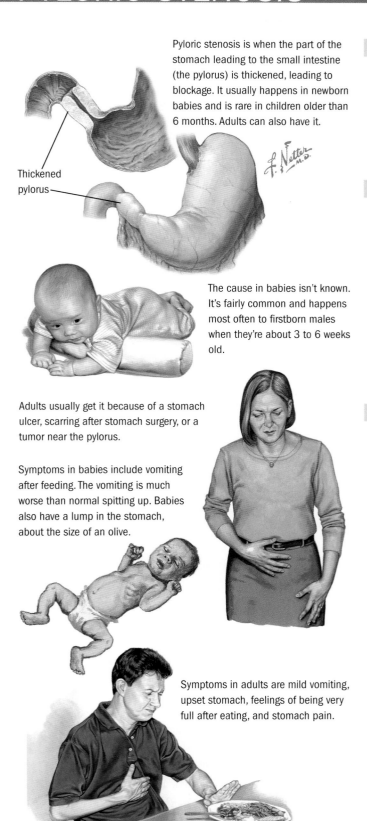

Pyloric stenosis is when the part of the stomach leading to the small intestine (the pylorus) is thickened, leading to blockage. It usually happens in newborn babies and is rare in children older than 6 months. Adults can also have it.

Thickened pylorus

The cause in babies isn't known. It's fairly common and happens most often to firstborn males when they're about 3 to 6 weeks old.

Adults usually get it because of a stomach ulcer, scarring after stomach surgery, or a tumor near the pylorus.

Symptoms in babies include vomiting after feeding. The vomiting is much worse than normal spitting up. Babies also have a lump in the stomach, about the size of an olive.

Symptoms in adults are mild vomiting, upset stomach, feelings of being very full after eating, and stomach pain.

What Is Pyloric Stenosis?

In pyloric stenosis, the part of the stomach that leads to the small intestine (called the pylorus) is thickened, leading to blockage. It usually happens in newborn babies and is rare in children older than 6 months. It can sometimes happen in adults.

What Causes Pyloric Stenosis?

Pyloric stenosis in infants is fairly common but the cause isn't known. The muscle of the pylorus gets too large and thick and blocks the tube leading out of the stomach (the stomach outlet). Liquids and solid foods can't go from the stomach to the small intestine. Stenosis happens most often to firstborn boys when they are about 3 to 6 weeks old and can also occur at 4 or 5 months.

Adults usually get pyloric stenosis because of a stomach ulcer, scarring after stomach surgery, or a tumor near the pylorus.

What Are the Symptoms of Pyloric Stenosis?

Babies vomit after feeding because milk can't drain from the stomach into the small intestine. This vomiting is much worse than normal spitting up and becomes more forceful as time passes. Babies may not get enough fluids because of the vomiting and become dehydrated and thirsty. They may be constipated. They may have trouble gaining weight and may even lose weight. Babies also have a lump in the stomach, about the size of an olive. This lump is the muscle that got too large.

Adults have only mild vomiting, upset stomach, feelings of being very full after eating, or stomach pain.

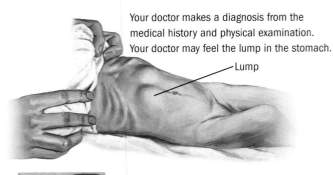

Your doctor makes a diagnosis from the medical history and physical examination. Your doctor may feel the lump in the stomach.

Lump

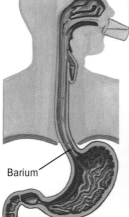

Barium x-rays or ultrasonography may also be done. An x-ray is a picture of the body's insides. For the x-ray, a chalky liquid called barium is given. The barium makes it easier to see the stomach and bowel in the x-ray.

Barium

X-ray

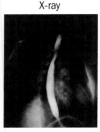

Ultrasound

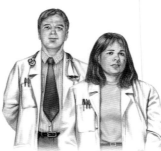

Surgery will be needed. In babies, a surgery called pyloromyotomy is done where the large, thickened muscle is cut. In adults, surgery depends on the condition causing your stenosis.

Call your doctor if your baby has pain, swelling, redness, bleeding, or drainage at the incision site. Also call your doctor if your baby develops a fever after surgery.

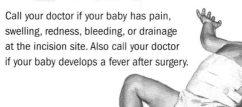

How Is Pyloric Stenosis Diagnosed?

The doctor makes a diagnosis from the medical history and physical examination. During the examination, the doctor may feel the lump in the stomach. The doctor may order barium x-rays or ultrasonography. These tests take pictures of inside the body.

How Is Pyloric Stenosis Treated?

Babies need surgery. During surgery (called pyloromyotomy), the large, thick muscle is cut. Babies are given intravenous fluids until after surgery. They can usually feed again in about 6 to 8 hours. A mild aspirin-like medicine may be given for pain.

Adults also need surgery and treatment for the condition that caused the stenosis. Sometimes, the pylorus can be opened without surgery (called endoscopic balloon dilation). In this procedure, the doctor puts a tube with a balloon on its tip through the mouth and into the stomach. The balloon is inflated and stretches the pylorus open.

Both babies and adults usually do well after surgery.

DOs and DON'Ts in Managing Pyloric Stenosis:

✔ **DO** apply warm compresses to the incision site if your baby seems uncomfortable.

✔ **DO** call your doctor if your baby keeps vomiting, has weight loss or poor weight gain, seems too tired, or has few or no stools for 1 or 2 days.

✔ **DO** call your doctor if your baby has pain, swelling, redness, bleeding, or drainage at the incision site. Also call your doctor if your baby develops a fever after surgery.

🚫 **DON'T** forget follow-up doctor appointments.

FROM THE DESK OF

NOTES

FOR MORE INFORMATION

Contact the following sources:

• American Pediatric Surgical Association
Tel: (847) 480-9576
Website: http://www.eapsa.org

• American Academy of Family Physicians
Tel: (913) 906-6000, (800) 274-2237
Website: http://www.aafp.org

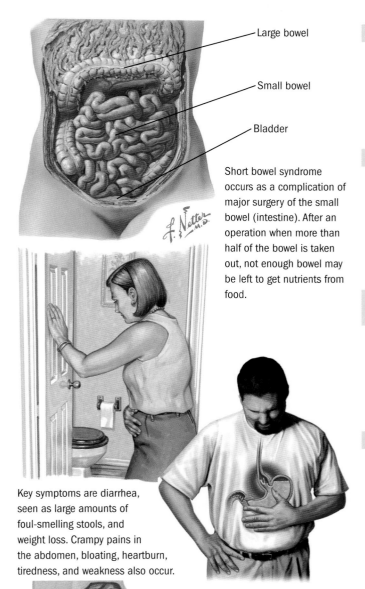

Large bowel

Small bowel

Bladder

Short bowel syndrome occurs as a complication of major surgery of the small bowel (intestine). After an operation when more than half of the bowel is taken out, not enough bowel may be left to get nutrients from food.

Key symptoms are diarrhea, seen as large amounts of foul-smelling stools, and weight loss. Crampy pains in the abdomen, bloating, heartburn, tiredness, and weakness also occur.

Your doctor will do blood tests and an upper gastrointestinal (GI) barium x-ray study. For this study, you swallow a chalky substance, barium, that moves quickly through the small bowel. X-rays can show what the small bowel looks like.

Barium

Barium swallow

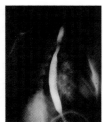

Barium contrast study

What Is Short Bowel Syndrome?

Short bowel syndrome occurs as a complication of major surgery of the small bowel (intestine). After surgery, not enough bowel is left to get nutrients from food. The result is that people can become malnourished.

What Causes Short Bowel Syndrome?

If more than half of the bowel is taken out during surgery, the risk of small bowel syndrome is great. Disorders of the small bowel that may need surgical treatment include congenital abnormalities and necrotizing enterocolitis in infants and Crohn's disease in adults.

What Are the Symptoms of Short Bowel Syndrome?

The key symptoms are diarrhea, seen as large amounts of foul-smelling stools, and weight loss. Painful cramps in the abdomen (belly), bloating, heartburn, tiredness, and weakness also occur. Symptoms usually begin a few days after abdominal surgery.

How Is Short Bowel Syndrome Diagnosed?

The doctor makes a diagnosis by taking a medical history and doing blood tests and an upper gastrointestinal (GI) barium x-ray study. For this x-ray, a chalky substance, barium, is swallowed and moves quickly through the stomach and small bowel. X-rays are then taken to show what the small bowel looks like.

Nutritional support in the form of intravenous hyperalimentation (TPN) is usually the first step in treatment. Liquid mixtures with all required nutrients are given through a vein. This type of feeding allows the bowel to rest and somewhat recover. A hospital stay may be needed.

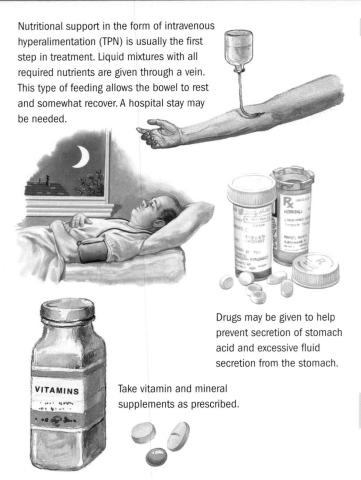

Drugs may be given to help prevent secretion of stomach acid and excessive fluid secretion from the stomach.

Take vitamin and mineral supplements as prescribed.

Close monitoring of the diet is key to successful treatment. You should eat a high-calorie, low-fat, low-residue diet. Be patient. This condition takes months to slowly get better and may need lifelong treatment.

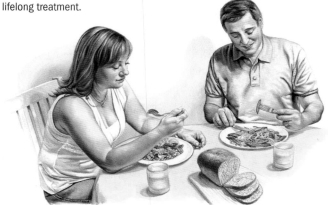

How Is Short Bowel Syndrome Treated?

Treatment involves nutritional support. The treatment at first is usually intravenous hyperalimentation (TPN, or total parenteral nutrition). Liquid mixtures with all required nutrients are given through a vein. This type of feeding allows the bowel to rest and somewhat recover. Hospitalization may be needed.

Medicines may be given to help prevent secretion of acid and excessive fluids by the stomach.

Usually after 1 to 4 weeks, the diarrhea will go away and the appetite will return. At this time, enteral feedings are started. For these feedings, mixtures are put through a tube directly into the stomach. This is a slow process while the intestine learns to work again. After weeks to months of this, feedings by mouth are slowly given.

Close monitoring of the diet is key to successful treatment. A high-calorie, low-fat, low-residue diet is needed. In some cases, people use TPN for the rest of their life. Fat-soluble vitamins and mineral supplements are also taken.

Symptoms may get better over time but will always mean close attention to diet.

DOs and DON'Ts in Managing Short Bowel Syndrome:

✔ **DO** be patient. This condition takes months to slowly get better and may need lifelong treatment.
✔ **DO** take vitamin and mineral supplements as prescribed.
✔ **DO** call your doctor if you have diarrhea after bowel surgery.
✔ **DO** call your doctor if you're being treated for short bowel syndrome and your symptoms worsen or return.

⊘ **DON'T** eat high-fat foods.

FROM THE DESK OF

NOTES

FOR MORE INFORMATION

Contact the following sources:

• Gastro-Intestinal Research Foundation
  Tel: (312) 332-1350
  Website: http://www.girf.org

• American College of Surgeons
  Tel: (800) 621-4111
  Website: http://www.facs.org

Stomach cancer refers to a cancerous growth in the stomach. Most cases are diagnosed in people older than 65.

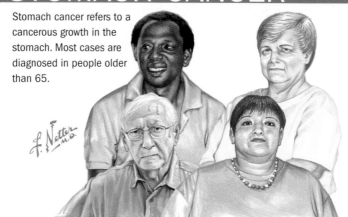

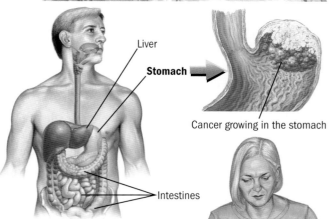

Liver

Stomach

Cancer growing in the stomach

Intestines

The cause isn't known, but people who have diets high in nitrates and infections with *Helicobacter pylori* bacteria have increased chances of getting it.

Pain in the abdomen, nausea, and loss of appetite are common symptoms.

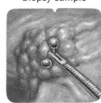

Biopsy sample

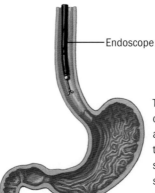

Endoscope

The best way to diagnose stomach cancer is by a biopsy. Your doctor uses a small lighted tube (endoscope) passed through the mouth and down into the stomach (upper endoscopy). Then, a small piece of stomach is taken for study with a microscope.

What Is Stomach Cancer?

Stomach (gastric) cancer refers to a cancerous (malignant) growth in the stomach.

These cancers occur in about 7 people per 100,000 in the United States. They are more common in Japan (more than 80 people per 100,000). Most cases are diagnosed in people older than 65.

What Causes Stomach Cancer?

The cause is unknown, but certain things increase chances of getting this disease. Diets high in nitrates may make this cancer more likely. Nitrates (found in smoked and salted foods) are converted to nitrites by bacteria, and nitrites are cancer-causing substances. Also, people whose stomach is infected with bacteria called *Helicobacter pylori* may have greater chances of getting stomach cancer. There is also a slight increase in risk if there is a family history of stomach cancer

What Are the Symptoms of Stomach Cancer?

People with early stomach cancers may not have symptoms. As the tumor grows, people have abdominal (belly) pain, nausea, and loss of appetite. Other complaints are abdominal bloating after eating, trouble swallowing, heartburn, weight loss, blood in stools, a mass that can be felt, fullness in the stomach after meals, and fluid in the abdomen (ascites).

How Is Stomach Cancer Diagnosed?

The only sure way to diagnose stomach cancer is with a biopsy. The doctor uses a small lighted tube (scope) passed through the mouth, down the esophagus, and into the stomach (upper endoscopy). If the doctor finds abnormal areas, a sample is taken and studied with a microscope.

Treatment depends on how far the cancer spread (its stage). For the best care, you'll want a team of specialists, including an oncologist and surgeon, in addition to your primary care doctor.

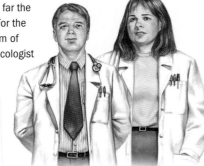

Surgery gives the only chance for cure. The part of the stomach with the cancer is removed. In this operation, a subtotal gastrectomy, up to three fourths of the stomach can be removed. The whole stomach may also be taken out.

Dashed lines show the part that may be removed depending on where the cancer is located.

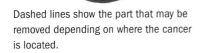

Eat a healthy diet.

Talk to your doctor if you need emotional support. Find a support group if you think that would help.

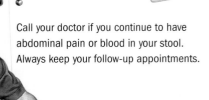

Call your doctor if you continue to have abdominal pain or blood in your stool. Always keep your follow-up appointments.

How Is Stomach Cancer Treated?

Treatment depends on how far the cancer spread (its stage). Surgery is the only chance for cure. Surgery includes complete removal of the cancer by taking out part of the stomach (subtotal gastrectomy) or near-total removal of the stomach with nearby lymph glands.

People with advanced cancer may have chemotherapy, usually a combination of different drugs. The doctor will recommend other doctors including an oncologist (specialist in cancer) be involved in care.

Radiation therapy doesn't work well for stomach cancer and may be used only to help reduce pain.

DOs and DON'Ts in Managing Stomach Cancer:

✔ **DO** tell your doctor about a family history of stomach cancer and recurrent *H. pylori* infection, which may be linked to stomach cancer.

✔ **DO** keep your follow-up doctor appointments. A team of doctors including your primary care doctor, surgeon, oncologist, and radiation oncologist will care for you.

✔ **DO** call your doctor if you have abdominal pain or blood in your stool.

✔ **DO** call your doctor if you have a fever during chemotherapy.

✔ **DO** call your doctor if you have pain or abnormal drainage around the incision after surgery.

✔ **DO** call your doctor if you need emotional support.

⊘ **DON'T** ignore stomach pain or blood in the stool. These may be signs of serious problems.

⊘ **DON'T** be afraid to ask for second opinions.

FROM THE DESK OF

NOTES

FOR MORE INFORMATION

Contact the following source:

• National Cancer Institute
Tel: (800) 422-6237
Website: http://www.cancer.gov

MANAGING YOUR
ULCERATIVE COLITIS

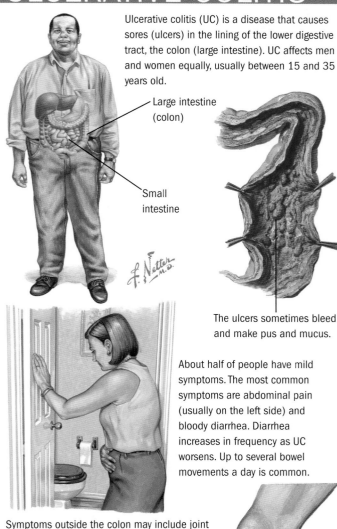

Ulcerative colitis (UC) is a disease that causes sores (ulcers) in the lining of the lower digestive tract, the colon (large intestine). UC affects men and women equally, usually between 15 and 35 years old.

Large intestine (colon)

Small intestine

The ulcers sometimes bleed and make pus and mucus.

About half of people have mild symptoms. The most common symptoms are abdominal pain (usually on the left side) and bloody diarrhea. Diarrhea increases in frequency as UC worsens. Up to several bowel movements a day is common.

Symptoms outside the colon may include joint pains, usually in knees, ankles, and wrists, and eye problems. UC can cause complications such as bleeding, bowel perforation, and abdominal infections.

Colonoscopy is done to confirm diagnosis. A lighted flexible tube (colonoscope) is put into the rectum to look at the rectum and lower colon and collect tissue samples.

Your doctor will do a physical exam and get blood and stool samples for study.

What Is Ulcerative Colitis?

Ulcerative colitis (UC) is a disease that causes sores in the lining of the digestive tract. Irritation in the lower part of the tract, the colon (large intestine), makes open sores or wounds called ulcers. These ulcers sometimes bleed and make pus and mucus. The colon also empties often, which causes diarrhea.

UC affects men and women equally and seems to run in families. About 250,000 Americans have UC. People between 15 and 35 years old are affected most often. Most people have UC for their whole lives. About half have mild symptoms. Others have more frequent, severe attacks.

What Causes UC?

The cause is unknown.

What Are the Symptoms of UC?

Most common symptoms are pain in the abdomen (belly) and bloody diarrhea with mucus. Bowel movements may relieve the pain, which is usually on the left side. As UC worsens, diarrhea increases, and several bowel movements daily is common. Periods of remission occur, but more than 75% of people have relapses.

Other symptoms include fatigue, weight loss, loss of appetite, and fever. Symptoms outside the colon include joint pains, usually in knees, ankles, and wrists. Eye problems may also occur. Complications include severe bleeding, perforation of the bowel, megacolon (dilation of the colon), and peritonitis (infection in the abdomen). People with UC also have greater chances of having colon cancer.

How Is UC Diagnosed?

The doctor will review the medical history and do a complete physical examination. The doctor will take blood and stool samples to check for bleeding and infection. UC is confirmed by colonoscopy. In this procedure, a lighted flexible tube is put into the rectum to look at the rectum and lower part of the colon. Colon tissue samples are taken and sent for study with a microscope.

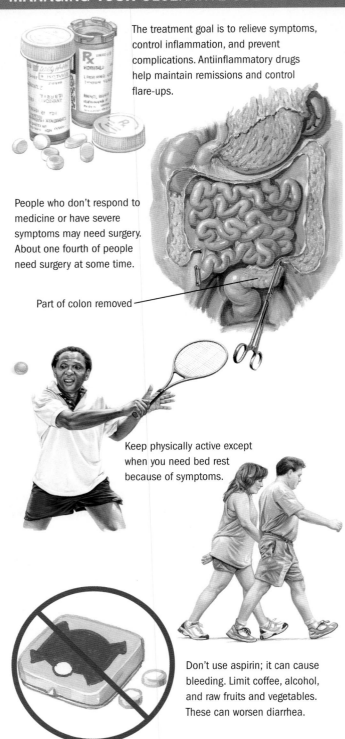

The treatment goal is to relieve symptoms, control inflammation, and prevent complications. Antiinflammatory drugs help maintain remissions and control flare-ups.

People who don't respond to medicine or have severe symptoms may need surgery. About one fourth of people need surgery at some time.

Part of colon removed

Keep physically active except when you need bed rest because of symptoms.

Don't use aspirin; it can cause bleeding. Limit coffee, alcohol, and raw fruits and vegetables. These can worsen diarrhea.

How Is UC Treated?

The goal is to relieve symptoms, control inflammation, and prevent complications.

The main medicines are antiinflammatory drugs, including mesalamine, sulfasalazine, olsalazine, and steroids. Mesalamine is used to maintain remissions and control minor to moderate symptom flare-ups. Steroids are for major flare-ups and to maintain remissions. Severe symptoms may mean hospitalization so the bowel can rest (no food by mouth), and intravenous food is given.

About one quarter of people need surgery, when medicines don't work or disease is severe. Surgery involves removing part of the colon.

DOs and DON'Ts in Managing UC:

- ✔ **DO** take medicine as prescribed.
- ✔ **DO** ask your doctor if you should take vitamins, minerals, or iron replacement.
- ✔ **DO** try to keep to normal physical activity.
- ✔ **DO** see your doctor regularly. Periodic colonoscopy is important to watch for cancerous changes.
- ✔ **DO** call your doctor if you get fever or chills, increased number of bowel movements, or increased bleeding.
- ✔ **DO** call your doctor if your abdomen becomes swollen, pain increases, or vomiting starts.

- ⊘ **DON'T** use aspirin. It increases the risk of bleeding.
- ⊘ **DON'T** drink coffee and alcohol in excess. Limit roughage (raw fruits and vegetables). These can make diarrhea worse.

FROM THE DESK OF

NOTES

FOR MORE INFORMATION

Contact the following sources:

- Crohn's and Colitis Foundation of America
  Tel: (800) 343-3637
  Website: http://www.ccfa.org

- National Digestive Diseases Information Clearinghouse
  Tel: (800) 891-5389
  Website: http://www.niddk.nih.gov/health/digest/digest.htm

Wilson's disease is a rare inherited disorder of copper metabolism. Copper is an essential metal for production of hemoglobin in red blood cells and for bone development and connective tissues. Wilson's disease causes too much copper to collect in the body. This copper gets into vital organs, mainly the liver and brain. The untreated disease is fatal.

A mutation of a gene that passes from parents to children causes the disease. Both parents must have the mutation for the child to have the disease.

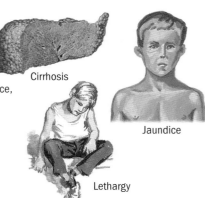

Symptoms usually start after a child is 3 years old, usually with hepatitis. Jaundice, fluid in the stomach, mental confusion, and lethargy can occur. Liver cirrhosis may also develop.

Cirrhosis

Jaundice

Lethargy

Effects on the brain lead to spastic muscle movements, tremors, trouble swallowing and speaking, and psychiatric problems (neurosis, psychosis, schizophrenia, and bipolar disorder).

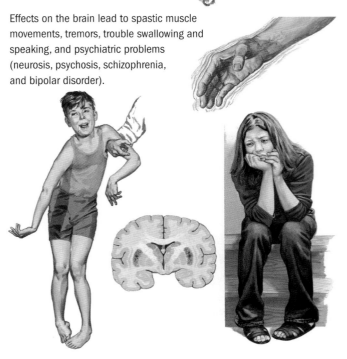

What Is Wilson's Disease?

Wilson's disease is a rare inherited disorder of copper metabolism. Copper is a metal found in small amounts in the blood. Copper plays an essential role in production of hemoglobin. Hemoglobin is a large protein molecule in red blood cells that attaches to oxygen and takes it to body tissues. Copper is also important for bone development and connective tissues.

Wilson's disease causes too much copper to collect in the body due to insufficient or defective copper excretion in the liver. The excess copper accumulates in vital organs, mainly the liver and brain. Untreated Wilson's disease is usually fatal. The disease affects 1 in 30,000 people.

What Causes Wilson's Disease?

A mutation of a gene that passes from parents to children causes the disease. The disease is autosomal recessive, which means that both parents must have the mutation and give it to a child for the child to have the disease. It's not contagious.

What Are the Symptoms of Wilson's Disease?

Symptoms don't usually start until after a child is 3 years old and may not start until the teenage years or later. Usually, the liver is affected first. Liver inflammation (hepatitis) develops and can be mistaken for hepatitis caused by a virus. Other possible symptoms are jaundice (yellow skin), fluid in the belly (ascites), mental confusion, and lethargy. Liver cirrhosis may also develop. Effects on the brain lead to spastic muscle movements, tremors, and trouble swallowing and speaking.

Copyright © 2010 by Saunders, an imprint of Elsevier, Inc.

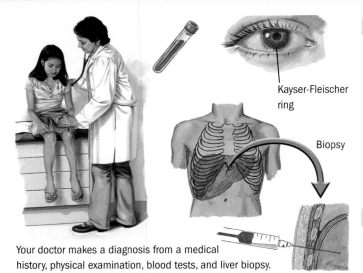

Kayser-Fleischer ring

Biopsy

Your doctor makes a diagnosis from a medical history, physical examination, blood tests, and liver biopsy. High blood ceruloplasmin and liver copper levels confirm the diagnosis. A key effect in the eye is a brownish Kayser-Fleischer ring.

Treatment goals are to remove excess copper and prevent it from reaccumulating by using medications. The chelating agents penicillamine and trientine remove the copper. Zinc acetate prevents absorption of copper from the gut. This drug shouldn't be used with penicillamine or trientine.

Keep follow-up doctor appointments. Once treatment begins, your doctor needs to watch your condition and test your blood (blood counts, liver function tests, and copper levels).

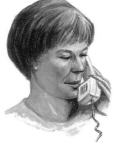

Call your doctor if you have side effects from your medicine. Don't stop taking your medicine. Treatment must continue for life. If you must stop taking it, your doctor should supervise this and can change the drug to another one.

How Is Wilson's Disease Diagnosed?

The doctor makes a diagnosis from a medical history, physical examination, blood tests, and liver biopsy. High blood ceruloplasmin and liver copper levels confirm the diagnosis. Ceruloplasmin is an oxygen-carrying protein in the blood. A key effect in the eye is a brownish color where the cornea and sclera (white part of the eye) meet, called a Kayser-Fleischer ring. Psychiatric problems may occur, including neurosis, psychosis, and bipolar disorder.

How Is Wilson's Disease Treated?

The doctor must suspect the disease in anyone younger than 40 with abnormal liver blood tests, abnormal behavior, and unexplained liver cirrhosis and nervous system symptoms. Treatment goals are to remove excess copper and prevent it from reaccumulating by using medications. Penicillamine is a chelating agent, which means a drug that binds to copper, so it can remove it. It's usually given for life. Drug side effects may include rash, fever, swollen lymph glands, kidney problems, and lower red and white blood cell counts. If penicillamine cannot be tolerated, another chelating drug called trientine can be used. Zinc acetate also helps, by preventing absorption of copper from the gut. This drug shouldn't be used with penicillamine or trientine.

DOs and DON'Ts in Managing Wilson's Disease:

✔ **DO** keep follow-up doctor appointments. Once treatment begins, your doctor needs to monitor your condition and blood tests (blood counts, liver function tests, and copper levels).

✔ **DO** call your doctor if you have side effects from your medicine.

⊘ **DON'T** stop taking the medicine. Treatment must continue for life. If you must stop taking it, your doctor should supervise this and can change the drug to another medicine.

FROM THE DESK OF

NOTES

FOR MORE INFORMATION

Contact the following source:

• Wilson's Disease Association International
Tel: (888) 264-1450
Website: http://www.wilsonsdisease.org

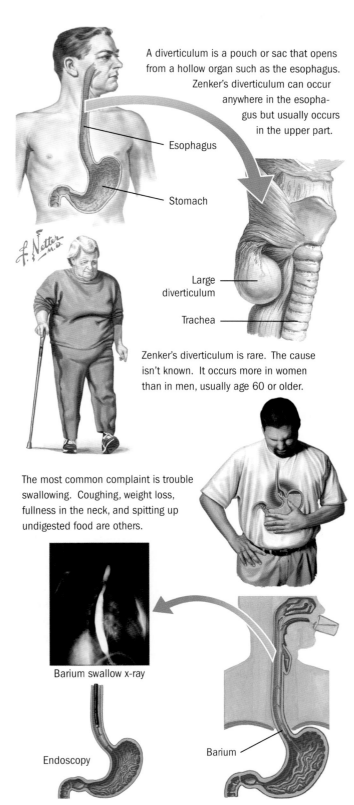

A diverticulum is a pouch or sac that opens from a hollow organ such as the esophagus. Zenker's diverticulum can occur anywhere in the esophagus but usually occurs in the upper part.

Esophagus

Stomach

Large diverticulum

Trachea

Zenker's diverticulum is rare. The cause isn't known. It occurs more in women than in men, usually age 60 or older.

The most common complaint is trouble swallowing. Coughing, weight loss, fullness in the neck, and spitting up undigested food are others.

Barium swallow x-ray

Endoscopy

Barium

Your doctor makes a diagnosis by taking a medical history and ordering a barium swallow, a kind of x-ray. Endoscopy may also be done.

What Is Zenker's Diverticulum?

A diverticulum is a pouch or sac that opens from a hollow organ such as the esophagus. The esophagus is the tube connecting the mouth with the stomach. Zenker's diverticulum can occur anywhere in the esophagus but is usually found in the upper part. The lining of the esophagus pushes backward, so food stays in the pouch.

Zenker's diverticulum is rare, occurring in less than 0.01% of the population. It's found more often in women than in men, usually those 60 years old or more.

This disorder can be associated with hiatal hernias, esophageal spasm, gastroesophageal reflux disease, and, rarely, cancer of the esophagus.

What Causes Zenker's Diverticulum?

The cause is unknown, but it may result from increased pressure in the esophagus. This pressure may occur if the esophagus doesn't relax completely when food is swallowed. The pressure leads to a tear or break (herniation) in muscle tissues lining the esophagus. The result is a diverticulum. Zenker's diverticulum isn't passed from parents to children and isn't contagious.

What Are the Symptoms of Zenker's Diverticulum?

The most common complaint is trouble swallowing (called dysphagia) solids and liquids. Coughing, bad breath (halitosis), weight loss, fullness in the neck, and spitting up undigested food are others.

An untreated diverticulum becomes larger and can lead to complications. These include food getting into lungs (aspiration), shortness of breath, fever, and pneumonia.

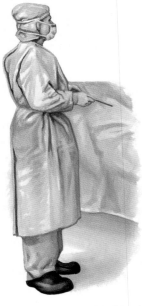

If you have symptoms, you will likely need surgery. If you have no symptoms and a small diverticulum (less than ¼ inch), your doctor may wait for symptoms to occur before doing surgery.

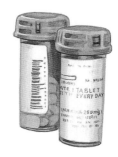

No drugs can get rid of the diverticulum. However, your doctor may prescribe medicines for heartburn, acid indigestion, or pneumonia from aspiration.

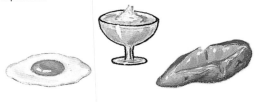

If treatment is conservative, you should eat soft foods (e.g., mashed potatoes, eggs, custards) that can be easily chewed and swallowed. Don't eat seeds, skins, or nuts.

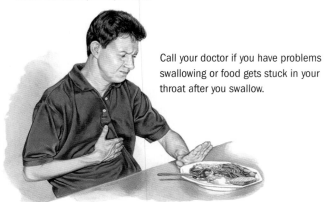

Call your doctor if you have problems swallowing or food gets stuck in your throat after you swallow.

FROM THE DESK OF

NOTES

How Is Zenker's Diverticulum Diagnosed?

The doctor makes a diagnosis by taking a medical history and ordering a barium swallow. In this test, barium contrast material is swallowed and x-rays are taken to get pictures of the esophagus.

The doctor may suggest seeing a gastroenterologist (doctor specializing in disorders of the esophagus, stomach, and intestines). The gastroenterologist may want to do a test called endoscopy. In this test, a scope with a lighted end is inserted into the mouth and passed through the esophagus into the stomach. Endoscopy helps find ulcers, abnormal tissue, and cancer in the esophagus.

How Is Zenker's Diverticulum Treated?

Surgery is the recommended treatment for people with symptoms. For people without symptoms and with a small diverticulum (less than ¼ inch), treatment may be conservative. This means that the doctor will wait for symptoms to occur before doing surgery.

Surgery helps dysphagia, cough, and aspiration in almost all people.

DOs and DON'Ts in Managing Zenker's Diverticulum:

✔ **DO** realize that Zenker's diverticulum can sometimes return after surgery (less than 4% of cases).

✔ **DO** understand that if treatment is conservative, you should eat soft foods (e.g., mashed potatoes) that can be easily chewed and swallowed.

✔ **DO** call your doctor if you have problems swallowing, develop a fever, or food gets stuck after swallowing.

✔ **DO** call your doctor if you have shortness of breath.

✔ **DO** call your doctor if you need a referral to a gastroenterologist or surgeon.

🚫 **DON'T** eat seeds, skins, or nuts. These foods can lead to retaining food in the esophagus and maybe aspirating it.

🚫 **DON'T** forget that drugs cannot get rid of the diverticulum. However, medicines may be prescribed for heartburn, acid indigestion, or pneumonia from aspiration.

FOR MORE INFORMATION

Contact the following source:
• American College of Gastroenterology
  Tel: (703) 820-7400
  Website: http://www.acg.gi.org

Women have two sweat glands in the area of the vagina called Bartholin glands. A Bartholin cyst can form when one of the sweatglands is blocked. Several different kinds of bacteria can cause infection and promote development of the cyst.

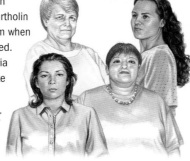

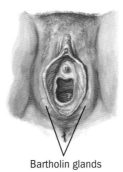

Bartholin glands

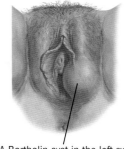

A Bartholin cyst in the left sweat gland. Cysts can be painless, unless they're infected.

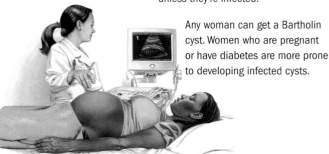

Any woman can get a Bartholin cyst. Women who are pregnant or have diabetes are more prone to developing infected cysts.

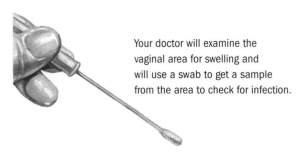

Your doctor will examine the vaginal area for swelling and will use a swab to get a sample from the area to check for infection.

Women with sexually transmitted diseases (STDs) have a greater chance of getting cysts, so blood tests to check for STDs may be done.

What Are Bartholin Cysts?

A Bartholin cyst is a swelling or bulge on one or both sides of the vagina. Cysts can form when one of the sweat glands (Bartholin glands) is blocked. Bartholin cysts that aren't infected may go away without treatment.

What Causes Bartholin Cysts?

Many times, the cause is unknown. Several different kinds of bacteria can cause infection and promote development of the cyst. Any woman can develop a Bartholin cyst. However, pregnant women or women with diabetes are more likely to develop them. Infected cysts are also more common in women who have sexually transmitted diseases or who are very sexually active.

What Are the Symptoms of Bartholin Cysts?

Main symptoms are swelling near the vagina (which can be painless) and painful swelling if a cyst becomes infected, which makes walking and having sex difficult.

How Are Bartholin Cysts Diagnosed?

The doctor will examine the vaginal area for swelling. The doctor may use a swab to get a sample to see whether an infection is present. Blood tests may be done to check for sexually transmitted infections. The doctor may suggest seeing a gynecologist (a doctor who specializes in female genital problems).

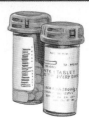

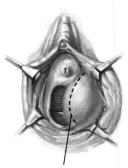

Some cysts clear up on their own. Infected cysts are treated with hot baths, applying moist heat, and taking antibiotics.

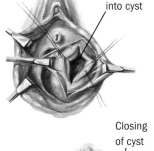

Opening into cyst

Place of cut for drainage

Closing of cyst

The goal is to make the cyst drain itself and clear the infection. If this doesn't work, your doctor may open up the cyst surgically (incision and drainage).

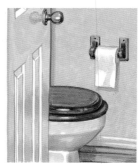

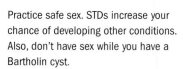

Practice good hygiene to prevent infections. After using the toilet, wipe from front to back to stop bacteria around the anus from getting to the vagina.

Condom

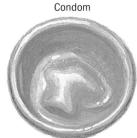

Practice safe sex. STDs increase your chance of developing other conditions. Also, don't have sex while you have a Bartholin cyst.

How Are Bartholin Cysts Treated?

The doctor may simply want regular examinations to watch the cyst. Women can do this themselves. The doctor will want a return visit in 2 to 3 months if the cyst doesn't go away or if symptoms worsen.

Infected cysts are treated with hot baths, applying moist heat, and taking antibiotics. It's important to follow the doctor's instructions exactly and take the medicine for as long as prescribed.

If these steps don't work, the doctor (or a gynecologist or surgeon) may drain the cyst. For this procedure, a small cut is made in the cyst, and stitching is done around the edge. This lets fluid drain out.

It's unusual to have a Bartholin cyst more than once. If it occurs again, surgical removal may be needed.

DOs and DON'Ts in Managing Bartholin Cysts:

✔ **DO** follow your doctor's instructions about applying heat, taking antibiotics, and returning for follow-up visits.
✔ **DO** practice good hygiene to prevent infections. After using the toilet, always wipe from the front to the back to stop bacteria around the anus from entering the vagina.
✔ **DO** practice safe sex to help prevent sexually transmitted diseases.
✔ **DO** make sure your blood sugar levels are controlled if you have diabetes.
✔ **DO** examine yourself, so that you can spot another cyst right away.
✔ **DO** call your doctor if you have fever and swollen glands in the groin.
✔ **DO** call your doctor if you have pus draining from the cyst.

⊘ **DON'T** squeeze the cyst. Squeezing may spread the infection.
⊘ **DON'T** have sex while you have a Bartholin cyst; it may be painful and worsen the infection.

FROM THE DESK OF

NOTES

FOR MORE INFORMATION

Contact the following sources:

• American College of Obstetricians and Gynecologists
Tel: (202) 638-5577
Website: http://www.acog.org

• National Women's Health Information Center
Tel: (800) 994-9662
Website: http://www.4woman.gov

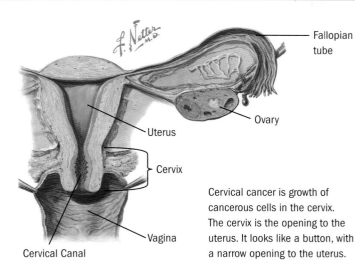

Uterus

Fallopian tube

Ovary

Cervix

Vagina

Cervical Canal

Cervical cancer is growth of cancerous cells in the cervix. The cervix is the opening to the uterus. It looks like a button, with a narrow opening to the uterus.

What Is Cervical Cancer?

The cervix is at the outer end of the uterus (womb). It looks like a button with a narrow opening that leads into the uterus. Cervical cancer is growth of malignant cells in the cervix. Finding cervical cancer early by using Pap tests has increased chances for cure.

What Causes Cervical Cancer?

Risks include having sex before age 18, having many sexual partners, smoking, using birth control pills, having a mother who took diethylstilbestrol (DES) during pregnancy, and being infected with human papillomavirus (HPV), which is a sexually transmitted disease (STD).

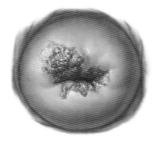

Early cervical cancer

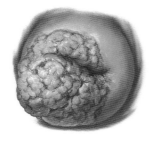

Advanced cervical cancer

What Are the Symptoms of Cervical Cancer?

Women usually have no symptoms until cancer has reached nearby tissue. The most common symptom is vaginal bleeding or bleeding after sex. Discharge from the vagina may occur. Cancer that invades nearby tissues can cause back pain, the need to urinate often, and bowel changes.

Women usually have no symptoms until the cancer spreads to nearby tissues. The most common symptom is vaginal bleeding or bleeding after sex. Later symptoms include back pain and bowel and urinary changes.

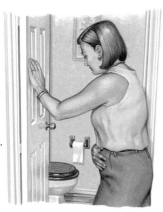

How Is Cervical Cancer Diagnosed?

Pap smears are 95% accurate in finding early cervical cancer. All women older than 20 (or younger, if sexually active) should have Pap tests, usually yearly, at least until age 65.

If a Pap smear is abnormal, the gynecologist will use colposcopy (checking the cervix with a microscope. If needed, a cone biopsy may be done. In this biopsy, a cone-shaped sample of tissue is removed for study.

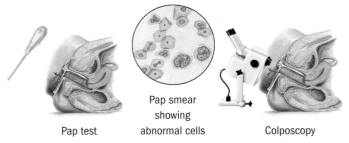

Pap test

Pap smear showing abnormal cells

Colposcopy

Pap tests are 95% accurate in finding early cervical cancer. Your gynecologist will do a colposcopy if your Pap smear is abnormal.

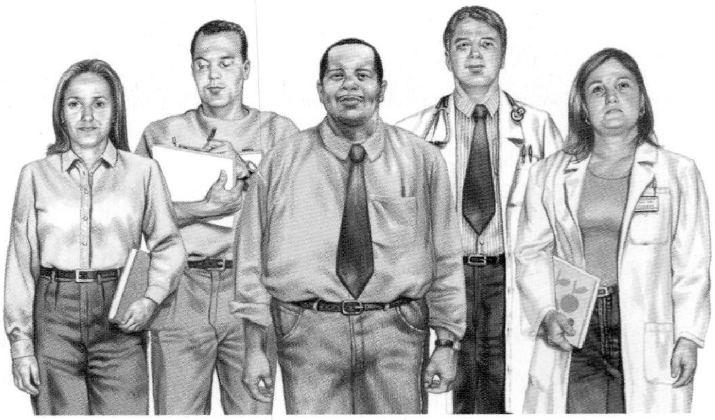

After you're diagnosed, more tests will be done to find out the cancer stage (if and where it spread). A team of doctors, including a primary care doctor, gynecologist, oncologist, and radiation oncologist, will be involved in care.

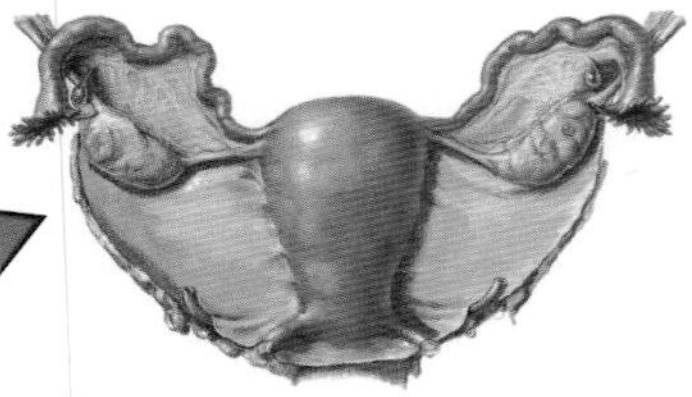

Hysterectomy is the removal of the uterus and ovaries.

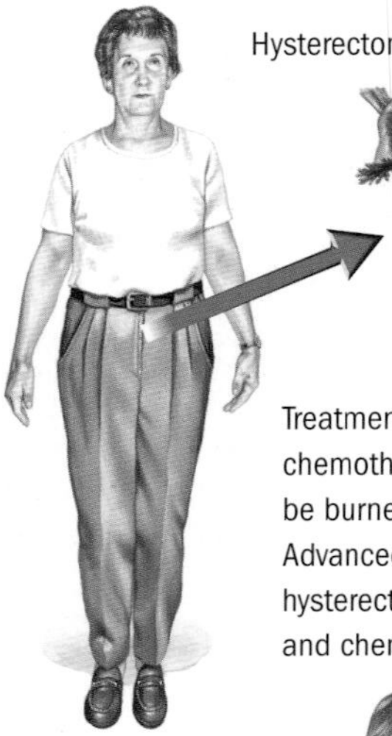

Treatment may include surgery, radiation, and chemotherapy (anticancer drugs). Early cancer can be burned away by laser, frozen, or cut out. Advanced cancer needs surgery such as hysterectomy, radiation therapy, and chemotherapy.

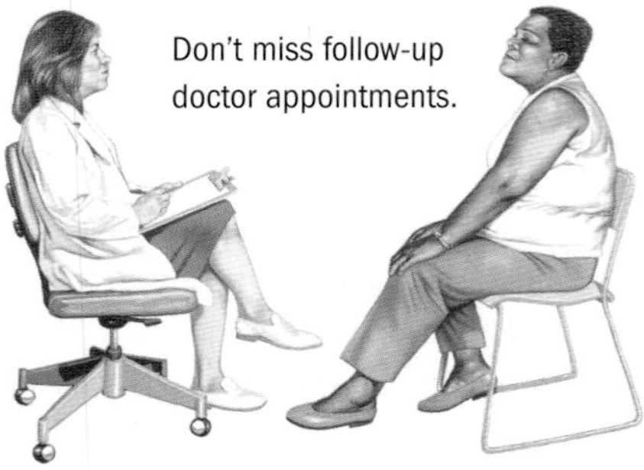

Don't miss follow-up doctor appointments.

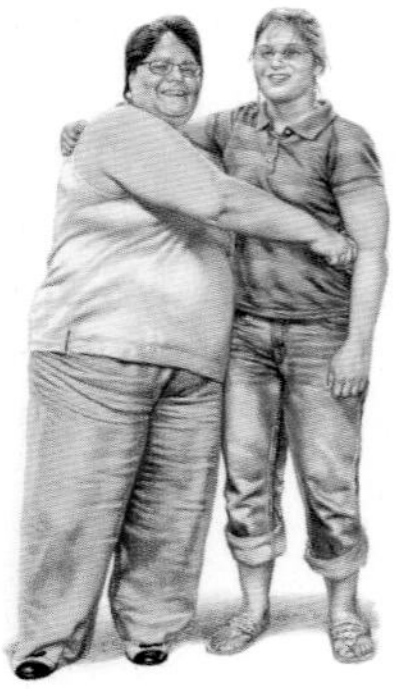

Help young girls around you reduce their risk of cervical cancer by teaching them about dangers of STDs and vaccination with HPV vaccine (Gardasil®) to reduce the risk of cervical cancer.

How Is Cervical Cancer Treated?

Treatment depends on the cancer stage. Staging means finding out whether cancer has spread, and if so, how much. Stages are numbered 0 to IV, depending on how far it has spread. A doctor uses a pelvic examination, blood and urine tests, x-rays, and computed tomography (CT) for staging. Additional tests such as cystoscopy and proctosigmoidoscopy (examinations with lighted tubes put into the bladder and rectum, respectively) may also be done.

Treatment may include surgery, radiation, and chemotherapy (anticancer drugs). Early cancer can be burned away by laser, frozen (cryotherapy), or cut out. Advanced cancer needs surgery such as hysterectomy, radiation therapy, and chemotherapy.

DOs and DON'Ts in Managing Cervical Cancer:

✔ **DO** understand that good nutrition after surgery, radiation, or chemotherapy is important.
✔ **DO** understand that a team of doctors, including a primary care doctor, gynecologist, oncologist, and radiation oncologist, can be involved in care.
✔ **DO** call your doctor if you have abnormal bleeding.
✔ **DO** call your doctor if you have pain, bowel or urinary problems, vaginal drainage, or fever after surgery.
✔ **DO** call your doctor if you have hot flashes, vaginal dryness, or vaginal pain with sex.

🚫 **DON'T** miss follow-up doctor appointments.
🚫 **DON'T** forget to stay active. Exercising daily helps you deal with the disease.
🚫 **DON'T** be afraid to ask about emotional support groups.
🚫 **DON'T** forget about social workers who can help with services such as rehabilitation, home care, finances, and transportation.

FROM THE DESK OF

NOTES

FOR MORE INFORMATION

Contact the following sources:

• National Cancer Institute (NCI)
  Tel: (800) 4-CANCER (422-6237)
  Website: http://www.cancer.gov
• American Cancer Society
  Tel: (800) ACS-2345 (227-2345)
  Website: http://www.cancer.org

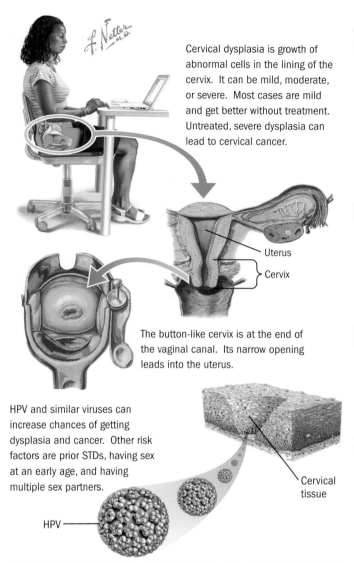

Cervical dysplasia is growth of abnormal cells in the lining of the cervix. It can be mild, moderate, or severe. Most cases are mild and get better without treatment. Untreated, severe dysplasia can lead to cervical cancer.

The button-like cervix is at the end of the vaginal canal. Its narrow opening leads into the uterus.

HPV and similar viruses can increase chances of getting dysplasia and cancer. Other risk factors are prior STDs, having sex at an early age, and having multiple sex partners.

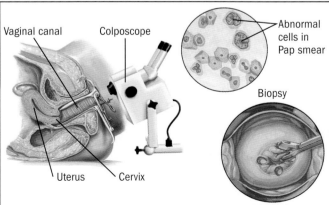

Cervical dysplasia causes no symptoms. It's usually found after an abnormal Pap smear. If a Pap smear is abnormal, your doctor will take a closer look with a colposcope. During colposcopy, your doctor takes a sample of tissue for study (biopsy).

What Is Cervical Dysplasia?

The button-like cervix is at the end of the vaginal canal. Its narrow opening leads into the uterus (womb). Cervical dysplasia, sometimes called precancerous changes or abnormal Pap smear, is growth of abnormal cells in the lining of the cervix. It can be mild, moderate, or severe. Most cases are mild and get better without treatment. Untreated, severe dysplasia can lead to cervical cancer.

What Causes Cervical Dysplasia?

Human papillomavirus (HPV), which is sexually transmitted, and similar viruses can increase chances of getting dysplasia and cancer. Other risk factors include history of STDs, having sex at a young age, and having multiple sex partners.

What Are the Symptoms of Cervical Dysplasia?

Symptoms don't occur. Cervical dysplasia is usually found by a Pap smear. Rarely, in very advanced dysplasia, abnormal bleeding occurs.

How Is Cervical Dysplasia Diagnosed?

Pap screening may show an abnormal Pap smear, but actual abnormal tissue may or may not be present. The only way to diagnose this condition is to do an office procedure called colposcopy. The doctor checks the cervix closely with a colposcope. This tool is a large microscope that magnifies the view of the cervix. If colposcopy shows an abnormal-looking area, the doctor does a biopsy. In a biopsy, the doctor removes a small piece of the cervical tissue without anesthesia. A sharp pinch or cramp is felt, only for a moment. The tissue is sent to a laboratory to see whether dysplasia is present and whether it's mild, moderate, or severe.

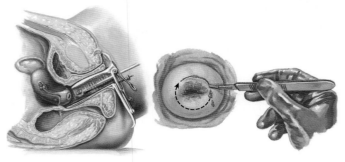

The most common ways to remove the abnormal tissue are loop cone biopsy (shown here) and freezing the abnormal cervical cells. These procedures are quick, are done in the doctor's office, and don't cause much discomfort.

Vaccination

Get vaccinated with HPV vaccine (Gardasil®). It works for HPV types 6, 11, 16, and 18 and minimizes the risk of cervical cancer from HPV.

Pap smear

Keep your follow-up doctor appointments. It's better to treat cervical dysplasia early, and cervical dysplasia can come back. Get regular Pap smears.

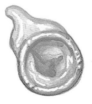

Practice safe sex. Use condoms. Protecting yourself from sexually transmitted diseases, especially HPV, can reduce your risk of getting cervical dysplasia agian.

How Is Cervical Dysplasia Treated?

The most common method is the loop cone biopsy. The doctor does this procedure in the office with local anesthesia. It's very successful. After the procedure, women may have mild cramping for 1 to 2 days afterward and increased vaginal discharge for 1 to 2 weeks.

Cryosurgery, or freezing the cervix, is also used. When the cervix is frozen, abnormal tissue dies and falls off. Women usually have mild-to-moderate cramping after this office procedure. Vaginal discharge usually increases for 2 to 4 weeks afterward.

DOs and DON'Ts in Managing Cervical Dysplasia:

✔ **DO** keep your follow-up doctor appointments. It's better to treat cervical dysplasia early.

✔ **DO** practice safe sex. Protecting yourself from sexually transmitted diseases, especially HPV, can reduce your risk of getting cervical dysplasia.

✔ **DO** use latex condoms when having sex, especially if your partner has had multiple sex partners.

✔ **DO** call your doctor if your bleeding lasts longer than a week after a cervical biopsy.

✔ **DO** call your doctor if you have more bleeding or vaginal discharge than expected after a loop cone biopsy.

✔ **DO** call your doctor if you have fever after a loop cone biopsy.

✔ **DO** get vaccinated with HPV vaccine (Gardasil®), which is for females 13 to 26 years old. It works for HPV types 6, 11, 16, and 18. It minimizes the risk of cervical cancer from HPV.

✔ **DO** get regular Pap smears.

⊘ **DON'T** miss follow-up doctor appointments if you had a cone biopsy or you were told that you have dysplasia. Cervical dysplasia can come back, so it's very important to have follow-up Pap smears and colposcopy.

FROM THE DESK OF

NOTES

MANAGING YOUR
CERVICAL POLYPS

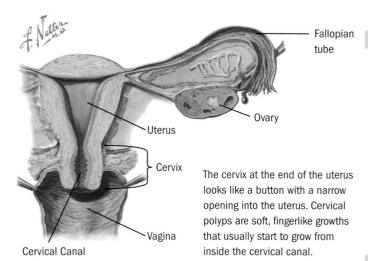

The cervix at the end of the uterus looks like a button with a narrow opening into the uterus. Cervical polyps are soft, fingerlike growths that usually start to grow from inside the cervical canal.

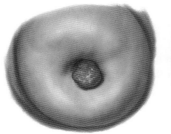

Small polyp

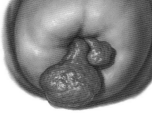

Small and large polyps

An inflammation causes the polyps, but the reason for the inflammation isn't known. Polyps don't usually cause pain or other symptoms but may sometimes cause abnormal spotting or bleeding.

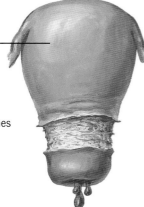

Bleeding through cervix

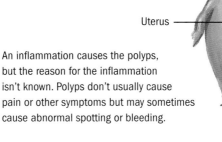

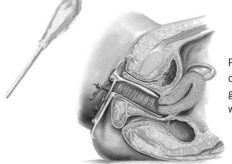

Polyps are often found during a routine gynecologic examination when a Pap test is done.

What Are Cervical Polyps?

The cervix is at the end of the uterus (womb). It looks like a button with a narrow opening that leads into the uterus. Cervical polyps are soft, fingerlike growths of tissue that usually start to grow from inside the cervical canal (entrance to the uterus). They hang from a stalk and often push through the opening.

Cervical polyps are common, especially in women older than 20 who have had children. Almost all are benign (not cancerous). They aren't contagious and seldom grow back. No specific ways to prevent them are known.

What Causes Cervical Polyps?

Cervical polyps are believed to grow because of inflammation. The reason for the inflammation isn't known, but cervical infections are suspected.

What Are the Symptoms of Cervical Polyps?

Many polyps don't cause symptoms. Sometimes a polyp will cause abnormal spotting or bleeding after sex or heavier bleeding during periods. An abnormal discharge from the vagina may also be seen. Polyps don't cause pain or discomfort.

How Are Cervical Polyps Diagnosed?

Polyps are often found during a routine gynecologic examination when a Pap test is done.

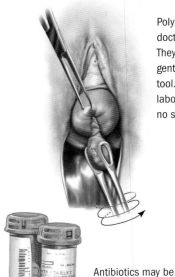

Polyps are easily removed in the doctor's office, without anesthesia. They're simply held and twisted off gently or taken off with a biopsy tool. They're then sent to the laboratory to make sure that there's no sign of cancer.

Antibiotics may be prescribed because many polyps are infected.

Call your doctor if you have pain the pelvic area or bleeding after menopause, between periods, or after sex.

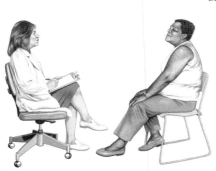

Visit your gynecologist each year. Like polyps, some other conditions don't cause symptoms, so your annual checkup is important to make sure that you're healthy.

How Are Cervical Polyps Treated?

Cervical polyps are easily removed in the doctor's office. No anesthesia or pain medicine is needed. The polyp is simply held and twisted off gently or taken off with a special tool called a biopsy instrument. The procedure only takes a few minutes and usually is painless. It may sometimes cause mild cramping. The polyp is sent to the laboratory for study, to make sure that there's no sign of cancer or any precancerous abnormality.

DOs and DON'Ts in Managing Cervical Polyps:

✔ **DO** keep your doctor's appointment to have the polyp removed. Even though the vast majority of polyps are benign (not cancerous), cancerous polyps do sometimes occur.

✔ **DO** continue your usual daily activities after the polyps are removed but avoid sexual intercourse and use of tampons until the follow-up visit with your doctor.

✔ **DO** call your doctor if you have vaginal bleeding after menopause (change of life), between periods, or after you have resumed sex.

✔ **DO** call your doctor if you have pain in the pelvic area.

✔ **DO** call your doctor if you have long or unusually heavy periods.

🚫 **DON'T** have sex until the polyp is removed if you've had bleeding after sex and were diagnosed with a polyp.

FROM THE DESK OF

NOTES

FOR MORE INFORMATION

Contact the following source:

• American College of Obstetricians and Gynecologists
Tel: (202) 638-5577
Website: http://www.acog.org

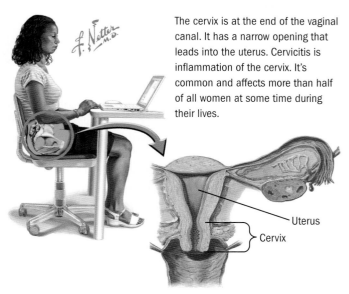

The cervix is at the end of the vaginal canal. It has a narrow opening that leads into the uterus. Cervicitis is inflammation of the cervix. It's common and affects more than half of all women at some time during their lives.

Uterus

Cervix

What Is Cervicitis?

The button-like cervix is at the end of the vaginal canal. It has a narrow opening that leads into the uterus (womb). Cervicitis is inflammation of the cervix. It's common and will affect more than half of all women at some time during their lives.

What Causes Cervicitis?

Causes include infections such as gonorrhea, chlamydia, and trichomoniasis (infection with the parasite *Trichomonas vaginalis*). Infections with viruses such as herpes simplex virus or human papillomavirus (HPV), the virus that causes genital warts, can also cause cervicitis. Bacteria such as staphylococcus and streptococcus are other causes. Sometimes a foreign body such as an intrauterine device (IUD) or a forgotten tampon, diaphragm, or pessary can lead to cervicitis. Risk factors include being younger than 25 years old, being single, having many sex partners, and having a history of sexually transmitted disease.

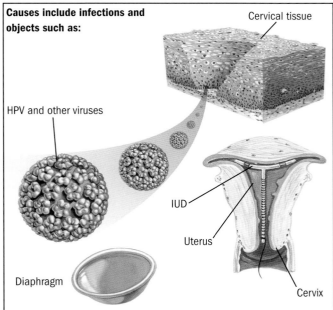

Causes include infections and objects such as:

Cervical tissue

HPV and other viruses

IUD

Uterus

Diaphragm

Cervix

What Are the Symptoms of Cervicitis?

Cervicitis may not cause symptoms and may be found only during a routine gynecological examination. Some women can have increased yellow or cream-colored vaginal discharge. Also, very slight vaginal bleeding may occur, as a pinkish or brownish discharge. Pain in the vagina or during sex may occur.

If cervicitis is caused by chlamydia or gonorrhea and the infection spreads to fallopian tubes, pelvic pain and infertility can result. Itching, irritation, and increased vaginal discharge can occur if *Trichomonas* is the cause. Herpes simplex virus may cause symptoms only if the infection is outside the body, on the vulva.

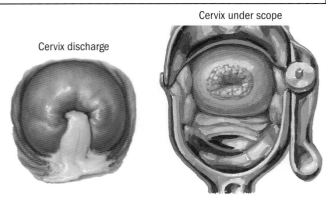

Cervix under scope

Cervix discharge

Women may have no symptoms, or they may have increased yellow or cream-colored vaginal discharge or very slight vaginal bleeding.

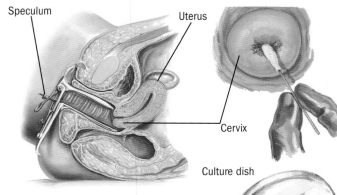

Speculum

Uterus

Cervix

Culture dish

Your doctor makes a diagnosis from a pelvic examination, cultures of the vaginal discharge, and blood tests to check for infections.

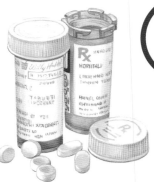

Treatment depends on the cause. Cervicitis caused by bacteria or *Trichomonas* needs antibiotics. Viral infections can't be cured, but medicines can make them less severe. Don't drink alcohol if taking metronidazole. You could have severe nausea.

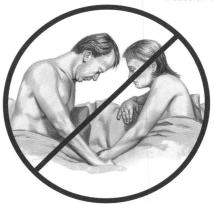

Avoid sex until you finish the antibiotic treatment and your vaginal discharge has stopped.

Protect yourself from STDs by using condoms.

How Is Cervicitis Diagnosed?

The doctor makes a diagnosis from a pelvic examination, cultures of the vaginal discharge, and blood tests to check for infections.

How Is Cervicitis Treated?

Treatment depends on the cause. Cervicitis caused by chlamydia, gonorrhea, or *Trichomonas* needs antibiotics. Taking antibiotics can make it more likely that a yeast infection will develop because the antibiotic kills healthy, protective bacteria, so yeast can grow.

Viral infections causing cervicitis cannot be cured, but antiviral medicines can make them less severe and shorten the duration of symptoms.

DOs and DON'Ts in Managing Cervicitis:

✔ **DO** take all your medicines as prescribed, even if your symptoms go away.

✔ **DO** protect yourself from sexually transmitted diseases such as gonorrhea, chlamydia, *Trichomonas*, herpes, and human immunodeficiency virus (HIV) and HPV infections. Know your partner. Use condoms.

✔ **DO** avoid sex until you finish the antibiotic treatment and your vaginal discharge has stopped.

✔ **DO** avoid douches or vaginal sprays. They can irritate the cervix.

✔ **DO** have regular Pap smears.

✔ **DO** call your doctor if you continue to have symptoms, such as vaginal discharge or bleeding, after you finish taking your medicine.

✔ **DO** call your doctor if you get a fever or pelvic pain while you're taking medicine.

✔ **DO** call your doctor if you cannot tolerate the medicine (e.g., you have nausea), or you have allergic symptoms (e.g., you get a rash).

⊘ **DON'T** drink alcoholic beverages if you're taking metronidazole for *Trichomonas* infection. Combining metronidazole and alcohol can cause severe nausea.

FROM THE DESK OF

NOTES

FOR MORE INFORMATION

Contact the following source:

• American College of Obstetricians and Gynecologists
  Tel: (202) 638-5577
  Website: http://www.acog.org

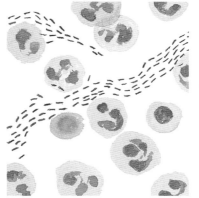

Haemophilus ducreyi

Chancroid is a sexually transmitted disease (STD) that causes painful ulcers involving skin of the genital area. It's very contagious but curable. The kind of bacteria named *Haemophilus ducreyi* causes the infection. It's transmitted by direct contact with open lesions.

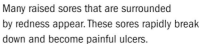

Many raised sores that are surrounded by redness appear. These sores rapidly break down and become painful ulcers.

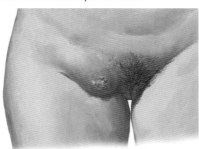

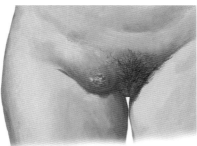

Lymph nodes in the groin may get large on one side. Fever, headache, chills, and fatigue are other symptoms.

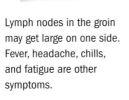

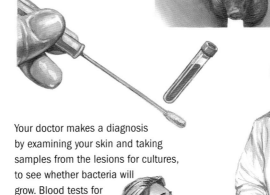

Your doctor makes a diagnosis by examining your skin and taking samples from the lesions for cultures, to see whether bacteria will grow. Blood tests for other STDs will be done. Your sexual contacts should also be tested.

What Is Chancroid?

Chancroid is a sexually transmitted disease (STD) that causes painful ulcers involving skin of the genital area. It's very contagious but curable.

Chancroid is rare in the United States but common in other parts of the world. Most people in the United States with chancroid have traveled to countries where it more commonly occurs.

What Causes Chancroid?

A kind of bacteria named *Haemophilus ducreyi* causes chancroid, which is spread by direct contact with open sores.

What Are the Symptoms of Chancroid?

Symptoms appear 4 to 7 days after exposure. Many raised sores that have red skin around them appear. These sores rapidly break down and become painful ulcers. Women most often have ulcers on the outer part of the vagina. Lymph glands (nodes) on one side of the groin area, in the fold between the leg and lower abdomen (belly), may get larger. Fever, headache, chills, and fatigue may occur. Women may have no obvious signs of infection, but the most common symptoms they have are pain with urination and with sex.

How Is Chancroid Diagnosed?

The doctor makes a diagnosis by examining the skin and taking samples of the lesions for culture (to see whether the bacteria will grow).

The doctor will test blood for other STDs. Sexual contacts should also be tested.

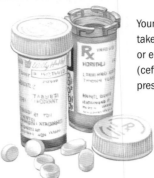

Your doctor will prescribe antibiotics to be taken by mouth (azithromycin, ciprofloxacin, or erythromycin) or to be given by injection (ceftriaxone). Pain medicine may also be prescribed.

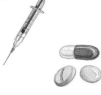

Wash the infected areas with soap and water three times a day and dry thoroughly.

Avoid sexual relations until an examination by your doctor shows that it's safe.

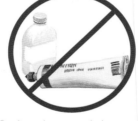

Don't apply creams, lotions, or oils on or near the lesions.

Call your doctor right away if you have painful blisters or sores on or near the genitals or a fever.

How Is Chancroid Treated?

The doctor will prescribe antibiotics to be taken by mouth (azithromycin, ciprofloxacin, or erythromycin) or to be given by one injection (ceftriaxone). Pain medicine may also be prescribed. Lesions should be washed three times a day with soap and water and kept dry. No creams, lotions, or oils should be used on or near the sores, because they increase the chance of spreading the lesions. Sexual relations should be avoided until a follow-up examination shows complete healing, which usually occurs in 2 to 3 weeks.

DOs and DON'Ts in Managing Chancroid:

✔ **DO** take your prescribed antibiotics until they're gone.

✔ **DO** take pain medicine if needed.

✔ **DO** wash infected areas with soap and water three times a day and dry completely.

✔ **DO** tell your sexual contacts about your infection so that they can get treatment.

✔ **DO** avoid sexual relations until an examination by your doctor shows that it is safe to do so. Avoid STDs by using condoms during sex.

✔ **DO** get tested for other STDs.

✔ **DO** call your doctor if you still have a fever after you finish your antibiotics.

✔ **DO** call your doctor if over-the-counter pain medicine doesn't help your pain.

✔ **DO** call your doctor if any lesion appears infected.

⊘ **DON'T** skip doses or stop taking your antibiotics before they're finished, even if you feel better.

⊘ **DON'T** put creams, lotions, or oils on or near the lesions.

⊘ **DON'T** have sexual relations until your doctor says you can.

FROM THE DESK OF

NOTES

FOR MORE INFORMATION

Contact the following sources:

• Centers for Disease Control and Prevention
National Center for HIV/AIDS, Viral, Hepatitis, STD, and TB Prevention
Website: http://www.cdc.gov/std

• American Social Health Association
STI Resource Center Hotline: (800) 227-8922
Website: http://www.ashastd.org

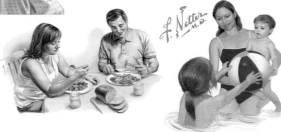

A number of contraceptive methods are available. Each person (or couple) should choose a method that fits with your lifestyle, frequency of sex, and personal preference. You will likely use different forms of contraception over your lifetime.

What Is Contraception?

Contraception is prevention of pregnancy by any method.

How Pregnancy Occurs

Each month, approximately 2 weeks after a woman bleeds (menstrual period), the ovary releases an egg (called ovulation). The egg travels to the fallopian tube, which connects to the uterus. If sex occurs near the time of ovulation and the man ejaculates (climaxes), sperm are released into the vagina. Sperm travel through the opening of the uterus (cervix) into the uterus and then into fallopian tubes. If a sperm fertilizes the egg, pregnancy occurs.

Options include:

Birth Control Pills

- Most common method used
- Very effective when taken as directed (one pill every day at same time)
- Do *not* protect against STDs

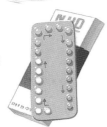

How Pregnancy Can Be Prevented

Pregnancy can be prevented in three ways: stop ovulation, stop sperm from getting to eggs in the fallopian tube, and change the uterine lining (endometrium) so it won't support pregnancy.

Pills

Birth control pills, the most common method, contain hormones similar to ovarian hormones and stop ovulation. Pills plus smoking, high blood pressure, obesity, or family history of clotting disorders may lead to increased chance of stroke, heart attack, or blood clots.

Implants and Injections

- Implants, a newer method, use capsules containing hormone placed under the skin on the arm
- For injections, contraceptive containing progesterone is injected every 3 months

Implants

Implants are capsules containing a certain hormone that are surgically placed under the skin on the arm.

Progesterone Injections

A contraceptive containing only the hormone progesterone is injected every 3 months and stops ovulation.

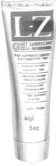

Condoms

- Placed on penis before sex to prevent sperm from entering the vagina
- Should use with spermicide
- Help reduce risk of contracting STDs

Barriers

Condoms, diaphragms, and cervical caps are barriers that stop sperm from getting to the egg. All should be used with a spermicide (chemical that kills sperm).

A condom is a thin rubber or animal membrane covering that is put on the penis. A rubber, dome-shaped diaphragm is put in the vagina over the cervix. A cervical cap (small rubber cap) fits right on the cervix. It works like the diaphragm but is smaller.

Diaphragms

- Placed into vaginal canal over the cervix before sex
- Should use with spermicide
- Do *not* prevent STDs

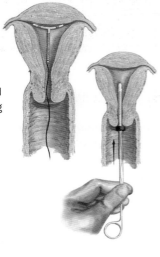

IUD

- Inserted and removed by doctor
- Replaced every year
- Alters the lining of your uterus and makes it hard for the fertilized egg to attach to the uterine wall
- Not for women who haven't had children, because they increase chances of pelvic infection

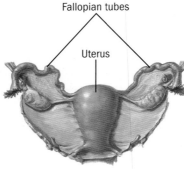

Fallopian tubes

Uterus

Tubal Ligation

- Permanent method, because in many cases it cannot be reversed
- Fallopian tubes are sealed by burning (cauterized) or closed by a clip so sperm cannot get to eggs

Vasectomy

- Permanent method because in many cases it cannot be reversed
- Tubes in the scrotum (vas deferens) are tied off so sperm cannot become part of ejaculate fluid

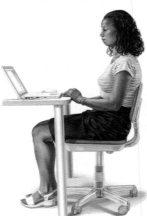

When deciding on birth control, remember to think of STDs too! Does your method of birth control prevent STDs? If not, consider another one or double up!

Intrauterine Devices (IUDs)

IUDs are small devices inserted into the uterus by a doctor. They change the uterus or fallopian tube so pregnancy cannot occur. The Copper T is a small T-shaped plastic IUD with wrapping of copper. Another IUD produces progesterone.

Permanent Surgical Methods

The two methods are tubal ligation (tying the tubes) in a woman and vasectomy in a man. A tubal ligation is done by special (laparoscopic) surgery. Very small cuts are made and fallopian tubes are sealed or closed. In vasectomy, which is minor surgery, tubes called vas deferens in the scrotum are tied off.

Abstinence (Rhythm) Method

Not having sex around the time of ovulation prevents pregnancy. This method works only if the woman has regular cycles. It is not recommended for young women whose cycles are still changing.

How Do You Choose a Contraception?

Some couples may use more than one form of birth control. Things to think about when choosing a method include how each is used, age, health, frequency of sex, and partner's feelings about methods.

DOs and DON'Ts in Deciding About Contraception:

- ✔ **DO** think about protection from sexually transmitted diseases (STDs) when choosing a method. Certain methods prevent both pregnancy and STDs.
- ✔ **DO** try a new method if you don't like your current one.
- ✔ **DO** talk with your partner to figure out the best method
- ✔ **DO** talk with your doctor about the benefits and risks of your chosen methods.

- ⊘ **DON'T** assume that your partner is taking care of it.

FROM THE DESK OF

NOTES

FOR MORE INFORMATION

Contact the following sources:

- American College of Obstetricians and Gynecologists
  Tel: (202) 638-5577
  Website: http://www.acog.org
- WebMD
  Website: http://www.webmd.com

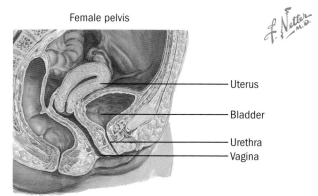

Female pelvis

- Uterus
- Bladder
- Urethra
- Vagina

Cystitis is inflammation of the bladder. The top of the urethra also becomes inflamed. It's much more common in women, but men can also have it. Sometimes, cystitis can become chronic and hard to treat.

The cause is often an infection, usually with bacteria (named *Escherichia coli*). Other causes are friction during sex, tight underwear, catheters, and irritants such as feminine hygiene spray and spermicidal jelly.

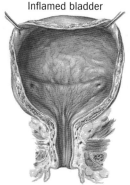

Inflamed bladder

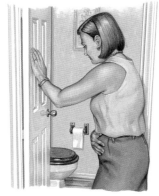

Symptoms include pain or burning when urinating, pain or pressure in the lower abdomen, cloudy or fishy-smelling urine, blood in the urine, and need to urinate often.

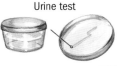

Urine test

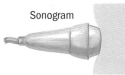

Sonogram

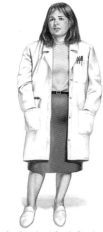

Your doctor will take a sample of urine and have it checked for infection. If you get infections often, your doctor may want a sonogram of the bladder and kidneys. A urologist may do more tests such as cystoscopy.

What Is Cystitis?

Cystitis is a condition in which the bladder becomes inflamed (red and swollen). The top of the urethra (the tube that takes urine from the bladder to outside the body) also becomes inflamed. It's much more common in women, but men can also have it. Sometimes, cystitis can become chronic (occur over and over) and become hard to treat.

What Causes Cystitis?

The cause is most often an infection, usually with bacteria (named *Escherichia coli*). Other causes are friction during sex, wearing tight underwear, drugs, foreign bodies such as catheters, and irritants such as feminine hygiene spray and spermicidal jelly. Cystitis can be a complication of another illness, and pregnant women can have greater chances of having cystitis.

What Are the Symptoms of Cystitis?

Common symptoms include pain or burning when urinating, pain or pressure in the lower abdomen (belly), cloudy or fishy-smelling urine, blood in the urine, frequent and urgent need to urinate, and low-grade fever.

How Is Cystitis Diagnosed?

The doctor will take a sample of urine and send it to a laboratory to check for infection.

If infections occur often, the doctor may want a sonogram of the bladder and kidneys and may suggest seeing a urologist (doctor specializing in urinary disorders). The urologist may do more tests, such as cystoscopy. In cystoscopy, a small flexible tube is put into the urethra and then the bladder. The tube has a camera so the doctor can see inside the urethra and bladder.

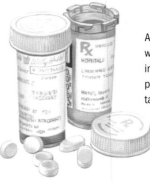

Antibiotic medicine, usually as pills, will be prescribed to stop the bacterial infection. Typically the pills are prescribed for 3 to 10 days; always take medicine as prescribed by doctor.

Drink plenty of fluids, especially water.

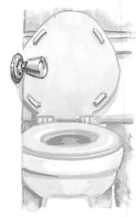

Follow good hygiene: empty your bladder completely when urinating. Urinate right after having sex. Wipe from front to back after a bowel movement.

Call your doctor if you develop a fever or if symptoms continue even with taking antibiotics.

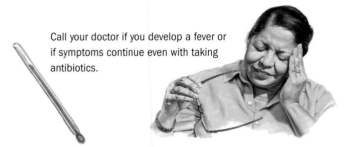

How Is Cystitis Treated?

Antibiotic medicine, usually as pills, will be prescribed to stop a bacterial infection. The pills are taken for 3 to 10 days. The doctor may want to do another examination after 1 to 2 weeks, or earlier, to make sure that the infection is gone. If infections occur often, medicine may be needed for up to 6 months.

Causes other than infections need other treatments, including avoiding certain products, such as bubble bath and spermicides, nerve stimulation, and other drugs.

DOs and DON'Ts in Managing Cystitis:

✔ **DO** take your medicine exactly as prescribed.
✔ **DO** drink plenty of fluids, especially water.
✔ **DO** empty your bladder completely when urinating.
✔ **DO** urinate right after having sex.
✔ **DO** wear cotton clothing. Women should wear cotton pantyhose. Avoid tight-fitting undergarments and clothing.
✔ **DO** keep your genital area clean. Take showers instead of tub baths.
✔ **DO** avoid perfumed or deodorant products in the genital area.
✔ **DO** keep other medical conditions under control. For example, if you have diabetes, keep your blood sugar under control.
✔ **DO** call your doctor if you develop a fever or if symptoms continue even with antibiotics.
✔ **DO** wipe from front to back after a bowel movement.

⊘ **DON'T** wear tight-fitting undergarments and clothing.
⊘ **DON'T** ignore symptoms. Untreated infection can spread to the kidneys and cause serious illness.

FROM THE DESK OF

NOTES

FOR MORE INFORMATION

Contact the following source:

• Interstitial Cystitis Association
Tel: (301) 610-5300, (800) 435-7422
Website: http://www.ichelp.org

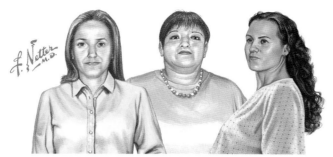

An ectopic pregnancy is one that develops outside the uterus. It is a medical emergency for the mother.

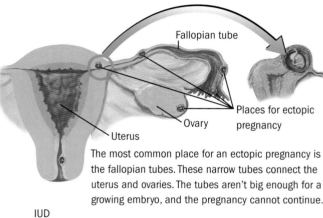

The most common place for an ectopic pregnancy is the fallopian tubes. These narrow tubes connect the uterus and ovaries. The tubes aren't big enough for a growing embryo, and the pregnancy cannot continue.

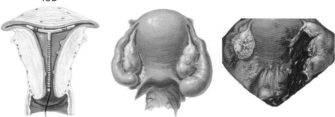

Most often, fallopian tubes are blocked or too narrow, so the egg cannot get to the uterus from the ovary. Usually, an infection called PID causes the blocked or narrowed tubes. Using an IUD for birth control and endometriosis are other causes.

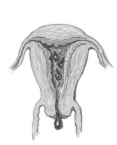

Symptoms include abnormal vaginal bleeding, often after a missed period; sharp pain or cramping in the lower abdomen; dizziness or fainting; and an abdomen that's tender to touch.

What Is an Ectopic Pregnancy?

An ectopic pregnancy is one that develops outside the uterus. The most common place for it is the fallopian tubes, so it's also called a tubal pregnancy. These narrow tubes connect the uterus and ovaries. In a normal pregnancy, the fertilized egg travels through fallopian tubes to the uterus.

Fallopian tubes aren't big enough for a growing embryo, and the pregnancy cannot continue normally. If the pregnancy continues, the tube will stretch and burst. This situation is an emergency. It's life-threatening for the mother.

Less often, an ectopic pregnancy develops in an ovary, the cervix, or the abdomen (belly).

What Causes an Ectopic Pregnancy?

Most often, fallopian tubes are blocked or too narrow, so the egg can't get to the uterus from the ovary. Usually, an infection called pelvic inflammatory disease (PID) causes the blocked or narrow tubes. Other risk factors are having an ectopic pregnancy before, surgery on the fallopian tubes or uterus, using an intrauterine device (IUD) for birth control, and endometriosis. Endometriosis is inflammation caused by the presence of the lining of the uterus outside the uterus.

What Are the Symptoms of an Ectopic Pregnancy?

Symptoms include abnormal bleeding from the vagina, often after a missed period; sharp pain or cramping in the lower abdomen; dizziness or fainting; and an abdomen that is tender to touch.

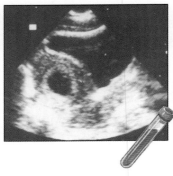

Diagnosis can be difficult because symptoms are often similar to a regular pregnancy. Your doctor will do a pregnancy test (through blood test) to confirm pregnancy. Your doctor may order an ultrasound scan of your abdomen. An ultrasound scan lets the doctor see your uterus and ovaries and whether you have an ectopic pregnancy.

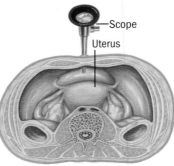

Scope

Uterus

Laparoscopy

Your doctor may also want to do a laparoscopy in the hospital with anesthesia. A scope with an attached light is put into your abdomen and lets the doctor see inside your body. If your doctor finds an ectopic pregnancy, it can be removed.

If the embryo is very small, a drug (methotrexate) can be used to end the pregnancy. However, major surgery may be needed to open the fallopian tube, remove the embryo, and stitch the tube closed. If the tube can't be fixed, it will be removed.

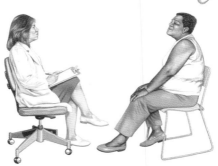

Talk to your doctor about future pregnancies and counseling.

How Is an Ectopic Pregnancy Diagnosed?

An ectopic pregnancy can be hard to diagnose because symptoms are at first like those of a regular pregnancy. The doctor first does a pregnancy test. The best one is a blood test, so the doctor will take a blood sample from a vein.

The doctor may also order ultrasonography of the abdomen. Ultrasonography is similar to an x-ray, because it lets the doctor see the uterus and ovaries inside the body. The doctor may also want to do laparoscopy, done in the hospital with anesthesia. An instrument with a light attached is put into the abdomen for a very close look at the organs. An ectopic pregnancy can be removed at the same time.

How Is an Ectopic Pregnancy Treated?

If the embryo is very small, a drug (methotrexate) can be used to end the pregnancy. The embryo can sometimes be flushed out of the tube by salpingostomy. In this procedure, the tube is surgically opened, so high-pressure fluid can flush out the embryo.

Surgery is often needed and may be a laparoscopy. In a laparoscopy, a very small abdominal cut is made. The fallopian tube is opened, the embryo is removed, and the tube is stitched closed. If the tube cannot be fixed, it's also removed.

For a ruptured fallopian tube, emergency surgery is done, and the tube is almost always removed.

DOs and DON'Ts in Managing Ectopic Pregnancy:

✔ **DO** avoid using an IUD for birth control.
✔ **DO** treat vaginal or pelvic infections right away.
✔ **DO** remember that having one ectopic pregnancy puts you at risk for having others in the future.

🚫 **DON'T** have many sexual partners, have sex without condoms, or get sexually transmitted diseases—all risk factors for PID.

FROM THE DESK OF

NOTES

FOR MORE INFORMATION

Contact the following source:

• National Women's Health Information Center
  Tel: (800) 994-9662
  Website: http//www.4woman.gov

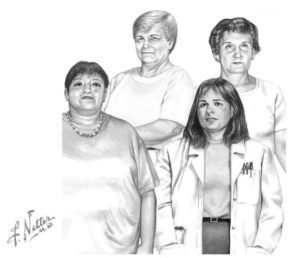

Endometrial cancer usually occurs in women between the ages of 55 and 70 after menopause. In the United States, about 300,000 new cases are diagnosed each year.

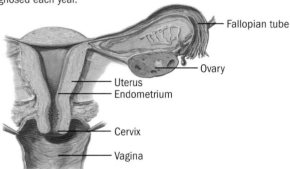

The inner layer of your uterus is called the endometrium. The reason cancer cells grow in the endometrium is unknown.

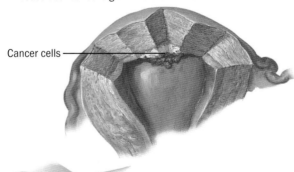

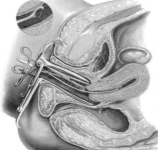

To confirm the diagnosis, your doctor will do a dilation and curettage (D&C), meaning opening and scraping. In the D&C, your doctor removes a tissue sample for study under a microscope.

What Is Endometrial Cancer?

The uterus, or womb, lies between the bladder and rectum. The inner layer of the uterus is the endometrium. Endometrial cancer is cancer of this layer.

Untreated endometrial cancer spreads and causes problems in the pelvic area, including bowel and urinary disorders. If the spread continues, swollen glands (lymph nodes), an abdominal (belly) mass, and eventually liver, lung, and bone disease can result.

More than 30,000 new cases cancer are diagnosed each year in the United States.

What Causes Endometrial Cancer?

The cause is unknown. It usually occurs in women between 55 and 70 years old, but can occur in younger women before they go through menopause. Women at increased risk are overweight, have diabetes, have never been pregnant or given birth, or took estrogen for effects of menopause.

What Are the Symptoms of Endometrial Cancer?

Bleeding from the vagina after menopause is the main symptom. For women who haven't gone through menopause, abnormal vaginal bleeding—heavy bleeding, minimal bleeding, bleeding between menstrual cycles—is the main symptom.

How Is Endometrial Cancer Diagnosed?

The doctor will ask about symptoms and do a physical examination, including a pelvic examination. Vaginal ultrasonography may also be done.

To confirm the diagnosis, the doctor may take a biopsy specimen from the uterus by dilation and curettage (D&C). To do this, the cervix is dilated (widened) and a curette (a small spoon-shaped instrument) is inserted into the uterus to remove tissue.

The cancer is then classified into stages. Staging tells whether and how much the cancer spread. Stage I means tumor is only in the uterus; stage II, tumor invaded the cervix; stage III, tumor involved the vagina, ovary, or abdomen; and stage IV, tumor invaded the bladder and intestine. Blood tests, chest x-rays, and computed tomography (CT) of the abdomen and pelvis are studied to look for cancer spread.

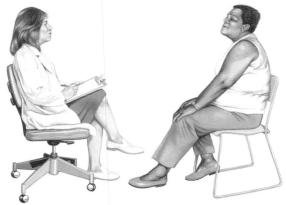

Your doctor will discuss treatment options with you. Treatment depends on how far the cancer has advanced. Tumors are classified as stage I, II, III, or IV. Most endometrial cancers are diagnosed in early stages—I or II.

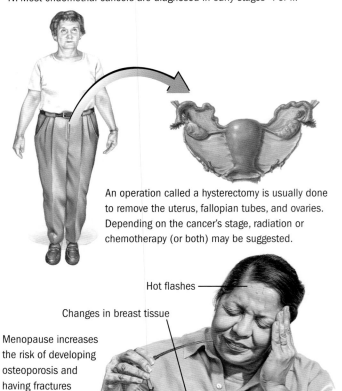

An operation called a hysterectomy is usually done to remove the uterus, fallopian tubes, and ovaries. Depending on the cancer's stage, radiation or chemotherapy (or both) may be suggested.

Hot flashes

Changes in breast tissue

Menopause increases the risk of developing osteoporosis and having fractures (e.g., in the wrist).

If you haven't yet gone through menopause, symptoms will start after surgery because the ovaries are removed. Talk to your doctor and other women about what you can expect and for support.

FROM THE DESK OF

NOTES

How Is Endometrial Cancer Treated?

Surgery, radiation, hormones, and chemotherapy are used for treatment, which depends on the cancer's stage. Most endometrial cancers are diagnosed in early stages (I or II), and an operation to remove the uterus, fallopian tubes, and ovaries (hysterectomy and bilateral salpingo-oophorectomy) is usually suggested. Radiation may then be given if needed. Both surgery and radiation have side effects.

Hormones or chemotherapy may be recommended for cancer that has spread or returned after other treatment. Both these treatments also have side effects.

DOs and DON'Ts in Managing Endometrial Cancer:

✔ **DO** remember that hysterectomy doesn't affect sexual intercourse and desire.
✔ **DO** remember you won't have periods. You can have hot flashes, sweating, and other symptoms if your ovaries are surgically removed or hurt by radiation.
✔ **DO** keep follow-up doctor visits during and after treatment to watch for treatment responses or cancer recurrence.
✔ **DO** call your doctor if you have vaginal bleeding or abnormal vaginal discharge.
✔ **DO** ask your doctor about services and support groups for emotional support.
✔ **DO** call your doctor if you have treatment side effects.

⊘ **DON'T** ignore vaginal bleeding after menopause.
⊘ **DON'T** ignore abnormal vaginal bleeding (excess, between periods) before menopause.

FOR MORE INFORMATION

Contact the following sources:

• American Cancer Society
Tel: (800) 227-2345
Website: http://www.cancer.org

• American College of Obstetricians and Gynecologists
Tel: (202) 638-5577
Website: http://www.acog.org

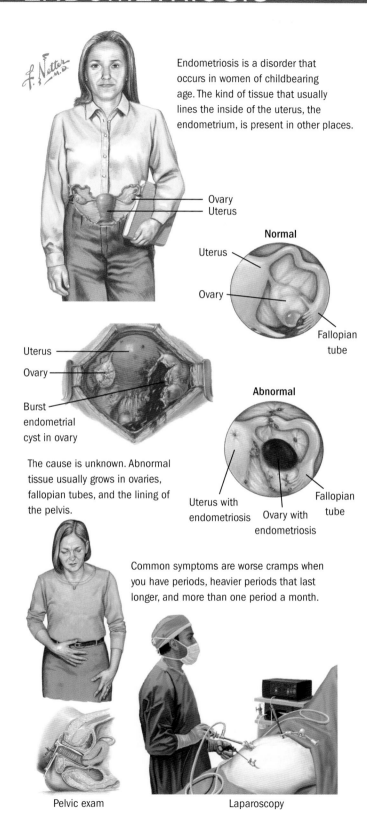

Endometriosis is a disorder that occurs in women of childbearing age. The kind of tissue that usually lines the inside of the uterus, the endometrium, is present in other places.

Ovary
Uterus

Normal
Uterus
Ovary
Fallopian tube

Uterus
Ovary
Burst endometrial cyst in ovary

Abnormal
Uterus with endometriosis
Ovary with endometriosis
Fallopian tube

The cause is unknown. Abnormal tissue usually grows in ovaries, fallopian tubes, and the lining of the pelvis.

Common symptoms are worse cramps when you have periods, heavier periods that last longer, and more than one period a month.

Pelvic exam   Laparoscopy

Your doctor will do a pelvic examination for diagnosis, but only laparoscopy can prove the presence of extra tissue.

What Is Endometriosis?

The uterus (womb) is between the bladder and rectum. The inner layer of the uterus is the endometrium. In the disorder endometriosis, the kind of tissue that usually lines the inside of the uterus is present in other places. The most common places are ovaries, fallopian tubes, and lining of the pelvis (peritoneum), especially behind the uterus.

Hormones that affect the uterine lining also affect the extra tissue. Each month, during a period, this extra lining also bleeds, which causes pain. This blood can't go anywhere, so cysts and scar tissue form.

About 5% to 15% of women of childbearing age get endometriosis. It can be managed but not prevented.

What Causes Endometriosis?

The cause is unknown. It may run in families. Scar tissue from endometriosis around pelvic organs can cause pain and infertility by blocking fallopian tubes. This scar tissue can sometimes block the intestines (bowel) or ureters (tubes that connect kidneys and bladder).

What Are the Symptoms of Endometriosis?

Endometriosis may cause no symptoms and be found only because of abdominal or pelvic surgery for something else. Symptoms include abdominal (belly) cramps during periods that are worse than normal, dull constant pain in the lower abdomen and back, pain during sex or bowel movements, a period more than once a month, heavier periods that last longer than usual, and trouble getting pregnant.

How Is Endometriosis Diagnosed?

The doctor will do a pelvic examination and a pregnancy test. The doctor may also do blood and urine tests to see if infection may be causing symptoms. Ultrasound, CT, or MRI may also be done to show organs inside the body. However, laparoscopy is the only way to have a definite diagnosis. In this operation, a telescope-like tool is put through a small cut into the abdomen to see the extra tissue. Laparoscopy can also be used as treatment. Biopsy samples (small pieces of tissue) may be taken for the diagnosis.

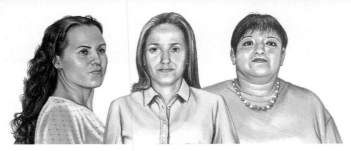

Endometriosis can be treated effectively in many ways. Your treatment depends on how bad your symptoms are, how old you are, and if you want to get pregnant.

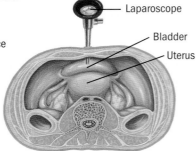

Birth control pills and other hormone pills can help symptoms. Ibuprofen or similar drugs can relieve painful periods.

Laparoscopic surgery can reduce pain and improve chances of getting pregnant. Tissue is removed through small cuts made in the abdomen.

- Laparoscope
- Bladder
- Uterus

Cross-section of abdomen

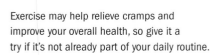

Exercise may help relieve cramps and improve your overall health, so give it a try if it's not already part of your daily routine.

FROM THE DESK OF

NOTES

How Is Endometriosis Treated?

The treatment chosen depends on symptoms, the woman's age, and if children are wanted.

Medicines work well. Pills for pain include nonsteroidal antiinflammatory drugs (NSAIDs) such as ibuprofen. Birth control pills or other hormones can help relieve symptoms.

In laparoscopic surgery, another treatment, the doctor can remove some endometriosis tissue by cauterizing (burning) or using a laser. Endometriosis can return, but this surgery may reduce pain and help chances of getting pregnant.

Surgery to remove the uterus and ovaries (total hysterectomy) is done only if the woman is older and doesn't want to have more children.

Problems can continue until menopause (change of life) and estrogen levels fall. At that time, lower levels of this hormone won't stimulate endometriosis.

DOs and DON'Ts in Managing Endometriosis:

✔ **DO** take pills as instructed by your doctor.
✔ **DO** see your doctor regularly.
✔ **DO** exercise and take ibuprofen or similar drugs to help relieve painful periods and cramps.
✔ **DO** call your doctor if treatment isn't helping symptoms.
✔ **DO** call your doctor if you cannot take your medicine or birth control pills.

⊘ **DON'T** forget to keep follow-up doctor appointments.
⊘ **DON'T** take herbal therapies without checking with your doctor.

FOR MORE INFORMATION

Contact the following sources:

- National Women's Health Information Center
  Tel: (800) 994-9662
  Website: http://www.4woman.gov

- American Society of Reproductive Medicine
  Tel: (205) 978-5000
  Website: http://www.asrm.org

- American College of Obstetricians and Gynecologists
  Tel: (202) 638-5577
  Website: http://www.acog.org

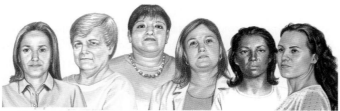

About 40% of women have sexual dysfunction at some time in their lives. Sexual dysfunction means any disorder that interferes with sexuality and causes marked distress. The four types of disorders are desire, arousal, orgasm, and sexual pain. Symptoms include loss of desire, painful sex, and difficulty achieving orgasms.

Female sexual dysfunction has many causes, including:

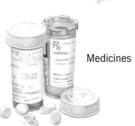

Recovering from pregnancy

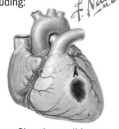

Chronic conditions such as heart disease

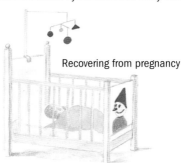

Medicines

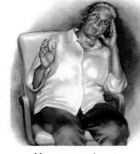

Menopause changes

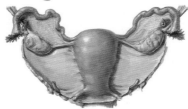

Gynecologic conditions

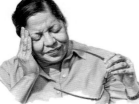

Depression

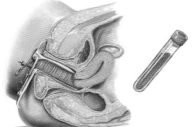

Your doctor will ask about your medical history and examine you (including a pelvic exam) to find the cause. Blood tests may also be done to rule out other factors.

What Is Female Sexual Dysfunction?

Female sexual dysfunction refers to any disorder that interferes with sexuality and causes marked distress in that woman. These disorders can usually be divided into four types: disorders of desire, disorders of arousal, disorders of orgasm, and disorders related to sexual pain.

What Causes Female Sexual Dysfunction?

The more common of the many causes are chronic medical conditions, such as diabetes, heart disease, arthritis, and urinary disorders. Drugs such as antidepressants and blood pressure medicines can interfere with orgasm. Also, gynecologic and hormonal conditions, such as after pregnancy, after menopause, and cancer of the cervix, uterus, or breast, can lead to dysfunction. Possible psychological issues include religion, taboos, guilt, relationship problems, abuse or rape, depression, and stress.

What Are the Symptoms of Female Sexual Dysfunction?

Symptoms include loss of desire, painful sex, no orgasms, feeling guilt or shame, depression, anxiety, and insomnia.

How Is Female Sexual Dysfunction Diagnosed?

The doctor will make a diagnosis on the basis of a medical history and physical examination (including a pelvic exam). Blood tests may be done to rule out factors such as diabetes and thyroid problems.

The doctor may suggest seeing a gynecologist for conditions that can be treated with surgery, a psychologist or psychiatrist if emotional issues are causing the dysfunction, and social services for issues of abuse.

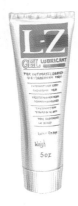

Treatment depends on the cause. Nonpetroleum lubricant and estrogen creams help with painful sex caused by vaginal dryness, seen often in women after menopause.

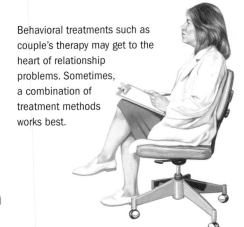

Behavioral treatments such as couple's therapy may get to the heart of relationship problems. Sometimes, a combination of treatment methods works best.

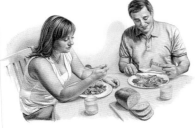

If a medicine is the cause, your doctor may suggest a change in dose or using another drug.

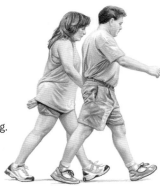

Talk to your partner about what you feel, both emotionally and physically, so you can work together to solve the problem. Get counseling if you need it.

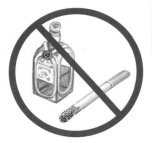

Follow a healthy lifestyle. Start exercising. Take time for fun and relaxation. Don't smoke, and don't abuse alcohol.

How Is Female Sexual Dysfunction Treated?

Treatment depends on the cause. If a medicine is the cause, a change in dose or to another drug may be suggested. Women who have gone through menopause (change of life) and have painful intercourse because of dryness of the vagina can use lubricants (not petroleum-based) and estrogen creams. Women with severe arthritis may change positions used during sex and try naproxen or ibuprofen before sex. Education, psychotherapy, and activities for better stimulation and changing routines also usually help.

Behavioral treatments such as couple's therapy can often get to the heart of relationship problems. Sometimes, a combination of treatment methods works best.

DOs and DON'Ts in Managing Female Sexual Dysfunction:

✔ **DO** talk and listen to your partner. Be open and honest.

✔ **DO** follow a healthy lifestyle. Start exercising. Take time for fun and relaxation.

✔ **DO** exercise your pelvic floor muscles (Kegel exercises) to strengthen them. This can help with some arousal and orgasm problems. To do these exercises, tighten your pelvic muscles as if you're stopping the stream of urine. Hold for a count of five, relax, and repeat.

✔ **DO** get counseling if needed. Your doctor can refer you to a sex therapist or counselor specializing in sexual and relationship problems.

✔ **DO** learn more about your body and how it works. Talk to your doctor about how many things can affect sex. These include medicines, illnesses, surgery, age, pregnancy, and menopause.

✔ **DO** remember that many things together make the sexual response work. These factors include emotions, experiences, beliefs, lifestyle, and relationships. Problems with any one of these can affect sexual arousal or satisfaction.

⊘ **DON'T** abuse alcohol.
⊘ **DON'T** smoke.

FROM THE DESK OF

NOTES

FOR MORE INFORMATION

Contact the following sources:

• American College of Obstetricians and Gynecologists
Tel: (202) 638-5577
Website: http://www.acog.org

• American Psychiatric Association
Tel: (888) 357-7924
Website: http://www.psych.org

MANAGING YOUR
FIBROCYSTIC BREAST CHANGES

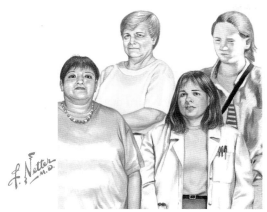

About 60% to 75% of women have changes in fibrous tissues of their breast. It's most common in women 30 to 50 years old.

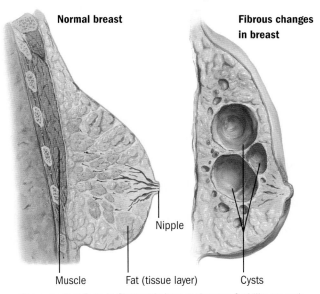

Normal breast

Fibrous changes in breast

Nipple

Muscle

Fat (tissue layer)

Cysts

The cysts that form in fibrocystic breast changes feel like smooth, firm, movable lumps.

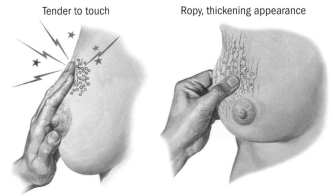

Tender to touch

Ropy, thickening appearance

Half of women don't have symptoms. Symptoms that do occur can be mild to severe and include a feeling of fullness, with dull, heavy pain and tenderness. Breast tissue can also feel dense and lumpy, as if it contains pebbles.

What Are Fibrocystic Breast Changes?

The newer term fibrocystic breast changes refers to many different conditions and includes older names such as fibrocystic breast disease. It's the most common benign (noncancerous) breast condition. The breast tissue forms cysts (sacs filled with fluid), which feel like smooth, firm, movable lumps. These changes also lead to thickening throughout the breast, pain, and tenderness. The cysts may spread through the breast, be in one area, or appear as one or more large lumps.

About 60% to 75% of all women will have changes in fibrous tissue in their breasts. Fibrocystic changes occur most often in women 30 to 50 years old. Only 10% of women younger than 21 are affected.

What Causes Fibrocystic Breast Changes?

The cause isn't clear, but hormones made by the ovaries may be important. Also, they usually stop after menopause (change of life).

What Are the Symptoms of Fibrocystic Breast Changes?

Symptoms can be mild to severe. Almost half of women have no symptoms. Most common symptoms are cyclic general pain and swelling in both breasts, with the worst symptoms just before periods. Breasts feel full, with dull, heavy pain and tenderness to pressure or touch. Breast tissue is dense and feels lumpy, as if it contains pebbles. A ropy thickening, especially in the upper outer parts of the breast, may also be present.

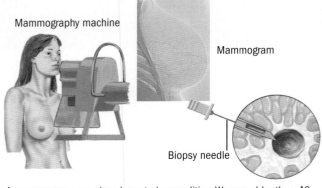

A mammogram can show breast abnormalities. Women older than 40 should have a regular mammogram, every 1 to 2 years. Your doctor may do a biopsy to rule out other conditions.

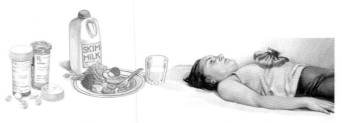

Wearing a well-fitting bra, heat or cold compresses, and over-the-counter pain relievers may help discomfort. Avoiding caffeine (coffee, tea, cola, chocolate) and eating a low-fat diet also help control the condition.

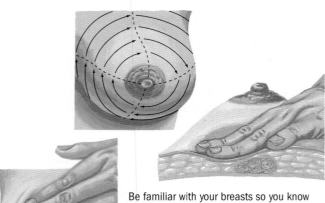

Be familiar with your breasts so you know when something changes. Do a monthly breast self-exam. Use finger pads to check the breast, in circles, firmly, carefully, and thoroughly. Feel for unusual lumps under the skin. Do this both standing and lying down.

FROM THE DESK OF

NOTES

How Are Fibrocystic Breast Changes Diagnosed?

The doctor makes a diagnosis on the basis of symptoms and examination. The doctor will order mammography and ultrasound examinations. Rarely, a biopsy may be needed to make sure that no other conditions are present.

How Are Fibrocystic Breast Changes Treated?

Good support (a well-fitting bra worn day and night) and pain relievers such as acetaminophen and nonsteroidal anti-inflammatory drugs (NSAIDs) are all that's needed by most women. Other things that may help include avoiding caffeine (coffee, tea, cola, chocolate), lowering fat in the diet, using heat (heating pad or hot water bottle), and taking vitamins and herbal preparations. Cold compresses or ice may also work. A monthly breast self-examination is important.

The doctor may prescribe stronger pain relievers, diuretics, or hormones (such as birth control pills) for severe symptoms. Sometimes, the doctor may treat cysts in the office by a method called aspiration, done with a needle. The needle removes the fluid, which will make the lump disappear. If it doesn't go away completely, a biopsy may be needed to rule out cancer.

DOs and DON'Ts in Managing Fibrocystic Breast Changes:

✔ **DO** become familiar with the normal feel of your breasts by monthly breast self-examinations.
✔ **DO** contact your doctor if you have changes in symptoms or feel something different during your self-examination.
✔ **DO** wear a well-fitting support bra, especially during exercise or vigorous activity.

⊘ **DON'T** use too much caffeine.
⊘ **DON'T** skip mammograms or other routine breast health care.

FOR MORE INFORMATION

Contact the following sources:

• American College of Obstetricians and Gynecologists
Tel: (202) 638-5577
Website: http://www.acog.org

• WebMD
Website: http://www.webmd.com

• American Cancer Society
Website: http://www.cancer.org

• Susan G. Komen Breast Cancer Foundation
Website: http://www.komen.org

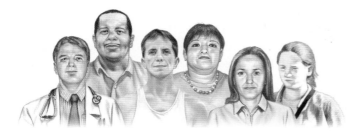

Genital herpes is a very contagious infection, and most people become infected through sex. There is no cure for genital herpes and breakouts vary from person to person.

Types of herpes simplex virus

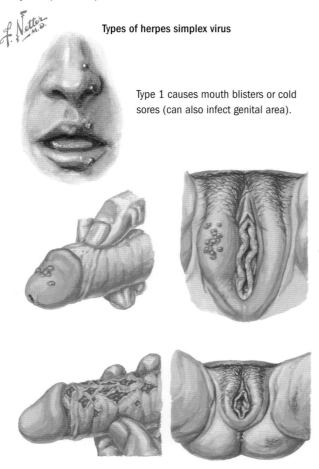

Type 1 causes mouth blisters or cold sores (can also infect genital area).

Type 2 causes lesions the in genital area. Condoms are not 100% protective against infection because lesions can break out on buttocks and thighs.

What Is Genital Herpes?

Genital herpes is a very contagious infection caused by the herpes simplex virus, or HSV. There are two types of HSV, type 1 and type 2. Type 1 usually causes mouth blisters or cold sores but can also infect the genital area. Type 2 causes most genital herpes cases.

How Is Genital Herpes Transmitted?

Most people get genital herpes from having sex with someone who is infected. The virus settles in a nerve in the body and remains there permanently. Condoms are not a complete barrier because the virus and lesions can also be on thighs and buttocks.

What Are the Symptoms of Genital Herpes?

Many people never have symptoms and don't know that they have herpes until the first outbreak. Symptoms of a first outbreak may include pain and itching in the lip or genital area. Sometimes, during a first outbreak, there may be a feeling of pressure in the abdomen, discharge from the vagina, headache, fever, and difficulty urinating. The first outbreak is the longest and most painful. It may last several days.

HSV starts as small red bumps, which develop into blisters. These blisters become painful open sores. After several days, the sores crust and in time disappear completely. About 50% of people who have a first outbreak of herpes will have more blisters. These outbreaks are usually milder and shorter and usually end in 7 to 10 days. Symptoms vary, so some people may have only one or two outbreaks in a lifetime, but others may have several per year. The cause of repeated outbreaks is unclear. Emotional stress, fatigue, illness, and menstruation may trigger them. As time goes on, the number of outbreaks usually decreases.

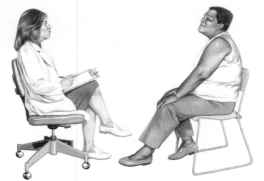

Your doctor will ask you about your sexual history and do a physical exam.

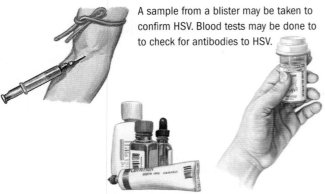

A sample from a blister may be taken to confirm HSV. Blood tests may be done to to check for antibodies to HSV.

Treatment includes use of antiviral drugs, acetaminophen, and topical medicines

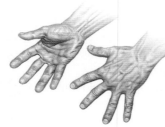

Wash your hands thoroughly after touching a sore to avoid spreading it to another part of your body or another person. You should always avoid touching sores.

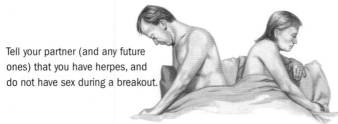

Tell your partner (and any future ones) that you have herpes, and do not have sex during a breakout.

How Is Genital Herpes Diagnosed?

The doctor usually makes a diagnosis from a physical examination. The doctor asks questions about symptoms and sexual activity.

Sometimes a sample may be taken from the blisters and sent to a laboratory to confirm that HSV is in the blister or to rule out other illnesses. A blood test can be done to check for antibodies to HSV, which indicate a current or past infection.

How Is Genital Herpes Treated?

No cure exists at this time. Antiviral drugs including acyclovir, famciclovir, and valacyclovir can be prescribed to shorten and prevent outbreaks. The antiviral medicines may be taken at the beginning of symptoms or daily to help prevent frequent outbreaks.

Over-the-counter pain medicine, such as acetaminophen or topical preparations, can be used to relieve discomfort.

DOs and DON'Ts in Managing Genital Herpes:

✔ **DO** take medication as directed.
✔ **DO** keep the infected area clean and dry.
✔ **DO** avoid touching the sores. If you touch them, wash your hands immediately to avoid spreading the infection to another part of your body or to someone else.
✔ **DO** tell sexual partners if you have symptoms for the first time.

⊘ **DON'T** pick at the sores. This may cause them to become infected.
⊘ **DON'T** allow the sores to be in direct contact with another person.
⊘ **DON'T** have sex during an outbreak to avoid infecting your partner.

FROM THE DESK OF

NOTES

FOR MORE INFORMATION

Contact the following sources:

- National Herpes Resource Center
  Tel: (919) 361-8400
  Website: http://www.ashastd.org

- American Academy of Dermatology
  Tel: (847) 330-0030
  Website: http://www.aad.org

Gestational diabetes (GD) is a common condition affecting 1 in 20 pregnant women. Gestational means during pregnancy. Diabetes causes high blood sugar (glucose) levels that can harm pregnancy. GD usually goes away after you give birth.

Insulin is a hormone, made by the pancreas, that helps break down sugar. Some hormones produced by pregnant women block insulin's effect, so more insulin than normal is needed.

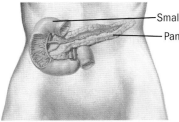

— Small intestine
— Pancreas

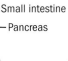

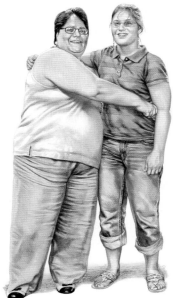

Symptoms include thirst and hunger. These may occur in any pregnancy, so you may not suspect anything unusual. Risk factors of developing GD include being overweight, having family members with diabetes, and being older than 35.

A simple test will give your blood sugar levels. Every pregnant woman should have her blood sugar level checked, by the doctor or by using a kit at home.

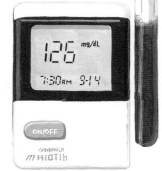

What Is Gestational Diabetes?

Diabetes is a condition in which blood glucose (sugar) levels are too high. Gestational means during pregnancy, so gestational diabetes (GD) occurs when diabetes is first found during pregnancy. GD usually goes away after the birth of the child. However, some women develop diabetes or prediabetes (impaired glucose tolerance) after delivery.

GD is common. About 1 in 20 pregnant women have it. It can cause problems in babies such as a higher birth weight (leading to a cesarean, or C-section, delivery), damage during birth (e.g., to shoulders), breathing problems, low blood sugar levels after birth, and higher risk of obesity and diabetes in later life. For women, GD increases the chance of getting preeclampsia late in pregnancy.

What Causes GD?

GD develops when women cannot make enough insulin. Insulin is a hormone that helps the body to break down sugar for energy. Without enough insulin, blood sugar levels rise and diabetes occurs. Certain hormones produced by women during pregnancy block insulin's effect, so more insulin than normal is needed.

What Are the Symptoms of GD?

GD has no clear symptoms. Pregnant women without GD may also have symptoms such as greater thirst, need to urinate, and hunger.

Women at greatest risk include those with diabetic family members, who are overweight or older than 35, or who already gave birth to a large baby, a baby born with an abnormality, or a stillbirth (dead baby). Also, women who had GD in another pregnancy or are Hispanic, African American, Native American, or Pacific Islander have a greater risk.

How Is GD Diagnosed?

It's hard to rely on symptoms to diagnose GD, so blood sugar levels should be tested during pregnancy, especially in high-risk women. If tests show high levels, the doctor will do frequent blood sugar tests for the rest of the pregnancy. Also, testing blood sugar levels at home will help monitor the condition.

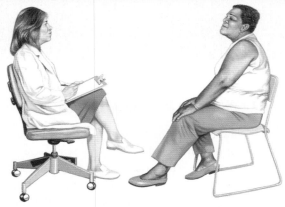

If you have GD, having your blood sugar level checked will be part of your regular pregnancy checkup. Special meals, moderate exercise, and insulin shots help keep blood sugar levels normal. Your doctor will discuss these plans with you.

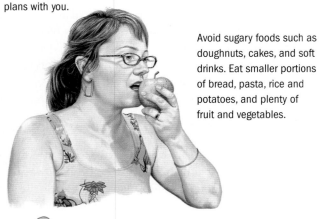

Avoid sugary foods such as doughnuts, cakes, and soft drinks. Eat smaller portions of bread, pasta, rice and potatoes, and plenty of fruit and vegetables.

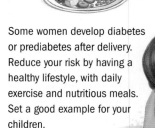

Some women develop diabetes or prediabetes after delivery. Reduce your risk by having a healthy lifestyle, with daily exercise and nutritious meals. Set a good example for your children.

FROM THE DESK OF

NOTES

How Is GD Treated?

Treatment is aimed at keeping blood sugar in the normal range. Special meal plans, moderate exercise, regular (e.g., daily) blood sugar testing, and insulin injections will do this.

DOs and DON'Ts in Managing GD:

✔ **DO** follow your doctor's advice about when to test blood sugar. It's important to check it after delivery.

✔ **DO** take insulin as prescribed.

✔ **DO** avoid sugary foods such as cakes, biscuits, and soft drinks.

✔ **DO** limit bread, pasta, rice and potatoes to smaller portions, and eat plenty of fruit and vegetables.

✔ **DO** regular moderate exercise such as walking.

✔ **DO** keep a snack handy if you are taking insulin. Test your blood sugar if you start to feel dizzy, faint, or tired.

✔ **DO** understand that GD will probably go away after birth.

🚫 **DON'T** eat high-fat foods such as butter, cream, fatty meat, burgers, and sausages.

🚫 **DON'T** cook your food with fat or oil. Try grilling, steaming, or microwaving.

🚫 **DON'T** skip meals when you're hungry.

🚫 **DON'T** get too tired when exercising. Stop if you feel tired, dizzy, faint, or very hungry.

FOR MORE INFORMATION

Contact the following sources:

• National Institute of Child Health and Human Development
Tel: (800) 370-2943
Website: http://www.nichd.nih.gov

• American Diabetes Association
Tel: (800) 342-2383
Website: http://www.diabetes.org

• National Institute of Diabetes and Digestive and Kidney Diseases
Tel: (800) 860-8747
Website: http://www.niddk.nih.gov/health/diabetes/ndic.htm

• American Dietetic Association
Tel: (800) 877-1600
Website: http://www.eatright.org

MANAGING YOUR
GRANULOMA INGUINALE

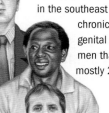

Granuloma inguinale is an STD that's common in tropical and developing countries. It also occurs more frequently in the southeast United States. It's a chronic infection affecting genital and groin areas. More men than women have it, mostly 20 to 40 years old.

The cause is the bacterium named *Calymmatobacterium granulomatis.*

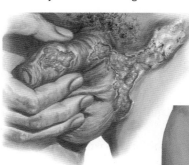

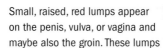

Small, raised, red lumps appear on the penis, vulva, or vagina and maybe also the groin. These lumps are first painless, but then they grow bigger and become ulcers. The area becomes dark red and may form large scars.

Your doctor diagnoses your condition from your history of exposure, physical examination, and finding bacteria in the ulcers. A biopsy or scrapings of the area are used to find the bacteria.

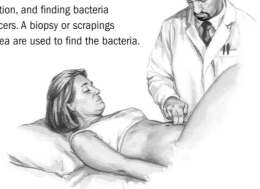

What Is Granuloma Inguinale?

Granuloma inguinale is a sexually transmitted disease (STD) that is common in tropical areas and developing countries. It does occur in the United States, usually in the Southeast. It's a chronic infection affecting genital and groin areas. More than twice as many men have it as women. Most infections occur in people 20 to 40 years old.

What Causes Granuloma Inguinale?

The cause is the kind of bacteria named *Calymmatobacterium granulomatis.*

What Are the Symptoms of Granuloma Inguinale?

Symptoms can take 1 to 2 weeks to occur after exposure. Small, raised, red lumps appear on the penis, vulva, or vagina and maybe also in the groin area. These lumps are painless, but then the lumps grow bigger and break down (become ulcers). As this happens, the area becomes dark red and may have raised edges that heal with formation of large scars.

How Is Granuloma Inguinale Diagnosed?

The doctor makes a diagnosis on the basis of the history of exposure, physical examination, and finding bacteria in the ulcers. The doctor does a biopsy or takes scrapings of the area to find the bacteria.

Testing for other STDs will be done.

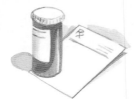

Antibiotics such as doxycycline, ciprofloxacin, or azithromycin must be taken for 3 weeks, until healing is complete.

Keep the infected areas clean and dry.

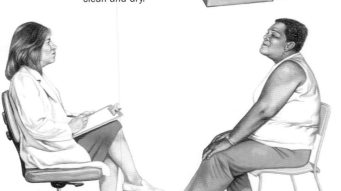

Keep follow-up appointments with your doctor to make sure that the infection is gone.

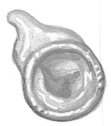

Practice safe sex. Use a latex condom. But don't have sex until your doctor says that you can, and avoid sexual partners whose health practices may be unknown.

Call your doctor if a fever develops during treatment or if ulcers become painful and infected.

How Is Granuloma Inguinale Treated?

Antibiotics such as doxycycline, ciprofloxacin, or azithromycin must be taken for 3 weeks, until healing is complete. The areas should be kept clean and dry. Sexual activities should be restricted until treatment is completed. No special diet is needed.

A follow-up examination with the doctor is important to make sure that no other treatment is necessary.

DOs and DON'Ts in Managing Granuloma Inguinale:

✔ **DO** take the antibiotics until they're finished.
✔ **DO** keep the lesions clean and dry.
✔ **DO** keep follow-up appointments with your doctor to make sure that the infection is over.
✔ **DO** tell your sexual contacts so that they can be examined and treated if needed.
✔ **DO** get tested for other STDs.
✔ **DO** avoid sexual partners whose health practices may be unknown.
✔ **DO** practice safe sex. Use a latex condom.
✔ **DO** call your doctor if ulcers become painful or have increased drainage.
✔ **DO** call your doctor if you get a fever during treatment.
✔ **DO** call your doctor if you cannot take the antibiotic medicine.

🚫 **DON'T** skip or stop the antibiotics until the treatment course is finished.
🚫 **DON'T** skip follow-up appointments with your doctor. If the infection isn't completely gone, it can come back.
🚫 **DON'T** apply creams or lotions to the lesions unless your doctor tells you to.
🚫 **DON'T** have sex until your doctor says that it's OK.

FROM THE DESK OF

NOTES

FOR MORE INFORMATION

Contact the following source:

• Centers for Disease Control and Prevention
Tel: (800) 311-3435
Website: http://www.cdc.gov

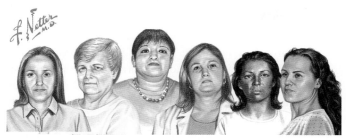

Many women have one or two periods a year when an ovary doesn't produce an egg (called anovulation). This hormonal irregularity is the usual cause of irregular bleeding, called dysfunctional uterine bleeding (DUB).

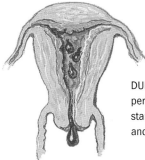

DUB includes continuous bleeding from one period to the next or having a long period; starting, stopping, and starting to bleed again; and heavier bleeding with clots.

DUB is common and not usually a problem, but it can be a sign of another disorder, so your doctor may do tests to rule out other causes like:

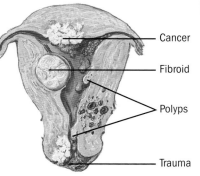

Cancer

Fibroid

Polyps

Trauma

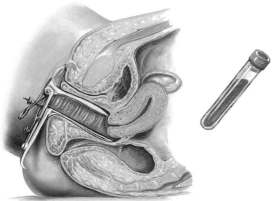

Your doctor will diagnose DUB from your medical history and physical (pelvic) examination. Your doctor may also do blood tests and ultrasonography.

What Is Dysfunctional Uterine Bleeding?

Dysfunctional uterine bleeding (DUB) is abnormal bleeding unrelated to your normal period. This very common problem doesn't have any single cause.

What Causes DUB?

A common cause is hormonal irregularities, most often because an ovary did not produce an egg during that one cycle. This cycle is called anovulatory. Anovulation is very common. Many women have one or two anovulatory cycles each year.

Abnormal bleeding might have other causes, including uterine fibroids (benign tumors of the uterus), endometrial polyps, cervical abnormalities, miscarriage, and uterine cancer (mostly in women before or after menopause, or change of life).

What Are the Symptoms of DUB?

Bleeding sometimes continues from one period to the next; other times it may be a heavy flow or just spotting. DUB may occur as bleeding between periods—bleed for a few days, stop for a few days, then bleed again—until the next period.

How Is DUB Diagnosed?

The doctor will diagnose DUB on the basis of a medical history and physical examination. Blood tests and ultrasonography may be done to rule out other causes.

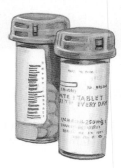

DUB usually may need no treatment. If symptoms persist, you may need a progestin hormone such as medroxyprogesterone. Side effects may include breast tenderness, backache, irritability, and mild depression.

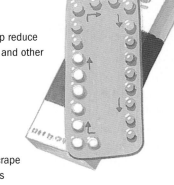

Taking birth control pills may help reduce bleeding but may cause nausea and other side effects.

Instrument used to scrape the lining of the uterus

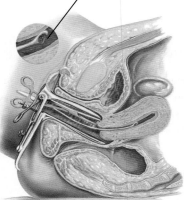

A minor procedure called dilation and curettage (D&C) is rarely needed to control bleeding. During a D&C, the lining of the uterus is scraped out, which stops the bleeding.

Call your doctor if you bleed heavily and feel dizzy or weak. These feelings may be symptoms of severe anemia.

How Is DUB Treated?

Most DUB is self-limiting and needs no treatment. Abnormal bleeding will often stop after the next period. However, sometimes very heavy bleeding can cause significant blood loss and does need treatment. Heavy flow can usually be reduced by taking a progestin hormone, such as medroxyprogesterone. Side effects include feeling bloated, breast tenderness, lower backache, increased irritability, and mild depression. However, usually progestin is taken for 7 to 10 days, so they last for only a short while. Birth control pills can be used temporarily to control heavy bleeding. They may cause mild nausea. A minor procedure called dilation and curettage (D&C) is rarely needed to control bleeding. During a D&C, the lining of the uterus (endometrium) is scraped out.

DOs and DON'Ts in Managing DUB:

✔ **DO** take your medicine as directed.
✔ **DO** call your doctor if your period lasts longer than 7 or 8 days, you bleed between periods, or bleeding doesn't slow or stop as expected.
✔ **DO** call your doctor if your period is much heavier than usual, such as soaking through maxi pads or super tampons every 2 hours, or passing large (walnut size or larger) clots.
✔ **DO** call your doctor if you bleed heavily and feel dizzy or weak. These feelings may be symptoms of severe anemia.
✔ **DO** call your doctor if you may be pregnant.

⊘ **DON'T** stop your medicine early (even if bleeding stops) unless your doctor tells you to do so.

FROM THE DESK OF

NOTES

FOR MORE INFORMATION

Contact the following source:

• American College of Obstetricians and Gynecologists
Tel: (202) 638-5577
Website: http://www.acog.org

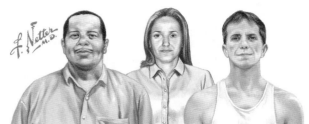

Lymphogranuloma venereum (LGV) is an infectious disease spread through sexual contact—an STD. It's found mostly in subtropical and tropical areas and is rather rare in the United States. It affects men much more than women, usually 20 to 40 years old.

The cause is the kind of bacteria named *Chlamydia trachomatis*. LVG usually involves lymph glands and genitals but may also affect the rectum and mouth.

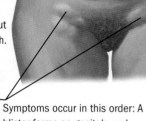

Symptoms occur in this order: A blister forms on genitals and ulcerates but heals quickly. Lymph glands in the groin become large, red, and tender. Abscesses form and drain thick pus and bloody fluid.

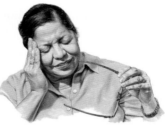

Fever, muscle aches, headache, loss of appetite, nausea, vomiting, and joint pain can also occur.

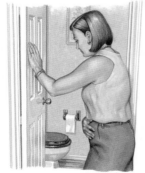

Dish for growing bacteria

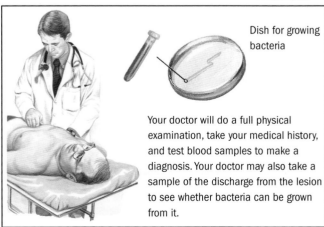

Your doctor will do a full physical examination, take your medical history, and test blood samples to make a diagnosis. Your doctor may also take a sample of the discharge from the lesion to see whether bacteria can be grown from it.

What Is Lymphogranuloma Venereum (LGV)?

Lymphogranuloma venereum (LGV) is an infectious disease spread through sexual contact—a sexually transmitted disease (STD). It usually involves lymph glands and genitals but may also affect the rectum and mouth. It's found mostly in subtropical and tropical areas and is rather rare in the United States. It generally affects men much more than women, 20 to 40 years old.

What Causes LGV?

The cause is the kind of bacteria named *Chlamydia trachomatis*. In addition to sexual spread, contact with items that carry the bacteria and nonsexual personal contact can spread the bacteria.

What Are the Symptoms of LGV?

Symptoms start 1 to 4 weeks after exposure and occur in the following order. A blister forms on the genitals and ulcerates but heals quickly. Then lymph glands in the groin area become large, red, and tender. Abscesses (pockets containing pus) form and drain thick pus and bloody fluid. Fever, muscle aches, headache, loss of appetite, nausea, vomiting, and joint pain also occur.

How Is LGV Diagnosed?

The doctor makes a diagnosis on the basis of a history of recent exposure, physical examination, and blood tests, including tests for other STDs. The doctor may also take a sample of the discharge from the lesion to see whether bacteria can be grown from it. Growth of the *Chlamydia* organisms proves the diagnosis. The presence of antibodies against the bacteria also means LGV. Antibodies are proteins that are part of the immune (infection-fighting) system.

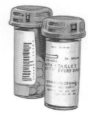

Antibiotics must be taken for 3 weeks. Take all your medicine as your doctor prescribes. Don't stop early just because you feel better. Nonprescription pain medicines (acetaminophen, ibuprofen) and local heat can help minor discomfort.

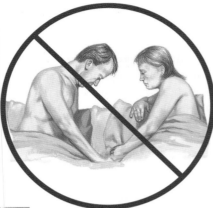

Avoid sex until you're completely healed. Tell your partners about your condition so that they can be tested and treated if needed.

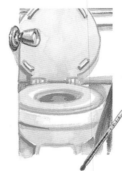

Call your doctor if you get a fever or diarrhea during treatment.

Always use condoms to protect against STDs.

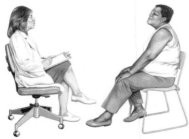

Remember that you can have this infection more than once, so keep follow-up appointments with your doctor to make sure that the infection is gone.

How Is LGV Treated?

Antibiotics are needed to fight the infection and must be taken for 3 weeks. Nonprescription pain medicines, such as acetaminophen and ibuprofen, and local heat can be used for minor discomfort. No special diet is needed, but good nutrition is important to promote healing. In some cases, surgery may be necessary to drain the affected lymph glands or remove the abscesses. Complications include chronic infection, impotence, and bowel and bladder disorders.

DOs and DON'Ts in Managing LGV:

✔ **DO** take medicines as directed by your doctor. Take them until they are all gone.
✔ **DO** rest during the acute phase of the infection. Then slowly return to your normal activities.
✔ **DO** practice safe sex—use condoms with new partners.
✔ **DO** keep follow-up appointments with your doctor.
✔ **DO** tell your sexual contacts about your disease so that they can be examined for infection and treated if needed.
✔ **DO** call your doctor if you have a high temperature during treatment.
✔ **DO** call your doctor if you have severe pain that over-the-counter medicines don't help.
✔ **DO** call your doctor if you get diarrhea while taking the antibiotics.
✔ **DO** call your doctor if you cannot tolerate the medicine.
✔ **DO** remember that you can catch this infection more than once.

🚫 **DON'T** have unprotected sex.
🚫 **DON'T** touch your eyes without washing your hands first, to prevent spreading the infection to your eyes.
🚫 **DON'T** skip doses or stop taking the antibiotics, even if you feel better, unless your doctor tells you to.
🚫 **DON'T** resume sex until your doctor says you can.

FOR MORE INFORMATION

Contact the following sources:

• Sexually Transmitted Diseases
  Centers for Disease Control and Prevention
  Tel: (800) 232-4636
  Website: http://www.cdc.gov/std

• American Social Health Association
  Hotline: (800) 227-8922
  Website: http://www.ashastd.org

FROM THE DESK OF

NOTES

Breast pain (mastodynia) can be cyclic or noncyclic, depending on whether it occurs with each period (cyclic) or not. Cyclic pain usually occurs in young women who haven't gone through menopause. Noncyclic pain occurs more in women older than 40.

Some causes of breast pain are

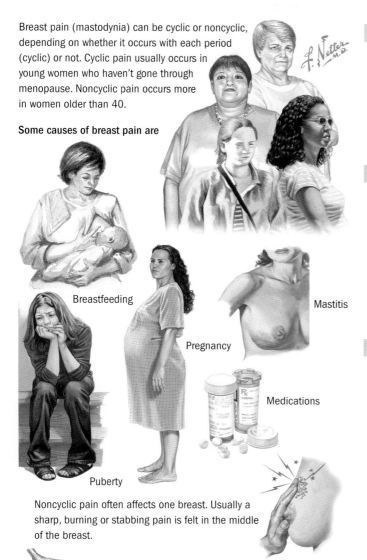

Breastfeeding

Pregnancy

Mastitis

Medications

Puberty

Noncyclic pain often affects one breast. Usually a sharp, burning or stabbing pain is felt in the middle of the breast.

Ovary releasing egg

Cyclic pain seems related to female hormones and periods. Pain starts when the ovary releases the egg, continues until the period begins, and stops at the end of the period. A dull ache is felt in the whole breast but more near the armpit.

Your doctor makes a diagnosis from a medical history and breast examination.

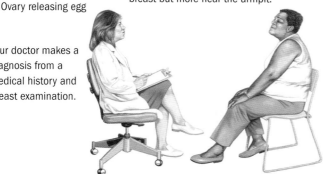

What Is Breast Pain?

Mastodynia is the medical term for breast pain. Pain can be cyclic or noncyclic, depending on whether it occurs with each period (cyclic) or not. Cyclic pain usually occurs in young women who haven't gone through menopause (change of life). Noncyclic pain occurs more in women older than 40.

What Causes Breast Pain?

The many causes include fibrocystic breast disease; use of estrogen hormones; infection of the breast (mastitis); pregnancy; puberty; normal hormonal changes before puberty or menopause; breastfeeding; and drugs, including digoxin, cimetidine, spironolactone, and methyldopa.

It's not contagious or passed from one generation to another.

What Are the Symptoms of Breast Pain?

Cyclic pain appears to be related to female hormones (estrogen, progesterone, and prolactin). A dull ache is felt in the whole breast but more on the upper outer area next to the armpit. Pain starts when the ovary releases the egg, continues until the period begins, and stops at the end of the period. Pain usually affects both breasts but sometimes one breast will be more painful than the other.

Noncyclic pain usually affects only one breast and isn't related to periods. Usually a sharp, burning, or stabbing pain is felt in the middle, around the nipple area.

Breast pain rarely means breast cancer.

How Is Breast Pain Diagnosed?

The doctor makes a diagnosis from a medical history and breast examination.

Also, the doctor may order mammography (a special x-ray examination of the breast). If the mammogram shows a lump, the doctor may order ultrasound (a test using sound waves to see whether the lump is solid or fluid-filled).

Breast pain rarely means breast cancer. For most women with breast pain unrelated to breast cancer, pain stops on its own. Symptoms that interfere with normal daily activities can be helped with pain medicines.

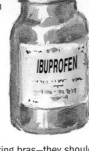

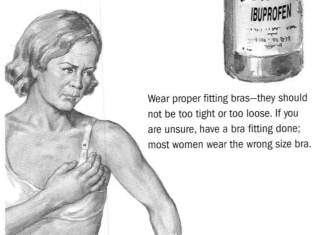

Wear proper fitting bras—they should not be too tight or too loose. If you are unsure, have a bra fitting done; most women wear the wrong size bra.

Don't use too much caffeine.

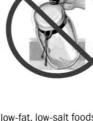

Eat low-fat, low-salt foods, and whole grains instead of processed grains. Avoid foods that trigger breast pain.

Although breast pain rarely means breast cancer, you should always do monthly self breast exams to check for lumps. Encourage the other women in your life to do the same.

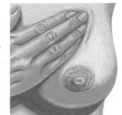

How Is Breast Pain Treated?

Treatment is conservative, including dietary limits (e.g., low-fat, low-cholesterol foods and less caffeine).

For most women with breast pain unrelated to breast cancer, pain stops on its own. Symptoms that interfere with normal daily activities can be helped with pain medicines such as antiinflammatory drugs (e.g., ibuprofen, naproxen).

DOs and DON'Ts in Managing Breast Pain:

✔ **DO** remember that breast cancer very rarely (<10%) causes breast pain

✔ **DO** eat low-fat foods, free of hydrogenated fats such as those in margarine. Eat whole grains instead of processed grains.

✔ **DO** call your doctor if you feel a lump in your breast.

✔ **DO** call your doctor if you see a discharge from your nipple.

✔ **DO** call your doctor if you see irregular dimpling of the breast or nipple.

✔ **DO** call your doctor if you have fever, fatigue, or nausea.

✔ **DO** call your doctor if you have long-lasting breast pain.

⊘ **DON'T** wear tight or loose-fitting bras.

⊘ **DON'T** use too much caffeine. Avoid foods that trigger breast pain. Avoid margarine, trans fats, and salt.

FROM THE DESK OF

NOTES

FOR MORE INFORMATION

Contact the following source:

• American College of Obstetricians and Gynecologists
Tel: (202) 638-5577
Website: http://www.acog.org

MANAGING YOUR
MENORRHAGIA

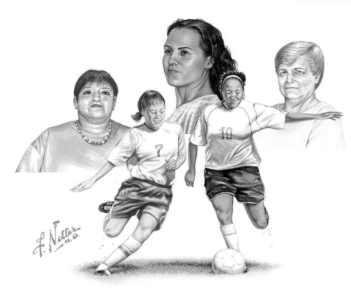

About 9% to 14% of women have unusually heavy menstrual bleeding, or menorrhagia. It occurs more often in young women and in older women who are close to menopause.

The cause is usually a buildup of too much of the uterine lining. The lining is shed by bleeding. Very heavy blood flow can mean soaking through at least one pad or tampon hourly for several hours.

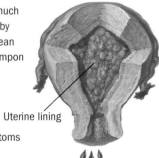

Uterus

Uterine lining

To figure out what's causing your symptoms and rule out other causes, your doctor may do some of these tests, in addition to doing a physical exam and blood tests:

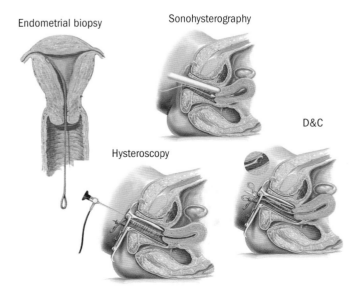

Endometrial biopsy

Sonohysterography

Hysteroscopy

D&C

What Is Menorrhagia?

Menorrhagia is the term for unusually heavy bleeding during otherwise normal menstruation (periods).

About 9% to 14% of all women have it, about 10% during childbearing years.

What Causes Menorrhagia?

Menorrhagia occurs more often in young women. It can also occur in older women who are close to menopause (change of life). Other causes are polyps, fibroids, certain drugs, cancer, and infection.

What Are the Symptoms of Menorrhagia?

Very heavy blood flow means soaking through at least one pad or tampon every hour for several hours, bleeding for more than 7 days or heavy periods regularly lasting 10 or more days, and unusually heavy bleeding for two periods in a row.

How Is Menorrhagia Diagnosed?

The doctor will make a diagnosis from the medical history, physical examination, and blood tests (to check for anemia). Anemia occurs when blood loss is so great that your blood count is too low. Anemia causes tiredness and feeling weak. Other special tests include a Pap test, biopsy of the lining of the uterus, ultrasound tests, hysteroscopy, laparoscopy, hysterosalpingography, and D&C (dilation and curettage). For the biopsy, a tissue sample is removed and looked at with a microscope. Ultrasound uses sound waves to take pictures of the uterus, ovaries, and pelvis. For hysteroscopy, a thin metal tube with a tiny camera in it is passed through the cervix into the uterus to look inside. Laparoscopy also lets the doctor look in the abdomen (belly) through a small cut. For hysterosalpingography, dye that is put into the uterus and fallopian tubes lets the doctor see the uterus on x-ray. The doctor uses a D&C to dilate the cervix and take samples of the lining of the uterus for study.

Treatment depends on the cause of heavy bleeding, the severity, and your preference (for example, if you're young and want children or are older and have had children).

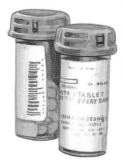

Your doctor may suggest hormones (to reduce blood flow) and iron supplements (for anemia).

Birth control pills may help make periods lighter and shorter.

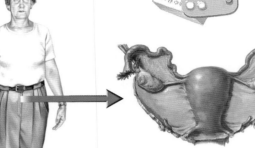

Certain outpatient and inpatient operations can treat menorrhagia. One is a hysterectomy (your uterus is removed), so it's usually for older women who are not planning to become pregnant.

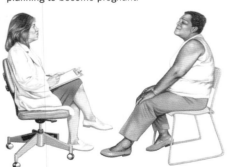

Tell your doctor about all your medicines (both prescription and over-the-counter). Also, don't delay getting care. Heavy, long-lasting bleeding can cause severe anemia.

How Is Menorrhagia Treated?

Treatment choice depends on the cause, side effects, and the woman's preference. Different treatments such as medicine and surgery can reduce heavy bleeding. Medicines include birth control pills, hormones (e.g., progesterone), and iron supplements. If medicines don't work, outpatient surgery may be done, which includes D&C and operative hysteroscopy. Other operations can cause infertility and are usually for older women who are not planning to get pregnant. These operations include endometrial ablation (the lining of the uterus is destroyed permanently), endometrial resection (removing the lining), and hysterectomy (removing the uterus and usually the cervix). A hysterectomy involves a hospital stay.

DOs and DON'Ts in Managing Menorrhagia:

✔ **DO** tell your doctor about medicines you take, including over-the-counter drugs.

✔ **DO** return for follow-up care when needed.

✔ **DO** call your doctor if symptoms worsen after treatment starts.

✔ **DO** eat iron-rich foods.

🚫 **DON'T** delay getting care. Prolonged bleeding can result in severe anemia.

FROM THE DESK OF

NOTES

FOR MORE INFORMATION

Contact the following sources:

• American College of Obstetricians and Gynecologists
Tel: (202) 638-5577
Website: http://www.acog.org

• National Women's Health Resource Center
Tel: (877) 986-9472
Website: http://www.healthywomen.org

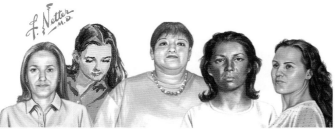

Up to 50% of women have pain before or during menstrual periods. For about 15% of them, the pain is so bad that it interferes with normal activities. This pain is called dysmenorrhea.

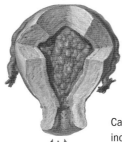

Uterus

Primary dysmenorrhea is caused by high levels of prostaglandin (a substance made by the uterus), which causes abnormal contractions in the uterus.

Causes of secondary dysmenorrhea include fibroids and endometriosis.

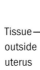
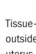

Fibroids (growths in or on walls of your uterus)

Endometriosis (tissue that normally lines the uterus is present in other places)

Tissue outside uterus

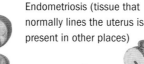

Symptoms

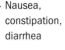

Sweating, chills

Nausea, constipation, diarrhea

Cramping in lower abdomen

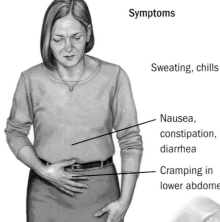

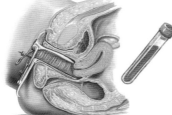

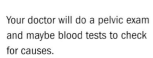

Your doctor will do a pelvic exam and maybe blood tests to check for causes.

What Is Dysmenorrhea?

Dysmenorrhea is pain in the abdomen (belly) or back occurring during periods (menstruation).

Up to 50% of all women have menstrual pain. For about 15% of them, the pain is so severe that they cannot continue with normal activities. This kind of pain is dysmenorrhea. It can disappear by itself or become less bothersome as you age or after delivery of a baby. Women usually develop menstrual pain 1 to 2 years after periods start or in their early 20s. It usually improves with time, but some women can have it into their 40s.

What Causes Dysmenorrhea?

The cause is thought to be high levels of prostaglandin (a substance produced by the uterus). In other women, fibroids or endometriosis may cause it. Endometriosis is a condition in which tissue from the lining of the uterus (endometrium) occurs in places where it's not normally found, such as on the ovaries.

Women with mothers and sisters with menstrual pain are slightly more likely to develop dysmenorrhea.

What Are the Symptoms of Dysmenorrhea?

Symptoms are cramping, tenderness, and sharp or dull pain in the lower abdomen that may spread to the lower back and inner thighs. Nausea, vomiting, diarrhea or constipation, bloating, needing to urinate often, chills, sweating, and feeling irritable and depressed may occur.

These symptoms usually begin the day blood flow begins and last 1 to 3 days. Symptom severity can vary, with cramping sometimes being mild and other times, severe.

How Is Dysmenorrhea Diagnosed?

The doctor will do a pelvic examination to make sure reproductive organs (uterus, ovaries, fallopian tubes) are normal. Blood tests and ultrasound of the uterus and ovaries may also be done. The doctor may suggest seeing a gynecologist, who will check for other problems. A gynecologist is a specialist in diseases of the female reproductive system.

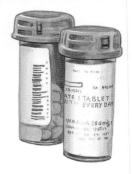

Over-the-counter pain relievers such as ibuprofen and naproxen can help reduce pain. If those don't work, your doctor may prescribe other medications.

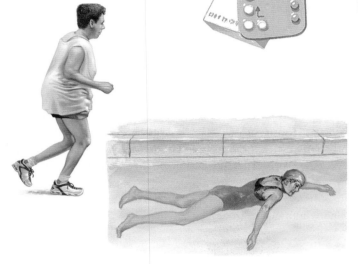

Some women find birth control pills help pain and make periods lighter, but they can't be used if you're trying to get pregnant.

Exercise to help strengthen muscles in your lower abdomen. Make exercise part of your daily routine.

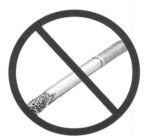

Smoking increases your chances of having menstrual pain as well as developing many other serious conditions. Don't smoke!

How Is Dysmenorrhea Treated?

Over-the-counter or prescription pain relievers help with pain. If one doesn't work, another may. Over-the-counter drugs include ibuprofen and naproxen. Taking birth control pills works well and makes bleeding lighter. It can take up to 3 months to notice a decrease in symptoms.

Applying a heating pad or hot water bottle to the lower abdomen, taking hot baths, or massaging the area may help.

Other treatments may include transcutaneous electrical nerve stimulation (TENS) and acupuncture. For TENS, a gentle electric current is applied to the skin. Acupuncture uses needles inserted through the skin into muscles.

DOs and DON'Ts in Managing Dysmenorrhea:

✔ **DO** exercise regularly, especially activities to strengthen lower abdominal muscles.
✔ **DO** lose weight if you are overweight.
✔ **DO** limit drinking of alcohol.
✔ **DO** try using heat, such as a heating pad, hot water bottle, or soaking in a hot tub.
✔ **DO** call your doctor if medicine doesn't relieve symptoms or if you don't tolerate the medicine.
✔ **DO** call your doctor if your dysmenorrhea becomes worse, even with treatment.

○ **DON'T** smoke.
○ **DON'T** take ibuprofen or similar medicines if you had stomach problems such as ulcers or gastritis.
○ **DON'T** use someone else's medicines.

FROM THE DESK OF

NOTES

FOR MORE INFORMATION

Contact the following sources:

• American College of Obstetricians and Gynecologists
Tel: (202) 638-5577
Website: http://www.acog.org

• National Women's Health Resource Center
Tel: (877) 986-9472
Website: http://www.healthywomen.org

MANAGING YOUR
OVARIAN CANCER

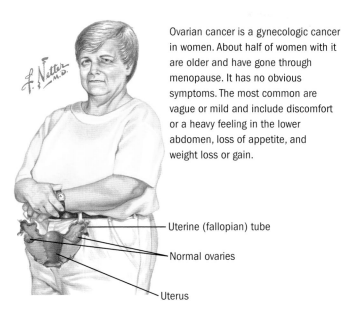

Ovarian cancer is a gynecologic cancer in women. About half of women with it are older and have gone through menopause. It has no obvious symptoms. The most common are vague or mild and include discomfort or a heavy feeling in the lower abdomen, loss of appetite, and weight loss or gain.

— Uterine (fallopian) tube

— Normal ovaries

— Uterus

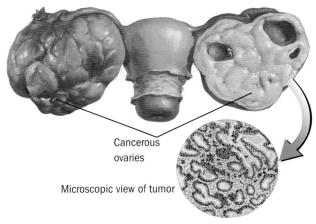

Cancerous ovaries

Microscopic view of tumor

An ovarian tumor detected in a physical exam can be tested to determine if it is cancerous. Your doctor can use the surgery to stage the tumor, which will help decide treatment.

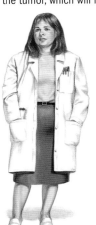

Your doctor may also use ultrasound and blood tests for diagnosis.

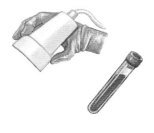

What Is Ovarian Cancer?

Ovarian cancer is a malignant tumor in the ovary, the woman's reproductive organ that releases eggs and female hormones, such as estrogen. It's the second most common women's cancer (after cancer of the uterus). About half of women with this cancer are older (average age of 59) and have gone through menopause (change of life), so their ovaries no longer work.

What Causes Ovarian Cancer?

The cause isn't clear, but certain things can increase chances of getting it. The most important are age and having relatives who had it. Others are obesity, having breast cancer, starting periods early, and going through menopause late. Some other factors, such as having children, breast feeding, and using birth control pills, can lower the chances.

What Are the Symptoms of Ovarian Cancer?

The most common symptoms are vague or mild and include discomfort or a heavy feeling in the lower abdomen (belly), loss of appetite, and weight loss or gain. Others are abnormal periods, back pain, nausea, and loss of appetite.

How Is Ovarian Cancer Diagnosed?

The doctor may suspect cancer because of symptoms and physical examination. Imaging tests (such as ultrasonography) can suggest the possibility of cancer. Biopsy is the only way to tell whether a mass in the ovary is cancer. In a biopsy, a small piece of tissue is surgically removed and studied with a microscope. The doctor also uses the surgery to find out the stage (extent) of a cancer. The stage relates to how far the cancer spread. Sometimes, tumor markers (CA-125, a substance found in blood) may help diagnosis.

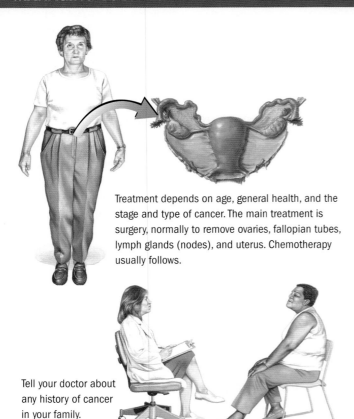

Treatment depends on age, general health, and the stage and type of cancer. The main treatment is surgery, normally to remove ovaries, fallopian tubes, lymph glands (nodes), and uterus. Chemotherapy usually follows.

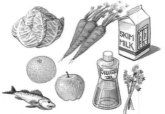

Tell your doctor about any history of cancer in your family.

Live a healthy lifestyle, with increased fruits, vegetables, and whole grains and less fat in your diet. Keep to your ideal weight, and exercise.

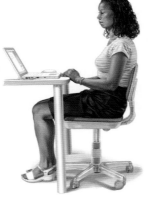

If your diagnosis has been confirmed or you are anxious as you wait for results, find out about local or online support groups you can join.

How Is Ovarian Cancer Treated?

Treatment depends on the location and stage of disease, type of cancer, and age and general health. The main treatment is surgery, usually to remove ovaries, fallopian tubes, lymph glands (nodes), and uterus. Special doctors called gynecologic oncologists are the best doctors for treatment.

Drugs (chemotherapy) and radiation therapy are other choices.

DOs and DON'Ts in Managing Ovarian Cancer:

✔ **DO** tell your doctor about relatives with ovarian cancer.

✔ **DO** remember, if you have not yet gone through menopause, that removing your ovaries and uterus means that you cannot become pregnant. You'll also go through menopause.

✔ **DO** ask your doctor about emotional and social support groups in your community.

✔ **DO** tell your doctor about medicine side effects.

✔ **DO** live a healthy lifestyle. Eat more fruits, vegetables, and whole grains and less fat. Keep to your ideal weight. Exercise.

⊘ **DON'T** miss follow-up doctor appointments.

FROM THE DESK OF

NOTES

FOR MORE INFORMATION

Contact the following sources:

• American College of Obstetricians and Gynecologists
  Website: http://www.acog.org

• WebMD
  Website: http://www.webmd.com

• U.S. Department of Health and Human Services
  Websites: http://womenshealth.gov
  http://www.4women.gov/faq/ovarian.htm

Ovarian cysts are fluid-filled growths on or in the ovary. Most are harmless. They're usually found during a routine pelvic examination or tests for something else.

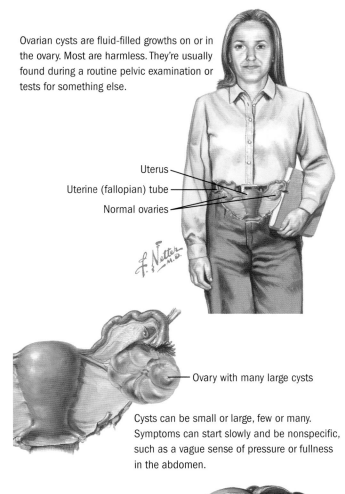

Uterus
Uterine (fallopian) tube
Normal ovaries

Ovary with many large cysts

Cysts can be small or large, few or many. Symptoms can start slowly and be nonspecific, such as a vague sense of pressure or fullness in the abdomen.

Symptoms can start suddenly, such as severe stabbing pain after a cyst bursts. When a cyst ruptures, the blood or other fluids inside it leak out.

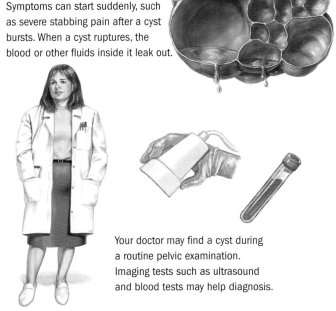

Your doctor may find a cyst during a routine pelvic examination. Imaging tests such as ultrasound and blood tests may help diagnosis.

What Are Ovarian Cysts?

Ovarian cysts are fluid-filled growths on or in the ovary, the woman's reproductive organ that releases eggs and female hormones such as estrogen. They may occur during normal ovulation. Most are harmless, benign growths, and are rarely cancer. Types of cysts include functional (normal, not disease related), dermoid, endometrioma, cystadenoma, or part of a disorder called polycystic ovarian syndrome (PCOS). Cysts occur more often in younger women than in women who have gone through menopause (change of life). Complications include twisting (torsion), bursting (rupture), and bleeding.

What Causes Ovarian Cysts?

Chances of having ovarian cysts increase with certain risk factors, including previous cysts, irregular periods (menstruation), increased upper body fat, and family history.

What Are the Symptoms of Ovarian Cysts?

Most ovarian cysts, especially those found during a regular pelvic examination, cause no symptoms or problems. When symptoms do occur, they can start suddenly, such as severe stabbing pain after a cyst bleeds or bursts. They can also start slowly and be nonspecific, such as a vague sense of pressure or fullness in the abdomen (belly). Abnormal bleeding, pain with intercourse or bowel movements, nausea, and fever may also occur.

How Are Ovarian Cysts Diagnosed?

The doctor may find a cyst during a routine pelvic examination. Ultrasonography, CT, or MRI may help diagnosis. For some special cysts, blood tests may also be done. Large or long-lasting cysts, or cysts that may be cancerous may need a biopsy. In a biopsy, a small piece of tissue is surgically removed and studied with a microscope.

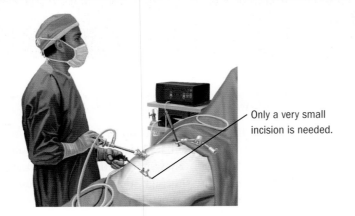

Only a very small incision is needed.

Most cysts go away on their own. If surgery is needed, a minimally invasive method (laparoscopy) may be used.

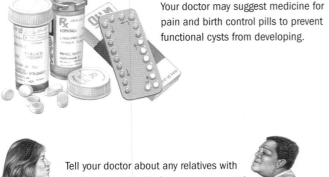

Your doctor may suggest medicine for pain and birth control pills to prevent functional cysts from developing.

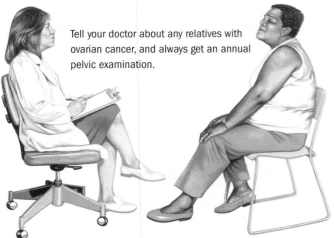

Tell your doctor about any relatives with ovarian cancer, and always get an annual pelvic examination.

How Are Ovarian Cysts Treated?

Treatment depends on the type of cyst and why it started. About 90% of ovarian cysts in younger women are noncancerous and need little or no therapy. Functional cysts need no therapy. They'll go away on their own. The doctor may prescribe birth control pills so that normal periods start and functional cysts don't develop as often. The doctor may also prescribe medicine for pain. Other cysts that don't go away or could be cancerous may need surgery to remove all or part of the ovary. Surgery can sometimes be done by using methods such as laparoscopy that use only small incisions (cuts into the abdomen).

DOs and DON'Ts in Managing Ovarian Cysts:

✔ **DO** tell your doctor about any relatives with ovarian cancer.

✔ **DO** get regular gynecologic care, including a pelvic examination, even if you're older.

✔ **DO** be aware of any changes in your periods.

⊘ **DON'T** panic if you have an ovarian cyst. Most aren't cancer, but all need to be checked by a doctor.

FROM THE DESK OF

NOTES

FOR MORE INFORMATION

Contact the following sources:

• American College of Obstetricians and Gynecologists
  Website: http://www.acog.org

• WebMD
  Website: http://www.webmd.com

• U.S. Department of Health and Human Services
  Websites: http://womenshealth.gov
  http://www.4women.gov/faq/ovarian.htm

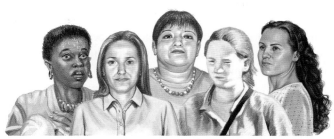

Paget's disease of the breast is a rare breast cancer. It's curable if found early, before it spreads. Paget's disease usually affects the nipple and the area under it. The cause is unknown.

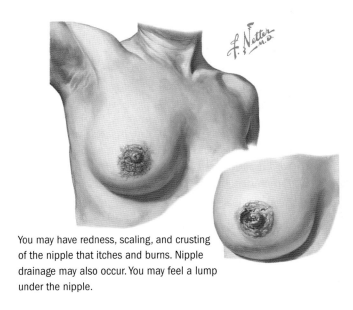

You may have redness, scaling, and crusting of the nipple that itches and burns. Nipple drainage may also occur. You may feel a lump under the nipple.

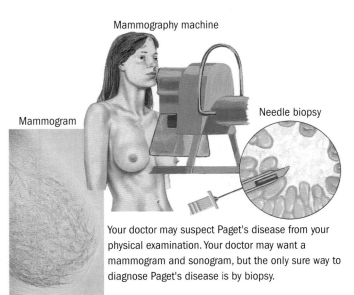

Mammography machine

Mammogram

Needle biopsy

Your doctor may suspect Paget's disease from your physical examination. Your doctor may want a mammogram and sonogram, but the only sure way to diagnose Paget's disease is by biopsy.

What Is Paget's Disease of the Breast?

Paget's disease of the breast is a rare breast cancer. It usually affects the nipple and the area below. This disease, like other breast cancer, spreads to lymph glands (nodes) nearby and then through the blood stream to other parts of the body, such as bones, lungs, and liver. The cancer is curable if found early, before it spreads.

What Causes Paget's Disease of the Breast?

The cause isn't known, but Paget's disease isn't contagious.

What Are the Symptoms of Paget's Disease of the Breast?

Redness, scaling, and crusting of the nipple that itches and burns may occur. Nipple drainage may also occur. A lump under the nipple may be felt.

How Is Paget's Disease of the Breast Diagnosed?

The doctor may suspect Paget's disease from the physical examination. A mammogram and sonogram may be done, but the only sure way to diagnose Paget's disease is by biopsy. In a biopsy, a small piece of tissue from the area is removed and studied with a microscope.

After diagnosis, the cancer must be staged, to find out the extent of disease. Blood tests; computed tomography (CT) of the head, chest, and abdomen; and bone scans are used for this. If these studies don't show cancer spread, surgery is done. The surgeon can tell the tumor size, whether it has spread to lymph nodes, and whether the cancer has a certain hormone receptor. This information is critical for treatment.

Therapy is similar to that for other breast cancers, except that the nipple and tissue just under it must be removed. Surgery, radiation therapy, chemotherapy, hormonal therapy, or a combination of all these can be used.

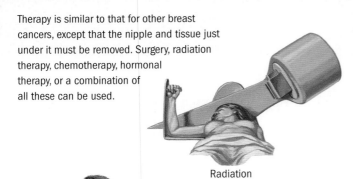

Radiation

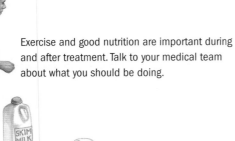

Exercise and good nutrition are important during and after treatment. Talk to your medical team about what you should be doing.

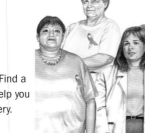

You are not alone. Find a support group to help you through your recovery.

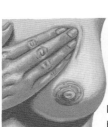

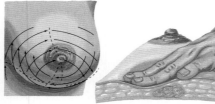

If you don't have your breasts removed, do monthly breast self-examinations and remind other women you know to do the same.

How Is Paget's Disease of the Breast Treated?

Therapy is similar to that for other breast cancers, except that the nipple and tissue just under it are removed. Surgery, radiation therapy, chemotherapy, hormonal therapy, or a combination of all these are used. Treatment involves a team of many specialists, including an oncologist (doctor specializing in cancer), surgeon, radiation oncologist (doctor specializing in radiation treatments), nutritionist, and social worker.

Side effects of surgery depend on the type of operation and how much breast tissue is removed (mastectomy or breast conserving operation). Removal of lymph nodes under the armpit may cause the arm to swell. Radiation side effects include red, dry, itchy skin over the radiation site; shortness of breath; coughing; and arm swelling.

Chemotherapy can cause nausea, vomiting, hair loss, easy bruising, bleeding, and infections.

Hormonal treatment can cause hot flashes, nausea, vomiting, irregular periods, vaginal bleeding, and rash.

DOs and DON'Ts in Managing Paget's Disease of the Breast:

✔ **DO** keep your doctor appointments during and after treatment so your doctor can check your response to treatment and look for cancer that may recur.
✔ **DO** remember the importance of exercise and good nutrition during and after treatment.
✔ **DO** call your doctor if you feel a lump, see nipple drainage, or feel swollen lymph glands under your armpits.
✔ **DO** call your doctor if you have fever, nausea, and vomiting after chemotherapy.
✔ **DO** call your doctor if you have back pain, leg weakness, stool or urine incontinence (leaking), or bone pain.
✔ **DO** find a support group if you think that would help you handle your disease.

⊘ **DON'T** ignore lumps, nipple discharge, or changes in nipple skin.

FROM THE DESK OF

NOTES

FOR MORE INFORMATION

Contact the following sources:
• American Cancer Society
  Tel: (800) 227-2345
  Website: http://www.cancer.org
• American College of Surgeons
  Tel: (312) 202-5000, (800) 621-4111
  Website: http://www.facs.org

MANAGING YOUR
PAINFUL INTERCOURSE

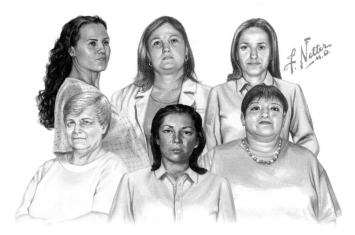

Painful intercourse is also called dyspareunia or coital pain. About 60% of women have pain with sex but don't tell their doctor about it.

Types of pain
- Primary: always pain with sex
- Secondary: sex is sometimes painful and sometimes not

Types of pain
- Superficial: pain in or around vaginal entrance
- Deep: pain from strong pelvic thrusting

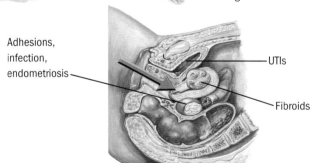

Adhesions, infection, endometriosis — UTIs — Fibroids

The many causes include infection, scars or adhesions, fibroids, dry vagina, menopause, and allergy to birth control substances. Others are endometriosis, STDs, pelvic inflammatory diseases, UTIs, and depression.

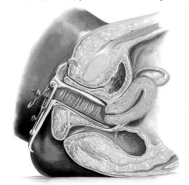

Your doctor will take a medical history and do a pelvic exam and blood tests for diagnosis. Other tests may be done to confirm the diagnosis.

What Is Painful Intercourse?

Painful intercourse is also called dyspareunia or coital pain. Some women have pain during or after sexual intercourse. It can be primary or secondary. Primary means that sex is always painful. Secondary means that sex is only sometimes painful. It can be superficial (pain in or around the vaginal opening) or deep (pain from strong thrusting). Up to 60% of women have pain with intercourse but don't tell their doctor.

What Causes Painful Intercourse?

The many causes include spasms at the vaginal opening, infection, scars or adhesions after giving birth or surgery, growths (fibroids) in the womb (uterus), dry vagina (from medicines or too little sexual arousal), menopause (change of life), and first time having sex (with torn hymen). Also, an allergy to birth control foam or jelly, diaphragms, or condoms can cause pain.

Other causes are endometriosis, radiation, trauma, sexually transmitted diseases (STDs), pelvic inflammatory diseases, urinary tract infections (UTIs), depression, and sexual injury.

What Are the Symptoms of Painful Intercourse?

The symptom is mild or severe pain during foreplay, sex, or attempted sex. Superficial pain occurs on entry into the vagina. Pain can be stinging, burning, itchy, and constant. Deep pain occurs over the lower abdomen (belly) or deep in the vagina. This pain feels like cramping, muscle spasms, or tight feeling before, during, or after sex.

How Is Painful Intercourse Diagnosed?

The doctor will take a medical history, do a physical examination, and maybe order blood tests and take a sample with a swab to check for infection.

Other tests include ultrasonography (uses harmless sound waves), cystoscopy, and colonoscopy. Cystoscopy uses a lighted tube put into the urinary bladder to look for cancer and infections. Colonoscopy uses a lighted tube that is put into the rectum and large intestine (colon), to check for inflammation (swelling), obstruction, and tumors.

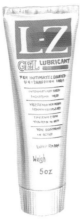

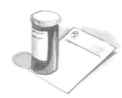

Treatment depends on the cause. The most common cause of superficial pain is not enough lubrication. Increasing foreplay can help stimulate natural lubrication. Or you can go to your local drug store and buy lubricant. Antibiotics are used for UTIs and STDs.

Talk to your partner about your pain. Pain caused by vigorous thrusting can be managed by stopping the forceful thrusting or trying different positions (for example, woman on top).

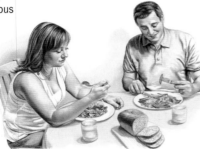

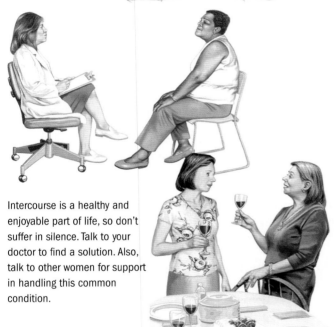

Intercourse is a healthy and enjoyable part of life, so don't suffer in silence. Talk to your doctor to find a solution. Also, talk to other women for support in handling this common condition.

How Is Painful Intercourse Treated?

Treatment depends on the cause and includes using more foreplay or store-bought lubricants for a dry vagina to antibiotics for UTIs or STDs. Adhesions from surgery, radiation, or endometriosis may need surgery. Deep pain can be prevented by simply changing position (woman on top) or stopping forceful thrusting.

DOs and DON'Ts in Managing Painful Intercourse:

✔ **DO** use sitz baths to help pain. Sit in a tub of hot water for 10 to 15 minutes.

✔ **DO** use a proper lubricant.

✔ **DO** get information about foreplay and exercises that help relax your vagina.

✔ **DO** try different sexual positions. Talk to your partner.

✔ **DO** avoid perfumed soaps.

✔ **DO** stop using foam or jelly for birth control if you may have an allergy.

✔ **DO** talk to a counselor about fears from past sexual trauma.

✔ **DO** call your doctor if you have a fever, vaginal bleeding or discharge, worsening vaginal pain, symptoms that don't go away after 3 months of treatment, or abdominal pain with nausea or vomiting.

⊘ **DON'T** use vaginal perfumes and avoid douching.

⊘ **DON'T** put up with the pain. Tell your doctor about it.

FROM THE DESK OF

NOTES

FOR MORE INFORMATION

Contact the following sources:

• Office on Women's Health, U.S. Department of Health and Human Services
Tel: (800) 994-9662
Website: http://www.4woman.gov/

• American College of Obstetricians and Gynecologists
Tel: (202) 638-5577
Website: http://www.acog.org

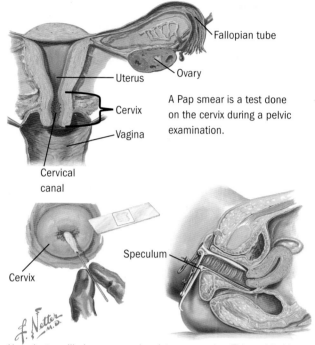

A Pap smear is a test done on the cervix during a pelvic examination.

Your doctor will place a speculum into your vagina. This tool holds open the vaginal walls and lets the doctor see inside. Your doctor will gently rub a swab or spatula around and inside the cervix to get a sample of cells. The sample is smeared onto a glass slide and sent to a laboratory for testing.

Types of cells in a normal cervix and in inflammation, precancer, and cancer

An abnormal Pap smear means that you may have inflammation, infection, or cancer of the cervix.

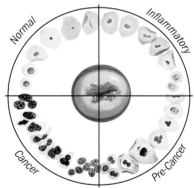

After one abnormal Pap smear, your doctor will probably do another in a few weeks. Other tests such as colposcopy may be done. In this test, your doctor uses a colposcope (which has a magnifying lens) to look closely at the cervix through the vagina. Small pieces of abnormal tissue may be removed and sent for study.

What Are Pap Smear Abnormalities?

The Pap smear is a test done during a pelvic examination. Cells from the cervix, which is the opening of the uterus, are removed and checked at a laboratory. To do this test, the doctor places a small tool called a speculum into the vagina. This tool holds open the vaginal walls and lets the doctor see the cervix and vagina. The doctor gently rubs a swab or spatula around and inside the cervix to get a sample. The sample is smeared onto a glass slide and sent for testing. The Pap smear test shows how the female hormone estrogen affects the cervix and vagina. It also shows whether the cervix has an infection or abnormal cells.

What Causes Pap Smear Abnormalities?

An abnormal Pap smear may be caused by inflammation, infection, or cancer of the cervix.

What Are the Symptoms of Pap Smear Abnormalities?

An abnormal Pap smear doesn't cause symptoms, but some discomfort may be felt during the pelvic examination.

How Are Pap Smear Abnormalities Diagnosed?

After one abnormal Pap smear, the doctor will probably do another in a few weeks. Other tests such as colposcopy may also be done. In a colposcopy, the doctor uses a colposcope (an instrument with a magnifying lens) to look closely at the cervix through the opening of the vagina. Small samples of tissue that looks abnormal may be removed and sent for testing.

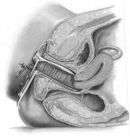

Your doctor may freeze, burn, or use a laser to destroy abnormal tissue, or use the loop electrosurgical excisional procedure (LEEP). LEEP uses a thin wire loop attached to an electrical unit. All these treatments can be done in your doctor's office.

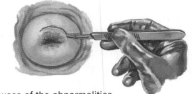

For more serious cases, your doctor may do a cone biopsy. A cone-shaped piece of the cervix, with all abnormal cells, is removed and checked for causes of the abnormalities. Your doctor cuts the tissue out with a surgical knife, cautery (burning) tool, laser, or wire loop.

Use a condom during sex to protect yourself against infection.

Don't smoke. Smoking may increase your risk of getting cancer of the cervix.

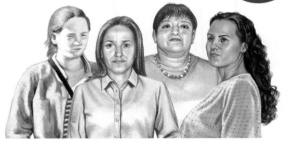

Have a regular Pap smear. If you are sexually active or are 18 or older, you should have a Pap smear every year, at least until age 65.

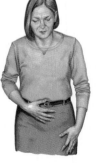

Call your doctor if you have severe pain or bleeding after the Pap smear.

How Are Pap Smear Abnormalities Treated?

A few women need treatment, which depends on the cause of the abnormalities. To destroy abnormal tissue, the doctor may use freezing, burning, a laser, or the loop electrosurgical excisional procedure (LEEP). LEEP uses a thin wire loop attached to an electrical unit.

For more serious abnormalities, the doctor may do a cone biopsy. A cone-shaped piece of the cervix, with all abnormal cells, is removed and checked for causes of the abnormality. The doctor cuts the tissue out with a surgical knife, cautery (burning tool), laser, or wire loop.

DOs and DON'Ts in Managing Pap Smear Abnormalities:

✔ **DO** have a regular Pap smear. If you're sexually active or are 18 years old or older, you should have a Pap smear yearly, or more often if you're at high risk for getting cervical cancer, at least until age 65. This way, you can find abnormalities very early, when treatment is most effective.

✔ **DO** call your doctor if you have severe pain or bleeding after the Pap smear.

✔ **DO** schedule your Pap smear between your periods. Menstrual blood can make the Pap smear less accurate. Also, don't douche before you have a Pap smear. Douching can change Pap smear results.

✔ **DO** use a condom during sex to avoid infection. A diaphragm doesn't protect you as well.

⊘ **DON'T** douche before having your Pap smear.

⊘ **DON'T** smoke. Smoking may increase your risk of getting cervical cancer.

FOR MORE INFORMATION

Contact the following sources:

- American College of Obstetricians and Gynecologists
  Tel: (202) 638-5577
  Website: http://www.acog.org

- National Cancer Institute
  Tel: (800) 4-CANCER (422-6237)
  Website: http://www.cancer.gov

- National Women's Health Network
  Tel: (202) 628-7814
  Website: http://www.nwhn.org

FROM THE DESK OF

NOTES

MANAGING YOUR
PELVIC ABSCESSES

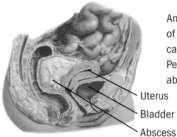

An abscess is a walled-off collection of pus caused by an infection that can occur in any part of the body. Pelvic abscesses occur in the lower abdomen, the pelvis.

Uterus
Bladder
Abscess

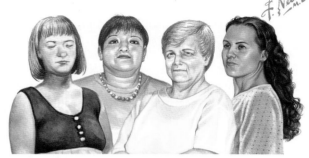

Pelvic abscesses can also be a complication of a hysterectomy or childbirth. They are seen in about one third of women admitted to the hospital with pelvic inflammatory disease. They are most common in women between 30 and 40 years old.

IUD   Appendicitis

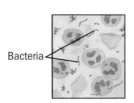
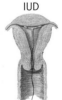
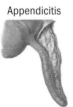

Bacteria

Bacteria are most often the cause. In elderly women, a common cause is diverticular disease. Infections that spread from one organ to another, such as in appendicitis, can cause abscesses. Risk factors include multiple sex partners, vaginal douching, using an IUD, and gonorrhea.

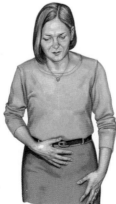

Almost all people complain of pain in the abdomen. Other symptoms include fever, chills, nausea, vomiting, abdominal bleeding, discharge from the vagina, and pain during examination.

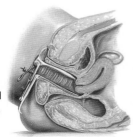

Your doctor will make a diagnosis from your medical history, physical examination, blood tests, cultures, and x-ray studies and maybe ultrasonography and CT.

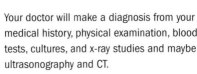

What Are Pelvic Abscesses?

An abscess is a walled-off collection of pus caused by an infection that can occur in any part of the body. Pelvic abscesses occur in the pelvis. They can be a complication of a hysterectomy or childbirth. They are seen in about one third of women admitted to the hospital with pelvic inflammatory disease (PID). It occurs most frequently in women between 30 and 40 years old.

What Causes Pelvic Abscesses?

Bacteria (aerobic and anaerobic) are most often the cause. Aerobic bacteria grow only when oxygen is present. Anaerobic bacteria grow without oxygen. Common bacteria include *Escherichia coli*, *Bacillus fragilis*, *Prevotella* species, streptococci, *Peptococcus*, and *Peptostreptococcus*. Sometimes, sexually transmitted bacteria causing PID, including *Neisseria gonorrhoeae* (gonorrhea), and nongonorrhea *Chlamydia* cervicitis (infection of the cervix), can also lead to pelvic abscess formation.

In elderly women, a common cause is diverticular disease (a condition affecting the intestine).

Infections that spread from one organ in the pelvic cavity to a nearby organ. Infections such as appendicitis or diverticulitis, can also cause pelvic abscesses.

Risk factors include multiple sexual partners, vaginal douching, use of an intrauterine device, and previous gonorrhea.

What Are the Symptoms of Pelvic Abscesses?

Almost all people complain of pain in the abdomen (belly). Other symptoms include fever, chills, nausea, vomiting, abdominal bleeding, discharge from the vagina, and pain during examination.

How Are Pelvic Abscesses Diagnosed?

The doctor will make a diagnosis from the medical history and physical examination. Blood tests, cultures, and x-ray studies will be done to confirm the diagnosis. The doctor may also order pelvic ultrasonography and computed tomography.

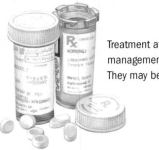

Treatment at first may be medical management—using antibiotics. They may be given in the hospital.

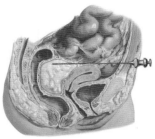

If antibiotics don't help, a surgeon can drain the abscess. A long needle is put into the abscess with the help of CT to drain the abscess. In some cases, the abscess and infected organs are removed surgically. Drainage can prevent rupture, which is life-threatening and needs immediate surgery.

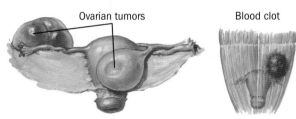

Ovarian tumors

Blood clot

Don't forget that a pelvic abscess may be hard to diagnose because it mimics other diseases, such as tumors (e.g., ovarian tumors) or blood clots in the pelvic cavity.

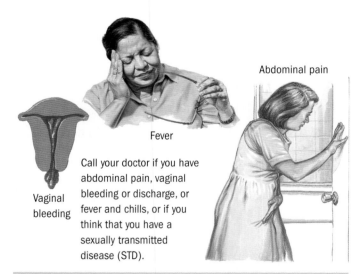

Fever

Abdominal pain

Vaginal bleeding

Call your doctor if you have abdominal pain, vaginal bleeding or discharge, or fever and chills, or if you think that you have a sexually transmitted disease (STD).

FROM THE DESK OF

NOTES

How Are Pelvic Abscesses Treated?

Treatment can be medical or surgical. Medical management includes using antibiotics, which may be given in the hospital. Antibiotic treatment alone may not be effective in people with large pelvic masses (larger than 3 inches) or severe infections, high fever, high white blood cell count, and larger abscesses. If medical treatment doesn't help, a surgeon can drain the abscess. Drainage can often be done with a long needle put into the abscess with the help of CT. In some cases, surgery is needed to drain or remove the abscess and infected organs. Rupture of a pelvic abscess is life-threatening and needs immediate surgery.

DOs and DON'Ts in Managing Pelvic Abscesses:

✔ **DO** remember that about three quarters of people treated with antibiotics get better with antibiotics alone. Those who don't are usually treated with drainage or surgery.

✔ **DO** call your doctor if you have abdominal pain, vaginal bleeding or discharge, or fever and chills.

✔ **DO** call your doctor if you think you have a sexually transmitted disease.

🚫 **DON'T** forget that a pelvic abscess may be hard to diagnose because it acts like other diseases, such as tumors (e.g., ovarian tumors) and blood clots in the pelvic cavity.

🚫 **DON'T** forget that the people with pelvic abscesses have greater chances of abscess rupture that can lead to sepsis (major infection), peritonitis (inflammation of abdominal and pelvic lining), shock, and death. Another complication in young women with PID is problems getting pregnant, because of scarring of fallopian tubes.

FOR MORE INFORMATION

Contact the following source:

• American College of Obstetricians and Gynecologists
Tel: (202) 638-5577
Website: http://www.acog.org

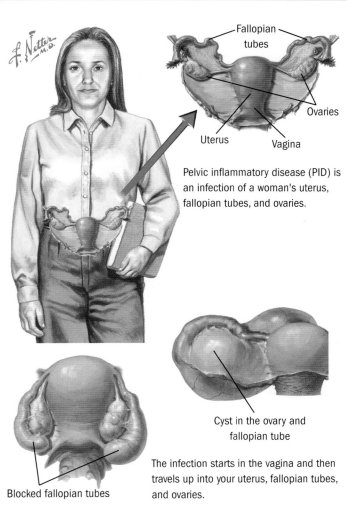

Fallopian tubes

Ovaries

Uterus

Vagina

Pelvic inflammatory disease (PID) is an infection of a woman's uterus, fallopian tubes, and ovaries.

Cyst in the ovary and fallopian tube

The infection starts in the vagina and then travels up into your uterus, fallopian tubes, and ovaries.

Blocked fallopian tubes

Common symptoms

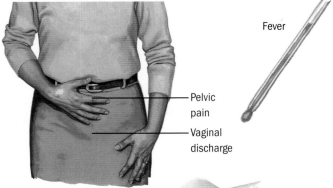

Fever

Pelvic pain

Vaginal discharge

Your doctor will do a pelvic exam, blood tests, and maybe cervical culture, uterine biopsy, ultrasound, or CT.

What Is Pelvic Inflammatory Disease?

Pelvic inflammatory disease (PID) is an infection of a woman's reproductive organs. The infection spreads up through the cervix (opening of the uterus), into the uterus, fallopian tubes, ovaries, and lowest part of the abdomen (belly, pelvic area). Infection tends to spread most easily during a period.

PID diagnosed and treated early usually has no long-term complications. However, PID can scar fallopian tubes and ovaries, making it hard to get pregnant or causing an ectopic pregnancy (fetus grows in a fallopian tube).

What Causes PID?

The cause is usually having sex with a person infected with gonorrhea or chlamydia, or other sexually transmitted diseases (STDs). Chances of getting PID increase with a new sexual partner, or more than one partner, and using an intrauterine device (IUD) for birth control.

What Are the Symptoms of PID?

The most common symptoms are pelvic pain, with or without fever and increased vaginal discharge.

How Is PID Diagnosed?

The doctor makes a diagnosis from symptoms plus a physical and pelvic examination and laboratory tests. Blood tests will show if an infection is present. In premenopausal women, a pregnancy test should be done before starting treatment. Sometimes, symptoms of an ectopic pregnancy are the same as PID symptoms, and the doctor needs to know which is causing symptoms. Other tests to check for infection include a culture from the cervix. For a culture, the cervix is swabbed, as for a Pap smear, and tested.

Imaging tests may also be done to get pictures of inside the body and exclude other medical disorders causing similar symptoms. These tests include ultrasonography (uses sound waves), magnetic resonance imaging (MRI), and computed tomography (CT that uses x-rays).

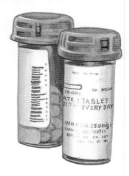

Antibiotics are started right away to stop the infection from spreading. Antibiotics may be given as injections (directly into muscle) followed by oral medicines or just oral antibiotic.

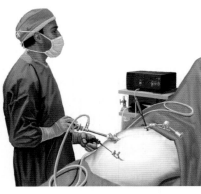

If pus remains around the fallopian tubes or ovaries after antibiotics, your doctor may suggest laparoscopic surgery to drain the pus. This surgery is done with a special lighted tube put into a small cut in the belly.

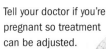

New sexual partners can increase your risk of getting PID. Condoms can help reduce that risk.

Tell your doctor if you're pregnant so treatment can be adjusted.

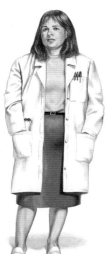

Call your doctor if your symptoms don't get better within 48 hours after starting antibiotics.

FROM THE DESK OF

NOTES

How Is PID Treated?

Early treatment is best, before the infection spreads.

The doctor may prescribe a combination of antibiotics given by injection and taken by mouth (oral), or just oral antibiotic. Severe infections may first need a hospital stay and antibiotics given intravenously.

For a pocket of pus around a fallopian tube or an ovary that doesn't get better with antibiotics, the doctor may operate (usually laparoscopic surgery) to drain the pus. Laparoscopic surgery is done through a special lighted tube put into a small cut in the belly.

DOs and DON'Ts in Managing PID:

✔ **DO** take all antibiotics as directed.
✔ **DO** have your sexual partner get treatment so you don't infect each other.
✔ **DO** call your doctor if your symptoms aren't better in 48 hours or symptoms worsen even with treatment, for example, if fever is higher or pelvic pain is worse.
✔ **DO** call your doctor if you cannot take the antibiotic (e.g., you throw up afterward).
✔ **DO** call your doctor if you think that you're allergic to the medicine.

⊘ **DON'T** have unprotected sex. Use condoms for protection against STDs.
⊘ **DON'T** have sex until symptoms are gone completely or until your doctor says you can.

FOR MORE INFORMATION

Contact the following sources:

• National Institute of Allergy and Infectious Diseases
Tel: (866) 284-4107
Website: http://www3.niaid.nih.gov

• American Academy of Family Physicians
Tel: (800) 274-2237
Website: http://www.aafp.org

• American College of Obstetricians and Gynecologists
Tel: (202) 638-5577
Website: http://www.acog.org

Normal location of organs

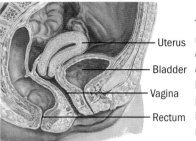

— Uterus

— Bladder

— Vagina

— Rectum

The uterus, bladder, and rectum near the vaginal canal can push through (prolapse, or bulge) into this canal. A bulging uterus is called uterine prolapse. A bladder prolapse is a cystocele. A prolapsed rectum is a rectocele.

Kinds of prolapses

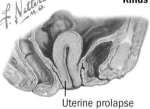

Uterine prolapse

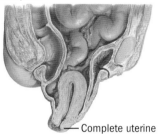

Complete uterine prolapse

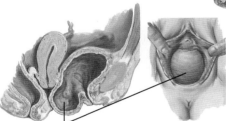

Bladder prolapse (cystocele)

Symptoms include pelvic pressure or pain, low backache, feeling that something is falling out or bulging, and bowel movement or bladder problems. Most rectoceles occur in women, but men may also have them.

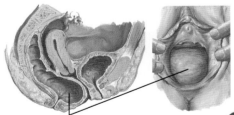

Rectal prolapse (rectocele)

The most common cause is childbirth, because it stretches muscles that support pelvic organs. Other causes are aging, menopause, being overweight, heavy lifting, long-lasting cough, straining during bowel movements, and cancers.

What Is Pelvic Organ Prolapse?

The uterus, bladder, and rectum near the vaginal canal can push through (prolapse) into this canal. A bulging uterus is called uterine prolapse. A bladder prolapse is a cystocele. A prolapsed rectum is a rectocele. The prolapsed organ can cause tissue to bulge out of the vagina. Women may first notice something like a ball of tissue coming out of the vagina. Most rectoceles occur in women. Rarely, men may have rectoceles.

What Causes Pelvic Organ Prolapse?

The most common cause is childbirth because it stretches muscles that support pelvic organs. Normal aging and menopause (change of life) contribute to prolapse. Levels of estrogen, which strengthen muscles near the bladder, rectum, and vagina, decrease. Being overweight, lifting heavy objects, having long-lasting cough, straining during bowel movements (from constipation), and cancers also cause prolapses.

What Are the Symptoms of Pelvic Organ Prolapse?

Mild or moderate prolapses may cause pelvic pressure, low backache, pain, or feeling that something is falling out. Urine may leak, especially with coughing, sneezing, or laughing. Rectoceles can cause bowel movement problems.

Severe prolapses also cause a feeling of fullness in the abdomen (belly) or a bulge that may go away when lying down. Other symptoms are problems emptying the bladder or having bowel movements, pelvic pain, abdominal discomfort, urgent or painful urination, and problems during sex.

How Is Pelvic Organ Prolapse Diagnosed?

The doctor will make a diagnosis from a physical examination, including a pelvic exam. Urine and blood tests may be done. Ultrasonography and voiding cystogram (cystourethrogram) may also be done. The cystogram is an x-ray taken during urination to show bladder shape.

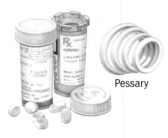

Pessary

Mild to moderate prolapses without symptoms need no treatment. Kegel exercises can be done to tighten pelvic floor muscles and strengthen muscles supporting the bladder and vagina. More severe prolapses with organ bulges need treatment, such as a pessary, hormone replacement therapy, and surgery.

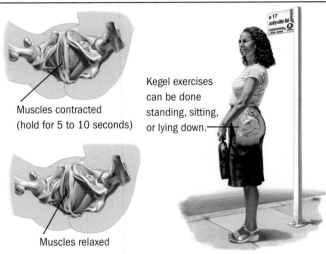

Muscles contracted (hold for 5 to 10 seconds)

Muscles relaxed

Kegel exercises can be done standing, sitting, or lying down.

Kegel exercises: Squeeze (for 5 to 10 seconds) and release your pelvic floor muscles (these are the muscles you would clench to stop urinating midstream). Do 30 to 50 Kegels each day. Your doctor should check to make sure you are doing your Kegel exercises correctly.

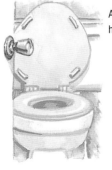

Avoid straining during bowel movements, heavy lifting, coughing, and constipation.

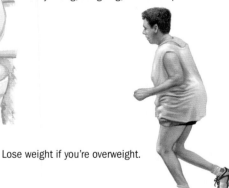

Lose weight if you're overweight.

How Is Pelvic Organ Prolapse Treated?

More severe prolapses with pelvic organ bulges need treatment. Mild to moderate prolapses (no organ bulges) and no symptoms need no treatment, just watching. Straining during bowel movements, heavy lifting, coughing, and constipation should be avoided. Eating high-fiber foods can help constipation. Kegel exercises involve tightening pelvic floor muscles and can help symptoms. These exercises strengthen muscles supporting the bladder and vagina. If Kegel exercises don't help, physical therapy (biofeedback, electrical stimulation) may. If all these treatments don't work, a pessary (plastic or rubber ring fitted into the vagina) can hold the bladder in place. Women after menopause may take hormone replacement therapy to help strengthen muscles. Surgery can be done when the pessary doesn't fit properly or if there is more than one prolapsed organ. Surgery may hold the bladder in the correct position.

DOs and DON'Ts in Managing Pelvic Organ Prolapse:

✔ **DO** Kegel exercises as directed. Do them when you lift anything heavy (books, luggage, groceries, baby) or when you cough, sneeze, or laugh.

✔ **DO** call your doctor if you have trouble emptying your bladder, you see vaginal bleeding, or your pessary falls out or isn't comfortable.

✔ **DO** eat a healthy diet with lots of fiber, fruits, and vegetables and drink plenty of liquids to prevent constipation.

✔ **DO** treat chronic cough. Don't smoke. Smoking can cause chronic cough.

✔ **DO** keep to a healthy body weight.

🚫 **DON'T** lift heavy objects (more than 20 to 25 pounds).

FROM THE DESK OF

NOTES

FOR MORE INFORMATION

Contact the following source:

• American College of Obstetricians and Gynecologists
Tel: (202) 638-5577
Website: http://www.acog.org

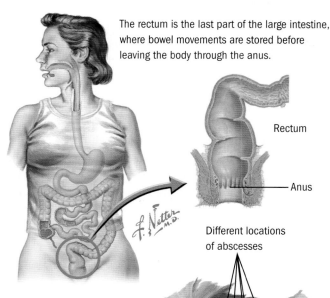

The rectum is the last part of the large intestine, where bowel movements are stored before leaving the body through the anus.

Rectum

Anus

Different locations of abscesses

When bacteria infect the rectal space and glands in the rectum that make mucus, small cavities form and fill with pus. These are perirectal abscesses. These bacteria are normally in the intestine and on skin outside the anal canal. Men get these abscesses more often than women.

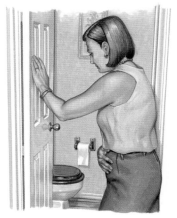

Symptoms include lasting rectal pain that is throbbing and often made worse with movement or straining. Other symptoms are fever, constipation, and trouble urinating.

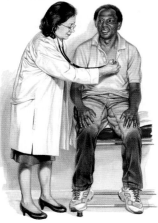

Your doctor makes a diagnosis from checking your symptoms and doing a physical examination.

What Is a Perirectal Abscess?

The rectum is the last part of the large intestine, where stools (bowel movements) are stored before leaving the body through the anal canal and anus. When the rectal space (the perirectal space) and glands in the rectum that make mucus are infected by bacteria, small hollow cavities or holes that fill with pus form. These collections of pus-filled cavities in this area are called perirectal abscesses. Abscesses can also form around the anus and are called perianal abscesses.

Anyone can have a perirectal abscess, but men get them more often than women.

What Causes a Perirectal Abscess?

The most common cause is a bacterial infection from the anal canal into one of the perirectal spaces. All these bacteria are normally found in the bowel (large intestine) and on skin outside the anal canal.

What Are the Symptoms of a Perirectal Abscess?

Symptoms include rectal pain that is lasting, throbbing, and often made worse with movement or straining. Others are fever, constipation, and trouble urinating. Sometimes, a rectal mass can be felt that is red, hot, tender, and swollen.

How Is a Perirectal Abscess Diagnosed?

The doctor makes a diagnosis from symptoms and doing a physical examination. Blood tests and urine tests may also be done.

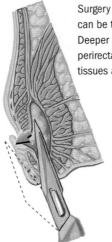

Surgery is usually needed. People with surface abscesses can be treated as an outpatient with local anesthesia. Deeper abscesses usually need a hospital stay. Untreated perirectal abscesses can spread infection into other tissues and be dangerous.

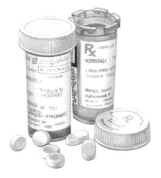

Antibiotics are often given but don't substitute for prompt surgery and draining the abscess. Pain after surgery is usually treated by sitting in warm water (sitz baths) and by taking pain medicines.

Complications after surgery can include incomplete healing, return of the abscess, and formation of a fistula. A fistula is a tunnel connecting the skin with the gland that the abscess started from. A fistula usually needs surgery.

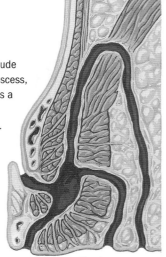

Fistula

Call your doctor if you have rectal pain and high temperature, a mass in your rectum, pus draining from your anus, or after surgery you have drainage from your incision.

How Is a Perirectal Abscess Treated?

The main treatment is surgery. People with surface abscesses can be treated as an outpatient with local anesthesia. Deeper abscesses usually need hospitalization. A general surgeon or surgeon who specializes in diseases of the colon and rectum does the operation.

Antibiotics are often given but don't substitute for prompt surgery and draining the abscess. Pain after surgery is usually treated by sitting in warm water (called sitz baths) three or four times daily. Medicines can also help relieve pain.

Stool softeners are used to prevent getting constipated and stop straining with bowel movements.

Complications that can occur after surgery include incomplete healing, having the abscess come back, and formation of a fistula. A fistula is a tunnel connecting the skin with the anal gland that the abscess started from. A fistula usually occurs 4 to 6 weeks after abscess drainage and needs surgery to fix it.

DOs and DON'Ts in Managing a Perirectal Abscess:

✔ **DO** get treatment. Untreated perirectal abscesses can spread into other tissues and make the problem worse.
✔ **DO** call your doctor if you have rectal pain and high temperature.
✔ **DO** call your doctor if you notice a mass in your rectum or drainage of pus from your anus.
✔ **DO** call your doctor if you have lasting drainage from your incision, fever, or pain after surgery.

⊘ **DON'T** ignore symptoms. The earlier surgery is done, the less the chances for complications (such as the abscess spreading to nearby tissues).
⊘ **DON'T** miss follow-up doctor appointments. The surgical wound should be checked frequently to make sure that it heals properly.

FROM THE DESK OF

NOTES

FOR MORE INFORMATION

Contact the following source:
• American College of Surgeons
  Tel: (312) 202-5000, (800) 621-4111
  Website: http://www.facs.org

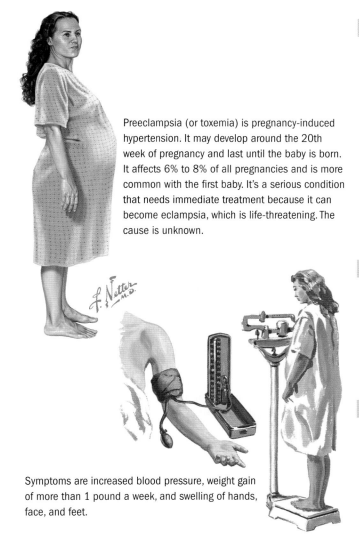

Preeclampsia (or toxemia) is pregnancy-induced hypertension. It may develop around the 20th week of pregnancy and last until the baby is born. It affects 6% to 8% of all pregnancies and is more common with the first baby. It's a serious condition that needs immediate treatment because it can become eclampsia, which is life-threatening. The cause is unknown.

Symptoms are increased blood pressure, weight gain of more than 1 pound a week, and swelling of hands, face, and feet.

Your doctor will make a diagnosis from your symptoms—increased blood pressure and large weight gain. Blood tests are done and urine is checked for protein, which indicates preeclampsia.

What Is Preeclampsia?

Preeclampsia is also called toxemia and pregnancy-induced hypertension (high blood pressure). It can cause swelling, sudden weight gain, and kidney problems. It may develop around the 20th week of pregnancy and last until the baby is born.

Preeclampsia affects about 6% to 8% of all pregnancies. It's more common with the first baby. Preeclampsia is a serious condition that needs immediate treatment because it can become a serious problem called eclampsia. Eclampsia is life-threatening and may lead to convulsions or coma. In rare cases, the mother or baby can die.

What Causes Preeclampsia?

The cause is unknown. Some believe that a problem with the placenta may be the trigger. Women who are carrying twins, have chronic high blood pressure, diabetes, kidney disease, or poor nutrition have greater chances of getting it. It seems to run in families.

What Are the Symptoms of Preeclampsia?

Symptoms are a major increase in blood pressure, sudden weight gain of more than a pound a week, and swelling of hands, face, and feet.

Severe preeclampsia causes these symptoms to get worse, along with abdominal pain, blurred vision, and headache. If it isn't treated and becomes eclampsia, symptoms will continue to get worse.

How Is Preeclampsia Diagnosed?

No specific test is done for preeclampsia. The doctor will make a diagnosis from the symptoms, such as increased blood pressure and large weight gain. Blood tests are done and urine is checked for protein, which indicates preeclampsia. Key signs are increased blood pressure and protein in urine.

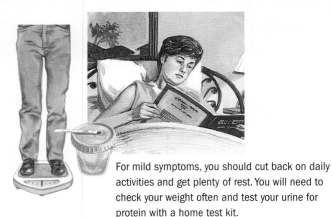

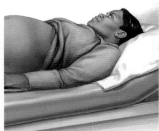

For mild symptoms, you should cut back on daily activities and get plenty of rest. You will need to check your weight often and test your urine for protein with a home test kit.

If you have more severe symptoms, you may need to stay in the hospital until the baby is born. The baby may need to be delivered early by cesarean section if symptoms continue to get worse.

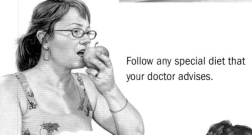

Follow any special diet that your doctor advises.

Tell your doctor if your hands, legs, or face swells, or if you have vision changes, headaches, or pain in your abdomen.

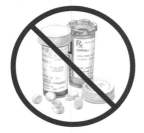

Don't take any medicines—including over-the-counter drugs—during pregnancy without talking to your doctor first.

FROM THE DESK OF

NOTES

How Is Preeclampsia Treated?

Treatment depends on the age of the fetus and how severe symptoms are. Home treatment is enough for mild symptoms. Daily activities are cut back. Resting in bed, preferably on the left side, is recommended. Measuring body weight frequently and keeping a record of these weights are important. A home kit is used to test urine for protein.

Women with more severe symptoms need a hospital stay, maybe even until the baby is born. Medicines may be given intravenously to prevent convulsions.

The baby may need to be delivered early by cesarean section if symptoms continue to get worse, if the preeclampsia becomes eclampsia.

Preeclampsia usually starts to go away 4 to 6 hours after the baby is born. Most women don't have high blood pressure after pregnancy.

DOs and DON'Ts in Managing Preeclampsia:

✔ **DO** get plenty of rest.
✔ **DO** lie on your left side.
✔ **DO** follow any special diet that your doctor advises.
✔ **DO** check your urine as instructed.
✔ **DO** tell your doctor if your hands, legs, or face swells, or if you have vision changes, headaches, or pain in your abdomen (belly).
✔ **DO** call your doctor if you have a weight gain of more than 3 pounds in 24 hours.

⊘ **DON'T** use medicines of any kind during pregnancy without first asking your doctor.

FOR MORE INFORMATION

Contact the following sources:

• Preeclampsia Foundation
  Tel: (800) 665-9341
  Website: http://www.preeclampsia.org

• National Women's Health Information Center
  Tel: (800) 994-9662
  Website: http://www.4woman.gov

• American College of Obstetricians and Gynecologists
  Tel: (202) 638-5577
  Website: http://www.acog.org

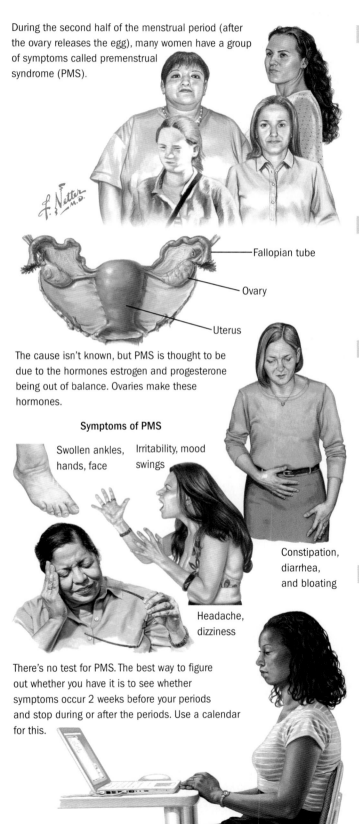

During the second half of the menstrual period (after the ovary releases the egg), many women have a group of symptoms called premenstrual syndrome (PMS).

Fallopian tube

Ovary

Uterus

The cause isn't known, but PMS is thought to be due to the hormones estrogen and progesterone being out of balance. Ovaries make these hormones.

Symptoms of PMS

Swollen ankles, hands, face

Irritability, mood swings

Constipation, diarrhea, and bloating

Headache, dizziness

There's no test for PMS. The best way to figure out whether you have it is to see whether symptoms occur 2 weeks before your periods and stop during or after the periods. Use a calendar for this.

What Is Premenstrual Syndrome?

Premenstrual syndrome (PMS) is a common group of symptoms that may occur during the second half of a woman's period (after the ovary releases the egg). About 50% of women have PMS, sometimes during their 20s and 30s, or not until their 40s. Emotional, mental, and physical symptoms vary from very mild to very severe. Most women cope with mild symptoms. Severe symptoms can affect family life, relationships, and work.

What Causes PMS?

The cause isn't known. PMS may be due to an imbalance of female hormones, estrogen and progesterone, which the ovaries produce. Other body chemicals, such as prostaglandin, may also cause PMS.

What Are the Symptoms of PMS?

The most common symptoms are being nervous and irritable; dizziness or fainting; wide mood swings; having less sex drive; headache; tender swollen breasts; feeling bloated; constipation or diarrhea; swelling of ankles, hands, and face; and acne.

Other behavioral symptoms are being depressed, crying easily, tension, anxiety, and trouble concentrating. Other physical symptoms are swelling in the lower abdomen (belly), and fatigue.

Sometimes, PMS may be mild and barely noticeable, but other times PMS may be more severe.

How Is PMS Diagnosed?

PMS can be diagnosed by keeping a calendar of periods and when symptoms occur. If symptoms always occur within 2 weeks before the period and always stop during or after the period, PMS is likely. No tests are used for diagnosis.

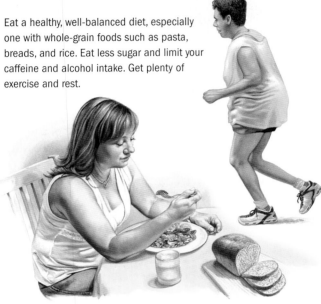

Eat a healthy, well-balanced diet, especially one with whole-grain foods such as pasta, breads, and rice. Eat less sugar and limit your caffeine and alcohol intake. Get plenty of exercise and rest.

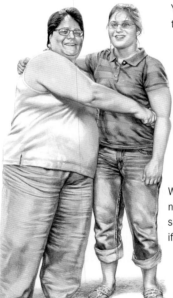

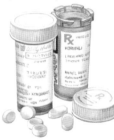

Your doctor may suggest medicine to help balance your hormones.

What works for one woman may not work for another. Join a support group or get counseling if you think that would help.

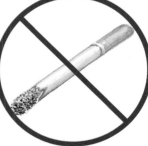

Don't smoke! Smoking may contribute to heavier periods.

How Is PMS Treated?

Helpful treatments include eating a healthy, well-balanced diet and getting plenty of exercise and rest. A diet especially high in complex carbohydrates (whole-grain foods such as pasta, breads, and rice) may help. Other lifestyle changes may be reducing or not drinking caffeinated beverages and not scheduling too many activities during PMS. Medicines that may help include drugs for depression; water pills (for fluid retention); pain medicine; antianxiety drugs, tranquilizers, or sedatives; medicines to change the balance of female hormones or control their effect; and birth control pills.

Try to reduce stress by using relaxation techniques such as yoga or meditation. Stop smoking if you smoke.

Join a support group or get counseling if you think that would help.

DOs and DON'Ts in Managing PMS:

✔ **DO** eat less salt just before your period.
✔ **DO** stop smoking and using alcohol.
✔ **DO** eat frequent, small meals. Eat a healthy, well-balanced diet, especially whole-grain breads and pastas. Eat less sugar and fewer carbohydrates.
✔ **DO** limit your intake of chocolate and caffeine (coffee, soft drinks, tea).
✔ **DO** call your doctor if symptoms don't get better with treatment, or if new, unexplained symptoms develop.
✔ **DO** exercise on a regular basis.
✔ **DO** call your doctor if your symptoms interfere with daily activities or your ability to work or do things at home.

⊘ **DON'T** drink alcohol.
⊘ **DON'T** smoke. Smoking may be related to heavier, more painful periods.

FROM THE DESK OF

NOTES

FOR MORE INFORMATION

Contact the following sources:

• American Academy of Family Physicians
Tel: (800) 274-2237
Website: http://www.aafp.org

• American College of Obstetricians and Gynecologists
Tel: (202) 638-5577
Website: http://www.acog.org

MANAGING YOUR
SYPHILIS

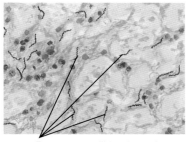

Treponema pallidum bacteria

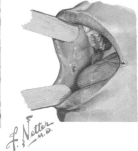

Syphilis is an STD caused by bacteria (*Treponema pallidum*) that can infect the skin, mouth, sex organs, and nervous system.

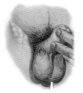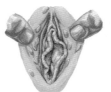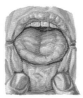

Syphilis has three stages. Stage one symptoms, starting 2 to 4 weeks after infection, include a painless sore (chancre) where bacteria entered the body, often on genitals but also in the mouth or rectum.

Stage two symptoms, 6 to 12 weeks after infection, include:

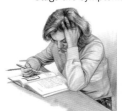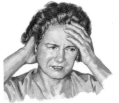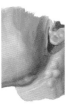

Tiredness, joint pain | Fever, headache, rash | Swollen lymph glands

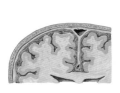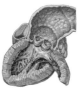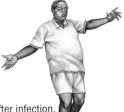

Stage three symptoms appear 10 to 40 years after infection. They include brain and heart damage, memory problems, paralysis, and balance problems.

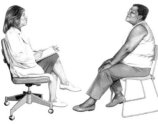

Your doctor makes a diagnosis from your medical history and examination, with attention to genitals, mouth, and anus. A very small piece of the sore will be biopsied or fluid from the sore will be removed to look for bacteria. Blood tests (such as VDRL) are done.

What Is Syphilis?

Syphilis is a sexually transmitted disease (STD) caused by bacteria that can infect the skin, mouth, sex organs, and nervous system.

If found early, syphilis is easy to cure and doesn't cause any lasting damage. Untreated syphilis can cause serious damage to the brain or nervous system and other organs, including the heart.

What Causes Syphilis?

The cause is a bacteria called *Treponema pallidum*. The infection is usually passed by sexual contact. Very rarely, bacteria can be passed through a break or cut in the skin, after a sore on an infected person is touched. If bacteria get near any moist areas or on any cuts or breaks in the skin, syphilis may occur.

Having syphilis once does not make people immune to the infection. They can get it again.

What Are the Symptoms of Syphilis?

Syphilis has three stages. Stage one symptoms occur 2 to 4 weeks after infection and include a painless sore (chancre) where bacteria entered the body. This sore often occurs on genitals but can also be seen in the mouth or rectum. It usually heals on its own in 1 to 5 weeks. If the infection is not treated, stage two symptoms begin 6 to 12 weeks later. They include fever, headache, joint pain, loss of appetite, rash (small, red scaly bumps on the penis, vagina, or mouth, and especially on palms and soles), sore throat, swollen lymph glands (armpit, groin, neck), and tiredness. This latent stage may last for years with no symptoms.

Stage three symptoms appear 10 to 40 years after the initial infection. They include brain and heart damage, memory problems, paralysis, and balance problems.

Some people with stage two or three syphilis may not have symptoms.

How Is Syphilis Diagnosed?

The doctor makes a diagnosis from the medical history and examination, with attention to sex organs, mouth, and anus. A very small piece of the sore or fluid from the sore will be removed to look for bacteria. A blood test (known as VDRL) will be done. The doctor will also want to test recent sexual partners.

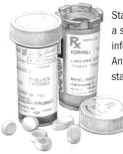

Stage one is easy to cure with antibiotics, given as a shot or taken by mouth and will prevent the infection from reaching more serious stages. Antibiotics, used for a longer time, are given for stage two and stage three disease.

Tell your doctor if you're pregnant or trying to become pregnant.

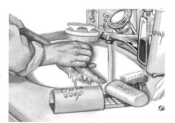

Penicillin

Also tell your doctor if you have a drug allergy, especially to penicillin.

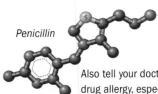

Wash your hands often to avoid spreading the infection.

Avoid sex for at least 2 weeks after treatment or until cleared by your doctor. Always practice safe sex—use condoms.

Call your doctor if you have a rash, fever, sore throat, or swelling in any joint after treatment.

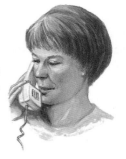

How Is Syphilis Treated?

Stage one is easy to cure with antibiotics, given as a shot or taken by mouth. People with stage two and stage three disease are given antibiotics for a longer time. Blood is tested after treatment to make sure that the infection is gone.

DOs and DON'Ts in Managing Syphilis:

✔ **DO** tell your doctor if you're pregnant.
✔ **DO** tell your doctor if you have a drug allergy, especially to penicillin.
✔ **DO** wash your hands often to avoid spreading the infection.
✔ **DO** practice safe sex. Use condoms.
✔ **DO** tell your sexual contacts that you have been treated for syphilis so that they can get tested.
✔ **DO** avoid sex for at least 2 weeks after treatment or until cleared by your doctor.
✔ **DO** get tested for other STDs.
✔ **DO** call your doctor if you have a rash, fever, sore throat, or joint swelling after treatment.

⊘ **DON'T** stop taking your medicine or change the dosage because you feel better unless your doctor says to.
⊘ **DON'T** have sex with anyone until your doctor tells you that you can.

FROM THE DESK OF

NOTES

FOR MORE INFORMATION
Contact the following sources:
• Infectious Diseases Society of America
Tel: (703) 299-0200
Website: http://www.idsociety.org
• Centers for Disease Control and Prevention
Tel: (800) 311-3435
Website: http://www.cdc.gov

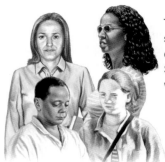

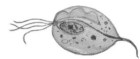

Trichomoniasis is an infection of the sex organs that spreads by sexual contact. It's one of the most common STDs. It affects both sexes, but mainly women aged 16 to 35 years.

The cause is a single-celled, microscopic parasite named *Trichomonas vaginalis*, found worldwide.

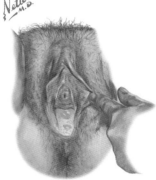

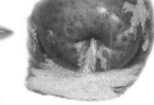

Vaginal itching, redness   Vaginal discharge

Women can have no symptoms or many symptoms. Typical ones include foul-smelling or frothy green discharge from the vagina and vaginal itching or redness. Others are pain during sex, lower abdominal discomfort, and need to urinate.

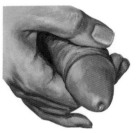

Most men don't have symptoms. When symptoms occur, they are usually discharge from the urethra, need to urinate, and burning feeling during urination.

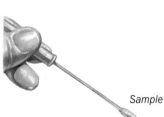

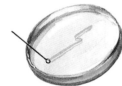

Culture

Sample

Your doctor will do a pelvic examination and collect samples from the vagina (women) or the urethra (men) for study. Diagnosis is confirmed by finding the parasite in the sample with a microscope and growing the parasite in a culture.

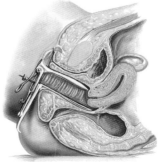

What Is Trichomoniasis?

Trichomoniasis is an infection of the sex organs that spreads by sexual contact. It's one of the most common sexually transmitted diseases (STDs). It affects both sexes, but mainly women aged 16 to 35 years. In the United States, about 2 million women become infected each year. Infection isn't fatal but can lead to complications, such as infertility; infection of the vaginal skin tissue (cellulitis); and, in men, blockage of the urethra (the tube in the penis that carries urine out of the body). Infection during pregnancy may lead to premature labor and low birth weight.

What Causes Trichomoniasis?

The cause is the single-celled, microscopic parasite named *Trichomonas vaginalis*, found worldwide.

What Are the Symptoms of Trichomoniasis?

Women can have no symptoms (asymptomatic) or many symptoms. Typical symptoms include foul-smelling or frothy green discharge from the vagina, vaginal itching, and vaginal redness. Other symptoms are pain during sex, lower abdominal discomfort, and need to urinate.

Most men don't have symptoms. When symptoms occur, they most often are discharge from the urethra, need to urinate, and a burning feeling during urination.

How Is Trichomoniasis Diagnosed?

The doctor will do a pelvic examination to collect samples from the vagina for study. Diagnosis is confirmed by finding the parasite in the sample with a microscope. Growing the parasite in a culture is another way to diagnose infection. Culture results may take 3 to 7 days. Blood tests can also be done to diagnose the parasite.

In men, the doctor collects samples from the urethra and looks for the parasite with a microscope. The parasite is harder to find in men.

Antibiotics are prescribed for treatment. Metronidazole is the best one. Both partners should be treated at the same time.

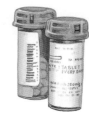

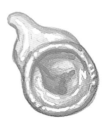

Don't drink alcohol while using metronidazole, because of side effects (flushing, headache, abdominal pain, nausea, and vomiting).

Avoid sexual contact during treatment. Once cured, always practice safe sex by using latex condoms. Remember birth control pills, diaphragms, and IUDs do not protect against STDs.

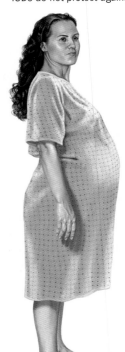

Metronidazole can cross the placenta, so it's not usually used during pregnancy. Babies born to mothers with trichomoniasis may get the infection during delivery, but this is rare.

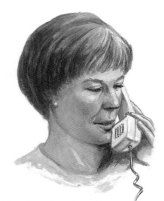

Call your doctor if you have burning with urination, vaginal discharge, pain with sex, or side effects from your medicines.

How Is Trichomoniasis Treated?

The doctor will prescribe antibiotics for treatment. Metronidazole is the best one and can be taken for 7 days. Both partners should be treated at the same time. Metronidazole can cross the placenta, so it isn't usually used during pregnancy. Side effects include nausea, vomiting, diarrhea, abdominal cramping, metallic taste in the mouth, seizures, and peripheral neuropathy. People should not drink alcohol while taking metronidazole, because flushing, headache, abdominal pain, nausea, and vomiting may occur.

DOs and DON'Ts in Managing Trichomoniasis:

✔ **DO** follow your doctor's instructions.

✔ **DO** avoid sex during treatment.

✔ **DO** practice safe sex. Use latex condoms if you think there's a chance of catching an STD. You could catch this infection from your partner.

✔ **DO** limit your sex partners. The more you have, the greater your chance of having sex with someone with an STD.

✔ **DO** call your doctor if you have burning with urination, vaginal discharge, pain with sex, or side effects from your medicines.

⊘ **DON'T** forget, if you have trichomoniasis, your sex partner should also be treated.

⊘ **DON'T** forget that even though you were infected with *Trichomonas* once, you're not immune. You can get infected again. Take all precautions to prevent another infection.

⊘ **DON'T** forget that babies born to infected mothers may get the infection during delivery, although this is rare.

FROM THE DESK OF

NOTES

FOR MORE INFORMATION

Contact the following sources:

- Centers for Disease Control and Prevention
  Tel: (800) 311-3435
  Website: http://www.cdc.gov

- Infectious Diseases Society of America
  Tel: (703) 299-0200
  Website: http://www.idsociety.org

- National Institute of Allergy and Infectious Diseases
  Tel: (301) 496-5717
  Website: http://www.niaid.nih.gov

MANAGING YOUR
GONOCOCCAL URETHRITIS

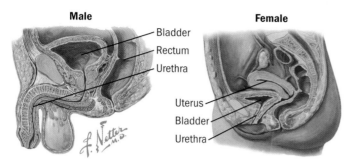

Male
- Bladder
- Rectum
- Urethra

Female
- Uterus
- Bladder
- Urethra

Urethritis is an inflammation of the urethra, the tube that takes urine from the bladder to outside the body. Gonococcal urethritis results from infection with bacteria—named *Neisseria gonorrhoeae*—that cause gonorrhea. It occurs most often in people 15 to 24 years old.

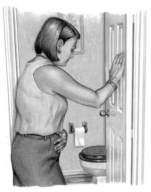

Many women have no symptoms. Symptoms, if they occur, may be frequent and painful urination; pain in the lower abdomen; pain with sex; urgent urination; and thick, smelly, vaginal discharge.

Some men may not have any symptoms, but others have pus or thick yellow discharge from the penis, frequent and painful urination, and swollen lymph glands in the pelvic area.

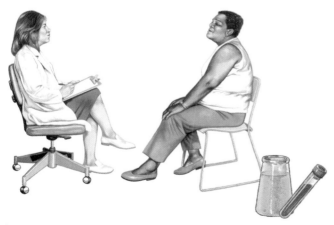

Your doctor will diagnose urethritis from your medical history and examination (especially the urethra, anus, and genitals). Blood and urine tests will be done. Fluid from the urethra will be tested for infection. Women will have a pelvic examination.

What Is Gonococcal Urethritis?

Urethritis is inflammation (swelling, redness) of the urethra, the tube that takes urine from the bladder to the outside of the body. Gonococcal urethritis results from infection with the bacteria causing gonorrhea. It occurs most often in people 15 to 24 years old.

What Causes Gonococcal Urethritis?

Infections with the bacteria named *Neisseria gonorrhoeae* (and *Chlamydia trachomatis*) cause most cases of urethritis. Some infections may be passed by sexual contact. Having had gonococcal urethritis does not protect against future infections.

What Are the Symptoms of Gonococcal Urethritis?

The most common symptom is pain with urination.

Some men don't have symptoms but others have pus or thick yellow discharge from the penis, frequent and painful urination, rash over the penis, and swollen lymph glands (nodes) in the pelvic area.

Some women also may not have symptoms. Symptoms, if they occur, may be frequent and painful urination; pain in the lower abdomen (belly); pain with sex; urgent urination; and thick, smelly, vaginal discharge.

How Is Gonococcal Urethritis Diagnosed?

The doctor makes a diagnosis from the medical history and examination, with attention to the urethra, anus, and genitals. The doctor will collect fluid from the urethra and test blood and urine samples for infection. Women will have a pelvic examination.

If gonococcal urethritis is diagnosed, the doctor will want to test sexual partners for infection.

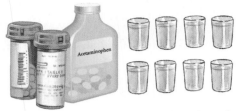

Antibiotics are used to treat the infection. Sitz baths and over-the-counter drugs (acetaminophen, ibuprofen) can help the pain. No special diet is needed, but drink several glasses of water a day. Make the urine more acidic by drinking cranberry juice.

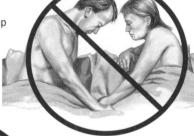

Avoid sex until your follow-up culture tells the doctor that your infection is gone.

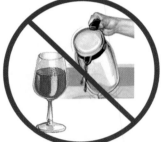

Avoid alcohol and caffeine during treatment because they irritate the urethra.

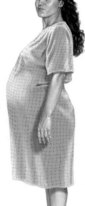

Tell your doctor if you're pregnant. The infection can be passed to babies during birth.

Remember, many birth control methods don't protect against STDs. But barrier methods, such as condoms, do protect. Practice safe sex by using condoms.

FROM THE DESK OF

NOTES

How Is Gonococcal Urethritis Treated?

Antibiotics will be used to treat the infection. Sitz baths several times a day may help ease pain. Over-the-counter drugs (acetaminophen, ibuprofen) can also help the pain.

No special diet is needed, but fluid intake should be increased to several glasses of water a day. Make the urine more acid by drinking cranberry juice. Acid urine may help with infection. Avoid alcohol and caffeine because they irritate the urethra.

Avoid sexual intercourse until the infection is gone.

DOs and DON'Ts in Managing Gonococcal Urethritis:

✔ **DO** tell your doctor about medicines you take, including prescription and over-the-counter drugs.
✔ **DO** tell your doctor if you're pregnant. The infection can be passed to babies during birth.
✔ **DO** wash your hands often so you don't spread the infection.
✔ **DO** increase your fluid intake to several glasses of water per day during treatment.
✔ **DO** avoid sex until the infection is gone.
✔ **DO** avoid bubble baths and bath oils that may irritate the urethra.
✔ **DO** keep the genital area clean, but use unscented plain soaps.
✔ **DO** call your doctor if you get a high temperature or see blood in your urine.
✔ **DO** call your doctor if symptoms don't improve in 1 week.
✔ **DO** practice safe sex. Use condoms.
✔ **DO** make sure your partner is tested and treated so you don't get infected again.

⊘ **DON'T** stop taking your medicine or change your dosage because you feel better, unless your doctor tells you to.
⊘ **DON'T** have sex until you have been treated and your doctor tells you that you can. Be sure that you use condoms to protect against sexually transmitted diseases.

FOR MORE INFORMATION

Contact the following sources:

• Centers for Disease Control and Prevention
Tel: (800) 311-3435
Website: http://www.cdc.gov

• American Social Health Association
Tel: (800) 230-6039
Website: http://www.ashatd.org

• National Kidney and Urologic Diseases Information Clearinghouse
Tel: (800) 891-5390
Website: http://kidney.niddk.nih.gov

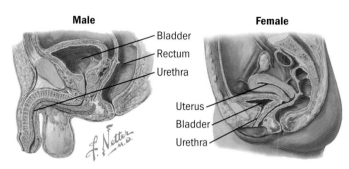

Male — Bladder, Rectum, Urethra

Female — Uterus, Bladder, Urethra

Urethritis is an inflammation of the urethra, the tube that takes urine from the bladder to outside the body. Nongonococcal urethritis (NGU) is most often due to infection with the kind of bacteria named *Chlamydia trachomatis*. It's the most common STD in the United States. NGU occurs most often in males, 15 to 30 years old.

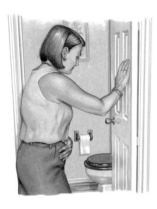

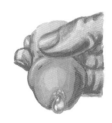

Symptoms start 1 to 5 weeks after infection (if experienced at all). The most common symptom is pain with urination. Others are whitish to clear discharge, frequent urination, urgent urination, itching or burning during urination, and pain with sex.

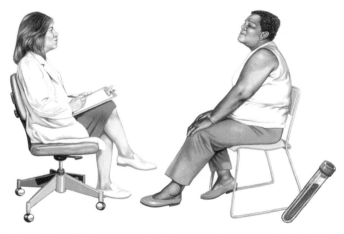

Your doctor will take your medical history, examine you, and collect fluid coming from the urethra to test for infection. Blood tests can confirm the diagnosis. Many people have both NGU and syphilis, so tests for syphilis should also be done.

What Is Nongonococcal Urethritis (NGU)?

Urethritis is inflammation (swelling, redness) of the urethra, the tube that takes urine from the bladder to outside the body. Nongonococcal urethritis (NGU) is most often due to infection with *Chlamydia*. It's the most common sexually transmitted disease (STD) in the United States and can be prevented by having safe sex. Males 15 to 30 years old with multiple sex partners have the greatest chance of getting NGU.

What Causes NGU?

The most common cause (more than 50% of cases) is infection with the kind of bacteria named *Chlamydia trachomatis*, the organism that causes chlamydia. The infection spreads almost always by sexual contact. Other causes are another bacterium named *Ureaplasma urealyticum* (15% to 30% of cases), a one-celled parasite named *Trichomonas vaginalis*, and herpes simplex virus. In up to 20% of cases, the cause isn't known.

What Are the Symptoms of NGU?

Symptoms appear 1 to 5 weeks after infection, but some men never have symptoms and women almost never have them. The most common symptom is pain with urination. Other symptoms are whitish to clear discharge, frequent urination, urgent urination, itching or burning during urination, and pain with sex. People can get NGU more than once; having the infection doesn't provide immunity.

How Is NGU Diagnosed?

After taking a medical history, the doctor will do an examination. The doctor will collect fluid coming from the urethra to test for infection. Blood tests can confirm the diagnosis. Many people have both NGU and syphilis at the same time, so tests for syphilis should be done before treatment for NGU begins.

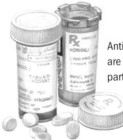

Antibiotics such as doxycycline and azithromycin are needed to cure the infection. Both sexual partners should be treated at the same time.

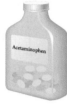

Over-the-counter medicines (such as acetaminophen and ibuprofen) can also be taken for pain.

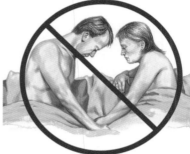

Avoid sex until your follow-up culture tells the doctor that your infection is gone.

Call your doctor if you have a high temperature or see blood in your urine.

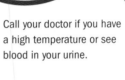

Bloody urine

Tell your doctor if you're pregnant. The infection can be passed to babies during birth.

Remember, many birth control methods don't protect against STDs. Barrier methods, such as condoms, do protect. Practice safe sex by using condoms.

How Is NGU Treated?

Antibiotics such as doxycycline and azithromycin are needed to cure the infection. Both sexual partners should be treated at the same time.

Sitz baths several times a day will help ease the pain.

Over-the-counter medicines (such as acetaminophen and ibuprofen) can be taken for pain.

People should avoid sex until the infection is gone. Men should use a condom during treatment if having sex.

In men, if blood and urine tests show that the infection is gone but symptoms continue, the doctor may check for prostate inflammation.

DOs and DON'Ts in Managing NGU:

✔ **DO** tell your doctor if you're pregnant. The infection can be passed to babies during birth.
✔ **DO** take antibiotics as prescribed until they are all gone.
✔ **DO** call your doctor if you have a high temperature.
✔ **DO** call your doctor if you see blood in your urine.
✔ **DO** call your doctor if symptoms don't get better in 1 week.

⊘ **DON'T** ever have unprotected sex. Either you or your partner should wear a condom to protect against STDs.
⊘ **DON'T** have sex until the infection is gone.
⊘ **DON'T** stop taking your medicine or change your dosage because you feel better unless your doctor tells you to.

FROM THE DESK OF

NOTES

FOR MORE INFORMATION

Contact the following source:
• Centers for Disease Control and Prevention
  Tel: (800) 311-3435
  Website: http://www.cdc.gov

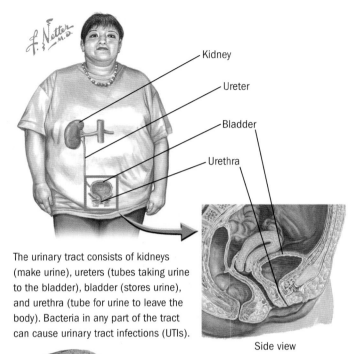

Kidney

Ureter

Bladder

Urethra

The urinary tract consists of kidneys (make urine), ureters (tubes taking urine to the bladder), bladder (stores urine), and urethra (tube for urine to leave the body). Bacteria in any part of the tract can cause urinary tract infections (UTIs).

Side view

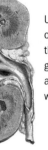

UTIs can start because of kidney stones, catheters, or bacteria on genital or anal skin that get inside the body because of wiping the wrong way after going to the toilet or because of sex. Women have a shorter urethra than men, so it's easier for women to get UTIs.

Kidney stones

Symptoms include needing to urinate often, painful urination, urinating only small amounts, cloudy or foul-smelling urine, and blood or pus in urine.

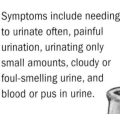

Cloudy urine

To confirm that you have a UTI, your doctor will test a urine sample.

What Are Urinary Tract Infections?

The urinary tract consists of organs that make, store, and get rid of urine: kidneys, ureters, bladder, and urethra.

Kidneys make urine. Urine then flows in tubes called ureters to the bladder. From the bladder, urine leaves the body through the urethra. Urinary tract infections (UTIs) are bacterial infections in any part of this tract.

What Causes UTIs?

The most common cause is a kind of bacteria named *Escherichia coli*, which is found in the intestines. Bacteria on the skin or near the anus can get into the urinary tract and move up. Women have a shorter urethra than men, so they get UTIs more often.

Bacteria also get into the tract through catheters (tubes) used during medical treatment, when stones or congenital abnormalities block the tract, or after vigorous sex. UTIs can also occur when another infection travels to the kidneys.

UTIs aren't usually contagious, but sex can be painful during an infection and should be avoided.

What Are the Symptoms of UTIs?

Symptoms include feeling the need to urinate often, painful urination, urinating only small amounts of urine, no control of the urine flow, cloudy or foul-smelling urine, and blood or pus in urine.

If the kidneys are infected, fever and back pain may occur.

How Are UTIs Diagnosed?

The doctor may want to test the urine (urinalysis). A clean-catch urine sample is needed. To get this sample, special cleaning methods are used and urination is started, stopped, and started again.

How Are UTIs Treated?

Antibiotics are usually needed for 3 to 10 days. Fluid intake should be increased to help flush the urinary tract. Caffeine and alcohol should be avoided. The doctor may prescribe pain medicine such as phenazopyridine. This drug will turn urine orange. Over-the-counter pain relievers (acetaminophen, ibuprofen) may help. Sitz baths may ease discomfort. Rest until fever and pain are gone.

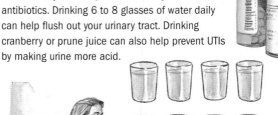

A UTI usually clears up in 3 to 10 days with antibiotics. Drinking 6 to 8 glasses of water daily can help flush out your urinary tract. Drinking cranberry or prune juice can also help prevent UTIs by making urine more acid.

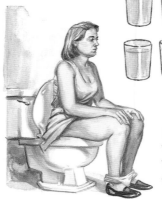

Use good hygiene. Women should wipe from front to back after using the toilet. Try to urinate often and empty your bladder completely.

If you use a diaphragm, consider switching to birth control pills to reduce risk of future UTIs. Discuss options with your doctor.

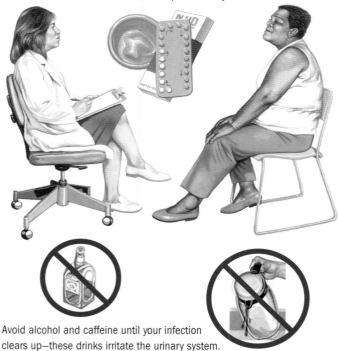

Avoid alcohol and caffeine until your infection clears up—these drinks irritate the urinary system.

No special diet is needed, but drinking juices (cranberry or prune juice) to make urine more acid can help, as can taking vitamin C.

DOs and DON'Ts in Managing UTIs:

✔ **DO** drink 6 to 8 glasses of water daily. Drinking water and cranberry juice helps the treatment of UTIs.

✔ **DO** use good hygiene. Women should wipe from front to back after using the toilet. Avoid douches and sprays (increase chances of getting UTIs). Showers may be better than baths. Wear cotton underwear and avoid tight pants.

✔ **DO** lower the risk of UTIs. Women can urinate just before and just after sex. Avoid using a diaphragm or spermicide.

✔ **DO** try to urinate often and empty your bladder completely.

✔ **DO** tell your doctor if you take birth control pills. Some antibiotics interfere with birth control pills.

✔ **DO** take antibiotics until they're gone. If you get UTIs often, your doctor may give you antibiotics to prevent them.

✔ **DO** call your doctor if your fever continues after 48 hours of antibiotic therapy or symptoms return after you finish your antibiotics.

⊘ **DON'T** skip doses or stop taking antibiotics before they're gone.

⊘ **DON'T** have sex until fever and symptoms stop.

⊘ **DON'T** hold your urine for long periods.

⊘ **DON'T** drink caffeinated beverages or alcohol.

FROM THE DESK OF

NOTES

FOR MORE INFORMATION

Contact the following sources:

• American Academy of Family Physicians
Tel: (800) 274-2237
Website: http://www.familydoctor.org

• American Urological Association
Tel: (866) 746-4282
Website: http://www.urologyhealth.org

• National Kidney and Urologic Diseases Information Clearinghouse
Tel: (800) 891-5390
Website: http://kidney.niddk.nih.gov

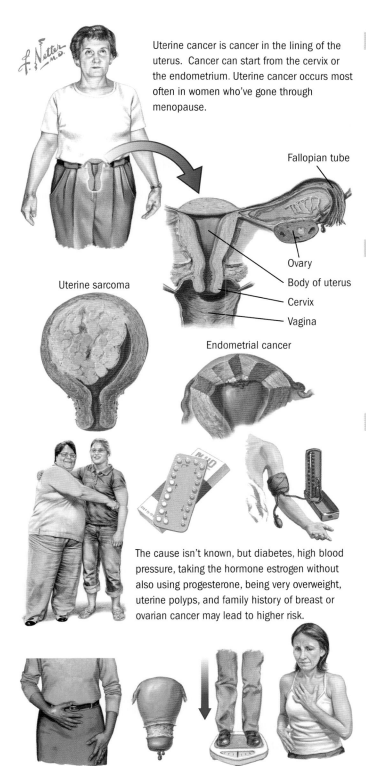

Uterine cancer is cancer in the lining of the uterus. Cancer can start from the cervix or the endometrium. Uterine cancer occurs most often in women who've gone through menopause.

Fallopian tube

Ovary

Body of uterus

Cervix

Vagina

Uterine sarcoma

Endometrial cancer

The cause isn't known, but diabetes, high blood pressure, taking the hormone estrogen without also using progesterone, being very overweight, uterine polyps, and family history of breast or ovarian cancer may lead to higher risk.

Early symptoms include bleeding and spotting, especially after sex, and watery or blood-streaked vaginal discharge. The uterus may get large. Later symptoms, after spread to other organs, include pain in the abdomen and chest and weight loss.

What Is Uterine Cancer?

A woman's uterus (womb), between the bladder and rectum, includes the cervix and the body. The cervix connects the uterus and vagina, and the body is connected to the fallopian tubes. Uterine cancer is cancer that grows in the lining of the uterus. Cancer can start from the cervix or the inner layer of the uterus (endometrium). It can also start from the body of the uterus; these rare tumors are uterine sarcomas.

Uterine cancer occurs most often in women who went through menopause (change of life).

What Causes Uterine Cancer?

The cause isn't known, but many things can increase the risk. Diabetes, high blood pressure, taking the hormone estrogen without also using progesterone, and being very overweight may lead to higher risk.

Other conditions that increase risk are family history of breast or ovarian cancer, uterine polyps, hormone imbalance, and going through menopause later than usual.

What Are the Symptoms of Uterine Cancer?

Early symptoms include bleeding and spotting, especially after sex. Watery or blood-streaked vaginal discharge can happen just before bleeding or spotting. Often bleeding occurs after periods have stopped for 12 months or more. The uterus may get larger, large enough to feel low in the abdomen (belly).

Later symptoms, after cancer spreads to other organs, include pain in the abdomen and chest and weight loss.

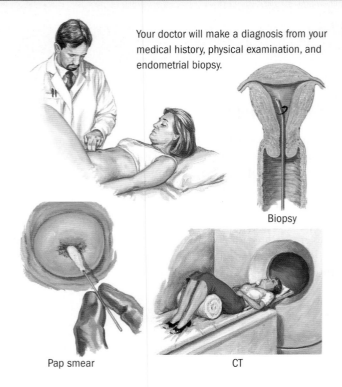

Your doctor will make a diagnosis from your medical history, physical examination, and endometrial biopsy.

Biopsy

Pap smear

CT

Tests done to stage the cancer include Pap smears, CT, MRI, ultrasonography, and scraping the uterine wall.

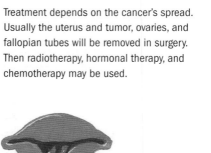

Treatment depends on the cancer's spread. Usually the uterus and tumor, ovaries, and fallopian tubes will be removed in surgery. Then radiotherapy, hormonal therapy, and chemotherapy may be used.

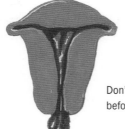

Don't ignore abnormal vaginal bleeding before or after menopause. Call your doctor.

How Is Uterine Cancer Diagnosed?

The doctor will make a diagnosis from the medical history, physical examination, and endometrial biopsy. In this biopsy, the doctor will take a tissue sample from the uterus and test it for cancer. Uterine cancer can spread to the bladder, rectum, and other organs. Other tests will be done to stage the cancer—find out whether it has spread and how far. Tests include Pap smears, mammography, blood tests, computed tomography (CT), magnetic resonance imaging (MRI), ultrasonography, and scraping the uterine wall.

How Is Uterine Cancer Treated?

Treatment depends on the cancer's spread. Usually the uterus and tumor, ovaries, and fallopian tubes will be removed in surgery.

Then radiotherapy, hormonal therapy, cortisone drugs, and chemotherapy may be used to shrink remaining cancer and prevent spread of cancer. An oncologist (doctor specializing in cancer) will help in your care.

DOs and DON'Ts in Managing Uterine Cancer:

✔ **DO** find a surgeon and oncologist with experience in uterine cancer treatment.

✔ **DO** keep doctor appointments during and after treatment to watch for side effects and return of cancer.

✔ **DO** resume sex and normal activities 4 to 8 weeks after surgery.

✔ **DO** realize that if you haven't gone through menopause, you won't have periods after your operation. You may have symptoms such as hot flashes if your ovaries were not removed during surgery.

✔ **DO** call your doctor if you have abnormal vaginal discharge (smell, amount, color).

✔ **DO** call your doctor if you need emotional support.

✔ **DO** call your doctor if you have side effects of treatment, signs of infection (fever, muscle aches, headache), or new, unexplained symptoms.

⊘ **DON'T** ignore vaginal bleeding before or after menopause.

FROM THE DESK OF

NOTES

FOR MORE INFORMATION

Contact the following source:

• American Cancer Society
Tel: (800) 227-2345
Website: http://www.cancer.org

MANAGING YOUR
UTERINE FIBROIDS

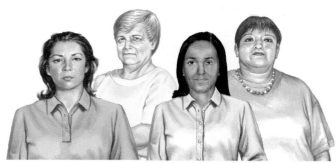

Fibroids are common noncancerous growths in or on the walls of the uterus. Almost half of women older than 50 have them.

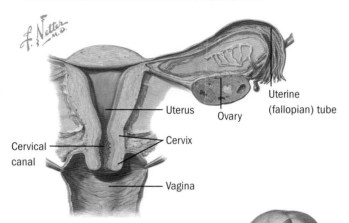

Fibroids can be one growth or a number of growths of different sizes. They can get large and make you look pregnant.

Possible locations and sizes of fibroids

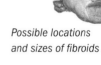

Symptoms depend on location and size of fibroids. Most fibroids cause no symptoms.

Possible symptoms of fibroids:

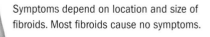

Painful periods, and needing to go to the bathroom often

Heavy bleeding during periods, and bleeding between periods

What Are Fibroids?

Fibroids, or leiomyomata (myomas), are common noncancerous growths that usually occur in or on the muscle walls of the uterus. One cell divides repeatedly and grows into a firm, rubbery mass separate from the rest of the uterine wall. Almost half of women older than 50 have these growths. They're more common in African American women than in Caucasian women. They can grow as a single mass or more often as a number of masses of different sizes.

What Causes Fibroids?

The cause isn't clear. Several factors probably work together to produce fibroids. These factors may be hormones such as estrogen, genetics (runs in families), and environmental. Being overweight, never having had a child, and getting periods before age 10 also may have an effect. The fibroids usually, but not always, shrink after menopause (change of life).

What Are the Symptoms of Fibroids?

Most fibroids (30% to 50%) cause no symptoms. Problems, when they occur, are related to the size and location of the fibroids. Fibroids may grow to be quite large so that a woman may look pregnant and have symptoms of pregnancy: pressure in the pelvic area (lower belly), heaviness, and need to go to the bathroom often to urinate. Fibroids in the uterine wall or in the cavity of the uterus may cause bleeding between periods or heavier and more painful periods. Constipation, backache, pain during sex, and leg pains may occur. Rarely, fibroids cause sudden pain or bleeding.

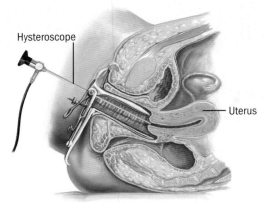

Your doctor may diagnose fibroids by a pelvic examination. Your doctor may do hysteroscopy, usually right in the doctor's office, for bleeding problems. A hysteroscope is a thin telescope put through the cervix to look into the uterus.

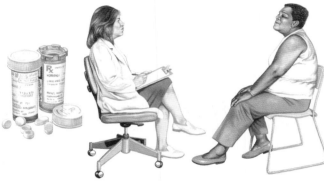

Most fibroids don't need treatment, but you need regular checkups to watch them. Medicines can help symptoms. If fibroids need treatment, surgery (hysterectomy) is an option.

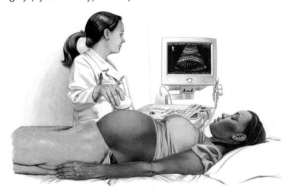

Don't delay having children because of fibroids. Fibroids usually don't cause problems in pregnancy.

How Are Fibroids Diagnosed?

The doctor will do an examination of the pelvic area. Ultrasound or x-rays may be used but aren't always needed for diagnosis. The doctor may do a special procedure (hysteroscopy) for women with bleeding symptoms. This simple procedure lets the doctor look into the uterus to find the cause of the bleeding or to plan or carry out therapy.

How Are Fibroids Treated?

Most fibroids need no treatment and only regular checks to be sure that they're not growing too large or causing problems. Medicines including hormones and drugs that act against hormones can be tried. If fibroids continue to be a problem, hysterectomy (surgery to remove the uterus) is an option. Sometimes, fibroids alone may be surgically removed (myomectomy), which saves the uterus if children are wanted. Another newer method is uterine artery embolization. In this method, arteries to the uterus are blocked so they don't feed the fibroids. Myolysis (electric current destroys fibroids and shrinks blood vessels feeding them) and cryomyolysis (liquid nitrogen is used instead of electric current) are other methods. However, fibroids can return and mean more surgery later. Newer medicines may shrink fibroids, but this change is only temporary.

DOs and DON'Ts in Managing Fibroids:

✔ **DO** get regular doctor checkups.
✔ **DO** tell your doctor your concerns and describe your symptoms.

🚫 **DON'T** delay having children just because you have fibroids. They usually won't get in the way of pregnancy. If you do need treatment for fibroids, some treatments can temporarily or permanently prevent you from becoming pregnant.
🚫 **DON'T** worry about getting cancer from fibroids. Typical fibroids are not cancerous.

FOR MORE INFORMATION

Contact the following sources:

• American College of Obstetricians and Gynecologists
  Website: http://www.acog.org

• WebMD
  Website: http://www.webmd.com

• U.S. Department of Health and Human Services
  Websites: http://womenshealth.gov
  http://www.4women.gov/faq/fibroids.htm

FROM THE DESK OF

NOTES

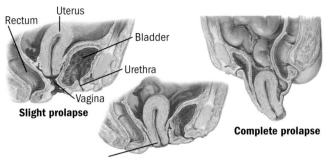

Rectum · Uterus · Bladder · Urethra · Vagina

Slight prolapse

Further prolapse, with cervix at vaginal opening

Complete prolapse

The uterus is located above the vagina. Uterine prolapse is a bulging of the uterus into the vagina.

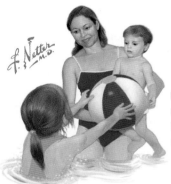

Pregnancy and childbirth are the usual cause. Large babies and long labors increase chances of having a uterine prolapse.

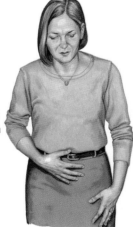

Common symptoms include a feeling of pressure, fullness, or heaviness and pain in your lower belly. Others are a backache that worsens during heavy lifting and pain with sex.

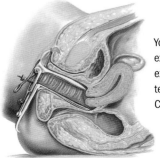

Your doctor makes a diagnosis by examining you (including a pelvic examination and Pap smear). Other tests, including ultrasonography and CT, may be done.

What Is Uterine Prolapse?

Uterine prolapse is a bulging of the uterus (womb) into the vagina.

Normally, the uterus is held just above the vagina by muscles and ligaments. With uterine prolapse, these muscles and ligaments stretch and get too weak to hold the uterus. The uterus slowly sags and moves out of its normal position, so that it bulges into the vagina. In severe cases, the uterus bulges so much that it protrudes outside the vagina, in between the legs. The bladder (which stores urine), urethra (which carries urine to outside the body), and rectum (muscle that controls bowel movements) may bulge out with the uterus.

An untreated prolapse can cause sores on the cervix (opening to the uterus) and increase chances of infection or injury to other pelvic organs.

What Causes Uterine Prolapse?

The cause is often pregnancy and childbirth. The more pregnancies, the more likely it will happen. Large babies, long labors, and use of forceps during delivery can make it even more likely.

Other causes include older age, being overweight or not physically fit, and heavy lifting. It can also happen if a condition puts extra pressure in the belly. Such conditions include a growth, a lot of coughing (such as from smoking), and constipation.

What Are the Symptoms of Uterine Prolapse?

Symptoms include feelings of pressure, fullness, or heaviness; pelvic pain (low in the belly); a backache that worsens during heavy lifting; and pain with sex. Other symptoms are a lump in the front or back of the vagina; bulging outside of the vagina, between the legs; pain when urinating; leaking urine during laughing, sneezing, or coughing; and problems with bowel movements.

How Is Uterine Prolapse Diagnosed?

The doctor makes a diagnosis by a physical examination (including a pelvic examination and Pap smear). The doctor may do other tests, including pelvic ultrasonography, computed tomography (CT), and biopsy (to check for growths inside the uterus).

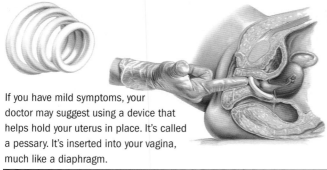

If you have mild symptoms, your doctor may suggest using a device that helps hold your uterus in place. It's called a pessary. It's inserted into your vagina, much like a diaphragm.

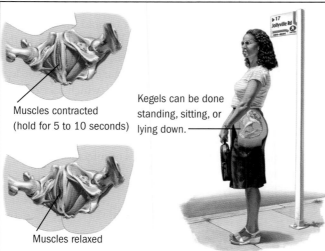

Muscles contracted (hold for 5 to 10 seconds)

Kegels can be done standing, sitting, or lying down.

Muscles relaxed

Kegel exercises can tighten the pelvic floor muscles and relieve symptoms enough so no further treatment is necessary in many cases. Squeeze (for 5 to 10 seconds) and release your pelvic floor muscles (these are the muscles you would clench to stop urinating midstream). Do 30 to 50 Kegels each day.

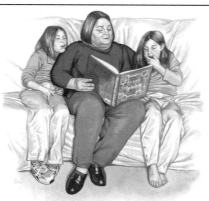

Carrying extra weight increases your chances of getting a uterine prolapse. Try to lose extra weight. It will help your overall health, too.

How Is Uterine Prolapse Treated?

Treatment depends on how bad the prolapse is, age, sexual activity, if other pelvic problems exist, and if pregnancy is desired.

Mild symptoms may mean using exercises (Kegel), hormone therapy, or a device called a pessary. Kegel exercises strengthen muscles and ligaments holding the uterus and vagina in place. Hormone creams also make these muscles and ligaments stronger. A pessary is a small ring-shaped device put into the vagina to hold the uterus in place.

More severe prolapse, may mean surgery. Sometimes the uterus must be removed (hysterectomy).

DOs and DON'Ts in Managing Uterine Prolapse:

✔ **DO** Kegel exercises daily. Do general exercises regularly for good overall muscle tone.

✔ **DO** lose weight if you're overweight.

✔ **DO** eat a well-balanced, high-fiber diet to avoid getting constipated.

✔ **DO** call your doctor if you have unusual vaginal bleeding, discomfort, or trouble urinating.

✔ **DO** call your doctor if symptoms don't get better after 3 months of treatment or exercise.

✔ **DO** avoid heavy lifting.

⊘ **DON'T** ignore pain or bleeding from your vagina.
⊘ **DON'T** smoke.

FROM THE DESK OF

NOTES

FOR MORE INFORMATION

Contact the following source:

• American College of Obstetricians and Gynecologists
  Tel: (202) 638-5577
  Website: http://www.acog.org

Vaginal yeast infections are very common, with up to 75% of women likely to have one at some time. They can occur in women of any age.

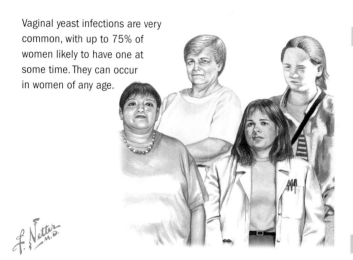

The cause is the fungus named *Candida albicans*. Women who take antibiotics, are diabetic, take birth control pills, or douche too often have more chances of getting these infections.

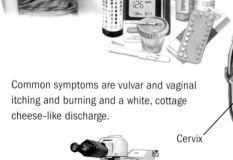

Common symptoms are vulvar and vaginal itching and burning and a white, cottage cheese–like discharge.

Cervix

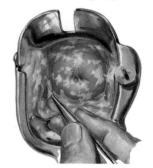

Your doctor will do a pelvic exam and may take a sample of the vaginal discharge to look at with a microscope.

What Is a Vaginal Yeast Infection?

Vaginitis is inflammation (swelling, redness) of the vagina that can have different causes, including infections. Infection with the yeast named *Candida albicans*, which is a kind of fungus, is one cause. They're very common, with up to 75% of women likely to have a vaginal yeast infection. Women of all ages can get these infections. When many *Candida* yeast organisms are present, they cause symptoms.

In most cases, *Candida* vaginitis is easily treated. A few women have yeast infections that come back frequently.

What Causes a Vaginal Yeast Infection?

The fungus *Candida* is the cause. Women are more likely to have vaginal yeast infections if they take antibiotics, because antibiotics kill healthy, protective bacteria in the vagina. Lack of healthy bacteria allows yeast to grow. Women who are diabetic, are pregnant or taking birth control pills, or are receiving long-term steroid treatment may also be more likely to get yeast infections. Other reasons for getting them include douching too often, poor diet, lack of sleep, or weakened immune (infection-fighting) systems.

What Are the Symptoms of a Vaginal Yeast Infection?

The most common symptoms are vulvar and vaginal itching and burning and a white, often clumpy discharge, sometimes described as cottage cheese–like. Yeast infections can also be present with minimal discharge.

How Is a Vaginal Yeast Infection Diagnosed?

The doctor makes a diagnosis by doing a pelvic examination and examining the vaginal discharge under a microscope. The doctor may send a sample of the discharge to a laboratory for culture, to see if *Candida* yeast will grow.

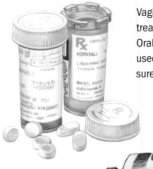

Vaginal creams and suppositories for treatment include over-the-counter drugs. Oral prescription medicines may also be used. Finish all your medicine, to make sure that the infection doesn't come back.

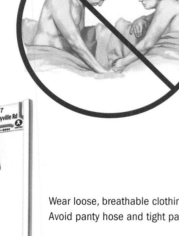

Don't have sex until your treatment is complete.

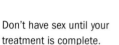

Wear loose, breathable clothing. Avoid panty hose and tight pants.

Eat 8 ounces of yogurt with acidophilus bacteria daily. Yogurt may help stop future yeast infections. It's also a good source of calcium!

How Is a Vaginal Yeast Infection Treated?

Vaginal creams, suppositories, and oral medicines are used for treatment.

Vaginal creams and suppositories are available over-the-counter; medicine taken by mouth usually requires a doctor's prescription. Common antifungal drugs include clotrimazole, miconazole, nystatin, and terconazole. Fluconazole is given orally. The over-the-counter medicines are often just as effective as prescription medicines, but some women find the pills easier to use. Side effects from any of the drugs are rare, but some women may have vaginal or vulvar burning.

DOs and DON'Ts in Managing a Vaginal Yeast Infection:

✔ **DO** take or use all your medicine as directed. If you don't finish a complete course, the infection may not be completely gone and may come back.

✔ **DO** use sitz baths if you have itching and discomfort. Soak the vulvar area for 10 to 15 minutes in plain water at a comfortable temperature, then pat the area dry.

✔ **DO** eat 8 ounces of yogurt with live acidophilus bacteria daily. Yogurt may help stop yeast infections from coming back and is a good source of calcium anyway!

✔ **DO** call your doctor if you still have symptoms after you finish the complete course of medicine.

✔ **DO** call your doctor if you have medicine side effects, such as vaginal or vulvar burning.

⊘ **DON'T** have sex while you're being treated.

⊘ **DON'T** wear tight, nonbreathing clothing (for example, panty hose and tight pants).

FROM THE DESK OF

NOTES

FOR MORE INFORMATION

Contact the following source:

• American College of Obstetricians and Gynecologists
Tel: (202) 638-5577
Website: http://www.acog.org

MANAGING YOUR
BACTERIAL VAGINAL INFECTION

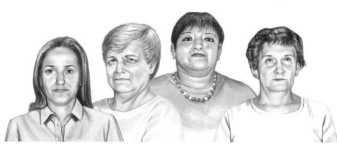

In bacterial vaginal infection, the balance of normal vaginal bacteria is upset. Women of all ages can get it.

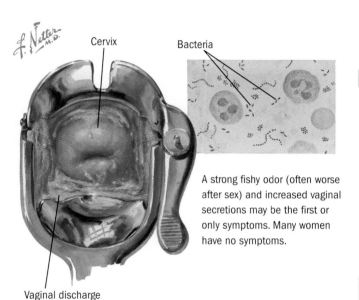

Cervix

Bacteria

A strong fishy odor (often worse after sex) and increased vaginal secretions may be the first or only symptoms. Many women have no symptoms.

Vaginal discharge

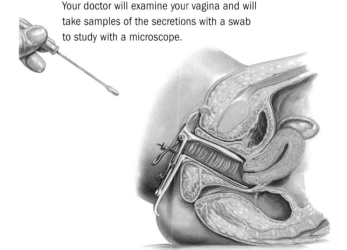

Your doctor will examine your vagina and will take samples of the secretions with a swab to study with a microscope.

What Is Bacterial Vaginal Infection?

Overgrowth of normal or abnormal bacteria in the vagina can result in irritation, inflammation (swelling), odor (especially after sex), and other symptoms. The balance of bacteria normally found in the vagina is upset and there is overgrowth of other types of bacteria. This common disorder accounts for about half of all vaginal infections. The urethra (opening of the bladder), the bladder, and skin in the genital area may also be affected.

Bacterial vaginal infection occurs most during years when women can have children. However, women of all ages can get it.

What Causes Bacterial Vaginal Infection?

The cause of the upset in the balance of bacteria isn't clear. Factors that may be related to bacterial vaginal infection include a new or many sex partners, douching, hot weather, poor health, and poor hygiene. However, women who never had sex can get it too. The risk of getting it can increase if you have diabetes or a weakened immune (infection-fighting) system.

It can't be caught from toilet seats, linens, or swimming pools.

What Are the Symptoms of Bacterial Vaginal Infection?

A strong fishy odor (often worse after sex) or increased vaginal secretions may be the first or only symptoms. The secretions may be clear, white, or gray and may be thin or heavy. Burning during urination and itching around the vagina may occur. Irritation, swelling, redness, and pain with sex are all common. Many women have no symptoms.

How Is Bacterial Vaginal Infection Diagnosed?

The doctor will examine the pelvic area, especially the vagina. The doctor will also take samples of the secretions with a swab to study with a microscope and perform additional tests.

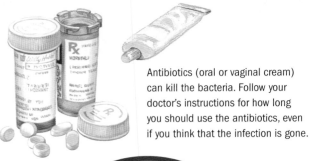

Antibiotics (oral or vaginal cream) can kill the bacteria. Follow your doctor's instructions for how long you should use the antibiotics, even if you think that the infection is gone.

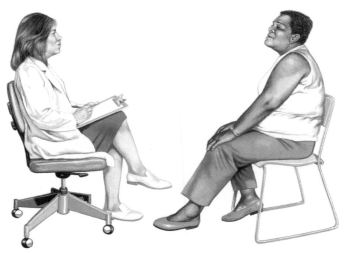

Avoid sex until your infection clears up. Limiting the number of sexual partners is one way to prevent future infections. Another may be to avoid douching.

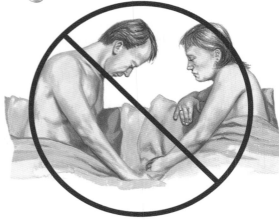

Always visit your doctor if you think you have a vaginal infection. Untreated infections may lead to complications, such as pelvic inflammatory disease (PID), pregnancy problems, and other infections.

FROM THE DESK OF

NOTES

How Is Bacterial Vaginal Infection Treated?

Antibiotics are given either by mouth or as a vaginal cream or suppository.

Untreated bacterial vaginal infection may lead to complications, such as pelvic inflammatory disease (PID), endometritis, cervicitis, pregnancy problems, and postoperative infections.

DOs and DON'Ts in Managing Bacterial Vaginal Infection:

✔ **DO** see a doctor if you think that you have an infection.
✔ **DO** follow your doctor's instructions.
✔ **DO** finish all your antibiotic medicine even though you may feel better.
✔ **DO** limit your number of sexual partners, to prevent future infections.

🚫 **DON'T** use over-the-counter medicines, leftover drugs, or medicines that you get from friends to treat your infection.
🚫 **DON'T** douche or rinse away your vaginal secretions before your doctor's appointment. Your doctor will want to see the secretions to make a correct diagnosis. For that matter, don't douche at all.

FOR MORE INFORMATION

Contact the following sources:

• American College of Obstetricians and Gynecologists
Tel: (202) 638-5577
Website: http://www.acog.org

• WebMD
Website: http://www.webmd.com

• U.S. Department of Health and Human Services
Websites: http://womenshealth.gov
http://www.4women.gov

Vulvar cancer affects the outer part of a woman's reproductive system: opening of the vagina, labia (vaginal lips), clitoris, and skin and tissue covering the pubic bone. This rare cancer usually occurs in women older than 50.

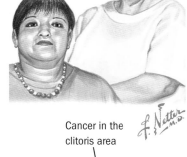

Cancer in the labia area

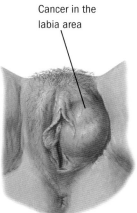

Cancer usually affects inner edges of vaginal lips but can occur in other spots.

Cancer in the clitoris area

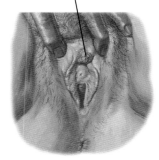

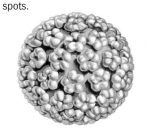

HPV

The cause is unknown, but risk factors include a history of cervical cancer, vaginal cancer, and HPV.

Common symptoms include pain during sex or with urination, vulvar itching, thickening or lump on the labia, and blood or discharge unrelated to periods.

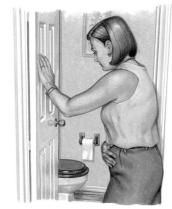

Your doctor can see early changes in the vulva during a routine pelvic exam. Your doctor will likely do a biopsy to get a small piece of tissue to check. An instrument called a colposcope may be used to do the biopsy.

Colposcopy

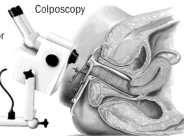

What Is Vulvar Cancer?

Cancer of the vulva affects the outer part of a woman's reproductive system. This area includes the opening of the vagina, labia (vaginal lips), clitoris, and skin and tissue covering the pubic bone. Most often, the cancer occurs on inner edges of vaginal lips.

This cancer is rather rare. Less than 1% of all cancers in women are vulvar cancers, usually in women older than 50 years.

What Causes Vulvar Cancer?

The cause is unknown, but some things can give women greater chances of getting this cancer. These things are long-term inflammation (swelling, redness) of the vulva, human papillomavirus (HPV) infection, and prior cervical or vaginal cancer. HPV causes genital warts, a sexually transmitted disease (STD).

What Are the Symptoms of Vulvar Cancer?

Common symptoms may include pain during sex or with urination, long-lasting itching in the vulva region, thickening or lump on the labia, rough white area on the vulva, and blood or discharge that isn't related to normal menstrual periods.

How Is Vulvar Cancer Diagnosed?

The doctor can often see early changes in the vulva during a routine pelvic examination. Because of the examination and symptoms, the doctor may order a biopsy to confirm the diagnosis. A biopsy involves taking a small piece of tissue for study with a microscope. An instrument called a colposcope may be used to do the biopsy. This tool has magnifying lenses for looking at the vagina and lets the doctor pick the best spot for a biopsy.

If biopsy results show cancer cells, other tests may be done to see if the cancer spread and how far.

Treatment depends on the type and size of cancer and its spread. For very small cancers, a laser beam can burn off the top layer of skin with cancer cells. An operation called excision or simple partial vulvectomy, or complete vulvectomy, may be done. You and your medical team will decide the best approach.

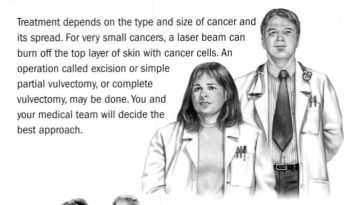

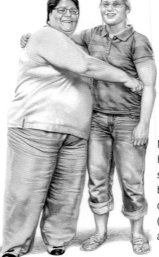

Many women with vulvar cancer have had an HPV infection. Practice safe sex by using condoms. Remember, birth control pills don't protect against disease. Consider vaccination for HPV (Gardasil®) if you're between ages 13 and 26.

Have regular check-ups with your gynecologist to catch problems early. Call your doctor if you have vaginal bleeding that's not related to your period or if you see skin changes on your labia.

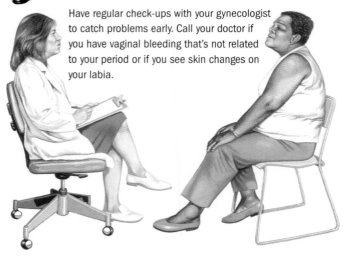

How Is Vulvar Cancer Treated?

Treatment depends on the type and size of cancer and its spread.

For very small cancers that are in only one spot, a laser beam can be used to burn off the top layer of skin that contains the cancer cells.

Surgery called excision or simple partial vulvectomy is often used to remove abnormal cells and some healthy tissue nearby. For large cancers, an operation called a vulvectomy may be needed. In this operation, all or part of the vulva is removed.

DOs and DON'Ts in Managing Vulvar Cancer:

✔ **DO** have regular check-ups, to catch problems early.

✔ **DO** reduce your risk factors as much as possible. A large percentage of women with vulvar cancer have HPV infection. Practice safe sex. Use condoms if you think that there's any chance of catching an STD.

✔ **DO** talk to your doctor about getting vaccinated for HPV (Gardasil®) if you are between ages 13 and 26.

✔ **DO** call your doctor if you notice skin changes on your labia.

✔ **DO** call your doctor if you have vaginal bleeding that's not related to your period.

🚫 **DON'T** ignore thickening of the skin or sores on your labia.

FROM THE DESK OF

NOTES

FOR MORE INFORMATION

Contact the following source:

• American Cancer Society
Tel: (800) 227-2345
Website: http://www.cancer.org

MANAGING YOUR
ACUTE MYELOGENOUS LEUKEMIA

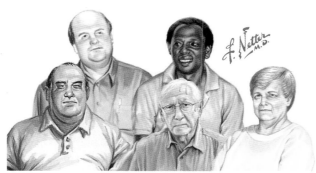

AML is the most common leukemia in adults, occurring in about 12 people per 100,000 population older than 65.

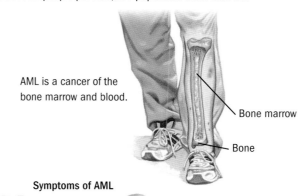

AML is a cancer of the bone marrow and blood.

Bone marrow

Bone

Symptoms of AML

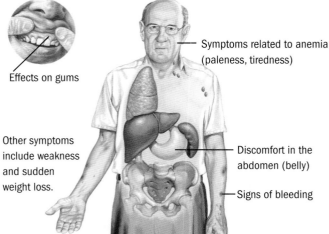

Effects on gums

Other symptoms include weakness and sudden weight loss.

Symptoms related to anemia (paleness, tiredness)

Discomfort in the abdomen (belly)

Signs of bleeding

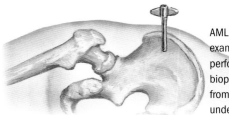

AML is usually found by examining the blood and performing a bone marrow biopsy. Marrow is removed from the bone and studied under a microscope.

What Is Acute Myelogenous Leukemia?

Leukemia is a cancer of the blood and bone marrow. Bone marrow is spongy tissue in the middle of bones. Blood cells form and develop in marrow and then move into the bloodstream. Leukemia can be acute and chronic. Acute leukemia affects cells in bone marrow before they fully develop. Chronic leukemia affects fully grown cells. The four subcategories are acute myelogenous leukemia (AML), acute lymphocytic leukemia (ALL), chronic lymphocytic leukemia (CLL), and chronic myelogenous leukemia (CML). AML, the most common leukemia in adults, affects one type of white blood cells (these cells help fight infection).

What Causes AML?

The cause is unknown. An increased risk of developing AML occurs after exposure to high doses of radiation, the chemical benzene, and drugs used to treat cancers and in people with certain genetic disorders. No effective way to prevent AML is known.

What Are the Symptoms of AML?

Common symptoms include paleness, weakness, shortness of breath, weight loss, and discomfort in the belly (abdomen). Tiredness, easy bleeding, bruising, and frequent infections result from fewer red blood cells (anemia), white blood cells, and platelets. Too many young white cells invade lymph nodes, liver, and spleen and cause swollen glands and enlargement of these organs. Bleeding from lungs, digestive tract, and brain can occur. AML can affect skin, gums, and linings of the spinal cord and brain.

How Is AML Diagnosed?

The doctor will use blood tests and perform a bone marrow biopsy. The biopsy involves removing marrow from bone and examining it under a microscope.

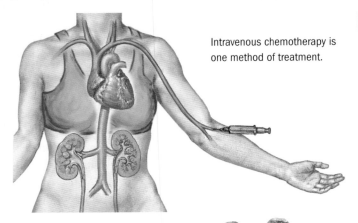

Intravenous chemotherapy is one method of treatment.

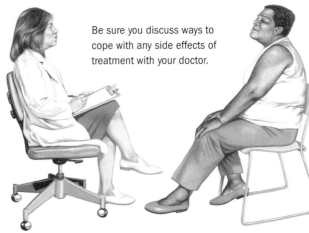

Talk to your doctor about bone marrow transplantation. Close relatives should be tested first because they are typically the best match.

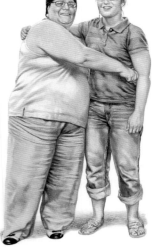

Be sure you discuss ways to cope with any side effects of treatment with your doctor.

How Is AML Treated?

A cancer specialist called an oncologist manages treatment. The goal is complete remission, so that no leukemia cells remain in blood or bone marrow after treatment. First, combination chemotherapy (induction therapy) is given. If needed, additional chemotherapy is used. Chemotherapy also affects normal cells, which can lead to anemia, easy bleeding, and frequent infections.

The doctor will examine the bone marrow after therapy. After complete remission, more chemotherapy is given to prevent leukemia's return.

The doctor may consider bone marrow transplantation, also called stem cell transplantation, at this point. Stem cells are the source of all blood cells. For a bone marrow transplant, healthy marrow containing stem cells is given to replace the abnormal marrow. Donors of healthy marrow are usually close relatives. Stem cells start to produce new blood cells without any leukemia cells.

DOs and DON'Ts in Managing AML:

✔ **DO** understand that treatments vary and depend on factors such as age, genetics, and availability of donor marrow.

✔ **DO** get treated in a center with experienced blood specialists (hematologists).

✔ **DO** ask your doctor for help in coping with side effects.

✔ **DO** tell your doctor if you feel chest pain or shortness of breath during treatment.

✔ **DO** call your doctor if you are bleeding or have a fever after you start chemotherapy.

🚫 **DON'T** miss follow-up appointments. They are extremely important to check for complete remission and for return of leukemia.

FOR MORE INFORMATION

Contact the following sources:

- The Leukemia and Lymphoma Society, Inc.
  Tel: (914) 949-5213, (800) 955-4572
  Website: http://www.leukemia-lymphoma.org

- National Cancer Institute
  Website: http://www.cancer.gov

- National Comprehensive Cancer Network
  Website: http://www.nccn.org

- Children's Oncology Group/National Childhood Cancer Foundation
  Website: http://www.curesearch.org

FROM THE DESK OF

NOTES

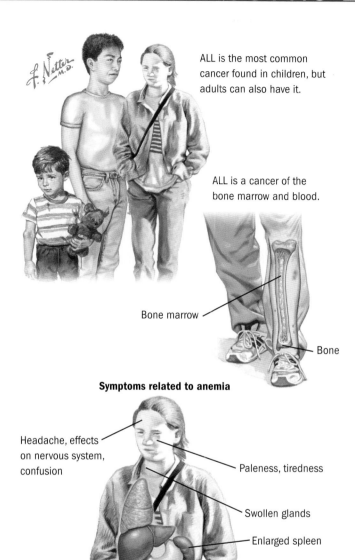

ALL is the most common cancer found in children, but adults can also have it.

ALL is a cancer of the bone marrow and blood.

Bone marrow

Bone

Symptoms related to anemia

Headache, effects on nervous system, confusion

Paleness, tiredness

Swollen glands

Enlarged spleen

Discomfort in the abdomen (belly)

Other symptoms include frequent infections, signs of bleeding, low-grade fever, and generally feeling sick.

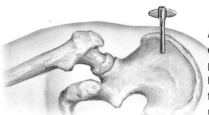

ALL is usually found by examining the blood and performing a bone marrow biopsy. Marrow is removed from the bone and studied under a microscope.

What Is Acute Lymphocytic Leukemia?

Leukemia is a cancer of the blood and bone marrow. Bone marrow is spongy tissue in the middle of bones. Blood cells form and develop in marrow and then move into the bloodstream. Leukemia can be divided into acute and chronic types. Acute leukemia affects cells in bone marrow before they fully develop. Chronic leukemia affects fully grown cells. The four subcategories are acute lymphocytic leukemia (ALL), acute myelogenous leukemia (AML), chronic lymphocytic leukemia (CLL), and chronic myelogenous leukemia (CML).

ALL prevents the body from making normal blood cells and causes production of abnormal young white blood cells. Normal white blood cells help fight infection, whereas leukemic cells are ineffective. ALL cells come from white blood cells called B cells or T cells. ALL usually occurs in children, especially boys, younger than 15. It is the most common cancer in children. Adults can also have ALL.

What Causes ALL?

The cause is unknown, and ALL can't be prevented.

What Are the Symptoms of ALL?

Symptoms include low fever, tiredness, increasing paleness, feeling sick, easy bruising and bleeding, enlarged spleen, pain in the belly (abdomen), frequent infections, and headache. Swollen glands, enlarged liver and spleen, and confusion can occur.

How Is ALL Diagnosed?

The doctor examines the blood and performs a bone marrow biopsy. The biopsy involves removing marrow from bone and examining it under a microscope. The doctor will check to see whether B or T cells are involved. The doctor also tests spinal fluid and may order a chest x-ray, CT (computed tomography) scan, and ultrasound.

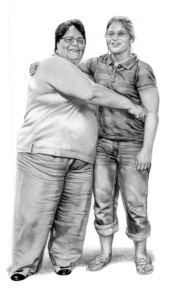

Talk to your doctor about bone marrow transplantation. Close relatives should be tested first because they are typically the best match.

How Is ALL Treated?

ALL can be cured; chemotherapy (anticancer drugs) is the main reason for better survival. At first, hospitalization is needed for blood transfusions, chemotherapy, and radiation.

Treatment usually involves four steps. The first two (using drugs for induction and consolidation) also remove normal blood cells, which can lead to serious complications.

After complete remission, the third step is radiation of the brain and chemotherapy, to get rid of leukemia cells.

Maintenance therapy uses drugs to prevent return of leukemia.

The doctor may consider bone marrow transplantation, also called stem cell transplantation. Healthy marrow containing stem cells (the source of all blood cells) is given, and stem cells produce new healthy cells to replace abnormal ones.

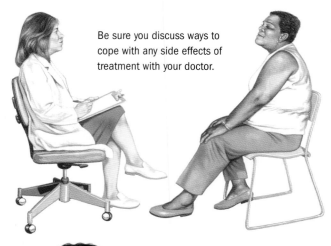

Be sure you discuss ways to cope with any side effects of treatment with your doctor.

DOs and DON'Ts in Managing ALL:

✔ **DO** take good care of your mouth. Rinse often with warm saltwater, and use a soft toothbrush.

✔ **DO** drink extra fluids.

✔ **DO** eat and drink high-calorie foods and beverages if you are getting chemotherapy.

✔ **DO** apply pressure and ice and call your doctor for abnormal bleeding.

✔ **DO** understand that treatments depend on age, genetics, and availability of donor marrow.

✔ **DO** call your doctor if you have a fever during treatment.

✔ **DO** avoid sick people, because your resistance to infection is low.

✔ **DO** go to a center where doctors treat people with ALL.

🚫 **DON'T** take aspirin or any medicine that contains it.

🚫 **DON'T** miss follow-up appointments. They are extremely important to check for complete remission and for return of leukemia.

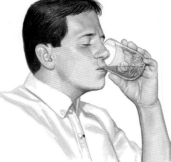

Rinse your mouth often with a warm saltwater solution, and make sure your mouth is in good condition.

FROM THE DESK OF

NOTES

FOR MORE INFORMATION

Contact the following sources:

- The Leukemia & Lymphoma Society, Inc.
  Tel: (914) 949-5213, (800) 955-4572
  Website: http://www.leukemia.org

- National Childhood Cancer Foundation
  Website: http://www.curesearch.org

- American Academy of Pediatrics
  Website: http://www.aap.org

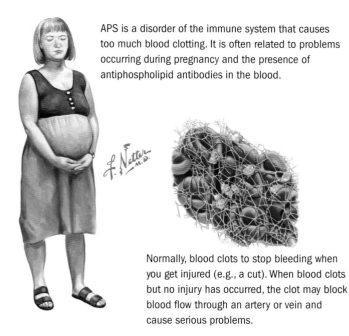

APS is a disorder of the immune system that causes too much blood clotting. It is often related to problems occurring during pregnancy and the presence of antiphospholipid antibodies in the blood.

Normally, blood clots to stop bleeding when you get injured (e.g., a cut). When blood clots but no injury has occurred, the clot may block blood flow through an artery or vein and cause serious problems.

Antiphospholipid antibodies interact with the clotting system so that people can get deep vein thrombosis and arterial thrombosis, which can lead to heart attacks and strokes.

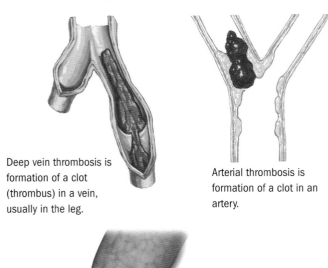

Deep vein thrombosis is formation of a clot (thrombus) in a vein, usually in the leg.

Arterial thrombosis is formation of a clot in an artery.

Clots in deep veins in the legs cause pain, swelling, redness, and warmth.

What Is Antiphospholipid Antibody Syndrome?

In antiphospholipid antibody syndrome (abbreviated APS), people have too much blood clotting and have antiphospholipid antibodies in the blood. Problems with pregnancy, such as miscarriage or premature birth may occur.

What Causes APS?

The cause is unknown. It can't be caught or passed from generation to generation. Antiphospholipid antibodies are thought to interact with the body's clotting system, so people are prone to getting deep vein thrombosis (formation of a blood clot, or thrombus, usually in leg veins) and arterial thrombosis (clots in arteries). These clots can lead to heart attacks and strokes.

The antiphospholipid antibodies are called lupus anticoagulant and anticardiolipin antibodies. They are found in people with systemic lupus erythematosus (an autoimmune disease, meaning the body's immune system attacks itself). Other risk factors for development of APS include rheumatoid arthritis, Behçet's syndrome, and Sjögren's syndrome. Medicine including hydralazine (for blood pressure), quinine (for leg cramps), and certain antibiotics can sometimes cause APS.

What Are the Symptoms of APS?

Clots in both veins and arteries can occur. Most often, venous thrombosis occurs in deep veins of legs. The clots cause leg swelling, pain, redness, and warmth. The most common site for thrombosis in arteries is cerebral (brain) blood vessels. Stroke, with slurred speech, paralysis, numbness, weakness, loss of vision, and swallowing problems, can result.

Other parts of the body involved include the heart, lungs, gastrointestinal tract, kidneys, and skin. Pregnant women can suffer spontaneous abortions, and the blood system can be affected, so anemia (low red blood cell count) or thrombocytopenia (low platelet count) results.

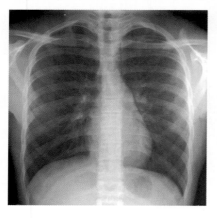

Blood tests and x-rays are used for diagnosis.

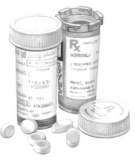

Blood thinners such as warfarin are usually prescribed as treatment in nonpregnant patients. Another blood thinner called heparin is used during pregnancy.

Call your doctor if you have signs of excessive blood thinning.

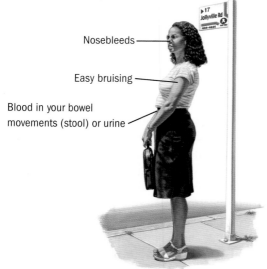

Nosebleeds

Easy bruising

Blood in your bowel movements (stool) or urine

How Is APS Diagnosed?

The doctor may suspect APS because of blood clots, and will order blood tests and x-rays to aid diagnosis and rule out complications.

At least one clinical feature and one laboratory feature are needed for diagnosis. Clinical features are clots or complications in pregnancy (death of a fetus, premature birth, or spontaneous abortions). Laboratory features include presence of anticardiolipin antibodies or lupus anticoagulant.

How Is APS Treated?

Blood thinners are used to prevent clots from forming. Common drugs are heparin and warfarin. If APS is caused by another disease, the doctor will treat that condition.

Regular blood tests are needed to monitor the level of blood thinner. Physical activity such as playing contact sports should be avoided.

DOs and DON'Ts in Managing APS:

✔ **DO** understand that although aspirin is a blood thinner, aspirin alone is not a useful APS treatment.
✔ **DO** understand that you can have antiphospholipid antibodies without having blood clotting, and blood thinners may not be needed.
✔ **DO** call your doctor if you think that you're pregnant or if you have a history of APS and you're pregnant.
✔ **DO** call your doctor if you have symptoms of APS.
✔ **DO** call your doctor if you are using blood thinners and have signs of too much blood thinning, such as easy bruising and bleeding.

🚫 **DON'T** miss your warfarin dose. Its blood level must be kept at the recommended range to reduce clotting risk.
🚫 **DON'T** use oral contraceptives if you already have antiphospholipid antibodies.

FROM THE DESK OF

NOTES

FOR MORE INFORMATION

Contact the following sources:

* National Heart, Lung, and Blood Institute
  Tel: (800) 575-9355
  Website: http://www.nhlbi.nih.gov

* National Stroke Association
  Tel: (800) 787-6537
  Website: http://www.stroke.org

MANAGING YOUR
ASTROCYTOMA

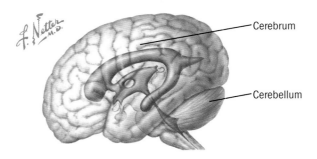

The brain has two major parts, the cerebrum and cerebellum. Astrocytomas can occur in both parts. Children more often have tumors in the cerebellum, at the bottom of the brain.

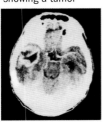

Glioblastoma, a type of astrocytoma

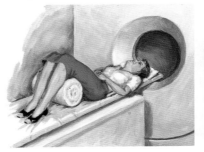

A common symptom is a headache. Some people have new seizures. Other symptoms include vision and speech problems, confusion, disorientation, memory problems, and irritability.

CT scan of the brain showing a tumor

Your doctor may do a CT scan (shown here) or an MRI scan of your brain. These scans can show brain tumors.

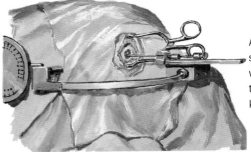

A biopsy is the only sure way to find out whether you have a tumor and what kind it is.

What Are Astrocytomas?

The brain is the major organ of your central nervous system and is made up of nerve cells (neurons) and supportive (glial) tissue. Different cells make up glial tissue, astrocytes and oligodendrocytes being the most numerous. Astrocytomas are brain cancers formed from astrocytes.

Astrocytomas are the most common brain tumors in adults. Children can also have them.

What Causes Astrocytomas?

The cause is unknown. Astrocytomas cannot be caught and aren't passed on from generation to generation.

What Are the Symptoms of Astrocytomas?

Symptoms are headaches (perhaps with nausea and vomiting) or new seizures. Other symptoms include weakness of arms or legs on one side of the body, vision and speech problems, and a change in mental abilities, such as confusion, disorientation, memory problems, and irritability.

How Are Astrocytomas Diagnosed?

The doctor makes a diagnosis on the basis of symptoms, but the first symptoms may be vague and often confused with tension headaches or sinus infections, so it's hard to diagnose. The doctor also uses magnetic resonance imaging (MRI) and computed tomography (CT). If MRI or CT scans show a mass, the only way to prove the diagnosis is to perform a biopsy. For a biopsy, a small piece of the mass is removed and studied under the microscope.

Astrocytomas can be grades I, II, III, or IV. Grades I and II are low-grade tumors, and grades III and IV are high-grade tumors. This system helps doctors decide about treatment and prognosis.

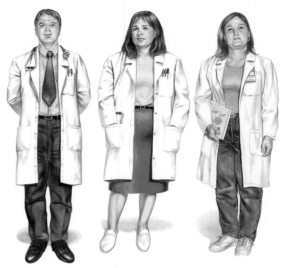

Treatment involves different specialists, including a neurosurgeon (doctor who operates on the nervous system), an oncologist (doctor who treats cancer), and a radiation oncologist (doctor who uses radiation to treat cancer).

After your doctor makes a diagnosis, it's important to have treatment as soon as possible. Surgery is the first treatment of almost all astrocytomas. It also helps the doctor make a diagnosis and decide on the tumor grade.

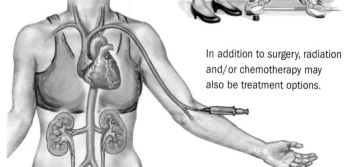

In addition to surgery, radiation and/or chemotherapy may also be treatment options.

FROM THE DESK OF

NOTES

How Are Astrocytomas Treated?

Rapid treatment, with surgery, radiation therapy, or chemotherapy, is very important. Treatment involves different specialists, including a neurosurgeon (a doctor specializing in nervous system surgery), oncologist (a doctor specializing in cancer treatment), and radiation oncologist (a doctor specializing in treating cancer with radiation).

Surgery is used first for almost all astrocytomas, to remove all or as much of the tumor as possible. Complications include bleeding, infection, and permanent nervous system problems.

Most people have radiation therapy after surgery. Complications include dry, red, itchy skin over the radiation site.

People with low-grade astrocytomas don't usually have chemotherapy. People with high-grade astrocytomas can be given chemotherapy with some good results. Side effects are nausea, vomiting, infections, hair loss, easy bruising, and easy bleeding.

DOs and DON'Ts in Managing Astrocytomas:

✔ **DO** realize that about 10% to 35% of astrocytomas (usually grade I) can be completely removed and cured.

✔ **DO** know that treatment of low-grade astrocytomas depends partly on tumor location.

✔ **DO** understand that astrocytomas are hard to remove completely.

✔ **DO** call your doctor if you have a severe headache with nausea and vomiting, muscle weakness on one side of your body, a seizure, or speech or vision problems.

✔ **DO** call your doctor if you have side effects from treatments, such as fever after chemotherapy.

✔ **DO** call your doctor if you need a referral to a specialist.

⊘ **DON'T** miss follow-up appointments with your doctor.

⊘ **DON'T** be afraid to ask for a second opinion. Ask for the opinion of doctors who are experienced in the treatment of people with astrocytomas.

⊘ **DON'T** forget to take your medicines prescribed by your doctor.

FOR MORE INFORMATION

Contact the following source:

• American Cancer Society
  Tel: (800) ACS-2345 (227-2345)
  Website: http://www.cancer.org

MANAGING YOUR
BLADDER CANCER

Normal male bladder

Bladder

Urethra

Bladder cancer may be very small or large, growing deep into the muscle of your bladder.

Small tumor   Large tumor

Muscle

Bladder cancer can be caused by many things, but most often the cause is cigarette smoking.

You may have pain low in your belly (in the pelvic area). One first sign is blood in the urine.

The doctor will examine you and order urine and blood tests to help make a diagnosis.

What Is Bladder Cancer?

The bladder is the organ that stores urine before it leaves the body. The bladder lining consists of transitional cells. Nearly 95% of all bladder cancers start from these cells (transitional cell carcinoma). Bladder cancer is a malignant tumor in this organ and may be small or large, growing deep into the bladder muscle, and it may spread (metastasize).

The other two types are squamous carcinoma and adeno-carcinoma. These tumors are usually larger and often go into the bladder wall and may metastasize.

Bladder cancer develops most often in people older than 50. Men have bladder cancer more often than women do.

What Causes Bladder Cancer?

Many things can cause bladder cancer, most often cigarette smoking. Usually the exact cause is unknown. Chemicals used at jobs in dye, textile, tire, rubber, and petroleum industries are another cause.

What Are the Symptoms of Bladder Cancer?

Very small cancers usually cause no symptoms, but blood in the urine, burning when urinating, or needing to urinate small amounts are possible symptoms.

Larger tumors cause more symptoms, such as pain low in the belly or losing weight.

How Is Bladder Cancer Diagnosed?

The doctor will do an examination and order a urine test to see if the urine shows blood, signs of infection, or abnormal (cancerous) cells.

The doctor may also order blood tests and tests of the kidneys and liver function.

X-rays of the bladder and urinary tract, ultrasound or computed tomography (CT) scans, and cystoscopy (using a lighted tube to see inside the bladder) may also be done. If abnormal areas are found, a piece of tissue (biopsy specimen) is taken for study under a microscope.

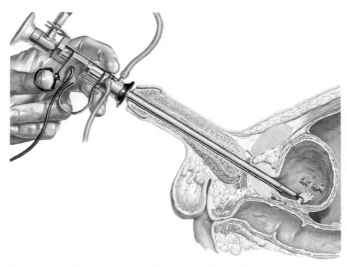

Surgery is needed to remove bladder cancer. The doctor can use endoscopy (using a lighted tube inserted through your urethra into your bladder) to remove the tumor.

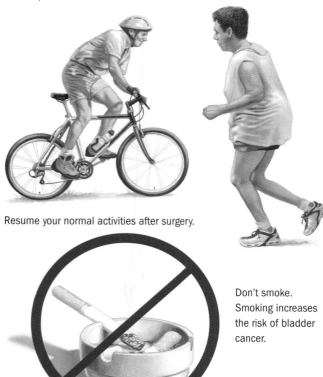

Resume your normal activities after surgery.

Don't smoke. Smoking increases the risk of bladder cancer.

How Is Bladder Cancer Treated?

Surgery is needed to remove the cancer. The operation depends on the type of cancer and whether it has spread.

A small or large tumor is removed by endoscopy (using a lighted tube inserted into the bladder). For a very large cancer, the whole bladder may need to be taken out (radical cystectomy). After this operation, urine will empty out through a pouch through the skin (urostomy), which needs special care.

Pain pills, radiation treatment, and anticancer medicine (chemotherapy) may also be needed.

DOs and DON'Ts in Managing Bladder Cancer:

✔ **DO** take pills as your doctor prescribes.
✔ **DO** resume normal activities (including sexual relations) after surgery or other treatment when your doctor says you can.
✔ **DO** call your doctor if you had surgery and have new symptoms of infection (back pain, fever, and vomiting).
✔ **DO** call your doctor if you have blood in your urine; you feel the need to urinate frequently, with urgency, or with hesitancy; or if urination is painful.
✔ **DO** call your doctor if you have pain or trouble with erections after surgery.
✔ **DO** call your doctor if you have excess bleeding, fever, and chills after cystoscopy.

⊘ **DON'T** smoke.
⊘ **DON'T** be frustrated if superficial cancer returns. The cancer can be controlled with close follow-up care and tumor removal.
⊘ **DON'T** miss follow-up doctor appointments, including cystoscopy every few months for the first year.

FROM THE DESK OF

NOTES

FOR MORE INFORMATION

Contact the following sources:

• The American Cancer Society
  Tel: (800) ACS-2345 (227-2345)
  Website: http://www.cancer.org

• The National Cancer Institute Cancer Information Service
  Tel: (800) 4-CANCER (422-6237)

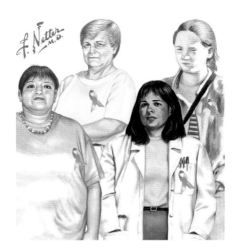

Early detection and treatment of breast cancer increases chances of successful recovery.

The cancer might be detected as a lump that you can feel under the skin of your chest or armpits.

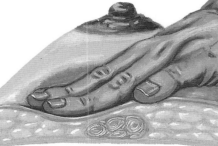

As cancer grows, it can change how your breast looks.

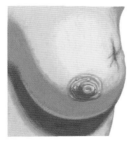

Dimpling of skin

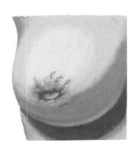

Nipple inversion

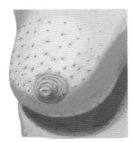

Orange peel appearance

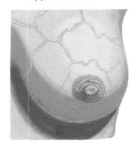

Enlargement and dilation of blood vessels

What Is Breast Cancer?

Breast cancer is abnormal growth of cells in the breast (ducts, lobules, or other tissues). It is the most common cancer in women in the United States. It is the second most common cause of cancer-related death in women, and the main cause of death in women aged 45 to 55. Each year, about 200,000 American women are diagnosed with breast cancer, and more than 40,000 die of this disease. Breast cancer occurs 100 times more often in women than in men.

Even though the number of new cases of breast cancer is rising, the death rate dropped about 20% in the past 20 years. This drop is partly because increased screening catches the disease earlier, so chances of recovery are higher.

Women with a strong family history of breast or ovarian cancer should talk with the doctor about whether blood testing for familial breast cancer is a good idea, to check for genes called BRCA1 and BRCA2.

A higher risk of breast cancer may be related to, among other factors, having previous breast cancer, age (especially older than 50), first menstrual period at a young age (12 or younger), menopause (when periods stopped) after age 55, and taking high-dose estrogen after menopause.

What Are the Symptoms of Breast Cancer?

Early breast cancer usually does not cause pain and may cause no symptoms. About 10% of people have no pain or lumps or any other sign of a problem with the breasts.

A growing breast tumor, however, can cause changes that both women and men should watch for:

- A lump or thickening (mass, swelling, skin irritation, or distortion) in or near the breast or under the arms
- A change in breast size or shape
- A change in color or feel of the skin of the breast, areola, or nipple (dimpled, puckered, or scaly)
- Nipple discharge, erosion, inversion, or tenderness

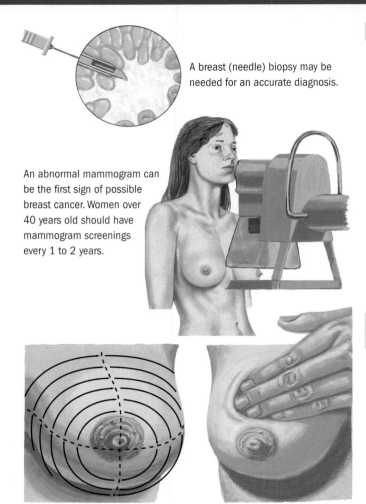

A breast (needle) biopsy may be needed for an accurate diagnosis.

An abnormal mammogram can be the first sign of possible breast cancer. Women over 40 years old should have mammogram screenings every 1 to 2 years.

A monthly breast self-exam is critical for detecting breast cancer before it spreads. Use the pads of the fingers to check the breast, in increasing or decreasing circles, firmly, carefully, and thoroughly. Feel for any unusual lump or mass under the skin. Check your breasts in both standing and lying down positions.

How Is Breast Cancer Diagnosed?

In many cases, a woman or her doctor feels a lump or discovers a change in the breast.

The doctor often suspects breast cancer because of an abnormal mammogram (a low-dose x-ray of breasts). Some women at high risk of developing breast cancer now have magnetic resonance imaging (MRI) to screen for it, in addition to mammograms.

A lump should not be ignored, even if mammogram results are normal. A mammogram doesn't show up to 20% of new breast cancers.

If cancer is suspected, the next step is to confirm the diagnosis by taking a biopsy, or removing a small piece of the abnormal area, for study. The biopsy may be done in the office.

DOs and DON'Ts in Diagnosing and Preventing Breast Cancer:

✔ **DO** have a regular screening mammogram, every 1 to 2 years if older than 40.

✔ **DO** a careful breast self-exam (BSE) monthly.

✔ **DO** get to know how your breasts normally feel so that you can better notice any change.

✔ **DO** call your doctor if you notice lumps or skin changes in your breasts.

✔ **DO** take medicine, if suggested by your doctor.

⊘ **DON'T** smoke.

⊘ **DON'T** drink alcohol in excess.

FROM THE DESK OF

NOTES

FOR MORE INFORMATION

Contact the following sources:

• American Cancer Society
  Website: http://www.cancer.org

• National Comprehensive Cancer Network
  Website: http://www.nccn.org

• Susan G. Komen Breast Cancer Foundation
  Website: http://www.komen.org

MANAGING YOUR
CHRONIC LYMPHOCYTIC LEUKEMIA

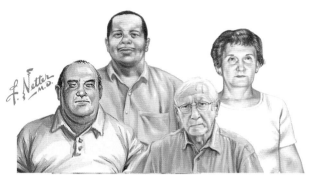

CLL is a very common type of leukemia. It usually occurs among people older than 60, in women twice as often as men.

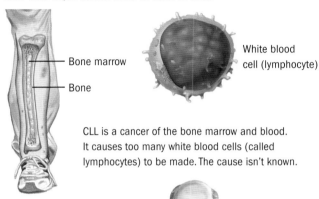

Bone marrow

Bone

White blood cell (lymphocyte)

CLL is a cancer of the bone marrow and blood. It causes too many white blood cells (called lymphocytes) to be made. The cause isn't known.

The most common symptoms are feeling sick and extremely tired, and sometimes infections and swollen glands (enlarged lymph nodes).

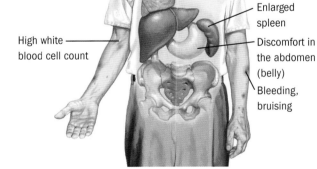

Symptoms related to anemia (paleness, weakness)

Swollen glands

Enlarged spleen

High white blood cell count

Discomfort in the abdomen (belly)

Bleeding, bruising

CLL is usually found by checking blood and urine and doing a bone marrow biopsy. In a biopsy, marrow is removed from the bone and studied under a microscope. Chest x-rays and computed tomography may also be done.

What Is Chronic Lymphocytic Leukemia?

Leukemia is cancer of the blood and bone marrow. Bone marrow is spongy tissue in the middle of bones. Blood cells form and develop in marrow and then move into the bloodstream. Leukemia can be acute or chronic. Acute leukemia affects cells in bone marrow before they fully develop. Chronic leukemia affects fully grown cells.

Chronic lymphocytic leukemia (CLL) causes too many white blood cells to be produced. These cells don't work normally, so people have greater chances of getting serious infections and bleeding.

CLL is the most common type of leukemia in Western countries. It usually occurs among people older than 60, in women twice as often as men. People have a normal lifespan in the early stages. CLL cannot be prevented.

What Causes CLL?

The cause of CLL is unknown. It cannot be caught but does seem to run in families. Also, one third of people with CLL have an extra chromosome 13 (producing trisomy 13). Farmers exposed to certain pesticides and people who work with rubber or asbestos may have an increased risk.

What Are the Symptoms of CLL?

The most common symptoms are feeling sick and extremely tired. Swollen glands (enlarged lymph nodes) or recurrent infections due to a weakened immune system can sometimes be the first symptom. People also have nosebleeds, easy bruising, or other bleeding problems, and weakness from anemia (low red blood cell count) or thrombocytopenia (low platelet count). Other symptoms in advanced stages are shortness of breath, weight loss, discomfort in the abdomen (belly), joint pain and swelling, and fever. Problems with the body's immune (infection-fighting) system lead to special types of blood problems (anemia, thrombocytopenia) and increased chances for bacterial, fungal, and unusual viral infections.

How Is CLL Diagnosed?

About one quarter of people have no symptoms. CLL is often found from blood tests done for another reason. These people have too many white blood cells, swollen glands, or enlarged spleen (the spleen makes and stores blood cells). The doctor may order more blood tests, bone marrow sample, chest x-rays, and computed tomography to determine the stage of CLL.

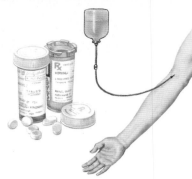

People with no symptoms may need no treatment. People with symptoms have chemotherapy and maybe radiation therapy.

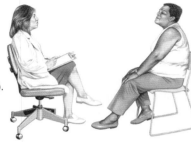

Talk to your doctor about what is the best treatment for you. Ask your doctor for a referral to a hematologist (specialist in blood diseases).

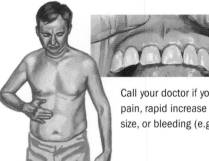

Call your doctor if you have fever, abdominal pain, rapid increase in spleen or lymph gland size, or bleeding (e.g., from gums).

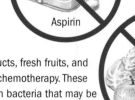

Aspirin

Don't take aspirin or aspirin-containing products.

Avoid dairy products, fresh fruits, and vegetables after chemotherapy. These foods can contain bacteria that may be dangerous to people with low white blood cell counts.

FROM THE DESK OF

NOTES

How Is CLL Treated?

People with no symptoms may need no treatment, but the doctor will watch them carefully. The doctor will suggest seeing a hematologist, a specialist in leukemia treatment.

People with symptoms receive chemotherapy. Chemotherapy can cause side effects, including nausea, vomiting, diarrhea, mouth sores, weakness, bleeding, greater chance of getting more infections, and other cancers.

Radiation therapy to the spleen and lymphoid tissue can help control symptoms. Sometimes the spleen is removed, but this doesn't affect normal living.

Bone marrow transplantation may cure younger people with CLL. Transplantation replaces diseased marrow with healthy marrow. It is not commonly done in CLL due to the advanced age of most patients.

DOs and DON'Ts in Managing CLL:

✔ **DO** take medicine as directed for infections.
✔ **DO** avoid being cut or injured, and use a soft toothbrush to avoid scraping your gums.
✔ **DO** avoid dairy products, fresh fruits, and vegetables after chemotherapy.
✔ **DO** call your doctor if you have fever, abdominal pain, rapid increase in spleen or lymph gland size, or bleeding (e.g., from gums).

⊘ **DON'T** use aspirin or aspirin-containing products without consent from your doctor.
⊘ **DON'T** eat uncooked vegetables, fruits, and milk products.

FOR MORE INFORMATION

Contact the following sources:

• The American Cancer Society
Tel: (800) ACS-2354 or (404) 320-3333
Website: http://www.cancer.org

• The Leukemia and Lymphoma Society
Tel: (914) 949-5213 or (800) 955-4572
Website: http://www.leukemia-lymphoma.org

• Cancer Care Inc.
Tel: (800) 813-HOPE (813-4673)
Website: http://www.cancercare.org

• National Comprehensive Cancer Network
Tel: (888) 909-6226
Website: http://www.nccn.org

CHRONIC MYELOGENOUS LEUKEMIA

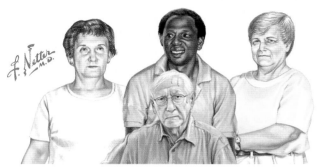

CML occurs among people of all ages but is most common after age 60.

White blood cells

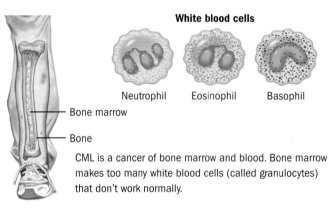

Neutrophil   Eosinophil   Basophil

Bone marrow

Bone

CML is a cancer of bone marrow and blood. Bone marrow makes too many white blood cells (called granulocytes) that don't work normally.

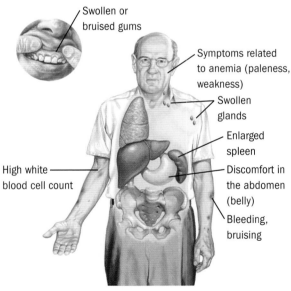

Swollen or bruised gums

Symptoms related to anemia (paleness, weakness)

Swollen glands

Enlarged spleen

Discomfort in the abdomen (belly)

High white blood cell count

Bleeding, bruising

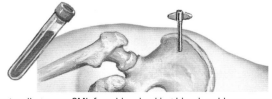

Your doctor diagnoses CML found by checking blood and bone marrow. In a bone marrow biopsy, marrow is removed from the bone for study with a microscope. Finding the Philadelphia chromosome confirms the diagnosis.

What Is Chronic Myelogenous Leukemia?

Leukemia is cancer of the blood and bone marrow. Bone marrow is spongy tissue in the middle of bones. Blood cells form and develop in marrow and then move into the bloodstream. Leukemia can be acute or chronic. Acute leukemia affects young (immature) cells in bone marrow. Chronic leukemia affects fully grown cells. About 20% of adult leukemia cases are chronic myelogenous leukemia (CML).

CML causes bone marrow to make too many white blood cells. These cells don't work normally.

In chronic CML, white blood cells become more immature and cannot fight infection. In advanced CML, most white blood cells are myeloblasts, the most immature cell, and people can get serious infections. CML occurs among people of all ages but is most common after age 60. CML cannot be caught or prevented and usually isn't passed on from parents to children.

What Causes CML?

The cause is unknown, but benzene and high radiation doses may be involved. Also, CML cells contain a chromosome abnormality (Philadelphia chromosome, found in over 95 percent of people with CML).

What Are the Symptoms of CML?

Many people with chronic CML have no or few symptoms. Some feel fullness in the abdomen (belly) from a large spleen. Some people may have tiredness, loss of appetite and weight, sweating, swollen or bruised gums, shortness of breath, bleeding, and bone pain.

Anemia (low red blood cell count) and thrombocytopenia (low platelet count) occur later. People with advanced CML may have severe headaches or shortness of breath (high numbers of myeloblasts get stuck in the lungs and brain).

How Is CML Diagnosed?

The doctor diagnoses chronic CML by blood and bone marrow tests that show a high white blood cell count, high platelet count, and Philadelphia chromosomes in marrow cells. For a bone marrow biopsy, a long hollow needle is inserted into the bone to remove a marrow sample for study with a microscope.

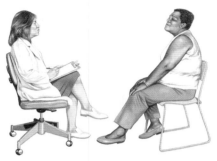

A hematologist (specialist in blood diseases) or oncologist (specialist in cancer) will treat you with medicine or bone marrow transplantation. More than half of people with chronic CML who get transplants are well and disease-free 5 years later.

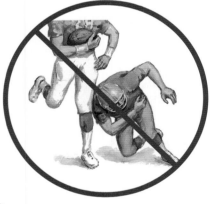

Tell your doctor if you have new symptoms; feel tired; lose weight; or have pain in the left side of your belly, bleeding, fever, sudden severe headaches, or shortness of breath.

Don't play contact sports if your platelet count is low (you may not have enough platelets to stop bleeding). Stop exercising if you get dizzy or short of breath or have pain.

Don't eat uncooked fruits, vegetables, and milk products during or immediately after chemotherapy. These foods can contain bacteria that may be dangerous to people with low white blood cell counts.

FROM THE DESK OF

NOTES

How Is CML Treated?

Hematologists (specialists in blood diseases) or oncologists (specialists in cancer) treat people with CML.

Abnormal bone marrow is replaced with healthy marrow or is treated with medicine. Replacement of marrow is called transplantation. Marrow donors are usually close relatives (brother, sister) or volunteers whose marrow is a close match. Transplantation has many side effects or complications including hair loss and mouth sores, infections, and life-threatening graft-versus-host disease.

The best drug treatment is imatinib (Gleevec).

DOs and DON'Ts in Managing CML:

✔ **DO** keep an active lifestyle, but exercise with caution.
✔ **DO** ask your doctor about diet limits.
✔ **DO** get a flu shot every fall.
✔ **DO** brush your teeth with a soft toothbrush.
✔ **DO** shave only with an electric razor if you have accelerated or advanced CML.
✔ **DO** tell your doctor if you have new symptoms or unexplained tiredness, weight loss, pain in the left side of your abdomen, bleeding, fever, sudden severe headaches, or shortness of breath.

🚫 **DON'T** eat uncooked fruits, vegetables, and milk products during or immediately after chemotherapy.
🚫 **DON'T** play contact sports if your platelet count is low.

FOR MORE INFORMATION

Contact the following sources:

• American Cancer Society
Tel: (800) ACS-2345 or (403) 320-3333
Website: http://www.cancer.org

• The Leukemia and Lymphoma Society
Tel: (800) 955-4572
Website: http://www.leukemia-lymphoma.org

• National Marrow Donor Program
Tel: (800) 627-7692
Website: http://www.marrow.org

• National Cancer Institute
Tel: (800) 4-CANCER (422-6237)
Website: http://www.cancer.gov

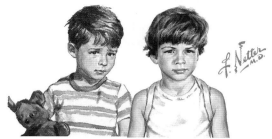

Hemophilia is an inherited blood disorder that causes bleeding. Factor VIII (hemophilia A) or factor IX (hemophilia B), both important blood clotting proteins, are too low. About 80% of people with hemophilia have hemophilia A, the rest have hemophilia B.

What Is Hemophilia?

Hemophilia is an inherited blood disorder that causes bleeding. Factor VIII or factor IX, which are important proteins in the blood for clotting, are too low. Hemophilia A (lack of factor VIII) is much more common than hemophilia B (lack of factor IX). About 80% of people have hemophilia A. Most hemophiliacs lead normal lives. Hemophilia is rather rare, occurring in 1 per 10,000 to 30,000 newborn boys.

What Causes Hemophilia?

Hemophilia is genetically passed to children, usually males, by their mothers. It's called a sex-linked disorder.

DNA

X-chromosome carries defect

Hemophilia is genetically passed to children, usually males, by their mothers. It's called a sex-linked disorder. Women usually have no symptoms because they have two X chromosomes, so one can be affected but the other one has normal genes. Men have only one X chromosome, so if that one is affected, hemophilia results.

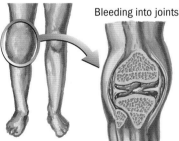

Bleeding into joints

Easy bruising and bleeding are the most common symptoms. Muscle and joint stiffness and slow healing are also symptoms.

What Are the Symptoms of Hemophilia?

Bleeding and easy bruising are the most common symptoms and can be mild to severe. Some people bleed after a minor injury, others rarely bleed, and sometimes bleeding starts without an injury. Bleeding can occur anywhere, but many bleeds start in a muscle or joint such as the knee and may cause pain or swelling. Bleeding gums and bloody urine are also common. Other symptoms include joint and muscle pain or stiffness and slow wound healing. Hemophilia can cause joints to tighten and lose the ability to move.

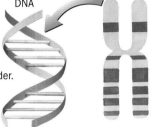

Bleeding after minor dental procedures, such as tooth extraction, and bleeding gums are other signs.

How Is Hemophilia Diagnosed?

Hemophilia is usually found in childhood, but sometimes people are diagnosed in early adulthood, such as after a tooth is pulled and bleeding can't be stopped.

The doctor will take a medical history, do a physical examination, and test blood for levels of factor VIII and factor IX. The doctor may suggest seeing a hematologist (specialist in blood problems).

Hemophilia is usually found in childhood, but sometimes people are diagnosed in early adulthood. Your doctor will take a medical history, examine you, and test blood for levels of factor VIII and factor IX. Your doctor may suggest seeing a hematologist.

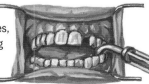

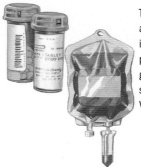

Treatment depends on levels of factors VIII and IX. Treatment is aimed at preventing injuries and increased levels of clotting proteins. Blood factors or medicines are given. When bleeding starts, treatment must start also, usually as self-infusion of factor VIII. Serious bleeding needs hospital care.

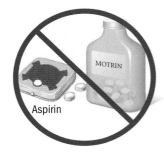

Don't use aspirin, ibuprofen (e.g., Motrin®, Advil®), naproxen (e.g., Aleve®), or other nonsteroidal antiinflammatory drugs.

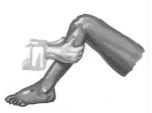

Physical therapy may help muscle and joint stiffness.

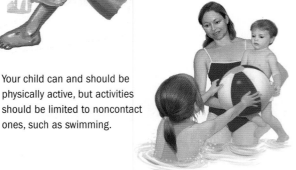

Your child can and should be physically active, but activities should be limited to noncontact ones, such as swimming.

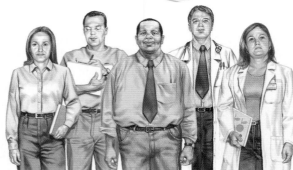

With help of an informed team, a person with hemophilia can live a normal life. Contact your hematologist before dental procedures or surgery. Keep your child's teachers and babysitters aware of the condition, so that they can act quickly if something happens.

FROM THE DESK OF

NOTES

How Is Hemophilia Treated?

Treatment involves replacing blood factors or using medicine. When bleeding starts, treatment must start also, usually as self-infusion of factor VIII. If started at home, infusion can continue at the hospital. Serious bleeding needs hospital treatment. To prevent damage, bleeding into a muscle or joint must be stopped as soon as possible. Surgery is sometimes needed to fix damaged joints or muscles. Special physical therapy exercises may help heal joints. Pain medicine is given. People who suffer trauma should go to the hospital immediately.

People who need surgery get factor replacement before and after surgery. Medicine such as desmopressin or aminocaproic acid can be used in mild cases.

DOs and DON'Ts in Managing Hemophilia:

✔ **DO** follow your doctor's directions about what to do if you bleed or are injured.
✔ **DO** tell your doctor about medicines you take, prescription and nonprescription.
✔ **DO** see your dentist twice yearly.
✔ **DO** exercise but avoid contact sports such as football. Swimming is OK.
✔ **DO** tell your doctor if you're going to the dentist or having surgery.
✔ **DO** go to the emergency room if you bleed from your rectum, cough up blood, suddenly have a bad headache, or cannot stop bleeding.
✔ **DO** avoid intramuscular injections.
✔ **DO** accident-proof your home. Wear a seatbelt and drive safely.

🚫 **DON'T** take medicine unless your doctor tells you to.
🚫 **DON'T** use aspirin, ibuprofen (e.g., Motrin®, Advil®), naproxen (e.g., Aleve®), or other nonsteroidal antiinflammatory drugs. These medications will increase the risk of bleeding.

FOR MORE INFORMATION

Contact the following sources:

• National Hemophilia Foundation
  Tel: (212) 328-3700
  Website: http://www.hemophilia.org

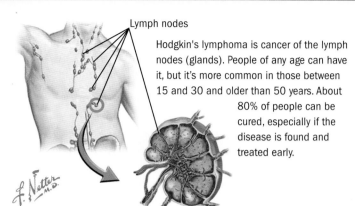

Lymph nodes

Hodgkin's lymphoma is cancer of the lymph nodes (glands). People of any age can have it, but it's more common in those between 15 and 30 and older than 50 years. About 80% of people can be cured, especially if the disease is found and treated early.

F. Netter M.D.

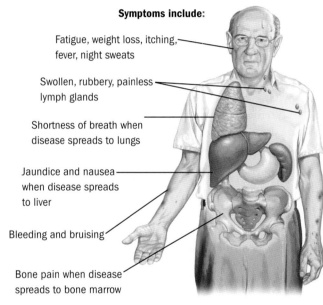

Symptoms include:

Fatigue, weight loss, itching, fever, night sweats

Swollen, rubbery, painless lymph glands

Shortness of breath when disease spreads to lungs

Jaundice and nausea when disease spreads to liver

Bleeding and bruising

Bone pain when disease spreads to bone marrow

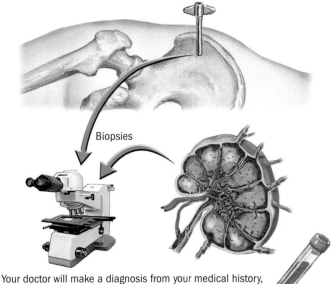

Biopsies

Your doctor will make a diagnosis from your medical history, physical examination, blood tests, lymph gland and bone marrow biopsies, x-rays, CT, and PET scan.

What Is Hodgkin's Lymphoma?

Hodgkin's lymphoma (or Hodgkin's disease) is cancer of the lymph nodes (lymph glands). Lymph glands and lymph vessels are part of the immune system that filter infection from the body. The disease usually affects lymph glands, white blood cells, and the spleen. People of any age can have it, but those between 15 and 30 and older than 50 years most often get it. It can range from mild to severe. About 80% of people can be cured, especially if the disease is found and treated early.

What Causes Hodgkin's Lymphoma?

The cause is unknown. People with impaired immune systems have greater risk.

What Are the Symptoms of Hodgkin's Lymphoma?

The most common symptom is swollen, painless, rubbery lymph glands, usually in the armpit, groin, and neck. Others include bleeding or easy bruising, fatigue, fever, itching, night sweats, pain in lymph glands after drinking alcohol, weakness, and weight loss. Certain symptoms relate to where the disease spreads.

How Is Hodgkin's Lymphoma Diagnosed?

The doctor will make a diagnosis from a medical history, physical examination, blood tests, and lymph gland and bone marrow biopsies. Biopsies involve getting bone marrow (with a needle) or small pieces of lymph node tissue for study with a microscope. Other tests may in some cases include laparotomy, which is surgery on the abdomen (belly) for disease staging. Staging shows how far the disease has spread. Chest x-ray, computed tomography (CT), and positron emission tomography (PET, a kind of x-ray) may also be done for staging. The doctor may suggest seeing an oncologist (cancer treatment specialist) and radiation oncologist (specialist in treating cancer with radiation).

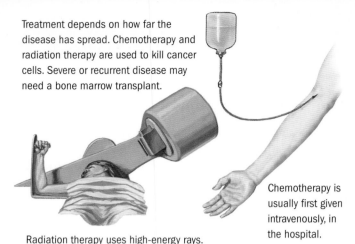

Treatment depends on how far the disease has spread. Chemotherapy and radiation therapy are used to kill cancer cells. Severe or recurrent disease may need a bone marrow transplant.

Radiation therapy uses high-energy rays.

Chemotherapy is usually first given intravenously, in the hospital.

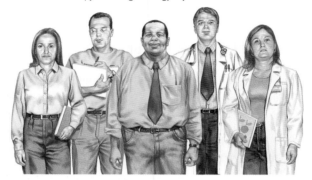

Remember that treatment involves a team: your primary doctor, oncologist, radiation oncologist, surgeon, nutritionist, and social service workers. Talk to someone about the stress of having cancer. Call your doctor if you feel depressed. Find support groups.

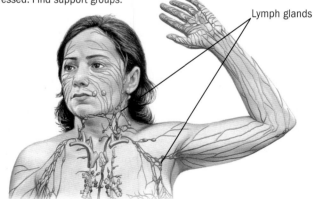

Lymph glands

Don't ignore swollen lymph glands. Don't miss follow-up doctor appointments to check your response to treatment and to watch for new symptoms.

How Is Hodgkin's Lymphoma Treated?

Treatment depends on how far the disease has spread. Chemotherapy (using drugs) and radiation therapy (or radiotherapy) are used to kill the cancer cells. Chemotherapy is usually first given intravenously (directly into vein), in the hospital. Pain medicine will also be given. Severe or recurrent disease may need a bone marrow transplant. Some treatments may affect the ability to have children.

DOs and DON'Ts in Managing Hodgkin's Lymphoma:

✔ **DO** tell your doctor about your medicines, including prescription and over-the-counter ones.
✔ **DO** tell your doctor if you're pregnant or breastfeeding.
✔ **DO** talk to someone about the stress of having cancer. Call your doctor if you feel depressed. Find support groups.
✔ **DO** take care of your teeth and mouth to prevent mouth sores.
✔ **DO** consider placing sperm in a sperm bank or eggs in an egg bank if you are planning to have children.
✔ **DO** remember that treatment involves a team: primary care doctor, oncologist, radiation oncologist, surgeon, nutritionist, and social service workers.
✔ **DO** call your doctor if you have pain, fever, or drainage from the incision after surgery.
✔ **DO** call your doctor if you have shortness of breath, chest pain, or coughing with a fever after radiation.
✔ **DO** call your doctor if you have bleeding, bruising, fever, nausea, or vomiting after chemotherapy.

⊘ **DON'T** ignore swollen lymph glands.
⊘ **DON'T** miss follow-up appointments during or after treatment.
⊘ **DON'T** be afraid to ask for medicine for pain, nausea, or vomiting.

FROM THE DESK OF

NOTES

FOR MORE INFORMATION

Contact the following sources:

• Leukemia and Lymphoma Society
Tel: (800) 955-4572
Website: http://www.leukemia-lymphoma.org

• National Cancer Institute
Tel: (800) 422-6237
Website: http://www.cancer.gov

MANAGING YOUR
THROMBOPHILIA

Thrombophilia is a condition related to the increased tendency of blood to clot (thrombosis). People can inherit it or have it because of another illness (an acquired disorder). Antiphospholipid antibody syndrome is the most common cause of the acquired disorder. Serious and life-threatening complications can result.

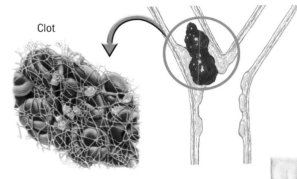

Clot

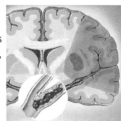

People can get blood clots in veins or arteries. Venous clots occur most often in deep veins of the legs and cause swelling, pain, redness, and warmth. Arterial thrombosis occurs most often in vessels in the head. They cause symptoms of stroke.

Stroke

Deep vein clot

Clotting trouble in antiphospholipid antibody syndrome is usually related to problems in pregnancy.

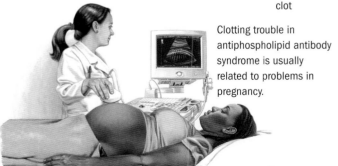

For diagnosis, the doctor usually does blood tests to find clotting disorders. Also, imaging studies can find locations of clots. For example, ultrasonography will show clots in deep veins of the leg.

What Is Thrombophilia?

Thrombophilia, or a hypercoagulable state, is a condition related to the increased tendency of blood to clot (thrombosis). People can inherit it or have it because of another illness (an acquired disorder). Sometimes, serious and life-threatening complications result.

What Causes Thrombophilia?

Inherited causes involve mutations in certain genes. People get these genes from their parents. The most common is factor V Leiden mutation. Others are a prothrombin mutation, hyperhomocysteinemia, and increased factor VIII activity. Prothrombin is a clotting protein in blood. Hyperhomocysteinemia means that there is too much of the amino acid homocysteine in the blood, which is related to not having enough of certain vitamins. Other rare inherited disorders include deficiency (not enough) of protein C, protein S, and antithrombin III (another protein that helps blood clotting). These disorders are often related to complications in pregnancy.

Antiphospholipid antibody syndrome is the most common cause of acquired thrombophilia. Antiphospholipid antibody is thought to be an abnormal blood protein. The cause of this syndrome is unknown, but it's not contagious or passed from parents to children.

What Are the Symptoms of Thrombophilia?

People can get blood clots in veins (venous thrombosis) or arteries (arterial thrombosis). Venous clots occur most often in deep veins of the legs and cause swelling, pain, redness, and warmth in the leg. Arterial thrombosis occurs most often in vessels in the head. They cause symptoms of stroke (e.g., slurred speech, paralysis, numbness, weakness, loss of vision, swallowing problems). People with antiphospholipid antibody syndrome have too much blood clotting. The clotting is usually related to problems with pregnancy (e.g., miscarriage, premature birth) and having antiphospholipid antibodies in the blood.

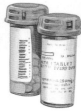

Medicine will be prescribed to thin the blood. Common drugs include heparin (given intravenously), low-molecular-weight heparin (given by injections under the skin), and warfarin (taken orally). Other diseases causing thrombophilia (e.g., systemic lupus erythematosus, rheumatoid arthritis) should be treated.

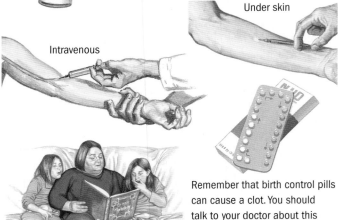

Under skin

Intravenous

Remember that birth control pills can cause a clot. You should talk to your doctor about this and consider an alternate birth control method.

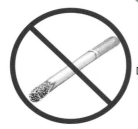

Consider screening family members for thrombophilia.

Call your doctor immediately you have swelling of one of your arms or legs, shortness of breath, or symptoms of a stroke.

Don't smoke.

How Is Thrombophilia Diagnosed?

For diagnosis, the doctor looks for clotting disorders, especially clots occurring in people younger than 50, repeated clots without an obvious cause, clots in unusual places, clots during or after pregnancy, and loss of a baby during pregnancy. The doctor will order tests to rule out the inherited and acquired disorders. Usually, these are blood tests (e.g., Factor V Leiden, protein C, protein S, lupus anticoagulant). Imaging studies can be used to locate clots. For example, ultrasonography will show clots in deep veins of the leg.

How Is Thrombophilia Treated?

Medicine will be prescribed to thin the blood. Common drugs include heparin (given intravenously), low-molecular-weight heparin (given by injections under the skin), and warfarin (taken orally). If thrombophilia is caused by another disease, such as systemic lupus erythematosus or rheumatoid arthritis, that condition will be treated. For hyperhomocysteinemia, vitamins such as folic acid, vitamin B6, and vitamin B12 may be given.

DOs and DON'Ts in Managing Thrombophilia:

✔ **DO** remember that oral birth control pills can cause a clotting event. You may have to avoid taking these pills. Check with your doctor.

✔ **DO** consider screening family members for thrombophilia.

✔ **DO** call your doctor immediately if you have swelling of one of your arms or legs, shortness of breath, or symptoms of a stroke.

⊘ **DON'T** smoke. Tobacco can increase your chances of having a clotting disorder.

⊘ **DON'T** forget that lifelong blood-thinning medicine may be needed.

FROM THE DESK OF

NOTES

FOR MORE INFORMATION

Contact the following source:

• National Heart, Lung, and Blood Institute
Tel: (301) 592-8573
Website: http://www.nhlbi.nih.gov

Red blood cells

Iron deficiency anemia occurs when the body doesn't have enough iron to make a normal supply of red blood cells. Usual causes are blood loss and having too little iron in the diet.

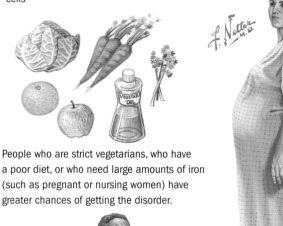

People who are strict vegetarians, who have a poor diet, or who need large amounts of iron (such as pregnant or nursing women) have greater chances of getting the disorder.

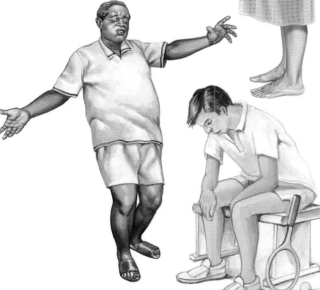

Symptoms are feeling tired and dizzy and having trouble with normal daily activities. Others are shortness of breath, palpitations, chest pain, and pale skin.

Your doctor makes a diagnosis by doing blood tests to measure the iron and hemoglobin content and the different kinds of blood cells. A bone marrow test may also be done.

What Is Iron Deficiency Anemia?

Iron deficiency anemia occurs when the body doesn't have enough iron to make a normal supply of red blood cells.

What Causes Iron Deficiency Anemia?

The cause is usually loss of blood or having too little iron in the diet. Normally, the body saves iron. As old red blood cells break down, iron inside is reused to make new red blood cells.

Iron-rich foods are animal products such as meat, milk, and eggs. Vegetables such as spinach and broccoli are iron rich, but the intestine can't absorb them as well. In developing countries, poor nutrition is the main cause of anemia. In Europe and the United States, chronic blood loss is more often the cause of iron deficiency.

People who are vegetarians (don't eat animal products), have a poor diet, or need large amounts of iron (such as pregnant or nursing women) have greater chances of getting the disorder. Also at risk are people with celiac disease, gastric ulcers, or intestinal tumors.

What Are the Symptoms of Iron Deficiency Anemia?

Symptoms are feeling tired and dizzy and having trouble doing normal daily activities. Severe disease may cause shortness of breath and pale skin. Long-lasting disease causes sore mouth, trouble swallowing, and soft, curling fingernails.

Another symptom is craving crunchy foods or ice cubes or eating odd things such as dirt or clay (called pica).

How Is Iron Deficiency Anemia Diagnosed?

The doctor makes a diagnosis by doing blood tests to measure the iron and hemoglobin content. Finding the reason for iron loss is important, especially for babies, teens, and pregnant women. Blood loss from the intestinal tract due to cancer or bleeding ulcers must be ruled out.

If the diagnosis remains unclear, the doctor may do a bone marrow test. A blood specialist will get a small sample of bone marrow from a spot near the hip and will study it with a microscope to determine the iron content and rule out other blood disorders that can cause anemia.

Treatment depends on the severity of the anemia. Extra iron as pills or liquid will likely be needed daily. Severe anemia may mean a blood transfusion.

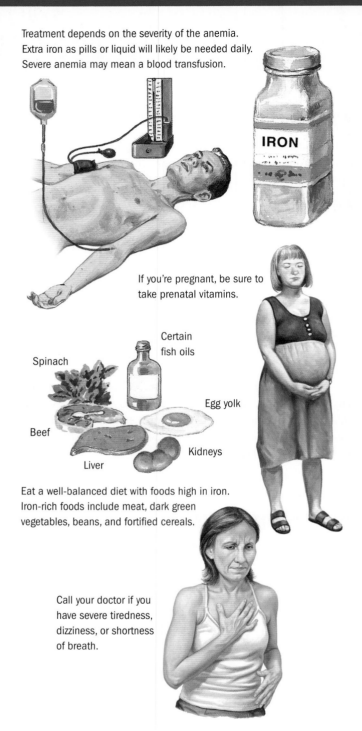

If you're pregnant, be sure to take prenatal vitamins.

Certain fish oils

Spinach

Beef

Liver

Egg yolk

Kidneys

Eat a well-balanced diet with foods high in iron. Iron-rich foods include meat, dark green vegetables, beans, and fortified cereals.

Call your doctor if you have severe tiredness, dizziness, or shortness of breath.

How Is Iron Deficiency Anemia Treated?

Treatment depends on how severe the anemia is. Usually, people need to take extra iron as pills or liquids. Iron is taken at least once daily for 3 to 6 months. Severe anemia may mean a blood transfusion. Recovery is slow. An iron supplement may be needed for several months or years, but people start feeling better in a few weeks.

DOs and DON'Ts in Managing Iron Deficiency Anemia:

✔ **DO** take your iron supplement as directed by your doctor.
✔ **DO** take prenatal vitamins if you're pregnant. Keep taking them if you breast-feed.
✔ **DO** eat a well-balanced diet with foods high in iron, such as meat, beans, and leafy green vegetables.
✔ **DO** watch for and report symptoms of worsening anemia. Call your doctor if you have severe tiredness, dizziness, chest pain, or shortness of breath.
✔ **DO** call your doctor if you have bleeding or chronic bleeding increases.
✔ **DO** call your doctor if you have abdominal pain from the iron supplement. A lower dose or changing the supplement may help.

⊘ **DON'T** overexert yourself.

FROM THE DESK OF

NOTES

FOR MORE INFORMATION

Contact the following sources:

• The American Society of Hematology
Tel: (202) 776-0544
Website: http://www.hematology.org

• Centers for Disease Control and Prevention
Tel : (800) 311-3435
Website: http://www.cdc.gov

• National Heart, Lung, and Blood Institute Health Information Center
Tel: (301)592 8573
Website: http://www.nhlbi.nih.gov/health/index.htm

CARING FOR YOUR NEWBORN WITH
JAUNDICE

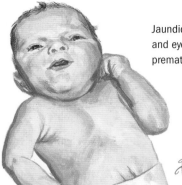

Jaundice, a yellowing of a newborn's skin and eyes, is common, especially in premature babies.

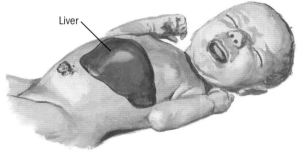

The yellow color results from too much of a substance called bilirubin. Bilirubin forms when red blood cells break down. The body usually gets rid of bilirubin through the liver. Because newborn babies have an immature liver, sometimes bilirubin builds up faster than the body can get rid of it.

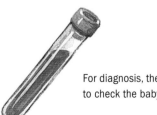

For diagnosis, the doctor will do a simple blood test to check the baby's bilirubin level.

What Is Jaundice?

Jaundice, also called icterus, is yellowing of the skin and whites of the eyes. It's a very common condition in newborns. Jaundice usually gets better by itself and disappears in a few days.

What Causes Jaundice?

A substance called bilirubin can build up in the blood. Bilirubin forms when red blood cells break down. The body usually gets rid of bilirubin through the liver. Because the liver in newborns is immature, sometimes bilirubin builds up faster than the body can get rid of it. Jaundice is the result. Very high levels of bilirubin can hurt the baby's nervous system. This condition is called kernicterus. Premature babies are more likely to get jaundice than are full-term babies.

Other causes include infection, a blood type conflict between mother and baby, and breast milk. Sometimes, breast milk interferes with the ability of a baby's liver to process bilirubin. This type of jaundice develops later than the others and can last for several weeks.

What Are the Symptoms of Jaundice?

The most common symptom is yellowing of the skin and whites of the eyes. Other symptoms, with very high bilirubin levels, are being drowsy and not eating well.

How Is Jaundice Diagnosed?

The doctor will do a simple blood test to check the bilirubin level.

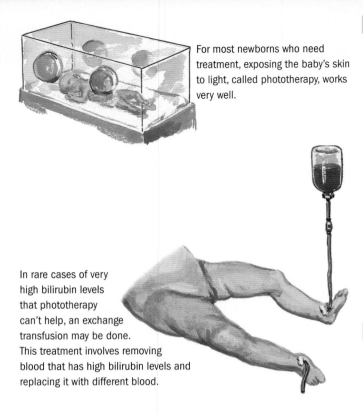

For most newborns who need treatment, exposing the baby's skin to light, called phototherapy, works very well.

In rare cases of very high bilirubin levels that phototherapy can't help, an exchange transfusion may be done. This treatment involves removing blood that has high bilirubin levels and replacing it with different blood.

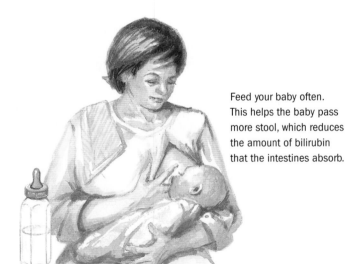

Feed your baby often. This helps the baby pass more stool, which reduces the amount of bilirubin that the intestines absorb.

How Is Jaundice Treated?

Many babies don't need treatment.

When treatment is needed, the best is phototherapy. The baby lies naked under fluorescent lights. The baby has eye patches to protect the eyes during the treatment. The lights help break down excess bilirubin so it can be removed more easily. An "ultraviolet blanket" can also be used. Bilirubin blood levels are checked regularly. Phototherapy usually lowers bilirubin levels in 2 days. Sometimes, the bilirubin level goes up after phototherapy, but only temporarily. The yellow color may last for a few days or even a week or two, even with low bilirubin blood levels.

In rare cases of extremely high bilirubin levels that can't be lowered by phototherapy, exchange transfusion may be done. This treatment involves removing blood with high levels of bilirubin and replacing it with different blood.

DOs and DON'Ts in Managing Jaundice:

✔ **DO** feed your baby often. This helps the baby pass more stool, which reduces the amount of bilirubin that the intestines absorb.

✔ **DO** see your doctor right away if your baby seems to be getting jaundice again, because it can mean that there's a different problem. Once newborn jaundice clears up, it usually doesn't come back.

⊘ **DON'T** panic. Most babies recover completely without treatment.

FROM THE DESK OF

NOTES

FOR MORE INFORMATION

Contact the following source:

• American Academy of Pediatrics
Tel: (847) 434-4000
Website: http://www.aap.org

MANAGING YOUR
LARYNGEAL CANCER

Your larynx is an organ that lies in front of your neck just above your windpipe. Laryngeal carcinoma is cancer of the larynx. Men are four times more likely to have it than women. The exact cause isn't known.

Larynx
Artery
Thyroid gland
Windpipe

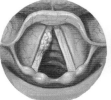
Open

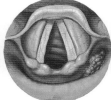
Closed

When you breathe, the vocal cords relax and open. When you hold your breath, the vocal cords close.

Places and types of laryngeal cancer

Early carcinoma, left vocal cord

Carcinoma in space near vocal cords

Carcinoma near cartilage

A common symptom is hoarseness or change in the voice. Other symptoms are a cough that doesn't go away, pain and trouble swallowing, loss of appetite and weight, and swollen neck lymph glands.

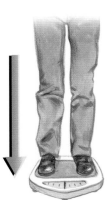
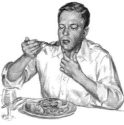
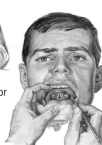

For diagnosis, your doctor uses a long-handled mirror to look down your throat. Your doctor may also do direct laryngoscopy and put a tool called a laryngoscope through your nose or mouth to look at your throat.

What Is Laryngeal Cancer?

The larynx lies in front of the neck just above the windpipe (trachea). It's used to make voice sounds and is also called the voice box. It helps breathing and swallowing. During breathing, vocal cords relax and open. The vocal cords close when holding the breath. With swallowing, the larynx stops foods and liquids from going down the windpipe into the lungs. Laryngeal carcinoma is cancer of the larynx.

More than 10,000 new cases are diagnosed in the United States each year. More men than women get it, but in the past 30 years women have been getting it more often, maybe because of increasing tobacco and alcohol use.

What Causes Laryngeal Cancer?

The exact cause is unknown. Some things that increase chances of getting it include age (older than 55), sex (men more than women), smoking, drinking alcohol, gastroesophageal reflux disease (GERD), and work exposures to substances such as sulfuric acid and asbestos. Smoking with drinking means even higher risk. Laryngeal caner is not contagious.

What Are the Symptoms of Laryngeal Cancer?

A common symptom is lasting hoarseness or change in the voice. Other symptoms are a cough that doesn't go away, trouble swallowing, pain with swallowing, loss of appetite and weight, swollen lymph glands in the neck, and shortness of breath.

How Is Laryngeal Cancer Diagnosed?

For diagnosis, the doctor may do indirect laryngoscopy. The doctor uses a long-handled mirror to look down the throat to see whether vocal cords move properly. The doctor may also do direct laryngoscopy and put a thin lighted tube (laryngoscope) through the nose or mouth to look down the throat. Biopsy may be done. In a biopsy, a small piece of tissue is removed to look for cancer cells with a microscope.

Laryngeal cancer must be staged to find out how far it has spread. Staging is usually done with computed tomography (CT) or magnetic resonance imaging (MRI).

You need a team of doctors—oncologist, radiation oncologist, and surgeon—and other health care workers to help with treatment.

Treatment includes surgery, radiation therapy, and chemotherapy. Surgery to remove the larynx is called laryngectomy. All or part of the larynx may be removed. After surgery, you may need a new airway in your neck (tracheostomy).

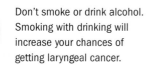

Don't smoke or drink alcohol. Smoking with drinking will increase your chances of getting laryngeal cancer.

Call your doctor if you see swollen lymph glands in your neck, you're hoarse or have voice changes, have neck or ear pain, or have trouble swallowing.

How Is Laryngeal Cancer Treated?

Treatments includes surgery, radiation therapy, and chemotherapy. Surgery to remove the larynx is called laryngectomy, either total (removing the whole larynx) or partial (removing only part). Sometimes, lymph nodes are removed. After laryngectomy, a new airway through the front of the neck (tracheostomy) may be needed.

Radiation therapy uses high-energy x-rays to kill cancer cells. It may be used alone to kill small tumors, before surgery to shrink large tumors, or with chemotherapy.

Chemotherapy (drugs that kill cancer cells) may be used before or after surgery or radiation.

DOs and DON'Ts in Managing Laryngeal Cancer:

✔ **DO** ask about loss of voice after treatment and different approaches for learning to speak again.

✔ **DO** call your doctor if you have hoarseness or changes in your voice.

✔ **DO** call your doctor if you have neck or ear pain with hoarseness or swollen lymph glands in your neck.

✔ **DO** call your doctor if you have pain with swallowing or trouble swallowing.

🚫 **DON'T** smoke or drink alcohol.

🚫 **DON'T** forget that you need a team of doctors, including an oncologist (specialist in diagnosing and treating cancer), radiation oncologist (specialist in radiation treatment), and surgeon.

FROM THE DESK OF

NOTES

FOR MORE INFORMATION

Contact the following source:

• National Cancer Institute
Tel: (800) 422-6237
Website: http://www.cancer.gov

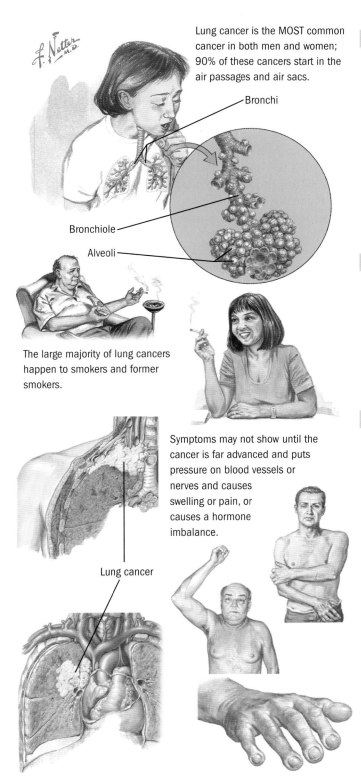

Lung cancer is the MOST common cancer in both men and women; 90% of these cancers start in the air passages and air sacs.

Bronchi

Bronchiole

Alveoli

The large majority of lung cancers happen to smokers and former smokers.

Symptoms may not show until the cancer is far advanced and puts pressure on blood vessels or nerves and causes swelling or pain, or causes a hormone imbalance.

Lung cancer

What Is Lung Cancer?

Lung cancer occurs when cells in the lung grow out of control and form a mass. Nearly 90% of lung cancers start in the lining of air passages or air sacs. Air passages are tubes called bronchi (main tubes) and bronchioles (smaller tubes). Air sacs (alveoli) are at the ends of the tubes.

Lung cancer is usually divided into two types: non–small cell and small cell.

Lung cancer is the most common cancer among both men and women. Every year, more than 170,000 new cases are diagnosed in the United States.

What Causes Lung Cancer?

Almost 90% of lung cancers occur among smokers or former smokers. Therefore use of tobacco (cigarettes, cigars, pipes) is the main cause.

Other causes include exposure to asbestos (especially for smokers), radon and radiation, and secondhand smoke (other people's smoke).

What Are the Symptoms of Lung Cancer?

Some people may have no symptoms until the cancer is advanced.

In others, symptoms include a cough that doesn't go away, coughing up bloody phlegm, shortness of breath, wheezing, continuing problems with pneumonia, tiredness, difficulty swallowing, loss of appetite, and weight loss.

A tumor may press on a large blood vessel, which causes swelling of the face and neck (called superior vena cava syndrome).

A tumor pressing on nerves near the lung can lead to pain in the shoulder, arm, and hand (called Pancoast's tumor).

Some types of lung cancer can produce certain chemicals (hormones) that lead to abnormal blood test results, such as a high calcium level; weakness; and other problems (e.g., Lambert-Eaton syndrome, clubbing of fingers or toes, and syndrome of inappropriate secretion of antidiuretic hormone [SIADH]).

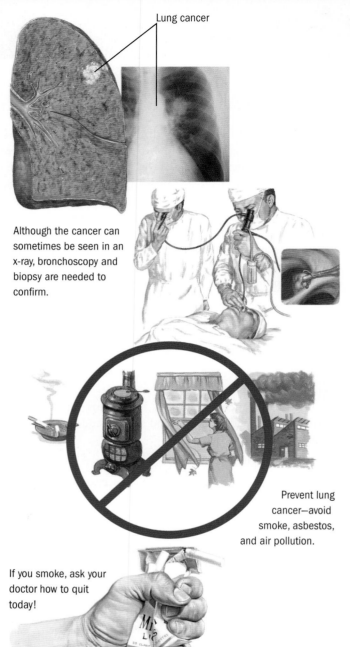

Lung cancer

Although the cancer can sometimes be seen in an x-ray, bronchoscopy and biopsy are needed to confirm.

Prevent lung cancer—avoid smoke, asbestos, and air pollution.

If you smoke, ask your doctor how to quit today!

How Is Lung Cancer Diagnosed?

Early diagnosis can be hard because people may have no symptoms until the cancer is advanced. In these people, a tumor may be found on a routine chest x-ray or computed tomography (CT) scan.

The only sure way to diagnose lung cancer is by taking and studying a sample of lung tissue (biopsy) or fluid from the lungs that contains cancer cells.

The doctor gets these samples in different ways, depending on the location of the problem area. One technique is bronchoscopy, or examination with a lighted scope (a thin, flexible tube) that passes through the mouth into the air passages. If this method doesn't work, needle aspiration can be done. In this procedure, a needle is passed through the chest into the tumor to get the cells.

Sometimes, the space surrounding the lungs has fluid in it. This fluid can be removed with a needle (thoracentesis) to check for cancer cells.

If none of these techniques works, surgery (thoracotomy) can be done to open the chest and get tissue samples directly.

DOs and DON'Ts in Preventing Lung Cancer:

✔ **DO** understand the effects of smoking and its major role in causing lung cancer.

✔ **DO** eat a healthy diet, including fruits and vegetables.

✔ **DO** avoid exposure to hazards such as radon and air pollution.

🚫 **DON'T** smoke—the most important lifestyle change.

🚫 **DON'T** ignore signs of lung cancer such as persistent cough or bloody phlegm. Early diagnosis is important.

FROM THE DESK OF

NOTES

FOR MORE INFORMATION

Contact the following sources:

• American Lung Association
Tel: (212) 315-8700
Website: http://www.lungusa.org

• American Cancer Society
Tel: (800) 227-2345
Website: http://www.cancer.org

MANAGING YOUR
MENINGIOMA

Meningiomas are slow-growing tumors in membranes covering the surface of the brain, spinal cord, or spinal nerve root. Almost all are benign, but they still cause problems by pressing on the brain or spinal cord. Meningiomas occur more often in women than in men, usually after age 40.

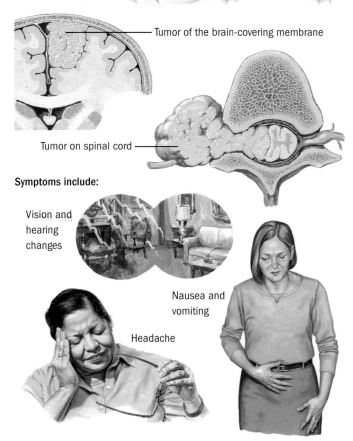

Tumor of the brain-covering membrane

Tumor on spinal cord

Symptoms include:

Vision and hearing changes

Nausea and vomiting

Headache

Your doctor may think that you have a meningioma from your medical history and physical examination. CT (shown here) or MRI of the brain, and maybe angiography will be done to find the tumor.

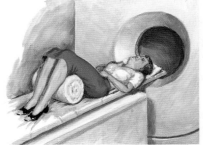

Tumor

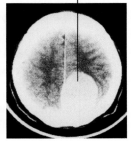

What Is a Meningioma?

Meningiomas are slow-growing tumors in membranes (meninges) that cover the surface of the brain, spinal cord, or spinal nerve root. About one-fifth of all brain tumors are meningiomas. Almost all meningiomas are benign (not cancerous), but they still cause problems because they press on the brain or spinal cord. Meningiomas occur nearly twice as often in women as in men, the most common age at time of diagnosis being 45. They are rare in children and adolescents. About 80% of people are cured if the tumor can be completely removed. Rarely, meningiomas are cancerous (malignant) and may recur quickly and destroy normal tissues nearby.

What Causes a Meningioma?

Meningiomas are caused by abnormal growth of cells on surface coverings of the brain, spinal cord, or spinal nerve roots. The cause of the abnormal growth is unknown.

What Are the Symptoms of a Meningioma?

Symptoms include headaches, vision changes, hearing changes, nausea and vomiting, weakness (especially on one side of the body), numbness or tingling, and loss of memory and the ability to think clearly. Meningiomas may sometimes irritate the brain's surface and cause epilepsy (seizures).

How Is a Meningioma Diagnosed?

The doctor may suspect a meningioma on the basis of the medical history and physical examination. The doctor will order computed tomography (CT) or magnetic resonance imaging (MRI) of the brain. A special x-ray of the blood vessels in the brain called angiography may be done if surgery is necessary.

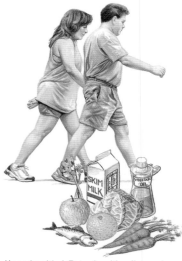

Some people without symptoms need no treatment but will be checked regularly with CT or MRI to watch the tumor. Otherwise, treatment is usually surgery to remove the tumor.

Follow your doctor's treatment instructions, and keep follow-up appointments. Take your medicines as prescribed.

Keep healthy! Eat a healthy diet, reduce your stress, get enough sleep, and exercise daily if you can.

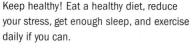

Call your doctor if you have new or repeating symptoms or if symptoms become much worse.

How Is a Meningioma Treated?

Some people with small, slow-growing meningiomas and no symptoms need no treatment but will be checked regularly with CT or MRI to monitor the growth of the tumor. Otherwise, treatment is surgery. After the tumor is removed, it will be examined to see whether it's cancerous. If it is cancer, more treatment with radiation may be used. In some cases, non-invasive radiosurgery (focused radiation [gamma knife]) may be used to treat deep tumors that are hard to reach surgically. For seizures before or after surgery, antiseizure medicine may be taken to prevent more seizures.

DOs and DON'Ts in Managing a Meningioma:

✔ **DO** follow treatments as prescribed by your doctor.
✔ **DO** keep all follow-up appointments to monitor growth of your tumor.
✔ **DO** return to activity and take medicines as prescribed by your doctor. Exercise daily if your doctor says you can.
✔ **DO** eat a healthy diet.
✔ **DO** get enough sleep and reduce your stress.
✔ **DO** call your doctor if you have new or repeating symptoms, or if symptoms become much worse.
✔ **DO** call your doctor if you have problems with your medicines.
✔ **DO** look for a support group if you think that will help you cope.

⊘ **DON'T** panic. In most cases, your illness can be cured with surgery.
⊘ **DON'T** drive if you've had a seizure, unless your doctor says that you can.

FROM THE DESK OF

NOTES

FOR MORE INFORMATION

Contact the following sources:

• National Brain Tumor Foundation
Tel: (800) 934-2873
Website: http://www.braintumor.org

• Mayo Clinic
Website: http://www.mayoclinic.com/

Mesothelioma is a rare cancer that affects the mesothelium. About 3000 new cases are diagnosed in the United States each year. More men than women get this illness, and risks increase with age.

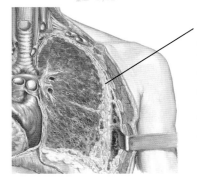

The mesothelium is a sac covering and protecting most internal organs. In most cases, cancer begins in the pleura (membrane around lungs and lining the chest wall) or peritoneum (membrane lining the abdomen).

Working with asbestos is the major risk factor. A history of asbestos exposure at work is reported in about 70% to 80% of all cases.

Symptoms may not appear until 30 to 50 years after exposure. Symptoms include:

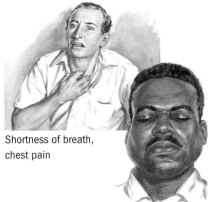

Shortness of breath, chest pain

Swelling of neck and face

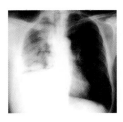

Your doctor will check your medical history (especially history of asbestos exposure), examine you, and order x-rays, lung function tests, CT, or MRI. A biopsy is needed to confirm the diagnosis.

What Is Mesothelioma?

Mesothelioma is a rare cancer that affects the mesothelium. The mesothelium is a sac that covers and protects most of the internal organs. In most cases, the cancer begins in the pleura (membrane around the lungs and lining the wall inside the chest) or peritoneum (membrane lining the abdominal cavity). About 3000 new cases are diagnosed in the United States each year. More men than women get this illness, and risks increase with age.

What Causes Mesothelioma?

Working with asbestos is the major risk factor. However, it can occur in some people without any asbestos exposure. The combination of smoking and asbestos exposure increases the risk.

What Are the Symptoms of Mesothelioma?

Symptoms may not appear until 30 to 50 years after asbestos exposure. Symptoms of pleural mesothelioma include shortness of breath and chest pain. Signs and symptoms of peritoneal mesothelioma include weight loss, abdominal pain and swelling, bowel obstruction, blood clotting abnormalities, anemia, and fever.

If cancer spreads to other body parts, pain, trouble swallowing, or neck or face swelling may occur.

How Is Mesothelioma Diagnosed?

Diagnosing this illness is often hard, because symptoms are similar to those of other conditions. The doctor will check the medical history (especially history of asbestos exposure), do a physical examination, and order x-rays, lung function tests, computed tomography (CT), or magnetic resonance imaging (MRI).

A biopsy is needed to confirm the diagnosis. In a biopsy, a surgeon removes a sample of tissue for study with a microscope.

The doctor may do thoracoscopy for cancer in the chest. The doctor makes a small cut through the chest and puts in a thin, lighted tube (thoracoscope) to look inside.

The doctor may do peritoneoscopy for cancer in the abdomen (belly). In this case, a similar instrument, called a peritoneoscope, is used.

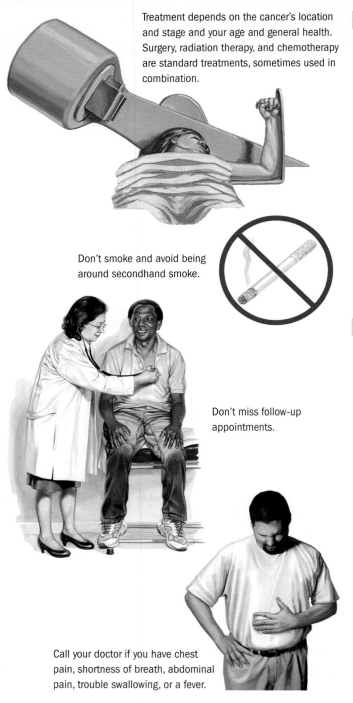

Treatment depends on the cancer's location and stage and your age and general health. Surgery, radiation therapy, and chemotherapy are standard treatments, sometimes used in combination.

Don't smoke and avoid being around secondhand smoke.

Don't miss follow-up appointments.

Call your doctor if you have chest pain, shortness of breath, abdominal pain, trouble swallowing, or a fever.

How Is Mesothelioma Treated?

The doctor will also want to learn the stage of the disease, or how far it has spread. Knowing the stage helps the doctor plan treatment. Mesothelioma can be localized (found only on the membrane) or advanced (spread to lymph nodes, lungs, chest wall, or abdominal organs).

Treatment depends on the cancer's location and stage and your age and general health.

Surgery, radiation therapy, and chemotherapy are sometimes combined. The doctor may remove part of the lining of the chest or abdomen and some tissue around it. Radiation therapy involves using high-energy x-rays to kill cancer. Radiation may come from a machine or from putting materials that produce radiation where cancer cells are found. Chemotherapy uses drugs to kill cancer cells. Most drugs are injected into a vein (intravenous, or IV).

DOs and DON'Ts in Managing Mesothelioma:

✔ **DO** report symptoms to your doctor.
✔ **DO** call your doctor if you have chest pain, shortness of breath, abdominal pain, trouble swallowing, or a fever.

⊘ **DON'T** smoke.
⊘ **DON'T** miss follow-up appointments.
⊘ **DON'T** be afraid to ask for pain medicine, especially after surgery.

FROM THE DESK OF

NOTES

FOR MORE INFORMATION

Contact the following source:

• National Cancer Institute Information
Cancer Information Service
Tel: (800) 422-6237
Website: http://cis.nci.nih.gov/

MANAGING YOUR
MULTIPLE MYELOMA

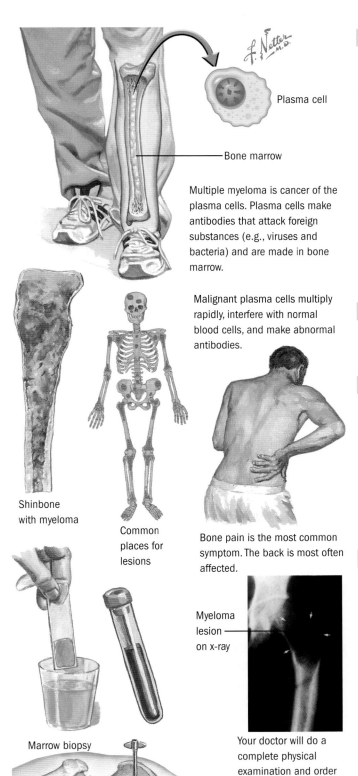

Plasma cell

Bone marrow

Multiple myeloma is cancer of the plasma cells. Plasma cells make antibodies that attack foreign substances (e.g., viruses and bacteria) and are made in bone marrow.

Malignant plasma cells multiply rapidly, interfere with normal blood cells, and make abnormal antibodies.

Shinbone with myeloma

Common places for lesions

Bone pain is the most common symptom. The back is most often affected.

Myeloma lesion on x-ray

Marrow biopsy

Your doctor will do a complete physical examination and order blood and urine tests, x-rays, and bone marrow biopsy for diagnosis.

What Is Multiple Myeloma?

Multiple myeloma is cancer of the plasma cells, which are special types of white blood cells (B lymphocytes). Lymphocytes are produced in bone marrow (the soft substance in the middle of bones). Plasma cells are involved in the immune system. They make antibodies that attack foreign substances (antigens such as viruses and bacteria) in the body. When plasma cells become abnormal and malignant, they multiply rapidly, interfere with normal blood cells, and make abnormal antibodies that can't fight disease. Overgrowth of these malignant cells can weaken bones and cause pain and fractures.

This disorder is uncommon, but more than 14,000 new cases are diagnosed yearly in the United States. Most cases occur after age 60.

What Causes Multiple Myeloma?

The cause is unknown. The disease isn't contagious.

What Are the Symptoms of Multiple Myeloma?

Bone pain is the most common symptom, with the back and ribs most often affected. Pain is worse with movement. Low blood count (anemia) and infections are common.

Myeloma cells destroy the bone and release calcium into blood, which leads to complications such as nerve compression, lower leg weakness, and kidney failure. High blood calcium levels can cause increased urination, weakness, and confusion.

How Is Multiple Myeloma Diagnosed?

The doctor will do a complete physical examination and order blood and urine tests, x-rays, and bone marrow biopsy for diagnosis. In a biopsy, marrow is removed from the bone and checked with a microscope. An abnormal protein in the blood, x-rays results, and abnormal plasma cells in the biopsy confirm the diagnosis.

Treatment depends on the stage of disease. Stem cell transplantation, chemotherapy, biologic therapy, blood transfusions, radiation therapy, and surgery are used.

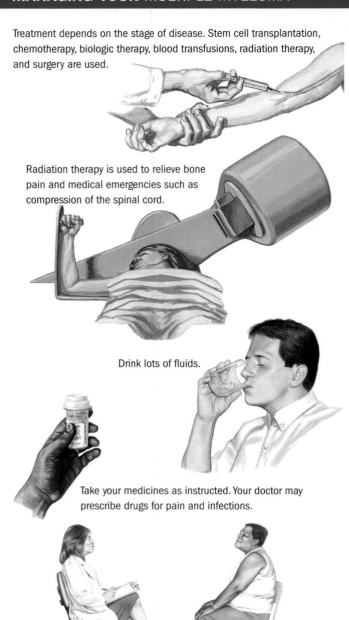

Radiation therapy is used to relieve bone pain and medical emergencies such as compression of the spinal cord.

Drink lots of fluids.

Take your medicines as instructed. Your doctor may prescribe drugs for pain and infections.

Don't miss follow-up appointments. Your doctor needs to repeat blood tests, x-rays, and urine tests to check responses to treatment or to decide to start treatment.

FROM THE DESK OF

NOTES

How Is Multiple Myeloma Treated?

Staging of the cancer is done to give a prognosis. Staging involves finding out the extent of disease. Many people with very early stage disease live longer than 5 years, but people with advanced disease have a shorter life expectancy.

An oncologist (doctor specializing in cancer) will be involved in treatment, which depends on the stage of disease. Stem cell transplantation, chemotherapy, biologic therapy, blood transfusions, radiation therapy, and surgery are used.

Radiation therapy is used for bone pain and medical emergencies (spinal cord compression).

Operations are needed for bone fractures. Supportive treatments, such as antibiotics (for infections), medications to lower the calcium level, and narcotic pain medicines, help well-being.

DOs and DON'Ts in Managing Multiple Myeloma:

✔ **DO** drink lots of fluids (for elevated calcium blood levels).

✔ **DO** take your medicines as prescribed.

✔ **DO** ask your doctor about counseling and support groups.

✔ **DO** call your doctor if you have fevers, back pain, leg numbness or weakness, and problems with bowel movements or urination. These can be caused by spinal cord compression.

✔ **DO** call your doctor if you see blood in stools, urine, phlegm, or vomit.

✔ **DO** call your doctor if you feel depressed.

⊘ **DON'T** be sedentary. This can lead to higher calcium levels.

⊘ **DON'T** lift heavy items. It can increase the risk of bone fractures.

⊘ **DON'T** suffer. Ask for pain medicines if you are in pain.

⊘ **DON'T** miss follow-up appointments. Your doctor needs to repeat blood tests, x-rays, and urine collections to check responses to treatment or decide to start treatment.

FOR MORE INFORMATION

Contact the following sources:

• International Myeloma Foundation
Tel: (800) 452-2873
Website: http://www.myeloma.org

• National Cancer Institute
Tel: (800) 422-6237
Website: http://www.cancer.gov

• American Cancer Society
Tel: (800) 227-2345
Website: http://www.cancer.org

MANAGING YOUR
NON-HODGKIN'S LYMPHOMA

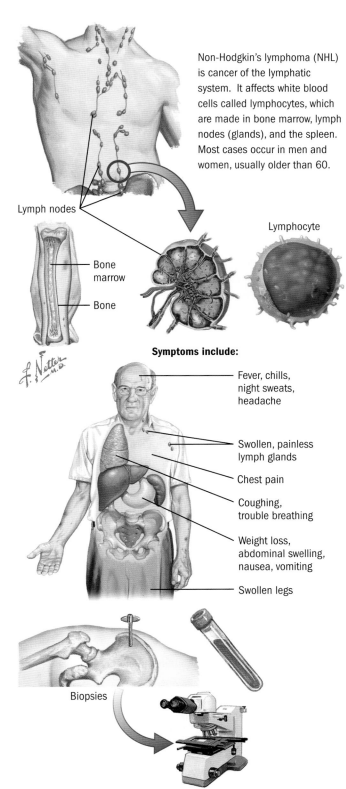

Non-Hodgkin's lymphoma (NHL) is cancer of the lymphatic system. It affects white blood cells called lymphocytes, which are made in bone marrow, lymph nodes (glands), and the spleen. Most cases occur in men and women, usually older than 60.

Lymph nodes

Bone marrow

Bone

Lymphocyte

Symptoms include:

Fever, chills, night sweats, headache

Swollen, painless lymph glands

Chest pain

Coughing, trouble breathing

Weight loss, abdominal swelling, nausea, vomiting

Swollen legs

Biopsies

Your doctor will make a diagnosis from your medical history, physical examination, blood tests, lymph gland and bone marrow biopsies, x-rays, CT, MRI, and PET scan.

What Is Non-Hodgkin's Lymphoma NHL?

Non-Hodgkin's lymphoma (NHL) is cancer of the lymphatic system, which is part of the body's immune (infection-fighting) system. It affects white blood cells called lymphocytes. Lymphocytes are made in bone marrow, lymph nodes (lymph glands), and spleen. NHL is more common than Hodgkin's lymphoma.

Most cases occur in men and women, usually older than 60.

What Causes NHL?

The cause is unknown. Weakening of the immune system by viruses such as human immunodeficiency virus (HIV) and Epstein-Barr virus (EBV), organ transplantation medicines, and too much radiation increase risks.

What Are the Symptoms of NHL?

The most common symptoms are swollen, painless lymph glands in the neck, armpits, and groin. Others include fever, chills, soaking night sweats, coughing, trouble breathing, chest pain, weakness, tiredness, weight loss, swollen legs and face, and abdominal pain and swelling. Nausea, vomiting, loss of appetite, headache, and itching can occur.

How Is NHL Diagnosed?

The doctor will make a diagnosis from a medical history, physical examination, blood tests, and lymph gland and bone marrow biopsy. In a biopsy, tissue taken from a gland or bone marrow is studied with a microscope. Other tests may include laparotomy, which is surgery on the abdomen (belly). X-rays, computed tomography (CT), and positron emission tomography (PET) may be done for staging.

An oncologist (specialist in cancer treatment) will be involved in the care.

How Is NHL Treated?

Low-grade lymphomas cannot be cured. With aggressive treatment, some intermediate and high-grade lymphomas can be cured. About 60% of NHLs can be cured.

Some NHLs grow so slowly that treatments are given only if symptoms occur. This is called watching and waiting.

Treatment depends on the type of NHL and how far the disease has spread. Medicines, radiation, and maybe bone marrow transplantation are used for treatment. About 60% of NHLs can be cured.

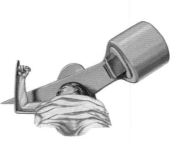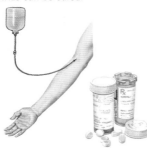

Radiation therapy uses high-energy x-rays from machines.

Chemotherapy may be given by mouth or through a vein in the hospital, or at home, or the doctor's office.

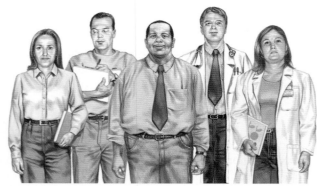

Remember that treatment is complex and involves a team: your primary care doctor, oncologist, radiation oncologist, surgeon, nutritionist, and social worker.

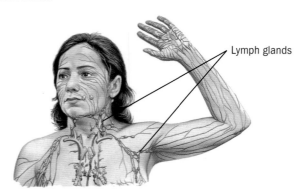

Lymph glands

Don't miss follow-up appointments and call your doctor if you notice any swollen lymph nodes.

FROM THE DESK OF

NOTES

Medicines, radiation, and maybe bone marrow transplantation are used for treatment. Chemotherapy may be given by mouth or through a vein in the hospital, or at home or the doctor's office. Biological treatment uses medicines made from substances produced by the body's immune system. Radiation therapy uses high-energy x-rays from machines or injections.

DOs and DON'Ts in Managing NHL:

✔ **DO** tell your doctor about your medicines, including prescription and over-the-counter ones.

✔ **DO** tell your doctor if you're pregnant or breastfeeding.

✔ **DO** talk to someone about the stress of having cancer. Call your doctor if you feel depressed. Find support groups.

✔ **DO** take care of your teeth and mouth to prevent mouth sores.

✔ **DO** consider placing sperm in a sperm bank or eggs in an egg bank if you plan to have children.

✔ **DO** remember that treatment is complex and involves a team: primary care doctor, oncologist, radiation oncologist, surgeon, nutritionist, and social worker.

✔ **DO** call your doctor if you have swollen lymph glands or low back pain with numbness or pain down your legs.

✔ **DO** call your doctor if you have cough, nausea, vomiting, shortness of breath, diarrhea, bloody stools, fever, or bruising after radiation.

✔ **DO** call your doctor if you have fever after chemotherapy.

⊘ **DON'T** ignore swollen lymph glands.

⊘ **DON'T** miss follow-up appointments during and after treatments.

⊘ **DON'T** be afraid to ask questions about infertility, stress, fear, life insurance, and job discrimination.

FOR MORE INFORMATION

Contact the following sources:

• Leukemia and Lymphoma Society
  Tel: (800) 955-4572
  Website: http://www.leukemia-lymphoma.org

• Lymphoma Research Association
  Tel: (212) 349-2910, (800) 235-6848
  Website: http://www.lymphoma.org

• National Cancer Institute, Cancer Information Service
  Tel: (800) 4-CANCER
  Website: http://www.cancer.gov

• American Cancer Society
  Tel: (800) ACS-2345 (227-2345)
  Website: http://www.cancer.org

Mouth cancer is a malignant tumor growing inside the mouth. It usually grows on the tongue or floor of the mouth, but gums, lips, jaw, and roof of the mouth may have the tumor. This cancer is highly curable when it's very small and found early.

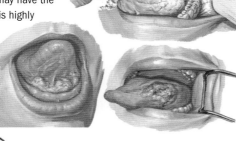

Most often, mouth cancer occurs in older men who used tobacco.

Using alcohol with tobacco greatly increases your chances of getting mouth cancer. Other causes include anything that irritates the inside of the mouth, poor oral care, poorly fitting dentures, and sun exposure (lip cancer).

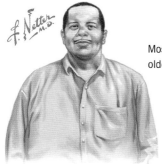

The first sign is usually a small sore—a small red or white bump or patch or an open sore (or ulcer) that it doesn't heal. Other symptoms are tongue pain, trouble swallowing, and voice changes.

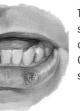

Your doctor will examine your mouth. A small piece of tissue will be removed (biopsied) and sent for study.

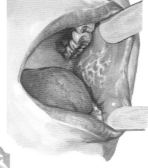

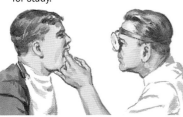

What Is Mouth Cancer?

Mouth cancer is a malignant tumor growing inside the mouth. It usually grows on the tongue or floor of the mouth but may grow on the gums, lips, jaw, and roof of the mouth. Most often, this cancer occurs in older men who used tobacco and drank alcohol in excess.

When found early, mouth cancer is highly curable with surgery or radiation therapy. Treatment is much less effective if smoking and drinking alcohol continue.

What Causes Mouth Cancer?

Chances of getting mouth cancer are greater with use of any kind of tobacco—cigarettes, cigars, pipe tobacco, and chewing tobacco. Using alcohol with tobacco greatly increases chances of getting it. Other causes include anything that irritates the inside of the mouth, poor oral care, poorly fitting dentures, and sun exposure (lip cancer).

What Are the Symptoms of Mouth Cancer?

The first sign is usually a small sore in the mouth or on the lip. It may be a small red or white bump or patch or an open sore (or ulcer) that doesn't heal.

Symptoms include tongue pain, feeling that something is caught in the throat, trouble swallowing, swollen jaw, and voice changes.

How Is Mouth Cancer Diagnosed?

The doctor will examine your mouth, maybe with a small, long-handled mirror to see the back of the tongue. A small piece of tissue will be removed (biopsy) and sent to the laboratory for study. The doctor may also do a chest x-ray.

If the biopsy shows mouth cancer, other tests will include computed tomography (CT) and magnetic resonance imaging (MRI), to see the size of the cancer and how far it spread, which is called staging.

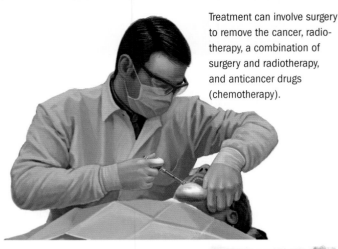

Treatment can involve surgery to remove the cancer, radiotherapy, a combination of surgery and radiotherapy, and anticancer drugs (chemotherapy).

How Is Mouth Cancer Treated?

Treatment can involve surgery, radiotherapy, a combination of surgery and radiotherapy, and anticancer drugs (chemotherapy).

Surgery will depend on where the cancer is, its size, and how far it has spread. For very large tumors, the surgeon may remove part of the jaw bone. Mouth surgery may cause swelling that makes it hard to cough, spit, eat, and even breathe. Sometimes a temporary opening is made through the skin in the low part of the neck into the windpipe. This opening, a tracheostomy, makes it easier to breathe and cough and clear fluid from the lungs.

Mouth surgery may cause swelling that makes it hard to cough, spit, eat, and even breathe. Sometimes a temporary opening is made through the skin in the neck into the windpipe. This opening, a tracheostomy, makes it easier to breathe and cough.

DOs and DON'Ts in Managing Mouth Cancer:

✔ **DO** follow all directions from your doctor.

✔ **DO** call your doctor if you have breathing problems, bleeding, or infection.

✔ **DO** avoid tobacco products and heavy alcohol drinking to prevent mouth cancer.

✔ **DO** have poorly fitting dentures repaired so that they don't irritate the inside of your mouth.

✔ **DO** see your doctor if you have a new sore in your mouth or on your lip that doesn't heal. Mouth cancer is highly curable when it's very small and is found early.

⊘ **DON'T** use tobacco or drink alcohol.

⊘ **DON'T** drive a car after surgery until your doctor says you can.

To prevent mouth cancer, don't use any type of tobacco and don't drink alcohol.

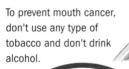

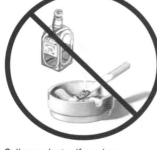

Call your doctor if you have breathing problems, bleeding, or infection. Symptoms of infection include a red or swollen incision, a temperature higher than 100° F, and drainage.

FROM THE DESK OF

NOTES

FOR MORE INFORMATION

Contact the following sources:

- National Cancer Institute
  Tel: (800) 422-6237
  Website: http://www.cancer.gov

- American Academy of Otolaryngology—Head and Neck Surgery
  Tel: (703) 836-4444
  Website: http://www.entnet.org

- American Cancer Society
  Tel: (800) ACS-2345 (227-2345)
  Website: http://www.cancer.org

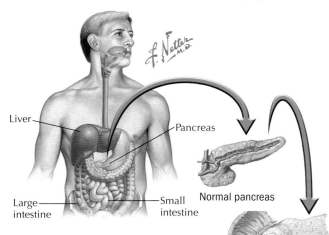

The pancreas is in the abdomen, surrounded by the stomach, intestines, and other organs.

Liver

Pancreas

Large intestine

Small intestine

Normal pancreas

Carcinoma of the pancreas

Pancreatic cancer is called a silent disease because it usually doesn't cause symptoms early on. Growing cancer causes pain in the upper abdomen and sometimes the back. Pain can get worse after eating or lying down.

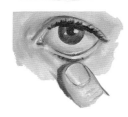

If cancer blocks the bile duct so that bile cannot pass into the intestines, the skin and whites of the eyes may become yellow. This condition is called jaundice.

Your doctor makes a preliminary diagnosis from symptoms and imaging tests (CT, MRI, ultrasound, ERCP). The best way to diagnose cancer is with a biopsy. A piece of pancreas is removed and checked with a microscope to detect any cancer cells.

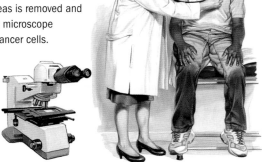

What Is Pancreatic Cancer?

Cancer of the pancreas refers to growth of cancer cells in the pancreas. The pancreas is in the abdomen (belly), with the stomach, intestines, and other organs around it. It makes juices used in digestion and several hormones, including insulin, which controls blood sugar (glucose) level. It releases these substances into ducts (tubes). Pancreatic cancer starts from cells lining these ducts.

Almost 30,000 people in the United States are diagnosed with this cancer each year. Early detection is best for a cure, but this cancer is hard to find early because most symptoms do not occur until the cancer has spread.

What Causes Pancreatic Cancer?

Causes are unclear, but smoking, alcoholism, and chronic inflammation (swelling) of the pancreas (pancreatitis) are related to this disease. Pancreatic cancer isn't contagious or hereditary.

What Are the Symptoms of Pancreatic Cancer?

Because pancreatic cancer doesn't cause symptoms early, it's called silent. Symptoms depend on the cancer's location and size. If the bile duct is blocked so that bile cannot pass into the intestines, jaundice may occur. The skin and whites of the eyes become yellow and urine may become dark.

Growing cancer causes pain in the upper abdomen and sometimes the back. Pain becomes worse after eating or lying down. Other symptoms are nausea, reduced appetite, weight loss, and weakness.

How Is Pancreatic Cancer Diagnosed?

The doctor makes a preliminary diagnosis from symptoms and special imaging tests called computed tomography (CT), magnetic resonance imaging (MRI), and ultrasound. They help decide the stage (extent) of disease by showing whether cancer affects other organs.

The doctor may also order a test called endoscopic retrograde cholangiopancreatography (ERCP). This test uses dye and a flexible tube passed down the throat and into the intestine to get x-rays. The best way to diagnose cancer is with a biopsy. A piece of pancreas is taken and checked with a microscope to detect cancer cells.

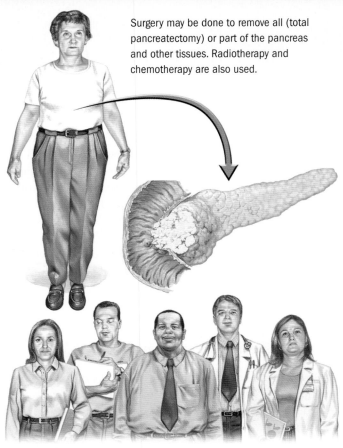

Surgery may be done to remove all (total pancreatectomy) or part of the pancreas and other tissues. Radiotherapy and chemotherapy are also used.

Understand that diagnosis and treatment of pancreatic cancer will need a team of doctors and health care workers.

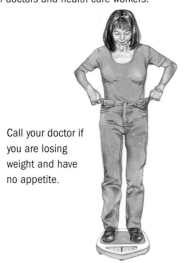

Call your doctor if you are losing weight and have no appetite.

How Is Pancreatic Cancer Treated?

Surgery may be done to remove all (total pancreatectomy) or part of the pancreas and other tissues. In the Whipple procedure, the surgeon removes the head of the pancreas, parts of the small intestine and stomach, and other tissues. Sometimes cancer cannot be completely removed, but surgery can help relieve symptoms.

Radiotherapy and chemotherapy are also used. Radiotherapy uses high-energy rays to kill cancer cells. Chemotherapy (drugs to kill cancer cells) may be given alone or with radiotherapy if cancer cannot be removed. Doctors sometimes give chemotherapy after surgery to control cancer cell growth.

DOs and DON'Ts in Managing Pancreatic Cancer:

✔ **DO** understand that you'll need a team of doctors for care. The team will include a primary care doctor, surgeon, oncologist (a doctor specializing in cancer), and maybe a radiation oncologist (a doctor specializing in using radiotherapy for cancer).

✔ **DO** call your doctor if you have jaundice, abdominal pain, weight loss, or no appetite.

✔ **DO** call your doctor if you have fever or see drainage from the incision site after surgery.

🚫 **DON'T** forget that treatments have side effects, such as pain and infection (surgery) and nausea, vomiting, and hair loss (chemotherapy).

🚫 **DON'T** be afraid to ask for a second opinion.

FROM THE DESK OF

NOTES

FOR MORE INFORMATION

Contact the following sources:

• National Cancer Institute
  Phone: (800) 4-CANCER (422-6237)
  Website: http://www.cancer.gov

• American Cancer Society
  Tel: (800) ACS-2345 (227-2345)
  Website: http://www.cancer.org

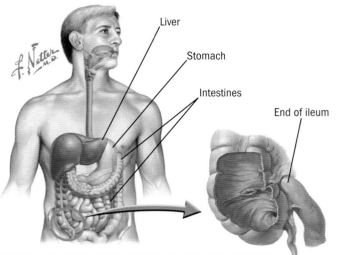

Pernicious anemia is a lack of red blood cells and hemoglobin because the body doesn't have enough of the essential vitamin B_{12} (also called cobalamin). The part of the small intestine called the ileum absorbs vitamin B_{12}. Absorption needs a specific protein (intrinsic factor) made in the stomach.

Absence of intrinsic factor is the usual cause. Cells lining the stomach can't make this factor. Other causes include absence of part of the stomach after surgery for ulcers or cancer, as well as certain stomach and small intestinal diseases.

Dashed lines show the part removed

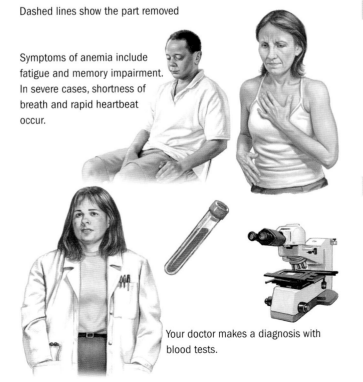

Symptoms of anemia include fatigue and memory impairment. In severe cases, shortness of breath and rapid heartbeat occur.

Your doctor makes a diagnosis with blood tests.

What Is Pernicious Anemia?

Pernicious anemia is a lack of sufficient red blood cells and hemoglobin because the body doesn't have enough cobalamin (vitamin B12). This vitamin is essential for normal growth and development of red blood cells, other blood cells, and cells in the nervous system. Absorption of vitamin B12 occurs in the part of the small intestine called the ileum. Absorption needs a specific protein (intrinsic factor) made in the stomach.

Pernicious anemia is uncommon. Both sexes are affected equally, most often after age 30. It's more common among people of northern European descent.

What Causes Pernicious Anemia?

Most often, absence of intrinsic factor is the cause, not poor intake of the vitamin. The immune system attacks cells lining the stomach and prevents them from making intrinsic factor. Other ways that people may not have intrinsic factor include absence of part of the stomach after surgery for ulcers or cancer, and certain stomach diseases that interfere with how vitamin B12 is made. Diseases of the small intestine (where vitamin B12 is absorbed), such as tapeworm infestation, Crohn's disease, or tropical sprue, can also cause lack of vitamin B12.

What Are the Symptoms of Pernicious Anemia?

Symptoms of anemia include fatigue and neurological problems. In severe cases, memory impairment, sensory impairment, shortness of breath, and rapid heartbeat occur. Lack of vitamin B12 can also cause problems with feeling and numbness in feet and hands. Severe deficiency can result in severe neurological problems, such as confusion and being disoriented.

How Is Pernicious Anemia Diagnosed?

The doctor makes a diagnosis with blood tests. Special tests (such as the Schilling test) may be needed to check for abnormal absorption of the vitamin and the presence of specific antibodies.

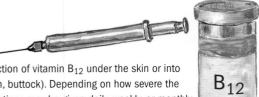

Therapy is injection of vitamin B_{12} under the skin or into a muscle (thigh, buttock). Depending on how severe the anemia is, injections may be given daily, weekly, or monthly, usually lifelong. People with poor intake can take oral vitamin B_{12} supplements.

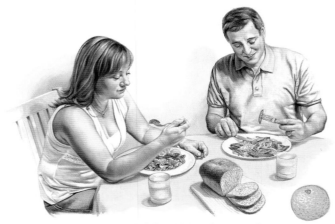

Eat a well-balanced diet, rich in folic acid (another vitamin important for blood cells) and other essential nutrients. Such foods may include oranges, bananas, broccoli, and peas, but ask your doctor for guidelines.

Discuss a vitamin supplement schedule with your doctor if you plan on becoming or are pregnant.

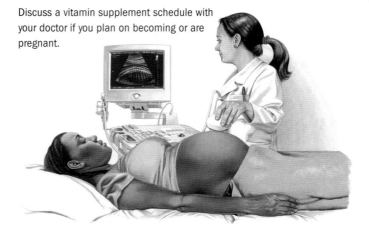

How Is Pernicious Anemia Treated?

Therapy is injection of vitamin B12 under the skin or into a muscle. Treatment of severe deficiency first involves daily injections followed by weekly and then monthly injections. It takes 4 to 8 weeks to see increased hemoglobin concentration. Treatment is lifelong.

People with poor intake can take oral vitamin B12.

A gel solution of vitamin B12 can also be given by the nose via a metered dose nasal inhaler, once weekly instead of monthly injections. This method should be used only after first giving vitamin B12 injections until levels are normal.

Vitamin B12 replacement leads to full correction of anemia. People who cannot absorb the vitamin need long-term treatment.

DOs and DON'Ts in Managing Pernicious Anemia:

✔ **DO** continue monthly injections, even if anemia is corrected.

✔ **DO** talk with your doctor if you're pregnant.

✔ **DO** eat a well-balanced diet, rich in folic acid (another vitamin important for the blood cells) and other essential nutrients.

✔ **DO** supplement your diet with oral vitamins if you eat a special diet, such as a vegetarian (especially vegan) diet.

✔ **DO** call your doctor if you have signs of severe anemia, such as chest pain, palpitations, or shortness of breath.

⊘ **DON'T** stop treatment. This lets anemia and all symptoms return.

FROM THE DESK OF

NOTES

FOR MORE INFORMATION

Contact the following source:

• National Heart, Lung, and Blood Institute
Tel: (301) 592-8573
Website: http://www.nhlbi.nih.gov

PROSTATE CANCER
SCREENING AND PREVENTION

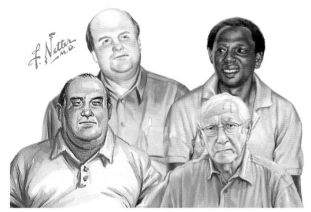

The survival rate for all stages of prostate cancer has risen in the past 20 years due to early detection and treatment.

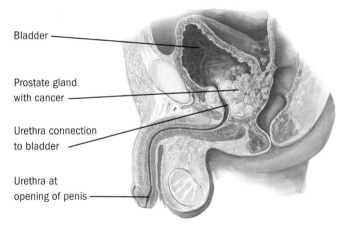

Bladder

Prostate gland with cancer

Urethra connection to bladder

Urethra at opening of penis

The prostate gland is at the base of the urethra near the bladder. A growing cancer may cause pain or interfere with urination or erections, but there may be no symptoms.

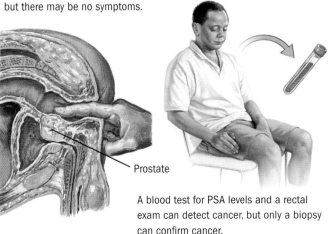

Prostate

A blood test for PSA levels and a rectal exam can detect cancer, but only a biopsy can confirm cancer.

What Is Prostate Cancer?

Prostate cancer is a growth of abnormal cells in the prostate gland. The prostate is a walnut-shaped gland in the male reproductive tract that makes seminal fluid, which mixes with sperm and other fluids. This gland surrounds the urethra, near its connection to the bladder. The urethra is the tube that carries urine from the bladder, through the penis, to outside the body. Cancer develops when cells mutate and begin to multiply out of control. These cells may spread (metastasize) from the prostate to other parts of the body, especially bones and lymph nodes. In the past 20 years, the survival rate for all stages of prostate cancer has improved because of early detection and treatment.

A higher risk of developing prostate cancer may be related to age (especially older than 65), race (African American), and family history (father, brother).

What Are the Symptoms of Prostate Cancer?

Early prostate cancer may not cause symptoms. Some men, however, may have pain, difficulty urinating, and rarely problems with erections (erectile dysfunction).

Other symptoms include a weak or interrupted flow of urine, need to urinate often (especially at night), difficulty holding back urine, inability to urinate, pain or burning when urinating, blood in the urine or semen, and nagging pain in the back, hips, or pelvis.

It is important to realize that these symptoms may have other less serious causes, such as benign prostatic hypertrophy (BPH) or infection. Always see your doctor for a diagnosis.

How Is Prostate Cancer Diagnosed?

The doctor will take a complete medical history and do a physical examination. Other diagnostic tests may include a digital rectal examination (DRE) and a blood test called prostate-specific antigen test (PSA test).

The doctor will usually recommend that a DRE and a PSA be done every year for men older than 50. Men in high-risk groups, such as African Americans or those with a strong family history of prostate cancer, should ask about being tested at a younger age. The diagnosis of cancer can be confirmed only with a biopsy (a tissue sample of the prostate).

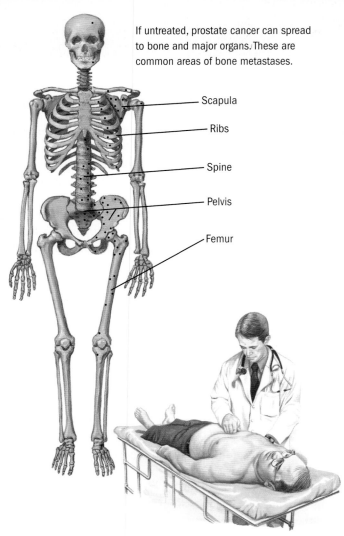

If untreated, prostate cancer can spread to bone and major organs. These are common areas of bone metastases.

- Scapula
- Ribs
- Spine
- Pelvis
- Femur

Get an annual physical including PSA test and rectal exam if you are over 50 or in a higher risk group.

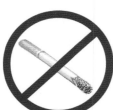

Don't smoke.

What Are the Complications of Prostate Cancer?

Many prostate cancers don't cause death, but some can spread outside the prostate gland and metastasize through the blood and lymph nodes to bones and major organs. This is known as extracapsular spread.

DOs and DON'Ts in Preventing Prostate Cancer:

✔ **DO** have a yearly DRE as recommended by your doctor.
✔ **DO** have a yearly PSA test as recommended by your doctor.

⊘ **DON'T** ignore possible symptoms of prostate cancer such as pain or difficulty urinating.
⊘ **DON'T** smoke.

FOR MORE INFORMATION

Contact the following sources:

- American Cancer Society
  Tel: (800) 227-2345
  Website: http://www.cancer.org

- National Cancer Institute
  Tel: (800) 422-6237
  Website: http://www.nci.nih.gov

- American Urological Association
  Tel: (866) RING-AUA
  Website: http://www.auanet.org/patients/

FROM THE DESK OF

NOTES

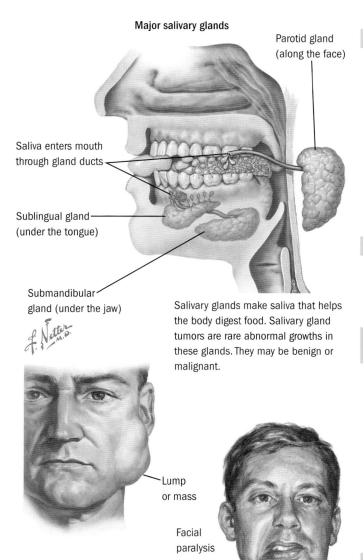

Major salivary glands

Parotid gland (along the face)

Saliva enters mouth through gland ducts

Sublingual gland (under the tongue)

Submandibular gland (under the jaw)

f. Netter M.D.

Salivary glands make saliva that helps the body digest food. Salivary gland tumors are rare abnormal growths in these glands. They may be benign or malignant.

Lump or mass

Facial paralysis

The cause is unknown. The first sign is a lump or mass. If the facial nerve is involved, paralysis in the face, with facial droop, can result.

Your doctor may suspect a salivary gland tumor from a physical exam and imaging tests (CT or MRI). The only sure way to diagnose the tumor is to biopsy or surgically remove the tumor and check it with a microscope.

Submandibular gland

What Are Salivary Gland Tumors?

Salivary glands are in the back of the mouth and make saliva that helps the body digest food. The major glands are parotid glands (along both sides of the face), submandibular glands (below the jaw bone), and sublingual glands (under the tongue).

Salivary gland tumors are rare abnormal growths in these glands. They may be benign or malignant (cancerous). In the parotid gland, 80% of tumors are benign; in the minor salivary glands, 80% of tumors are malignant.

What Causes Salivary Gland Tumors?

The cause is unknown. They aren't contagious or passed on from one generation to the next.

What Are the Symptoms of Salivary Gland Tumors?

A lump or mass is the usual first sign. Salivary gland cancers tend to spread by invading nearby tissue. Local spread of parotid tumors may involve the facial nerve. This tumor can lead to paralysis in the face, with facial droop and inability to close the eye on the affected side. Other salivary gland cancers spread into muscles at the floor of the mouth and base of the skull, and to local lymph glands (nodes). Facial pain, ear pain, headache, and swollen lymph glands result.

Advanced cancer can spread by blood to lungs and bones.

How Are Salivary Gland Tumors Diagnosed?

The doctor uses computed tomography (CT) or magnetic resonance imaging (MRI) and physical examination to diagnose the tumor. The only sure way to confirm the diagnosis is to biopsy the mass and check the tissue for cancer cells with a microscope.

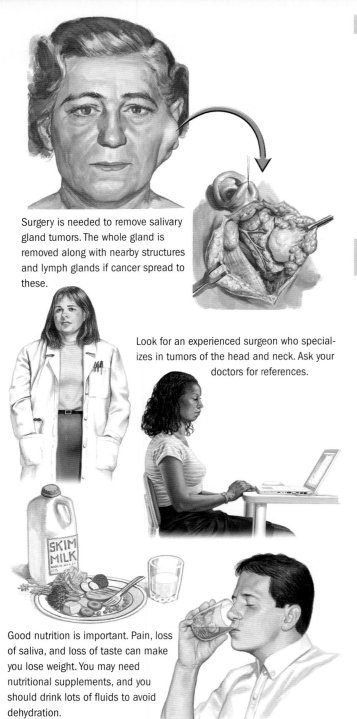

Surgery is needed to remove salivary gland tumors. The whole gland is removed along with nearby structures and lymph glands if cancer spread to these.

Look for an experienced surgeon who specializes in tumors of the head and neck. Ask your doctors for references.

Good nutrition is important. Pain, loss of saliva, and loss of taste can make you lose weight. You may need nutritional supplements, and you should drink lots of fluids to avoid dehydration.

How Are Salivary Gland Tumors Treated?

Salivary gland tumors can be cured if found and removed before they spread. Treatment is removal of the entire gland and nearby structures and lymph glands, if these are involved. Complications of surgery include cutting important nerves, such as the facial nerve and the nerve that goes to the tongue.

Radiation therapy can be used for advanced inoperable tumors or tumors that return. Complications may be dry, red, itchy skin; loss of ability to produce saliva, which causes dry mouth, sore throat, and trouble swallowing; loss of facial hair growth; and loss of taste.

DOs and DON'Ts in Managing Salivary Gland Tumors:

✔ **DO** look for an experienced surgeon who specializes in tumors of the head and neck.

✔ **DO** understand that good nutrition is important. Pain, loss of saliva, and loss of taste can make you lose weight. You may need nutritional supplements and lots of fluids.

✔ **DO** remember to keep all doctor appointments to watch for side effects or cancer that may return.

✔ **DO** remember that the earlier the cancer is found, the better the prognosis. The 10-year survival rate is 90% for very small tumors with no spread, but only 25% for larger tumors with spread to a lymph gland.

✔ **DO** call your doctor if you find a lump in your head or neck or have facial or ear pain.

✔ **DO** call your doctor if you suddenly have facial droop and can't close your eye on the same side.

✔ **DO** call your doctor if you need emotional support.

⊘ **DON'T** ignore lumps in your mouth, cheek, or neck.
⊘ **DON'T** ignore swollen lymph glands.

FROM THE DESK OF

NOTES

FOR MORE INFORMATION

Contact the following sources:

• National Cancer Institute
  Tel: (800) 422-6237 (800-4-CANCER)
  Website: http://www.cancer.gov

• American Academy of Otolaryngology—Head and Neck Surgery
  Tel: (703) 836-4444
  Website: http://www.entnet.org

MANAGING YOUR
SICKLE CELL ANEMIA

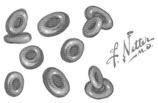

Normal red blood cells

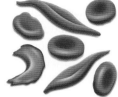

Red blood cells with sickle cell anemia

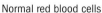

Sickle cell anemia is a hereditary blood disease that affects red blood cells. Red blood cells have abnormal hemoglobin-S and become crescent or sickle shaped. They can't pass through small blood vessels, which get blocked. Tissues and organs can't get enough blood and are damaged.

More than 50,000 people in the United States have the disease, mostly African Americans. The cause is a mutation in DNA for beta-globin, a protein in hemoglobin.

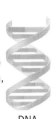

DNA

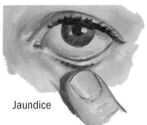

Jaundice

Common symptoms are anemia, fast heartbeat, jaundice, tiredness, and severe bone pain during a crisis.

Pregnancy, surgery, infection, and high altitudes can make symptoms worse.

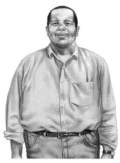

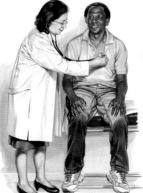

Your doctor makes a diagnosis from your family history and blood tests to look for sickle-shaped red blood cells and abnormal hemoglobin. A simple screening test in early pregnancy or after birth can check for the disease in a baby.

What Is Sickle Cell Anemia?

Sickle cell anemia is a hereditary blood disease that's passed from parents to children. It affects red blood cells. Normal red blood cells are soft and round and contain hemoglobin. Hemoglobin helps carry oxygen to parts of the body. People with sickle cell anemia have red blood cells with abnormal hemoglobin-S (Hb-S). Red blood cells become crescent or sickle shaped and cannot pass through small blood vessels. Vessels get blocked, tissues and organs may become damaged because they cannot get enough blood, and acute illness (crisis) results. Problems can affect every organ.

People may have sickle cell trait. Sickle cell trait means having one sickle cell gene and one normal gene, so both abnormal and normal hemoglobin are made. People with the trait are healthy but can have children with sickle cell anemia if their sexual partner also has sickle cell trait.

More than 50,000 people in the United States have the disease, which is lifelong.

What Causes Sickle Cell Anemia?

The cause is a mutation in DNA for beta-globin, a protein that makes up hemoglobin. The disease is most common among African Americans but people of Mediterranean, Caribbean, South and Central American, Arabian, and East Indian descent can have it.

What Are the Symptoms of Sickle Cell Anemia?

Common symptoms include chronic anemia (low blood cell count), fast heartbeat, yellow skin (jaundice), tiredness, and severe bone pain during a crisis. Symptoms get worse during a crisis. Pregnancy, surgery, infection, and high altitudes make symptoms worse. Complications include kidney and eye disease, heart disease, leg ulcers, and strokes. Infections such as osteomyelitis (bone infection) and pneumonia (acute chest syndrome) can occur. In aplastic crisis, bone marrow stops making red blood cells.

How Is Sickle Cell Anemia Diagnosed?

The doctor makes a diagnosis from a family history of the disease and blood tests. Blood tests look for sickle-shaped red blood cells and abnormal hemoglobin. A simple screening test in early pregnancy or after birth can check for the disease in a baby.

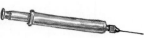

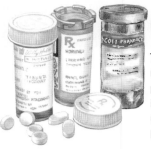

Treatment involves controlling pain. Oral medicine can help mild crises. Severe pain may need intramuscular or intravenous shots of narcotics. Children usually receive penicillin to prevent bacterial infection.

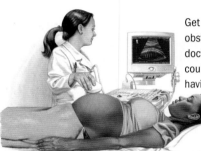

Drink plenty of fluids to avoid dehydration, especially during a crisis.

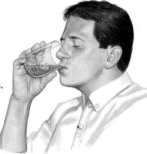

Get prenatal care from your obstetrician and primary care doctor. Consider genetic counseling to check your risk for having an affected child.

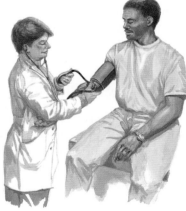

Call your doctor if you have fever, shortness of breath, severe abdominal pain, neurological symptoms (such as trouble speaking), or a painful crisis that doesn't get better with home treatment.

How Is Sickle Cell Anemia Treated?

Treatment involves controlling pain. Oral medicine can help mild crises. Severe pain may need intramuscular or intravenous narcotics. Hydroxyurea is a medication that can reduce the number of crises. Fluids are given to prevent dehydration. Sometimes, blood transfusion is needed. Abnormal blood cells are replaced with normal cells.

Children usually receive penicillin to prevent bacterial infection.

Bone marrow transplantation from a brother or sister may cure the disease, but this treatment is experimental.

DOs and DON'Ts in Managing Sickle Cell Anemia:

✔ **DO** drink fluids to avoid dehydration.

✔ **DO** eat a healthy diet with plenty of green, leafy vegetables (high in folate). Take a daily folate supplement.

✔ **DO** mild to moderate exercise. Rest if you feel tired and drink enough fluids.

✔ **DO** consider genetic counseling to check your risk for having an affected child.

✔ **DO** get prenatal care from your obstetrician and primary care doctor.

✔ **DO** call your doctor if you have fever, shortness of breath, severe abdominal pain, or neurological symptoms (such as trouble speaking).

🚫 **DON'T** fly on airplanes without pressurized cabins.

🚫 **DON'T** overuse pain drugs.

🚫 **DON'T** drink alcohol in excess.

FROM THE DESK OF

NOTES

FOR MORE INFORMATION

Contact the following sources:

• Sickle Cell Disease Association of America, Inc.
Tel: (800) 421-8453
Website: http://www.sicklecelldisease.org

• National Heart, Lung, and Blood Institute Information Center
Tel: (301) 592-8573
Website: http://www.nhlbi.nih.gov

Testicles are male sex glands. Testicular malignancies are cancers of the testicles. Most cases occur in men 20 to 40 years old.

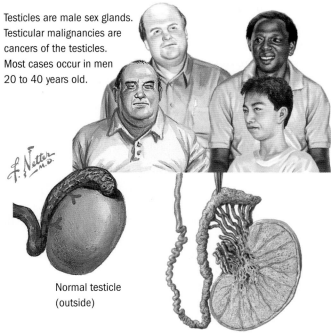

Normal testicle (outside)

Normal testicle (inside)

Types of cancers:

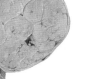

Seminoma

Teratoma

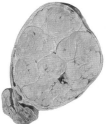

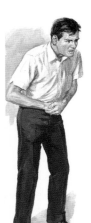

The most common first symptom is a painless lump or swelling on or around the testicle. Another common symptom is pain in the pelvis, groin, or lower back.

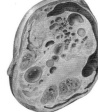

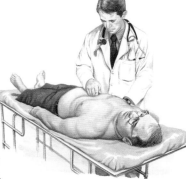

The best way to find testicular cancer is by self-examination of the testicles. Your doctor will then examine you and order ultrasound to make a diagnosis.

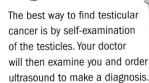

What Is Testicular Cancer?

Testicles (testes) are male sex glands that make and store sperm. Testicular malignancies are cancers of the testicles. About 7500 new cases are diagnosed each year in the United States. Most occur in men between 20 and 40 years old.

What Causes Testicular Cancer?

The cause is unknown. Men with a greater chance of getting it include those born with an undescended testicle and those who have fathers or brothers with testicular cancer. Testicular cancer isn't contagious.

What Are the Symptoms of Testicular Cancer?

The most common first symptom is a painless lump or swelling on or around the testicle. Other symptoms are a feeling of fullness or heaviness in the scrotum (the sac or pouch that holds the testicles), swollen lymph glands (nodes) in the groin or thigh, back pain, and testicular or scrotal pain.

How Is Testicular Cancer Diagnosed?

The best way to find testicular cancer is by doing self-examination of the testicles. A doctor will diagnose testicular cancer by doing a physical examination (including testicles) and ordering an ultrasound scan to find the mass. Ultrasound uses sound waves to see inside testicles; it's painless and harmless. If ultrasound shows a mass (lump), a urologist will operate to remove the testicle.

Then, staging is done to find out how far the disease has spread. Staging involves blood tests, computed tomography (CT), and maybe surgery to remove lymph nodes (called retroperitoneal lymph node dissection, or RPLND).

Stage I disease means the cancer is only in the testicle. Stage II disease has spread to nearby lymph nodes. Stage III disease has spread far from the testicles.

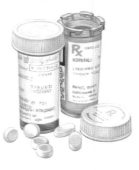

Treatment depends on the type of cancer (seminomatous or nonseminomatous) and its stage. Radiation, chemotherapy, and surgery are used. Your doctor will discuss treatment options with you.

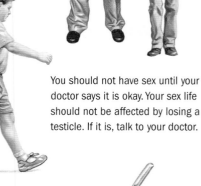

In most cases, if a testicle has to be removed it doesn't affect ability to have children.

You should not have sex until your doctor says it is okay. Your sex life should not be affected by losing a testicle. If it is, talk to your doctor.

Call your doctor if you have a fever after chemotherapy or if you have swelling or pain in your testicle, back pain, or shortness of breath.

How Is Testicular Cancer Treated?

Treatment depends on the type of cancer (seminomatous or nonseminomatous) and its stage. Seminomatous tumors without spread are treated with radiation. With distant spread, chemotherapy is used.

Surgery (RPLND) is used for early-stage nonseminomatous tumors. For more advanced disease, chemotherapy is added.

Having one testicle removed shouldn't affect having sex or children.

Almost 90% of newly diagnosed testicular cancers are curable. Even cancers that spread have very good cure rates of 70% to 80%.

DOs and DON'Ts in Managing Testicular Cancer:

✔ **DO** ask your doctor if you need to save sperm for the future.

✔ **DO** learn and perform testicular self-examinations twice monthly.

✔ **DO** ask about emotional support groups.

✔ **DO** call your doctor if you feel a lump on your testicle.

✔ **DO** call your doctor if you have swelling or pain in your testicle.

✔ **DO** call your doctor if you have a fever after chemotherapy.

✔ **DO** call your doctor if you have excess drainage from the surgical area.

⊘ **DON'T** stop taking medicine or change dosage because you feel better unless your doctor says to.

⊘ **DON'T** have sex until your doctor says you can.

⊘ **DON'T** miss follow-up doctor appointments. These are important to monitor for recurrence of the cancer.

⊘ **DON'T** forget to do self-examinations on the remaining testicle; it may also get cancer.

⊘ **DON'T** be afraid to ask about sex.

FROM THE DESK OF

NOTES

FOR MORE INFORMATION

Contact the following sources:

• American Cancer Society
Tel: (800) ACS-2345 (227-2345)
Website: http://www.cancer.org

• National Cancer Institute
Tel: (800) 422-6237
Website: http://www.cancer.gov

MANAGING YOUR
THYROID CANCER

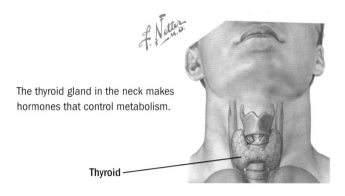

The thyroid gland in the neck makes hormones that control metabolism.

Thyroid

Thyroid cancers are abnormal growths that start from either thyroid follicular cells or thyroid parafollicular cells. The papillary type from follicular cells is the most common and occurs among young people.

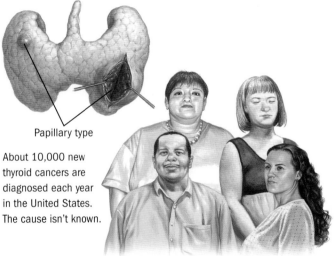

Papillary type

About 10,000 new thyroid cancers are diagnosed each year in the United States. The cause isn't known.

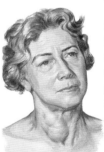

Usually, a thyroid nodule (lump) in the neck is the first symptom. As the cancers grow, they spread to nearby areas and cause hoarseness, trouble swallowing, swollen lymph glands, and neck pain.

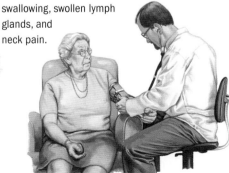

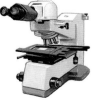

Your doctor may suspect thyroid cancer by finding a lump on your thyroid during a physical examination. For proof of cancer, your doctor can take cells from the lump by FNAB and study them with a microscope.

What Is Thyroid Cancer?

The thyroid gland in the neck makes hormones that control metabolism. Cells in the thyroid gland are called follicular and parafollicular cells. Thyroid cancers are abnormal growths of these cells. These cancers start from either follicular cells (papillary, follicular, and anaplastic cancers) or parafollicular cells (medullary carcinoma). The papillary type is the most common. It occurs among young people. The follicular type occurs in older people. The medullary type can occur as isolated cancers or in families, as a hereditary form. The anaplastic type is aggressive and hard to treat.

About 10,000 new thyroid cancers are diagnosed each year in the United States.

What Causes Thyroid Cancer?

The cause is unknown. Radiation exposure is a risk for this cancer, especially in children who have radiation therapy to the head, neck, or upper chest during infancy or childhood. Thyroid cancer isn't contagious.

What Are the Symptoms of Thyroid Cancer?

Usually, a thyroid nodule (lump) is the first symptom. As the cancers grow, they usually spread to nearby areas and cause hoarseness, trouble swallowing, swollen lymph glands, and neck pain.

How Is Thyroid Cancer Diagnosed?

The doctor may suspect thyroid cancer by finding a lump on the thyroid during a physical examination. For proof of cancer, cells are taken from the lump by fine-needle aspiration biopsy (FNAB) and studied with a microscope. In this type of biopsy, the doctor uses a needle to get a sample.

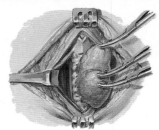

The type of treatment depends on whether the cancer has spread. Treatment can be surgery, radiation therapy, or chemotherapy. Surgical removal of the thyroid is called thyroidectomy. Radioactive iodine can be used after surgery or to treat spread of cancer.

Thyroidectomy

If the whole thyroid is removed, you'll need to take thyroid replacement hormone for the rest of your life. If only part is removed, you may also need hormone to stop growth of remaining thyroid tissue.

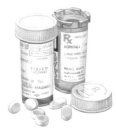

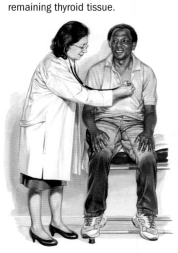

Don't miss follow-up doctor appointments. Careful neck examinations, blood tests, and thyroid scans are done to make sure that the cancer hasn't returned.

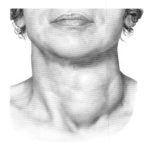

Call your doctor if you find a lump in your neck or are hoarse; have hand tremors, diarrhea, sweats, and palpitations; can't tolerate cold or have a raspy voice or constipation; or have numbness around your mouth, tips of your fingers, and feet with muscle spasms.

How Is Thyroid Cancer Treated?

Treatment can be surgery, radiation therapy, or chemotherapy. Type of treatment depends on whether the cancer has spread.

Removal of the thyroid, either part or the whole gland, is called thyroidectomy. Complications of surgery include injury to vocal cords.

If the whole thyroid is removed, thyroid replacement medicine is taken for the rest of life. If only part is removed, hormone may also be given to stop growth of remaining thyroid tissue.

Radioactive iodine can be used after surgery or to treat spread of cancer. Radioactive iodine kills normal and cancer cells.

Chemotherapy is used if other treatments don't work.

DOs and DON'Ts in Managing Thyroid Cancer:

✔ **DO** take your prescribed medicines.
✔ **DO** find a surgeon with experience in thyroid operations.
✔ **DO** remember that the earlier the cancer is found, the better the chances of cure.
✔ **DO** call your doctor if you find a lump in your neck or are hoarse.
✔ **DO** call your doctor if you have hand tremors (shaking), diarrhea, sweats, and palpitations. You may be taking too much thyroid medicine after surgery.
✔ **DO** call your doctor if you cannot tolerate cold, have a raspy voice, are constipated, lose eyebrow hair, or gain weight. You may be taking too little thyroid medicine.
✔ **DO** call your doctor if after surgery you have numbness around your mouth, tips of your fingers, and feet, with muscle spasms of your hands, legs, or face. You can have a low calcium level.

⊘ **DON'T** miss follow-up doctor appointments. Careful neck examinations, blood tests, and thyroid scans are done to make sure the cancer hasn't returned.

FROM THE DESK OF

NOTES

FOR MORE INFORMATION

Contact the following sources:
• National Cancer Institute
  Tel: (800) 4-CANCER (422-6237)
  Website: http://www.cancer.gov
• American Cancer Society
  Tel: (800) 227-2345
  Website: http://www.cancer.org

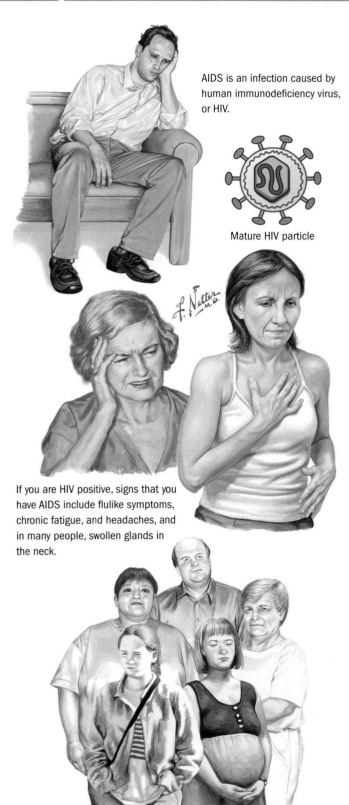

AIDS is an infection caused by human immunodeficiency virus, or HIV.

Mature HIV particle

If you are HIV positive, signs that you have AIDS include flulike symptoms, chronic fatigue, and headaches, and in many people, swollen glands in the neck.

AIDS affects many people in the world. If you've been diagnosed, don't forget that you're not alone!

What Is Acquired Immunodeficiency Syndrome?

Acquired immunodeficiency syndrome (AIDS) is an infection caused by human immunodeficiency virus (HIV), which kills or damages the body's immune cells. The body can't fight infections and certain cancers. People with AIDS may get life-threatening opportunistic infections, which are caused by viruses or bacteria that usually don't make healthy people sick.

What Causes AIDS?

HIV infection can result from sexual activity, using an infected needle, or blood transfusion. It can also pass from a mother to her unborn child or to a baby through breastfeeding. AIDS develops when the immune system is so weak that it cannot fight infection, usually months or years after infection with HIV.

What Are the Symptoms of AIDS

Many people have no symptoms when first infected with HIV. Most people stay symptom-free for months or years, even though the virus is still active.

Some people have a flulike illness, with fever, headache, tiredness, and enlarged lymph nodes, called swollen glands. Blood levels of CD4-positive T cells (also called T4 cells), key infection-fighting cells, drop. Other symptoms seen before full-blown AIDS include lack of energy, weight loss, frequent fevers and sweats, long-lasting or frequent yeast infections, and short-term memory loss. Some people develop herpes infections that cause shingles or mouth, genital, or anal sores.

The most common symptoms of AIDS include infection of the lungs, brain, or eyes. Additional symptoms include trouble thinking, diarrhea, and loss of appetite. Thrush, a fungal infection that causes painful swallowing and a white coating on the tongue, may occur. AIDS increases the risk of getting skin cancer and lymphoma (cancer of lymphatic tissue, part of the immune system).

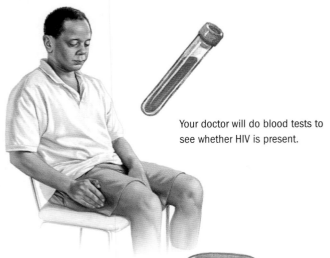

Your doctor will do blood tests to see whether HIV is present.

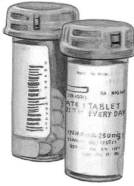

If you've been diagnosed with AIDS, you will have to take medicine that will strengthen your immune system.

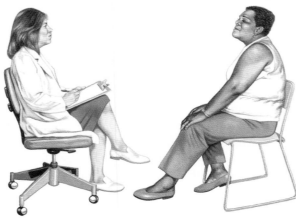

Be sure to talk to your doctor if you've been diagnosed with AIDS. Look for an AIDS support group in your area if you feel alone. Although AIDS has no cure as yet, better treatments let people live longer and healthier lives.

How Is AIDS Diagnosed?

The doctor will take a medical history, do a physical examination, and test blood for HIV and for the presence of other infections. A chest x-ray and other tests may be done.

How Is AIDS Treated?

Medicine will help the immune system fight HIV. A specialist in infectious deseases will help coordinate your care. Several medicines may keep HIV from growing. Other medicines may treat additional symptoms. A nutritionist can help plan a healthy diet.

DOs and DON'Ts in Managing AIDS:

✔ **DO** practice safe sex (always use a latex condom).
✔ **DO** limit the number of sexual partners.
✔ **DO** follow your doctor's directions.
✔ **DO** tell your doctor about all your medicines and medical problems.
✔ **DO** tell your sexual partner about having AIDS so that he or she can be tested.
✔ **DO** avoid being with people with colds or stomach flu.
✔ **DO** call your doctor right away or go to the emergency room if you have a severe headache, fever, cough, severe diarrhea or vomiting, or bad stomach pain, or if bright lights bother you.
✔ **DO** talk to someone about your stress.
✔ **DO** call your doctor if you have shortness of breath, new pain or skin lesions, new cough, changes in vision, worse fatigue or weakness, temperature higher than 101°F, trouble staying awake, or confusion.

⊘ **DON'T** skip medicine doses or doctor's appointments.
⊘ **DON'T** stop taking your medicine because you feel better unless your doctor says you should.
⊘ **DON'T** drink too much alcohol or use drugs.
⊘ **DON'T** share needles or use injection drugs.
⊘ **DON'T** eat foods such as raw eggs, raw oysters, or unpasteurized milk (may have harmful bacteria).
⊘ **DON'T** donate blood, sperm, or organs.

FROM THE DESK OF

NOTES

FOR MORE INFORMATION

Contact the following sources:

• Centers for Disease Control
  Tel: (800) 232-4636

• Internet Sites
  http://www.healthfinder.gov
  http://www.healthanswers.com
  http://www.niaid.nih.gov/factsheets/hivinf.htm

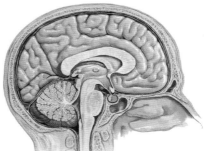

The brain is part of the central nervous system of your body. It acts like the central processing unit of your computer.

What Is a Brain Abscess?

The brain is part of the central nervous system of your body. It works like the central processing unit of your computer. It receives, accepts, and inputs outside data, stores data, and organizes responses to data. The immune system, skull, and tissue layers around the brain protect it against infection. However, bacteria and other organisms can get through this protection and cause infection. The brain sometimes responds to infection by forming small hollow cavities filled with pus, called abscesses.

Brain abscesses are rare and can occur at any age, but they usually occur in people between 30 and 45. The risk increases with head injury, drug abuse, diabetes, cancer, AIDS, severe illness, and infections of the face, ears, nose, and eyes. Emergency hospital care is needed. Almost half of people affected continue to have nerve or behavioral effects after treatment. Since the use of antibiotics and computed tomography (CT) and magnetic resonance imaging (MRI), the death rate from brain abscesses has decreased to 10%.

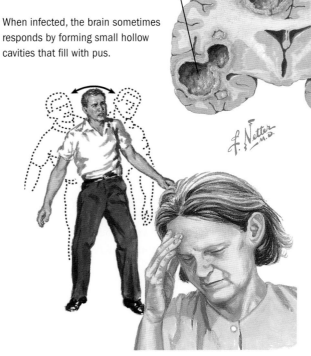

Abscesses

When infected, the brain sometimes responds by forming small hollow cavities that fill with pus.

What Causes a Brain Abscess?

Bacteria are the usual cause. Fungi are a common cause in people with poor immune system protection (e.g., with AIDS). Brain abscesses usually result from spreading of other infections, such as sinusitis or middle ear or dental infections, or from surgery for brain tumors.

What Are the Symptoms of a Brain Abscess?

The most common symptoms are fever, headache, and nervous system problems. Such problems may be confusion, disorientation, speech or walking difficulties, change in mental status, or arm and leg weakness on one side. Other symptoms include nausea, vomiting, stiff neck, and seizures.

The most common symptoms are fever, headache, and nervous system changes, such as confusion, disorientation, speech or walking problems, or arm and leg weakness on one side.

How Is a Brain Abscess Diagnosed?

The doctor finds brain abscesses by obtaining a medical history, performing a physical exam, and looking at results from MRI or CT of the brain.

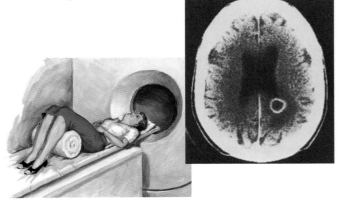

The doctor makes a diagnosis by checking your symptoms and results of CT (shown here) or MRI.

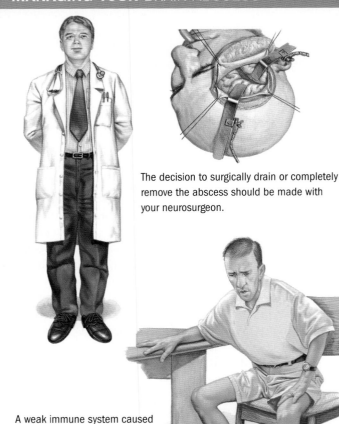

The decision to surgically drain or completely remove the abscess should be made with your neurosurgeon.

A weak immune system caused by diabetes, cancer, AIDS, or severe illness will increase the risk of having a brain abscess.

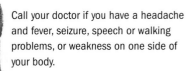

Call your doctor if you have a headache and fever, seizure, speech or walking problems, or weakness on one side of your body.

How Is a Brain Abscess Treated?

Treatment involves antibiotics and surgical drainage or removal of the abscess. The decision to surgically drain or remove the abscess should be made with a neurosurgeon. Sometimes antibiotics alone may offer a cure, but surgery is usually needed. Complications from surgery include a worsening condition, stroke, and infection. Most people have antibiotics given intravenously and then by mouth. Special drugs are available for brain abscesses caused by a fungus.

DOs and DON'Ts in Managing a Brain Abscess:

✔ **DO** follow your doctor's instructions about antibiotics. Finish the full course of medicine.

✔ **DO** realize that the earlier the diagnosis is made the better the prognosis for remaining nervous system and behavioral effects.

✔ **DO** follow up with your appointments, including doctor visits and repeated CT or MRI, to be sure that the infection is gone.

✔ **DO** call your doctor if you have a headache and fever or a seizure or notice changes in your mental state (e.g., confusion or disorientation), speech or walking problems, or weakness on one side of your body.

⊘ **DON'T** ignore symptoms. Remember that most brain abscesses result from other infections that spread to the brain. Report all symptoms to your doctor.

⊘ **DON'T** do drugs! Drug abuse increases the risk of infections.

FROM THE DESK OF

NOTES

FOR MORE INFORMATION

Contact the following source:

• American Academy of Otolaryngology—Head and Neck Surgery
Tel: (703) 836-4444
Website: http://www.entnet.org

MANAGING YOUR
BREAST ABSCESS

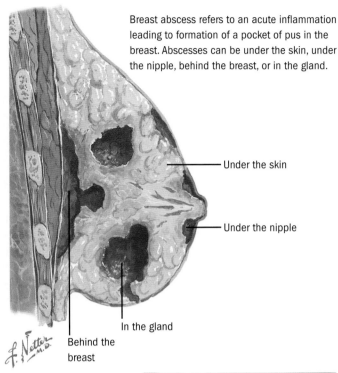

Breast abscess refers to an acute inflammation leading to formation of a pocket of pus in the breast. Abscesses can be under the skin, under the nipple, behind the breast, or in the gland.

— Under the skin

— Under the nipple

In the gland

Behind the breast

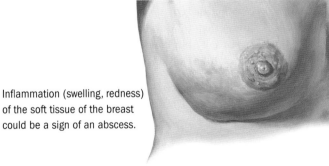

Inflammation (swelling, redness) of the soft tissue of the breast could be a sign of an abscess.

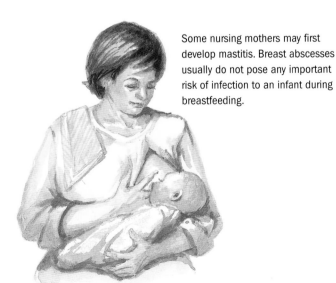

Some nursing mothers may first develop mastitis. Breast abscesses usually do not pose any important risk of infection to an infant during breastfeeding.

What Are Breast Abscesses?

An abscess is a pocket containing pus that can occur in any part of the body. Breast abscess refers to an inflammation (swelling, redness) that results in such a collection of pus in the breast.

What Causes Breast Abscesses?

Bacteria most often cause breast abscesses. The most common types of bacteria are named *Staphylococcus aureus* and *Streptococcus*. Sometimes anaerobic bacteria (which grow without oxygen) can cause breast abscesses.

Breast abscesses usually occur in women of childbearing age. About 10% to 30% of all breast abscesses occur after pregnancy, when nursing mothers breastfeed newborns. Nursing mothers may first develop a condition called mastitis, or inflammation of the breast's soft tissue. About 1 in 15 of these women can develop breast abscesses.

Blockage of nipple ducts because of scarring can also cause breast abscesses.

Breast abscesses are not inherited and cannot be passed from one person to another. They usually present no risk of infection to a newborn.

What Are the Symptoms of Breast Abscesses?

A painful, swollen, hot red mass on the breast is usual. Sometimes, drainage through the skin over the abscess or nipple duct opening may be present. Other symptoms include fever, chills, nausea, and vomiting. Sometimes, the nipple may be inverted (pointing inward), and the abscess can look like other conditions, such as breast cancer or an infected cyst.

How Are Breast Abscesses Diagnosed?

The doctor makes a diagnosis by means of a physical examination. The doctor may in some cases consult a general surgeon to cut, drain, and perform a biopsy of the area. In a biopsy, a small piece of breast tissue is taken for study under the microscope. Pus can be studied to identify the bacteria, which helps the doctor select the right antibiotic for treatment.

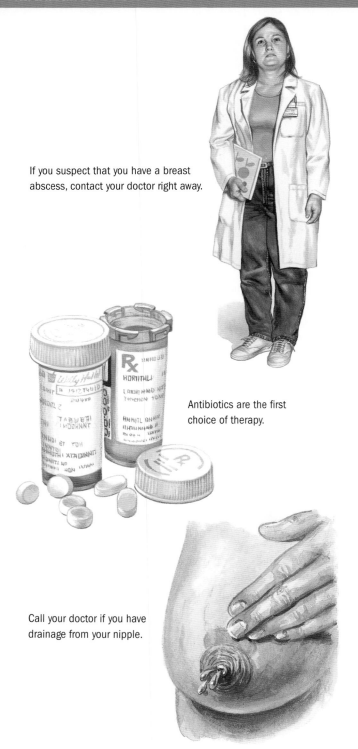

If you suspect that you have a breast abscess, contact your doctor right away.

Antibiotics are the first choice of therapy.

Call your doctor if you have drainage from your nipple.

How Are Breast Abscesses Treated?

Antibiotics are the first therapy used. If mastitis is found early, antibiotic therapy may cure the problem without surgery. However, most women with a breast abscess will need an incision (cutting) and drainage. Complications of incision and drainage include formation of a new abscess, scarring of ducts, and formation of fistulas. A fistula is a passage leading from the abscess to the outside skin.

DOs and DON'Ts in Managing Breast Abscesses:

✔ **DO** remember that you can use warm, moist compresses on the infected breast tissue.

✔ **DO** remember that up to 40% to 50% of breast abscesses can come back.

✔ **DO** call your doctor immediately if you feel a lump or have redness or pain in your breast. Prompt diagnosis and treatment with antibiotics may prevent the need for surgery.

✔ **DO** call your doctor if you notice nipple inversion or drainage from your nipple.

✔ **DO** call your doctor if you have fever or chills.

✔ **DO** call your doctor if you have pain with breastfeeding.

🚫 **DON'T** forget to tell your doctor if you are allergic to penicillin or other drugs.

🚫 **DON'T** forget that good nipple hygiene if you're breastfeeding can prevent skin cracking and abrasions that can lead to mastitis and breast abscesses.

FROM THE DESK OF

NOTES

FOR MORE INFORMATION

Contact the following sources:

• American College of Obstetricians and Gynecologists
Tel: (202) 638-5577
Website: http://www.acog.org

• American College of Surgeons
Tel: (800) 621-4111

MANAGING YOUR
ACUTE BRONCHITIS

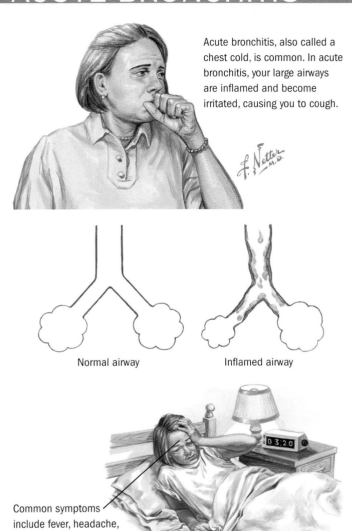

Acute bronchitis, also called a chest cold, is common. In acute bronchitis, your large airways are inflamed and become irritated, causing you to cough.

Normal airway   Inflamed airway

Common symptoms include fever, headache, and shortness of breath.

The usual cause is a viral infection, most likely after cold or flu symptoms.

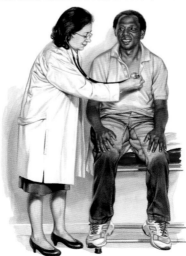

The doctor will ask about your symptoms, do a physical examination, and listen to your lungs with a stethoscope. X-rays may be done for long-term or severe symptoms.

What Is Acute Bronchitis?

Acute bronchitis is inflammation (swelling) of the large airways (or bronchial tubes) in the lungs. Acute means that the bronchitis starts suddenly. This common condition is sometimes called a chest cold.

Coughing results from this inflammation and irritation of the lining of these large airways. Also, glands in the airways produce too much mucus (slimy, thick fluid that moistens and protects many passages in the body). This inflammation and mucus cause airways to narrow, resulting in noisy breathing.

Complete recovery can occur within 10 to 14 days, but the cough may last longer. Smokers have a slower recovery time. Acute bronchitis can sometimes lead to the more serious pneumonia. Repeated attacks of acute bronchitis may mean the presence of long-standing (chronic) bronchitis, asthma, or another lung disorder.

What Causes Acute Bronchitis?

The usual cause is a viral infection, most likely after cold or flu symptoms. Other causes include bacteria and irritation of the large airways by chemicals, fumes, dust, or pollutants.

Smokers and people with lung problems, such as chronic bronchitis, asthma, or cystic fibrosis, are more likely to get acute bronchitis.

What Are the Symptoms of Acute Bronchitis?

Symptoms include those of the common cold, such as runny nose and sore throat, fever, headache, aches and pains, cough with mucus, wheezing, shortness of breath, and chest pain when breathing deeply or coughing.

How Is Acute Bronchitis Diagnosed?

The doctor will ask about symptoms, do a physical examination, and listen to the lungs with a stethoscope.

For long-term or severe symptoms, the doctor may order a chest x-ray to exclude more serious infections such as pneumonia. Blood tests aren't normally needed.

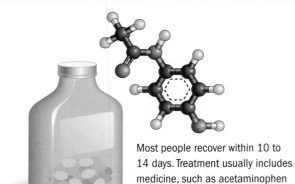

Most people recover within 10 to 14 days. Treatment usually includes medicine, such as acetaminophen or ibuprofen to reduce fever and pain.

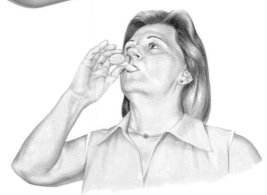

Your doctor may recommend use of bronchodilators, given by inhalers, to open up your airways and help breathing.

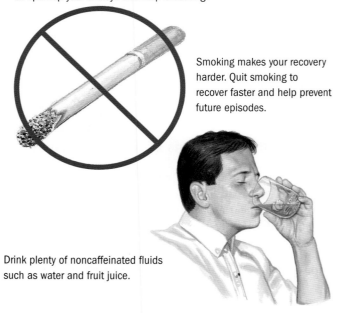

Smoking makes your recovery harder. Quit smoking to recover faster and help prevent future episodes.

Drink plenty of noncaffeinated fluids such as water and fruit juice.

How Is Acute Bronchitis Treated?

Antipyretic medicines reduce body temperature and analgesic drugs ease chest discomfort and body aches. These drugs include acetaminophen and ibuprofen.

Cough syrups may or may not work, and some make people drowsy.

Decongestants can help with cold symptoms.

Bronchodilators, usually given by inhaler, open the airways and help with breathing.

People with acute bronchitis don't usually need antibiotics because the cause is a virus and antibiotics treat bacterial infections. However, if the doctor suspects bacteria as the cause, antibiotics may be given.

DOs and DON'Ts in Managing Acute Bronchitis:

✔ **DO** quit smoking if you smoke.
✔ **DO** avoid smoky environments.
✔ **DO** drink plenty of noncaffeinated fluids, such as water and fruit juices.
✔ **DO** get plenty of rest.
✔ **DO** use a room humidifier or damp towels for increased humidity in your room.
✔ **DO** wash your hands often to prevent spread of infection.
✔ **DO** call your doctor if you become short of breath or cough up blood.
✔ **DO** call your doctor if your cough lasts longer than 3 weeks.

⊘ **DON'T** go out in cold or damp weather.
⊘ **DON'T** delay in getting medical care if your symptoms worsen, don't improve, or you get new symptoms.

FROM THE DESK OF

NOTES

FOR MORE INFORMATION

Contact the following source:

• Medline Plus
U.S. National Library of Medicine
8600 Rockville Pike
Bethesda, MD 20894
Website: http://medlineplus.gov/

MANAGING YOUR
CAT-SCRATCH DISEASE

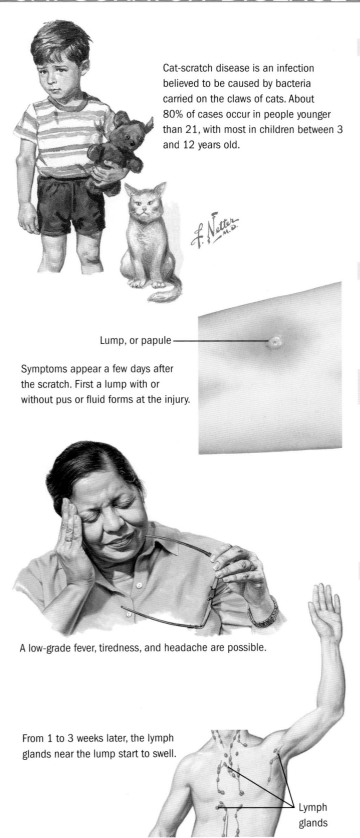

Cat-scratch disease is an infection believed to be caused by bacteria carried on the claws of cats. About 80% of cases occur in people younger than 21, with most in children between 3 and 12 years old.

Lump, or papule —

Symptoms appear a few days after the scratch. First a lump with or without pus or fluid forms at the injury.

A low-grade fever, tiredness, and headache are possible.

From 1 to 3 weeks later, the lymph glands near the lump start to swell.

Lymph glands

What Is Cat-Scratch Disease?

Cat-scratch disease is an infection that is believed to be caused by bacteria carried on the claws of cats. The infection spreads to lymph glands (nodes) nearest the scratch. Lymph glands are masses of tissue that are part of the body's immune system, which fights infection.

Cat-scratch disease is rather rare. Most cases seem to happen in early autumn and the middle of winter. It occurs more often in children and young adults. About 80% of cases occur in people younger than 21, with most between 3 and 12 years old.

What Causes Cat-Scratch Disease?

The cause of the infection is a type of bacteria called *Bartonella henselae*. Most domestic cats have the infection but rarely show any signs of being infected.

What Are the Symptoms of Cat-Scratch Disease?

Symptoms appear a few days after the scratch. First a lump with or without pus or fluid forms at the injury. From 1 to 3 weeks later, lymph glands near the lump begin to swell. The swelling means that the number of white blood cells (lymphocytes), which are the infection-fighting cells, is increasing and they are attacking the bacteria. There may be a low-grade fever, fatigue, and headache.

How Is Cat-Scratch Disease Diagnosed?

The doctor will diagnose the disease on the basis of the history of a recent cat scratch and the look of the scratch, with reddened crusted blisters. The doctor may also see swollen lymph nodes filled with pus and draining through the skin near the scratch.

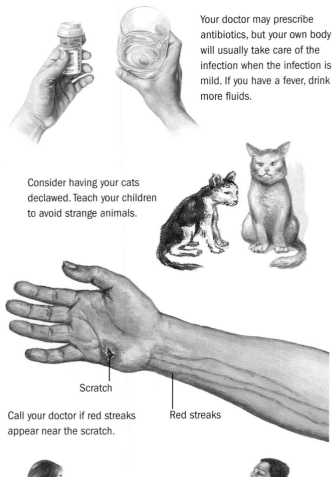

Your doctor may prescribe antibiotics, but your own body will usually take care of the infection when the infection is mild. If you have a fever, drink more fluids.

Consider having your cats declawed. Teach your children to avoid strange animals.

Scratch

Call your doctor if red streaks appear near the scratch.

Red streaks

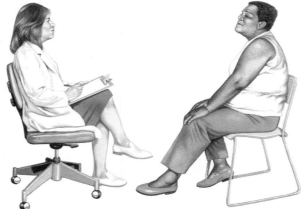

Your doctor will diagnose cat-scratch disease on the basis of a recent cat scratch, blisters at the site of the scratch, and swollen glands.

How Is Cat-Scratch Disease Treated?

Unless the body's immune system isn't working well, the infection usually goes away with antibiotic treatment in 1 to 2 weeks. The body's own immune system may take care of the infection without antibiotics in very mild cases. People with poor infection-fighting ability (e.g., with HIV or AIDS) may develop a more severe infection and generally need antibiotics. Rest is best until the fever subsides and energy returns. No special diet is needed, but drinking more fluids during the fever helps. Using heat on the blisters and taking pain relievers also help symptoms.

DOs and DON'Ts in Managing Cat-Scratch Disease:

✔ **DO** rest until the fever subsides and energy returns.
✔ **DO** take antibiotics, if they're prescribed, until they're gone.
✔ **DO** watch scratches from a cat for signs of infection.
✔ **DO** use care when handling cats. Teach young children to avoid strange animals.
✔ **DO** have cats declawed, if possible.
✔ **DO** call your doctor if a high fever occurs (temperature of 102° F or above).
✔ **DO** call your doctor if a lymph gland becomes red and painful.
✔ **DO** call your doctor if red streaks appear near the scratch.

⊘ **DON'T** skip doses or stop antibiotics if they were prescribed.
⊘ **DON'T** isolate the infected person because the disease is not spread from person to person.
⊘ **DON'T** handle strange animals.

FROM THE DESK OF

NOTES

FOR MORE INFORMATION

Contact the following source:

• National Institute of Allergy and Infectious Diseases
Tel: (301) 496-5717
Websites: http://www.healthfinder.gov (Choose SEARCH to search by topic.)
http://www.healthanswers.com

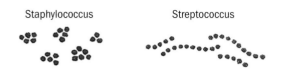

Staphylococcus   Streptococcus

Cellulitis is an infection in the skin and soft tissues under the skin. It is caused by bacteria called staphylococcus (staph) and streptococcus (strep).

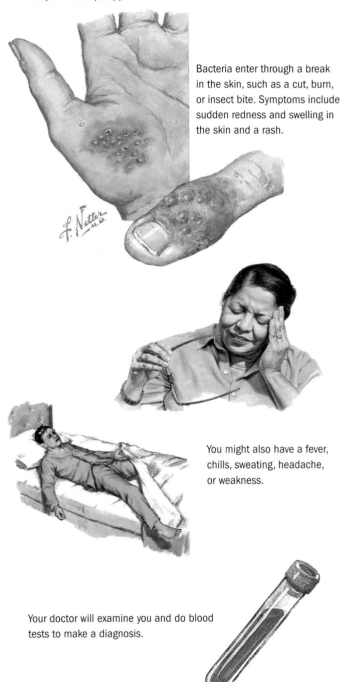

Bacteria enter through a break in the skin, such as a cut, burn, or insect bite. Symptoms include sudden redness and swelling in the skin and a rash.

You might also have a fever, chills, sweating, headache, or weakness.

Your doctor will examine you and do blood tests to make a diagnosis.

What Is Cellulitis?

Cellulitis is an infection in the skin and soft tissue layers under the skin. People with diabetes, blood circulation problems, and weakened immune systems can easily develop cellulitis. Also, people who had recent medical procedures, such as heart or lung surgery, can get cellulitis, as can people who work on farms or in gardens or who handle fish.

What Causes Cellulitis?

Cellulitis is caused by bacteria, usually kinds of bacteria called staphylococcus (staph) and streptococcus (strep). Bacteria enter through a break in the skin, such as a cut, burn, insect bite, open sore, or crack (for example, between toes).

What Are the Symptoms of Cellulitis?

Symptoms include sudden redness, swelling, and tenderness in the skin and a rash. Sometimes a red line extends toward the closest lymph nodes (glands). Other signs of infection include fever, chills or sweating, headache, rapid heartbeat, and weakness.

Most often cellulitis affects lower legs and feet, but it can also occur on the face (especially cheeks), hands, or scalp, and in children, around the rectum. Cellulitis can also occur as an eye infection, with swollen eyelids, loss of sight, and problems with eye movement.

How Is Cellulitis Diagnosed?

The doctor will examine the area and do blood tests. Sometimes, a tiny sample of skin (biopsy) may also be taken when the diagnosis is unclear.

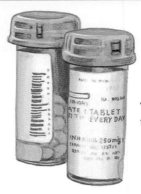

Your doctor will give you medicine to fight the infection and stop the pain.

How Is Cellulitis Treated?

Medicine (antibiotics) will fight the infection and relieve pain. People with mild infections can take medicine by mouth and don't need to be hospitalized. People with cellulitis that is hard to treat are sometimes hospitalized and given intravenous antibiotics. In most people, the infection clears up in 7 to 10 days. People with diabetes or other medical problems may have a longer recovery.

DOs and DON'Ts in Managing Cellulitis:

✔ **DO** take medicine for as long as your doctor tells you, even if you feel better, unless your doctor says you can stop.

✔ **DO** elevate your leg if it has cellulitis, but wiggle your toes or flex your ankle frequently to prevent blood clots.

✔ **DO** apply cool, wet cloth dressings.

✔ **DO** tell your doctor at once if the infection spreads or you develop high fevers, vomiting, headache, or red streaks that don't go away.

✔ **DO** call your doctor at once if you notice areas of infection starting nearby, your skin becomes dark or discolored, or blisters appear.

✔ **DO** avoid injuring your skin by wearing protective clothing or equipment.

✔ **DO** clean a cut or injury and use an antibiotic ointment. If it seems to be infected (red or warm), call your doctor.

⊘ **DON'T** skip doses or stop taking antibiotics until finished.

⊘ **DON'T** resume normal activities until swelling and pain stop.

⊘ **DON'T** swim if you have a skin wound.

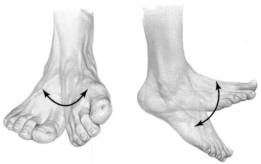

Put up your leg if it has cellulitis, but don't keep it completely immobile. Occasionally wiggle your toes and flex your ankle.

Call your doctor immediately if you have a high fever.

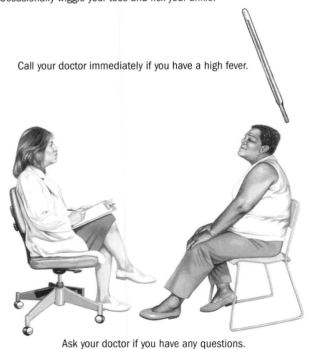

Ask your doctor if you have any questions.

FROM THE DESK OF

NOTES

FOR MORE INFORMATION

Contact the following sources:

• American Academy of Dermatology
Tel: (888) 462-3376
Website: http://www.aad.org

• National Health Info Center
Tel: (800) 336-4797
Website: http://www.health.gov/nhic/

MANAGING YOUR
COMMON COLD

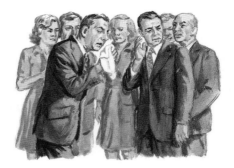

The common cold is an infection of airways of the nose, throat, upper windpipe, and ears. Colds are most common in winter, when viruses spread easily among people indoors.

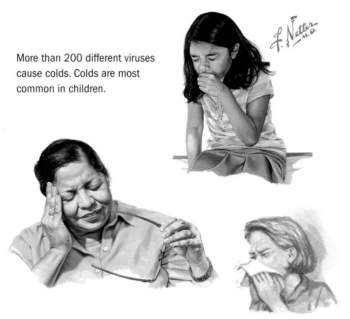

More than 200 different viruses cause colds. Colds are most common in children.

Symptoms include sore throat, dry cough, low fever, watery eyes, hoarse voice, and stuffy, runny nose. Sneezing, headache, no appetite, and feeling tired are others.

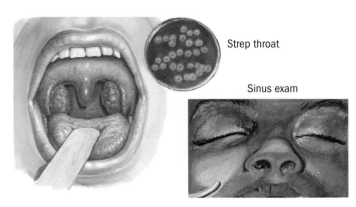

Strep throat

Sinus exam

You don't need to see your doctor for a cold. Symptoms that are severe or last more than a week might need tests to check for strep throat or sinus infection.

What Is a Common Cold?

The common cold, also called an acute upper respiratory tract infection (URI), is an infection of airways of the nose, throat, upper windpipe, and ears.

People in the United States have 1 billion colds yearly. They're most common in children, who usually have 6 to 10 colds yearly. Adults average two to four. Women, especially 20 to 30 years old, have more colds than men. People older than 60 average less than one cold a year.

What Causes a Common Cold?

More than 200 different viruses cause colds. The ones called rhinoviruses cause about one third of adult colds. Coronaviruses cause a large percentage of adult colds. Causes of 30% to 50% of adult colds aren't clear. Colds are most common in winter, when viruses spread easily among people indoors.

Being very tired or stressed (weakened immune system) and having allergies can increase chances of getting a cold.

What Are the Symptoms of a Common Cold?

Symptoms usually start 2 to 3 days after infection and last 2 to 14 days. Most are in the nose, throat, and ears and include sore throat, dry cough, low fever, watery eyes, hoarse voice, and stuffy, runny nose. Sneezing, headache, no appetite, and feeling tired are others.

How Is a Common Cold Diagnosed?

Seeing a doctor isn't needed for a cold. Symptoms that are severe or last more than a week might need tests to check for strep throat or sinus infection.

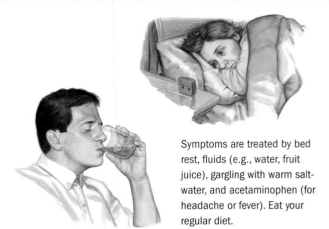

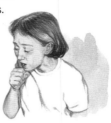

Symptoms are treated by bed rest, fluids (e.g., water, fruit juice), gargling with warm salt-water, and acetaminophen (for headache or fever). Eat your regular diet.

Call your doctor if you have constant coughing, trouble breathing between coughing bouts, high fever, and painful, swollen neck glands.

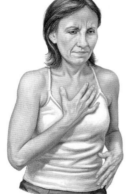

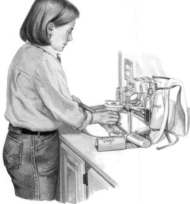

Hand washing is the easiest and best way to avoid getting colds. Sneeze or cough into a facial tissue and throw it right away.

How Is a Common Cold Treated?

Only symptoms are treated, by bed rest, fluids (water, fruit juice, tea, carbonated beverages), gargling with warm saltwater, and use of acetaminophen for headache or fever. Eat a regular diet.

Over-the-counter cold remedies (decongestants, cough suppressants) may relieve symptoms but won't prevent, cure, or shorten colds. Most also have side effects. Over-the-counter antihistamines may help a runny nose and watery eyes.

Sometimes people may get a bacterial infection following the cold that the doctor will need to treat.

DOs and DON'Ts in Managing a Common Cold:

✔ **DO** use saltwater drops for a stuffy nose.
✔ **DO** use a rubber bulb syringe to clean a really stuffy baby's nose. Loosen thick sticky nasal drainage with drops of saltwater solution.
✔ **DO** remember that cold weather has little or no effect on whether you get a cold.
✔ **DO** understand that hand washing is the easiest and best way to avoid getting colds. Not touching the nose or eyes is another. Sneeze or cough into a facial tissue and throw it right away. Stay away from people who have colds.
✔ **DO** eat a well-balanced, healthy diet with citrus fruits and other sources of vitamin C.
✔ **DO** realize that antibiotics don't kill viruses, so antibiotics aren't useful for colds.
✔ **DO** call your doctor if you have symptoms of a secondary bacterial infection.
✔ **DO** call your doctor if your baby won't drink fluids.

⊘ **DON'T** put cotton swabs into a child's nose. Use a tissue or swab outside the nose.
⊘ **DON'T** give aspirin to children and teenagers with a viral illness, because of the risk of Reye's syndrome, a serious illness.
⊘ **DON'T** forget that taking large doses of vitamin C is not effective to prevent colds.

FROM THE DESK OF

NOTES

FOR MORE INFORMATION

Contact the following source:

• American Academy of Family Physicians
Tel: (800) 274-2237
Website: http://www.aafp.org

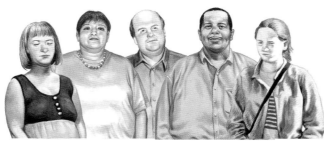

Condyloma acuminatum is the medical term for warts that occur in the genital area. Genital warts are thought to be one of the most common sexually transmitted disease (STD). People who are 17 to 33 years old are at greatest risk of getting these warts.

Genital warts – female   **Genital warts – male**

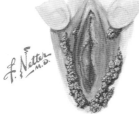

People usually have no symptoms, but itching, burning, and discharge can occur. Warts grow in clusters, as small pink or white nodules. The clusters can quickly become very large.

Cervix

Vagina

Cervical
tissue

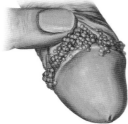

Virus

The cause is the virus HPV that causes other warts. About 90% of cases are caused by HPV-6 and HPV-11. Having prior history of STD and multiple sex partners are risk factors.

Your doctor will diagnose genital warts by a physical examination. Testing may also be done for other STDs.

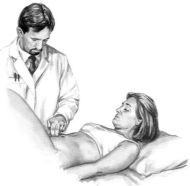

What Are Genital Warts?

Condyloma acuminatum is the medical term for warts that occur in the genital area, including the urethra (the tube taking urine from the bladder to outside the body) and anus. Genital warts are thought to be one of the most common sexually transmitted disease (STD). People who are 17 to 33 years old are at greatest risk of getting genital warts.

What Causes Genital Warts?

The cause is the same human papillomavirus (HPV) that causes other warts. About 90% are caused by HPV-6 and HPV-11. These warts are much more contagious than other warts and are easily passed from skin of infected people. After exposure, warts appear in 1 to 6 months. Having multiple sex partners and prior history of STD are risk factors for getting these warts.

What Are the Symptoms of Genital Warts?

People usually have no symptoms, but itching, burning, and discharge can occur if the warts become irritated or infected. These warts appear on moist surfaces, such as the penis and the entrance to the vagina and rectum. They grow in clusters, as small pink or white nodules. The warts are small, but the clusters can quickly become very large, cauliflower-like masses. Complications of untreated warts can include cervical cancer in females and urinary blockage in males if they occur on the urethra.

How Are Genital Warts Diagnosed?

The doctor will make a diagnosis by the look of the warts at physical examination. The doctor may also do a culture or biopsy of the area. Testing may also be done for other STDs.

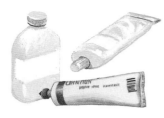

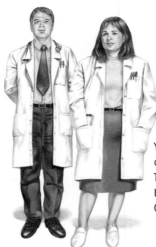

Your doctor should treat your condition—don't use over-the-counter wart removers. Topical medicines are put on small warts. Larger warts may need liquid nitrogen. Other treatments are lasers and surgery.

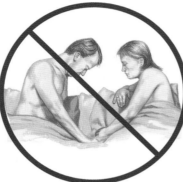

Don't have sex until warts are completely gone. Protect yourself—always use latex condoms during sex.

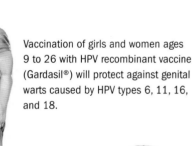

Vaccination of girls and women ages 9 to 26 with HPV recombinant vaccine (Gardasil®) will protect against genital warts caused by HPV types 6, 11, 16, and 18.

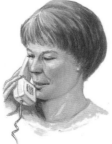

Call your doctor when you have signs of recurring warts or if treated areas show signs of infection: redness, swelling, tenderness, or foul smell.

How Are Genital Warts Treated?

A doctor should treat genital warts. Don't use over-the-counter wart removers. Topical medicines such as imiquimod, 5-fluoro-uracil, podofilox, and trichloroacetic acid cream can be applied to small warts. Larger warts may be treated with liquid nitrogen. Laser treatment or surgical removal may be needed. Warts commonly come back, so treatment may need to be repeated. The doctor may prescribe ointment to apply at home.

DOs and DON'Ts in Managing Genital Warts:

✔ **DO** apply medicine as instructed.
✔ **DO** keep follow-up doctor appointments until all warts are gone.
✔ **DO** tell sexual partners about your condition so that they can be examined and treated.
✔ **DO** avoid sex until warts are completely gone.
✔ **DO** use proper hygiene.
✔ **DO** get tested for other STDs.
✔ **DO** always use latex condoms during sex.
✔ **DO** get vaccinated if you are female (all girls and women ages 9 to 26) with HPV recombinant vaccine (Gardasil®). It will protect against genital warts caused by HPV types 6, 11, 16, and 18.
✔ **DO** call your doctor if warts come back.
✔ **DO** call your doctor if treated areas show signs of infection: redness, swelling, tenderness, or foul smell.

⊘ **DON'T** apply medicine to moles, birthmarks, or warts that are bleeding.
⊘ **DON'T** have sex until warts are gone and healing is complete.
⊘ **DON'T** skip follow-up appointments. Warts can come back, and you may need a different treatment.

FROM THE DESK OF

NOTES

FOR MORE INFORMATION

Contact the following sources:

• The American Social Health Association
Tel: (800) 230-6039
Website: http://www.ashastd.org

• National Institute of Allergy and Infectious Diseases
Website: http://www3.niaid.nih.gov

MANAGING YOUR
CONJUNCTIVITIS

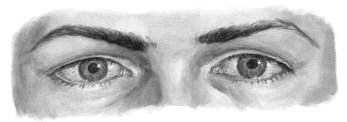

Conjunctivitis, or pinkeye, is the most common eye infection. It causes soreness and swelling (inflammation) of the skin lining the eyelid and the white part of the eyeball.

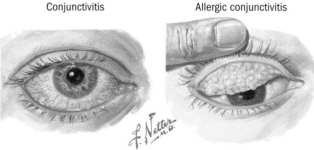

Conjunctivitis   Allergic conjunctivitis

The cause can be bacteria or virus (very contagious) or an allergy (e.g., to pollen). Viral conjunctivitis usually causes inflammation and very watery discharge.

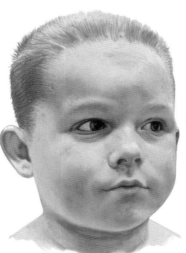

Bacterial conjunctivitis produces a slimy discharge that causes crusting of the eyelids. Bacterial conjunctivitis is most common in children.

Your doctor will examine you to make a diagnosis.

What Is Conjunctivitis?

Conjunctivitis (also called pink eye) is the most common eye infection. It causes soreness and swelling (inflammation) of the skin that lines the eyelid and the white part of the eyeball. One or both eyes can have it. People of any age can get conjunctivitis. It occurs most often in the fall.

Serious complications that threaten sight are very rare.

What Causes Conjunctivitis?

The cause can be infection with bacteria or virus (very contagious) or an allergy to something such as pollen.

The virus is usually the one that causes a common cold. Different bacteria (such as *Staphylococcus* and *Streptococcus*) can cause the infection. Direct contact with tears or the infected area, which occurs by placing towels, fingers, or handkerchiefs near the eye, will pass these infections to others.

What Are the Symptoms of Conjunctivitis?

Conjunctivitis produces a red irritated eye with a watery discharge (allergic and viral) or a discharge of mucus and pus (bacterial). Bacterial conjunctivitis also causes soreness and swelling in one eye, slight pain and feeling dirt or grit in the eye, and a slimy discharge that causes lids to crust. It's most common in children.

Viral conjunctivitis usually causes inflammation and discharge that is more watery than that in bacterial conjunctivitis.

Allergic conjunctivitis produces red, irritated, itchy eyes; small watery discharge; and inflammation of both eyes. Itching is characteristic of allergic conjunctivitis. Allergies can be to pollen, pets, and house dust.

How Is Conjunctivitis Diagnosed?

The doctor makes a diagnosis from an examination.

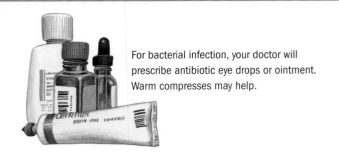

For bacterial infection, your doctor will prescribe antibiotic eye drops or ointment. Warm compresses may help.

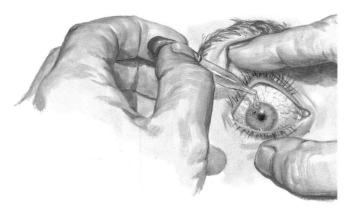

For viral conjunctivitis, your doctor will suggest eye drops that help increase moisture in the eye. Antibiotic eye drops or ointment won't work on viruses.

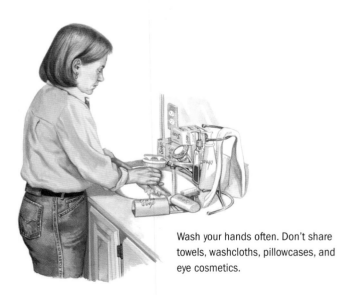

Wash your hands often. Don't share towels, washcloths, pillowcases, and eye cosmetics.

How Is Conjunctivitis Treated?

For bacterial infection, the doctor will prescribe antibiotic eye drops or ointment. Warm compresses on the eye may also be used.

For viral conjunctivitis, the doctor may suggest eye drops that help increase moisture in the eye. Antibiotic eye drops or ointment won't work. Warm compresses on the eye may help.

For allergic conjunctivitis, the doctor will prescribe eye drops for inflammation. Cold, not hot, compresses may soothe the eye. Decongestant and antihistamines may also be used.

Bacterial conjunctivitis is usually much better within 48 hours of starting therapy. It's usually over in about 1 week.

Viral conjunctivitis usually improves in 1 to 2 weeks but may take longer.

Symptoms of allergic conjunctivitis may be seasonal.

DOs and DON'Ts in Managing Conjunctivitis:

✔ **DO** avoid direct contact with anyone who has conjunctivitis.

✔ **DO** wash your hands often.

✔ **DO** use separate towels, washcloths, and pillowcases from other family members if you have conjunctivitis.

✔ **DO** throw away old eye cosmetics and don't share eye cosmetics with others.

✔ **DO** avoid the cause of the allergy, if possible.

✔ **DO** use medicines as directed. If using more than one eye drop, wait between use of each so that the second doesn't wash the first out.

✔ **DO** call your doctor if you have severe pain, fever, and blurred vision with conjunctivitis.

⊘ **DON'T** touch the infected area or rub your eye.

⊘ **DON'T** wear contact lenses until treatment is over. You may need to replace the contact lenses and the container normally used for storing them.

FROM THE DESK OF

NOTES

FOR MORE INFORMATION

Contact the following sources:

• American Academy of Ophthalmology
Tel: (415) 561-8500
Websites: http://www.aao.org
http://www.eyenet.org

• American Academy of Optometry
Tel: (301) 984-1441
Website: http://www.aaopt.org

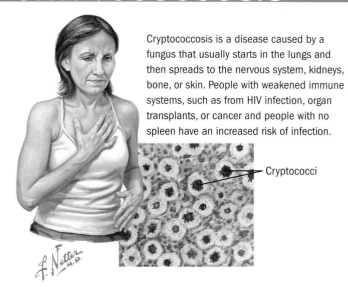

Cryptococcosis is a disease caused by a fungus that usually starts in the lungs and then spreads to the nervous system, kidneys, bone, or skin. People with weakened immune systems, such as from HIV infection, organ transplants, or cancer and people with no spleen have an increased risk of infection.

— Cryptococci

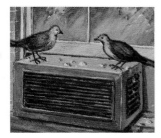

The fungus may spread through the air on dust particles contaminated by pigeon droppings.

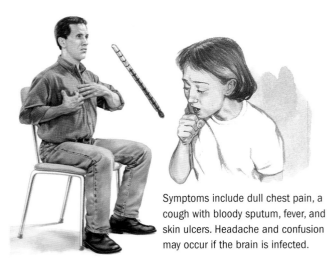

Symptoms include dull chest pain, a cough with bloody sputum, fever, and skin ulcers. Headache and confusion may occur if the brain is infected.

Your doctor will examine you and test your blood and urine. A spinal tap may be done to look for brain infection.

What Is Cryptococcosis?

Cryptococcosis is a disease caused by a fungus that usually starts in the lungs without symptoms and then spreads to the nervous system, kidneys, bone, or skin. It's more serious for people with disorders of the immune system. The fungus may spread through the air on dust particles contaminated by pigeon droppings. It isn't passed from person to person.

What Causes Cryptococcosis?

The fungus named *Cryptococcus* is the cause. People with human immunodeficiency virus (HIV) infection, organ transplants, cancer, or weakened immune systems from other diseases or people without a spleen (after it's removed) have an increased risk of infection. For these people, cryptococcosis may be life threatening.

What Are the Symptoms of Cryptococcosis?

Symptoms include dull chest pain, a cough that may produce bloody sputum, severe headache, fever, blurred vision, confusion, red facial rash, and skin ulcers.

How Is Cryptococcosis Diagnosed?

The doctor will do a physical examination and tests of blood and urine. A spinal tap may be done to look for infection in spinal fluid and membranes around the brain (meningitis). In a spinal tap, a sample of spinal fluid is taken by inserting a needle in the spine and removing fluid. Computed tomography or magnetic resonance imaging of the brain may also be done to check for brain infection.

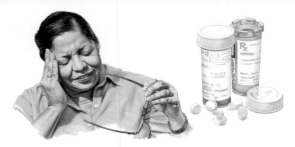

Most people with normal immune systems do well without treatment. People with weakened immune systems may need hospitalization and treatment with antifungal medicine. Drug side effects are nausea, vomiting, and headache.

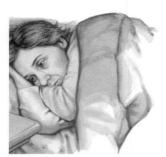

Rest until the fever and cough stop.

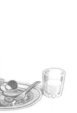

Drink enough liquids and eat a good diet. Try small frequent meals if nausea is a problem.

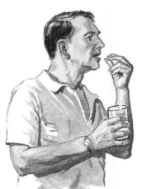

Don't skip doses or stop taking the antifungal medicine.

How Is Cryptococcosis Treated?

Most people with a normal immune system will do well. Mild cases in healthy people may need no treatment. Those with a weakened immune system may need hospitalization and life-long treatment.

The doctor will prescribe antifungal medicines. These may first be given intravenously and then given by mouth when the condition improves. Side effects of the medicine include nausea, vomiting, and headache. Acetaminophen can be used for minor pain and fever. No special diet is needed. Bed rest may be needed until fever and cough stop.

DOs and DON'Ts in Managing Cryptococcosis:

✔ **DO** avoid contact with areas with pigeon droppings, especially if you have a weak immune system.

✔ **DO** rest until fever and cough improve.

✔ **DO** take acetaminophen for minor pain and fever.

✔ **DO** drink enough and eat a good diet. Try small frequent meals if nausea is a problem.

✔ **DO** keep follow-up doctor appointments, to look for recurrence of the disease.

✔ **DO** call your doctor if you cannot take the medicine because of nausea and vomiting.

✔ **DO** call your doctor if you have unexplained weight loss, high fever, severe headache, neck stiffness, or blurred vision.

🚫 **DON'T** skip doses or stop taking the antifungal medicine.

FROM THE DESK OF

NOTES

FOR MORE INFORMATION

Contact the following sources:

• National Heart, Lung, and Blood Institute
Tel: (301) 592 8573
Website: http://www.nhlbi.nih.gov

• National Institute of Allergy and Infectious Disease
Tel: (301) 496-5717
Website: http://www3.niaid.nih.gov

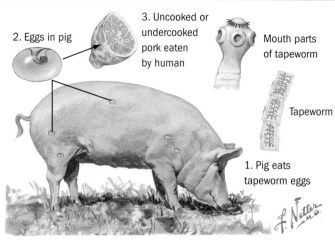

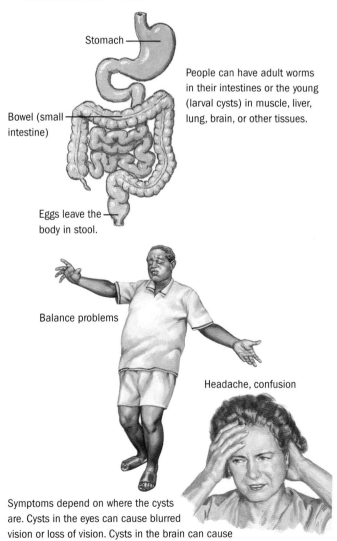

2. Eggs in pig

3. Uncooked or undercooked pork eaten by human

Mouth parts of tapeworm

Tapeworm

1. Pig eats tapeworm eggs

Cysticercosis is an infection caused by eating a tapeworm found in contaminated food or water.

Stomach

Bowel (small intestine)

People can have adult worms in their intestines or the young (larval cysts) in muscle, liver, lung, brain, or other tissues.

Eggs leave the body in stool.

Balance problems

Headache, confusion

Symptoms depend on where the cysts are. Cysts in the eyes can cause blurred vision or loss of vision. Cysts in the brain can cause seizures, headaches, confusion, and balance problems. Cysts in muscles may cause no symptoms.

What Is Cysticercosis?

Cysticercosis is an infection caused by eating the pork tapeworm, named *Taenia solium*, in contaminated food or water, or eating tapeworm eggs passed on by an infected person.

This tapeworm occurs worldwide, and cysticercosis affects about 50 million people, usually in rural developing countries. About 1000 new cases are diagnosed each year in the United States. Cysticercosis of the brain can cause seizures in adults.

What Causes Cysticercosis?

People can have adult tapeworms living in the intestine or the young stage (larval cysts) living in muscle, liver, lung, brain, or other tissues. Pigs usually become infected by eating eggs in contaminated human bowel movements (stools). People eat raw or undercooked meat from an infected pig and thus eat the eggs too. With poor hygiene, these eggs can spread to food, water, or other items.

What Are the Symptoms of Cysticercosis?

Tapeworm eggs hatch in the stomach, go into the intestine, through the bloodstream, and may develop into cysticerci (small cysts) in muscles, brain, or eyes. Symptoms can occur months to years after infection and depend on where cysts are found. Cysts in eyes can cause blurred vision, loss of vision, swelling, and detachment of the retina. Cysts in the brain and spinal cord can cause seizures, headaches, confusion, lack of attention, difficulty with balance, brain swelling, and even death. Cysts in the heart can cause heart rhythm abnormalities and rarely heart failure. Cysts in muscles may cause no symptoms.

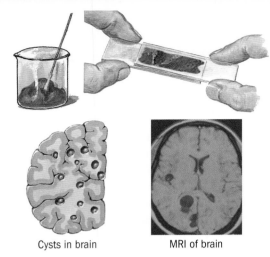

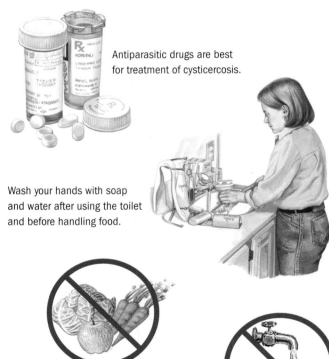

Cysts in brain   MRI of brain

Your doctor makes a diagnosis by looking at stool samples under a microscope for eggs and doing blood tests and x-rays. For brain symptoms, MRI or CT may be needed.

Antiparasitic drugs are best for treatment of cysticercosis.

Wash your hands with soap and water after using the toilet and before handling food.

To prevent infection in areas with poor sanitation, drink only bottled and boiled water and wash and peel raw vegetables and fruits before eating.

How Is Cysticercosis Diagnosed?

The doctor makes a diagnosis by looking at samples of stool under a microscope for tapeworm eggs. The doctor may also order blood tests and x-rays. For brain symptoms, magnetic resonance imaging (MRI) or CT of the head may be needed. A biopsy is sometimes done for diagnosis. In a biopsy, a piece of tissue is taken with a needle from a part of the body for study with a microscope.

How Is Cysticercosis Treated?

Cysticercosis is treated with antiparasitic medicines, which are safe and work well.

DOs and DON'Ts in Managing Cysticercosis:

✔ **DO** avoid eating raw or undercooked pork and other meats.

✔ **DO** wash your hands with soap and water after using the toilet and before handling food, especially when traveling in developing countries.

✔ **DO** wash and peel all raw vegetables and fruits before eating. Avoid food that may be contaminated with stool.

✔ **DO** drink only bottled water and water boiled for 1 minute to prevent cysticercosis.

✔ **DO** remember that family members of infected people should also have stool tested.

✔ **DO** remember that some antiparasitic medicines shouldn't be used during pregnancy.

✔ **DO** call your doctor if you or a family member may have cysticercosis and want to be tested.

🚫 **DON'T** forget that the tapeworm infection can be difficult to diagnose, so your doctor may ask for several stool specimens over several days to study them for signs of a tapeworm.

🚫 **DON'T** eat meat of pigs that are likely to be infected.

🚫 **DON'T** drink fountain drinks or drinks with ice cubes.

FROM THE DESK OF

NOTES

FOR MORE INFORMATION

Contact the following source:

• Website: http://www.cdc.gov/ncidod/dpd/parasites/cysticercosis/factsht_cysticercosis.htm

CARING FOR YOUR CHILD WITH AN EARACHE

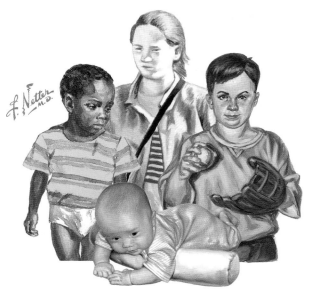

Earaches, called otitis media, are infections in the middle ear. They affect people of any age but are most common in babies and children.

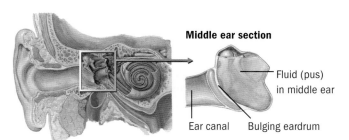

Middle ear section

Fluid (pus) in middle ear

Ear canal   Bulging eardrum

Infection occurs when germs causing colds, sore throats, and flu spread and cause inflammation of the eardrum and area around it.

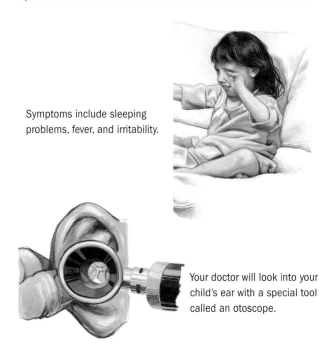

Symptoms include sleeping problems, fever, and irritability.

Your doctor will look into your child's ear with a special tool called an otoscope.

What Is an Earache?

An earache, called otitis media, is an infection in the middle ear (between the eardrum and auditory tube, which links the middle ear to the back of the nose). This area contains nerves and small bones for hearing. Earaches can affect people of any age but are most common in babies and children. Three fourths of children get earaches. Infection occurs when germs causing colds, sore throats, and flu spread and cause inflammation (swelling, redness) of the eardrum and area around it.

What Causes an Earache?

Causes include viruses, bacteria, allergies, and rupture of the eardrum. Allergies cause blockage of sinuses and eustachian tubes.

What Are the Symptoms of an Earache?

Usual symptoms or behaviors include fever, sleeping problems, irritability, pulling on the ears, fluid coming out of ears, loss of hearing and balance, headache, waking in the middle of the night crying in severe pain, and dizziness.

How Is an Earache Diagnosed?

The doctor will look into the child's ear with a special tool called an otoscope. This tool lets the doctor see signs of inflammation in the middle ear. A hearing test may also be done to see if the hearing has been affected.

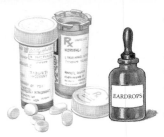

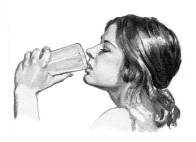

Treatments include antibiotics, pain relievers (such as acetaminophen), and eardrops. If a virus (such as the cold or flu virus) is the cause, antibiotics cannot help. To avoid Reye's syndrome, don't give aspirin to children with a virus.

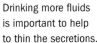

Drinking more fluids is important to help to thin the secretions.

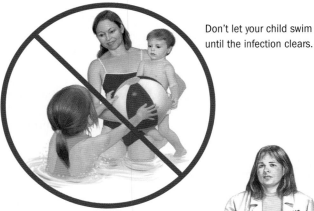

Don't let your child swim until the infection clears.

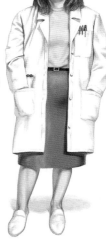

Call your doctor if your child has the earache for more than 2 days after treatment starts.

How Is an Earache Treated?

The doctor may prescribe an oral antibiotic that kills bacteria (such as penicillin) and pain relievers (such as acetaminophen). Eardrops containing an antibiotic and maybe steroids to reduce swelling may also be used. If a virus (such as the cold or flu virus) is the cause, antibiotics cannot help. Watchful waiting may be proper for some earaches.

Resting is suggested until fever and pain leave. No special diet is needed, but drinking more fluids is important to help thin secretions.

DOs and DON'Ts in Managing an Earache:

✔ **DO** follow your doctor's advice about pain relievers and antibiotics if prescribed.

✔ **DO** hold babies in the sitting position while feeding.

✔ **DO** keep a follow-up appointment for the doctor to re-check the ears.

✔ **DO** use nonaspirin medicines for fever and pain.

✔ **DO** use a heating pad or hot water bottle wrapped in a towel on the ear for pain.

✔ **DO** have your child drink more fluids.

✔ **DO** call your doctor if your child has the earache for more than 2 days after treatment starts.

✔ **DO** call your doctor if your child has a severe headache or fever after treatment starts.

✔ **DO** call your doctor if your child has redness or swelling behind the ear or dizziness.

⊘ **DON'T** let your child swim until the infection clears.

⊘ **DON'T** let your child be near cigarette smoke for long periods. In young children this can increase the chance of more infections.

⊘ **DON'T** put anything in the ear other than drops prescribed by your doctor.

⊘ **DON'T** give aspirin to children, to avoid the dangerous Reye's syndrome.

FROM THE DESK OF

NOTES

FOR MORE INFORMATION

Contact the following sources:

• American Academy of Otolaryngology—Head and Neck Surgery
Tel: (703) 836-4444
Website: http://www.entnet.org/

• American Academy of Pediatrics
Tel: (847) 228-5005

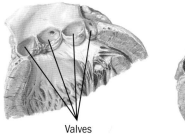

Early infection

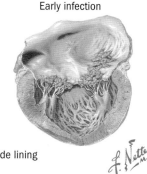

Valves

Endocarditis is inflammation, with or without infection, that affects the inside lining of the heart and heart valves.

What Is Endocarditis?

Endocarditis is inflammation, with or without infection, that affects the inside lining of the heart and heart valves.

What Causes Endocarditis?

Bacteria or fungi are the usual cause. Bacteria include *Staphylococcus* and *Streptococcus*. The bacteria or fungi can get to the heart by entering the bloodstream from infections somewhere else in the body (e.g., urinary or gastrointestinal tract or skin). Surgical or dental procedures can also let these organisms reach the heart.

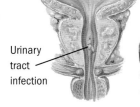

Skin infection

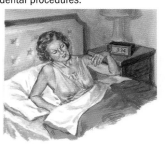

Dental infection

Urinary tract infection

Bacteria (such as *Staphylococcus* and *Streptococcus*) or fungi are the usual cause. Bacteria or fungi can get to the heart by entering the bloodstream from infections somewhere else in the body (e.g., urinary or gastrointestinal tract or skin) or after surgical or dental procedures.

What Are the Symptoms of Endocarditis?

Symptoms include fever, fatigue, weakness, chills and night sweats, muscle and joint pain, and heart murmur. Later symptoms are swelling of feet and legs and shortness of breath with an irregular heartbeat.

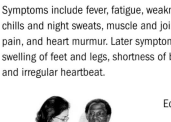

Symptoms include fever, fatigue, weakness, chills and night sweats, muscle and joint pain, and heart murmur. Later symptoms are swelling of feet and legs, shortness of breath, and irregular heartbeat.

How Is Endocarditis Diagnosed?

The doctor can make a diagnosis by taking a medical history, doing a physical examination, and getting blood cultures and an echocardiogram (ultrasound of the heart). The doctor usually finds a new heart murmur at the physical.

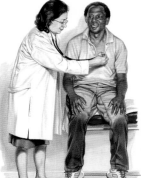

Echocardiography

Your doctor can make a diagnosis by taking your medical history, examining you, and ordering blood cultures and echocardiography. Your doctor may find a new heart murmur at the physical.

The first treatment goal is to get rid of the infection, usually with intravenous antibiotics. Nonaspirin drugs such as acetaminophen can be used for fever and minor pain. Another goal is to treat complications (e.g., congestive heart failure or blood clots).

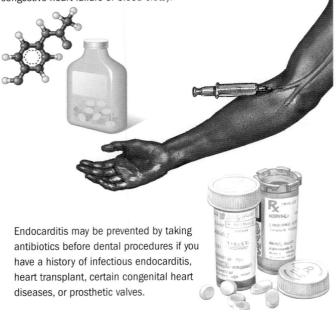

Endocarditis may be prevented by taking antibiotics before dental procedures if you have a history of infectious endocarditis, heart transplant, certain congenital heart diseases, or prosthetic valves.

Resume normal activity slowly as your strength allows.

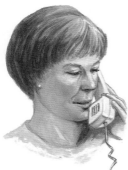

Call your doctor if, after your treatment, you have fever, loss of appetite or weight gain without diet changes, blood in your urine, chest pain, shortness of breath, or sudden weakness in muscles of your face or limbs.

How Is Endocarditis Treated?

Intravenous antibiotics, usually given for 4 to 6 weeks, are used to get rid of the infection. A home health nurse will help with intravenous antibiotic treatment at home. Nonaspirin medications such as acetaminophen can be used for fever and minor pain. A regular diet can be followed. Fluid intake should be increased for fever. Good dental hygiene is needed to prevent infection.

Another goal is to treat complications (e.g., congestive heart failure or blood clots). The doctor may suggest surgery in some cases. Surgery may be needed for congestive heart failure that doesn't respond to usual therapy, endocarditis caused by fungi, recurrent blood clots, abscesses leading to heart rhythm abnormalities, and lasting high fever or sepsis after 72 hours of antibiotics.

DOs and DON'Ts in Managing Endocarditis:

✔ **DO** take your antibiotics until they're gone. Endocarditis may be prevented by using antibiotics before dental procedures if you have a history of prior infectious endocarditis, heart transplant, certain congenital heart diseases, or prosthetic valves.

✔ **DO** use nonaspirin drugs for fever and minor pain.

✔ **DO** increase fluid intake, especially during fever.

✔ **DO** resume normal activity slowly as your strength allows.

✔ **DO** see your dentist regularly. Use a soft-bristled toothbrush.

✔ **DO** call your doctor if, after your treatment, you have fever, loss of appetite or weight gain without diet changes, blood in your urine, chest pain, shortness of breath, or sudden weakness in muscles of your face or limbs.

⊘ **DON'T** skip doses or stop taking antibiotics until you finish a complete treatment course, or until your doctor tells you to stop.

⊘ **DON'T** try to keep your normal schedule; you need rest for a full recovery.

⊘ **DON'T** have dental work or surgical procedures without telling your doctor of your history of endocarditis.

FROM THE DESK OF

NOTES

FOR MORE INFORMATION

Contact the following source:

• National Heart, Lung, and Blood Institute
 Tel: (301) 592-8573
 Website: http://www.nhlbi.nih.gov

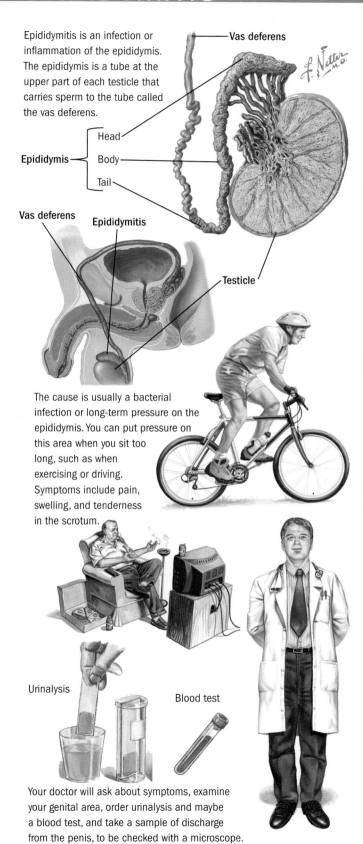

Epididymitis is an infection or inflammation of the epididymis. The epididymis is a tube at the upper part of each testicle that carries sperm to the tube called the vas deferens.

Vas deferens

Head
Epididymis — Body
Tail

Vas deferens

Epididymitis

Testicle

The cause is usually a bacterial infection or long-term pressure on the epididymis. You can put pressure on this area when you sit too long, such as when exercising or driving. Symptoms include pain, swelling, and tenderness in the scrotum.

Urinalysis

Blood test

Your doctor will ask about symptoms, examine your genital area, order urinalysis and maybe a blood test, and take a sample of discharge from the penis, to be checked with a microscope.

What Is Epididymitis?

Epididymitis is an infection or inflammation (swelling) of the epididymis. The epididymis is a tube at the upper part of each testicle that carries sperm to the tube called the vas deferens, which takes the sperm out. Epididymitis is curable with treatment.

What Causes Epididymitis?

The cause is usually a bacterial infection or long-term pressure on the epididymis. Bacteria from a urinary tract or prostate infection can spread to the testicles. In sexually active men, a sexually transmitted disease (STD) is often the cause. Pressure epididymitis occurs after sitting too long, such as when driving a car or riding a bicycle for long periods. Injury and urinary tract blockage are other causes. The cause is often unknown.

What Are the Symptoms of Epididymitis?

Symptoms include pain, swelling, and tenderness in the scrotum; a burning feeling when urinating; discharge from the penis; fever; and pain during sex. Swelling may last for several days.

How Is Epididymitis Diagnosed?

The doctor will ask about symptoms and examine the penis and scrotum. The doctor may order a urinalysis and a blood test to look for infection. The doctor may also take a sample of discharge from the penis, to be checked with a microscope. A sonogram (ultrasound) of the painful testicle may be done to exclude other causes of the pain and swelling.

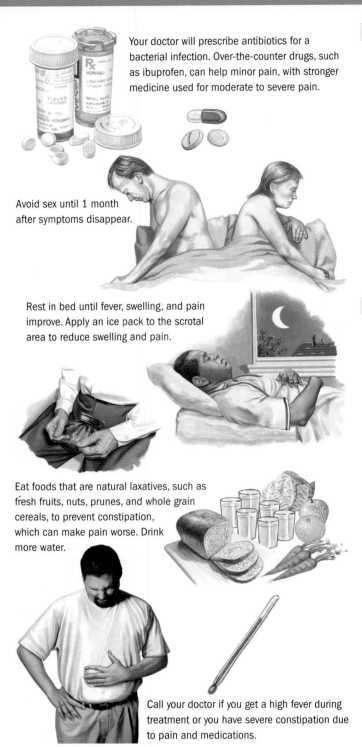

Your doctor will prescribe antibiotics for a bacterial infection. Over-the-counter drugs, such as ibuprofen, can help minor pain, with stronger medicine used for moderate to severe pain.

Avoid sex until 1 month after symptoms disappear.

Rest in bed until fever, swelling, and pain improve. Apply an ice pack to the scrotal area to reduce swelling and pain.

Eat foods that are natural laxatives, such as fresh fruits, nuts, prunes, and whole grain cereals, to prevent constipation, which can make pain worse. Drink more water.

Call your doctor if you get a high fever during treatment or you have severe constipation due to pain and medications.

FROM THE DESK OF

NOTES

How Is Epididymitis Treated?

Antibiotics will be given for a bacterial infection. Over-the-counter drugs, such as ibuprofen, can help pain. Stronger medicine may be needed for moderate to severe pain. Scrotal rest is advised. This means getting pressure off this area by leaning back, as if sitting in a lawn chair. An ice pack on the area will help swelling and discomfort. A rolled towel under the scrotum helps support and elevate it and reduces swelling and pain. Pain usually begins to go away 1 to 3 days after starting antibiotics or scrotal rest.

Sex should be avoided for several days after symptoms go away.

In rare cases, surgery may be needed for complications of infection.

DOs and DON'Ts in Managing Epididymitis:

✔ **DO** rest until fever, swelling, and pain improve.
✔ **DO** put a soft, rolled towel under the scrotum while in bed.
✔ **DO** apply an ice pack to the scrotal area.
✔ **DO** wear an athletic supporter when your activity increases.
✔ **DO** take antibiotics until they are finished.
✔ **DO** take nonprescription pain medicine.
✔ **DO** use condoms to prevent STD infection.
✔ **DO** call your doctor if you get a high fever during treatment, if nonprescription drugs don't control your pain, or if you become severely constipated.
✔ **DO** call your doctor if your symptoms don't improve in 3 or 4 days after you start treatment.

⊘ **DON'T** skip doses or stop your antibiotics even if you feel better.
⊘ **DON'T** have sex for several days after symptoms go away.

FOR MORE INFORMATION

Contact the following source:

• American Urological Association
  Tel: (866) 746-4282
  Website: http://www.auanet.org

Fever of unknown origin (FUO), as its name says, is a high temperature without any known cause after diagnostic tests. Infections, tumors, and collagen vascular diseases are the three major reasons for it.

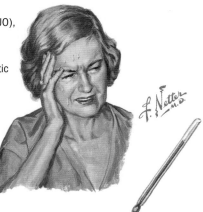

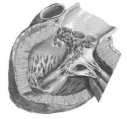

Infections, the most common cause, include endocarditis (infection of the heart's lining or valves).

Other causes include:

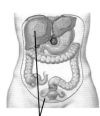

Growths in the abdomen or pelvis

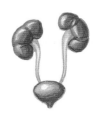

Urinary tract infection

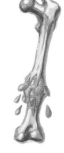

Osteomyelitis (an infection of bone or bone marrow)

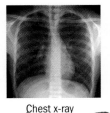

Chest x-ray

Abdominal CT scan

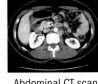

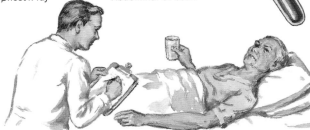

As part of your evaluation, your doctor will take a detailed history, do a physical examination, and order blood tests and maybe imaging studies, such as x-rays and CT.

What Is Fever of Unknown Origin?

Fever of unknown origin (FUO), as its name says, is a high temperature without any known cause after diagnostic tests have been done.

What Causes FUO?

Three major causes are infections, tumors, and collagen vascular diseases. Collagen-vascular diseases include systemic lupus, rheumatoid arthritis, and scleroderma. They're caused by the body's immune (infection-fighting) system attacking its own organs.

Infections, the most common cause, include endocarditis (infection of the heart's lining or valves), tuberculosis, abscesses, and viral infections such as cytomegalovirus infection. Tumors, the second most common cause, include Hodgkin's and non-Hodgkin's lymphomas. Other tumors are leukemia, multiple myeloma, and renal, liver, colon, and breast cancers. The most common collagen-vascular disease in young people is juvenile rheumatoid arthritis. In older people, it's inflammation of the temporal artery, found at the temple region of the head.

Other rare causes of FUO are drugs such as antibiotics, antihistamines, antiseizure drugs, antiinflammatory drugs, and medicines used for acid reflux and peptic ulcers.

What Are the Symptoms of FUO?

The medical definition describes the symptom: a temperature of 101° F (38.3° C) for more than 3 weeks and no diagnosis after 1 week of evaluation.

How Is FUO Diagnosed?

As part of the evaluation, the doctor will take a detailed history, do a physical examination, and order blood tests.

If the diagnosis remains unclear, the doctor may order imaging studies, such as x-rays and computed tomography (CT) of the chest, abdomen (belly), and pelvis.

If endocarditis may be the cause, echocardiography (an ultrasound test using sound waves to take pictures of the heart) will be done.

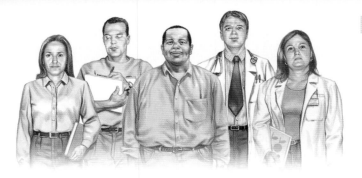

The disease causing the fever must be treated. Different specialists may be involved in your care and treatment.

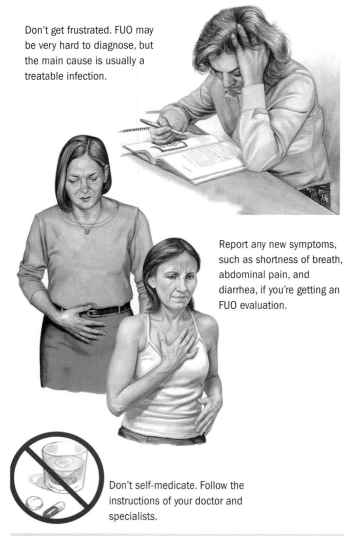

Don't get frustrated. FUO may be very hard to diagnose, but the main cause is usually a treatable infection.

Report any new symptoms, such as shortness of breath, abdominal pain, and diarrhea, if you're getting an FUO evaluation.

Don't self-medicate. Follow the instructions of your doctor and specialists.

How Is FUO Treated?

The disease causing the fever must be treated. A doctor who specializes in infections will help with diagnosis, evaluation, and treatment of infectious diseases. Antibiotics will be given for infections. If a tumor is found, an oncologist (a doctor specializing in cancer treatment) will be involved. For a collagen-vascular disease, a rheumatologist (a doctor specializing in joint and collagen-vascular diseases) will help.

DOs and DON'Ts in Managing FUO:

✔ **DO** remember that your doctor won't usually start using medicines without making a diagnosis. If the FUO remains undiagnosed, your doctor may just watch for more symptoms.

✔ **DO** report any new symptoms if you are being evaluated for FUO.

✔ **DO** call your doctor if you have a long-lasting fever (101° F or higher).

✔ **DO** call your doctor if you have symptoms that may help make the diagnosis (e.g., cough, sputum production, shortness of breath, abdominal pain, diarrhea, bloody stools, muscle aches, joint aches, joint swelling, bone pain, or burning with urination).

🚫 **DON'T** get frustrated. FUO may be very hard to diagnose. About 5% to 15% of cases don't have a diagnosis.

🚫 **DON'T** self-medicate. Follow the instructions of your doctor and specialists.

🚫 **DON'T** forget that infection is the main cause of FUO. Common infections include urinary tract infections, pneumonia, tuberculosis, endocarditis, osteomyelitis (infection of the bone), tick-borne diseases (e.g., Lyme disease), gonorrhea, syphilis, herpes, HIV, AIDS, and abdominal abscesses.

FROM THE DESK OF

NOTES

FOR MORE INFORMATION

Contact the following sources:

• American Academy of Family Physicians
  Tel: (800) 274-2237
  Website: http://www.aafp.org

• American Medical Association
  Tel: (312) 464-5000, (800) 621-8335
  Website: http://www.ama-assn.org

MANAGING YOUR
BOILS

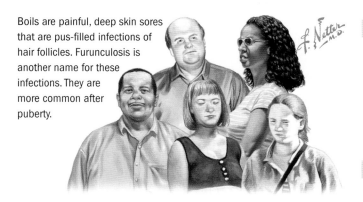

Boils are painful, deep skin sores that are pus-filled infections of hair follicles. Furunculosis is another name for these infections. They are more common after puberty.

What Are Boils?

Boils are painful, deep sores of the skin. They are pus-filled infections of hair follicles. Furunculosis is another name for these infections.

Boils are uncommon in young children and are more frequent after puberty.

What Causes Boils?

The usual cause is the type of bacteria named *Staphylococcus*. The infection begins in a hair follicle and goes into deeper skin layers. People can pass the infection to others if contact is made with pus from a boil.

People have greater chances of getting boils if they have infected wounds, poor hygiene, tight clothing, chafing, and exposure to certain chemicals and cosmetics. Some disorders such as diabetes and alcoholism can increase the risk of getting boils. Boils can follow folliculitis (inflammation of hair follicles) made worse by irritation or sweating.

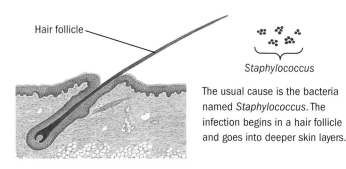

Hair follicle

Staphylococcus

The usual cause is the bacteria named *Staphylococcus*. The infection begins in a hair follicle and goes into deeper skin layers.

What Are the Symptoms of Boils?

A boil starts as a small, painful sore that quickly gets bigger and becomes a painful lump. Boils at first are usually ½ to 1 inch in diameter. They usually occur on the neck, face, waist, groin, underarms, and buttocks. Pain gets worse as the boils grow larger. Boils either remain deep in the skin and reabsorb or burst through at the skin surface. They may let out a white, bloody discharge. After the boils burst, pain gets better, but redness and swelling may last for days or weeks, and then scarring will occur. Without treatment, the infection may enter the bloodstream and spread to other body parts.

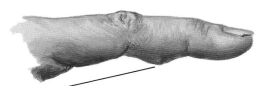

A boil starts as a small, painful sore that quickly gets bigger and becomes a painful lump. Boils usually occur on the neck, face, waist, groin, underarms, and buttocks.

How Are Boils Diagnosed?

The doctor will diagnose boils by examining the affected part of the skin. The doctor may want to take a sample of the pus to check for bacteria.

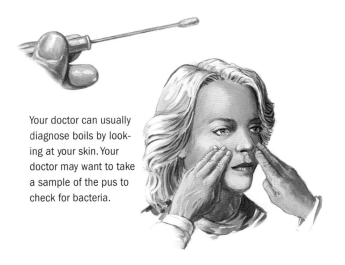

Your doctor can usually diagnose boils by looking at your skin. Your doctor may want to take a sample of the pus to check for bacteria.

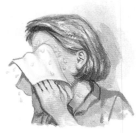

Warm moist compresses, three or four times daily for 20 minutes each time, provide comfort and help the boil drain. Your doctor may cut and drain the boil. Your doctor may also prescribe antibiotics for severe infections or ones that return.

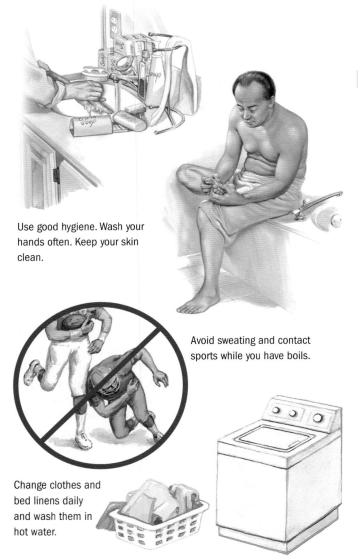

Use good hygiene. Wash your hands often. Keep your skin clean.

Avoid sweating and contact sports while you have boils.

Change clothes and bed linens daily and wash them in hot water.

How Are Boils Treated?

Warm moist compresses, three or four times daily for 20 minutes each time, provide comfort and help boils come to a head and drain.

The doctor may cut and drain a boil when the skin over it becomes thin and the mass below is soft. Without treatment, boils heal in 10 to 20 days, but they'll heal faster and have less severe symptoms with treatment. The doctor may prescribe antibiotics for severe infections or ones that return.

A complication is formation of new boils if pus that drains when the boil opens contaminates nearby skin.

DOs and DON'Ts in Managing Boils:

✔ **DO** use your prescribed antibiotics.

✔ **DO** reduce activity until the infection heals. Avoid sweating and contact sports while boils are present.

✔ **DO** keep your skin clean.

✔ **DO** change clothes and bed linens daily and wash them in hot water.

✔ **DO** call your doctor if you have a fever or symptoms don't get better in 3 or 4 days with treatment.

✔ **DO** call your doctor if you or family members get new boils.

⊘ **DON'T** use nonprescription antibiotic creams or ointments on the boil's surface. They usually don't work.

⊘ **DON'T** share towels, washcloths, or clothing with other household members.

⊘ **DON'T** try to squeeze the boil or manipulate it with objects. It may make the infection worse.

FROM THE DESK OF

NOTES

FOR MORE INFORMATION

Contact the following source:

• American Academy of Dermatology
Tel: (866) 503-7546
Website: http://www.aad.org

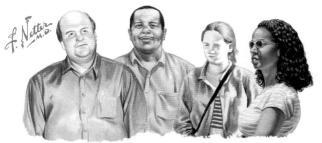

Rubella, also called German measles, is a mild viral illness. It was once common in childhood before widespread vaccination for measles, mumps, and rubella (MMR).

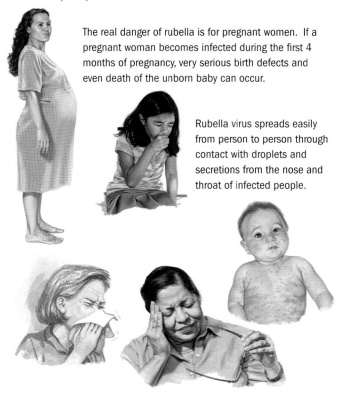

The real danger of rubella is for pregnant women. If a pregnant woman becomes infected during the first 4 months of pregnancy, very serious birth defects and even death of the unborn baby can occur.

Rubella virus spreads easily from person to person through contact with droplets and secretions from the nose and throat of infected people.

Symptoms include a rash lasting 2 to 3 days, headache, low-grade fever, stuffy or runny nose, and swollen glands in the neck or behind the ears. Adults and teenagers usually have more symptoms than children do.

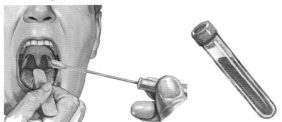

Rubella can be hard to diagnose because of its vague symptoms. Your doctor will take a medical history and examine you. The doctor may take a swab of throat secretions or get a sample of blood or urine, which will be sent to a laboratory for study.

What Is Rubella?

Rubella, also called German measles, is a viral illness. It was once common in childhood before widespread vaccination for measles, mumps, and rubella (MMR) in the United States.

In both children and adults, rubella tends to be brief and mild. Complications are rare. The real danger of rubella is for pregnant women. If a pregnant woman becomes infected with the virus during the first 4 months of pregnancy, very serious birth defects and even death of the unborn baby can occur.

What Causes Rubella?

Rubella virus is the cause. The virus is passed from person to person through contact with droplets and secretions from the nose and throat of infected people. It's highly contagious and spreads very easily. A person can pass the virus to others starting 1 week before the rash appears until 1 week after the rash goes away. A pregnant woman can pass the virus to her unborn baby through the bloodstream.

What Are the Symptoms of Rubella?

Some people have no symptoms at all. It usually takes 2 to 3 weeks after exposure before symptoms start. If symptoms do appear, they may include a rash on the head and body that usually lasts 2 to 3 days, headache, low-grade fever, stuffy or runny nose, and swollen glands in the neck or behind the ears. Adults and teenagers usually have more symptoms than children do. These other symptoms include loss of appetite, mild conjunctivitis (inflammation of the lining of the eyelids and eyeballs), and swelling and pain in joints (especially in young women). Symptoms are usually gone in several days. Sometimes, it may take a few days longer for the rash and symptoms to go away.

How Is Rubella Diagnosed?

Rubella can be difficult to diagnose because its symptoms are very vague. The doctor will take a medical history and do a physical examination. To make the diagnosis, the doctor may take a swab of throat secretions or get a sample of blood or urine. These are sent to a laboratory for study. These tests are usually done only if a woman thinks that she may be pregnant. Also, testing is advisable if someone with rubella has been in close contact with a pregnant woman and may have infected her.

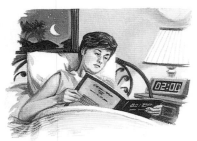

No treatment exists for rubella. Discomfort is generally minimal and can usually be helped with over-the-counter medicines. You may need to rest and adjust your activity level according to how you feel.

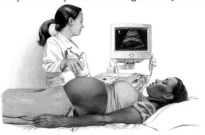

Call your doctor immediately if you're pregnant, were exposed to rubella, and haven't been vaccinated against it. If you have rubella, you should stay away from women who may be pregnant.

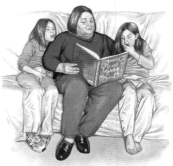

Rubella is highly contagious. A person is contagious starting 1 week before the rash appears until 1 week after the rash ends. Once you have rubella, you become immune to it.

Vaccinate your child with MMR to prevent rubella. Children 12 to 15 months old should receive the MMR vaccine.

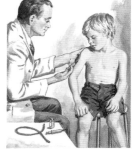

Don't give aspirin to children with rubella, because of the dangerous Reye's syndrome. Use acetaminophen for body aches or fever.

How Is Rubella Treated?

No treatment exists for rubella. Discomfort is generally minimal, and in most cases it can be relieved with over-the-counter medicines. Once people have rubella, they become immune to it. Children 12 to 15 months old should receive the MMR vaccine.

DOs and DON'Ts in Managing Rubella:

✔ **DO** take over-the-counter medicine (acetaminophen) for fever, headache, and joint pain as directed by your doctor.

✔ **DO** adjust your activity to how you feel.

✔ **DO** call your doctor if you or your child has a high temperature, severe headaches, or shortness of breath.

✔ **DO** call your doctor immediately if you are pregnant, were exposed to rubella, and have not been vaccinated against it.

✔ **DO** vaccinate your child with MMR to prevent rubella.

⊘ **DON'T** give aspirin to children with rubella, because of the dangerous Reye's syndrome. Use acetaminophen for body aches or fever.

FROM THE DESK OF

NOTES

FOR MORE INFORMATION

Contact the following source:

• Centers for Disease Control and Prevention
Tel: (800) 311-3435
Website: http://www.cdc.gov

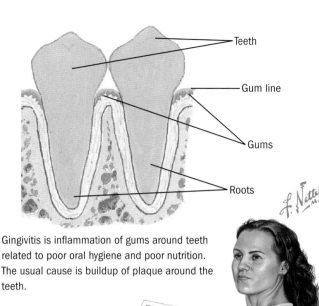

Teeth

Gum line

Gums

Roots

f. Netter
M.D.

Gingivitis is inflammation of gums around teeth related to poor oral hygiene and poor nutrition. The usual cause is buildup of plaque around the teeth.

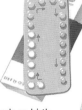

Some medicines, such as birth control pills, can increase the chance of getting gingivitis. Pregnancy and chronic diseases such as diabetes can also make you more likely to get it.

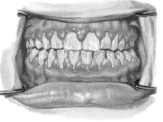

The most common symptoms of gingivitis are gums that bleed easily, especially when brushing the teeth; swollen and red gums; bad breath; and a bad taste in the mouth.

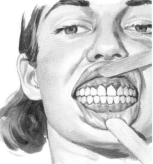

Your dentist or doctor examines your teeth and gums to diagnose gingivitis. X-rays may be taken to see whether infection spread below the gum line.

What Is Gingivitis?

Gingivitis is inflammation (swelling, redness) of the gums around the teeth caused by poor oral hygiene and poor nutrition. Most cases of simple gingivitis clear up quickly with treatment. Good mouth care is important at home. Recovery time can depend on medical conditions that may affect the mouth.

What Causes Gingivitis?

The usual cause is buildup of plaque around the teeth. Plaque is a sticky material made up of bacteria, food debris, and mucus. When plaque isn't removed, it hardens into a substance called calculus or tartar, which becomes trapped at the base of the teeth and irritates the gums. Certain medicines, such as birth control pills; pregnancy; and chronic diseases, such as diabetes, can increase the chance of getting gingivitis.

What Are the Symptoms of Gingivitis?

The most common symptoms are gums that bleed easily (especially when brushing the teeth), swollen and reddened gums, bad breath, and bad taste in the mouth.

How Is Gingivitis Diagnosed?

The dentist or doctor does an examination of the teeth and gums to diagnose gingivitis. X-rays may be taken to see whether infection has spread below the gum line.

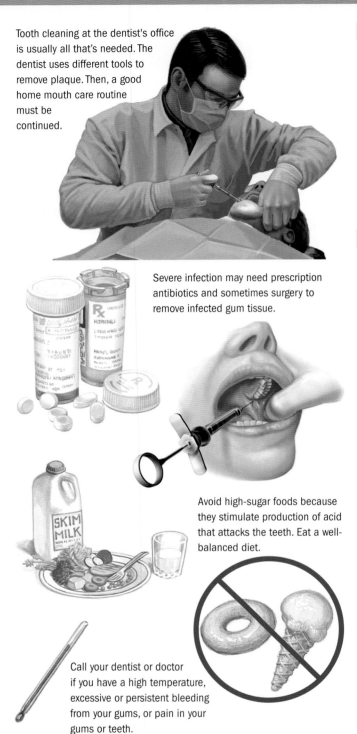

Tooth cleaning at the dentist's office is usually all that's needed. The dentist uses different tools to remove plaque. Then, a good home mouth care routine must be continued.

Severe infection may need prescription antibiotics and sometimes surgery to remove infected gum tissue.

Avoid high-sugar foods because they stimulate production of acid that attacks the teeth. Eat a well-balanced diet.

Call your dentist or doctor if you have a high temperature, excessive or persistent bleeding from your gums, or pain in your gums or teeth.

FROM THE DESK OF

NOTES

How Is Gingivitis Treated?

Cleaning at the dentist's office is usually all that's needed. Different tools are used to remove plaque. Then, a home mouth care routine must be continued. Careful brushing of teeth with a soft-bristled toothbrush and daily flossing are important. Fluoride mouthwash may be prescribed. Avoid high-sugar foods because they stimulate production of acid that attacks the teeth. Eat a well-balanced diet.

Severe infection may need prescription antibiotics and sometimes surgery to remove infected gum tissue.

DOs and DON'Ts in Managing Gingivitis:

✔ **DO** follow your dentist's advice for cleaning your teeth.
✔ **DO** use the right brushing method to get the area between the gums and teeth really clean. Brush and floss twice daily. Change your toothbrush often, even monthly. Use a fluoride toothpaste to reduce tooth decay.
✔ **DO** rinse your mouth after flossing with an antiseptic mouthwash.
✔ **DO** see your dentist regularly for examinations and cleanings.
✔ **DO** keep your appointments for follow-up visits.
✔ **DO** call your dentist if you have a high temperature, excessive bleeding from your gums, or pain in your gums or teeth.

🚫 **DON'T** brush with a hard-bristled brush that may irritate the gums.

FOR MORE INFORMATION

Contact the following sources:

• National Institute of Dental and Craniofacial Research
Tel: (301) 496-4261
Website: http://www.nidcr.nih.gov/OralHealth/

• American Dental Association
Tel: (312) 440-2500
Website: http://www.ada.org

• American Academy of Periodontology
Tel: (312) 787-5518
Website: http://www.perio.org/consumer/gingivitis.htm

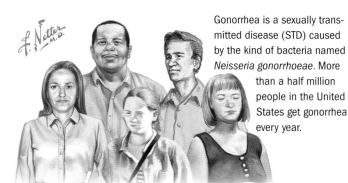

Gonorrhea is a sexually transmitted disease (STD) caused by the kind of bacteria named *Neisseria gonorrhoeae*. More than a half million people in the United States get gonorrhea every year.

Usually sex organs are infected, but gonorrhea may also affect other parts of the body, such as the eyes, throat, and joints. Infected mothers can pass it to their babies during childbirth.

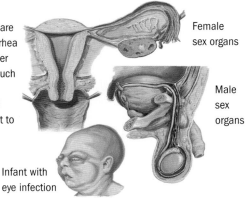

Female sex organs

Male sex organs

Infant with eye infection

Symptoms include creamy green-yellow discharge from the penis or vagina, and pain or burning when urinating. Men can have painful and swollen testicles. Women can have bleeding between periods and pain during sex.

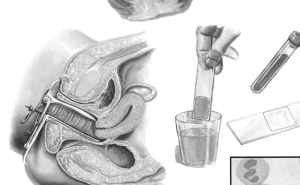

Your doctor will ask about symptoms and sexual activity and will examine you (including a pelvic exam in women). Your doctor will order blood and urine tests and send a sample of discharge to a laboratory for study with a microscope.

What Is Gonorrhea?

Gonorrhea is a sexually transmitted disease (STD) that is caused by bacteria. It usually affects the sex organs but may also occur in other parts of the body, such as the eyes, throat, and joints.

Untreated gonorrhea can lead to serious problems, including pharyngitis, tonsillitis, severe arthritis, and bloodstream infection. In women, it can cause pelvic inflammatory disease (PID) and can be passed from pregnant women to their babies during birth. In men, it can cause infections called urethritis and epididymitis. Urethritis is inflammation (swelling, redness) of the urethra, the tube that carries urine and semen through the penis. Epididymitis is inflammation or infection of the epididymis, a long tube above and behind each testicle.

More than half a million people in the United States get gonorrhea every year.

What Causes Gonorrhea?

The cause is a type of bacteria named *Neisseria gonorrhoeae*. It spreads very easily by having sex with an infected person.

What Are the Symptoms of Gonorrhea?

Most men have symptoms when first infected, but many women may have very mild or no symptoms. They often don't know that they have gonorrhea until they have other problems. Symptoms in men usually start within 2 weeks after exposure. They include creamy green-yellow discharge from the penis, pain when urinating, and painful and swollen testicles. Symptoms in women include pain or burning when urinating, yellow or green vaginal discharge that can be bloody, bleeding between periods, and pain during sex. Other symptoms may include sore throat, low-grade fever; tender lower abdomen (belly); pain in knees, ankles, or elbows; and a rash on the palms of the hands.

How Is Gonorrhea Diagnosed?

For diagnosis, the doctor asks about symptoms and sexual activity and examines the sexual organs, including the pelvic area for women. Blood and urine tests and tests for STDs will be done. A sample of discharge from the penis or cervix will be taken and sent to a laboratory for study. Throat, rectum, or eye discharges may also be tested.

Untreated gonorrhea can lead to serious problems:

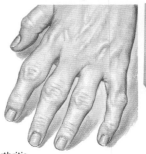

Arthritis

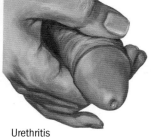

Urethritis

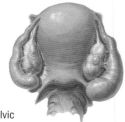

Pelvic inflammatory disease

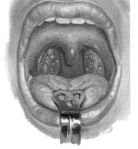

Gonococcal pharyngitis or tonsillitis

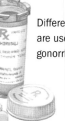

Different antibiotics are used to treat gonorrhea.

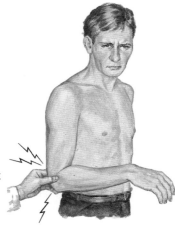

Practice safe sex. Use condoms if you think there's any chance of catching or spreading an STD.

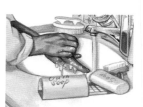

Wash hands thoroughly and often after using the bathroom.

Call your doctor if you get joint pain, genital sores, or swollen testicles.

How Is Gonorrhea Treated?

Treatment with antibiotics cures gonorrhea in 1 to 2 weeks. The antibiotic is either given by injection or taken by mouth.

DOs and DON'Ts in Managing Gonorrhea:

✔ **DO** practice safe sex. Use condoms if you think that there's any chance of catching an STD.

✔ **DO** get treatment as soon as possible.

✔ **DO** make sure your sexual partner visits a doctor to check for infection.

✔ **DO** realize that gonorrhea is often diagnosed with other STDs. Your doctor will also test you for other STDs.

✔ **DO** wash hands thoroughly and often after using the bathroom.

✔ **DO** use sitz baths for discomfort.

✔ **DO** remember that follow-up cultures should be done.

✔ **DO** call your doctor if you get fever, chills, and abdominal pain after treatment starts.

✔ **DO** call your doctor if you get joint pain, genital sores, or swollen testicles.

✔ **DO** call your doctor if you were told that a sexual contact has gonorrhea.

⊘ **DON'T** have unprotected sex until you finish treatment, are tested again, and your doctor says that you can. This is important to avoid spreading the infection.

FROM THE DESK OF

NOTES

FOR MORE INFORMATION

Contact the following sources:

• Infectious Diseases Society of America
Tel: (703) 299-0200
Website: http://www.idsociety.org

• Centers for Disease Control and Prevention
Tel: (404) 639-3534
Website: http://www.cdc.gov

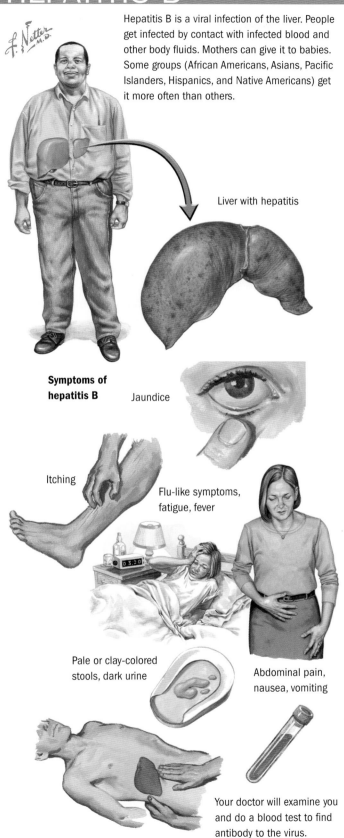

Hepatitis B is a viral infection of the liver. People get infected by contact with infected blood and other body fluids. Mothers can give it to babies. Some groups (African Americans, Asians, Pacific Islanders, Hispanics, and Native Americans) get it more often than others.

Liver with hepatitis

Symptoms of hepatitis B

Jaundice

Itching

Flu-like symptoms, fatigue, fever

Pale or clay-colored stools, dark urine

Abdominal pain, nausea, vomiting

Your doctor will examine you and do a blood test to find antibody to the virus.

What Is Hepatitis B?

Hepatitis B is infection of the liver with a virus. More than 1 million people in the United States are carriers of the virus. About 200,000 people get this disease each year. Certain racial and ethnic groups, including African Americans, Asians, Pacific Islanders, Hispanics, and Native Americans, have higher rates of infection.

About 90% of people recover completely in a few months. Others become carriers or chronically infected. Hepatitis B is a serious disease, and about 1% of people die during the acute stage.

What Causes Hepatitis B?

The cause is the hepatitis B virus. The virus is passed to others by sexual contact with infected people and using nonsterile needles. Infected blood and other body fluids (e.g., semen, vaginal secretions, breast milk, tears, saliva, and fluid in open sores) can spread the virus. Infected mothers can give it to babies.

What Are the Symptoms of Hepatitis B?

Not all people have symptoms. If they do occur they usually appear within 6 months from when the infection is acquired. First symptoms may be rashes, joint pains, fatigue, and other flu-like symptoms. Then, jaundice (yellow skin or whites of the eyes) may occur. Other symptoms are pale or clay-colored stools, dark urine, itching, loss of appetite, nausea, vomiting, low-grade fever, and pain in the abdomen (belly). Severe disease may lead to cirrhosis (liver scarring), fluid in the abdomen (ascites), and liver failure.

How Is Hepatitis B Diagnosed?

The doctor will do an examination and blood test to show the presence of the virus in the blood (hepatitis B antigens) and the body's response to the infection (hepatitis B antibodies). Liver function tests will also be abnormal.

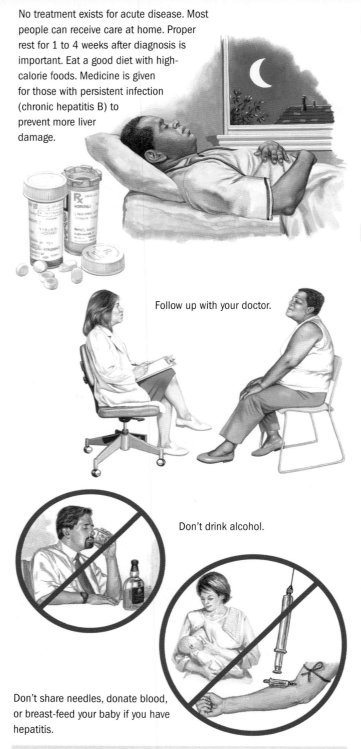

No treatment exists for acute disease. Most people can receive care at home. Proper rest for 1 to 4 weeks after diagnosis is important. Eat a good diet with high-calorie foods. Medicine is given for those with persistent infection (chronic hepatitis B) to prevent more liver damage.

Follow up with your doctor.

Don't drink alcohol.

Don't share needles, donate blood, or breast-feed your baby if you have hepatitis.

How Is Hepatitis B Treated?

No treatment exists for acute disease. Most people can receive care at home. Activity is as tolerated. Proper rest for 1 to 4 weeks after diagnosis is beneficial. During this time, intimate contact with other people should be avoided. The diet should be high in calories. People who come in contact with infected people and newborns of infected mothers should be given immune globulin plus hepatitis B vaccine within 2 weeks of exposure.

Medicine is given to those with persistent infection (chronic hepatitis B) to prevent more liver damage.

DOs and DON'Ts in Managing Hepatitis B:

✔ **DO** get plenty of rest and eat a well-balanced diet.
✔ **DO** use condoms when having sex.
✔ **DO** avoid exposing others to your blood and other body fluids.
✔ **DO** call your doctor if symptoms don't go away in 4 or 6 weeks or new symptoms develop.
✔ **DO** ask your doctor about vaccines for family members and others close to you.

🚫 **DON'T** drink alcohol or take medications such as acetaminophen that can further damage your liver.
🚫 **DON'T** share needles, donate blood, or breast-feed your baby.
🚫 **DON'T** have sex with an infected person or carrier.

FROM THE DESK OF

NOTES

FOR MORE INFORMATION

Contact the following sources:

• American Liver Foundation
Tel: (800) 465-4837
Website: http://www.liverfoundation.org/

• Hepatitis Foundation International
Tel: (800) 891-0707
Website: http://www.hepfi.org/

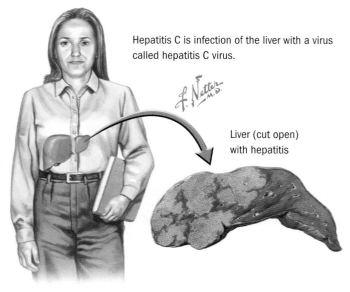

Hepatitis C is infection of the liver with a virus called hepatitis C virus.

Liver (cut open) with hepatitis

What Is Hepatitis C?

Hepatitis C is infection of the liver with a virus.

Some people never have serious health problems, but up to 20% get liver cirrhosis in 20 or 30 years. Cirrhosis means liver scarring, so the liver cannot work well. At least 50% of the people may have chronic disease, meaning liver inflammation (swelling) is long-lasting. About 1% to 5% of people die of liver disease.

What Causes Hepatitis C?

The cause is the hepatitis C virus.

The virus is passed to others by infected blood, as when people share needles to inject drugs. The next most common way is anal sex.

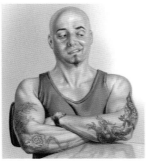

The virus is passed to others by infected blood, as when people share needles to inject drugs. You can also catch hepatitis C from sharp injuries and tattooing.

Other ways to get hepatitis C are by pricking a finger on a contaminated needle; tattooing, body piercing, or acupuncture with nonsterile equipment; mother-to-baby infection during birth; and blood transfusions or organ transplants done in the United States before July 1992 or in other countries with no blood screening.

Hugging, kissing, toilet seats, or sharing cups or kitchen utensils cannot transmit hepatitis C.

What Are the Symptoms of Hepatitis C?

Most people have no symptoms, but symptoms can be mild to severe and sometimes life-threatening. Symptoms of acute disease include headache, aches and pains, tiredness, and upset stomach. These can last for several weeks. The most common symptom of chronic hepatitis C is fatigue. Others are nausea, vomiting, diarrhea, loss of appetite, and pain in the upper abdomen (belly), under the ribs.

Symptoms of acute disease include headache, aches and pains, tiredness, and upset stomach. The most common symptom of chronic hepatitis C is fatigue.

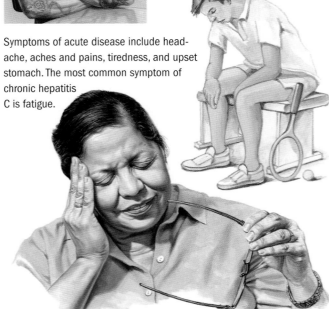

How Is Hepatitis C Diagnosed?

People often find out about hepatitis C by a routine blood test showing high liver enzyme levels or when donating blood and hepatitis C antibody is found. If your doctor suspects hepatitis C, blood tests will be done to look for the presence of antibodies to the hepatitis C virus. The antibody is a substance made by the immune, or infection-fighting, system in response to an infection.

Blood tests are used for diagnosis. More than one test will be done to confirm the disease.

Acute hepatitis C has no specific treatment. Most people can receive care at home, including rest and proper diet. People with chronic disease are treated with medicines, but some may cause flu-like symptoms and they don't work for everyone.

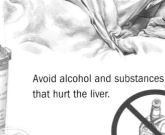

Avoid alcohol and substances that hurt the liver.

See your doctor right away if you get jaundice.

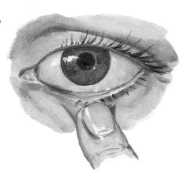

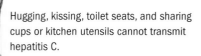

Hugging, kissing, toilet seats, and sharing cups or kitchen utensils cannot transmit hepatitis C.

How Is Hepatitis C Treated?

Acute hepatitis C generally has no specific treatment. Most people can receive care at home. Rest and proper diet are important for severe symptoms. Avoid alcohol and substances that hurt the liver.

People with chronic disease are treated with medicines such as interferon for 24 to 48 weeks, but they don't work for everybody and not everyone wants to take the drugs because of potential side effects. Success depends on which type of hepatitis C virus caused the infection. With genotypes 2 and 3, about 80% of people get well. The cure rates are lower in those with genotypes 1 and 4.

DOs and DON'Ts in Managing Hepatitis C:

✔ **DO** get help for a drug problem if you have one.
✔ **DO** follow a healthy lifestyle. Avoid alcohol, which strains the liver. If possible, give it up completely.
✔ **DO** get regular medical checkups.
✔ **DO** see your doctor right away if you get jaundice (yellow skin and dark-colored urine), pain in your abdomen, nausea or vomiting lasting more than 1 to 2 days, or blood in your vomit.
✔ **DO** call your doctor if hepatitis C symptoms persist after completion of treatment.

🚫 **DON'T** take medicines that can hurt the liver, such as acetaminophen.
🚫 **DON'T** share needles.
🚫 **DON'T** breast-feed your baby.

FOR MORE INFORMATION

Contact the following sources:

• Hepatitis Foundation International
  Tel: (800) 891-0707
  Website: http://www.hepfi.org

• American Gastroenterological Association
  Tel: (301) 654-2055
  Website: http://www.gastro.org

• National Digestive Diseases Information Clearinghouse
  Tel: (800) 891-5389
  Website: http://www.niddk.nih.gov/health/digest/ nddic.htm

FROM THE DESK OF

NOTES

Herpangina is a viral disease in which ulcers and sores form inside the mouth. The throat and mouth become inflamed. It's a common infection in children 1 to 10 years old, but people of any age can get it.

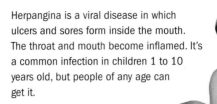

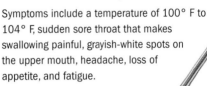

The coxsackievirus causes herpangina. It spreads from person to person by contact, such as kissing or sharing food, and by contamination with feces, such as when people go to the bathroom, don't wash their hands, and then touch their mouth or food.

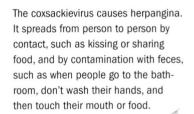

Symptoms include a temperature of 100° F to 104° F, sudden sore throat that makes swallowing painful, grayish-white spots on the upper mouth, headache, loss of appetite, and fatigue.

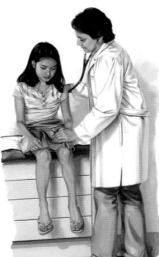

Your doctor will make a diagnosis on the basis of a medical history and physical examination. Other tests aren't needed.

What Is Herpangina?

Herpangina is a self-limited viral disease in which ulcers and sores form inside the mouth. The throat and mouth become inflamed (swollen, red). It's a common childhood infection in children 1 to 10 years old. It may be confused with strep throat or canker sores. It often occurs during the summer and fall. Recovery takes a few days to a week. Little treatment is needed.

What Causes Herpangina?

The cause is a virus called coxsackievirus. It spreads from person to person by the respiratory route or by close contact, such as kissing or sharing food. It also spreads by contamination with feces (bowel movements), such as when people go to the bathroom, don't wash their hands, and then touch their mouth or food.

What Are the Symptoms of Herpangina?

Symptoms usually appear 2 to 9 days after exposure. They include a temperature of 100° F to 104° F, a sudden sore throat that makes swallowing painful, grayish-white spots with red borders on the upper mouth, headache, loss of appetite, and fatigue. The feet, hands, and buttocks can have sores similar to those in the mouth.

How Is Herpangina Diagnosed?

The doctor will make a diagnosis on the basis of the medical history and physical examination. Blood tests are rarely needed.

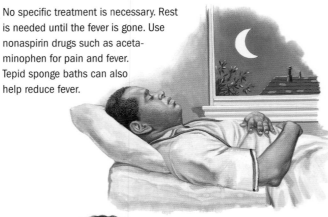

No specific treatment is necessary. Rest is needed until the fever is gone. Use nonaspirin drugs such as acetaminophen for pain and fever. Tepid sponge baths can also help reduce fever.

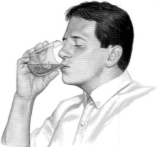

Increase fluid intake to prevent dehydration.

A soft or liquid diet should be given until the throat is no longer painful. Ice pops, ice cream, gelatin, and ice chips may ease mouth and throat pain. Avoid acidic fruit juices that may irritate the throat.

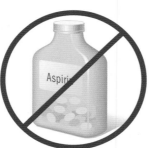

Don't give aspirin to a child younger than 16 years, because of the risk of the dangerous Reye's syndrome.

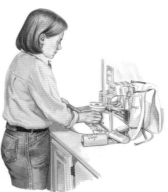

Everyone in the household should wash hands carefully to prevent spreading the infection.

FROM THE DESK OF

NOTES

How Is Herpangina Treated?

No specific treatment is needed. Fluid intake should be increased to prevent dehydration. Rest is needed until the fever is gone. A nonaspirin medicine, such as acetaminophen or ibuprofen, can be used for fever and pain. Tepid sponge baths can also be used to reduce fever.

A soft or liquid diet should be given until the throat is no longer painful. Ice pops, ice cream, gelatin, and ice chips may ease mouth and throat pain. Avoid acidic fruit juices that may irritate the throat. Sometimes a topical pain medicine such as lidocaine can help the sore throat or mouth.

DOs and DON'Ts in Managing Herpangina:

✔ **DO** rest until the fever is gone.
✔ **DO** use nonaspirin drugs such as acetaminophen for pain and fever. Use tepid sponge baths to reduce the fever.
✔ **DO** use ice pops or ice chips to decrease discomfort.
✔ **DO** wash hands carefully, to prevent spreading the disease. Avoid kissing and sharing food.
✔ **DO** call your doctor if symptoms don't go away in 1 week or if fever becomes very high or doesn't go away.
✔ **DO** call your doctor if fluids cannot be tolerated.
✔ **DO** call your doctor if signs of dehydration appear, such as dry, wrinkled skin; dark urine; or less need to urinate.
✔ **DO** call your doctor if anyone else in the family shows symptoms of the disease.

🚫 **DON'T** share food or kiss anyone until the infection has resolved.
🚫 **DON'T** give aspirin to a child younger than 16 years (because of the risk of Reye's syndrome).
🚫 **DON'T** give acidic fruit juices, which will irritate the mouth and throat.
🚫 **DON'T** eat spicy foods that may irritate the mouth.

FOR MORE INFORMATION

Contact the following sources:

• National Institute of Allergy and Infectious Diseases
Tel: (301) 496-5717, (866) 284-4107
Website: http://www3.niaid.nih.gov

• American Academy of Otolaryngology—Head and Neck Surgery
Tel: (703) 836-4444
Website: http://www.entnet.org

• American Academy of Pediatrics
Tel: (847) 434-4000
Website: http://www.aap.org

Human immunodeficiency virus (HIV) causes AIDS. This virus attacks the immune system and destroys white blood cells called lympho-cytes.

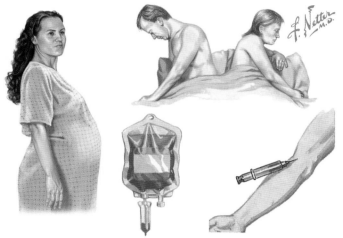

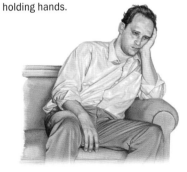

Sexual activity, use of an infected needle, and blood transfusion can spread HIV infection. An infected mother can pass it to her child in pregnancy or through breastfeeding. You can't get infected by casual contact such as holding hands.

Symptoms first include body aches, fatigue, fever, headache, nausea, vomiting, and rash. Then, people can have infections, diarrhea, loss of appetite and weight, memory loss, mouth sores, night sweats, skin cancer, swollen glands, and trouble thinking.

Your doctor makes a diagnosis from your medical history, physical examination, and blood tests.

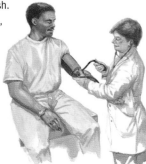

What Is Human Immunodeficiency Virus (HIV) Infection?

The human immunodeficiency virus (HIV) causes acquired immunodeficiency syndrome (AIDS). This virus attacks the immune (infection-fighting) system and destroys white blood cells called lymphocytes. People who are infected with HIV are HIV positive (HIV+). However, blood tests may be negative if done very early after being infected. After several months or years of being HIV+, AIDS may develop, when the immune system is very weak.

What Causes HIV Infection?

HIV is usually caught from sexual activity, use of an infected needle, or from blood transfusion. It may also be passed from an infected mother to her unborn child. People cannot get infected by casual contact such as holding hands.

What Are the Symptoms of HIV Infection?

People may at first have no symptoms, but 1 to 6 weeks after infection, many have flu-like symptoms. These may include body aches, fatigue, fever, headache, nausea, and rash. After these symptoms, most people may not have any others for several months or years until the virus significantly weakens the immune system. Then they get infections that can involve lungs, eyes, or skin and can be life threatening. Other symptoms may be diarrhea, fatigue, fever, loss of appetite and weight, memory loss, mouth sores, night sweats, skin cancer, swollen glands, and trouble thinking.

How Is HIV Infection Diagnosed?

The doctor makes a diagnosis from a medical history, physical examination, and blood tests.

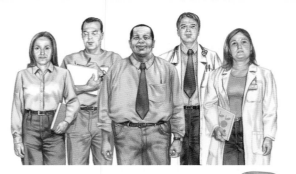

Today, many medicines help people with HIV live a longer, healthier life. The virus will always live in your body, but the prognosis and lifestyle have improved compared with just a few years ago.

Find a local support group, which can help you cope with being HIV+.

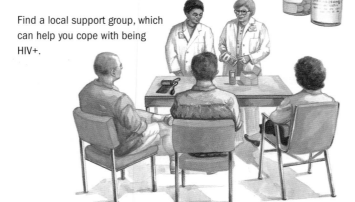

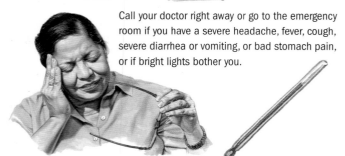

Call your doctor right away or go to the emergency room if you have a severe headache, fever, cough, severe diarrhea or vomiting, or bad stomach pain, or if bright lights bother you.

Always practice safe sex by using latex condoms. Other birth control methods, such as the pill, diaphragm, and IUD, don't prevent STDs. Tell your partners about being HIV+ so that they can be tested.

How Is HIV Infection Treated?

Treatment depends on the stage of infection. An infectious disease specialist will prescribe medicine to strengthen the immune system and fight the virus. Blood tests must be done often to see how well the medicines work. Life-long medicine will be needed.

Other medicines may be needed for loss of appetite. A nutritionist will help plan a healthy diet.

Exposure to other infections should be avoided. Support groups can help people deal with HIV. Activities aren't restricted, but rest and eating well are important. To avoid exposing others to HIV infection, use condoms and don't donate blood or sperm.

DOs and DON'Ts in Managing HIV Infection:

✔ **DO** follow your doctor's directions.

✔ **DO** practice safe sex. Use latex condoms. Tell your partners about being HIV+ so that they can be tested.

✔ **DO** avoid people who have colds or stomach flu.

✔ **DO** eat a healthy diet and get enough sleep and exercise.

✔ **DO** get help for the emotional stress of being HIV+.

✔ **DO** tell your doctor if you're pregnant or planning a pregnancy.

✔ **DO** call your doctor if you have signs of infection (fever, rash, cough, diarrhea, skin lesions).

✔ **DO** call your doctor right away or go to the emergency room if you have a severe headache, fever, cough, severe diarrhea or vomiting, or bad stomach pain or if bright lights bother you.

⊘ **DON'T** donate blood, sperm, or organs.

⊘ **DON'T** stop taking your medicine or change your dosage because you feel better unless your doctor tells you to.

⊘ **DON'T** have unprotected sex.

⊘ **DON'T** drink alcohol, use drugs, or share needles.

⊘ **DON'T** eat foods such as raw eggs, raw oysters, or unpasteurized milk that may contain harmful bacteria.

FROM THE DESK OF

NOTES

FOR MORE INFORMATION

Contact the following sources:

• American Social Health Association
Tel: (800) 227-8922
http://www.ashastd.org

• Centers for Disease Control and Prevention
Tel: (800) 232-4636
Website: http://www.cdc.gov

MANAGING YOUR
HUMAN PAPILLOMAVIRUS INFECTION

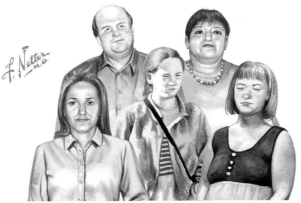

Warts are very common, and most aren't serious or dangerous, but they can spread. About 65% of cases clear up on their own in 2 years. Also, the human papillomavirus (HPV) causes genital warts, which occur most often in young sexually active men and women.

Genital warts—female   **Genital warts—male**

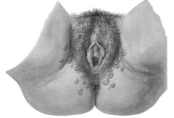

Genital HPV is a very common sexually transmitted infection from genital contact.

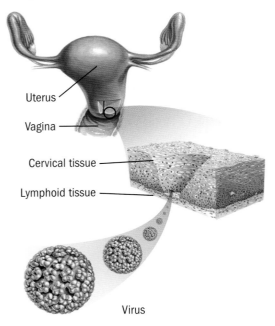

Uterus

Vagina

Cervical tissue

Lymphoid tissue

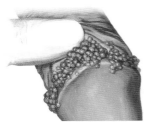

Virus

Genital HPV infection affects the cervix and then the uterus and can lead to cervical cancer. A doctor should always check for genital warts and treat them. Your partner should also be checked by a doctor, because you can give the infection to another person.

What Is Human Papillomavirus Infection?

The human papillomavirus (HPV) is a virus that causes warts, which are unsightly growths on the skin. Warts are very common and aren't serious or dangerous, but they aren't pretty and can spread. Most warts disappear without treatment in 2 years, but they often return. Genital warts in females need treatment because they can lead to cervical cancer. A vaccine (Gardasil) against the genital wart virus is recommended for girls and women 9 to 26 years old.

What Causes Human Papillomavirus Infection?

Viruses called human papillomavirus (HPV) cause warts. Types 6, 11, 16, and 18 cause genital warts and cervical cancer.

Because warts are a viral infection, they can be passed from one person to another or spread to different parts of the body. Moist skin and open skin are more likely to become infected.

What Are the Symptoms of Human Papillomavirus Infection?

Warts look different on different parts of the body. Common warts look like little rough cauliflowers and often occur on hands, arms, and legs. Periungual warts occur around fingernails. Flat warts, slightly raised and flesh colored, occur on the face, knees, and elbows of children and young women. Genital warts occur on genital and rectal areas and are often transmitted sexually. Plantar warts occur on bottoms of feet. Filiform warts are small with hairlike bulges.

How Is Human Papillomavirus Infection Diagnosed?

The doctor will do a physical examination and may order a biopsy of the wart or skin abnormality and blood tests to confirm the diagnosis. In a biopsy, a small piece of skin with the lesion is removed and studied under a microscope.

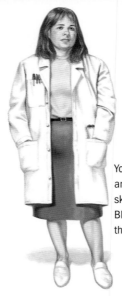

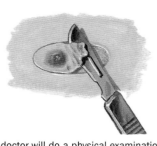

Your doctor will do a physical examination and may want to do a biopsy of the wart or skin abnormality if the diagnosis is unclear. Blood tests may also be needed to confirm the diagnosis.

How Is Human Papillomavirus Infection Treated?

Treatment isn't always successful, and not all warts need treatment. Treatment itself can cause problems, such as pain, infection, and scarring.

Treatment depends on wart location. Common warts can first be treated by a solution of salicylic and lactic acids. The solution is put on the wart each night, and the next morning dead skin is peeled off. Plantar warts can be treated with 40% salicylic acid plasters that are placed on the warts and removed weekly so dead skin can be taken off. The doctor can prescribe stronger medicine if these treatments don't work.

Genital warts almost always need a doctor's care. The doctor will use a blistering agent. Sexual partners will also need to be examined.

Other treatments include freezing, cutting, and burning (using a laser or electricity).

Treatments depend on where your warts are. A solution of salicylic and lactic acids is put on common warts at night, and the next morning dead skin is peeled off. Salicylic acid plasters are put on plantar warts and dead skin is taken off. Treatments for genital warts include taking medicines, cutting, freezing, and burning.

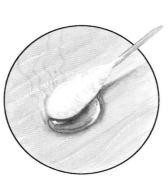

DOs and DON'Ts in Managing Human Papillomavirus Infection:

✔ **DO** treat warts early.
✔ **DO** wash hands after touching your warts, but try not to touch them.
✔ **DO** use salicylic acid solution on common warts and salicylic acid plasters on plantar warts as directed.
✔ **DO** call your doctor if your warts aren't better after several weeks of treatment.
✔ **DO** call your doctor if you have genital warts.

⊘ **DON'T** bite fingernails, pick cuticles, or soak hands for long periods.
⊘ **DON'T** pick at, dig at, or pull on warts.
⊘ **DON'T** cut or scrape warts.
⊘ **DON'T** let other body parts come in contact with warts.
⊘ **DON'T** shave or cut hair over warts.

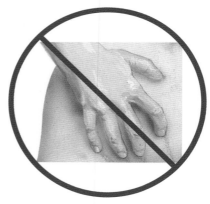

Don't scratch or pick at your warts.

To prevent spreading warts, always wash your hands after touching one, but try not to touch them at all.

FROM THE DESK OF

NOTES

FOR MORE INFORMATION

Contact the following sources:

- Centers for Disease Control and Prevention
  Tel: (800) 311-3435
  Website: http://www.cdc.gov
- American Academy of Dermatology
  Tel: (866) 503-SKIN (7546)
  Website: http://www.aad.org

Septic arthritis (or infectious arthritis) is a bacterial infection inside a joint. Infection usually affects only one joint at a time. Anyone can have a joint infection, but it's most common in children younger than 3 and adults older than 80.

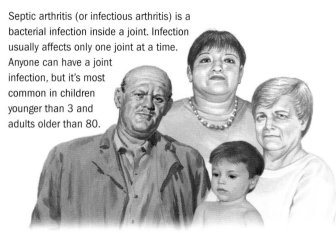

Joints that may be infected

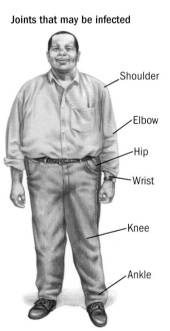

- Shoulder
- Elbow
- Hip
- Wrist
- Knee
- Ankle

Swollen joint with infection

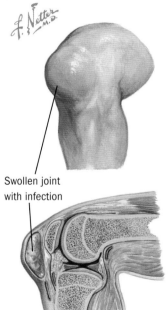

Usual causes are changes in a joint from other kinds of arthritis, an impaired immune system, and an artificial joint (joint replacement). Joints swell quickly and are very painful and hard to bend.

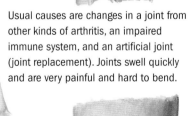

Your doctor may suspect septic arthritis after examining you. Diagnosis is confirmed by taking a sample of the joint fluid with a needle and testing it in a laboratory.

What Is Septic Arthritis?

Septic arthritis (or infectious arthritis) is a bacterial infection inside a joint. Joints are usually germfree (sterile). When bacteria get into a joint, they cause inflammation (swelling, redness) and pain. Infection usually affects only one joint at a time: knee, hip, wrist, shoulder, elbow, or ankle.

Anyone can have a joint infection, but it's most common in children younger than 3 and adults older than 80.

What Causes Septic Arthritis?

Usual causes are abnormal changes in a joint from other forms of arthritis, a poorly working immune (infection-fighting) system, and an artificial joint (joint replacement). The immune system problem may be caused by medicines and other conditions, such as diabetes, kidney disease, or cancer.

What Are the Symptoms of Septic Arthritis?

Infected joints swell quickly and are very painful and hard to bend. High temperature, chills, shakes, muscle aches, and fatigue occur. Depending on the joint, people may be unable to walk or use their arms.

How Is Septic Arthritis Diagnosed?

The doctor may suspect a joint infection on the basis of the medical history and physical examination. The doctor will diagnose a joint infection by removing fluid from the joint with a needle and testing it in the laboratory for evidence of infection.

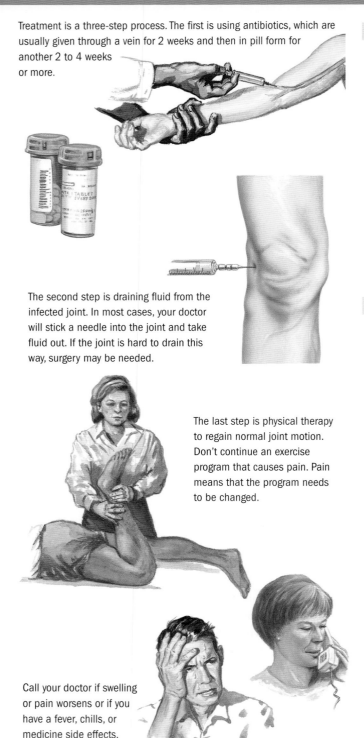

Treatment is a three-step process. The first is using antibiotics, which are usually given through a vein for 2 weeks and then in pill form for another 2 to 4 weeks or more.

The second step is draining fluid from the infected joint. In most cases, your doctor will stick a needle into the joint and take fluid out. If the joint is hard to drain this way, surgery may be needed.

The last step is physical therapy to regain normal joint motion. Don't continue an exercise program that causes pain. Pain means that the program needs to be changed.

Call your doctor if swelling or pain worsens or if you have a fever, chills, or medicine side effects.

FROM THE DESK OF

NOTES

How Is Septic Arthritis Treated?

Three stages of therapy are needed: antibiotics, joint drainage, and restoring normal motion to the joint.

Antibiotics are usually given through a vein for the first 2 weeks and then by mouth for 2 to 4 weeks or more.

Joint fluid should be drained to help resolve the infection. Most joints can be drained by sticking a needle into the joint and taking fluid out. Other joints are harder to drain this way and instead need drainage by an operation.

After the first few days of treatment, people with joint infections should start therapy to restore normal joint motion. Physical therapists help with restoring normal movement. Therapy should continue until after the pain leaves and the joint works normally.

DOs and DON'Ts in Managing Septic Arthritis:

✔ **DO** take your medicines as prescribed.
✔ **DO** ask your doctor which over-the-counter drugs you may take with your prescription medicines.
✔ **DO** exercises to maintain joint motion and preserve strength.
✔ **DO** call your doctor if you have drug side effects or if medicines and treatments don't help the pain.
✔ **DO** call your doctor if you have new fever, chills, and worsening pain or swelling.
✔ **DO** call your doctor if you need a referral for physical or occupational therapy.

🚫 **DON'T** wait to see whether medicine side effects will go away.
🚫 **DON'T** continue an exercise program that causes pain. If you have pain after exercise, the exercise program usually needs to be modified specifically for you.

FOR MORE INFORMATION

Contact the following sources:

• Arthritis Foundation
  Tel: (800) 283-7800
  Website: http://www.arthritis.org

• Centers for Disease Control and Prevention
  Tel: (800) 311-3435
  Website: http://www.cdc.gov

• Infectious Disease Society of America
  Tel: (703) 299-0200
  Website: http://www.idsociety.org

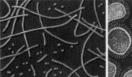

Many people get the flu every year, mostly during fall and winter. The virus infects cells of the respiratory tract (from the nose, down the throat, into the windpipe and the lungs). The virus is very small, visible only with a special microscope.

Virus seen with an electron microscope

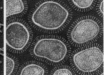 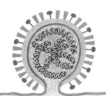

Magnified view   Even larger view   Virus budding (growing) on a cell

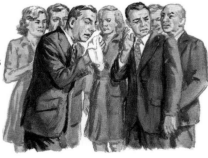

You get the virus by breathing in small droplets that an infected person sneezed into the air. These droplets contain virus.

What Is Influenza?

Influenza, or the flu, is a respiratory viral infection. It begins suddenly, lasts for 7 to 10 days, and goes away.

Influenza spreads quickly. People get it mostly in fall and winter.

What Causes Influenza?

People get the virus that causes influenza by breathing in small droplets that an infected person has coughed or sneezed into the air, or from touching something that an infected person touched. It's similar to the common cold but worse.

What Are the Symptoms of Influenza?

Symptoms come on suddenly. They usually start 24 to 48 hours after exposure to the flu virus. The worst symptoms and fever usually last 3 to 5 days. They include high temperature (as high as 104° F), chills, muscle aches, feeling very weak or tired, headache, eye pain in bright light, coughing, sneezing, sore throat, runny nose, and upset stomach (more in children than adults). A cough and feeling very weak and tired can last for up to 6 weeks.

How Is Influenza Diagnosed?

The doctor will make a diagnosis from the symptoms, especially during fall and winter. At other times of year, the doctor may do tests to confirm the diagnosis. Testing may involve taking a sample of liquid from a runny nose or using a blood sample. The doctor may also order a chest x-ray to check for pneumonia (a complication).

Symptoms include fever, chills, headache, feeling very weak or tired, and muscle aches. Your doctor will use symptoms and perhaps tests (of fluid from a runny nose) for diagnosis.

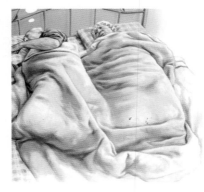

The best treatment is rest. Medicines can control symptoms. Nonaspirin medicines (such as acetaminophen), cough syrups, and decongestants can help you feel better. Don't give aspirin to children with the flu, it can cause Reye's syndrome.

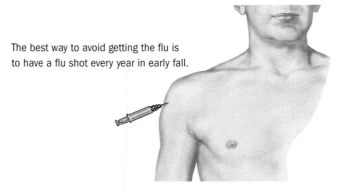

The best way to avoid getting the flu is to have a flu shot every year in early fall.

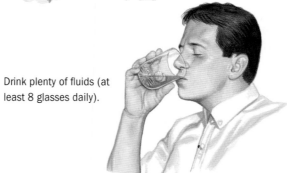

For up to some weeks after the flu, you may still feel weak, get tired easily, and have a cough.

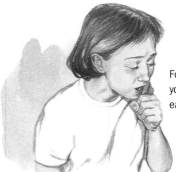

Drink plenty of fluids (at least 8 glasses daily).

FROM THE DESK OF

NOTES

How Is Influenza Treated?

The best treatment is rest. Influenza cannot be cured with antibiotics, but other medicines can control symptoms. For discomfort, nonaspirin medicines, such as acetaminophen and ibuprofen, cough syrups, and decongestants are used. Don't give aspirin to a child younger than 16 because of the risk of the serious Reye's syndrome.

Warm baths or heating pads can help muscle aches. A cool mist vaporizer may thin secretions, and gargling with warm salt water or mouthwash may ease a sore throat. Drinking lots of fluids is important.

DOs and DON'Ts in Managing Influenza:

✔ **DO** get a flu shot every year.
✔ **DO** drink plenty of fluids (at least 8 glasses daily) to thin lung secretions. Small children should avoid milk (it can thicken secretions).
✔ **DO** stop smoking to reduce the risk of complications.
✔ **DO** rest as much as possible. Continue to rest for 2 or 3 days after the fever goes away.
✔ **DO** wash hands often and have those who care for you wash their hands also. Throw away all tissues quickly.
✔ **DO** call your doctor if your fever or cough worsens, you get shortness of breath or chest pain, you cough up bloody sputum, or you have neck pain or stiffness.
✔ **DO** call your doctor if you have pain with a thick discharge from the ears or sinuses.

⊘ **DON'T** go to work or school if you think you have the flu. Avoid spreading the virus to others.
⊘ **DON'T** let anyone with a chronic illness or poor immune system (such as those with AIDS or getting chemotherapy) to come near a person with the flu.
⊘ **DON'T** share glasses or eating utensils.
⊘ **DON'T** give aspirin to a child younger than 16.

FOR MORE INFORMATION

Contact the following sources:

• Infectious Disease Society of America
Tel: (703) 299-0200
Website: http://www.idsociety.org

• National Institute for Allergy and Infectious Diseases
Tel: (301) 496-5717, (866) 284-4107
Website: http://www.niaid.nih.gov

• Centers for Disease Control and Prevention
Tel: (800) 311-3435
Website: http://www.cdc.gov

• WHO Collaborating Center for Influenza
CDC Influenza Branch
Tel: (800) 232-4636
Website: www.cdc.gov/flu/

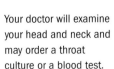

Cold or flu

Laryngitis is usually caused by a cold, the flu, or using the voice too much (e.g., singing). Allergies, sinus infections, smoking, and breathing in chemicals may cause chronic laryngitis.

Singing

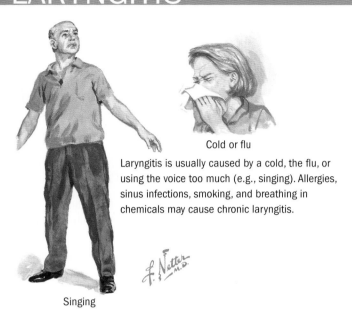

Roof of mouth

Vocal cords

Windpipe

Esophagus

**Looking down a
normal throat**

Laryngitis

Symptoms are a low, raspy, hoarse voice or loss of voice. Swollen vocal cords distorts sounds made by air passing over them, so your voice sounds hoarse. You may also have a dry cough or feel a lump in your throat.

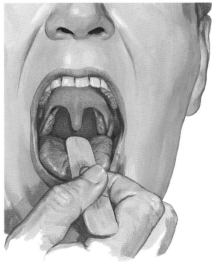

Your doctor will examine your head and neck and may order a throat culture or a blood test.

What Is Laryngitis?

Laryngitis is an inflammation (swelling, redness) of the vocal cords that results in hoarseness. Vocal cords are folds of mucous membrane in the larynx (voice box). When they're swollen, sounds made by air passing over the cords are distorted, so the voice sounds hoarse. Laryngitis usually goes away in 2 to 3 weeks, but when it lasts longer, it is said to be a chronic, or long-lasting, illness. Chronic laryngitis may take much longer to go away, depending on the cause.

What Causes Laryngitis?

Most often, a cold, the flu, or using the voice too much (singing or shouting) causes laryngitis, but viral or bacterial infections can also do so. Causes of chronic laryngitis include allergies, chronic sinusitis (sinus infection), smoking, alcohol, and breathing in irritating chemicals. Less often, heartburn or a sore on the vocal cords is the cause. More rarely, a growth causes the condition.

What Are the Symptoms of Laryngitis?

Main symptoms are a low, raspy hoarse voice or the loss of voice. Others include a dry cough, scratchy throat, stuffed nose, or feeling that there's a lump in the throat.

How Is Laryngitis Diagnosed?

The doctor will do a physical examination (head and neck) and maybe a throat culture or a blood test. For chronic laryngitis, a test called a laryngoscopy may be done. In this test, the doctor examines the throat with a mirror or viewing tube.

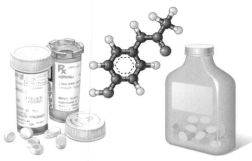

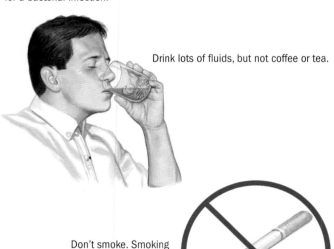

Resting the voice is usually enough treatment. Acetaminophen, ibuprofen, cough syrups, and lozenges can help minor pain. Antibiotics can be given for a bacterial infection.

Drink lots of fluids, but not coffee or tea.

Don't smoke. Smoking can cause laryngitis.

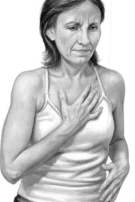

Call your doctor if you get a high fever or have trouble breathing.

How Is Laryngitis Treated?

For minor discomfort, a nonaspirin medicine such as acetaminophen or ibuprofen can be used. Cough syrups and lozenges can also help. Resting the voice by whispering or writing notes instead of talking is usually all that is needed. If a bacterial infection is causing laryngitis, the doctor will prescribe antibiotics. This medicine should be taken until it's completely finished. No special diet is needed, but liquids may be easier going down the throat. No activity restrictions are needed.

If the cause is a growth, a doctor may need to remove it.

DOs and DON'Ts in Managing Laryngitis:

✔ **DO** use a humidifier or breathe in warm steam.
✔ **DO** drink more fluids. Warm liquids, such as chicken soup, are best.
✔ **DO** call your doctor if you get a high fever or have trouble breathing.
✔ **DO** call your doctor if your symptoms last longer than 2 weeks.

⊘ **DON'T** take decongestants.
⊘ **DON'T** drink alcohol, coffee, or tea.
⊘ **DON'T** smoke or breathe in cigarette smoke. Smoking can cause laryngitis.
⊘ **DON'T** use your voice unless you absolutely have to.
⊘ **DON'T** skip doses or stop taking any prescribed antibiotic, even if you feel better. You must finish all the medicine for it to work well.

FROM THE DESK OF

NOTES

FOR MORE INFORMATION

Contact the following sources:

• American Academy of Family Physicians
  Tel: (800) 274-2237
  Website: http://www.aafp.org

• National Institute of Allergy and Infectious Disease
  Tel: (301) 496-5717
  Website: http://www.niaid.nih.gov

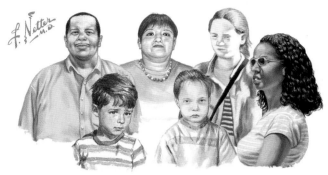

Tiny parasites (lice) that live on the body or in clothing cause skin inflammation called pediculosis. The three types are head lice, body lice, and pubic (crab) lice. Head lice are most common in children.

Lice live on the head, eyebrows, eyelashes, facial hair, pubic hair, and the back of the neck. Lice eggs, called nits, are white and are easier to see than are the small gray lice.

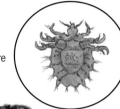

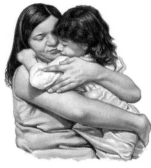

Sharing a brush, comb, or hat with someone who is infected spreads lice. They can also spread by close person-to person contact. Pubic lice spread by sexual contact.

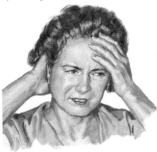

Symptoms include an itchy scalp (worse at night), a moving feeling in the hair, rash and sores on the scalp, and nits on the scalp and eyebrows.

Many times, a school nurse will find lice during routine checks of children. A magnifying glass helps show the nits. Your doctor may also use a special light called a Wood's lamp to see nits. Seeing them is all that's needed for diagnosis.

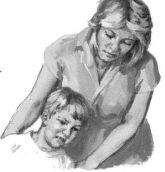

What Are Lice?

Lice are tiny parasites that live on the body or in clothing and cause skin inflammation (redness, itching, swelling) called pediculosis. The three types are head lice, body lice, and pubic (crab) lice. Head lice are most common in children. About 6 to 12 million cases per year occur in the United States.

What Causes Lice?

Lice live on the head, eyebrows, eyelashes, facial hair, pubic hair, and the back of the neck. Lice eggs, called nits, are white and are easier to see than the small gray lice. Sharing a brush, comb, or hat with someone who is infected spreads lice. They can also spread by close person-to-person contact. Pubic lice spread by sexual contact.

What Are the Symptoms of Lice?

Symptoms usually go away within a few days of treatment. They include an itchy scalp (worse at night), a moving feeling in the hair, rash and sores on the scalp, and nits on the scalp and eyebrows.

How Are Lice Diagnosed?

The doctor will take a medical history and do an examination, with special attention to the scalp and using a magnifying glass. The doctor may also use a special light called a Wood's lamp to see nits.

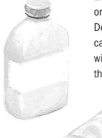

Lice are treated with medicated creams, lotions, or shampoos applied to affected body parts. Don't use more than recommended because that can cause side effects. Lice can also be removed with a special comb and by pulling out lice or nits that are left with fingers or tweezers.

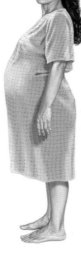

Don't use anti-lice shampoo and medicine if you're pregnant, unless your doctor says to.

All family members should be examined for lice. Keep your children out of school, day care, or camp until your doctor says that it's OK to go back.

Clean clothing, bedding, pillows, stuffed toys, and fabric furniture that was used during the infestation. Wash all clothes in hot water at 130° F for 20 minutes. Dry them in a hot dryer. Clean the house.

How Are Lice Treated?

Lice are treated with medicated creams, lotions, or shampoos applied to affected body parts. Some of these include permethrin (Nix®, Elimite®), applied once; pyrethrins (Rid®, R and C®, A-200®), reapplied in 7 days; and lindane (Kwell®, by prescription), reapplied in 7 days.

Lice can also be removed with a special comb and by pulling out lice or nits that are left with fingers or tweezers. A magnifying glass helps show the nits and lice. Eyelashes should be checked for lice and nits.

Side effects of treatments include skin irritation or body absorption of the medicine. These usually occur when medicine is applied more often than recommended. Keep all preparations out of the eyes and out of the reach of children.

DOs and DON'Ts in Managing Lice:

✔ **DO** tell your doctor if you're pregnant.
✔ **DO** check the heads of all family members.
✔ **DO** call your doctor if symptoms don't get better after 1 week.
✔ **DO** protect your eyes from the anti-lice shampoo.
✔ **DO** keep your child out of school, day care, or camp until your doctor says that it's OK to go back.
✔ **DO** clean clothing, bedding, pillows, stuffed toys, and fabric furniture that was used during the infection. Wash all clothes in hot water at 130° F for 20 minutes. Dry them in a hot dryer. Clean the house. Put clothes that cannot be washed in a sealed plastic bag for 2 weeks before drycleaning them.
✔ **DO** soak combs and brushes for at least 1 hour in anti-lice shampoo, disinfectant, hot water, or rubbing alcohol.
✔ **DO** call your doctor if family members or sexual partners have symptoms of lice or symptoms return after treatment.

⊘ **DON'T** use more anti-lice shampoo than recommended.
⊘ **DON'T** use anti-lice shampoo and medicine if you're pregnant unless your doctor says to.
⊘ **DON'T** use medicine around your eyes unless your doctor tells you to.

FROM THE DESK OF

NOTES

FOR MORE INFORMATION

Contact the following source:

• National Pediculosis Association
  Tel: (781) 449-6487, (866) 323-5465
  Website: http://www.headlice.org

MANAGING YOUR
LISTERIOSIS

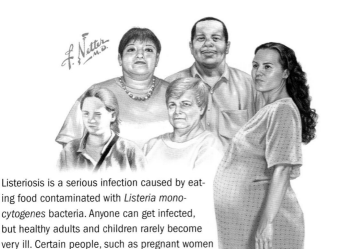

Listeriosis is a serious infection caused by eating food contaminated with *Listeria monocytogenes* bacteria. Anyone can get infected, but healthy adults and children rarely become very ill. Certain people, such as pregnant women and unborn babies, have a higher risk of serious illness.

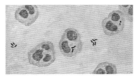

White blood cells with Listeria bacteria

These bacteria are found most often in undercooked and raw meat and in dairy products.

People with weak immune systems are also at high risk. These people include those with diseases such as cancer or AIDS, those who have organ transplants, and people over 70 years.

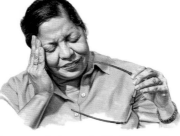

Some people have a flu-like illness, with fever, muscle aches, nausea, vomiting, diarrhea, and stomach pain.

Your doctor will do a physical examination and take a medical history. A blood culture and spinal tap may be done. A blood culture involves sending blood to a laboratory to see whether bacteria are in the blood and can grow.

What Is Listeriosis?

Listeriosis is a serious infection caused by eating food contaminated with bacteria. These bacteria are found most often in undercooked meat and in dairy products. Listeriosis is a serious public health problem but it's an uncommon infection.

Anyone can get infected, but healthy adults and children rarely become seriously ill. However, certain people, such as pregnant women and unborn babies, have a higher risk. Listeriosis cause a premature birth, miscarriage, or stillbirth. A newborn can also become seriously ill if infected before birth. People with weak immune (infection-fighting) systems are also at high risk. These people include those with diseases such as cancer or AIDS, those who have organ transplants, and elderly people.

What Causes Listeriosis?

The cause is eating food contaminated with the kind of bacteria named *Listeria monocyto0genes*. *Listeria* is found in soil and water and can get on raw vegetables from soil or from fertilizer (manure). *Listeria* can also get into raw meats and milk and processed foods (such as deli cheeses, cold cuts, and hot dogs).

What Are the Symptoms of Listeriosis?

Some people have a flu-like illness, with symptoms such as fever, muscle aches, nausea, vomiting, diarrhea, and stomach pain. If bacteria enter the nervous system, symptoms may be worse. Headache, stiff neck, seizures, loss of balance, and feeling confused or disoriented can occur.

How Is Listeriosis Diagnosed?

The doctor will do a physical examination and take a medical history. Tests done for diagnosis include a blood culture and spinal tap. A blood culture involves taking blood from a vein and sending it to a laboratory for study, to see whether bacteria are in the blood and can grow.

The spinal tap involves removing a small sample of fluid from around the spinal cord and having a laboratory test it for the presence of the *Listeria* bacteria.

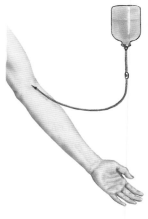

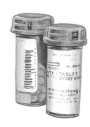

Treatment is antibiotics, which may be given for 2 weeks or more. People are often treated in the hospital, where antibiotics can be given intravenously.

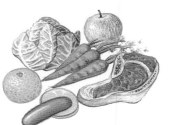

Thoroughly cook all animal products, including eggs, meat, and poultry. Wash fruits and vegetables before eating them.

Only drink pasteurized milk; it has been heated to kill bacteria.

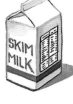

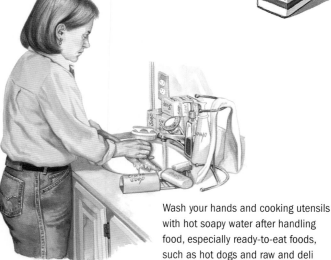

Wash your hands and cooking utensils with hot soapy water after handling food, especially ready-to-eat foods, such as hot dogs and raw and deli meats.

How Is Listeriosis Treated?

Treatment is with antibiotics. People are often treated in the hospital. Antibiotics can then be given intravenously (injected directly into the vein). This method is the fastest and most effective way of giving an antibiotic.

Antibiotic treatment usually lasts for 2 weeks. People with weak immune systems may need longer treatment, because the illness often comes back.

DOs and DON'Ts in Managing Listeriosis:

✔ **DO** tell your doctor about all your medicines (including over-the-counter drugs and herbal products).

✔ **DO** call your doctor if you still have symptoms after you finish the antibiotics.

✔ **DO** thoroughly cook all animal products including eggs, meat, and poultry.

✔ **DO** wash all fruits and vegetables before eating them.

✔ **DO** wash your hands and cooking utensils with hot soapy water after handling food, especially after contact with raw and deli meats.

⊘ **DON'T** stop taking your antibiotics without asking your doctor first.

⊘ **DON'T** drink unpasteurized milk. Pasteurized milk has been heated to kill bacteria.

FROM THE DESK OF

NOTES

FOR MORE INFORMATION

Contact the following source:

• Centers for Disease Control and Prevention
Tel: (800) 232-4636
Website: http://www.cdc.gov

MANAGING YOUR
LUNG ABSCESS

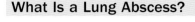

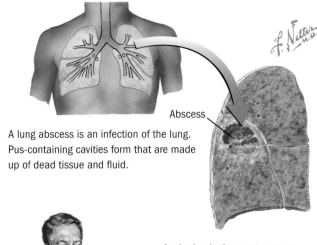

Abscess

A lung abscess is an infection of the lung. Pus-containing cavities form that are made up of dead tissue and fluid.

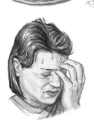

Aspiration is the most common reason for formation of lung abscesses. Aspiration means that foreign material (such as food, drink, vomit, or secretions from the mouth) is breathed into lungs.

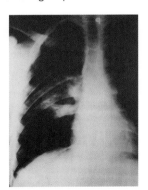

Symptoms include fever, chills, sweats, cough, tiredness, weakness, loss of appetite, weight loss, and chest pain made worse by coughing or taking deep breaths.

X-ray

Bronchoscopy

Your doctor makes a diagnosis from symptoms, chest x-rays, and CT. Sputum and blood cultures may help confirm the cause. Your doctor may order bronchoscopy to rule out lung cancer if you have signs and symptoms of recurrent obstruction.

What Is a Lung Abscess?

Lung abscess is an infection of the lung. Pus-containing cavities form that are made up of bacteria or other microorganisms, dead (necrotic) tissue, and fluid. People over age 60 have a greater risk of getting abscesses.

What Causes a Lung Abscess?

Aspiration is the most important reason for formation of lung abscesses. Aspiration means that foreign material (usually food, drink, vomit, or secretions from the mouth) is breathed into the lungs. Inflammation, pneumonia, and abscess formation can occur in 7 to 14 days. Stroke, seizure disorders, drug abuse, alcoholism, poor oral hygiene (gum disease), emphysema, lung cancer, and disorders of the esophagus (swallowing problems) can lead to aspiration.

Bacteria causing lung abscesses are usually anaerobes (don't need oxygen to grow) and originate from the mouth. Other microorganisms, such as parasites and fungi, can also infect lungs and cause abscesses.

What Are the Symptoms of a Lung Abscess?

Symptoms usually develop during weeks to months. Symptoms include fever, chills, sweats, and a cough with foul-smelling and bad-tasting sputum. People are often tired, are weak, lose their appetite, and lose weight. Sometimes, blood in the sputum and chest pain made worse by coughing or taking deep breaths occur. People may have rapid heart rate, rapid breathing, wheezing, and fluid in the lungs (pleural effusion).

How Is a Lung Abscess Diagnosed?

The doctor makes a diagnosis from symptoms and chest x-rays. The doctor may order computed tomography (CT) of the chest to see the abscess. Sputum and blood cultures may help confirm the bacteria or microorganism causing the abscess. The doctor may order bronchoscopy to rule out lung cancer if there are signs that something may be obstructing the airways. In this test, a lighted tube is passed through the mouth into the lungs to see in the lungs and get samples of lung tissue.

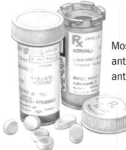

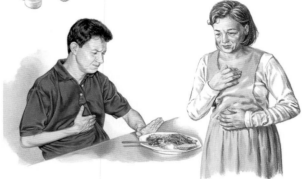

Most people usually need intravenous and oral antibiotics, given for 4 to 6 weeks. Finish all your antibiotics as prescribed by your doctor.

Tell your doctor about symptoms of relapse, such as chest pain, fever, or coughing up blood, or problems with medicines. Report pain with swallowing or food getting stuck when you swallow.

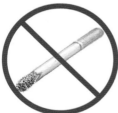

Don't smoke. Smoking can lead to lung abscess, emphysema, and lung cancer.

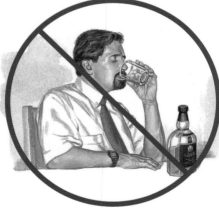

Don't drink alcohol. Lung abscesses are common in alcoholics, who have greater chances of aspiration.

How Is a Lung Abscess Treated?

First, the microorganism causing the abscess is treated. Second, the condition leading to aspiration (e.g., seizures, alcoholism, poor oral hygiene, or stroke) is treated.

Most people usually need intravenous and oral antibiotics, given for 4 to 6 weeks. Up to 95% of people are cured, but the cure will depend on the infection's cause.

DOs and DON'Ts in Managing a Lung Abscess:

✔ **DO** finish all your antibiotics as prescribed by your doctor.
✔ **DO** tell your doctor about symptoms of relapse, such as chest pain, fever, or coughing up blood, or problems with medicines (e.g., rash, diarrhea, tongue swelling, wheezing, or shortness of breath).
✔ **DO** report pain with swallowing or food getting stuck when you swallow.
✔ **DO** call your doctor if you have a drinking or drug problem.
✔ **DO** call your doctor if you have a seizure.
✔ **DO** call your doctor if your fever lasts for more than 7 days after starting antibiotics.

⊘ **DON'T** stop your antibiotics unless your doctor tells you to.
⊘ **DON'T** smoke. Smoking can lead to lung abscess, emphysema, and lung cancer.
⊘ **DON'T** use recreational drugs.
⊘ **DON'T** abuse sleeping pills, anxiety pills, and opiate narcotics. They can lead to aspiration.
⊘ **DON'T** drink alcohol in excess. Lung abscesses are common in alcoholics, who have greater chances of aspiration.

FROM THE DESK OF

NOTES

FOR MORE INFORMATION
Contact the following source:
• American Lung Association
Tel: (212) 315-8700, (800) 586-4872
Website: http://www.lungusa.org

The lymphatic system consists of organs, nodes, ducts, and vessels. It makes and moves a fluid called lymph from tissues through vessels to the blood. Lymphangitis is an inflammation of lymphatic vessels. It's a common complication of bacterial infections.

Lymphatic system

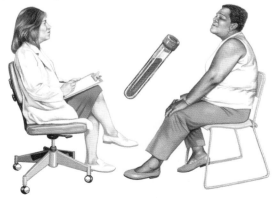

A wound that becomes infected with *Staphylococcus* (staph) or *Streptococcus* (strep) bacteria can cause lymphangitis.

Symptoms include red streaks near the wound that are moving toward the nearest lymph nodes. For example, if an arm is infected, armpit nodes are affected. Nodes get swollen and tender. Fatigue, throbbing pain at the wound, loss of appetite, headache, muscle aches, chills, and fever also may occur.

Your doctor makes a diagnosis from your medical history and physical examination, especially feeling the lymph nodes. The doctor will also order blood tests.

What Is Lymphangitis?

The lymphatic system consists of organs, nodes (glands), ducts, and vessels (channels) throughout the body. It's part of the immune system. It makes and moves a fluid called lymph from tissues through vessels to the blood. Lymphangitis is an inflammation (swelling) of the lymphatic vessels. It's a common complication of bacterial infections. Lymphangitis may suggest that an infection is quickly getting worse. Life-threatening infections and septicemia (blood poisoning) can result.

What Causes Lymphangitis?

A wound that becomes infected with *Staphylococcus* (staph) or *Streptococcus* (strep) bacteria can cause lymphangitis, as can most other infections.

What Are the Symptoms of Lymphangitis?

Symptoms include red streaks near the wound that move toward the nearest lymph nodes. For example, if the arm is infected, nodes in the armpit are affected. If the leg is infected, nodes in the groin are affected. Nodes will get swollen and tender. Fatigue, throbbing pain at the wound site, loss of appetite, headache, muscle aches, chills, and fever may also occur.

How Is Lymphangitis Diagnosed?

The doctor will make a diagnosis from a medical history and physical examination, especially feeling the lymph nodes. The doctor will also order blood tests to find out the type of bacteria involved and how severe the illness is.

Lymphangitis should be treated very quickly. Treatment includes antibiotics (intravenous or by mouth) and pain medicines.

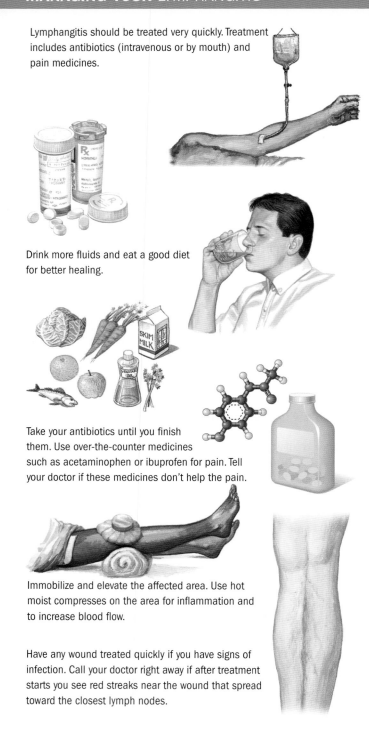

Drink more fluids and eat a good diet for better healing.

Take your antibiotics until you finish them. Use over-the-counter medicines such as acetaminophen or ibuprofen for pain. Tell your doctor if these medicines don't help the pain.

Immobilize and elevate the affected area. Use hot moist compresses on the area for inflammation and to increase blood flow.

Have any wound treated quickly if you have signs of infection. Call your doctor right away if after treatment starts you see red streaks near the wound that spread toward the closest lymph nodes.

How Is Lymphangitis Treated?

Lymphangitis should be treated very quickly. Treatment of an uncomplicated disorder is usually successful. Treatment includes antibiotics and pain medicines. People with symptoms of a serious illness (fever, chills, muscle pains) may need antibiotics given intravenously (directly into a vein). Hot moist compresses or a heating pad put on the wound site several times a day will help inflammation, as will anti-inflammatory drugs. The affected area should be elevated and immobilized if possible. Wound care, including drainage of the wound if needed, should be done only after antibiotics are started.

People with group A streptococcal infections should be treated aggressively. These illnesses can get worse very quickly and can have serious complications. Complications can be life-threatening.

DOs and DON'Ts in Managing Lymphangitis:

✔ **DO** take your antibiotics until you finish them.
✔ **DO** use over-the-counter medicines such as acetaminophen or ibuprofen for pain.
✔ **DO** tell your doctor if the medicines don't help the pain.
✔ **DO** drink more fluids and eat a good diet for better healing.
✔ **DO** immobilize and elevate the affected area.
✔ **DO** use hot moist compresses on the area for inflammation and to increase blood flow to the area.
✔ **DO** have any wound treated quickly if you see signs of infection.
✔ **DO** call your doctor if you continue to have a high temperature after you start antibiotics.
✔ **DO** call your doctor if red streaks continue to occur near the wound and spread toward the closest lymph node area after treatment starts.

⊘ **DON'T** skip doses or stop your antibiotics until they're all gone.
⊘ **DON'T** use the affected limb. Keep it raised.
⊘ **DON'T** ignore a wound if it looks infected.

FROM THE DESK OF

NOTES

FOR MORE INFORMATION

Contact the following sources:

• National Heart, Lung, and Blood Institute
Tel: (301) 592-8573
Website: http://www.nhlbi.nih.gov

• Centers for Disease Control and Prevention
Tel: (800) 232-4636
Website: http://www.cdc.gov

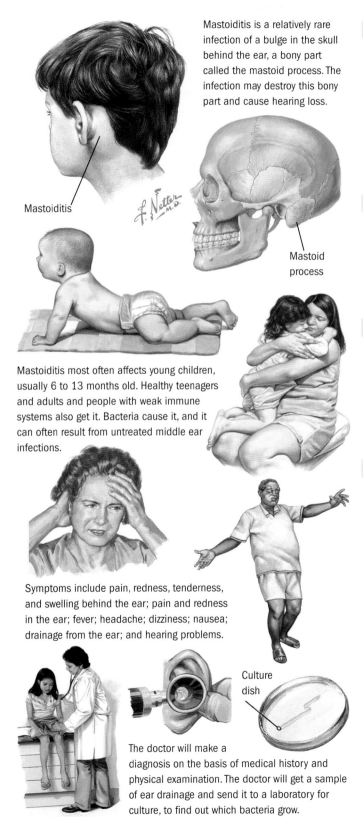

Mastoiditis is a relatively rare infection of a bulge in the skull behind the ear, a bony part called the mastoid process. The infection may destroy this bony part and cause hearing loss.

Mastoiditis

Mastoid process

Mastoiditis most often affects young children, usually 6 to 13 months old. Healthy teenagers and adults and people with weak immune systems also get it. Bacteria cause it, and it can often result from untreated middle ear infections.

Symptoms include pain, redness, tenderness, and swelling behind the ear; pain and redness in the ear; fever; headache; dizziness; nausea; drainage from the ear; and hearing problems.

Culture dish

The doctor will make a diagnosis on the basis of medical history and physical examination. The doctor will get a sample of ear drainage and send it to a laboratory for culture, to find out which bacteria grow.

What Is Mastoiditis?

Mastoiditis is a relatively rare infection of a bulge in the skull behind the ear, a bony part called the mastoid process. The infection may cause destruction of this bony part followed by hearing loss. Mastoiditis most often affects young children, usually those 6 to 13 months old. Also, healthy teenagers and adults can get it; so can people with weakened immune (infection-fighting) systems.

What Causes Mastoiditis?

Bacteria, most commonly the kind named *Haemophilus influenzae*, *Staphylococcus*, or *Streptococcus*, are the cause. Mastoiditis can be a complication of an untreated middle ear infection.

What Are the Symptoms of Mastoiditis?

Symptoms can appear 2 weeks or more after the start of an untreated middle ear infection. They include pain, redness, tenderness, and swelling behind the ear; increased pain and redness in the ear; fever; headache; dizziness; nausea; drainage from the ear; and hearing problems in the ear.

How Is Mastoiditis Diagnosed?

The doctor will make a diagnosis on the basis of the medical history and physical examination. The doctor will get a sample of the ear drainage and send it to a laboratory for culture, to find out which bacteria will grow. The doctor may also want to order x-rays, CT, or MRI.

Antibiotics are first given IV and then orally. Antibiotic treatment must continue for at least 2 weeks. If antibiotics and myringotomy (surgical drainage of the ear) don't help, an operation (mastoidectomy) is done. Mastoidectomy can involve removing infected bone cells, cleaning the area, and draining the middle ear.

Use nonaspirin products such as acetaminophen for fever and pain.

Don't miss follow-up appointments with your doctor. It's important to make sure that the infection is gone.

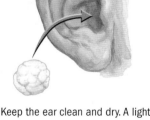

Keep the ear clean and dry. A light cotton ball placed on the outer ear canal may help absorb drainage.

How Is Mastoiditis Treated?

Treatment may be difficult because it's hard for medicine to go deep enough into the mastoid bone. Repeated or long-term treatment may be needed. More severe infections need intravenous (injected directly into a vein) antibiotics. Antibiotics are first given intravenously and then orally (by mouth). The antibiotic treatment must continue for at least 2 weeks. Complications include hearing loss (partial or complete), abscesses, facial paralysis or palsy, and spread of infection to the brain (meningitis) or other parts of the body. If an abscess occurs, an operation to drain the abscess may be needed. An operation called mastoidectomy is done if treatment with antibiotics and myringotomy (surgical drainage of the ear) don't help. Simple mastoidectomy involves removing infected bone cells, cleaning the area, and draining the middle ear. Then antibiotics are put into the ear. Other operations, rarely needed, are radical mastoidectomy (for serious or chronic infection) and modified radical mastoidectomy.

DOs and DON'Ts in Managing Mastoiditis:

✔ **DO** take your antibiotics until they're all gone.
✔ **DO** use nonaspirin products such as acetaminophen for fever and pain.
✔ **DO** keep the ear clean and dry. A light cotton ball placed on the outer canal may help absorb drainage.
✔ **DO** drink more fluids during your fever.
✔ **DO** call your doctor if you continue to have a fever while you take antibiotics.
✔ **DO** call your doctor if you have a severe headache, dizziness, weakness, or increased pain.
✔ **DO** call your doctor if you have nausea, vomiting, or diarrhea.
✔ **DO** call your doctor if you get a rash.

⊘ **DON'T** skip doses or stop taking antibiotics until you have finished all your medicine.
⊘ **DON'T** miss follow-up doctor appointments. It's important to make sure that the infection is gone.

FROM THE DESK OF

NOTES

FOR MORE INFORMATION

Contact the following source:

• American Academy of Otolaryngology—Head and Neck Surgery
 Tel: (703) 836-4444
 Website: http://www.entnet.org

MANAGING YOUR
MENINGITIS

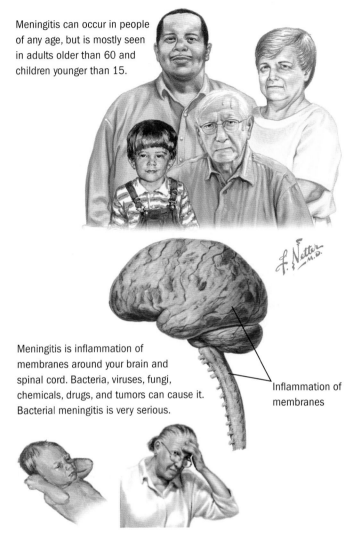

Meningitis can occur in people of any age, but is mostly seen in adults older than 60 and children younger than 15.

Meningitis is inflammation of membranes around your brain and spinal cord. Bacteria, viruses, fungi, chemicals, drugs, and tumors can cause it. Bacterial meningitis is very serious.

Inflammation of membranes

In adults, the most common symptoms are high temperature, severe headache, and stiff neck. Children are feverish, fretful, and tired; they cry and don't eat. Newborns may not have the common symptoms.

Your doctor will do a procedure called a spinal tap for diagnosis. Fluid is taken from your back through a needle to look at under a microscope. Blood tests and x-rays may also be done.

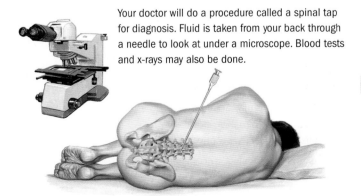

What Is Meningitis?

Meningitis is inflammation of membranes around the brain and spinal cord. It can be bacterial, viral, or fungal. People of any age can get meningitis, but most adults are older than 60 and most children younger than 15, and half are younger than 4.

People who have greater chances of getting bacterial meningitis include those who had their spleen removed, have poor immune (infection-fighting) systems, have suffered a head injury, or have cancer or diabetes mellitus. Those living in crowded camps or dormitories and alcoholics also have a greater chance of getting meningitis.

What Causes Meningitis?

The many causes include bacteria, viruses, fungi, chemicals, drugs, and tumors. The most common bacteria include *Neisseria meningitidis*, *Haemophilus influenzae*, *Streptococcus pneumoniae*, *Listeria monocytogenes*, *Escherichia coli*, *Klebsiella* species, and group B streptococcus. Bacteria spread through passing of respiratory and throat secretions (coughing, kissing).

What Are the Symptoms of Meningitis?

In adults common symptoms include high fever, severe headache, and stiff neck, which start over several hours. Others are nausea, vomiting, light sensitivity, feeling sick, muscle and joint aches, and seizure-like muscle jerks. Poor coordination, confusion, drowsiness, loss of consciousness, and rash also occur.

Children have fever, high-pitched moaning or crying, grunting, fretfulness, and tiredness. They don't eat, are sick, arch their back or neck, and have pale, blotchy skin and rash. Newborns and small babies may seem only slow or inactive, be irritable, vomit, or feed poorly. They may not have the common symptoms.

How Is Meningitis Diagnosed?

The doctor makes a diagnosis by looking for bacteria in a sample of spinal fluid. The doctor gets fluid by doing a spinal tap. A needle is put into a spot in the lower back where fluid in the spinal canal can be reached. The doctor may also order blood tests and x-ray imaging tests of the brain.

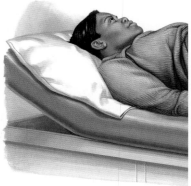

People need a hospital stay for treatment with intravenous antibiotics, plenty of fluids, and rest. Bacterial meningitis is usually fatal if untreated.

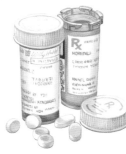

Antibiotics are given to treat bacterial meningitis but not viral meningitis.

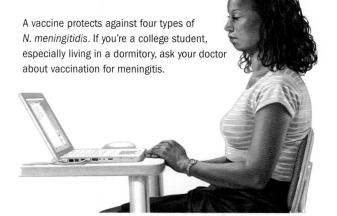

People who are close contacts of someone with bacterial meningitis caused by *N. meningitidis* should get antibiotics to prevent meningitis.

A vaccine protects against four types of *N. meningitidis*. If you're a college student, especially living in a dormitory, ask your doctor about vaccination for meningitis.

How Is Meningitis Treated?

People need a hospital stay for treatment with intravenous antibiotics, plenty of fluids, and rest. Bacterial meningitis is usually fatal if untreated. Other types of meningitis (viral) aren't as dangerous, and people don't usually need a hospital stay. Viral meningitis usually goes away on its own. Antibiotics can't help it.

A neurologist (specialist in brain diseases) or a doctor who treats infectious diseases may be involved in care.

Most people usually recover completely from meningitis. Recovery can take 2 to 3 weeks or longer.

A vaccine protects against four types of *N. meningitidis*. It's not routinely used in the United States, but is sometimes used for outbreaks. College students, especially those living in dormitories, have more chances of getting meningitis and should consider getting this vaccine.

DOs and DON'Ts in Managing Meningitis:

✔ **DO** understand the importance of bacterial meningitis. It's a medical emergency and needs immediate attention and treatment.

✔ **DO** call your doctor if you have symptoms of bacterial meningitis.

✔ **DO** call your doctor if you have questions about meningitis vaccines.

⊘ **DON'T** forget that people who are close contacts of someone with meningitis caused by *N. meningitidis* should get antibiotics to prevent meningitis.

FROM THE DESK OF

NOTES

FOR MORE INFORMATION

Contact the following sources:

• Meningitis Foundation of America
  Tel: (800) 668-1129
  Website: http://www.musa.org

• National Meningitis Association
  Tel: (866) 366-3662
  Website: http://www.nmaus.org

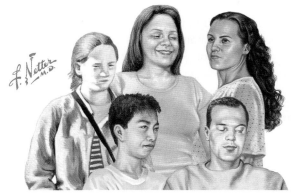

Mononucleosis, also called mono and kissing disease, is an acute infection affecting the respiratory system, liver, and lymphatic system. It spreads by close contact. It's common in adolescents and young adults. Children who have it often don't show many symptoms.

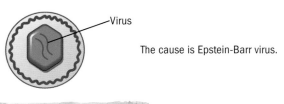

Virus

The cause is Epstein-Barr virus.

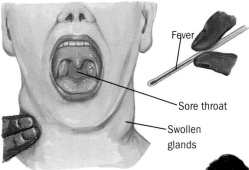

Fever

Sore throat

Swollen glands

The most common symptoms are fever, sore throat, and swollen and sore glands in the neck. Others are severe tiredness, general body aches, and maybe a swollen spleen and liver.

The doctor will take a medical history and do a physical exam, with special attention to the neck, throat, and abdomen when mono is suspected. Blood tests, throat cultures, and ultrasonography may be done.

What Is Mononucleosis?

Mononucleosis, also called mono and kissing disease, is an acute infection affecting the respiratory system, liver, and lymphatic system. It spreads by close contact. It's common in adolescents and young adults and rare in people older than 35. It's usually harmless and goes away by itself. Rarely, it becomes serious and causes major fatigue, so people miss weeks of school or work. The most serious complication is the spleen becoming swollen. It may burst if hit by direct contact, such as while playing contact sports.

What Causes Mononucleosis?

The cause is the Epstein-Barr virus (EBV). The virus spreads through saliva, such as by kissing, coughing, or sharing food or utensils with someone who's infected.

What Are the Symptoms of Mononucleosis?

Most important symptoms are fever, sore throat, and swollen and sore glands, especially in the neck. Headache, joint and muscle pain, general body aches, loss of appetite, feeling sick, puffy eyes, rash, stomach fullness or pain, severe tiredness (sleeping 12 to 16 hours daily), abdominal pain, and yellow skin may also occur.

Fever, body aches, and sore throat usually go away after 1 to 4 weeks. If the spleen got large, 6 weeks may be needed before it becomes normal and risk of bursting goes away. People may feel tired for several months after having mononucleosis. Sometimes tonsils get large and can cause breathing problems.

How Is Mononucleosis Diagnosed?

The doctor takes a medical history and does an examination, with special attention to the neck, throat, and abdomen. Blood tests and maybe throat cultures and ultrasonography are done to be sure of the diagnosis.

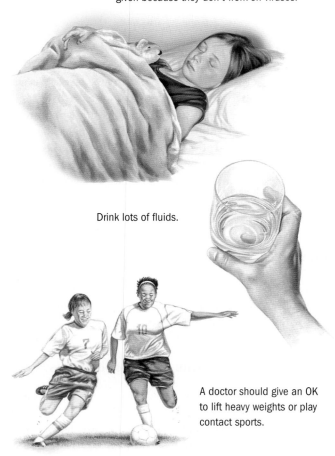

Bed rest and good nutrition are the best treatment. Most cases get better on their own. Antibiotics aren't given because they don't work on viruses.

Drink lots of fluids.

A doctor should give an OK to lift heavy weights or play contact sports.

Children should not be given aspirin because of the chance of Reye's syndrome. Reye's syndrome causes organ failure, especially affecting the brain and liver. Its symptoms usually start with vomiting.

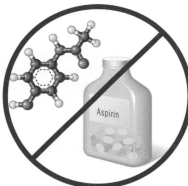

Aspirin

How Is Mononucleosis Treated?

Most cases get better by themselves. Antibiotics don't work because a virus is the cause. Bed rest and good nutrition are the best treatment. No special diet is needed. For muscle aches and minor discomfort, ibuprofen or naproxen is used. Children younger than 16 years shouldn't take aspirin because of the risk of Reye's syndrome. For severe throat inflammation, steroids may be prescribed. Recovery takes 10 days to months.

DOs and DON'Ts in Managing Mononucleosis:

✔ **DO** get plenty of rest and drink lots of fluids.
✔ **DO** tell your doctor about all your medicines, including prescription and nonprescription.
✔ **DO** tell your doctor if your symptoms get worse or don't get better after 2 weeks.
✔ **DO** tell your doctor if you have stomach or shoulder pain.
✔ **DO** get your doctor's OK to lift heavy weights or play contact sports.
✔ **DO** arrange for schoolwork to be done at home, if needed.
✔ **DO** avoid kissing or sharing food or utensils with someone who's sick. Wash your hands often.
✔ **DO** call your doctor if your temperature is higher than 102° F.
✔ **DO** call your doctor if you have trouble swallowing or breathing, are constipated and strain during bowel movements, or get sudden severe abdominal pain.
✔ **DO** call your doctor if you have a severe headache, neck pain, or stiffness.

⊘ **DON'T** drink alcohol.
⊘ **DON'T** play contact sports.
⊘ **DON'T** give your child aspirin because of the chance of Reye's syndrome. Reye's syndrome causes organ failure, especially affecting the brain and liver. Its symptoms usually start with vomiting.

FROM THE DESK OF

NOTES

FOR MORE INFORMATION

Contact the following sources:

• The Infectious Diseases Society of America
Tel: (703) 299-0200
Website: http://www.idsociety.org

• WebMD
Website: http://www.webmd.com

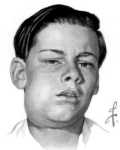

Mumps is a contagious infection that causes painful swelling of salivary glands. These glands, on both sides of the jaw, make saliva. Mumps is most often seen in children between 10 and 15 years old.

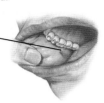

Infected salivary gland

What Is Mumps?

Mumps is a contagious viral infection that causes painful swelling of salivary glands. These glands, on both sides of the jaw, make saliva. Mumps is most often seen in children between 10 and 15 years old.

Before the mumps vaccine was developed, mumps was a common childhood illness. It's now much less common.

Complications can happen, usually in adults. Hearing can be lost temporarily. Organs can become swollen and irritated. These organs include testicles in boys who have gone through puberty and men (sometimes with infertility), ovaries or breasts in women and girls who have gone through puberty, pancreas, lining of the brain, heart, and joints.

A virus causes mumps. It spreads easily from person to person by airborne droplets or direct contact.

What Causes Mumps?

A virus causes mumps. It spreads easily from person to person by airborne droplets or direct contact. It takes 14 to 18 days to come down with mumps. People with mumps are contagious 48 hours before and up to 6 days after swelling begins.

Earliest symptoms before the swelling are feeling sick, no appetite, and often a headache. Then, symptoms include pain and swelling on one or both sides of the neck, in front of the ears at the corner of the jaw; trouble swallowing or talking; fever; and rash.

What Are the Symptoms of Mumps?

Earliest symptoms before the swelling are feeling sick, no appetite, and often a headache. Then, symptoms include pain and swelling on one or both sides of the neck, in front of the ears at the corner of the jaw; trouble swallowing or talking; fever; and rash. Fever is better in 3 or 4 days, and swelling and pain get better in about a week. About half the people don't have symptoms.

Complications can happen, usually in adults. Hearing can be lost temporarily. Organs such as testicles in older boys and men, ovaries or breasts in older girls and women, pancreas, brain, heart, and joints can become swollen and irritated.

How Is Mumps Diagnosed?

The doctor will make a diagnosis from the medical history and physical examination. Tests are also done on a throat swab and blood samples.

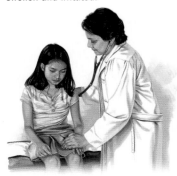

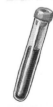

Your doctor will make a diagnosis from your medical history and physical examination. Tests are also done on a throat swab and blood samples.

Recovery usually takes 10 days and gives lifetime immunity to mumps. Take acetaminophen or ibuprofen to help fever and pain.

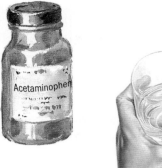

Drink more fluids, but not acidic or sour liquids. Avoid spicy foods or foods that make more saliva or need a lot of chewing.

Stay home to avoid exposing other people to mumps. Rest while you have fever and until strength returns.

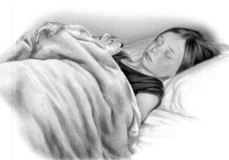

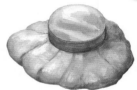

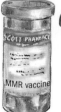

If the testicles are affected, use an ice pack near the testicles to help pain. Wear an athletic supporter.

Children should be vaccinated with the measles, mumps, rubella (MMR) vaccine, which will prevent mumps.

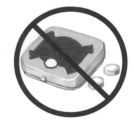

Don't give aspirin to children younger than 16 because of the risk of Reye's syndrome, a dangerous illness.

How Is Mumps Treated?

Recovery usually takes 10 days and gives lifetime immunity to mumps. Acetaminophen or ibuprofen can help reduce fever and pain. Cool compresses to the jaw can also ease pain. Tepid sponge baths can bring high temperature down. Drink more fluids, but not acidic or sour liquids. Avoid spicy foods and foods that make more saliva or need a lot of chewing. Rest until fever disappears and strength returns. Children shouldn't go to school until they're no longer contagious (8 to 9 days after swelling resolves).

DOs and DON'Ts in Managing Mumps:

✔ **DO** drink plenty of fluids (not sour or acidic).

✔ **DO** stay home to avoid exposing other people. Rest while you have fever and until strength returns.

✔ **DO** use an ice pack near the testicles to help pain if the testicles are affected. Wear an athletic supporter.

✔ **DO** use cool compresses on the jaw for discomfort.

✔ **DO** eat a soft diet without spicy irritating foods that may make more saliva or need a lot of chewing.

✔ **DO** call your doctor if you have vomiting, diarrhea, temperature more than 101° F, or severe headache that acetaminophen doesn't help.

✔ **DO** call your doctor if pain or swelling develops in your testicles.

✔ **DO** call your doctor if symptoms aren't better in about 7 days.

🚫 **DON'T** give aspirin to children younger than 16 because of the risk of Reye's syndrome, a dangerous illness.

🚫 **DON'T** send children to school until they're no longer contagious.

FROM THE DESK OF

NOTES

FOR MORE INFORMATION

Contact the following sources:

• Centers for Disease Control and Prevention
Tel: (800) 311-3435
Website: http://www.cdc.gov

• American Academy of Pediatrics
Tel: (847) 434-4000
Website: http://www.aap.org

MANAGING YOUR
NAIL FUNGUS

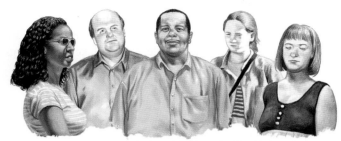

Nail fungus, or onychomycosis, is an infection of nails with fungal organisms, usually those called dermatophytes. More toenails than fingernails are affected. It's more common in people over 65, those with poor circulation, and diabetics.

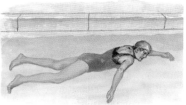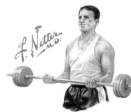

The infection spreads at public swimming pools and locker rooms, where people walk around barefoot. Infection can spread in families by sharing towels or shoes.

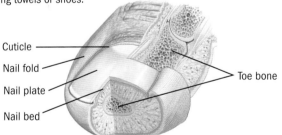

Cuticle

Nail fold

Nail plate

Nail bed

Toe bone

Signs of a fungal infection:

Nails separate from nail bed

Nails become thicker and change shape

Nails become brittle, split, and chip

Nails turn yellow, brown, or white

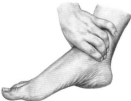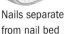

Your doctor makes a diagnosis by examining you nails. A scraping of the nail or nail clippings may be taken and sent to a laboratory for study.

What Is Nail Fungus?

Nail fungus, or onychomycosis, is an infection of nails with fungal organisms. More toenails than fingernails are affected. It's more common in elderly people with poor circulation and diabetics. People often have a fungal foot infection (athlete's foot), along with toenail fungus.

What Causes Nail Fungus?

The most frequent causes are fungi called dermatophytes. People often pick up and spread the infection at public swimming pools and locker rooms, where they walk around barefoot. Conditions there are warm and damp, which are best for fungi to grow.

Fungal infections can also spread in families by sharing towels and footwear. Damage to nails can make it easier to get infected.

What Are the Symptoms of Nail Fungus?

Symptoms include change in nail color to yellow, brown, or white; thicker nails with shape changes; brittle and flaky nails, with splits and chips; accumulation of fungus and dirt under nails, leading to a bad smell; separation of nails from toes or fingers; and, rarely, pain.

How Is Nail Fungus Diagnosed?

The doctor makes a diagnosis from an examination of the nails. A scraping of the nail or nail clippings may be taken and sent to a laboratory for study.

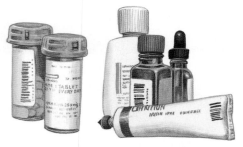

Early treatment is best, but getting rid of the fungus can be hard. Oral antifungal drugs, such as terbinafine, taken for 3 months for toenail fungus are the usual treatment. Topical medicine may also be used. It can take up to 6 months to cure fingernails, 1 year for toenails. Relapse is common.

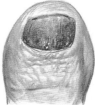

If antifungal treatments don't work, your doctor may want to discuss removing your nail. A podiatrist can do this surgically or with chemicals.

Wash and check your feet daily. Keep your feet dry. Call your doctor if your toes or fingers crack around the nails or become red and tender or if pus drainage, swelling, or redness occurs near nails.

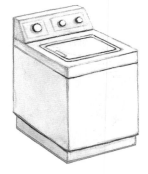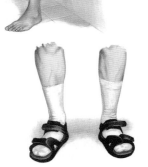

Wear clean socks that absorb moisture. Wash used socks, towels, and bathmats at 150°F or more. Wear shoes that fit well and let air circulate. Don't go barefoot in public places. Wear flip-flops at locker rooms and swimming pools.

How Is Nail Fungus Treated?

Early treatment is best, but getting rid of the fungus may be hard. Untreated, nails may have permanent damage and deformity, leading to problems wearing shoes or walking.

Oral antifungal drugs, such as terbinafine, are taken for 3 months for toenail fungus and 6 weeks for fingernail fungus are the usual treatment. Some people cannot take these drugs because of their other drugs or medical problems.

Antifungal drugs can also be put directly on infected nails (topical treatment) for up to 12 months. These topical drugs don't usually work very well.

Other treatments, not usually done, include removing the infected nail and scraping the nail to make it less thick. Usually, a foot doctor (podiatrist) does these.

DOs and DON'Ts in Managing Nail Fungus:

✔ **DO** follow directions for using your drugs.
✔ **DO** tell your doctor about your other medical problems and drugs.
✔ **DO** wear shoes that fit well and let air circulate.
✔ **DO** wear clean socks that absorb moisture. Wash used socks, towels, and bathmats at 150° F or more.
✔ **DO** go to a podiatrist for nail trimming.
✔ **DO** wash and check your feet daily. Keep your feet dry. Report signs of infection (swelling, drainage) to your doctor.
✔ **DO** call your doctor if your toes or fingers crack around the nails or become red and tender.
✔ **DO** call your doctor if pus drainage, swelling, or redness occurs near nails.
✔ **DO** call your doctor if nails become painful to touch.
✔ **DO** avoid going barefoot in public places, especially gyms, showers, and locker rooms.

⊘ **DON'T** wear shoes for too long if they make your feet sweat a lot.
⊘ **DON'T** use nail polish all the time. It prevents moisture from escaping from your nails.
⊘ **DON'T** share shoes, towels, or nail-trimming instruments.

FROM THE DESK OF

NOTES

FOR MORE INFORMATION

Contact the following source:

• American Academy of Dermatology
  Tel: (847) 330-0230, (866) 503-7546
  Website: http://www.aad.org

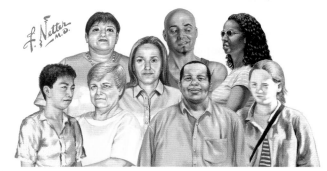

Oral herpes is also called herpes labialis, herpes simplex-1, or HSV-1. Most infections spread by contact during childhood, so 80% of adults have been exposed to HSV-1. HSV-1 is a virus in the family of viruses that cause chickenpox, shingles, cold sores, and mononucleosis.

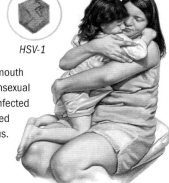

HSV-1

HSV-1 causes blisters around the mouth and gums. It spreads mainly by nonsexual intimate contact with saliva of an infected person, for example, to a child kissed by an adult who's shedding the virus. HSV-1 enters the body through a break in the skin.

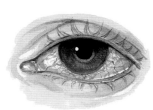

Most people never have symptoms. Those who do can have itching, pain, burning, or tingling before blisters form. Then small blisters start and form ulcers and crusts. Other symptoms are eye pain, red eyes, fatigue, fever, headache, itching, muscle aches, and tearing from the eyes.

Your doctor will make a diagnosis by checking the area for blisters. Doing blood tests for antibodies against HSV and taking fluid from a blister for study are usually not necessary.

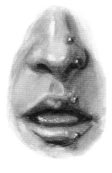

What Is Oral Herpes?

Oral herpes (also called herpes labialis, herpes simplex-1, or HSV-1) leads to blisters around the mouth and gums. This virus is in the family of viruses that causes chickenpox, shingles, cold sores, and mononucleosis. Most infections spread by contact during childhood, so 80% of adults have been exposed to HSV-1. The other HSV, HSV-2, spreads by sexual contact.

These infections cannot be cured.

What Causes Oral Herpes?

The cause, HSV-1, spreads mainly by nonsexual intimate contact with saliva of an infected person, for example, a child kissed by an adult who's shedding the virus but has no symptoms. The virus may enter the body through a break in the skin or through tender skin of the mouth.

What Are the Symptoms of Oral Herpes?

Most people never have symptoms. Blisters, if they appear, occur days or weeks after exposure to the virus. Blisters can return months or years after the initial infection. Some people have blisters once; others get them many times. Itching, pain, burning, or tingling can occur before blisters form. Then small blisters start and form ulcers and crusts. Other symptoms include eye pain (especially to bright light), red eyes, fatigue, fever, headache, itching, muscle aches, tearing from eyes, and tingling.

How Is Oral Herpes Diagnosed?

The doctor will make a diagnosis by examining the area. Blood tests for antibodies against HSV may also be done. The doctor may take fluid from a blister for study if the diagnosis is unclear.

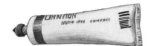
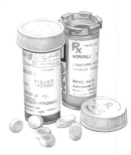

Drugs (acyclovir, valacyclovir, and famciclovir) can help shorten or prevent an attack. Aspirin, acetaminophen, or ibuprofen can help if pain is present.

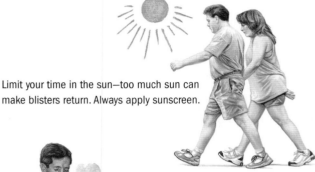

Limit your time in the sun—too much sun can make blisters return. Always apply sunscreen.

Avoid and learn how to deal with physical and emotional stress. Stress can make blisters return.

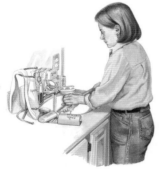

Wash your hands with soap and warm water often, especially after using the bathroom, to avoid spreading the infection.

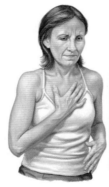

Call your doctor right away, or go to the emergency room, if you have a severe headache, shortness of breath, or eye pain, or bright lights bother you.

FROM THE DESK OF

NOTES

How Is Oral Herpes Treated?

Drugs (acyclovir, valacyclovir, and famciclovir) can help shorten or prevent an attack.

Penciclovir is a topical cream useful for herpes outbreaks. Popular remedies (such as moisturizing or anesthetic lip balms) may not work at all.

Aspirin, acetaminophen, or ibuprofen can help pain.

DOs and DON'Ts in Managing Oral Herpes:

✔ **DO** wash your hands with soap and warm water often, especially after using the bathroom.

✔ **DO** keep blistered skin clean and dry. Avoid shaving the affected area.

✔ **DO** understand that kissing or having oral sex will spread the infection.

✔ **DO** learn to recognize early symptoms (tingling, itching). Starting antiviral drugs early may abort or shorten the duration of an attack.

✔ **DO** avoid sharing personal hygiene items.

✔ **DO** call your doctor if your symptoms get worse, you have a fever, or pus drains from a blister.

✔ **DO** call your doctor right away, or go to the emergency room, if you have a severe headache, shortness of breath, or eye pain, or if bright lights bother you.

✔ **DO** call your doctor for infections that return more than four to six times a year. You may benefit from daily prophylactic therapy.

✔ **DO** avoid and learn how to deal with physical and emotional stress. Stress can weaken your immune system and make blisters return.

✔ **DO** eat healthy foods. Get enough sleep and exercise.

✔ **DO** avoid spending too much time in the sun or getting sunburned. Sun can make blisters return. Always apply sunscreen.

⊘ **DON'T** kiss anyone or share eating utensils or personal care items with others while you have symptoms.

⊘ **DON'T** have oral sex until you and your partner have no symptoms and your blisters are gone.

⊘ **DON'T** touch, rub, or scratch blisters. You can get a bacterial infection.

FOR MORE INFORMATION

Contact the following sources:

- National Herpes Resource Center
  American Social Health Association
  Tel: (800) 227-8922
  Website: http://www.ashastd.org/herpes/herpes_overview.cfm

- American Academy of Dermatology
  Tel: (866) 503-7546
  Website: http://www.aad.org

MANAGING YOUR
ORCHITIS

Orchitis is an inflammation of one or both testes in the scrotum. Most cases go away without complications. Very rarely, sterility can result. Being older than 45 increases chances of having orchitis.

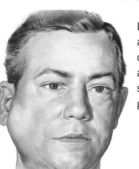

Different factors, including viruses and bacteria, cause orchitis. One common cause is mumps. Others are urinary tract infections, multiple sexual partners, and STDs such as gonorrhea and chlamydia.

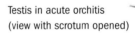

Testis in acute orchitis
(view with scrotum opened)

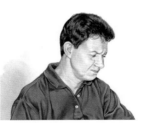

Common symptoms include pain and swelling in the scrotum, nausea, fever, pain when urinating, a heavy feeling on the affected side, scrotum that is tender to touch, and pain with sex.

Your doctor will do a full physical examination and take your medical history. Based on these results, your doctor may take blood and urine samples to test for infection.

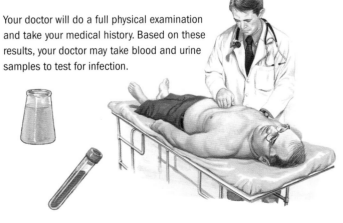

What Is Orchitis?

Orchitis is inflammation (swelling) of one or both testes in the scrotum.

Most cases go away without complications. Very rarely, sterility can result.

What Causes Orchitis?

Different factors, including viruses and bacteria, cause orchitis. One common cause is mumps, the childhood disease that involves swelling of glands that make saliva. However, when teenage boys get the mumps, they can also get orchitis. About 15% to 25% of adults and teenagers who get the mumps also get orchitis.

Urinary tract infections, multiple sexual partners, and sexually transmitted diseases (STDs) such as gonorrhea and chlamydia can also lead to orchitis. Being older than 45 also increases chances of having orchitis.

What Are the Symptoms of Orchitis?

Common symptoms include pain and swelling in the scrotum, nausea, fever, pain when urinating, a heavy feeling on the affected side, scrotum that is tender to touch, and pain with sex. Swelling may last for several weeks after the infection is gone.

How Is Orchitis Diagnosed?

The doctor will do a complete physical examination, take a medical history, and may do tests to check for infection. These tests may include urinalysis, urine culture, and blood tests.

If a discharge is coming from the penis, the doctor may take a sample of the discharge and send it to a laboratory for study. This test may also help find out if an STD is present.

Treatment depends on the cause. A bacterial infection usually responds to antibiotics within 2 to 3 days. If the cause is a virus such as the mumps virus, orchitis will just have to run its course. Antibiotics don't work against viruses. Your doctor may prescribe pain medicine for severe symptoms.

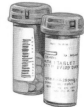

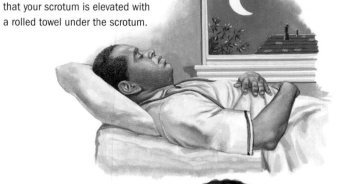

Apply ice packs to your scrotum and wear an athletic supporter to help reduce pain and swelling.

When resting in bed, lie down so that your scrotum is elevated with a rolled towel under the scrotum.

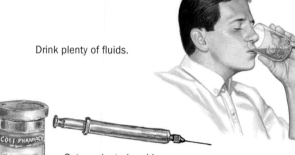

Drink plenty of fluids.

Get vaccinated and have your child vaccinated against mumps. It's given as part of the measles-mumps-rubella (MMR) vaccine.

Always wear condoms to protect yourself against STDs.

How Is Orchitis Treated?

Treatment depends on the cause. A bacterial infection usually responds to antibiotics within 2 to 3 days. If the cause is a virus, such as the mumps virus, orchitis will just have to run its course. Antibiotics don't work against viruses. The worst pain should lessen within a few days, but the doctor may prescribe pain medicine for severe symptoms. Using an athletic supporter and applying cool compresses or ice packs to the affected area may also help with pain.

DOs and DON'Ts in Managing Orchitis:

✔ **DO** apply ice packs to the scrotum to help relieve swelling and pain.

✔ **DO** wear an athletic supporter, which may help with the pain.

✔ **DO** drink plenty of fluids and take over-the-counter medicine for pain relief. If pain is severe, your doctor may prescribe something stronger.

✔ **DO** call your doctor if you have severe pain, high temperature, or trouble urinating.

✔ **DO** use latex condoms to prevent being infected with an STD.

✔ **DO** talk to your doctor if you are prone to getting urinary tract infections.

✔ **DO** get vaccinated and have your child vaccinated against mumps to prevent orchitis from mumps. It's given as part of the measles-mumps-rubella (MMR) vaccine during childhood.

⊘ **DON'T** put pressure on your scrotum while it's swollen.

⊘ **DON'T** have unprotected sex if an STD is suspected. Use a condom if you think there's any chance of catching an STD.

FROM THE DESK OF

NOTES

FOR MORE INFORMATION

Contact the following source:

• American Urological Association
Tel: (866) 746-4282
Website: http://www.auanet.org

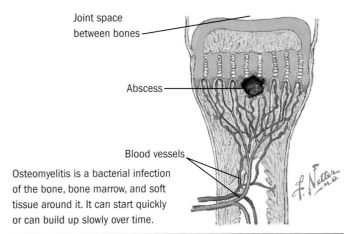

Joint space between bones

Abscess

Blood vessels

Osteomyelitis is a bacterial infection of the bone, bone marrow, and soft tissue around it. It can start quickly or can build up slowly over time.

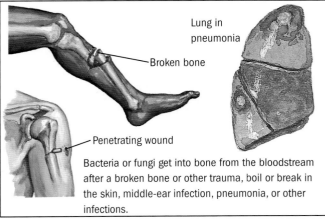

Lung in pneumonia

Broken bone

Penetrating wound

Bacteria or fungi get into bone from the bloodstream after a broken bone or other trauma, boil or break in the skin, middle-ear infection, pneumonia, or other infections.

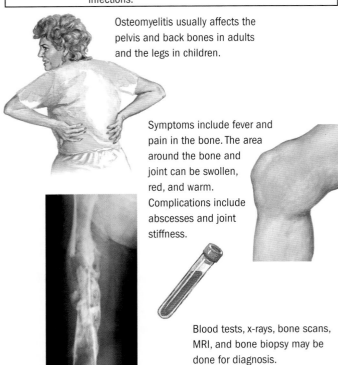

Osteomyelitis usually affects the pelvis and back bones in adults and the legs in children.

Symptoms include fever and pain in the bone. The area around the bone and joint can be swollen, red, and warm. Complications include abscesses and joint stiffness.

Blood tests, x-rays, bone scans, MRI, and bone biopsy may be done for diagnosis.

What Is Osteomyelitis?

Osteomyelitis is a bacterial infection of the bone, bone marrow, and soft tissue around the bone. Bacteria get into bone from the bloodstream after a broken bone or other trauma, boil or break in the skin, middle ear infection, pneumonia, or other infections.

Osteomyelitis can start quickly and be very painful, or it can build slowly and cause less pain. People are more likely to get osteomyelitis if they have diabetes, are having dialysis, or inject drugs into the body.

What Causes Osteomyelitis?

Microorganisms such as bacteria and fungi can cause the infection. The infection usually starts somewhere else in the body and moves through the blood to end up in bone.

What Are the Symptoms of Osteomyelitis?

Symptoms include high temperature and pain in the bone. The area around the bone and nearby joint can be swollen, red, and warm. Other symptoms are feeling sick, nausea, sweating, and chills. Complications include an abscess that won't heal until the bone heals and permanent joint stiffness.

How Is Osteomyelitis Diagnosed?

The doctor will do blood tests to check white blood cells for infection and look for bacteria or fungi causing the infection.

Other tests are x-rays of the bone, magnetic resonance imaging (MRI) or bone scan to find infected bone, and bone biopsy. In a biopsy, a needle is used to get a sample of bone for study.

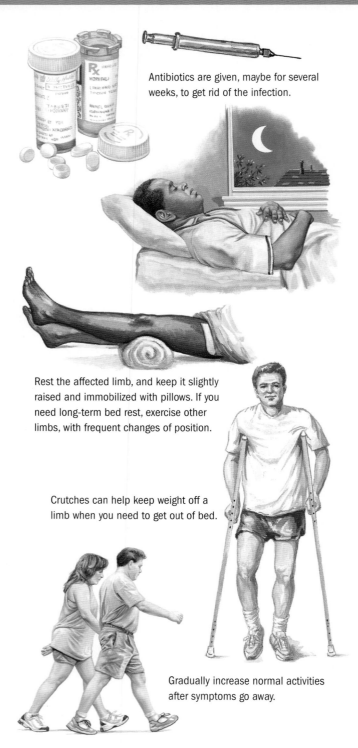

Antibiotics are given, maybe for several weeks, to get rid of the infection.

Rest the affected limb, and keep it slightly raised and immobilized with pillows. If you need long-term bed rest, exercise other limbs, with frequent changes of position.

Crutches can help keep weight off a limb when you need to get out of bed.

Gradually increase normal activities after symptoms go away.

How Is Osteomyelitis Treated?

Osteomyelitis can be cured with medicine. Antibiotics are given, maybe for several weeks, to get rid of infection.

A hospital stay may be needed to drain an abscess or give high doses of intravenous antibiotics. Pain relievers may be needed.

The affected limb should be rested, kept slightly raised, and immobilized with pillows. A lower limb shouldn't bear weight. If long bed rest is needed, other limbs should be exercised, with frequent changes of position.

In people with long-term infection, the bone may die. A surgeon will remove dead bone.

DOs and DON'Ts in Managing Osteomyelitis:

✔ **DO** take the full course of antibiotics.
✔ **DO** change position in bed often to prevent pressure sores. Check skin for redness at pressure points.
✔ **DO** isometric exercises often to prevent muscle weakness and maintain joint flexibility.
✔ **DO** increase normal activities slowly after symptoms go away.
✔ **DO** use sterile dressings if you have an open wound. Wash hands before and after changing dressings.
✔ **DO** call your doctor if fever increases during treatment.
✔ **DO** call your doctor if pain becomes intolerable.
✔ **DO** call your doctor if a new abscess forms or drainage increases from an old abscess.
✔ **DO** see your doctor if you have symptoms of an infection anywhere in your body. This is very important if you had a recent injury, have diabetes, are having dialysis, or inject drugs.

⊘ **DON'T** stop taking antibiotics or change your dosage because you feel better. If you stop too soon, infection can return.
⊘ **DON'T** dangle the affected limb. Keep it slightly raised.
⊘ **DON'T** put weight on an affected leg. Crutches may help for trips to the bathroom.

FROM THE DESK OF

NOTES

FOR MORE INFORMATION

Contact the following source:

• National Institute of Arthritis and Musculoskeletal and Skin Diseases
Tel: (877) 226-4267
Website: http://www.niams.nih.gov

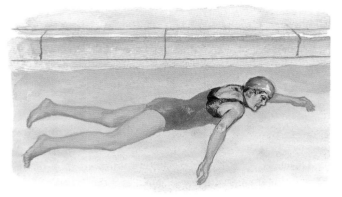

Otitis externa, called swimmer's ear, is an infection of the ear canal. Swimming in contaminated water or water that has insufficient chlorine can lead to swimmer's ear.

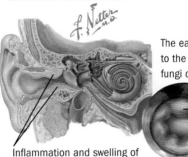

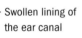

The ear canal goes from the eardrum to the outside of the ear. Bacteria or fungi can infect the ear canal.

Swollen lining of the ear canal

Inflammation and swelling of the walls in the ear canal

Symptoms include ear pain that gets worse when pulling on the ear or pushing on the little bump (tragus) in front of the ear, or itching in the ear.

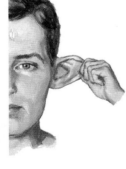

Tragus

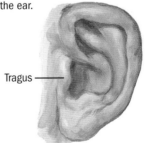

Your doctor will examine your ear to make a diagnosis.

What Is Otitis Externa?

Otitis externa, or swimmer's ear, is an infection of the delicate skin lining the ear canal. The ear canal goes from the eardrum to the outside of the ear.

People with diabetes mellitus or skin allergies and those whose ears don't make enough wax can also get this infection.

It usually lasts 7 to 10 days with treatment.

What Causes Otitis Externa?

The cause is bacteria or fungi that infect the lining of the ear canal. The infection can start after swimming in dirty water or in pools treated with insufficient chlorine or after having too much water in the ear for any reason. Inflammation (swelling) caused by an allergy to hair spray can also cause otitis externa, as can regular use of earphones, which can trap moisture in the ear canal. Sometimes injury to the ear canal, as from cleaning the ear too hard with a bobby pin, cotton swab, or other object, will cause the disorder. Such cleaning can push earwax and dirt back toward the eardrum. This material can trap water and lead to infection.

What Are the Symptoms of Otitis Externa?

Symptoms include ear pain that gets worse when pulling on the earlobe or outer ear or pushing on the little bump (tragus) in front of the ear, itching in the ear, slight fever (sometimes), pus coming from the ear, temporary loss of hearing in the ear, and sometimes a small painful lump or boil in the ear canal. These boils may cause severe pain. If they burst, a small amount of blood or pus may leak from the ear.

How Is Otitis Externa Diagnosed?

The doctor will examine the ear and in cases of severe or recurrent infection may take a sample of the fluid from inside the ear for study. The doctor may also suggest seeing an otolaryngologist, a doctor who specializes in diseases of the ears, nose, and throat.

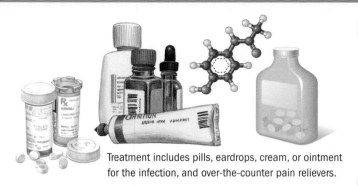

Treatment includes pills, eardrops, cream, or ointment for the infection, and over-the-counter pain relievers.

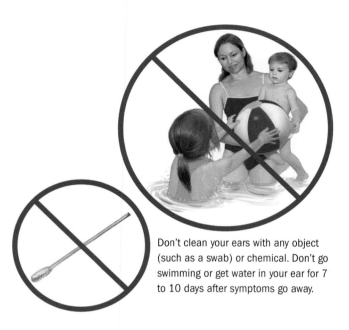

Don't clean your ears with any object (such as a swab) or chemical. Don't go swimming or get water in your ear for 7 to 10 days after symptoms go away.

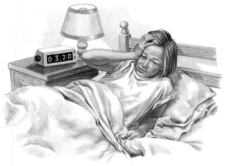

Call your doctor if pain continues after treatment starts.

How Is Otitis Externa Treated?

Treatment involves medicine as pills, eardrops, cream, or ointment for the infection. Over-the-counter medicine, such as aspirin or acetaminophen, and warm compresses may help with minor pain.

The ear canal shouldn't get wet for 7 to 10 days after all symptoms go away.

DOs and DON'Ts in Managing Otitis Externa:

✔ **DO** keep water out of your ear. Wear earplugs or a shower cap when showering.

✔ **DO** call your doctor if pain continues in spite of treatment or if your ears feel clogged, as if they need cleaning.

✔ **DO** use eardrops as directed.

✔ **DO** call your doctor if pain becomes severe and isn't helped by nonprescription drugs.

✔ **DO** call your doctor if you get a high temperature after treatment starts.

⊘ **DON'T** clean your ears with any object or chemical.

⊘ **DON'T** leave earplugs in too long.

⊘ **DON'T** use hairspray or hair dye near your ears.

⊘ **DON'T** go swimming or get any water in your ear for 7 to 10 days after symptoms go away.

FROM THE DESK OF

NOTES

FOR MORE INFORMATION

Contact the following source:

• American Academy of Otolaryngology
Tel: (703) 836-4444
Website: http://www.entnet.org

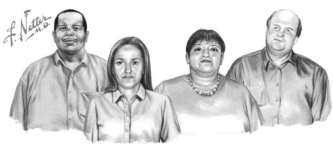

Thrombophlebitis (or phlebitis) is inflammation of a vein. When this happens, the blood circulation in that area becomes slow, and small blood clots can form in the vein. Leg veins are affected more often than arm or neck veins. The major danger is that clots can travel to veins deeper in the body and can cause larger clots to form DVT, which is very serious.

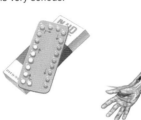

The usual cause is infection or injury to a vein. It happens most often in veins just under the skin after blood is taken for a blood test or intravenous medicine is injected. Other risk factors include having cancer, varicose veins, blood clotting disorders, being inactive for a long time (such as sitting in a car or an airplane), smoking, being pregnant, using birth control pills, and being overweight.

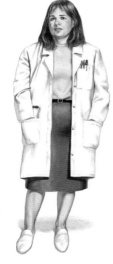

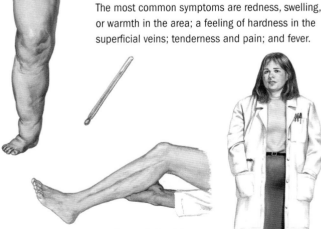

The most common symptoms are redness, swelling, or warmth in the area; a feeling of hardness in the superficial veins; tenderness and pain; and fever.

Your doctor will make a diagnosis by doing a physical examination that finds swelling and redness in the area and by noting symptoms. If clots in the deep veins may be present, the doctor may order ultrasonography.

What Is Thrombophlebitis?

Thrombophlebitis (or phlebitis) is inflammation of a vein. When this happens, the blood circulation in that area becomes slow and small blood clots (thrombi) can form in the vein. It happens most often in veins just under the skin after blood is taken for a blood test or intravenous medicine is injected. Inflammation of the vein and these small clots can cause pain, redness, and swelling of the affected arm or leg. Leg veins are affected more often than arm or neck veins.

Thrombophlebitis near the surface of the skin is called superficial thrombophlebitis. It's not life-threatening. The major danger from thrombophlebitis is that clots can travel to veins deeper in the body. These can cause larger clots to form (thrombosis) in the deep veins (called deep vein thrombosis, or DVT). DVT is a very serious condition because blood clots from the deep veins are likely to break off and go to the lungs. They can cause a life-threatening condition called pulmonary embolism.

What Causes Thrombophlebitis?

The usual cause is infection or injury to a vein from trauma. Other risk factors include having varicose veins in the legs, being inactive for a long time (such as sitting in a car or an airplane), smoking, being pregnant, using birth control pills, and being overweight. People with blood clotting abnormalities and those with cancer are also at increased risk for thrombophlebitis.

What Are the Symptoms of Thrombophlebitis?

The most common symptoms are redness, swelling, or warmth in the area; a feeling of hardness in the superficial veins of the leg or arms; tenderness and pain in the affected area; and fever.

How Is Thrombophlebitis Diagnosed?

The doctor will make a diagnosis by doing a physical examination that finds swelling and redness in the area and by noting the symptoms. If the doctor thinks that clots in the deep veins are present, the doctor may order ultrasonography to find them. Ultrasonography uses sound waves to see inside the vein and is painless and harmless. A blood test called D-dimer may also be done to check for DVT. This test isn't specific for thrombophlebitis.

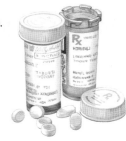

Treatment of superficial thrombophlebitis involves rest and raising the affected limb. A warm compress may also be used. Antiinflammatory medicine may help control the pain and reduce the inflammation. Antibiotics will be prescribed for an infection.

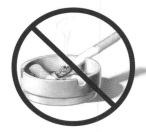

Stop smoking. Smoking increases your chance of having blood clots.

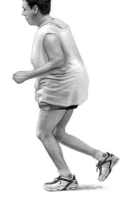

If you're overweight, lose weight. This will help your blood circulation and overall health.

Get up to walk around or stretch your legs if you take long car or plane trips.

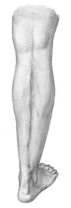

Call your doctor right away if you have redness, swelling, and pain in your leg. You could have DVT.

How Is Thrombophlebitis Treated?

Treatment of superficial thrombophlebitis involves rest and raising the affected limb. A warm compress may also be used. Prescription support stockings may be used to prevent DVT. The doctor may also prescribe antiinflammatory medicine to help control the pain and reduce the inflammation. Antibiotics will be prescribed for an infection.

People with thrombophlebitis usually feel better with treatment in 7 to 10 days.

DOs and DON'Ts in Managing Thrombophlebitis:

✔ **DO** stop smoking.
✔ **DO** lose weight if you are overweight or obese.
✔ **DO** call your doctor right away if you have redness, swelling, and pain in your leg.
✔ **DO** get up to walk around or stretch your legs if you take long car or plane trips.

⊘ **DON'T** wear garters or knee-high stockings that might squeeze your veins and slow the blood flow in them.
⊘ **DON'T** sit or stand for long periods without moving your legs.

FROM THE DESK OF

NOTES

FOR MORE INFORMATION

Contact the following source:

• National Heart, Lung, and Blood Institute
  Tel: (301) 592-8573
  Website: http://www.nhlbi.nih.gov

CARING FOR YOUR CHILD WITH
PINWORMS

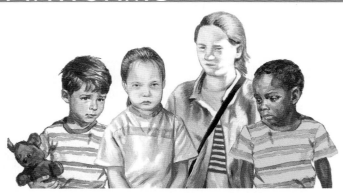

Pinworms are tiny worms that cause a common intestinal infection. It's often found in children 5 to 14 years old.

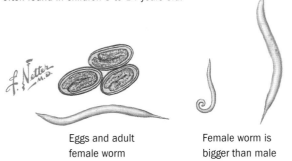

Eggs and adult female worm	Female worm is bigger than male

Children get pinworms by eating or drinking contaminated food and beverages. Eggs get passed to others when children touch their anus and then touch something else.

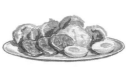

Food and water can become contaminated with eggs.

Baby worms hatch from eggs and grow in intestines.

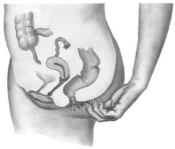

Itching around the anus or buttocks (especially at night) is the most common symptom. Scratching lets worms and eggs get on fingers and under nails.

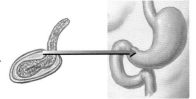

Diagnosis can involve using a piece of transparent adhesive tape on the anus to get worms that are then looked at with a microscope.

What Are Pinworms?

Pinworms are tiny worms that cause a common intestinal infection. It's often found in children 5 to 14 years old. Crowded living conditions increase chances of spread to family members. It is usually more a nuisance than a major health problem.

People get the worms by eating contaminated food or drinking contaminated beverages. Eggs hatch and baby worms grow in the intestine. Female worms travel to the anal area to lay more eggs. Eggs get to other people by direct contact.

What Causes Pinworms?

Worms named *Enterobius vermicularis*, about the length of a staple, usually spread when children touch their hands and anus and then touch something else.

What Are the Symptoms of Pinworms?

Itching around the anus or buttocks (especially at night) is the most common symptom. Others include irritated skin around the anus, restlessness in infants, trouble sleeping, and itching in the area of the vagina.

How Are Pinworms Diagnosed?

The doctor will take a medical history and do an examination. Because worms usually move around at night, the best time to check for worms is a couple of hours after children go to sleep and right after children wake in the morning. Parents can use a flashlight to better see the worms. A piece of transparent adhesive tape placed on the anus can get some worms that are then looked at with a microscope.

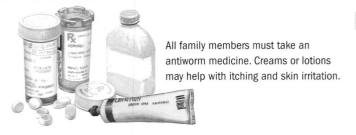

All family members must take an antiworm medicine. Creams or lotions may help with itching and skin irritation.

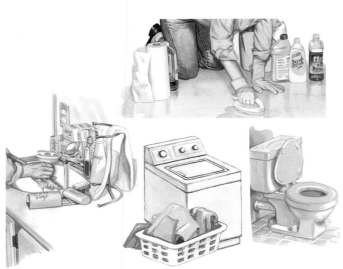

All eggs must be destroyed. To do this, cleaning everything—hands, fingernails, clothing, bedding, bathrooms, dishes, eating utensils—is important.

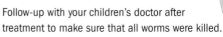

Follow-up with your children's doctor after treatment to make sure that all worms were killed.

How Are Pinworms Treated?

All family members will take an antiworm medicine. Creams or lotions may help with itching and irritation. Worms are killed in a couple of days, and itching should stop in 1 week.

All eggs must be destroyed. To do this, family members should wash hands and clean fingernails often. They should shower daily and wash the anal area carefully. Hands should be kept away from mouths. Hot water should be used to wash dishes, eating utensils, clothing, bedding, and towels. The house (especially toilet bowls, bathrooms, and bedrooms) and children's toys should be cleaned with a disinfectant.

DOs and DON'Ts in Managing Pinworms:

✔ **DO** tell your children's doctor about other medical problems and medicines.

✔ **DO** call your children's doctor if itching doesn't get better after 1 week.

✔ **DO** have your children take medicine as directed.

✔ **DO** teach children good hand-washing methods with soap after toileting and before eating.

✔ **DO** tell the school nurse or day care about the pinworms.

✔ **DO** keep your children's fingernails clean and short.

✔ **DO** bathe your children and change underwear and bed linens daily.

✔ **DO** use very hot water to wash dishes, scrub all washable toys with a bleach solution, and scrub toilets thoroughly.

✔ **DO** follow-up with your children's doctor after treatment to make sure all worms were killed.

✔ **DO** call your children's doctor if anyone has symptoms again after treatment or side effects from medicines that don't go away quickly.

🚫 **DON'T** let your children scratch their anal area, suck their fingers, or bite their nails.

🚫 **DON'T** let other children play or sleep over until treatment is over.

FROM THE DESK OF

NOTES

FOR MORE INFORMATION

Contact the following sources:

• National Center for Preparedness, Detection, and Control of Infectious Diseases
Tel: (800) 311-3435
Website: http://www.cdc.gov/ncpdcid/

• National Institute of Allergy and Infectious Diseases
Tel: (301) 496-5717, (866) 284-4107
Website: http://www3.niaid.nih.gov/

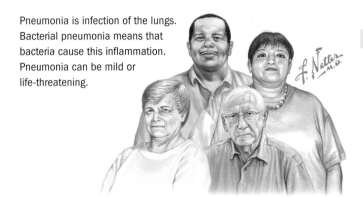

Pneumonia is infection of the lungs. Bacterial pneumonia means that bacteria cause this inflammation. Pneumonia can be mild or life-threatening.

What Is Bacterial Pneumonia?

Pneumonia is infection of the lungs. Bacterial pneumonia means that bacteria cause this infection. Bacteria get to lungs by breathing or by the bloodstream. Pneumonia can be mild or life-threatening.

Certain conditions may weaken the body's defense system and increase chances of getting bacterial pneumonia. These conditions include older age, smoking, drinking alcohol in excess, lung disease, congestive heart failure, diabetes, kidney failure, HIV infection, drugs such as anticancer agents and prednisone, and viral respiratory infections. Healthy people of all ages can also get pneumonia.

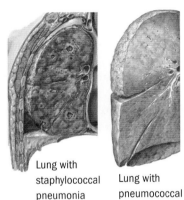

Lung with staphylococcal pneumonia

Lung with pneumococcal pneumonia

Bacteria enter the body by the bloodstream or by breathing. Bacteria that cause pneumonia include *Streptococcus, Mycoplasma, Staphylococcus, Haemophilus, Legionella,* and other bacteria found in the intestines and mouth.

What Causes Bacterial Pneumonia?

Common types of bacteria that cause pneumonia include *Streptococcus, Mycoplasma, Staphylococcus, Haemophilus, Legionella,* and bacteria normally found in the intestines and mouth.

Shortness of breath, pain when breathing, fever, chills, cough, and yellow or green phlegm are symptoms. Others are headache, muscle and body pain, and tiredness.

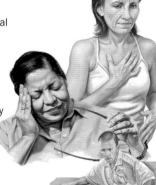

What Are the Symptoms of Bacterial Pneumonia?

Symptoms include chest pain, chills, confusion, cough, fever, headache, and muscle and body pain. Others are pain with breathing, yellow or green phlegm (more than usual, sometimes with blood), shortness of breath, sweating, and tiredness. People with severe pneumonia have rapid breathing, low blood pressure, temperature higher than 102° F, and confusion. Some people, such as the very old, may have few symptoms.

How Is Bacterial Pneumonia Diagnosed?

The doctor will take a medical history and do an examination. The doctor will order chest x-rays and sputum and blood tests, to find out which bacteria are causing pneumonia.

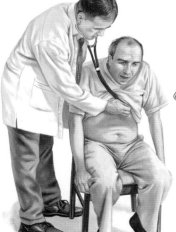

To find out the type and severity of your pneumonia, your doctor will examine you and order blood and sputum tests and chest x-rays.

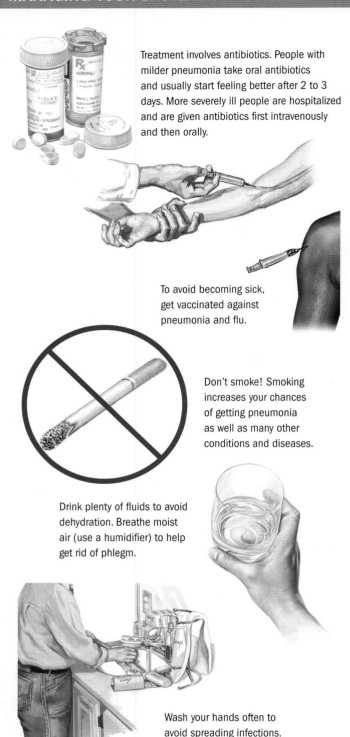

Treatment involves antibiotics. People with milder pneumonia take oral antibiotics and usually start feeling better after 2 to 3 days. More severely ill people are hospitalized and are given antibiotics first intravenously and then orally.

To avoid becoming sick, get vaccinated against pneumonia and flu.

Don't smoke! Smoking increases your chances of getting pneumonia as well as many other conditions and diseases.

Drink plenty of fluids to avoid dehydration. Breathe moist air (use a humidifier) to help get rid of phlegm.

Wash your hands often to avoid spreading infections.

FROM THE DESK OF

How Is Bacterial Pneumonia Treated?

Treatment involves antibiotics. People with milder pneumonia take oral antibiotics and usually start feeling better after 2 to 3 days. Most recover after 7 to 10 days. More severely ill people are hospitalized and are first given antibiotics intravenously. They may get oxygen and have special treatment to help clear phlegm. They may need mechanical ventilation in an intensive care unit. After they improve, they take oral antibiotics. People infected with certain types of bacteria or with chronic medical conditions may need antibiotics for 14 to 21 days or longer.

DOs and DON'Ts in Managing Bacterial Pneumonia:

✔ **DO** get pneumonia and flu shots.
✔ **DO** tell your doctor about medicines you take (prescription and over-the-counter).
✔ **DO** call your doctor if you're getting worse or don't feel better after 2 to 3 days.
✔ **DO** tell your doctor if you're pregnant or taking birth control pills.
✔ **DO** call your doctor right away or go to the emergency room if shortness of breath becomes worse.
✔ **DO** try to cough up as much phlegm as possible.
✔ **DO** wash your hands often, to avoid spreading infection.
✔ **DO** take antibiotics exactly as prescribed, until they're gone.
✔ **DO** use acetaminophen or aspirin (except in children) to reduce fever and pain.
✔ **DO** drink plenty of fluids to avoid dehydration.
✔ **DO** breathe moist air (use a humidifier) to help get rid of phlegm.
✔ **DO** call your doctor if you have fever, green or yellow sputum, increased shortness of breath, chest pain, or dusky-colored skin, lips, or fingernails.
✔ **DO** avoid air pollution and smoke, especially if you have lung problems.

⊘ **DON'T** stop taking your medicine just because you feel better.
⊘ **DON'T** smoke.
⊘ **DON'T** drink alcohol in excess.

FOR MORE INFORMATION

Contact the following source:

• American Lung Association
  Tel: (212) 315-8700, (800) 586-4872
  Website: http://www.lungusa.org

MANAGING YOUR
MYCOPLASMA PNEUMONIA

Pneumonia is an infection of the lungs. This pneumonia usually affects people younger than 40, most often those 5 to 20 years old. People may not be sick enough to go to the doctor or to stay in bed, so it's often called walking pneumonia. People may never even know that they had pneumonia.

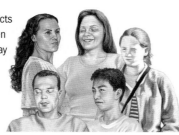

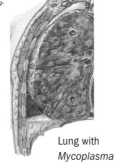

Mycoplasma pneumonia is caused by the kind of bacteria named *Mycoplasma pneumoniae.*

Lung with *Mycoplasma* pneumonia

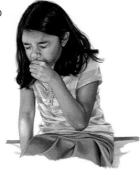

The infection is passed from person to person when someone who's infected coughs and the other person breathes in contaminated droplets.

Symptoms are mild and usually start 2 to 3 weeks after exposure. A dry, persistent cough is the most common symptom. Fever, headaches, chills, sweating, chest pain, and sore throat also occur.

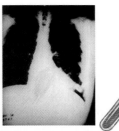

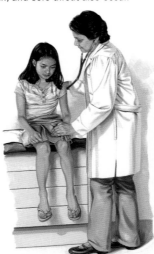

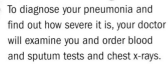

To diagnose your pneumonia and find out how severe it is, your doctor will examine you and order blood and sputum tests and chest x-rays.

What Is Mycoplasma Pneumonia?

Pneumonia is an infecton of the lungs. People of all ages can get this kind of pneumonia, but it usually affects people younger than 40, most often those who are 5 to 20 years old. People may not be sick enough to stay in bed or go to the doctor, and they may never even know that they had pneumonia. It's often called walking pneumonia. These infections occur throughout the year but are seen slightly more often during winter.

What Causes Mycoplasma Pneumonia?

Infection occurs after breathing in airborne droplets that someone who is infected cough into the air. These droplets are contaminated with the kind of bacteria named *Mycoplasma pneumoniae,* the cause of this pneumonia. *Mycoplasma* infections often spread quickly when people live or work in close quarters, such as within families or schools.

What Are the Symptoms of Mycoplasma Pneumonia?

Symptoms are mild and usually start 2 to 3 weeks after exposure to the bacteria. A dry, persistent cough is the most common symptom. Fever, headaches, chills, sweating, chest pain, and sore throat also occur. Exposure to *Mycoplasma* may also cause ear and throat infections.

How Is Mycoplasma Pneumonia Diagnosed?

The doctor will make a diagnosis from the medical history and physical examination. The doctor will order tests to find out how severe the pneumonia is. These tests include chest x-rays and blood and sputum tests. People who are in the emergency department of a hospital will have their blood oxygen level measured.

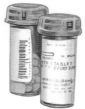

Oral antibiotics are given, usually for 5 to 14 days, to treat the infection.

Drink plenty of fluids. Rest and a high-protein diet are also important for recovery.

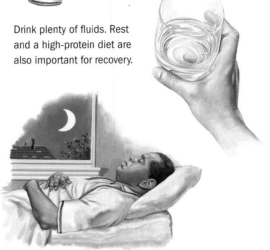

Avoid contact with anyone who has a chronic medical condition such as diabetes or heart disease. They can become very sick if they get *Mycoplasma* pneumonia.

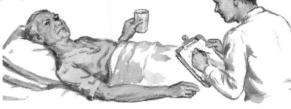

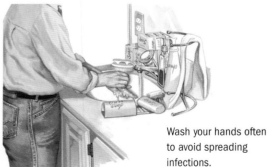

Wash your hands often to avoid spreading infections.

How Is Mycoplasma Pneumonia Treated?

Oral antibiotics are given, usually for 5 to 14 days, to treat the infection. Improvement usually begins within 1 or 2 days of starting antibiotics, but the cough may last for weeks. Nasal sprays and oral decongestants are often used for nasal symptoms. Rest, a high-protein diet, and drinking enough fluids are important for recovery.

DOs and DON'Ts in Managing Mycoplasma Pneumonia:

✔ **DO** take your antibiotic medicine exactly as the doctor prescribed. Take the pills as scheduled until they are all gone.

✔ **DO** use acetaminophen or aspirin (except in children) for relief of fever and pain.

✔ **DO** drink plenty of fluids to avoid dehydration.

✔ **DO** breathe moist air (use a humidifier) to help get rid of phlegm.

✔ **DO** call your doctor if you suspect *Mycoplasma* pneumonia because of a sense of being sick, fever, shortness of breath, or phlegm.

✔ **DO** call your doctor if your symptoms fail to go away or they get worse after 48 hours of antibiotic therapy.

✔ **DO** call your doctor if nausea prevents you from taking your prescribed antibiotics.

✔ **DO** call your doctor if you see blood in your sputum.

🚫 **DON'T** spend time with people who have chronic medical conditions if you are sick. They can become very sick if they get *Mycoplasma* pneumonia.

FROM THE DESK OF

NOTES

FOR MORE INFORMATION

Contact the following source:

• American Lung Association
Tel: (800) LUNG-USA (586-4872)
Website: http://www.lungusa.org

Pneumonia is an infection of the lungs. Pneumocystis pneumonia is a serious, possibly life-threatening illness. Survival is lower for people with severe immune system problems such as AIDS. This pneumonia can come back after treatment if preventive drugs aren't used.

Microscopic slide of lung tissue showing the fungus (black dots).

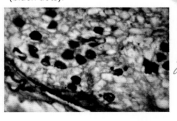

Pneumocystis jiroveci is a fungus that usually causes pneumonia in people with weak immune systems, such as those with HIV infection and those getting cancer chemotherapy, long-term prednisone therapy, or drugs to stop transplant rejection.

The most common symptoms are shortness of breath, dry cough, and fever.

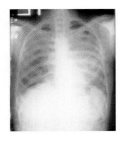

Your doctor will take chest x-rays and do blood tests to diagnose your pneumonia. Special tests include sputum tests for *Pneumocystis* and bronchoscopy.

For bronchoscopy, your doctor looks at your lungs with a lighted tube passed through your nose or mouth. Lung fluids are collected and biopsy samples may be taken.

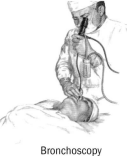

Biopsy

Bronchoscopy

What Is Pneumocystis Pneumonia?

Pneumonia is an infection of the lungs. Pneumocystis pneumonia is a serious, possibly life-threatening illness. More than half of people survive if treated, but survival is lower for people with severe immune (infection-fighting) system problems. Pneumocystis pneumonia can come back after treatment if preventive drugs aren't used.

What Causes Pneumocystis Pneumonia?

Pneumocystis jiroveci (formerly called *Pneumocystis carinii*) is a fungus that usually causes pneumonia in people with weak immune systems. Such people include those with human immunodeficiency virus (HIV) infection and those getting cancer chemotherapy, long-term prednisone therapy, or drugs to stop transplant rejection. It's unclear how this pneumonia develops. The fungus may spread person to person. It may also be inactive for years and then become active when the immune system is weak.

What Are the Symptoms of Pneumocystis Pneumonia?

Symptoms usually start slowly and become worse over time. The most common symptoms are shortness of breath, dry cough, and fever. Others are weight loss, chest discomfort, and chills.

How Is Pneumocystis Pneumonia Diagnosed?

The doctor uses chest x-rays and blood tests to decide the severity of the illness. Special tests may be needed, including sputum tests for *Pneumocystis* and bronchoscopy. For bronchoscopy, the doctor looks at the lungs with a lighted tube passed through the nose or mouth. Lung fluids are collected and biopsy samples may be taken.

The drug combination trimethoprim/sulfamethoxazole (TMP/SMX) is usually the first drug tried, given orally or intravenously.

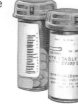

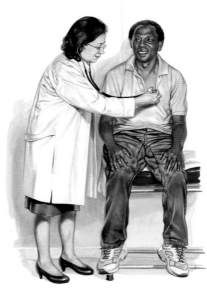

Severely ill patients are hospitalized for supportive treatments such as supplemental oxygen and possibly mechanical ventilation in an intensive care unit.

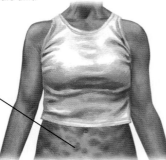

Call your doctor if you get a rash. It may be an allergic reaction to your drug treatment.

People at risk of getting pneumocystis pneumonia should have preventive treatment, such as oral TMP/SMX. If you have a condition affecting your immune system, talk to your doctor about this treatment.

How Is Pneumocystis Pneumonia Treated?

The combination trimethoprim/sulfamethoxazole (TMP/SMX) is usually the first drug tried. It's given orally or intravenously. Other drugs include pentamidine, for those allergic to sulfa or who don't get better with TMP/SMX. Therapy is usually given for up to 21 days. Steroids are used in severe cases to help reduce lung inflammation.

Severely ill patients are hospitalized for supportive treatments such as supplemental oxygen and mechanical ventilation in an intensive care unit. The most common side effects include rash, nausea, fever, and low white blood cell counts.

Oral TMP/SMX is effective for preventing this pneumonia. It can be given as one tablet three times per week or daily. People who are HIV-positive, have low CD4 counts, had previous pneumocystis pneumonia, or are using steroids or other immunosuppressant drugs should receive this preventive therapy.

Prognosis is worse for people with lung disease, with pneumothorax, needing mechanical ventilation, and when diagnosis and treatment are delayed.

DOs and DON'Ts in Managing Pneumocystis Pneumonia:

✔ **DO** take your prescription medicines exactly as prescribed. Finish all the antibiotics.

✔ **DO** use nonprescription cough suppressants as needed.

✔ **DO** use acetaminophen or aspirin (except in children) for fever and pain.

✔ **DO** see your doctor regularly to check your immune system if you're HIV-positive.

✔ **DO** call your doctor if you think that you have pneumonia because of a fever, cough, or shortness of breath.

✔ **DO** call your doctor if your symptoms get worse even with therapy.

✔ **DO** call your doctor if you get a rash (may mean a drug allergy).

✔ **DO** call your doctor if you cannot take your prescribed medicines because of nausea.

⊘ **DON'T** smoke!

⊘ **DON'T** stop taking your antibiotics just because you feel

FROM THE DESK OF

NOTES

FOR MORE INFORMATION

Contact the following source:

• American Lung Association
  Tel: (800) LUNG-USA (586-4872)
  Website: http://www.lungusa.org

MANAGING YOUR
VIRAL PNEUMONIA

Pneumonia is an infection of the lungs. With viral pneumonia, infection is caused by viruses. People of any age can be affected. Smokers, elderly people, and people with chronic lung diseases may be most likely to get it.

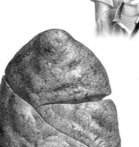

Lung with viral pneumonia

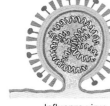

Influenza virus

The usual causes include influenza virus, respiratory syncytial virus, adenovirus, parainfluenza virus, and varicella virus.

Common symptoms include fever, chills, cough, shortness of breath, chest discomfort, muscle aches, tiredness, and poor appetite. Runny nose, irritated eyes, sore throat, and rashes may also occur.

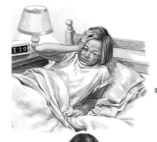

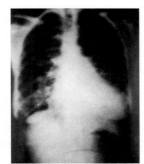

It's hard to tell whether a virus, and which virus, is causing pneumonia. Your doctor usually diagnoses pneumonia by using chest examinations, x-rays, and maybe blood and respiratory secretion tests.

What Is Viral Pneumonia?

Pneumonia is an infection of the lungs. In viral pneumonia, infection is caused by viruses. People of any age can be affected. Smokers, elderly people, and people with chronic lung diseases may be most likely to get it. People with weak immune (infection-fighting) systems because of chemotherapy or drug treatment after organ transplantation are especially at risk of getting cytomegalovirus pneumonia.

Bacterial pneumonias can follow viral pneumonias, especially those caused by influenza virus, because viruses can weaken lung defenses.

What Causes Viral Pneumonia?

Viral infections start after contaminated droplets from someone with an infection are breathed in. Virus can also be directly transferred to the nose, mouth, or eyes by hands that touched something contaminated with virus. The usual causes include influenza virus, respiratory syncytial virus, adenovirus, parainfluenza virus, and varicella virus.

What Are the Symptoms of Viral Pneumonia?

Usual symptoms include fever, chills, cough, shortness of breath, chest discomfort, muscle aches, tiredness, and poor appetite. Runny nose, irritated eyes, sore throat, and symptoms outside the respiratory tract (such as rashes) may occur.

How Is Viral Pneumonia Diagnosed?

It's hard to tell whether a virus, and which virus, is causing pneumonia. Many viruses produce similar symptoms, and few specific diagnostic tests exist. The doctor usually diagnoses pneumonia by using chest examinations, x-rays, and maybe tests of blood and respiratory secretions. Studies of blood and sputum are usually done to make sure a bacterial infection isn't also present.

Antiviral drugs may be prescribed, depending on which virus is the cause and how severe symptoms are. Acetaminophen can help reduce fever and pain.

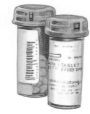

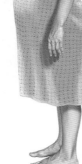

Call your doctor if nausea or vomiting stops you from taking your medicines or makes you dehydrated.

Tell your doctor if you're pregnant or taking birth control pills.

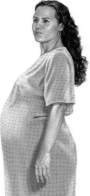

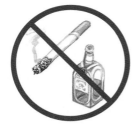

Drink plenty of fluids so you don't get dehydrated. Breathe moist air (use a humidifier) to help get rid of phlegm.

Don't smoke! Smoking increases your chances of getting pneumonia and many other conditions and diseases. Also don't drink alcohol in excess.

How Is Viral Pneumonia Treated?

Antiviral drugs may be prescribed, depending on the virus and how severe symptoms are.

Viral pneumonia in healthy people goes away in 1 to 2 weeks, but cough and fatigue may last for many weeks. Viral pneumonia can be serious and life-threatening in people with other medical illnesses.

DOs and DON'Ts in Managing Viral Pneumonia:

✔ **DO** tell your doctor about all your medical problems.
✔ **DO** tell your doctor about medicines you take, prescription and over-the-counter.
✔ **DO** call your doctor if you're getting worse or don't feel better after 2 to 3 days.
✔ **DO** tell your doctor if you're pregnant or taking birth control pills.
✔ **DO** call your doctor right away or go to the emergency room if shortness of breath gets worse.
✔ **DO** try to cough up as much phlegm as possible.
✔ **DO** put an air humidifier in your room so you can breathe moist air, which helps get rid of phlegm.
✔ **DO** drink plenty of fluids so you don't get dehydrated.
✔ **DO** use acetaminophen or aspirin (except in children) for fever and pain.
✔ **DO** call your doctor if you think that you have pneumonia because you have fever, too much sputum, increased shortness of breath, or chest pain.
✔ **DO** call your doctor if you have dusky-colored skin, lips, or fingernails.
✔ **DO** call your doctor if nausea or vomiting stops you from taking your medicines.
✔ **DO** call your doctor if you get dehydrated because of vomiting or diarrhea.

⊘ **DON'T** stop taking your medicine just because you feel better, unless your doctor tells you to.
⊘ **DON'T** smoke.
⊘ **DON'T** drink alcohol in excess.

FROM THE DESK OF

NOTES

FOR MORE INFORMATION

Contact the following source:

• American Lung Association
  Tel: (800) LUNG-USA (586-4872)
  Website: http://www.lungusa.org

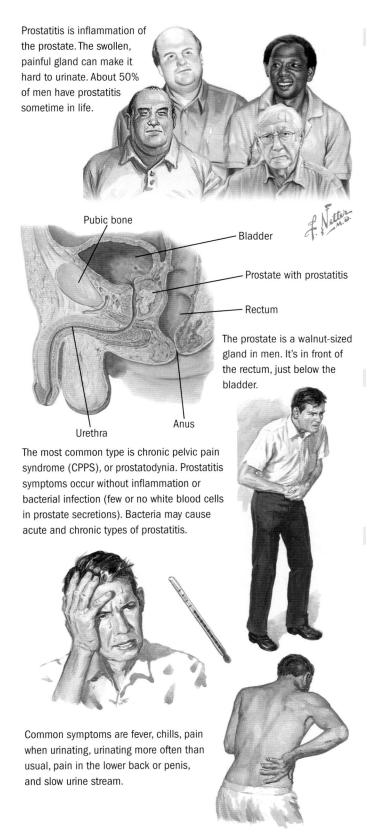

Prostatitis is inflammation of the prostate. The swollen, painful gland can make it hard to urinate. About 50% of men have prostatitis sometime in life.

Pubic bone

Bladder

Prostate with prostatitis

Rectum

The prostate is a walnut-sized gland in men. It's in front of the rectum, just below the bladder.

Urethra

Anus

The most common type is chronic pelvic pain syndrome (CPPS), or prostatodynia. Prostatitis symptoms occur without inflammation or bacterial infection (few or no white blood cells in prostate secretions). Bacteria may cause acute and chronic types of prostatitis.

Common symptoms are fever, chills, pain when urinating, urinating more often than usual, pain in the lower back or penis, and slow urine stream.

What Is Prostatitis?

The prostate is a walnut-sized gland in the male reproductive tract. It lies in front of the rectum, just below the bladder, which stores urine. The prostate surrounds the urethra (tube that takes urine out of the body). Prostatitis refers to inflammation of the prostate gland. The swollen, painful gland can make it hard to urinate. About 50% of men may have prostatitis sometime in life.

Prostatitis can be classed into four disorders. Acute bacterial prostatitis is least common, usually seen in young or middle-aged men. Chronic bacterial prostatitis is rather uncommon, usually found in men with a problem in the prostate. The most common is chronic pelvic pain syndrome (CPPS), or prostatodynia. Men have prostatitis symptoms but without inflammation or bacterial infection (few or no infection-fighting white blood cells in prostate secretions).

Nonbacterial prostatitis refers to inflammation with infection-fighting white blood cells but no bacterial infection.

What Causes Prostatitis?

Bacteria causing acute and chronic prostatitis get into the prostate from the urethra by backward flow of infected urine.

Prostatitis may also result from sexual contact, infection with chlamydia or mycoplasma, or chemical or immune reaction to urine.

Muscle spasm may cause CPPS.

What Are the Symptoms of Prostatitis?

Common symptoms are fever, chills, pain when urinating, urinating more often than usual, pain in the lower back or penis, and slow urine stream. Sometimes, symptoms are severe and start suddenly. Other times, symptoms are milder and start slowly. Chronic bacterial prostatitis may cause no symptoms, but bloody urine, incontinence, or bladder infection may occur. Additional symptoms of nonbacterial prostatitis or CPPS are pelvic pain and urgent, burning, or nighttime urination.

Your doctor will examine your prostate by doing a rectal exam. The gland may feel warm, tender, and swollen. A tender prostate suggests acute bacterial prostatitis. An enlarged prostate is common in chronic bacterial prostatitis. Men with other types of prostatitis can have a normal prostate.

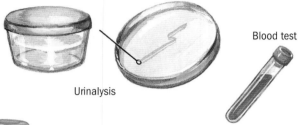

Your doctor will check samples of urine, prostate fluid, and blood for infection.

Blood test

Urinalysis

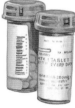

Antibiotics are usually given for acute bacterial prostatitis for 14 days to 4 weeks. Men with chronic bacterial prostatitis usually take antibiotics for 4 weeks. Don't stop taking your medicine, even if you start to feel better. Other types of prostatitis may be hard to treat but may need no specific treatment.

Don't ride a bike. It puts pressure on the prostate gland.

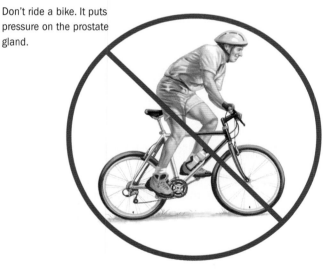

How Is Prostatitis Diagnosed?

The doctor will examine the prostate by doing a rectal exam (inserting a gloved finger into the rectum). The gland may feel warm, tender, and swollen. A tender prostate suggests acute bacterial prostatitis. An enlarged prostate is common in chronic bacterial prostatitis. Men with nonbacterial prostatitis or CPPS may have a normal prostate.

The doctor will check samples of urine, prostate gland fluid, and blood for infection.

How Is Prostatitis Treated?

Antibiotics are usually given for acute bacterial prostatitis for 14 days to 4 weeks. More serious infections may need intravenous antibiotics. Men with chronic bacterial prostatitis usually take antibiotics for 4 weeks. Relapses or infections that don't clear up may need long-term antibiotics. Nonbacterial prostatitis and CPPS may be hard to treat but may need no specific treatment.

DOs and DON'Ts in Managing Prostatitis:

✔ **DO** finish all the antibiotic medicine.

✔ **DO** tell your doctor about medicines you take for other illnesses.

✔ **DO** call your doctor if you have burning or pain with urination or you see blood in the urine.

✔ **DO** call your doctor if you have symptoms plus fever, chills, and sweats.

✔ **DO** call your doctor if you have urinary frequency, urgency, or nighttime urination or if you leak urine.

⊘ **DON'T** ride a bicycle. This puts pressure on the prostate gland.

⊘ **DON'T** eat foods or drink alcohol if they make symptoms worse.

⊘ **DON'T** stop taking your medicine even if you start to feel better.

FROM THE DESK OF

NOTES

FOR MORE INFORMATION

Contact the following source:

• The Prostatitis Foundation
  Tel: (888) 891-4200
  Website: http://www.prostatitis.org

Pyelonephritis is a kidney infection that usually starts as a urinary tract infection (UTI). UTIs are common, but pyelonephritis isn't. It's also serious. Repeated infections may lead to chronic pyelonephritis, which can cause kidney failure.

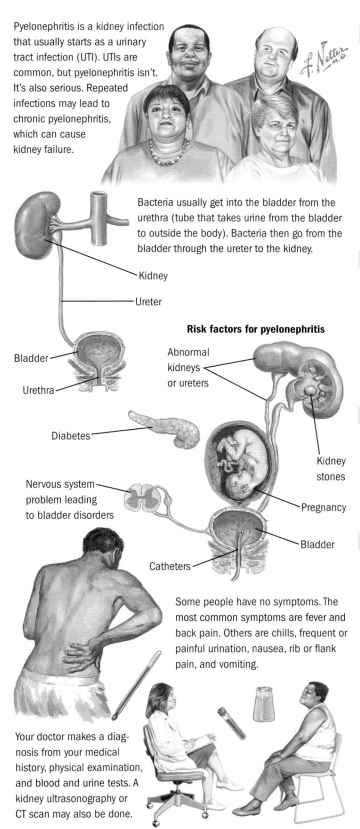

Bacteria usually get into the bladder from the urethra (tube that takes urine from the bladder to outside the body). Bacteria then go from the bladder through the ureter to the kidney.

Kidney

Ureter

Bladder

Urethra

Risk factors for pyelonephritis

Abnormal kidneys or ureters

Diabetes

Nervous system problem leading to bladder disorders

Kidney stones

Pregnancy

Bladder

Catheters

Some people have no symptoms. The most common symptoms are fever and back pain. Others are chills, frequent or painful urination, nausea, rib or flank pain, and vomiting.

Your doctor makes a diagnosis from your medical history, physical examination, and blood and urine tests. A kidney ultrasonography or CT scan may also be done.

What Is Pyelonephritis?

Pyelonephritis is a kidney infection. It usually starts as a urinary tract infection (UTI), which is an infection of the bladder with bacteria. The bladder stores urine before it leaves the body. These bacteria usually get into the bladder from the urethra (tube that takes urine from the bladder to outside the body). When bacteria get to the kidney, pyelonephritis results.

Kidney infections are less common than UTIs, but they're more serious. Repeated infections may lead to scarring. Infection that keeps damaging the kidneys can cause chronic pyelonephritis, which can cause kidney failure.

What Causes Pyelonephritis?

Bacteria first infect the urine and then reach the kidneys by traveling up the ureter or from the bloodstream.

People who have greater chances of getting pyelonephritis include women, older people, and people with catheters, diabetes, or urinary tract blocked because of stones or enlarged prostate gland.

What Are the Symptoms of Pyelonephritis?

Some people have no symptoms. The most common symptoms are fever and back pain. Other symptoms include chills, frequent urination, nausea, painful urination, rib or flank pain, sudden urge to urinate, and vomiting.

How Is Pyelonephritis Diagnosed?

The doctor makes a diagnosis from the medical history, physical examination, and tests of urine and blood for infection. Ultrasonography or CT of the kidneys may help find an infection. Ultrasonography uses sound waves to see kidneys and is painless and harmless.

The doctor may suggest seeing a urologist (doctor who specializes in urinary problems).

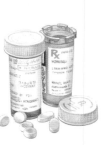

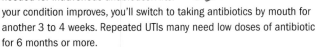

Typically, for treatment, a hospital stay is needed for intravenous antibiotics. After your condition improves, you'll switch to taking antibiotics by mouth for another 3 to 4 weeks. Repeated UTIs many need low doses of antibiotic for 6 months or more.

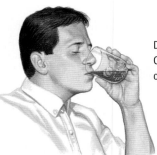

Drink plenty of fluids but avoid alcohol. Cranberry juice and water are great choices.

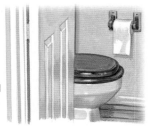

To prevent UTIs, women should wipe from front to back, away from the vagina, after going to the bathroom. Urinate before and after sex.

Men should have the prostate checked and get treated for an enlarged prostate.

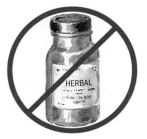

Don't take herbal preparations that you may find at health food stores. Some cause kidney disease.

How Is Pyelonephritis Treated?

Most people are admitted to the hospital and treated with antibiotics put directly into a vein. After symptoms improve, antibiotics given by mouth may be needed for 3 to 4 weeks.

Pain medicine and fluids are also given through a vein if dehydration is present. For repeated UTIs, low doses of antibiotic may be given daily for 6 months or more to prevent infections.

If a kidney stone caused the infection, a urologist may take the stone out.

DOs and DON'Ts in Managing Pyelonephritis:

✔ **DO** tell your doctor about your other medical problems, especially kidney problems.

✔ **DO** tell your doctor about your medicines, including prescription and over-the-counter medicines.

✔ **DO** tell your doctor if you're pregnant.

✔ **DO** drink plenty of water and cranberry juice.

✔ **DO** urinate when you need to. Don't hold your urine for prolonged periods.

✔ **DO** call your doctor if your symptoms get worse or don't get better with treatment.

✔ **DO** call your doctor right away or go to the emergency room if you have a temperature higher than 101° F or are vomiting.

✔ **DO** have kidney stones removed.

✔ **DO** urinate before and after sex.

✔ **DO** wipe away from the vagina, toward the back, after using the bathroom to prevent UTIs.

✔ **DO** have your prostate checked and get treated if you have an enlarged prostate.

⊘ **DON'T** stop taking your medicine or change your dosage because you feel better unless your doctor tells you to.

⊘ **DON'T** become dehydrated. Drink plenty of fluids, but don't drink alcohol.

⊘ **DON'T** take any herbal preparations that you may find at health food stores. Some cause kidney disease.

FROM THE DESK OF

NOTES

FOR MORE INFORMATION

Contact the following sources:

• National Kidney Foundation
Tel: (800) 622-9010
Website: http://www.kidney.org

• Centers for Disease Control and Prevention
Tel: (800) 311-3435
Website: http://www.cdc.gov

Reiter's syndrome is also called reactive arthritis, meaning it occurs as a reaction to something else that's happening in the body, such as an infection. It's most often found in men 20 to 40 years old. The cause is unknown.

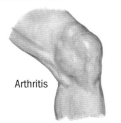

It causes three seemingly unrelated symptoms: a kind of arthritis, eye inflammation, and a urinary tract condition called urethritis.

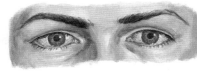

Arthritis

Eye inflammation

Other symptoms include:

Rashes (tip of the penis and soles of the feet)

Painless ulcers on the mouth and tongue

Heel pain and swelling

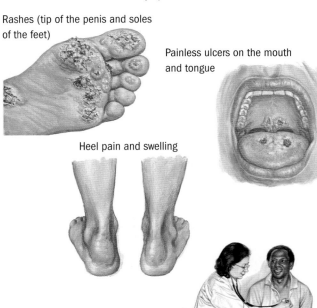

Your doctor makes a diagnosis from symptoms and a physical examination. Blood tests check the erythrocyte sedimentation rate (ESR) and HLA-B27 antigen. The doctor may also order x-rays of joints.

What Is Reiter's Syndrome?

Reiter's syndrome is an illness that causes three seemingly unrelated symptoms: a type of arthritis, eye inflammation called uveitis or conjunctivitis, and a urinary tract condition called urethritis. Another name for the illness is reactive arthritis. This term means that arthritis usually occurs as a reaction to something else that's happening in the body, usually an infection.

Reiter's syndrome is most often found in men 20 to 40 years old.

What Causes Reiter's Syndrome?

The cause is unknown, but symptoms often follow a bacterial infection. Most cases tend to occur after a sexually transmitted disease (STD), such as chlamydia; a stomach illness, such as food poisoning; or an intestinal infection. People may also inherit a tendency to get it.

What Are the Symptoms of Reiter's Syndrome?

The first symptoms usually involve the urinary tract and start a few days after an infection. Arthritis and eye symptoms (pinkeye or blurry vision) then develop in the next several weeks. Common symptoms are burning or stinging when urinating; discharge from the penis; red, itchy, burning eyes; joint pain and swelling, usually in large joints, such as knees, hips, and ankles; painless ulcers on the mouth and tongue; and rashes on the tip of the penis and soles of the feet. Other symptoms are low-grade fevers, fatigue, muscle aches, stiff joints, heel pain, and low back pain.

How Is Reiter's Syndrome Diagnosed?

The doctor makes a diagnosis from symptoms and a physical examination. No specific tests exist for this syndrome, but the doctor may order blood tests. One test is an erythrocyte sedimentation rate (ESR). People with arthritis usually have a high rate. Another test looks for specific substances in the blood known as antigens. About 80% to 90% of people with the syndrome have one substance, HLA-B27 antigen. The doctor may also order an x-ray of joints that may be affected. Your doctor may refer you to an eye specialist (ophthalmologist) for treatment of the eye inflammation.

Treatment involves medicines, exercises, and physical therapy. Antibiotics can treat an infection. NSAIDs such as ibuprofen or naproxen help pain, stiffness, and swelling.

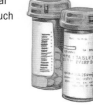

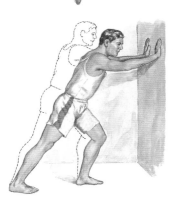

Physical therapy and exercises are very important parts of your treatment.

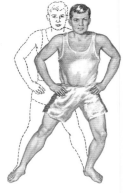

Daily stretching and strengthening exercises help keep your joints from getting stiff. A physical therapist can teach you how to do them.

Learn and maintain good sitting, standing, and sleeping postures.

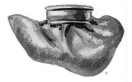

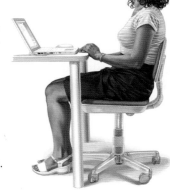

Using a heating pad or taking a hot shower can help stiffness and aches. Cold packs can reduce swelling.

How Is Reiter's Syndrome Treated?

Treatment involves medicines, exercises, and physical therapy. Antibiotics can treat an infection. Nonsteroidal antiinflammatory drugs (NSAIDs) such as ibuprofen or naproxen help pain, stiffness, and swelling. People with long-lasting arthritis may need other medicines for the immune system. Sometimes cortisone injections into joints help. Steroid eye drops may be needed for eye inflammation.

Physical therapy and exercises are very important. Physical therapists can teach simple stretching and strengthening exercises. Good posture reduces pain and keeps normal motion in the joints and spine.

Some people may recover fully, in 3 to 4 months. Symptoms never return. Even with treatment, however, many people have many bouts of arthritis, back pain, rashes, eye inflammation and urinary symptoms.

DOs and DON'Ts in Managing Reiter's Syndrome:

✔ **DO** take medicine to help pain and swelling.
✔ **DO** daily stretching exercises to keep your joints from getting stiff.
✔ **DO** use a heating pad or hot shower to help stiffness and aches. Applying ice or cold packs can reduce swelling.
✔ **DO** learn and maintain good sitting, standing, and sleeping postures.
✔ **DO** call your doctor if you have medicine side effects.
✔ **DO** call your doctor if medicines and other treatments don't help the pain.
✔ **DO** call your doctor if you need a referral to a physical or occupational therapist.

⊘ **DON'T** engage in unsafe sexual practices. Use latex condoms to help avoid spreading STDs.

FROM THE DESK OF

NOTES

FOR MORE INFORMATION

Contact the following sources:

• National Institute of Arthritis and Musculoskeletal and Skin Diseases
Tel: (301) 495-4484, (877) 226-4267
Website: http://www.niams.nih.gov

• Arthritis Foundation
Tel: (800) 283-7800
Website: http://www.arthritis.org

CARING FOR YOUR CHILD WITH
RHEUMATIC FEVER

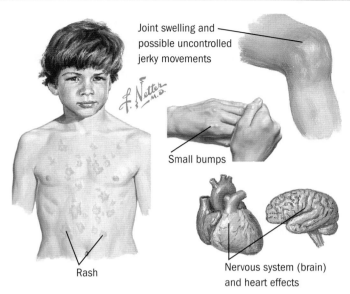

Rheumatic fever is an autoimmune disorder occurring after a *Streptococcus* bacterial infection. It usually occurs in children younger than 18. It affects the heart, nervous system, skin, and joints.

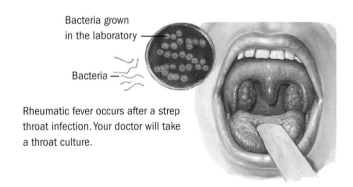

Rheumatic fever occurs after a strep throat infection. Your doctor will take a throat culture.

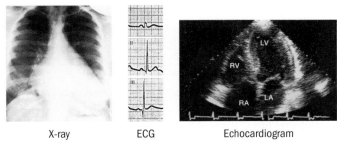

Your doctor will also look at a chest x-ray and test how your child's heart works. These tests are ECG and echocardiography (uses sound waves to get pictures of the heart).

What Is Rheumatic Fever?

Rheumatic fever is an inflammation of the heart, nervous system, skin, and joints after a recent bacterial infection. Rheumatic fever usually occurs in children younger than 18. It cannot be caught, but the infection that causes it can.

What Causes Rheumatic Fever?

Rheumatic fever is probably an autoimmune disorder, which means that the body reacts against its own cells or tissues. A recent strep throat infection triggers it. The infection with the bacteria named *Streptococcus* may have been mild or untreated. Substances called antibodies produced during the infection also attack and can destroy cells in the joints, the heart, and other body parts.

What Are the Symptoms of Rheumatic Fever?

Symptoms include fever, loss of appetite, mild rash, tiredness, paleness, small bumps under the skin over bony areas (such as hands, wrists, elbows, and knuckles), and joint inflammation with pain, swelling, and warmth.

If the heart is affected, shortness of breath, swelling of the ankles and around the eyes, and rapid heartbeat may occur. If the brain is affected, uncontrolled jerky movements may occur.

The most common complication is damage to heart valves that causes a heart murmur. Sometimes the damaged valves may need to be replaced.

How Is Rheumatic Fever Diagnosed?

The doctor will make a diagnosis from the medical history, physical examination, and laboratory tests. A chest x-ray, electrocardiography (ECG), and throat culture will be done. The doctor will order another test called echocardiography to look for heart valve damage.

If heart damage is present, you will be referred to a cardiologist (a doctor who specializes in heart treatment).

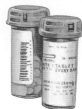

Antibiotics are needed to fight the infection. Antiinflammatory medicine will help muscle and joint pain.

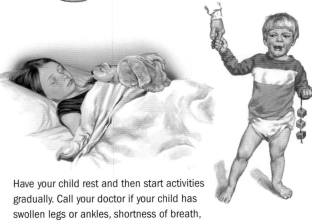

Have your child rest and then start activities gradually. Call your doctor if your child has swollen legs or ankles, shortness of breath, vomiting, diarrhea, severe belly pain, or high temperature.

Have your child drink plenty of fluids.

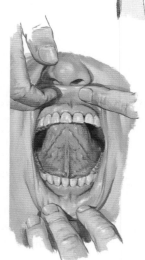

Tell doctors and dentists about your child's rheumatic fever.

How Is Rheumatic Fever Treated?

Children must limit their activity until symptoms are gone, which could take 2 to 5 weeks.

Antibiotics for the bacteria will be given for several days. Tell your doctor if your child is allergic to penicillin.

In the early stages a liquid or soft diet may be better. Later a normal diet that is high in calories, protein, and vitamins is followed.

Aspirin or other antiinflammatory drugs are given for muscle and joint pain.

DOs and DON'Ts in Managing Rheumatic Fever:

✔ **DO** have your child take antibiotics until the prescription is all gone.

✔ **DO** have your child with a fever drink enough fluids.

✔ **DO** have your child rest and then start activity gradually. Rest periods and naps should be scheduled.

✔ **DO** get prompt evaluation for future sore throats.

✔ **DO** tell doctors and dentists about your child's rheumatic fever.

✔ **DO** call your doctor if during treatment your child has swollen legs or ankles, shortness of breath, vomiting, diarrhea, dry hacking cough, severe pain in the abdomen (belly), or a temperature of 101°F or higher.

⊘ **DON'T** let your child resume activity until the fever and other symptoms are gone.

FROM THE DESK OF

NOTES

FOR MORE INFORMATION

Contact the following sources:

• National Heart, Lung, and Blood Institute Information Center
Tel: (301) 592-8573
Website: http://www.nhlbi.nih.gov

• American Heart Association
Tel: (800) 242-8721
Website: http://www.americanheart.org

MANAGING YOUR
SINUSITIS

Frontal sinus

Ethmoid sinuses

Maxillary sinus

Sinusitis is inflammation and swelling of one or more sinuses. It's very common. Sinuses are four hollow spaces in bones of the face. Each sinus has an opening to allow air and mucus in the nose to move in and out. If sinuses become blocked, sinusitis (also called sinus infection) results.

f. Netter. M.D.

The cause can be bacteria, allergies, pollution, or nasal polyps. It often occurs after a cold or allergic reaction.

Main symptoms are headache and pressure or pain in the forehead or face. The nose may be stuffed and runny, with a green or yellow-green discharge. Swollen eyes, with pain behind them and dark circles underneath, may occur.

Painful areas

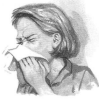

Children may be irritable, and have a long-lasting cough, in addition to sinus congestion.

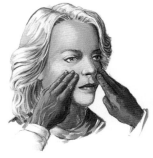

Your doctor will examine your face, nose, and ears and listen to your chest. X-rays or maybe other imaging tests of the sinuses may be done on rare occasions.

What Is Sinusitis?

Four hollow spaces in bones of the face are sinuses. Each sinus has an opening to allow air and mucus in the nose to move in and out. If sinuses become blocked, sinusitis, or sinus infection, results. Sinusitis is inflammation and swelling of one or more sinuses. Blocked sinuses can also lead to infection caused by bacteria.

Sinusitis is very common. Sinusitis can be sudden and short (acute) or long-lasting (chronic).

What Causes Sinusitis?

The cause can be bacteria, allergies, pollution, or nasal polyps. It often starts after a cold or allergic reaction.

What Are the Symptoms of Sinusitis?

Main symptoms are headache and pressure or pain in the forehead or face. The nose may be stuffed and runny, with a green or yellow-green discharge. Swollen eyes, with pain behind them and dark circles underneath, may occur. The throat may become sore. Children may be irritable, and have a long-lasting cough, in addition to sinus congestion. Symptoms usually go away in 7 to 21 days.

How Is Sinusitis Diagnosed?

The doctor will examine the face, nose, and ears, and listen to the chest. X-rays or maybe other imaging tests of the sinuses may be done on rare occasions. If sinusitis is due to an allergy or sinusitis occurs three times a year or more, the doctor may suggest seeing an allergist (specialist in allergies).

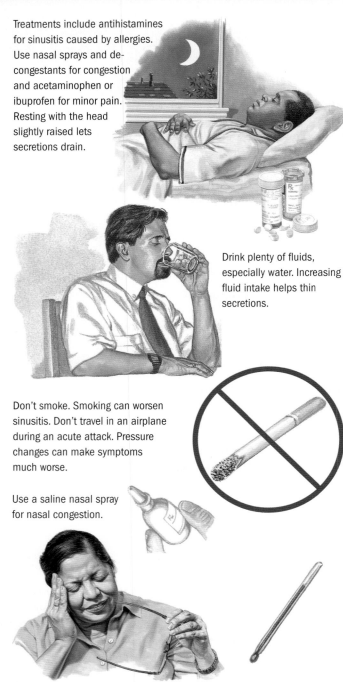

Treatments include antihistamines for sinusitis caused by allergies. Use nasal sprays and decongestants for congestion and acetaminophen or ibuprofen for minor pain. Resting with the head slightly raised lets secretions drain.

Drink plenty of fluids, especially water. Increasing fluid intake helps thin secretions.

Don't smoke. Smoking can worsen sinusitis. Don't travel in an airplane during an acute attack. Pressure changes can make symptoms much worse.

Use a saline nasal spray for nasal congestion.

Call your doctor if you have fever and chills, your face swells over the sinuses, or you have blurred vision or a severe headache that medicines don't help.

How Is Sinusitis Treated?

The doctor may prescribe antihistamines for sinusitis caused by allergies. Nasal sprays and decongestants help congestion. Increasing fluid intake helps thin secretions. Resting with the head slightly raised will let secretions drain easier. For minor pain, acetaminophen or ibuprofen can be used.

For sinusitis caused by bacterial infection, the doctor will prescribe an antibiotic. Most sinus infections are caused by viruses, and antibiotics don't work and shouldn't be taken.

Acute sinusitis usually goes away in 2 to 3 weeks with treatment.

DOs and DON'Ts in Managing Sinusitis:

✔ **DO** drink plenty of fluids, especially water.
✔ **DO** use a saline nasal spray for nasal congestion.
✔ **DO** quit smoking. Smoking can worsen sinusitis.
✔ **DO** use a vaporizer or inhale steam from a shower to relieve congestion.
✔ **DO** use warm compresses over the sinus area four times a day, for 1 or 2 hours.
✔ **DO** use a humidifier in the winter and an air conditioner in the summer.
✔ **DO** call your doctor if you have lasting fever and chills.
✔ **DO** call your doctor if your face swells over the sinuses.
✔ **DO** call your doctor if you have blurred vision or a severe headache that medicines don't help.
✔ **DO** avoid allergy triggers.

⊘ **DON'T** use over-the-counter nose sprays. They can make symptoms worse.
⊘ **DON'T** travel in an airplane during an acute attack. Pressure changes can make symptoms much worse. Check with your doctor first if you must fly.

FROM THE DESK OF

NOTES

FOR MORE INFORMATION

Contact the following source:

• American Academy of Otolaryngology—Head and Neck Surgery
Tel: (703) 836-4444
Website: http://www.entnet.org

Stomatitis is a general inflammation of the mouth. It involves the soft mucous membranes lining the mouth, lips, tongue, and palate. People of all ages can get it.

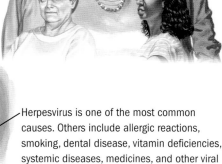

Herpesvirus is one of the most common causes. Others include allergic reactions, smoking, dental disease, vitamin deficiencies, systemic diseases, medicines, and other viral and bacterial infections.

Symptoms are pain, fever, tiredness, headache, and loss of appetite. Small sores occur on the lips, gums, tongue, roof of the mouth, or inside the cheeks. Sores are often red and may hurt, burn, or tingle. Eating and swallowing hurt. Sometimes, people have bad breath.

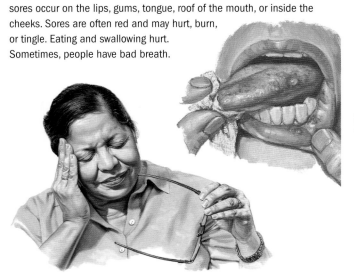

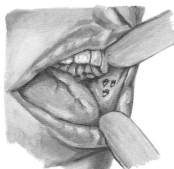

Your doctor makes a diagnosis by examining your mouth. The doctor may gently scrape a sample from the mouth and check it with a microscope.

What Is Stomatitis?

Stomatitis is a general inflammation (swelling, redness) of the mouth. It involves the soft mucous membranes lining the mouth (mucosa), lips, tongue, and palate. It's called herpetic stomatitis when caused by herpesvirus, and aphthous stomatitis (canker sores) when causes are unknown. Stomatitis is common in all ages.

What Causes Stomatitis?

Herpesvirus is one of the most common causes. Others include allergic reactions, smoking, dental disease, vitamin deficiencies, systemic diseases, medicines, and other viral and bacterial infections.

What Are the Symptoms of Stomatitis?

Inflammation of the mouth may cause pain, fever, tiredness, headache, and loss of appetite. Usually, people have one or more small sores on their lips, gums, tongue, roof of the mouth, or inside the cheeks. Sores are often red and may hurt, burn, or tingle. Eating and swallowing hurt. Sometimes, people have bad breath (halitosis).

How Is Stomatitis Diagnosed?

The doctor makes a diagnosis by examining the mouth. The doctor may gently scrape a sample from the mouth to check with a microscope. This sample will show if a yeast infection caused the stomatitis. If the cause isn't clear or treatment doesn't help, a biopsy is done. A biopsy involves taking a small sample of the sore for study with a microscope. Blood tests are not usually necessary but may be done in recurrent or persistent cases.

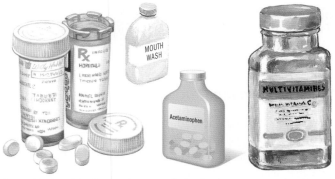

Stomatitis from irritating products usually heals after you stop using the product. Antibiotics are given for bacterial infections. Many medications for stomatitis can be liquids swished around in the mouth and then sometimes swallowed. Vitamin supplements and oral corticosteroids may be needed in more severe cases. Acetaminophen and topical anesthetic agents can relieve pain.

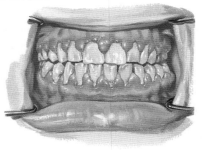

Very bad stomatitis can cause bleeding and infection of gums.

Use good oral hygiene. Brush with a soft toothbrush, floss your teeth, and clean your tongue after each meal. Avoid strong mouthwashes, but rinse your mouth well, especially before going to bed.

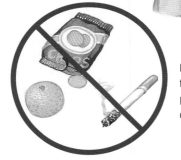

Don't smoke. Don't eat citrus foods, foods with sharp surfaces (such as potato chips), or foods that are spicy or acidic.

How Is Stomatitis Treated?

Stomatitis caused by irritation from foods, mouthwashes, or cigarettes usually heals after use of the product stops. Antibiotics are given for bacterial infections. Often, medicines for infections are liquids that are swished around in the mouth. Some need to be swallowed after swishing. Vitamin supplements are given for rare nutritional problems. For severe symptoms, oral corticosteroids may be needed. Canker sores and herpes sores usually heal in 1 or 2 weeks. Thrush heals quickly with medicine. Other types of stomatitis may take several weeks to heal.

Sometimes, complications such as bleeding and infection occur. Because of mouth pain, many people, especially babies, don't eat or drink enough. They lose weight and become dehydrated. This is especially dangerous for babies. Intravenous fluids may be needed for severe dehydration.

The key is to relieve symptoms. Pain medicine such as acetaminophen and topical anesthetic agents can do this. Mouth rinses with baking soda and warm water can help.

DOs and DON'Ts in Managing Stomatitis:

✔ **DO** see a dentist regularly.
✔ **DO** use good oral hygiene. Brush and floss teeth and clean the tongue after each meal. Use a soft-bristled toothbrush.
✔ **DO** avoid sharp-surfaced foods, such as peanuts, popcorn, and potato chips.
✔ **DO** take your dentures out at night. Have them adjusted so that they fit better.
✔ **DO** avoid strong mouthwashes, but rinse your mouth well, especially before going to bed.
✔ **DO** call your doctor if your symptoms don't go away after 7 to 14 days of treatment.

⊘ **DON'T** smoke.
⊘ **DON'T** eat citrus foods or foods that are spicy or acidic.

FOR MORE INFORMATION

Contact the following sources:

• National Institute of Dental and Craniofacial Research
  Tel: (301) 402-7364
  Website: http://www.nidcr.nih.gov/OralHealth/

• American Academy of Periodontology
  Tel: (312) 787-5518
  Website: http://www.perio.org

• American Dental Association
  Tel: (312) 440-2500
  Website: http://www.ada.org

FROM THE DESK OF

NOTES

MANAGING YOUR
TOXIC SHOCK SYNDROME

Toxic shock syndrome is a severe, life-threatening kind of blood poisoning caused by bacterial toxins. *Staphylococcus aureus* and *Streptococcus pyogenes* bacteria make these toxins.

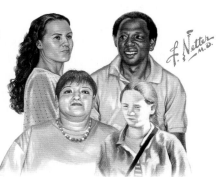

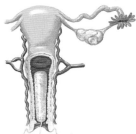

The best known type is related to tampon use during menstrual periods. However, both sexes can get it from wounds or infections of the skin, lungs, throat, or bones.

Symptoms of toxic shock syndrome

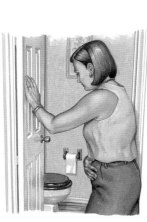

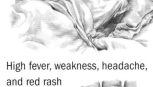

High fever, weakness, headache, and red rash

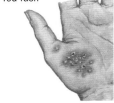

Vomiting, diarrhea, muscle pain

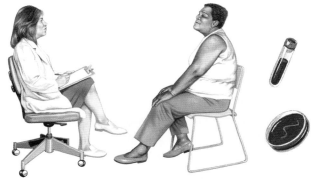

Your doctor makes a diagnosis from your medical history, symptoms, examination, and blood tests. Samples from infected areas may be checked for bacteria.

What Is Toxic Shock Syndrome?

Toxic shock syndrome is a severe, life-threatening form of blood poisoning caused by bacterial toxins. The best known type is related to tampon use during menstrual periods. However, both sexes can get it from wounds or infections of the skin, lungs, throat, or bones.

What Causes Toxic Shock Syndrome?

The cause is toxins made by *Staphylococcus aureus* bacteria. The syndrome is related to use of contraceptive sponge and diaphragm birth control methods as well as tampon use. The second type is caused by *Streptococcus pyogenes* bacteria after they enter the body through injured skin from wounds caused by surgery or minor trauma, such as cuts, scrapes, and chicken-pox blisters infected with bacteria.

What Are the Symptoms of Toxic Shock Syndrome?

Symptoms include sudden shaking and a fever (temperature often higher than 102° F), severe muscle pain or aches, vomiting, diarrhea, thirst, rapid pulse, deep red rash that looks like sunburn, severe weakness, headache, confusion, and low blood pressure. Symptoms of the streptococcal syndrome also include trouble breathing, dizziness, and weak and rapid pulse. The infected wound can look swollen and red, and liver and kidneys may stop working.

How Is Toxic Shock Syndrome Diagnosed?

The doctor makes a diagnosis from the medical history, symptoms, physical examination, and blood tests. The doctor may want samples from infected areas, such as wounds and vagina, to check for bacterial growth.

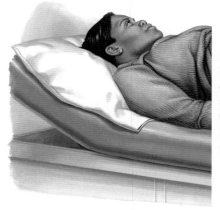

Early diagnosis and hospital treatment are essential, with intravenous antibiotics and fluids given. Complications can arise, so being at the hospital helps prevent and treat them.

You may still need antibiotics after you leave the hospital. Take the medicine as the doctor prescribes. Finish all your medicine. Don't stop taking antibiotics early just because you feel better.

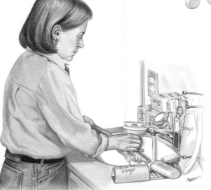

Wash your hands carefully before you insert tampons. Bacteria are on your skin, especially your hands, and can be transferred to the tampons.

Don't use superabsorbent tampons, especially overnight. Alternate tampons with sanitary napkins. Don't use tampons at all if you ever had toxic shock syndrome.

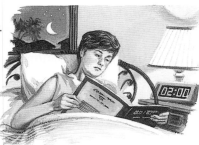

How Is Toxic Shock Syndrome Treated?

Early diagnosis and hospital treatment are essential. Complications often include peeling of skin on the hands and feet, loss of hair and nails, kidney failure, congestive heart failure, and respiratory distress.

Intravenous fluids and antibiotics will be given in the hospital. Breathing problems may need oxygen and mechanical ventilation. Dialysis will be used for kidney failure.

After symptoms are controlled and initial dangers are over, care can be given at home. Antibiotics may still be needed. Rest is important, with activities increased slowly. Drink more fluids, and follow a well-balanced diet.

DOs and DON'Ts in Managing Toxic Shock Syndrome:

✔ **DO** get treatment immediately for symptoms of toxic shock. It progresses rapidly and may be fatal if not treated.
✔ **DO** change tampons frequently.
✔ **DO** get medical treatment for wounds that look infected.
✔ **DO** finish all antibiotics.
✔ **DO** wash your hands carefully before you insert tampons. Bacteria are found on the skin, especially the hands.
✔ **DO** get immediate care if you have a fever or rash, especially during your period and when using tampons, or if you had recent surgery.
✔ **DO** realize that toxic shock syndrome can come back. People who have it once can get it again.

⊘ **DON'T** skip doses or stop antibiotics unless your doctor tells you.
⊘ **DON'T** ignore a wound if it looks red and swollen or has pus.
⊘ **DON'T** use superabsorbent tampons, especially overnight. Alternate tampons with sanitary napkins.
⊘ **DON'T** use tampons if you have a skin infection, especially in the genital area.
⊘ **DON'T** use tampons at all if you ever had toxic shock syndrome.

FROM THE DESK OF

NOTES

FOR MORE INFORMATION

Contact the following sources:

• Centers for Disease Control and Prevention
Tel: (404) 639-2215, (800) 232-4636
Website: http://www.cdc.gov

• National Institute of Allergy and Infectious Disease
Tel: (301) 496-5717
Website: http://www3.niaid.nih.gov

MANAGING YOUR
TOXOPLASMOSIS

Toxoplasmosis is an infection caused by a tiny organism that lives in birds, animals, and humans. It affects the gastrointestinal tract, heart, nerves, and skin. The disease is most dangerous for pregnant women and people with weak immune systems, such as those getting chemotherapy, with AIDS, and with organ transplants.

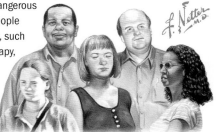

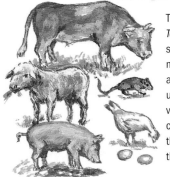

The cause is a parasite named *Toxoplasma gondii*. The disease spreads by eating undercooked meat (lamb, pork) from an infected animal; by eating contaminated, uncooked, unwashed fruits or vegetables; or by handling infected cat litter or feces. Mothers can pass the parasite to unborn babies through their bloodstream.

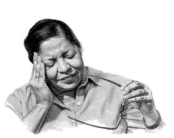

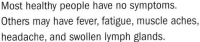

Most healthy people have no symptoms. Others may have fever, fatigue, muscle aches, headache, and swollen lymph glands.

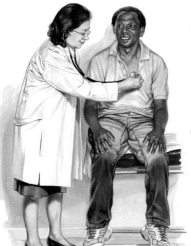

Your doctor makes a diagnosis from your medical history, physical examination, and blood tests.

What Is Toxoplasmosis?

Toxoplasmosis is an infection caused by a microscopic organism (protozoa) that lives in birds, animals, and humans. It affects the gastrointestinal tract (which includes the mouth, esophagus, stomach, intestines, and anus), heart, nerves, and skin. The disease is most dangerous for pregnant women and people with weak immune systems. This includes people who are receiving chemotherapy, have AIDS, and have an organ transplant.

Children younger than 5 need treatment to prevent eye complications. Other complications include inflammation (swelling) of the brain and heart and lung damage. If a pregnant woman has the infection early in pregnancy, she may miscarry or have a stillbirth, or the baby may be born with birth defects.

Over 30% of healthy people in the United States may have toxoplasmosis. Many don't know it because they don't have symptoms.

What Causes Toxoplasmosis?

The cause is a microscopic parasite named *Toxoplasma gondii*. The disease can spread by eating undercooked meat from an infected animal (especially lamb and pork) or by handling cat litter or feces if the cat has the infection. People who eat contaminated, uncooked, or unwashed fruits or vegetables that had contact with manure can also get it. Mothers can pass the parasite to unborn babies through the blood.

What Are the Symptoms of Toxoplasmosis?

Most healthy people have no symptoms. Others may have fever, fatigue, muscle aches, headache, and swollen lymph glands.

How Is Toxoplasmosis Diagnosed?

The doctor makes a diagnosis from a medical history, physical examination, and blood tests.

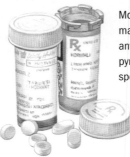

Most people don't need treatment. Others may need prescription drugs such as the antibiotic sulfadiazine or the antiparasitic pyrimethamine. Acetaminophen or tepid sponge baths can reduce fever.

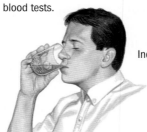

Your doctor will do blood tests often to watch for medicine side effects. Keep your doctor appointments for the follow-up blood tests.

Increase your fluid intake.

Rest until symptoms go away. Slowly increase your activity.

Wash your hands often with soap and water, especially when you handle meats, vegetables, and fruits. Wash vegetables and fruits before eating them. Cook meats well.

Use sunscreen when outdoors, because the medicine may make you more sensitive to the sun. Don't stay in the sun for long periods.

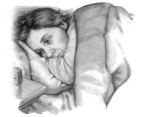

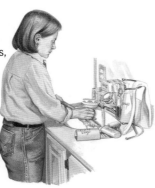

How Is Toxoplasmosis Treated?

Most people don't need treatment. Others may need prescription drugs such as the antibiotic sulfadiazine or antiparasitic pyrimethamine for 4 to 6 weeks or longer. These drugs can cause upset stomach, sun sensitivity, bleeding, or bruising. The doctor will do blood tests to watch for side effects.

Activity levels depend on the symptoms.

Acetaminophen or tepid sponge baths can be used to reduce fever. No special diet is needed, but fluid intake should be increased.

DOs and DON'Ts in Managing Toxoplasmosis:

✔ **DO** use acetaminophen for aches and fever.

✔ **DO** use tepid sponge baths to help reduce fever.

✔ **DO** rest until symptoms go away. Slowly increase your activity.

✔ **DO** keep doctor appointments for follow-up blood tests.

✔ **DO** use sunscreen when outdoors because the medicine may make you more sensitive to the sun.

✔ **DO** wash your hands often with soap and water, especially when you handle meats, vegetables, and fruits.

✔ **DO** cook meats well. Wash vegetables and fruits before eating them.

✔ **DO** call your doctor if your symptoms don't get better with treatment.

✔ **DO** call your doctor if you have bleeding, bruising, visual changes, or increased weakness.

🚫 **DON'T** eat undercooked meats, especially lamb and pork, uncooked eggs, or unpasteurized milk.

🚫 **DON'T** change the cat litter box if you're pregnant, had an organ transplant, are receiving chemotherapy, or have AIDS. If you must change the box, use gloves and wash your hands afterward.

🚫 **DON'T** stop taking your medicine before it's all gone unless your doctor tells you to.

🚫 **DON'T** stay in the sun for long periods or forget to use sunscreen.

FROM THE DESK OF

NOTES

FOR MORE INFORMATION

Contact the following sources:

• National Heart, Lung and Blood Institute
  Tel: (301) 592-8573
  Website: http://www.nhlbi.nih.gov

• National Institute of Allergy and Infectious Diseases
  Tel: (301) 496-5717
  Website: http://www3.niaid.nih.gov

MANAGING YOUR
TRAVELER'S DIARRHEA

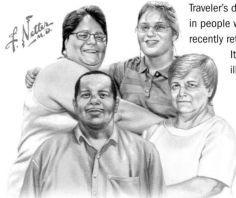

Traveler's diarrhea (TD) is diarrhea in people who are traveling or recently returned from traveling. It's the most common illness in travelers.

What Is Traveler's Diarrhea (TD)?

Travelers' diarrhea (TD) is diarrhea in people who are or recently returned from traveling. It's the most common illness in travelers. Each year between 20% and 50% of international travelers, about 10 million people, develop TD. Three or more unformed (meaning no separate pieces) stools (bowel movements) in 24 hours mean TD. In most cases, TD runs its course without complications, with 90% of cases going away within 1 week, and 98% within 1 month.

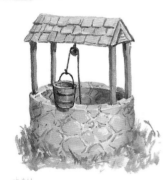

The usual cause is bacteria, but viruses and parasites can also cause TD. It's usually related to travel in developing countries or places with a contaminated water supply.

What Causes TD?

The usual cause is bacteria, but viruses and parasites can also cause TD. It's usually related to travel in developing countries with a contaminated water supply.

What Are the Symptoms of TD?

Most symptoms start suddenly. Symptoms include diarrhea (unformed bowel movements), cramps and tenderness in the abdomen (belly), and sometimes nausea or vomiting and fever. Stools are often large and watery, and may contain mucus or blood. Babies (who usually have frequent bowel movements) may have TD if they have stools twice as often or more often than normal over 2 to 3 days.

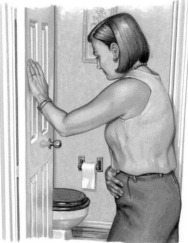

Symptoms, which start suddenly, include diarrhea, abdominal cramps and tenderness, and sometimes nausea or vomiting and fever.

How Is TD Diagnosed?

The doctor will suspect TD on the basis of the medical history, recent travel, and physical examination.

For severe TD or for bloody stool the doctor may order a stool culture. In this test, a small amount of stool is checked to find the cause. Additional tests may also be done.

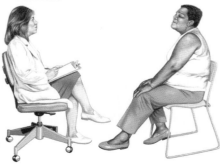

Your doctor will suspect TD on the basis of the medical history, recent travel, and physical examination. Your doctor may order a stool culture and additional tests for severe TD or bloody stool.

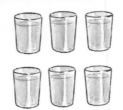

Prevention is best. Drink bottled water and avoid ice cubes when you travel. Drinking enough clear fluids is important, especially for babies and young children, because diarrhea can lead to dehydration.

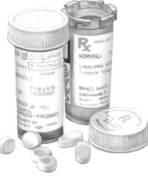

For severe or worsening symptoms, the doctor may prescribe an antibiotic or other drug.

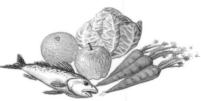

When you travel, wash all fruits and vegetables carefully in uncontaminated water. Be careful of tap water, ice, unpasteurized milk, dairy products, undercooked meat, and seafood.

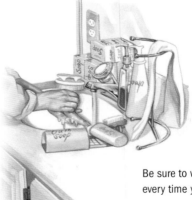

Be sure to wash your hands every time you use the toilet.

How Is TD Treated?

Prevention is best. Drink bottled water. Avoid ice cubes when traveling. TD usually stops after 5 to 7 days without lasting effects. Drinking enough clear fluids is important, because diarrhea can lead to dehydration. Fluids are especially important for infants and young children, who can easily become dehydrated. A liquid that contains added substances such as electrolytes in water may be suggested. Pregnant women, older people, and people who are ill with another disease need to be careful about replacing fluids.

For severe or worsening symptoms, the doctor may prescribe an antibiotic or other drug. Knowing the area of travel helps the doctor pick the best medicine.

Sometimes, the doctor may suggest seeing a gastroenterologist (specialist in bowel diseases) if the diarrhea persists.

DOs and DON'Ts in Managing TD:

✔ **DO** drink enough fluids.
✔ **DO** be careful about fluid intake in children, elderly people, pregnant women, and people with other illnesses.
✔ **DO** wash your hands every time you use the toilet.
✔ **DO** call your doctor if you get a high temperature, have blood in your bowel movement, or get severe abdominal pain.
✔ **DO** make sure that the water you drink isn't contaminated. In certain parts of the world, use only bottled water that is well sealed when you get it. Be careful of tap water, ice, unpasteurized milk, and dairy products.
✔ **DO** wash all fruits and vegetables carefully in uncontaminated water. Avoid undercooked meat and seafood.

🚫 **DON'T** wait to talk to your doctor if you have blood or mucus in your stools or have a high temperature.
🚫 **DON'T** swim in contaminated water.
🚫 **DON'T** take medicine that may be offered to you as a cure unless a doctor ordered it. Some of these drugs may make TD worse.

FROM THE DESK OF

NOTES

FOR MORE INFORMATION

Contact the following source:

• Centers for Disease Control and Prevention
  Tel: (800) 311-3435
  Website: http://www.cdc.gov

Trichinosis is an infection caused by a parasitic roundworm, *Trichinella spiralis,* that lives in intestines of pigs and other animals.

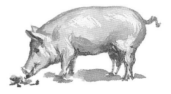

Roundworm

People get it by eating the meat of an infected animal when the meat hasn't been cooked enough. Worms are carried in the blood to muscles, where they curl into balls and become covered by a capsule (cyst).

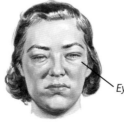

Early symptoms are diarrhea, low-grade fever, nausea, vomiting, and fatigue. Later ones are muscle pain, headache, weakness, and high temperature.

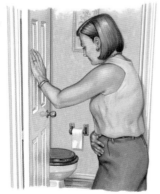

Eyelids and face may become puffy.

Skin may itch and burn.

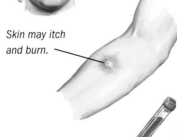

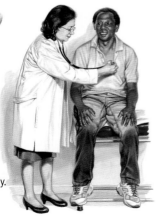

To confirm the diagnosis, your doctor will order blood tests and get a small piece of muscle tissue (muscle biopsy) for study.

What Is Trichinosis?

Trichinosis is an infection caused by a parasitic roundworm that lives in intestines of pigs and other animals. Today, pigs aren't as common a source of infection as they were. Bear meat is now the most common source of infection.

People get trichinosis by eating the meat of an infected animal when the meat hasn't been cooked enough to kill the worm cysts. Within 2 days of eating the infected meat, the worms mature and lay eggs, which become larvae (young immature worms). By the seventh day, larvae are carried in the blood to muscles. In muscles, the worms curl into balls and become covered by a capsule (cyst).

Complications of trichinosis can include congestive heart failure; respiratory failure; pneumonia; and kidney, heart, and brain damage.

What Causes Trichinosis?

The cause is the worm *Trichinella spiralis.*

What Are the Symptoms of Trichinosis?

Early symptoms are diarrhea, a low-grade fever, nausea, vomiting, fatigue, and discomfort in the abdomen (belly). Seven to 10 days later, the eyelids and face may become puffy. Muscle pain, aching joints, headache, weakness, shortness of breath, high temperature, chills, sensitivity to light, and itching and burning of the skin also occur. Fatigue, weakness, and diarrhea can last for months. Severe infections can lead to death.

How Is Trichinosis Diagnosed?

The doctor may suspect trichinosis from the medical history and physical examination. To confirm the diagnosis, the doctor will order blood tests and get a small piece of muscle tissue (muscle biopsy) for study. This tissue is checked with a microscope to identify the parasite.

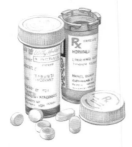

Medicines (anthelmintic, or antiworm, drugs) will kill the worms in your intestines. Acetaminophen and tepid sponge baths can help fever. Corticosteroid drugs may be prescribed for severe infection or infection involving the brain and nervous system.

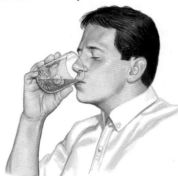

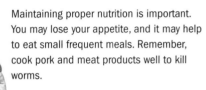

Drink more fluids to prevent dehydration.

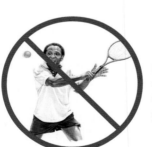

Maintaining proper nutrition is important. You may lose your appetite, and it may help to eat small frequent meals. Remember, cook pork and meat products well to kill worms.

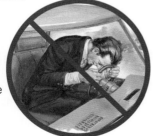

Rest is important until your symptoms are gone. Resume normal activities slowly after you have no more symptoms.

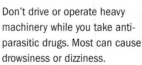

Don't drive or operate heavy machinery while you take antiparasitic drugs. Most can cause drowsiness or dizziness.

How Is Trichinosis Treated?

The doctor will prescribe medicines (anthelmintic, or antiworm, drugs) to kill the worms, if the parasites are in the intestines. Acetaminophen and tepid sponge baths can be used to reduce fever. Corticosteroid drugs such as prednisone may be prescribed if the infection is severe or if it involves the brain and nervous system.

Maintaining proper nutrition is important. Appetite loss occurs, so it may help to eat small frequent meals.

DOs and DON'Ts in Managing Trichinosis:

- ✔ **DO** take your medicine as directed.
- ✔ **DO** rest. Rest is important until your symptoms are gone. Resume your normal activities slowly after you have no more symptoms.
- ✔ **DO** use acetaminophen or ibuprofen for fever and pain.
- ✔ **DO** eat small, frequent meals for proper nutrition.
- ✔ **DO** increase your fluid intake to prevent dehydration.
- ✔ **DO** call your doctor if you have side effects from the medicine and cannot tolerate them.
- ✔ **DO** call your doctor if you have a high fever, shortness of breath, or an irregular heartbeat.
- ✔ **DO** cook pork and meat products well, to kill worms.

- ⊘ **DON'T** drive or operate heavy machinery while you're taking antiparasitic drugs. Most can cause drowsiness, dizziness, nausea, or diarrhea.
- ⊘ **DON'T** skip doses of medicine. Usually the course of treatment is short, but if you cannot tolerate the medicine, tell your doctor.
- ⊘ **DON'T** eat undercooked meat, to prevent future infections.

FROM THE DESK OF

NOTES

FOR MORE INFORMATION

Contact the following sources:

- National Institute of Allergy and Infectious Diseases
  Tel: (301) 496-5717
  Website: http://www3.niaid.nih.gov

- Centers for Disease Control and Prevention
  Tel: (800) 311-3435
  Website: http://www.cdc.gov

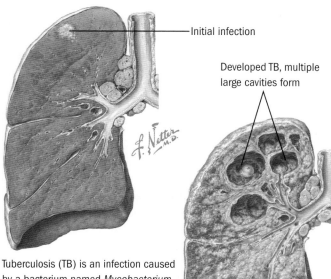

Initial infection

Developed TB, multiple large cavities form

Tuberculosis (TB) is an infection caused by a bacterium named *Mycobacterium tuberculosis* that destroys body tissues. TB affects lungs but can also spread to bones, lymph glands, brain, heart, and other organs.

Bacteria last for months in darkness and moisture.

People catch TB by close contact, such as breathing in bacteria that someone coughed into the air.

Symptoms of active TB include a cough lasting for weeks, coughing up sputum (phlegm) or blood, chest pain, and fever.

Chest x-rays may also be done.

Your doctor will do the tuberculin skin test to see whether you have TB. Swelling and redness mean a positive reaction.

What Is Tuberculosis?

Tuberculosis (TB) is an infection caused by a type of bacteria that attacks and destroys body tissues. It usually affects lungs but can also spread (disseminate) to bones, lymph glands (nodes), nervous system, heart, and other organs.

Many people first have inactive TB, called a latent infection. Later TB becomes active, especially if the immune (infection-fighting) system is weakened, such as by HIV, cancer, or chemotherapy.

What Causes TB?

The cause is a type of bacteria named *Mycobacterium tuberculosis*. People catch TB by close contact, such as breathing in bacteria in the air that someone spread by coughing.

What Are the Symptoms of TB?

People in early stages often feel normal. Symptoms include a cough lasting at least 3 weeks, coughing up sputum (phlegm) or blood, chest pain, fever, night sweats, losing weight and appetite, tiredness, and weakness.

How Is TB Diagnosed?

The doctor will suspect TB in people with an unexplained cough, weight loss, or fever. The doctor will ask about contact with places and people, history of TB or skin test results, risk factors (especially HIV), foreign travel, and job exposure. A tuberculin skin test (PPD) may be done. For this test, a tiny amount of fluid is injected under the skin on the arm and swelling that appears is measured 72 hours later. The size of swelling (induration) where the fluid was injected determines if the tuberculin test is positive. A positive test usually means that the person has been exposed to TB. A negative test may mean that another test is needed.

The doctor may also want to take chest x-rays and samples of sputum, blood, or urine for study and test for HIV.

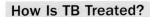

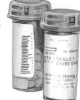

TB can nearly always be cured, usually by taking medicines. It's very important to finish the treatment, even if you feel better, to prevent bacteria from persisting and spreading later on.

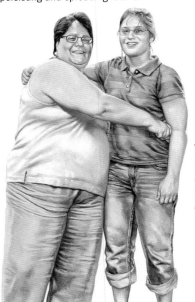

You should let close family members, friends, and other close contacts know you have been exposed to TB so that they get tested too.

If you smoke, you need to quit! You need your lungs to be as healthy as possible to fight the TB. Talk to you doctor about ways to stop if you don't think you can do it on your own.

Don't drink alcohol, or take other medicines unless your doctor says you can.

How Is TB Treated?

Active TB can nearly always be cured, usually by taking medicines for 6 months or longer. People should feel better after a few weeks. It's very important to finish the treatment, even if symptoms disappear. If medicines are stopped too soon, bacteria may stay in the body, and TB may return and spread to other parts of the body and to others. Family members and close contacts will need TB screening.

DOs and DON'Ts in Managing TB:

✔ **DO** take your medicines exactly as your doctor tells you.

✔ **DO** use a routine, such as a pill dispenser, that helps you remember to take your medicines.

✔ **DO** ask your doctor about medicine side effects.

✔ **DO** keep follow-up doctor appointments.

✔ **DO** be careful not to infect others. Follow your doctor's advice on hygiene.

✔ **DO** call your doctor if you have fever or chills, concerns about effects of medicines, or lasting or worsening symptoms despite taking medicines, or if you cough up discolored sputum or blood.

⊘ **DON'T** stop treatment early.

⊘ **DON'T** smoke.

⊘ **DON'T** assume you're not infective unless your doctor says so.

⊘ **DON'T** drink alcohol or take other medicine unless you talk with your doctor first. Alcohol is toxic to the liver and may interfere with medications you are taking for TB.

FROM THE DESK OF

NOTES

FOR MORE INFORMATION

Contact the following sources:

• Centers for Disease Control and Prevention
Tel: (800) 232-4636
Website: http://www.cdc.gov/tb/default.htm

• The American Lung Association
Tel: (800) 548-8252
Website: http://www.lungusa.org

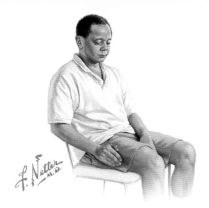

Chronic fatigue syndrome (CFS) is a condition in which you feel tired most or all of the time. It lasts longer than 6 months. The cause isn't known but may be related to an abnormal response to an infection.

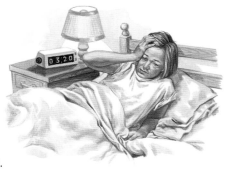

Other symptoms include headache, trouble sleeping, confusion, problems with concentration and memory, and muscle and joint pain.

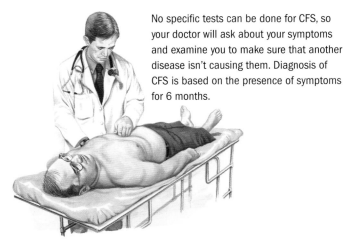

No specific tests can be done for CFS, so your doctor will ask about your symptoms and examine you to make sure that another disease isn't causing them. Diagnosis of CFS is based on the presence of symptoms for 6 months.

What Is Chronic Fatigue Syndrome?

Chronic fatigue syndrome (CFS) is a debilitating condition in which people feel tired most or all of the time. The symptoms often include muscle aches and difficulty concentrating and last at least 6 months. Symptoms can come and go over long periods, and many people can have serious problems, including being unable to work. With good lifestyle habits, many people, especially those with CFS that occurred after a viral infection, improve or recover completely after 2 to 3 years.

What Causes CFS?

The cause is unknown. Some believe that it is a complication of a viral infection, but no viruses have been identified. An abnormal response to an infection of the body's immune system (the system that fights infections) or stress may have a role in CSF.

What Are the Symptoms of CFS?

The most common complaints, apart from feeling tired, weak, or exhausted most of the time, include confusion and problems with concentration and memory, trouble sleeping, headache, sore throat, slight fever, vision changes, and pain in muscles, joints, and bones.

How Is CFS Diagnosed?

No specific test can diagnose CFS. The doctor makes a diagnosis after noting specific symptoms present for at least 6 months: lasting, unexplained fatigue that isn't the result of ongoing exertion, isn't helped by rest, and results in a considerable reduction in activities.

Other symptoms include problems with memory or concentration, sore throat, tender lymph nodes (swollen glands), muscle pain, headache, pain in many joints, and unrefreshing sleep.

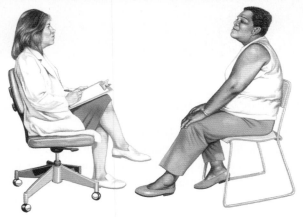

Stay positive, and talk to your doctor about changes you can make to feel better. If depression or another medical condition may make the symptoms of CFS worse, that condition needs treatment.

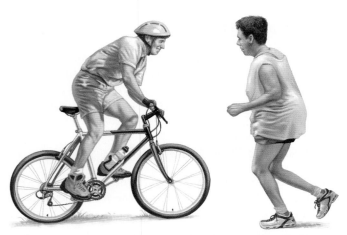

Start or keep up an exercise program based on your doctor's advice.

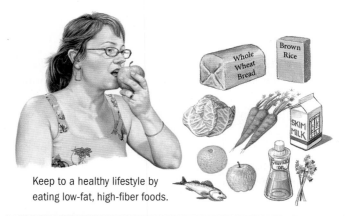

Keep to a healthy lifestyle by eating low-fat, high-fiber foods.

How Is CFS Treated?

No cure is available, but supportive care from the doctor is very important. The doctor may prescribe antiinflammatory medications to help with muscle aches. Antidepressants may also be prescribed. The doctor will likely suggest an exercise program and a balanced diet. Counseling and behavior therapy may help with coping with CFS symptoms.

DOs and DON'Ts in Managing CFS:

✔ **DO** follow your doctor's advice.

✔ **DO** take your medicine.

✔ **DO** keep a positive mental outlook, and remember that setbacks may occur.

✔ **DO** begin an exercise program based on your doctor's advice.

✔ **DO** eat a balanced, low-fat, high-fiber diet.

✔ **DO** call your doctor if symptoms get worse after treatment starts.

⊘ **DON'T** get discouraged about CFS and its treatment if you have setbacks.

⊘ **DON'T** exercise too hard.

FROM THE DESK OF

NOTES

FOR MORE INFORMATION

Contact the following source:

• Chronic Fatigue and Immune Dysfunction Syndrome Association of America
Tel: (800) 442-3437
Website: http://www.cfids.org

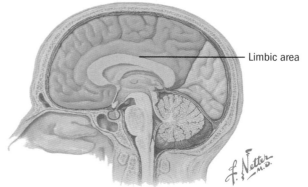

Limbic area

Cocaine causes high levels of a brain chemical called dopamine in the limbic area, which makes people feel good (the high).

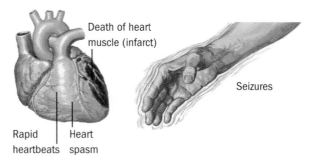

Death of heart muscle (infarct)

Seizures

Rapid heartbeats | Heart spasm

Cocaine abuse can cause heart problems, including rapid heartbeats and infarcts (death of heart muscle). Serious complications include seizures, stroke, kidney failure, and HIV infection.

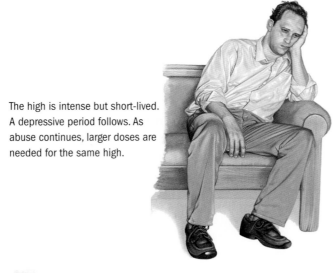

The high is intense but short-lived. A depressive period follows. As abuse continues, larger doses are needed for the same high.

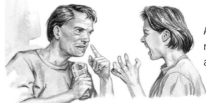

A cocaine binge can cause rapid heartbeat, irritability, and aggression.

What Are Cocaine Abuse and Dependence?

Cocaine is an illegal drug obtained from the coca plant, *Erythroxylon coca*. A strong stimulant, cocaine causes euphoria (makes people high). It can damage all organs but mostly affects the heart, brain, and lungs. Usually a white or off-white powder, it's called coke, C, snow, flake, or blow. People sniff it through a tube or straw, dissolve it in water and inject it, or burn it and breathe the smoke (crack).

Pregnant addicted women can have crack babies with major birth defects.

What Causes Cocaine Abuse and Dependence?

Cocaine causes high levels of a brain chemical called dopamine, which makes people feel good.

Because the high doesn't last long and a depressive period follows, people may need to use cocaine often, leading to addiction. As abuse continues, tolerance develops, so larger doses taken more often are needed for the same high.

What Are the Symptoms of Cocaine Abuse and Dependence?

Short-term effects include euphoria, high energy levels, and needing less food and sleep.

A binge can produce rapid heartbeat, high blood pressure, irritability, and aggression.

Regularly snorting can lead to loss of sense of smell, nosebleeds, trouble swallowing, hoarseness, being underweight, and runny nose. Serious complications of cocaine use and overdose include stroke, seizures, and heart attacks.

Cocaine overdose usually causes high blood pressure and fast pulse, as well as chest pain, tremors, convulsions, and even death.

How Are Cocaine Abuse and Dependence Diagnosed?

The doctor will ask questions about symptoms, medical conditions, work history, family medical history, and patterns of cocaine, tobacco, and alcohol use.

The doctor will also do a physical examination, order blood and urine tests, and check for nasal perforations and heart damage.

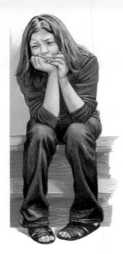
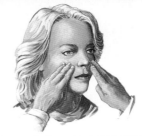

Regular snorting can cause loss of smell, nosebleeds, and being underweight.

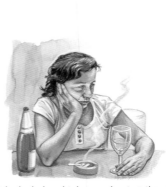

Behavioral therapy can help cocaine abuse and dependence. Quitting can be long and hard, and cravings for cocaine may last a long time.

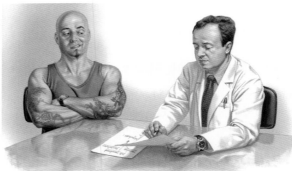

Don't drink alcohol and take cocaine together. Call your doctor if you're pregnant and using cocaine. Cocaine can cause your baby to have birth defects.

How Are Cocaine Abuse and Dependence Treated?

Cocaine-dependent people need a lot of help to quit. Behavioral therapy can help reduce or stop drug use.

Residential programs and outpatient substance abuse clinics can offer behavioral therapies and help with detoxification. Twelve-step recovery groups (Narcotics Anonymous) also help some people.

Cocaine overdose is an emergency. Treatment depends on symptoms and organs affected.

DOs and DON'Ts in Managing Cocaine Abuse and Dependence:

✔ **DO** admit that you have a cocaine problem.
✔ **DO** understand that a cocaine or crack habit can cost thousands of dollars weekly.
✔ **DO** understand that breaking a cocaine habit isn't easy. Cravings may last for a long time.
✔ **DO** call your doctor if you're pregnant and using cocaine.
✔ **DO** call your doctor if you share needles or have fevers and take cocaine intravenously.
✔ **DO** call your doctor if you have chest pain or passed out while using cocaine or you have abnormal heartbeats, new seizures, shortness of breath, or headaches.
✔ **DO** call your doctor if you want detoxification.

⊘ **DON'T** try to deal with your cocaine dependence on your own. Get medical help.
⊘ **DON'T** take alcohol and cocaine together.
⊘ **DON'T** be fooled that cocaine is a safe drug. All forms can lead to overdose and to life-threatening complications.
⊘ **DON'T** share needles. Sharing puts you at risk for HIV and AIDS.
⊘ **DON'T** use cocaine if you're pregnant.

FROM THE DESK OF

NOTES

FOR MORE INFORMATION

Contact the following sources:

• National Institute on Drug Abuse
 Tel: (301) 443-1124
 Website: http://www.nida.nih.gov/

• Narcotics Anonymous
 Tel: (818) 773-9999 / Fax: (818) 700-0700
 Website: http://www.na.org/

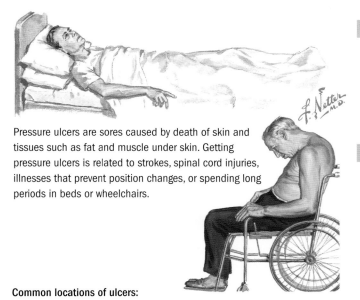

Pressure ulcers are sores caused by death of skin and tissues such as fat and muscle under skin. Getting pressure ulcers is related to strokes, spinal cord injuries, illnesses that prevent position changes, or spending long periods in beds or wheelchairs.

Common locations of ulcers:

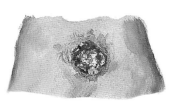

Ulcers can form on body parts that have pressure when people sit or lie still for long periods. The weight of the body part causes slow circulation over that point and less nutrition, so skin and tissues die and ulcers form.

There are four stages of ulcers. Stage 1: skin is red but not broken. Stage 2: outer skin is broken, with blistering and drain-age (shown here). Stage 3: tissue under skin affected, sores painful around the edges, with foul-smelling drainage. Stage 4: muscle or bone affected.

Your doctor will diagnose a pressure ulcer by examining skin and tissues under the skin.

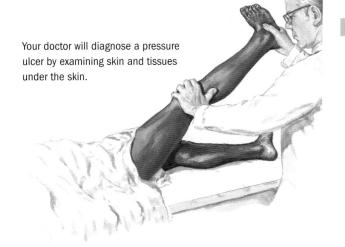

What Are Pressure Ulcers?

Pressure ulcers, also known as decubitus ulcers, are sores that result from injury to the skin and tissue below it. Skin dies over parts of the body that have pressure when people sit or lie still for long periods.

What Causes Pressure Ulcers?

The weight of the body or body part causes circulation in the skin over that pressure point to slow down. With less circulation and nutrition, skin and tissues such as fat and muscle die, and ulcers or sores develop.

Other things that contribute to ulcers are poor nutrition, wet skin from urine and stool, and friction from moving over clothes and bedding.

What Are the Symptoms of Pressure Ulcers?

Symptoms include red skin but not broken skin (stage 1 ulcers). In stage 2 ulcers, the outer skin layer is broken, with blistering and drainage. In stage 3 ulcers, tissue under the skin is affected. Sores may have a white or black base, can be painful around the edges, and have foul-smelling drainage. Stage 4 ulcers reach muscle or bone. They can be white or black at the base and have a bone infection and foul-smelling drainage. Greater risk of developing pressure ulcers is related to stroke, spinal cord injuries, or illnesses that prevent changing positions easily. Also, people who spend long periods in bed or wheelchairs, cannot control their bowels or bladder, or cannot tell caregivers that they're sore or need turning are more prone to getting pressure ulcers.

How Are Pressure Ulcers Diagnosed?

The doctor will make a diagnosis by examining the skin and tissues near the skin.

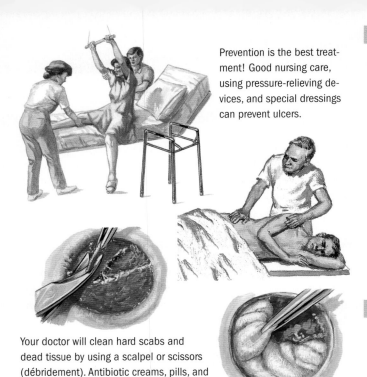

Prevention is the best treatment! Good nursing care, using pressure-relieving devices, and special dressings can prevent ulcers.

Your doctor will clean hard scabs and dead tissue by using a scalpel or scissors (débridement). Antibiotic creams, pills, and injections can help control infections.

Move bedridden people or encourage them to move at least every 2 hours. Know which pressure points may have ulcers and check them often.

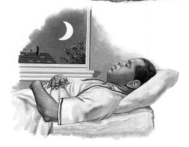

Use pressure relief devices, such as pillows, gel or foam cushions or mattresses, and foam or gel heel protectors.

How Are Pressure Ulcers Treated?

Prevention is by far the best treatment! Good nursing care, using pressure-relieving devices, and special dressings can prevent ulcers. Treatment depends on the ulcer's stage.

All ulcers must be kept clean with sterile saline and an irrigation tool. Don't use hydrogen peroxide, povidone-iodine solution, liquid detergents, and bleach.

The doctor cleans hard scabs and dead tissue by using a scalpel or scissors (débridement). Wet-to-dry dressings and moist wound dressings can be used to pull off scabs when they are changed. Enzymes on some of the medicated dressings can help remove dead tissue.

The doctor may prescribe antibiotic creams, pills, and injections to control infections.

DOs and DON'Ts in Managing Pressure Ulcers:

✔ **DO** call your doctor if drainage, pain, or redness around an ulcer increases.

✔ **DO** call your doctor if drainage smells foul and looks like pus.

✔ **DO** call your doctor if you get fever, chills, confusion, weakness, or rapid heartbeat.

✔ **DO** know which pressure points may have ulcers and check them often. These points usually don't have fat padding.

✔ **DO** use pressure relief devices, such as pillows, gel or foam cushions or mattresses, and foam or gel heel protectors.

✔ **DO** move bedridden people or encourage them to move at least every 2 hours.

✔ **DO** keep skin clean and lubricated but not moist.

✔ **DO** keep down friction when moving someone. Keep the head of a bed no higher than 30 degrees to prevent sliding and friction.

✔ **DO** promote good nutrition.

🚫 **DON'T** use a doughnut type of cushion, because they can cause pressure ulcers in other areas.

FOR MORE INFORMATION

Contact the following sources:

• American Academy of Dermatology
  Tel: (866) 503-7546, (847) 330-9239
  Website: http://www.aad.org

• MedlinePlus
  Website: http://nlm.nih.gov/medlineplus/pressuresores. html

• American College of Surgeons
  Tel: (800) 621-4111
  Website: http://facs.org

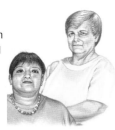

Fibromylagia causes pain in muscles, tendons, and ligaments and is most common in women.

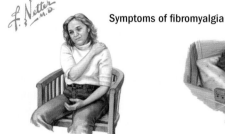

Symptoms of fibromyalgia

Chronic fatigue and general achiness

Not enough sleep and sleep is of poor quality

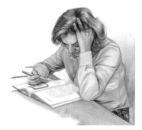

Poor concentration

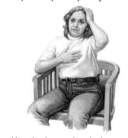

Headache and pain in the chest or abdomen

Fibromyalgia tender points

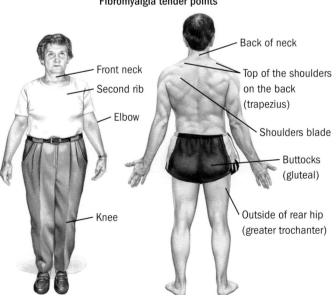

Front neck
Second rib
Elbow
Knee

Back of neck
Top of the shoulders on the back (trapezius)
Shoulders blade
Buttocks (gluteal)
Outside of rear hip (greater trochanter)

What Is Fibromyalgia?

Fibromyalgia (FM) is a chronic condition causing pain in muscles, tendons, and ligaments. In FM, specific places in the body where pain is felt are called *tender points*.

What Causes Fibromyalgia?

The cause is unknown, but it is not thought to be an infection. Possibilities include poor sleep, certain chemicals called serotonin and substance P, muscle abnormalities, and stress hormones.

FM is most common in women aged between 20 and 50 and is also common in women older than 60.

What Are the Symptoms of Fibromyalgia?

Pain and fatigue are the main symptoms and can affect activities at work and home.

Pain is usually worse in the upper back and neck and the lower back and hips. Pain can occur near any tender point, however.

Fatigue can be severe. Headaches, numbness or tingling in the hands or feet, and forgetfulness are other symptoms.

How Is Fibromyalgia Diagnosed?

A doctor uses a medical history and an examination of joints and muscles for diagnosis. For a diagnosis of FM, the doctor must find at least 11 of the 18 tender points.

Laboratory tests and x-rays may be done to rule out other diseases causing similar symptoms. Blood tests and x-rays are usually normal in fibromyalgia.

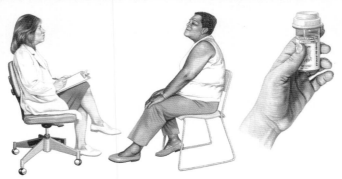

Treatment includes use of medicines, exercise, and counseling.

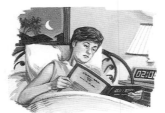

Get enough good sleep. Your doctor may prescribe medicine to help with this.

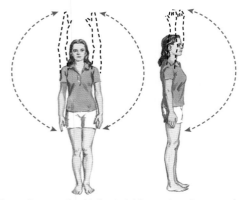

Every day, you should do stretching and posture exercises.

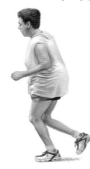

Four or five times a week, you should do endurance exercises.

How Is Fibromyalgia Treated?

No cure exists for FM, but people with FM can feel better with the right treatment. Medicines, exercise, reducing stress, and improving sleep to reduce fatigue can help people feel better.

Drugs can improve the amount and quality of sleep. Interrupted sleep prevents people from reaching the deepest sleep, but medicines can help them reach this deeper stage of sleep. As a result, pain decreases. The most common medicines include low doses of antidepressants (e.g., amitriptyline or duloxetine). Common side effects include grogginess, dry mouth, constipation, and weight gain.

Exercises help reduce pain. Stretching and posture exercises should be done daily for good body alignment and to prevent pain. Endurance exercises should be done three or four times a week; these include walking, biking, and water therapy. It is important to begin to exercise slowly and to increase gradually.

Often people with FM forget how to relax. A counselor can offer relaxation therapy as well as family counseling to see whether depression or family or financial problems are contributing to FM.

DOs and DON'Ts in Managing Fibromyalgia:

✔ **DO** call your doctor if you have drug side effects.
✔ **DO** ask your doctor what over-the-counter pain medications you may take.
✔ **DO** communicate and follow up with your healthcare workers.

⊘ **DON'T** expect medicines alone to reduce your pain and fatigue. Feeling better involves better sleep, exercise, and stress management.
⊘ **DON'T** take any diet supplement without discussing it first with your doctor.
⊘ **DON'T** stop exercising.

FROM THE DESK OF

NOTES

FOR MORE INFORMATION

Contact the following sources:

• Arthritis Foundation
Tel: (800) 283-7800
Website: http://www.arthritis.org

• American College of Rheumatology
Tel: (404) 633-3777
Website: http://www.rheumatology.org

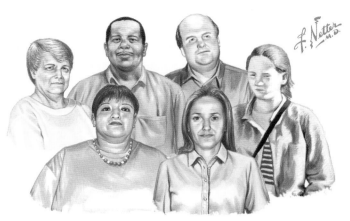

Hyperhidrosis, or too much sweat, is a rather common problem. It can also be related to abnormal sweat odor (called bromhidrosis). Hyperhidrosis often affects the feet, but it can also involve hands and armpits. It's usually not curable, but it can be treated.

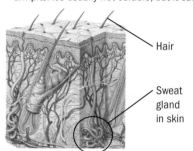

Hair

Sweat gland in skin

The cause is unknown but may be related to stress. Other less common causes include certain kinds of arthritis, nervous system disorders, blood system disorders, and medicines.

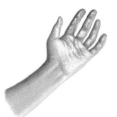 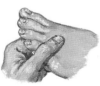 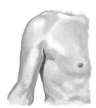

Symptoms are too much sweating of the feet, hands, or armpits, or all three. The sweating can cause embarrassment and sometimes a foul odor. Shirt, socks, and shoes can become stained.

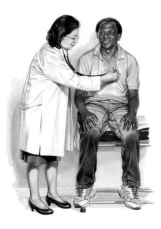

Your doctor makes a diagnosis from your medical history, physical examination. Blood tests may be done to rule out other disorders.

What Is Hyperhydrosis?

Hyperhydrosis, or too much sweat, is a rather common problem. It can also be related to abnormal sweat odor (called bromhidrosis). Hyperhydrosis often affects the feet, but can also involve hands and armpits. It's usually not curable, but it can be treated.

What Causes Hyperhydrosis?

The cause is unknown but may be related to stress in some people. Other less common causes include certain kinds of arthritis, nervous system diseases and trauma to the spinal cord, disorders of the blood system, and certain medicines.

What Are the Symptoms of Hyperhydrosis?

Symptoms are too much sweating of the feet, hands, or armpits, or all three. Sometimes other parts of the body are affected. The sweating can cause embarrassment and sometimes a foul odor. Shirt, socks, and shoes can become stained.

How Is Hyperhydrosis Diagnosed?

The doctor makes a diagnosis of hyperhydrosis from a medical history and physical examination. Blood tests may be done to rule out conditions, such as overactive thyroid, that may cause similar symptoms.

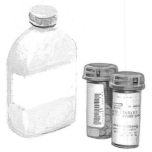

Treatment is often with small amounts of Drysol® (aluminum chloride). After symptoms are controlled, Drysol® should be used as little as possible, especially in armpits. Iontophoresis and Botox® may be tried for severe cases.

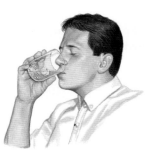

Drink plenty of water to avoid dehydration. Drink more during hot summer months, 8 to 10 glasses (8 ounces per glass) of water per day. Drink more if you're in hot sun.

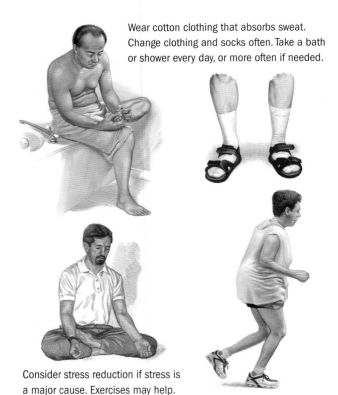

Wear cotton clothing that absorbs sweat. Change clothing and socks often. Take a bath or shower every day, or more often if needed.

Consider stress reduction if stress is a major cause. Exercises may help.

FROM THE DESK OF

NOTES

How Is Hyperhydrosis Treated?

Treatment is often with Drysol® (20% aluminum chloride hexahydrate). Before bedtime, affected areas are washed and dried and a small amount of Drysol® is applied. It's washed off in the morning. This treatment is repeated for 1 to 2 weeks, then once per week or as needed. Sensitive skin should have treatments less often. After symptoms are controlled, Drysol® should be used as little as possible, especially in armpits. Other medicines may also be prescribed if Drysol® doesn't work. Sometimes, oral medicines called anticholinergics are prescribed, but these may cause side effects, such as dry mouth, blurred vision, and dizziness.

Iontophoresis—use of a mild electric current in tap water—can be tried in some cases for about 30 minutes a day. Botox® (botulinum toxin) injections to the armpit sweat glands also work and are often used by dermatologists (specialists in skin diseases) in severe cases.

DOs and DON'Ts in Managing Hyperhydrosis:

✔ **DO** avoid other deodorants and antiperspirants when you first use Drysol® for armpit sweating. Dry the armpit with a hairdryer first, apply Drysol®, then immediately dry with the hairdryer again. After you use Drysol® once or twice a week, you can use other antiperspirants and deodorants during the day.

✔ **DO** drink plenty of water to avoid dehydration. Drink more during hot summer months, 8 to 10 glasses (8 ounces per glass) of water per day. Drink more if you're in hot sun.

✔ **DO** wear cotton clothing that absorbs sweat. Change clothing and socks frequently.

✔ **DO** take a bath or shower every day, more often if needed.

✔ **DO** consider stress reduction counseling if stress is a major cause.

✔ **DO** call your doctor if you see redness, swelling, or pus drainage.

✔ **DO** call your doctor if symptoms don't get better in 3 to 4 weeks of treatment.

⊘ **DON'T** wear nylon or manufactured fabrics.

⊘ **DON'T** use deodorants and antiperspirants on armpits during the first 1 to 2 weeks of Drysol® therapy. Use baking soda instead.

FOR MORE INFORMATION

Contact the following source:

• American Academy of Dermatology
  Tel: (847) 330-0230, (866) 503-7546
  Website: http://www.aad.org

WEIGHT CONTROL FOR WOMEN
TAKING CHARGE OF YOUR OBESITY

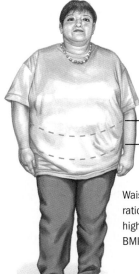

— Waist size (circumference)

— Hip size (circumference)

Waist size more than 35 inches or waist-to-hip ratio more than 0.85 is considered obese with high risks of diseases. Another measure is the BMI = weight (kg)/height^2 (m^2).

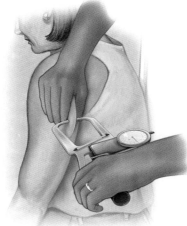

Your doctor uses a caliper to measure skinfold thickness, to determine relative obesity.

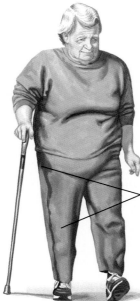

Obesity can strain lower weight-bearing joints and cause wear-and-tear arthritis in the hips and knees. It also increases risks for many other diseases such as diabetes and heart disease.

What Is Obesity?

Obesity is an increased percentage of total body fat compared with normal. Overweight is increased body weight relative to height. Both have important effects on health.

Body mass index (BMI) is one way to see whether someone is overweight. The formula for BMI is weight (kg)/height^2 (m^2). Women 19 to 35 years old should have a BMI of 19 to 25, and women older than 35, of 21 to 27.

Skinfold measurements are used to determine relative obesity. Waist and hip size are used to determine body fat distribution. Females with a body fat content higher than 33% are obese. An increased waist-to-hip ratio is a risk factor for diabetes and heart disease.

What Causes Obesity?

Obesity is caused by eating too many calories for the physical activities performed. Why certain people gain too much weight isn't known. Genetics (parents passing on a tendency to gain weight to children), psychological reasons (eating when stressed), culture, and society (people are encouraged to eat too much) may play a role.

What Are the Symptoms of Obesity?

A women with a BMI higher than 25 is overweight; a woman with a BMI of 30 or higher is obese; and a woman with a BMI of 40 or more is severely obese. Being overweight increases the chances of having serious health problems, such as high blood pressure, diabetes, coronary artery disease, and pulmonary hypertension. It strains arthritic joints and causes shortness of breath and tiredness.

How Is Obesity Diagnosed?

The doctor will do a physical examination (weight, BMI, blood pressure) and take a medical history. The doctor may use calipers (a tool that measures thickness) to find the amount of body fat. Blood and urine tests may also be done as part of the medical evaluation.

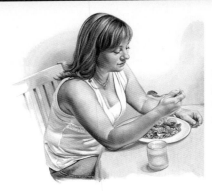

Make lifestyle changes to lose weight. Begin a medically supervised diet and exercise program.

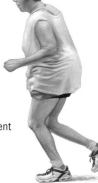

Different kinds of exercise appeal to different people. Find activities that you enjoy!

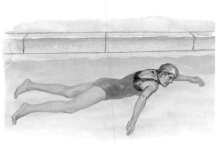

Surgery such as stomach stapling and medicines may be discussed with your doctor if other methods don't work.

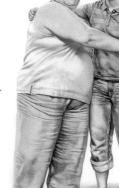

Children learn eating and exercise habits from the adults in their life—set a good example!

FROM THE DESK OF

NOTES

How Is Obesity Treated?

Diet, exercise, medicines, and surgery are all used. A registered dietitian and doctors can help plan a good low-fat, low-calorie diet. Exercise is very effective, and an individualized supervised program helps prevent complications. Few drugs (such as amphetamines) are available for weight loss, and they cause side effects. They should be tried only after diet and exercise and only under direct supervison of the doctor.

Morbidly obese women (more than 100% above ideal body weight or with a BMI higher than 40) who had no success with other methods may try surgery, such as gastric bypass or vertical band gastroplasty (stomach stapling).

DOs and DON'Ts in Managing Obesity:

✔ **DO** tell your doctor about other medical problems.
✔ **DO** tell your doctor about all your drugs. Call your doctor if you have side effects from medicines.
✔ **DO** tell your doctor if you're pregnant or nursing.
✔ **DO** consider joining a support group.
✔ **DO** some daily exercise activity.
✔ **DO** learn your current weight, body mass index, and body fat content.
✔ **DO** call your doctor if you gain weight even with diet and exercise.
✔ **DO** call your doctor if you have severe diarrhea or low blood sugar (glucose) after surgery.

○ **DON'T** try fad diets.
○ **DON'T** try to lose weight too quickly.
○ **DON'T** drink a lot of alcohol and soft drinks or eat fast food.
○ **DON'T** smoke to control body weight.
○ **DON'T** become discouraged if weight loss stops for a while.

FOR MORE INFORMATION

Contact the following sources:

• The Endocrine Society
Tel: (301) 941-0200
Website: http://www.endo-society.org

• National Institutes of Health
Tel: (301) 496-4000
Website: http://www.nih.gov

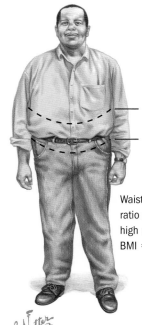

Waist size (circumference)

Hip size (circumference)

Waist size more than 40 inches or waist-to-hip ratio more than 1.0 is considered obese with high risks of diseases. Another measure is the BMI = weight (kg)/height^2 (m^2).

Your doctor uses a caliper to measure skinfold thickness, to determine relative obesity.

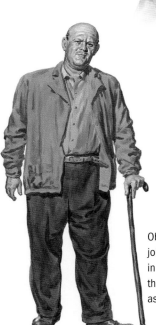

Obesity can strain lower weight-bearing joints and cause wear-and-tear arthritis in the hips and knees. It also increases the risk for many other diseases, such as diabetes and heart disease.

What Is Obesity?

Obesity is an increased percentage of total body fat compared with normal. Overweight is increased body weight relative to height. Both have important effects on health.

Body mass index (BMI) is one way to see whether someone is overweight. The formula for BMI is weight (kg)/height^2 (m^2). Men 19 to 35 years old should have a BMI of 19 to 25, and men older than 35, a BMI of 21 to 27.

Skinfold measurements are used to determine relative obesity. Waist and hip size are used to determine body fat distribution. Males with a body fat content higher than 25% are obese. An increased waist-to-hip ratio is a risk factor for diabetes and heart disease.

What Causes Obesity?

Obesity is caused by eating too many calories for the physical activities performed. Why certain people gain too much weight isn't known. Genetics (parents passing on a tendency to gain weight to children), psychological reasons (eating when stressed), culture, and society (people are encouraged to eat too much) may play a role.

What Are the Symptoms of Obesity?

A man with a BMI higher than 25 is overweight; a man with a BMI of 30 or more is obese; and a man with a BMI of 40 or more is severely obese. Being overweight increases the chances having serious health problems, such as high blood pressure, diabetes, coronary artery disease, and pulmonary hypertension. It strains arthritic joints and causes shortness of breath and tiredness.

How Is Obesity Diagnosed?

The doctor will do a physical examination (weight, BMI, blood pressure). The doctor will also take a medical history. The doctor may use calipers (a tool that measures thickness) to find the amount of body fat. Blood and urine tests may also be done as part of the medical evaluation.

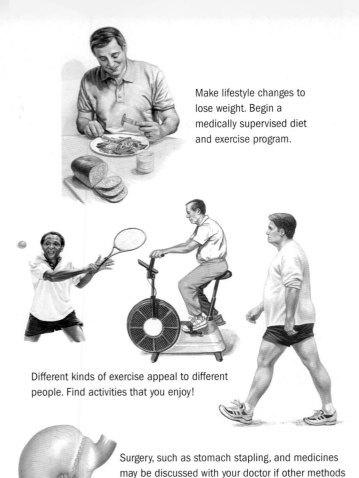

Make lifestyle changes to lose weight. Begin a medically supervised diet and exercise program.

Different kinds of exercise appeal to different people. Find activities that you enjoy!

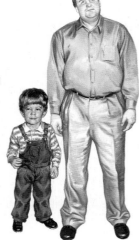

Surgery, such as stomach stapling, and medicines may be discussed with your doctor if other methods don't work.

Children learn eating and exercise habits from the adults in their life— take this opportunity to set a good example!

How Is Obesity Treated?

Diet, exercise, medicines, and surgery are all used. A registered dietitian and doctors can help plan a good low-fat, low-calorie diet. Exercise is very effective, and an individualized supervised program helps prevent complications. Few drugs (such as amphetamines) are available for weight loss, and they cause side effects. They should be tried only after diet and exercise and only under direct supervision of the doctor.

Morbidly obese men (more than 100% above ideal body weight or with a BMI higher than 40) who had no success with other methods may try surgery, such as gastric bypass or vertical band gastroplasty (stomach stapling).

DOs and DON'Ts in Managing Obesity:

✔ **DO** tell your doctor about other medical problems.
✔ **DO** tell your doctor about all your drugs. Call your doctor if you have side effects from medicines.
✔ **DO** consider joining a weight loss support group.
✔ **DO** some daily activity.
✔ **DO** learn your current weight, body mass index, and body fat content.
✔ **DO** call your doctor if you gain weight even with diet and exercise.
✔ **DO** call your doctor if you have severe diarrhea or low blood sugar (glucose) after surgery.

⊘ **DON'T** try fad diets.
⊘ **DON'T** try to lose weight too quickly.
⊘ **DON'T** spend spare time watching television or playing video games.
⊘ **DON'T** drink a lot of alcohol and soft drinks or eat fast food.
⊘ **DON'T** smoke to control body weight.
⊘ **DON'T** become discouraged if weight loss stops for a while.

FROM THE DESK OF

NOTES

FOR MORE INFORMATION

Contact the following sources:

• The Endocrine Society
Tel: (301) 941-0200
Website: http://www.endo-society.org

• National Institutes of Health (NIH)
Tel: (301) 496-4000
Website: http://www.nih.gov

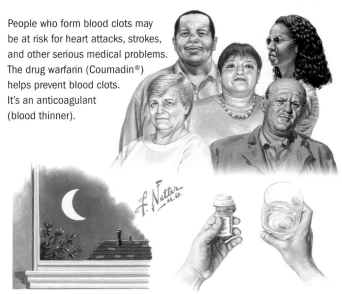

People who form blood clots may be at risk for heart attacks, strokes, and other serious medical problems. The drug warfarin (Coumadin®) helps prevent blood clots. It's an anticoagulant (blood thinner).

Pills are usually taken daily at the same time of day, usually evening. Never skip doses or take double doses unless instructed to do so by your doctor. If you miss a dose, take it as soon as you remember.

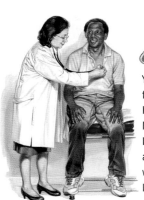

Your doctor decides the dose by seeing how fast your blood clots with a test called the INR (International Normalized Ratio). If the INR value is too high, bleeding may occur. If it's too low, clots may form. Illness such as a fever or flu can affect the INR and warfarin dose, as can diarrhea and vomiting lasting more than 1 day.

Side effects may include

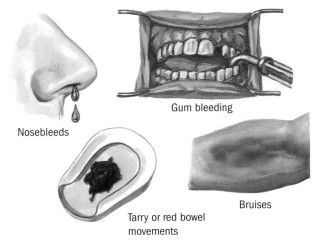

Nosebleeds

Gum bleeding

Tarry or red bowel movements

Bruises

What Is Warfarin and What Does It Do?

People who form blood clots may be at risk for heart attacks, strokes, and other serious medical problems. The drug warfarin (Coumadin®) helps prevent blood clots and is also used to treat blood clots. It's an anticoagulant (blood thinner).

How Should Warfarin Be Taken?

Pills are usually taken daily at the same time. The doctor bases the dose on a blood test called the INR (International Normalized Ratio). Never skip doses or take double doses unless instructed to do so by your doctor.

How Is the Dose Decided?

The doctor decides the dose by testing how fast the blood clots. If the INR result is too high, bleeding may occur. If it's too low, clots may form. Illness such as a fever or flu can affect the INR test and warfarin dose, as can diarrhea and vomiting lasting more than 1 day.

What Are the Side Effects?

Side effects include bleeding. A little bleeding may occur even with correct doses. Such bleeding includes easy bruising, slight gum bleeding when brushing teeth, nosebleeds, and menstrual periods that are a little heavier than normal. Major bleeding requires immediate care. This bleeding includes red or tarry bowel movements, gum bleeding or nosebleeds that don't stop quickly, coffee-colored or bright red vomit, or red, coffee-colored, or cola-colored urine. Other problems may include severe headaches or stomach aches, bruises for no reason, much heavier periods, cuts that don't stop bleeding in 10 minutes, dizziness, and weakness.

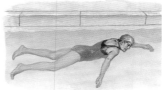

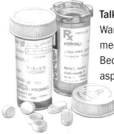

You need to avoid injury. Be careful using sharp objects, such as knives and scissors. Wear gloves when doing yard work. Use an electric razor, soft toothbrush, and waxed dental floss. Don't use toothpicks. Trim nails carefully. Avoid activities and risky sports that could cause injury. Safe activities are swimming and walking.

Talk with your doctor about all your other medicines. Warfarin can change the way they work, and other medicines, such as aspirin, can affect warfarin. Because over-the-counter medicines may contain aspirin, your doctor must approve all your drugs.

Foods can affect how warfarin works. High amounts of vitamin K can work against the drug, so talk to your doctor about foods you should avoid. Call your doctor if you can't eat for several days or have stomach problems, vomiting, or diarrhea.

Remember, you can bleed inside your body but not see blood. For example, a fall could cause bleeding under the skin, so you may see only a bruise. **Call your doctor or go to the hospital immediately if you have a severe fall or head trauma, even if you don't see blood.**

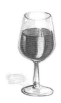

Limit alcohol. Drinking more than two drinks a day or changing your usual drinking pattern can affect warfarin dosage. Avoid binge drinking.

DOs and DON'Ts in Managing Warfarin Therapy:

✔ **DO** be careful using sharp objects, such as knives and scissors. Wear gloves when doing yard work. Use an electric razor, soft toothbrush, and waxed dental floss. Don't use toothpicks. Trim nails carefully. Avoid activities and risky sports that could cause injury. Safe activities are swimming and walking.

✔ **DO** remember that you can bleed but not see blood. For example, a fall could cause bleeding under the skin, so you see only a bruise. Call your doctor or go to the hospital immediately if you have a severe fall or head trauma, even if you don't see blood.

✔ **DO** talk to your doctor about wearing a medical alert bracelet or necklace.

✔ **DO** talk with your doctor about all your other medicines. Warfarin can change the way they work, and other medicines can affect warfarin.

✔ **DO** talk with your doctor before using aspirin. Aspirin interferes with warfarin and the blood's ability to clot. Because over-the-counter medicines may contain aspirin, your doctor must approve all drugs.

✔ **DO** talk to your doctor about diet and foods with high amounts of vitamin K. This vitamin may affect warfarin. Such foods include kiwi, blueberries, broccoli, cabbage, Brussels sprouts, green onions, asparagus, cauliflower, peas, lettuce, spinach, parsley, kale, endive, and turnip, collard, and mustard greens. Beef and pork liver, mayonnaise, margarine, canola and soybean oil, vitamins, soybeans, and cashews also have vitamin K.

✔ **DO** call your doctor if you cannot eat for several days or have vomiting or diarrhea for more than 1 day. These problems could affect warfarin dosage.

✔ **DO** limit alcohol. Drinking more than two drinks a day or changing your usual drinking pattern can affect warfarin dosage. Avoid binge drinking.

FROM THE DESK OF

NOTES

FOR MORE INFORMATION

Contact the following source:

• Agency for Healthcare Research and Quality
  Tel: (301) 427-1364
  Website: http://www.ahrq.gov/coumadin.htm

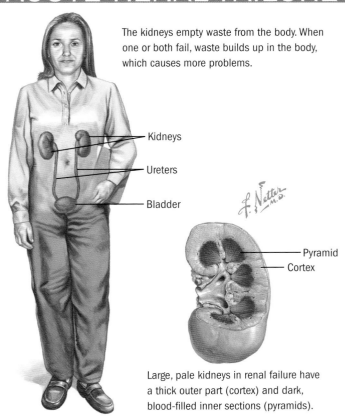

The kidneys empty waste from the body. When one or both fail, waste builds up in the body, which causes more problems.

Kidneys

Ureters

Bladder

Pyramid

Cortex

Large, pale kidneys in renal failure have a thick outer part (cortex) and dark, blood-filled inner sections (pyramids).

Many things can cause renal failure, such as kidney inflammation, kidney blockage, and chronic urinary tract infections. An early symptom of acute renal failure is often little or no urine output. Other symptoms include nausea, vomiting, appetite loss, and diarrhea.

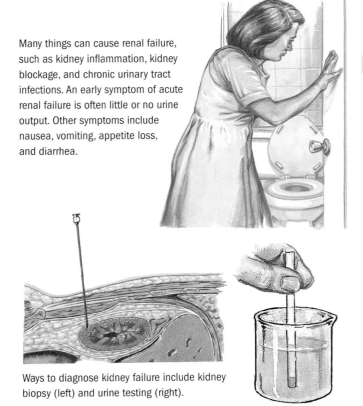

Ways to diagnose kidney failure include kidney biopsy (left) and urine testing (right).

What Is Acute Renal Failure?

Acute renal failure means that kidneys suddenly can't get rid of the body's waste. Kidneys normally do this by making urine. When they fail, waste products build up and are harmful.

What Causes Acute Renal Failure?

Conditions that reduce the blood supply to kidneys, block flow of urine after it leaves kidneys, or injure kidneys can cause renal failure. These include chronic urinary infections and kidney damage from congestive heart failure, diabetes, or high blood pressure.

Causes of acute renal failure include illnesses that have an indirect effect on kidneys (e.g., low blood pressure), kidney blockage, and direct kidney injury (e.g., by drugs and x-ray dyes).

What Are the Symptoms of Acute Renal Failure?

An early symptom is little or no urine output.

Later ones include nausea, vomiting, diarrhea, and appetite loss. Being irritable, not able to sleep, convulsions, stupor, coma, severe itching, high or low blood pressure, unexplained bruising, and bleeding for no reason are additional signs.

How Is Acute Renal Failure Diagnosed?

Blood and urine tests can measure how well kidneys work. A biopsy (taking a sample of tissue from kidneys) may be done, as may x-rays of the chest, belly, kidneys, and ureters (tubes taking urine from kidneys to the bladder).

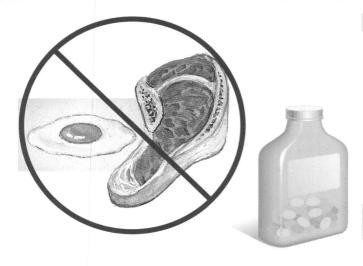

Because many things cause kidney failure, different treatments are possible. Your doctor may ask you to lower the amount of protein, salt, and potassium in your diet. You may also take medicines or have dialysis.

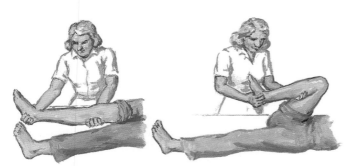

If you must stay in bed, flex your legs often to prevent blood clots from forming in your legs.

How Is Acute Renal Failure Treated?

Treatment depends on the reason for acute renal failure. However, most likely a hospital admission, may be necessary. Medicines may help increase the amount of urine made, and an artificial kidney machine may be used for dialysis. The doctor may suggest a reduced intake of protein, salt, and potassium and use of blood pressure pills and calcium supplements. In many cases, kidneys may recover completely, but recovery may take up to 6 weeks.

DOs and DON'Ts in Managing Acute Renal Failure:

✔ **DO** follow a low-protein diet if your doctor recommends it. A proper diet is critical to prevent complications. You may have to eliminate fruit, chocolate, and nuts because of high potassium levels. When kidneys don't work, high levels are dangerous for your heart.

✔ **DO** take medicines as prescribed.

✔ **DO** weigh yourself daily and keep a record of fluids you drink and the amount of fluid you pass if your doctor asks you to.

✔ **DO** flex your legs often, if you must stay in bed, to reduce the chance of getting blood clots.

✔ **DO** tell your doctor of any exposure to toxic chemicals or drugs.

✔ **DO** keep to your fluid restriction to avoid fluid buildup in your lungs.

✔ **DO** tell your doctor about all your medicines, including over-the-counter and herbal preparations.

✔ **DO** call your doctor if you have chills, fever, vomiting, headache, muscle aches, or diarrhea.

✔ **DO** avoid anything poisonous to kidneys, such as some drugs.

✔ **DO** treat anything that might damage kidneys, such as high blood pressure, diabetes, congestive heart failure, and infections.

🚫 **DON'T** stop taking your medicines before asking your doctor. Don't miss any doses.

🚫 **DON'T** take over-the-counter medicines or herbal preparations unless you check with your doctor.

FROM THE DESK OF

NOTES

FOR MORE INFORMATION

Contact the following sources:

• National Kidney Foundation, Inc.
Tel: (800) 622-9010, (212) 889-2210
E-mail: info@kidney.org
Website: http://www.kidney.org

• National Institute of Diabetes, Digestive, and Kidney Diseases
Website: http://www2.niddk.nih.gov

MANAGING YOUR
CHRONIC RENAL FAILURE

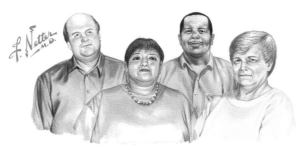

In renal failure, kidneys can't get rid of the body's waste. Waste products build up and are harmful. Chronic failure occurs slowly.

Kidneys are important in many ways. They get rid of waste products (make urine). They control the body's water, blood salt, and calcium levels.

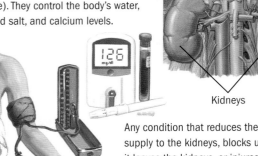

Kidneys

Any condition that reduces the blood supply to the kidneys, blocks urine after it leaves the kidneys, or injures kidneys can cause renal failure. Common causes include diabetes and high blood pressure.

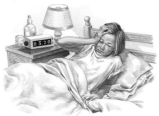

Chronic renal failure is a silent disease and may not have early symptoms. Later symptoms may include nausea, vomiting, diarrhea, and appetite loss.

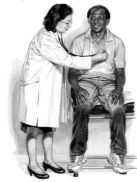

Your doctor diagnoses renal failure with physical examination, urine, and blood tests. Biopsy and x-rays may also be done.

What Is Chronic Renal Failure?

Kidneys are important in many ways. They control the amount of water and by-products of metabolism. They get rid of waste products (make urine). They control the body's water, blood salt, and calcium levels. In renal failure (or kidney failure), kidneys can't get rid of the body's waste products. Waste products build up in the body and are harmful. Acute failure occurs suddenly. Chronic failure occurs slowly.

What Causes Chronic Renal Failure?

The cause is any condition that reduces the blood supply to the kidneys, blocks urine after it leaves the kidneys, or injures the kidneys. Inflammation, urinary tract infections, congestive heart failure, diabetes, gout, and high blood pressure can cause it. Medications used for other medical disorders can also damage the kidneys.

What Are the Symptoms of Chronic Renal Failure?

Chronic renal failure is often a silent disease and has no early symptoms. Later signs and symptoms may include nausea, vomiting, diarrhea, and appetite loss. Others are listless feelings; shortness of breath; mouth problems; stomach pain; numbness, tingling, and burning in legs and feet; lower sex drive; loss of menstrual periods; anemia; and muscle and bone pain. Being irritable, not sleeping well, depression, convulsions, stupor, and coma, are seen; itching, abnormal blood pressure, and bleeding problems may also occur.

How Is Chronic Renal Failure Diagnosed?

The doctor often finds impaired renal function at a routine examination or urine or blood tests. Tests will then be done to see how well the kidneys work. X-rays may also be done. Your doctor may refer you to a kidney specialist (nephrologist) for additional evaluation.

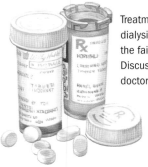

Treatment can involve diet, medicine, dialysis, controlling diseases causing the failure, and kidney transplantation. Discuss treatment options with your doctor and follow instructions.

Dialysis removes waste products from the blood when kidneys can't. Dialysis may be done temporarily or permanently.

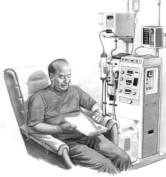

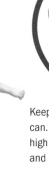

Keep your weight under control. Weigh yourself daily, and keep records of fluid intake and output.

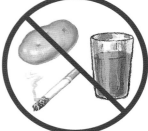

Keep healthy: exercise as much as you can. Stop smoking. Don't eat foods high in potassium such as bananas and orange juice.

How Is Chronic Renal Failure Treated?

Treatment can involve diet, medicine, dialysis, controlling diseases causing the failure, and transplantation. Foods containing potassium, phosphorous, and too much salt or protein should be avoided. Controlling blood pressure is important. Injections to correct anemia and calcium pills may be needed. Diuretics (water pills) can prevent gaining too much fluid. Your doctor may recommend a kidney transplant. Certain drugs that can affect the kidneys must be avoided. High blood pressure, diabetes, congestive heart failure, and infections must be treated.

Some people need dialysis if other treatments don't work. Dialysis removes waste products from the blood when kidneys can't. Dialysis may be done temporarily or permanently.

The doctor will suggest seeing a kidney specialist.

DOs and DON'Ts in Managing Chronic Renal Failure:

✔ **DO** follow the diet that your doctor suggests, including fluid restriction.

✔ **DO** take medicines exactly as prescribed. Don't miss doses.

✔ **DO** weigh yourself daily. Keep records of fluid intake and output.

✔ **DO** exercise as much as you can but limit strenuous activities.

✔ **DO** stop smoking.

✔ **DO** call your doctor if you have chills, fever, headache, muscle aches, shortness of breath, nausea, vomiting, or chest pains.

🚫 **DON'T** become dehydrated, but don't drink water or liquids in excess. Don't get overtired.

🚫 **DON'T** eat foods you should avoid. Too much potassium can make you very ill.

🚫 **DON'T** take over-the-counter drugs without checking with your doctor.

FOR MORE INFORMATION

Contact the following sources:

• National Kidney Foundation
Tel: (800) 622-9010
Website: http://www.kidney.org

• National Institute of Diabetes and Digestive and Kidney Diseases
Website: http://www.niddk.nih.gov

• National Kidney and Urological Diseases Information Clearinghouse
Tel: (800) 891-5390
Website: http://kidney.niddk.nih.gov

FROM THE DESK OF

NOTES

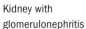
Normal kidney

Kidney with glomerulonephritis

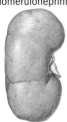

Glomerulonephritis refers to a group of diseases that cause inflammation of the part of the kidney that filters blood. Kidneys cannot get rid of waste products and extra body fluid. Kidneys may stop working completely. This disorder may occur in adults but is most common in children.

Strep throat

Hearing loss

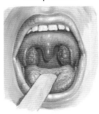
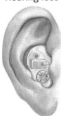

Acute glomerulonephritis may start after a throat or skin infection (strep) or other illnesses. Often the cause isn't known.

Mild glomerulonephritis usually has no symptoms. In severe cases, symptoms include:

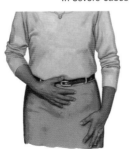

Bloody urine, urinating less often

Swollen face, eyelids, hands, and ankles

Feeling sick or nauseous, vomiting, losing your appetite

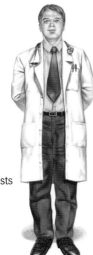

Your doctor makes a diagnosis from medical history, urine and blood tests, and imaging tests such as ultrasonography.

What Is Glomerulonephritis?

Glomerulonephritis is inflammation of the part of the kidney that filters blood; it is caused by several diseases. The kidney is damaged and cannot get rid of waste products and extra body fluid. Sometimes, kidneys may stop working completely. The two forms are acute and chronic. The acute form starts suddenly, but the chronic form may develop slowly, over many years, and produce no symptoms until severe damage has occurred.

Glomerulonephritis may occur in adults but is most common in children.

What Causes Glomerulonephritis?

Acute glomerulonephritis may start after a throat or skin infection. Other illnesses that may cause glomerulonephritis include lupus, erythematosus, Goodpasture's syndrome, Wegener's granulomatosis, Henoch-Schönlein purpura, polyarteritis nodosa, and immune system changes. Many times, the cause is unknown. Chronic disease can follow acute disease years later.

What Are the Symptoms of Glomerulonephritis?

Mild glomerulonephritis usually has no symptoms. More serious disease causes slightly red or bloody urine, drowsiness, nausea or vomiting, headaches, appetite loss, less urination, and sometimes fever. Face, eyelids, and hands swell in the morning, and ankles swell in the evening. Shortness of breath, cough, high blood pressure, and blistery, dry, or itchy skin are others. Nighttime muscle cramps may occur. Symptoms may last from weeks to several months.

How Is Glomerulonephritis Diagnosed?

The doctor makes a diagnosis from the medical history, urine tests showing protein and blood cells, blood tests, and imaging tests such as ultrasonography of the kidney. Sometimes, a kidney biopsy is needed to find the best treatment. In a biopsy, the doctor removes a tiny piece of kidney with a special needle.

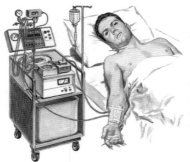

Glomerulonephritis may go away by itself, but medicines, special blood filtering, or using an artificial kidney machine may be needed. Chronic disease has no specific treatment except for following a special diet.

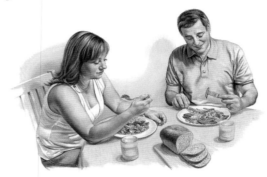

To prevent complications, keep to your special diet. Eat less protein, salt, and potassium.

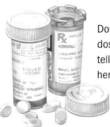

Don't stop taking your medicine or change your dosage because you feel better unless your doctor tells you to. Don't take over-the-counter drugs or herbal supplements without asking your doctor.

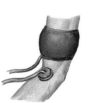

Control your blood pressure if you have chronic glomerulonephritis. This is the most important thing that may slow kidney damage. Do exercise but limit strenuous activities.

How Is Glomerulonephritis Treated?

Children usually recover more quickly than adults. A doctor who specializes in kidney treatment (nephrologist) will be involved in the care.

Sometimes, glomerulonephritis goes away by itself. However, high doses of medicines that affect the immune system or special filtering of the blood (plasmapheresis) may be needed. Temporary treatment with an artificial kidney machine may be needed to remove extra fluid and poisons that build up in the body.

No specific treatment is available for chronic glomerulonephritis. Following a special diet with less protein, salt, and potassium may be needed. Blood pressure pills and calcium supplements may also be taken.

DOs and DON'Ts in Managing Glomerulonephritis:

✔ **DO** follow dietary advice. It prevents complications.
✔ **DO** keep to your fluid restrictions. Fluid could build up in your lungs and could be dangerous.
✔ **DO** control your blood pressure if you have chronic glomerulonephritis. This is *the most important thing that may slow kidney damage.*
✔ **DO** exercise but limit strenuous activities.

⊘ **DON'T** stop taking your medicine or change your dosage because you feel better unless your doctor tells you to.
⊘ **DON'T** take any over-the-counter medicine or herbal supplements without checking with your doctor. Some herbal preparations at health food stores may cause kidney damage.

FROM THE DESK OF

NOTES

FOR MORE INFORMATION

Contact the following source:

• National Kidney Foundation, Inc.
Tel: (800) 622-9010
Website: http://www.kidney.org

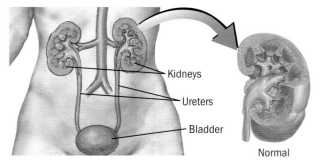

Kidneys

Ureters

Bladder

Normal

Hydronephrosis is the dilation or swelling of kidneys because of a blockage that stops urine from flowing out of the body.

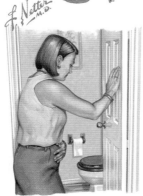

Kidneys with hydronephrosis

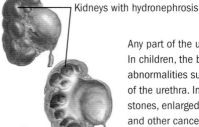

Any part of the urinary tract can be blocked. In children, the blockage is often due to abnormalities such as narrowing or pinching of the urethra. In adults, causes include kidney stones, enlarged prostate gland, and prostate and other cancers.

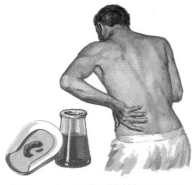

Symptoms depend on the cause. For example, people with kidney stones may have blood in the urine and severe pain in the side that travels to the groin. Men with prostate cancer or an enlarged prostate may have problems urinating. People with colon cancer may see blood in the stool or a change in bowel movements.

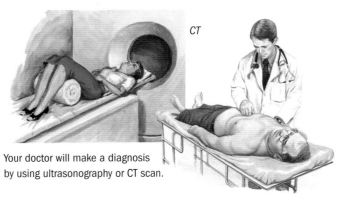

CT

Your doctor will make a diagnosis by using ultrasonography or CT scan.

What Is Hydronephrosis?

Hydronephrosis is the dilation or swelling of kidneys because of a blockage that stops urine from flowing out of the body.

Hydronephrosis can be cured, depending on the cause. Complications include urinary infections, high blood pressure, kidney failure, and dehydration.

What Causes Hydronephrosis?

The cause is a blockage of any part of the urinary tract. In children, the blockage is often due to abnormalities such as narrowing or pinching of the urethra. The urethra is the tube taking urine from the bladder to outside the body. Also narrowing at the opening of the ureters, the tubes carrying urine from the kidneys to the bladder, can cause a blockage.

In adults, causes often include kidney stones, enlarged prostate gland, and prostate cancer. Other causes are cancers of the bladder, uterus, ovary, and colon.

What Are the Symptoms of Hydronephrosis?

Symptoms depend on the cause. For example, people with kidney stones may have blood in the urine and severe pain in the side (flank) that travels to the groin. Men with prostate cancer or an enlarged prostate may have problems urinating, need to urinate at night, and be unable to completely empty the bladder. People with colon cancer may see blood in the stools (bowel movements) or change in bowel movements.

How Is Hydronephrosis Diagnosed?

In addition to the physical exam, the doctor will make a diagnosis by using ultrasonography or computed tomography (CT).

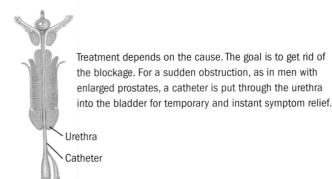

Treatment depends on the cause. The goal is to get rid of the blockage. For a sudden obstruction, as in men with enlarged prostates, a catheter is put through the urethra into the bladder for temporary and instant symptom relief.

— Urethra

— Catheter

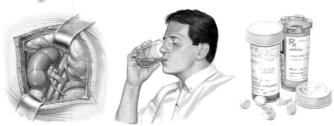

In people with kidney stones, treatments include pain control and increasing fluid intake. If the kidney stone is too large to pass, shock wave treatment (lithotripsy) to break up the stone or surgery may be needed.

Hydronephrosis can occur in children as well as in adults.

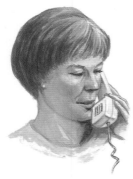

Call your doctor if you have abdominal or flank pain, you have blood in your urine, you see a drop in your urine output, or you cannot urinate.

How Is Hydronephrosis Treated?

Treatment depends on the cause. The goal is to get rid of the blockage. For a sudden obstruction, as in men with enlarged prostate glands, a catheter is put through the urethra into the bladder. The catheter gives temporary and instant relief of symptoms until more complete therapy, such as medicine or surgery, can be given.

People with kidney stones are usually treated by a urologist (a surgeon specializing in diseases of the genital and urinary tract) with medications for pain control and increasing fluid intake. Shock wave treatment (lithotripsy) or surgery can be done to remove the stones if they are too large to pass on their own.

The kidney can return to normal, depending on how long the blockage has been there; whether problems such as infections, stones, or other causes of the blockage are also present; and how severe the blockage is.

DOs and DON'Ts in Managing Hydronephrosis:

✔ **DO** understand that hydronephrosis is not a disease but is the result of many different diseases.

✔ **DO** realize that the longer hydronephrosis remains untreated, the more kidney function is lost.

✔ **DO** get advice from a urologist if hydronephrosis is found.

✔ **DO** call your doctor if you have abdominal or flank pain or blood in the urine.

✔ **DO** call your doctor if you see a drop in your urine output or you cannot urinate.

⊘ **DON'T** forget that hydronephrosis can occur in both children and adults.

⊘ **DON'T** miss follow-up doctor appointments. You may need more ultrasound scans to monitor the kidney size.

FROM THE DESK OF

NOTES

FOR MORE INFORMATION

Contact the following source:

• National Kidney Foundation
 Tel: (800) 622-9010
 Website: http://www.kidney.org

MANAGING YOUR
KIDNEY STONES

Location of kidneys

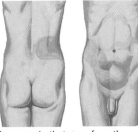

Normal kidney   Kidney with stones

Large stones can fill the tubes (ureters) carrying urine to the bladder. Stones cause problems in urine flow and can cause infections.

Severe pain that goes from the middle of the back to the lower belly is the most common symptom.

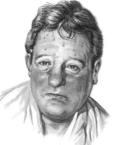

Fever, sweating, chills, and urgent urination are symptoms that your stones may have caused an infection.

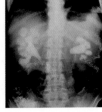
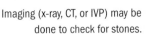

Imaging (x-ray, CT, or IVP) may be done to check for stones.

What Are Kidney Stones?

Kidney stones are hard deposits that form in kidneys. This process is called nephrolithiasis. Kidney stones can be tiny or up to several inches around. Very large stones that fill the tubes carrying urine from the kidneys to the bladder (ureters) are called staghorn stones.

What Causes Kidney Stones?

Stones may form if urine contains too much of certain chemicals, such as calcium, uric acid, cystine, or struvite (a mixture of phosphate, magnesium, and ammonium). Having a diet that is very high in protein and drinking too little water increase the risk of getting stones. About 85% of kidney stones are made from calcium. Uric acid stones occur more often if gout is present. Struvite stones form more often in infected urine (infection stones).

What Are the Symptoms of Kidney Stones?

About one-third of people have kidney stones, but only half of these have symptoms. Even without symptoms, stones may cause problems, such as infections and blocking urine flow. Stones getting stuck in ureters cause the symptoms.

The most common symptom is severe pain (urinary colic) that comes and goes and usually moves from the side of the back (flank) to the lower belly (abdomen). Other common symptoms include pain in the back, thigh, groin, and sex organs (genitals); blood in the urine; nausea; and vomiting.

If a stone causes an infection, additional symptoms may be chills; fever; painful, frequent, and urgent urination; and sweating.

How Are Kidney Stones Diagnosed?

The doctor takes a medical history, does a physical examination, and tests the urine. An x-ray or ultrasound study of your abdomen may be needed. These studies will uncover most stones (calcium, cystine, and struvite stones). X-rays cannot show uric acid stones. Computed tomography (CT) of the urinary tract may also be ordered. Rarely, if the diagnosis is still unclear, a special x-ray study (intravenous pyelogram, or IVP) may be done. In this study, dye is used to outline the stone.

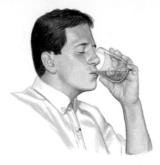

Drink plenty of fluids. Flushing small stones out of the body is the easiest treatment.

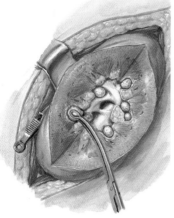

Surgery may be needed if stones are too large to pass.

Your doctor may prescribe antibiotics if you have an infection. Take all medications as prescribed and for as long as your doctor advises.

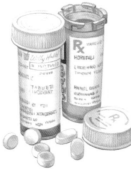

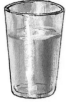

Drink at least 4 pints of water a day.

Follow your doctor's advice for a healthy diet; it may help prevent future stones.

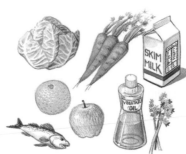

How Are Kidney Stones Treated?

Treatment depends on several things, such as the size and number of stones, where they are, and whether an infection is present.

The simplest way to treat a small stone is to flush it out by drinking lots of fluid. Medicine may help relieve pain. Antibiotics are given for an infection.

Stones that do not pass by themselves may need removal by a urologist. A urologist is a doctor who specializes in diseases of the urinary system. The urologist may use a long, thin tool (cystoscope) to do this.

Sometimes, shock waves are used to break the stone into smaller pieces that can be passed. This treatment is called lithotripsy.

DOs and DON'Ts in Managing Kidney Stones:

✔ **DO** take all your prescribed medicines.
✔ **DO** follow your doctor's advice about diet.
✔ **DO** drink plenty of fluids, at least 4 pints a day.
✔ **DO** call your doctor's office if you feel worse.
✔ **DO** call your doctor or go to the emergency room if you have severe vomiting, severe pain, or fever with severe back pain.

⊘ **DON'T** get dehydrated.
⊘ **DON'T** stop taking your medicine or change the dosage because you feel better unless your doctor tells you to.

FOR MORE INFORMATION

Contact the following sources:

- American Urological Association
  Tel: (866) 746-4282
  Website: http://www.urologyhealth.org

- National Kidney Foundation
  Tel: (800) 622-9010
  Website: http://www.kidney.org

- National Kidney & Urologic Diseases Information Clearinghouse
  Tel: (800) 891-5390
  Website: http://www.kidney.niddk.nih.gov

FROM THE DESK OF

NOTES

MANAGING YOUR
NEPHROTIC SYNDROME

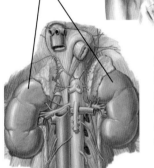

Nephrotic syndrome is a condition in which kidneys don't work well. This syndrome is most common in children 2 to 6 years old, but adults can have it.

Kidneys

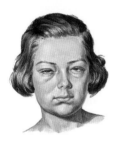

Kidneys clean the blood of poisons. Healthy kidneys also keep important chemicals called proteins in the blood. With nephrotic syndrome, kidneys get rid of proteins with other wastes that leave the body during urination.

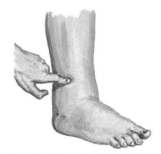

First symptoms are puffy eyes and ankles, then puffy skin, from water gain. The abdomen swells. Much less urine is made. Urine can look frothy.

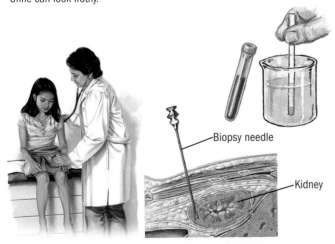

Biopsy needle

Kidney

Most people see the doctor because of swollen ankles, legs, or face. Blood tests that find excess protein in urine tests confirm the diagnosis. A kidney specialist may be seen for a biopsy. In a biopsy, a small piece of kidney tissue is removed with a special needle and sent to a laboratory.

What Is Nephrotic Syndrome?

Nephrotic syndrome, also called nephrosis, is a condition in which kidneys don't work well. It's most common in children, but adults can also have it.

Each kidney consists of 1 million fine filters to clean the blood of poisons. Healthy kidneys also keep important chemicals called proteins in the blood. The body needs proteins to grow and repair itself. With nephrotic syndrome, kidneys get rid of proteins with other wastes that leave the body during urination. This causes problems throughout the body.

What Causes Nephrotic Syndrome?

Various kidney problems can lead to nephrotic syndrome. The most common are primary inflammatory conditions of kidneys called glomerulonephritis. Others include diabetes. The condition isn't contagious. Sometimes, the cause is unknown.

What Are the Symptoms of Nephrotic Syndrome?

Nephrotic syndrome is usually painless. People gain excessive amounts of water weight, which causes distress and discomfort. Initial symptoms from this gain are puffy eyes and ankles. Skin then becomes puffy. The abdomen (belly) swells. Much less urine is made. Urine can look frothy. Other symptoms include weakness, loss of appetite, and a sense of feeling sick. High cholesterol levels result from kidney damage.

How Is Nephrotic Syndrome Diagnosed?

Most people go to the doctor because of swollen ankles or legs, or even a swollen face. The doctor will find high levels of protein in urine tests. Blood tests confirm the diagnosis. A kidney specialist (nephrologist) may be consulted for a biopsy. In a biopsy, a small piece of tissue is removed from the kidney with a special needle and studied in a laboratory.

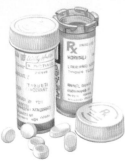

Diet and medicines are usually enough to control symptoms. The different medicines include immunosuppressants for inflammation, diuretics for swelling, ACE inhibitors for blood pressure, and statins for high cholesterol. You may need medicine for 3 months or more.

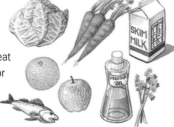

Eat a low-fat, low-salt diet. Don't eat prepared foods that contain salt or high-protein, high-fat foods.

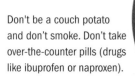

Stay out of bed and keep active to help fluid loss and prevent blood clots in your legs.

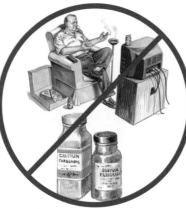

Don't be a couch potato and don't smoke. Don't take over-the-counter pills (drugs like ibuprofen or naproxen).

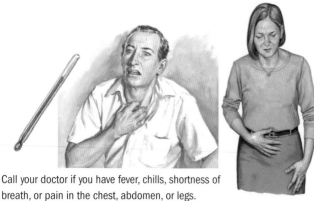

Call your doctor if you have fever, chills, shortness of breath, or pain in the chest, abdomen, or legs.

FROM THE DESK OF

NOTES

How Is Nephrotic Syndrome Treated?

Symptoms usually start to improve in 2 to 3 weeks after starting treatment with diet and medicines. Different medicines may be needed. Immunosuppressive drugs, such as prednisone and cyclophosphamide, may be needed to help kidney inflammation. Diuretics ("water pills" such as furosemide) reduce swelling. Medicine often must be taken for 3 months or more.

Because people with nephrotic syndrome tend to develop blood clots in the legs, keeping active is important. Anticoagulant medicines help prevent blood clots.

Other drugs such as angiotensin-converting enzyme (ACE) inhibitors lower protein loss and blood pressure. Cholesterol-lowering drugs such as statins are often used to lower very high cholesterol levels that occur with nephrotic syndrome.

DOs and DON'Ts in Managing Nephrotic Syndrome:

✔ **DO** eat a low-fat, low-salt diet.
✔ **DO** ask your doctor how much protein you should eat and about a recommended fluid intake.
✔ **DO** stay out of bed and keep active to help fluid loss and prevent clots.
✔ **DO** take medicines as prescribed.
✔ **DO** call your doctor if you have fever, chills, shortness of breath, or pain in the chest, abdomen, or legs.

⊘ **DON'T** eat prepared foods that contain excessive salt.
⊘ **DON'T** eat a high-protein, high-fat diet.
⊘ **DON'T** become a "couch potato."
⊘ **DON'T** smoke.
⊘ **DON'T** take over-the-counter pills (especially drugs such as ibuprofen or naproxen) that will complicate your treatment.

FOR MORE INFORMATION

Contact the following sources:

• National Kidney and Urologic Diseases Information Clearinghouse
Tel: (800) 891-5390
Website: http://www.niddk.nih.gov

• National Kidney Foundation
Tel: (800) 622-9010
Website: http://www.kidney.org

• American Association of Kidney Patients
Tel: (800) 749-2257
Website: http://www.aakp.org

MANAGING YOUR
RHABDOMYOLYSIS

Rhabdomyolysis is a condition that occurs when muscle is damaged. This damage releases the pigment myoglobin from muscle into the blood.

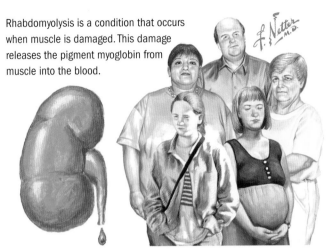

Kidneys normally filter myoglobin out of the blood. Substances from the muscle breakdown may harm the kidneys by blocking kidney filtering structures. The kidneys fail and release toxic waste products into the blood.

Causes include crushing injuries to muscles, seizures, and exercise-related heatstroke. Other causes are severe frostbite, severe burns, alcoholism, drug overdose, and cocaine use.

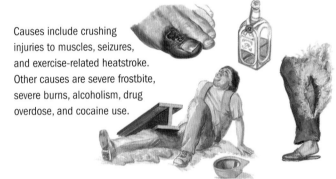

The main symptom is red or brown urine. Then, less urine or no urine may be produced. This serious symptom means kidney failure. Other symptoms are severe muscle aches, fatigue, lethargy, joint pain, extreme thirst, and fast or irregular heartbeat.

Your doctor will make a diagnosis from your medical history, physical examination, and laboratory tests of blood and urine.

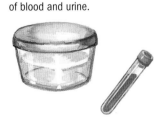

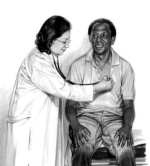

What Is Rhabdomyolysis?

Rhabdomyolysis is a condition that occurs when muscle is damaged. This damage releases the pigment myoglobin from muscle into the blood. Kidneys normally filter the pigment out of the blood. Substances from the muscle breakdown may harm the kidneys by blocking their filtering structures. The kidneys fail and release toxic waste products into the blood.

What Causes Rhabdomyolysis?

Causes include crushing injuries to muscle, seizures, and exercise-related heatstroke. Other causes are severe frostbite, severe burns, alcoholism, drug overdose, cocaine use, and side effects of medicines such as statins (used to treat high cholesterol). Sometimes, too much high endurance exercise by someone who isn't trained enough can cause excessive muscle breakdown and rhabdomyolysis.

What Are the Symptoms of Rhabdomyolysis?

The main symptoms are muscle pains and red or brown urine that may then turn into less urine or no urine being produced. This serious sign of being unable to urinate, a symptom of kidney failure, means that immediate medical care is needed. Other symptoms are fatigue, lethargy, joint pain, extreme thirst, and fast or irregular heartbeat.

How Is Rhabdomyolysis Diagnosed?

The doctor will make a diagnosis from the medical history, physical examination, and laboratory tests. Blood studies will show poor kidney function, high potassium levels, and other abnormalities of body fluids. Urine may be red or brown because of pigments and dehydration.

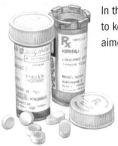

In the hospital, intravenous fluids are first given to keep a steady urine flow. This treatment is aimed at flushing pigments through the kidneys.

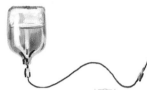

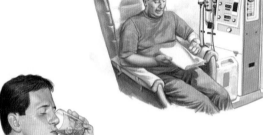

The main adverse effect of this treatment is fluid overload if kidneys already started to fail. In this case, dialysis (kidney machine) may be needed to remove fluid and wastes and to rest the kidneys until they can recover.

Drink plenty of fluids to stay well hydrated.

Call your doctor right away if you see red or brown urine, have general muscle aches, or cannot urinate.

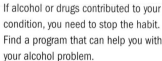

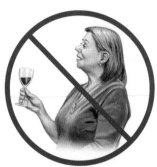

If alcohol or drugs contributed to your condition, you need to stop the habit. Find a program that can help you with your alcohol problem.

How Is Rhabdomyolysis Treated?

Treatment takes place in the hospital. Intravenous fluids are first given to keep a steady urine flow. This treatment is helpful to flush pigments through the kidneys. Medicines may be given to change the acidity of the urine, to make the urine alkaline, and to increase urination. This also flushes pigments out of the kidneys.

The main adverse effect of this treatment is fluid overload if kidneys already started to fail before treatment. In this case, dialysis (kidney machine) may be needed to remove fluid and wastes and to rest the kidneys until they can recover. Weeks to months may be needed, depending on how severe the problem is.

DOs and DON'Ts in Managing Rhabdomyolysis:

✔ **DO** get medical care right away if you see red or brown urine or have general muscle aches, if you had one of the causes of rhabdomyolysis, especially a crushing muscle injury or exercise-related heatstroke.

✔ **DO** also get medical care if after you had treatment of rhabdomyolysis you see colored urine or decrease in urine output. Get immediate medical care if you cannot urinate.

✔ **DO** stay well hydrated and drink plenty of fluids.

✔ **DO** stop using alcohol or drugs that may have contributed to your condition. Find a program that can help you with your alcohol problem.

⊘ **DON'T** let yourself become dehydrated if you are at risk of having rhabdomyolysis. Being dehydrated may let pigments build up in the kidney. This is especially important if you had exercise-induced heatstroke, because you're already dehydrated.

⊘ **DON'T** take part in high endurance sports without having had the proper training.

FROM THE DESK OF

NOTES

FOR MORE INFORMATION

Contact the following sources:

• American College of Emergency Physicians
  Tel: (800) 798-1822
  Website: http://www.acep.org

• American Association of Kidney Patients
  Tel: (800) 749-2257
  Website: www.aakp.org

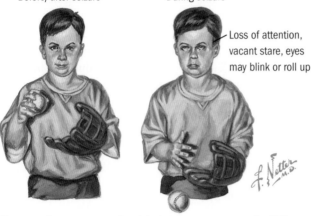

Before/after seizure   During seizure

Loss of attention, vacant stare, eyes may blink or roll up

Absence seizures may occur in adults but are more common in children. They are periods of altered consciousness. The person is alert and attentive before and after the seizure.

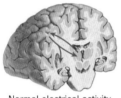

Normal electrical activity

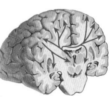

Abnormal signals in the brain cause absence seizures. A seizure involves impaired awareness and responsiveness for 2 to 15 seconds.

Electrical activity during seizure

Causes of seizures

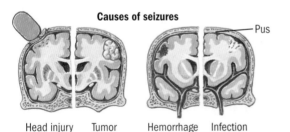

Pus

Head injury   Tumor   Hemorrhage   Infection

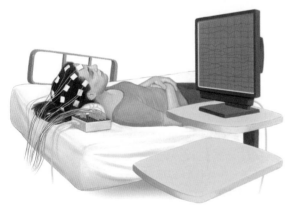

In addition to a family medical history and observation, your doctor may order a safe and painless test to record your brain's electrical activity, called an EEG, for diagnosis.

What Are Absence Seizures?

Absence seizures are seizures with periods of altered consciousness, which may be noted only as a blank stare. They may occur in adults but are more common in children. They may be mistaken for daydreaming. Warning signs such as a strange feeling, unusual taste or odor, or headache may come before the seizure.

What Causes Absence Seizures?

A seizure is caused by abnormal signals in the brain. Head injuries, strokes, brain infections, or tumors can cause these seizures, but often the reason for them is unknown.

What Are the Symptoms of Absence Seizures?

Symptoms in addition to those mentioned above include some fluttering of eyelids and twitching of muscles in the face. Seizures usually last less than 10 seconds and stop by themselves. People are completely unaware of these seizures and continue with their previous activity.

How Are Absence Seizures Diagnosed?

The doctor uses observations from eyewitnesses and the medical history to diagnose absence seizures. Also, an MRI or CT scan of the brain can tell whether there is a physical cause, such as damage to the brain from congenital defects, stroke, or trauma. The doctor may also order a brain wave study called an electroencephalogram (EEG). This safe and painless test records the brain's electrical activity with electrodes placed on the scalp.

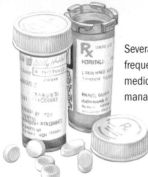

Several different medicines can reduce the frequency and severity of seizures. Take the medicine as prescribed by your doctor to manage your seizures.

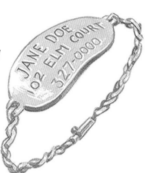

Although drugs can help, seizures may still occur. You can get medical ID bracelets to show that you can have seizures and the drugs that you take. You should wear it at all times so that you can get the proper care quickly.

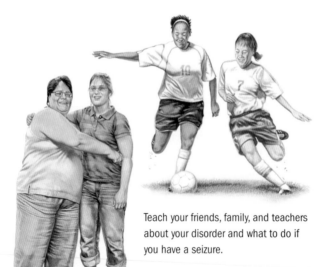

Teach your friends, family, and teachers about your disorder and what to do if you have a seizure.

How Are Absence Seizures Treated?

Until the seizure disorder is well controlled, precautions may be needed. People living alone should arrange to have help until the doctor believes that it is safe to resume living alone.

The main treatment is medicine. Sometimes more than one drug may be used. The doctor may have to take blood samples to make sure that the correct dose is given and may adjust the dose as needed. Often, the medicine will reduce the frequency and severity of the seizures, but some people, even with the medicine, will continue to have seizures. Also, all drugs have side effects.

DOs and DON'Ts in Managing Absence Seizures:

✔ **DO** call the doctor if you have any problems with your medicines.

✔ **DO** take the medicine prescribed by your doctor and have blood tests to measure levels of the drug.

✔ **DO** wear an ID bracelet indicating that you have a seizure disorder and listing the drugs you take.

✔ **DO** call the doctor if your seizures become more frequent or severe.

✔ **DO** teach your family and friends about your disorder and what to do if you have a seizure.

✔ **DO** tell someone near you that you feel a seizure coming on and lie down.

✔ **DO** arrange to have someone call the doctor if you are injured during a seizure, have difficulty breathing, or do not regain consciousness shortly after the seizure.

✔ **DO** arrange to have someone call 911 for an ambulance when continuous seizures occur.

⊘ **DON'T** operate dangerous machinery or drive unless your doctor approves.

⊘ **DON'T** swim alone.

⊘ **DON'T** climb on ladders or roofs or do anything that may be dangerous if you have a seizure.

FROM THE DESK OF

NOTES

FOR MORE INFORMATION

Contact the following source:

· Epilepsy Foundation of America
  Tel: (800) EFA-1000, (301) 459-3700
  Website: http://www.epilepsyfoundation.org

MANAGING YOUR
ACOUSTIC NEUROMA

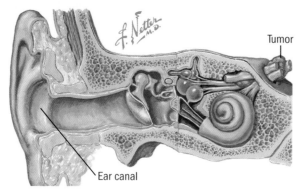

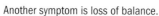

An acoustic neuroma is a benign tumor located inside the ear. It is most often seen in people between the ages of 30 and 60.

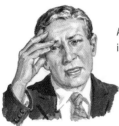

A common symptom of an acoustic neuroma is hearing loss in one or both ears.

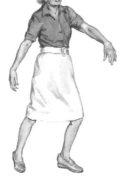

Another symptom is loss of balance.

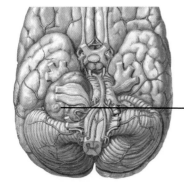

Looking down at a brain with an acoustic neuroma

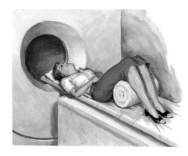

To help diagnose an acoustic neuroma, your doctor may do an MRI scan of your brain, or a CT scan (shown here).

What Is an Acoustic Neuroma?

An acoustic neuroma is a benign (noncancerous) tumor that starts from a nerve of the brain, the eighth cranial nerve, or the vestibular nerve. Cranial nerves are 12 pairs of nerves that come from the bottom surface of the brain. Cells wrapping around this nerve are called Schwann cells. Acoustic neuromas are also called vestibular schwannomas.

Neuromas can affect either one ear (unilateral) or both ears (bilateral). Most occur in people 30 to 60 years old.

What Causes an Acoustic Neuroma?

The cause is unclear, but the tumor results from production of too many Schwann cells around the vestibular nerve. Unilateral neuromas occur irregularly and are not inherited. Bilateral neuromas are associated with the genetic disorder neurofibromatosis. Acoustic neuromas are not contagious and cannot spread from one person to another. No way to prevent acoustic neuromas is known.

What Are the Symptoms of an Acoustic Neuroma?

The first symptom in more than 90% of people is one-sided hearing loss. The usually subtle hearing loss occurs slowly. However, sudden acute hearing loss can occur.

Other symptoms include loss of balance and tinnitus (a ringing or hissing sound in the ear).

A growing tumor may press on nerves and cause numbness and tingling in the face or facial muscle paralysis and loss of facial expression. A large tumor can squeeze part of the brain and lead to headaches, clumsy walking, and confusion.

How Is an Acoustic Neuroma Diagnosed?

If symptoms appear, the doctor will do complete neurological and ear examinations and hearing test (audiogram). Early diagnosis is critical.

The doctor may order an MRI or CT scan of the brain.

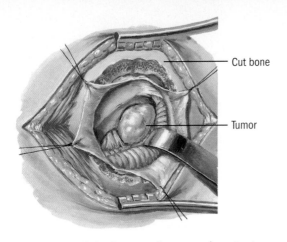

Cut bone

Tumor

The most common way to treat an acoustic neuroma is surgery to remove the neuroma and save your hearing. Other treatments include gamma knife radiosurgery and radiation therapy.

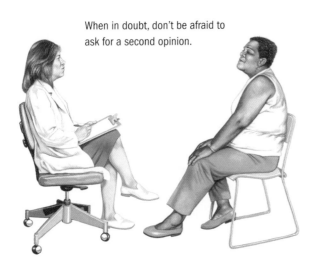

When in doubt, don't be afraid to ask for a second opinion.

How Is an Acoustic Neuroma Treated?

Treatments include surgery, radiation, and monitoring. Treatment is decided on the basis of tumor size and growth rate, degree of impairment, life expectancy, age, and surgical risk.

Surgery is the most reliable treatment. For very small tumors, hearing may be saved and symptoms may improve. Surgery for larger tumors is more complicated.

Another excellent choice, instead of traditional surgery, is gamma knife surgery. This method uses beams of high-energy gamma radiation aimed exactly at the tumor and leaves other areas alone.

Radiation therapy may reduce the size or limit the growth of a neuroma. This therapy is sometimes preferred for elderly people, people in poor health, people with tumors affecting both ears, or people with a tumor affecting their only hearing ear.

Just watching the tumor may be reasonable in some cases, usually people with other serious illnesses.

DOs and DON'Ts in Managing an Acoustic Neuroma:

✔ **DO** realize that one of the possible complications of tumor removal is that symptoms can worsen because pieces of nerves controlling hearing, balance, or facial nerves may also be removed.

✔ **DO** call your doctor if you notice hearing loss or have new balance problems.

✔ **DO** call your doctor if you have problems swallowing, tinnitus, one-sided facial numbness, and tingling, especially with dizziness, headache, or other symptoms.

⊘ **DON'T** be afraid to ask for a second opinion.

FOR MORE INFORMATION

Contact the following sources:

• National Institute on Deafness and Other Communication Disorders
Tel: (800) 241-1044
E-mail: nidcdinfo@nidcd.nih.gov
Website: http://www.nidcd.nih.gov

• Acoustic Neuroma Association
Tel: (770) 205-8211, (877) 200-8211
Fax: (770) 205-0239, (877) 202-0239
E-mail: info@anausa.org
Website: http://www.anausa.org

FROM THE DESK OF

NOTES

MANAGING YOUR
ALZHEIMER'S DISEASE

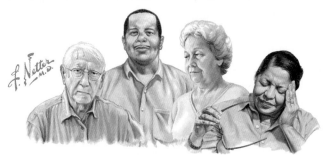

Alzheimer's disease is the most common form of dementia among older people. It affects memory, thinking, and language.

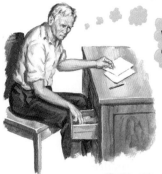

Where is my checkbook?

The first symptom is usually forgetfulness. Later, memory and thinking problems become worse.

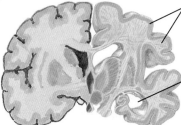

Deterioration of some brain parts (gyri, hippocampus)

Enlargement of ventricles (four fluid-filled cavities in the brain)

Normal brain   Alzheimer's brain

In Alzheimer's disease, brain cells die and the brain shrinks. Abnormal proteins form clumps and tangles around and inside these cells.

Language Test
Doctor: Write me a brief paragraph about your work.

Good   Concern

Thought Test
Doctor: Draw a clock face for me.

Good   Abnormal

Memory Test
Doctor: Here are 3 objects: a pipe, a pen, and a picture of Abraham Lincoln. I want you to remember them and in five minutes, I will ask you what they were.

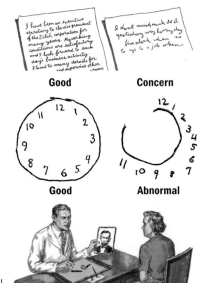

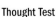

What Is Alzheimer's Disease?

Dementia is a serious brain disorder that affects a person's ability to carry out daily activities. Alzheimer's disease (AD) is the most common type of dementia among older people. It is a slow disease, starting with mild memory problems and ending with severe brain damage. It affects memory, thinking, and language.

The course of the disease and how fast changes occur vary from person to person. AD is usually not inherited.

What Causes Alzheimer's Disease?

The cause remains unknown. In AD, brain cells that store and process information begin to fail and die. Also, more abnormal proteins are made, which form clumps and tangles around and inside these cells.

What Are the Symptoms of Alzheimer's Disease?

The first symptom is usually increased forgetfulness. People forget names or where they put things. However, some forgetfulness is normal with aging; not everyone with these symptoms has AD or dementia.

Later, memory and thinking problems grow. People forget recent events and names of familiar people or objects, ask the same question or tell the same story over and over, and have trouble organizing everyday life (e.g., paying bills).

In middle and later stages of AD, people need help with everyday activities. Eventually they need total care. People become unable to get dressed, lose awareness of events, become easily disoriented or anxious, get lost, show emotional and personality changes, and have greater physical disability.

How Is Alzheimer's Disease Diagnosed?

No one test can show whether someone has AD. The doctor will diagnose it by checking general health, medical history, and mental abilities. The doctor will ask questions about a person's own life and wider world. The doctor may also test reasoning, hand-to-eye coordination, balance, and sensation, as well as look for depression. A brain scan may show other causes of dementia.

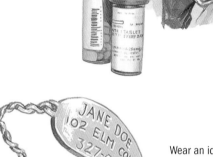

Although there is no cure for Alzheimer's, drugs may slow the progression of symptoms. Anti-depressant drugs may help if you are anxious, depressed, or agitated.

Wear an identification band so people can help you.

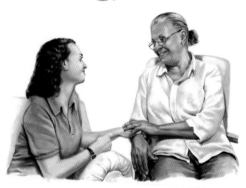

You are not alone. Find out about groups and organizations to help and support you. Also rely on family and friends.

How Is Alzheimer's Disease Treated?

There is no cure. Drugs can sometimes slow the worsening of symptoms. These drugs include cholinesterase inhibitors and memantine. Other medicines can help anxiety, depression, agitation, behavior problems, or psychotic symptoms.

People with AD have trouble adapting to changing living environments. Printing information that is often forgotten and putting it around the home can help. A medical alert bracelet or tag giving the home address helps people who get lost.

DOs and DON'Ts in Managing Alzheimer's Disease:

✔ **DO** find out about help and support.
✔ **DO** try to simplify daily routines and living spaces.
✔ **DO** think about home safety. Change objects or situations that could be dangerous (e.g., add handrails or door locks).
✔ **DO** join a support group.
✔ **DO** keep socially, physically, and mentally active. Understand that nursing home care will be likely.
✔ **DO** wear an identification band.
✔ **DO** arrange for breaks for caregivers.
✔ **DO** call the doctor if you have sudden marked worsening of symptoms, new health issues, or problems with medicines.

⊘ **DON'T** assume that you have AD. Mental changes have many causes that are reversible or treatable.
⊘ **DON'T** change your living environments any more than absolutely necessary. Unfamiliar experiences and confusing environments are hard to handle and often cause anxiety.

FROM THE DESK OF

NOTES

FOR MORE INFORMATION

Contact the following sources:

• Alzheimer's Association
Tel: (800) 272-3900 (24-hour helpline)
Website: http://www.alz.org

• Alzheimer's Disease Education and Referral Center
Tel: (800) 438-4380
Website: http://www.alzheimers.org

• The Alzheimer's Foundation of America
Tel: (866) 232-8484
Website: http://www.alzfdn.org

CARING FOR YOUR CHILD WITH
AUTISM

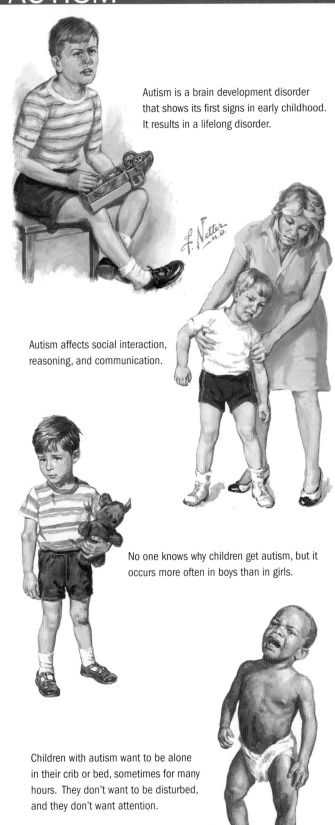

Autism is a brain development disorder that shows its first signs in early childhood. It results in a lifelong disorder.

Autism affects social interaction, reasoning, and communication.

No one knows why children get autism, but it occurs more often in boys than in girls.

Children with autism want to be alone in their crib or bed, sometimes for many hours. They don't want to be disturbed, and they don't want attention.

What Is Autism?

Autism is a brain development disorder that shows its first signs in early childhood. It results in a lifelong disorder with problems in reasoning, social interaction, and communication. Children with autism become self-focused, lose ability to relate to others, and have trouble with language, reasoning, and play.

What Causes Autism?

The cause is unknown, and autism cannot be prevented. It occurs more in boys than in girls and more in some families. Autism may result from chemical changes in the brain. Conditions (e.g., rubella in the mother, lack of oxygen at birth) affecting brain development before, during, or after birth may play a role.

It isn't due to bad parenting or a behavior disorder, however.

What Are the Symptoms of Autism?

Some children have mild symptoms, others have worse symptoms. Symptoms include turning inward and withdrawing from society. Some symptoms start when children are very young, even 1 to 2 years old. Children don't make eye contact, smile, or cuddle. They want to stay alone in a crib or bed, sometimes for many hours. They don't want to be disturbed. They don't want attention. They are quiet and passive. They may repeat gestures or behaviors, such as flicking fingers, arranging objects, and insisting on rituals. Autistic children have short attention spans.

Older children may be overly sensitive to sounds, smells, touch, or taste. They may lack imaginative play. They may not learn to speak when expected.

Children react to changes in the home or in the usual routine with temper tantrums. At about age 5 to 6, self-isolation, tantrums, and rituals tend to occur less often. Even then, children don't learn language and social skills normally. However, some children older than 10 have had a normal school education, and some adults with autism have lived alone and held jobs.

How Is Autism Diagnosed?

No specific test is available. A team of doctors and others makes the diagnosis. This team includes a neurologist (doctor specializing in nervous system diseases), psychologist, pediatrician, speech therapist, and learning consultant.

Tests may be done to rule out other illnesses.

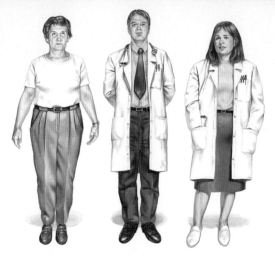

A team of doctors and others, including a neurologist (specialist in nervous system illness), pediatrician, and speech therapist, should be involved, because no test can tell whether a child has autism.

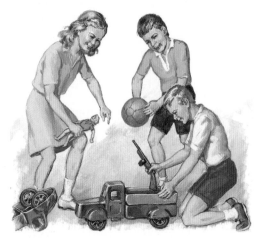

Therapy at an early age can help your child develop fine motor skills and speech and communication skills.

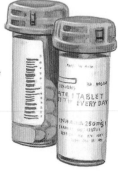

Your doctor might also prescribe medicine for your child, for specific symptoms.

How Is Autism Treated?

No cure exists, but with proper help children can learn to cope with symptoms.

Early intensive interventions are the most successful. Life-long follow-up care will be needed. Therapy may include speech and language, occupational, and physical therapies. Therapy can help children learn how to communicate better, improve fine muscle movement, and help develop strength, coordination, and movement.

The doctor and counselor may suggest music therapy, behavior modification, and specific diets.

There are no specific medicines to treat autism. Sometimes, the doctor may suggest medicine to treat specific symptoms.

DOs and DON'Ts in Managing Autism:

✔ **DO** provide a regular routine in your home to help reduce repetitive behaviors.

✔ **DO** enroll your child in a treatment program that is led by a team of doctors and counselors.

✔ **DO** check out support services and local support groups for parents or caretakers.

✔ **DO** call your doctor if you have questions about your child's health or need information about services for autistic children.

✔ **DO** call your doctor if your child has problems related to medicine, or if symptoms worsen.

⊘ **DON'T** deny your child the opportunity to reach full potential. Children with autism can be creative but need structure.

⊘ **DON'T** accept traditional therapies as the only methods.

FROM THE DESK OF

NOTES

FOR MORE INFORMATION

Contact the following sources:

• Autism Society of America
Tel: (800) 3AUTISM (328-8476), (301) 657-0881
Website: http://www.autism-society.org

• Autism Research Institute
Tel: (866) 366-3361
Website: http://www.autism.com

• Autism Collaboration
Website: http://www.autism.org

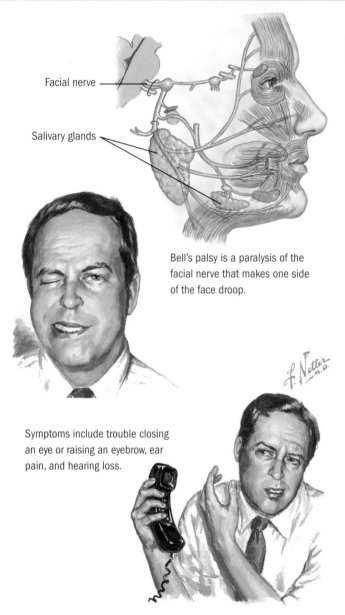

Bell's palsy is a paralysis of the facial nerve that makes one side of the face droop.

Facial nerve

Salivary glands

Symptoms include trouble closing an eye or raising an eyebrow, ear pain, and hearing loss.

A neurologist may need to study the nerve to see how it works and diagnose the problem. A test called electromyography may help diagnosis.

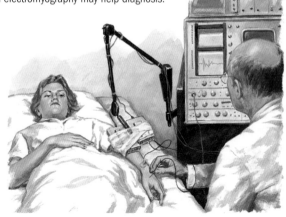

What Is Bell's Palsy?

Bell's palsy is paralysis of the facial nerve that causes one side of the face to droop. It is the most common cause of paralysis in the face.

Bell's palsy affects both men and women, most often between ages 15 and 45. Most people recover completely. It cannot be prevented.

What Causes Bell's Palsy?

The cause is a weak nerve in the face. It is unclear why it occurs, but an infection, such as with a virus, may lead to it. Sometimes, bites from ticks carrying Lyme disease can result in Bell's palsy.

What Are the Symptoms of Bell's Palsy?

Symptoms can start suddenly and be distressing. Some people have mild weakness in the face. Others have severe symptoms such as not being able to close the eye or move half of the face. Sometimes complete paralysis occurs in hours. Symptoms also include being unable to raise the eyebrows or having drooping eyebrows, chewing problems, drooling, drooping eyelid, dry eye, ear pain, facial droop, facial numbness, loss of hearing and taste, sounds heard as too loud, and tearing. For most people, symptoms go away completely; sometimes facial weakness remains.

How Is Bell's Palsy Diagnosed?

The doctor takes a medical history and checks the ears, nose, and mouth. The doctor may get a CT or MRI scan of the brain and blood tests to look for other causes of Bell's palsy. A doctor who treats nerve problems (neurologist) may order a special test called electromyography (EMG) to study how the nerve works and predict chances of recovery.

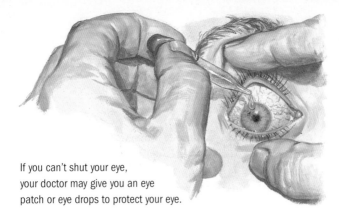

If you can't shut your eye, your doctor may give you an eye patch or eye drops to protect your eye.

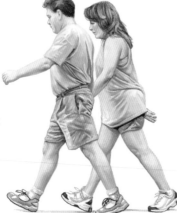

Your doctor will want to see you regularly to make sure that you're getting better.

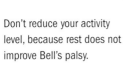

Don't reduce your activity level, because rest does not improve Bell's palsy.

How Is Bell's Palsy Treated?

Most people with mild symptoms get all better without medicine. Medicines can help severe symptoms. The medicines (e.g., corticosteroids such as prednisone) reduce inflammation (swelling) in the nerve. If an infection is suspected to be the cause of Bell's palsy, the doctor may give medicine to treat the infection. An eye patch or eye drops or ointment will protect an open eye, which is critical. Rarely, people who don't recover completely will have an operation to reduce pressure on the facial nerve or improve facial movements.

DOs and DON'Ts in Managing Bell's Palsy:

✔ **DO** follow your doctor's directions and take your medicines as prescribed.

✔ **DO** tell your doctor about other medical problems, especially diabetes.

✔ **DO** tell your doctor about your prescription and over-the-counter drugs.

✔ **DO** tell your doctor if you're pregnant.

✔ **DO** tell your doctor if you recently had a vaccine or a tick bite.

✔ **DO** call your doctor if your symptoms don't get better or get worse or if you have ringing, dizziness, or deafness in your ear.

✔ **DO** call your doctor right away or go to the emergency room if another part of your body becomes weak or numb.

✔ **DO** protect your eye.

✔ **DO** call your doctor if your eye stays red and irritated or becomes painful or if you cannot stop drooling.

✔ **DO** call your doctor if you have problems with medicines.

⊘ **DON'T** stop taking your medicines or change your dose because you feel better unless your doctor tells you to.

⊘ **DON'T** reduce your activity level. Rest doesn't help Bell's palsy.

⊘ **DON'T** stop corticosteroids abruptly; they must be tapered.

FROM THE DESK OF

NOTES

FOR MORE INFORMATION

Contact the following source:

• American Academy of Otolaryngology–Head and Neck Surgery
Tel: (703) 836-4444
Website: http://www.entnet.org

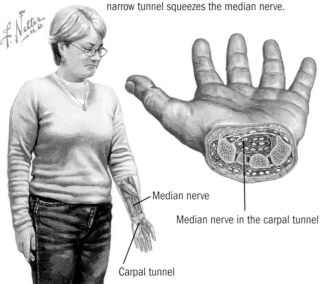

In carpal tunnel syndrome, the wrist swells and the narrow tunnel squeezes the median nerve.

Median nerve

Median nerve in the carpal tunnel

Carpal tunnel

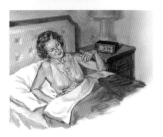

Tingling and/or pain in the fingers may interfere with sleep.

Wrist position and motion may cause or worsen carpal tunnel syndrome.

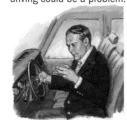

Gradual numbness of fingers while driving could be a problem.

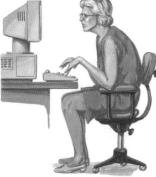

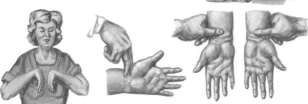

Tests for carpal tunnel syndrome include:
Bending the wrist (Phalen test),
Tapping the wrist (Tinel sign), and
Pressing the wrist to cause symptoms (tingling).

What Is Carpal Tunnel Syndrome?

Carpal tunnel syndrome (CTS) is an ailment affecting the wrist and hand. The nerve controlling feeling and movement in the wrist and hand involved in carpal tunnel syndrome is the median nerve. It lies in a passage in the wrist called the carpal tunnel.

What Causes Carpal Tunnel Syndrome?

In CTS, the tunnel becomes narrow because of swelling in the wrist. The smaller tunnel squeezes the median nerve, which causes pain and other symptoms.

Moving the hand and wrist repeatedly in the same way, such as typing, writing, and using a computer mouse, can cause CTS. Cashiers, butchers, and janitors have an increased risk of CTS. Pregnant women often get CTS because their hormones change and they retain fluid. Several illnesses, for example, muscle and bone disorders, underactive thyroid (hypothyroidism), and diabetes, can also increase risk of CTS.

What Are the Symptoms of Carpal Tunnel Syndrome?

In the wrist, hand, and fingers, CTS causes pain, tingling, numbness, and weak grip (a tendency to drop something). Symptoms often improve when the hand is wrung or shaken. Some people feel discomfort in the upper arm and shoulder.

Symptoms often worsen at night and can interfere with sleep.

How Is Carpal Tunnel Syndrome Diagnosed?

The doctor examines the wrist, and to cause symptoms, will tap it over the median nerve and will bend it and hold it there for a few seconds. Special tests (EMG) to check the wrist's nerves and muscles may also be done.

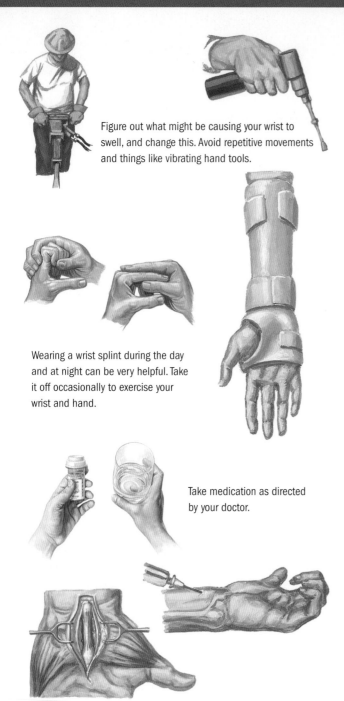

Figure out what might be causing your wrist to swell, and change this. Avoid repetitive movements and things like vibrating hand tools.

Wearing a wrist splint during the day and at night can be very helpful. Take it off occasionally to exercise your wrist and hand.

Take medication as directed by your doctor.

If pain does not improve, other treatments like wrist surgery or an injection of medicine may be recommended.

How Is Carpal Tunnel Syndrome Treated?

Treatment involves two steps. The first is a lifestyle change: stop doing whatever caused CTS. This change may be hard if it involves a job, but talk to your employer. Sometimes simple changes, such as using a wrist pad while typing so your wrist is in a better position, help. A physical therapist or occupational therapist can suggest ways to do things differently.

The second step is to take pressure off the median nerve. Medicine, wrist splints, and surgery are usually used. A wrist splint at night is best, but some people wear a splint during the day. Pills give relief for a short time by decreasing inflammation. Medicine can also be injected into the wrist and can help for a longer period.

Surgery to make more room for the nerve is the best way to reduce pressure on the nerve when other treatments are ineffective. With surgery, you usually get better quickly, but you should rest your wrist for at least 6 weeks to avoid new symptoms.

DOs and DON'Ts in Managing Carpal

Tunnel Syndrome:

✔ **DO** change what caused CTS.
✔ **DO** take pills as directed by your doctor.
✔ **DO** briefly take off a wrist splint, if you wear it during the day, to exercise your wrist and hand.

⊘ **DON'T** hit things with the butt of your palm. This may injure your median nerve.
⊘ **DON'T** delay getting treatment. If muscle wasting occurs, chances of full recovery are less.
⊘ **DON'T** use vibrating hand tools.
⊘ **DON'T** hold your hand or wrist in awkward positions.
⊘ **DON'T** use repetitive movements of the hand or wrist, especially forceful grasping or pinching.
⊘ **DON'T** use direct pressure over the palm and wrist.
⊘ **DON'T** completely stop using and exercising your hand.

FROM THE DESK OF

NOTES

FOR MORE INFORMATION

Contact the following sources:

• American Academy of Orthopaedic Surgeons
  Tel: (800) 346-AAOS
  Website: http://www.aaos.org

• Arthritis Foundation
  Tel: (800) 283-7800
  Website: http://www.arthritis.org

CARING FOR YOUR CHILD WITH
CEREBRAL PALSY

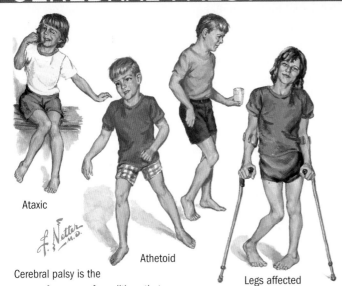

Ataxic

Athetoid

Legs affected

Cerebral palsy is the name of a group of conditions that affect muscles and nerves. It is not inherited, but it begins very early in life. Children with spastic CP have muscle tightness, with stiff movements, especially in the legs, arms, and back. Athetoid CP affects the whole body, so children have problems with balance and coordination.

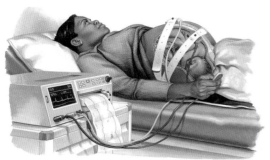

It is caused by injury to parts of the brain that control the ability to use muscles. The injury can take place during pregnancy, during birth, or early in childhood.

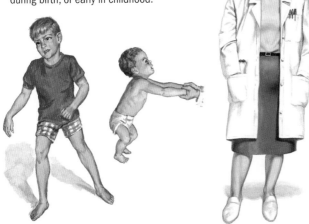

Your doctor will examine your child and carefully evaluate your child's movement.

What Is Cerebral Palsy?

Cerebral palsy (CP) is the name of a group of conditions affecting muscles and nerves. It isn't inherited but begins early in life. The three types of CP are spastic (most common), athetoid, and ataxic.

CP is a lifelong condition that doesn't get worse, and most children with CP have a normal life span.

Some people are mildly affected and can live fairly normal lives. Others are more severely disabled. Many people have normal intelligence despite their severe physical disabilities.

What Causes CP?

The cause is injury to parts of the brain that control the ability to use muscles. Cerebral means related to the brain. Palsy means weakness or problems using muscles. The injury can happen during pregnancy, during birth, or early in childhood. It can involve not having enough oxygen during or after birth, an infection (e.g., German measles) that spreads from mother to baby, or a serious infection early in life.

What Are the Symptoms of CP?

CP can be mild, moderate, or severe. Symptoms include abnormal movements of arms and legs, feeding problems in an infant, poor muscle tone early in life, slow development of walking and talking, abnormal body posture, muscle spasms, body stiffness, poor coordination, and crossed eyes.

Children with spastic CP have muscle tightness, with stiff movements, especially in the legs, arms, and back. Athetoid CP affects the whole body, so children have problems with balance and coordination. They have slow, uncontrolled movements and low muscle tone that makes it hard to sit straight and walk. Symptoms of mixed CP are a combination of these two types.

Sometimes children with CP can have problems learning, hearing, or seeing, or have mental retardation.

How Is CP Diagnosed?

The doctor will do a physical examination and carefully check your child's movement.

The doctor may order tests to confirm CP, including CT and MRI of the brain, ultrasound, and nerve conduction tests.

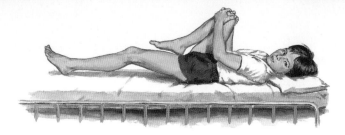

There is no cure for cerebral palsy. Physical therapy is one way to make things easier for your child.

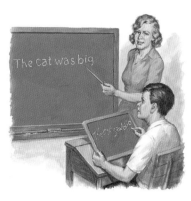

Occupational therapy will help your child with fine motor skills, such those needed for dressing, feeding, and writing.

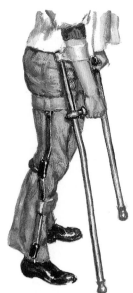

Special equipment, such as braces and crutches, may help your child.

How Is CP Treated?

CP cannot be cured, but symptoms and disabilities can be helped with physical therapy (PT), occupational therapy (OT), psychological counseling, and surgery. PT helps children develop stronger muscles and work on skills such as walking, sitting, and balance. Special equipment, such as braces and splints, may also benefit some children. With OT, children develop fine motor skills, such as those needed for dressing, feeding, and writing. Speech and language therapy helps children with speaking skills. Children and families are aided by support, special education, and related services.

DOs and DON'Ts in Managing CP:

✔ **DO** avoid preventable risks such as German measles during pregnancy.

✔ **DO** call your doctor about treatments that could help symptoms.

✔ **DO** remember that states must meet educational needs of children with disabilities, such as through early intervention services.

✔ **DO** make sure special education and related services are provided for school-age children and preschoolers through school systems.

✔ **DO** have a positive attitude about the person with CP.

⊘ **DON'T** smoke, use alcohol, or abuse drugs during pregnancy.

⊘ **DON'T** forget about assistive devices, such as voice synthesizers and computer technology.

⊘ **DON'T** give up hope. Progress in people with CP is usually slow.

FROM THE DESK OF

NOTES

FOR MORE INFORMATION

Contact the following sources:

• United Cerebral Palsy Foundation
Tel: (800) 872-5827
Website: http://www.ucp.org

• National Dissemination Center for Children with Disabilities
Tel: (800) 695-0285
Website: http://www.nichcy.org

MANAGING YOUR
CHARCOT-MARIE-TOOTH DISEASE

Charlot-Marie-Tooth disease is an inherited disease that affects nerves and causes muscles of the legs, hands, and feet to weaken and lose feeling. Males, usually 10 to 20 years old, are more likely than females to have it. It's named after three doctors who first diagnosed it.

One of the first signs is a high arched foot. In time, people can have foot deformities, hammer toes, foot drop, and a stork-like look of the lower legs.

Some patients have no symptoms; others experience:

Trouble walking

Foot sores that don't heal

Loss of muscle tone from knees down

Unusual feet (curled up toes)

Nerve conduction

Your doctor makes a diagnosis by doing nerve conduction studies, electromyography, and maybe a nerve biopsy.

Electromyography

What Is Charcot-Marie-Tooth Disease?

Charcot-Marie-Tooth disease has nothing to do with teeth. It's named after the three doctors who first diagnosed it. This inherited disease affects nerves and causes muscles of the legs, hands, and feet to weaken and lose feeling. The illness develops slowly and is usually noted between 10 and 20 years of age. It can also affect people 50 to 60 years old. Men are more likely than women to have it, by a ratio of 3 to 1. It doesn't usually shorten life.

What Causes Charcot-Marie-Tooth Disease?

The cause is mutations in genes affecting nerves going to and from the brain. The nerves don't send electrical signals to muscles to make them contract.

What Are the Symptoms of Charcot-Marie-Tooth Disease?

The most common symptoms are weak muscles, loss of muscle tone from knees down, unusual feet (high arches, curled-up toes), trouble walking, muscle cramping, bone and muscle pain, and foot sores that don't heal.

Foot deformities, hammer toes, and foot drop can occur. People can't feel hot, cold, vibration, and light touch. People also get numbness and feel off balance and unsteady. Loss of feeling can lead to cuts, infections, and ulcers.

How Is Charcot-Marie-Tooth Disease Diagnosed?

The doctor makes a diagnosis by doing nerve conduction studies. These tests record electrical responses of a muscle to stimulation of its nerve at two points along the nerve. Also, the doctor will order electromyography (EMG) to measure the pattern of electrical activity in the muscle. The doctor may also get a biopsy sample of a nerve. In a biopsy, a small piece of the nerve is removed for study with a microscope.

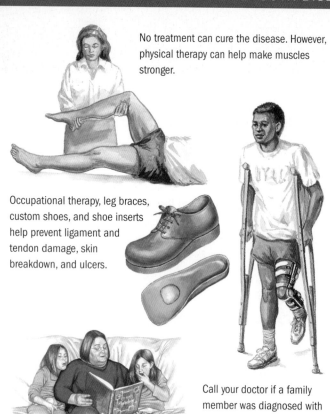

No treatment can cure the disease. However, physical therapy can help make muscles stronger.

Occupational therapy, leg braces, custom shoes, and shoe inserts help prevent ligament and tendon damage, skin breakdown, and ulcers.

Call your doctor if a family member was diagnosed with this disease. Get genetic counseling. The disease is inherited and can't be prevented.

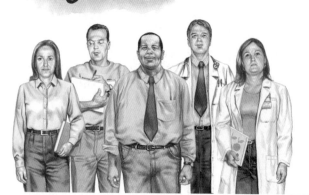

Have a positive attitude. Follow your doctor's suggestions for physical and occupational therapy. Vigorous physical therapy may help preserve muscle function. Get advice from people and facilities with experience in this disease. A neurologist is the best person to ask for advice.

How Is Charcot-Marie-Tooth Disease Treated?

No treatment can cure the disease. The disease can later affect hand muscles, usually stopping at elbows and midthighs. Physical therapy can help make muscles stronger. Occupational therapy, leg braces, custom shoes, and shoe inserts help prevent ligament and tendon damage, skin breakdown, and ulcer formation.

The doctor can prescribe pain relievers. Surgery can sometimes correct major foot deformities.

DOs and DON'Ts in Managing Charcot-Marie-Tooth Disease:

✔ **DO** have a positive attitude.
✔ **DO** follow your doctor's suggestions for physical and occupational therapy. Vigorous physical therapy may help preserve muscle function.
✔ **DO** get advice from people and facilities with experience in this disease. A neurologist (doctor specializing in diseases of the brain and spinal cord) is the best person to ask.
✔ **DO** call your doctor if you notice muscle weakness of your feet and hands.
✔ **DO** call your doctor if a family member was diagnosed with this disease. Get genetic counseling. The disease is inherited and cannot be prevented.

⊘ **DON'T** ignore symptoms. Early treatment may help preserve some muscle and nerve function.
⊘ **DON'T** forget that Charcot-Marie-Tooth disease is NOT muscular dystrophy or multiple sclerosis. Muscular dystrophy involves muscles directly. Multiple sclerosis involves the brain and spinal cord.
⊘ **DON'T** confuse this disease with Lou Gehrig's disease (amyotrophic lateral sclerosis [ALS]).

FROM THE DESK OF

NOTES

FOR MORE INFORMATION
Contact the following source:
• Charcot-Marie-Tooth Association
  Tel: (610) 499-9264, (800) 606-2682
  Website: http://www.charcot-marie-tooth.org

MANAGING YOUR CLUSTER HEADACHES

Cluster headaches are one of the more severe types of head pain. They are more common in men than women. They are rare, occurring in less than 1% of people, and are most common between adolescence and middle age.

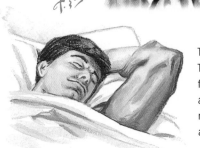

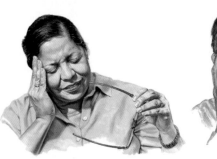

The exact cause is unknown. Triggers can include drugs, foods, smoking, drinking alcohol, and changing the normal sleep pattern, such as taking a nap.

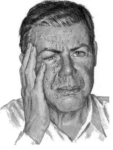

The pain is usually constant, intense, and nonthrobbing, deep in and around the eye on one side of the head. Pain often moves into the forehead, temple, and cheek. Other symptoms are watery eyes, drooping eyelids, and vision problems

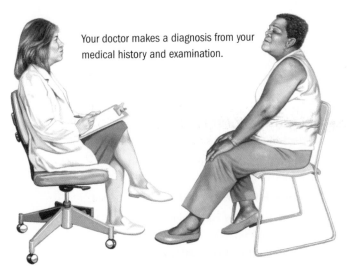

Your doctor makes a diagnosis from your medical history and examination.

What Are Cluster Headaches?

Cluster headaches are one of the more severe types of head pain. They are more common in men than women. The pain is usually constant, intense, and nonthrobbing, deep in and around the eye on one side of the head. Pain often moves into the forehead, temple, and cheek. Pain may leave as quickly as it began or fade slowly.

Cluster headaches are unpredictable. Several months can pass without headaches, but then they start again. They are rather rare, occurring in less than 1% of people, and are most common between adolescence and middle age.

What Causes Cluster Headaches?

The exact cause is unknown. Triggers can include drugs, certain foods, smoking, drinking alcohol, and changing the normal sleep pattern (such as taking a nap).

What Are the Symptoms of Cluster Headaches?

Headaches occur in groups or clusters. Each cluster usually begins in spring or fall and lasts about 2 to 3 months. Headaches may occur nightly after 1 to 2 hours of sleep or several times during the day and night. Each attack may last almost an hour. They often have a pattern, occurring at the same time each day for 6 to 12 weeks, followed by no headaches for many months or years. Other symptoms are watering eyes, drooping eyelids, and vision problems on the side of the headache.

How Are Cluster Headaches Diagnosed?

The doctor makes a diagnosis from the medical history and examination. No tests are needed. If the symptom pattern changes, the doctor may order additional tests such as magnetic resonance imaging (MRI) of the head.

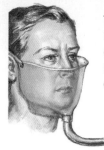

The goal is to help symptoms, because cluster headaches cannot be cured. Certain medicines can prevent more attacks. For breakthrough headaches, the best treatment is breathing pure oxygen.

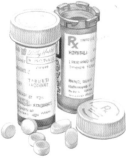

Take your medicines as prescribed. Check with your doctor before using over-the-counter pain relievers.

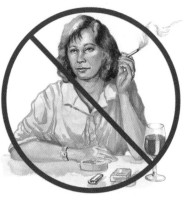

Avoid triggers of attacks, such as alcohol, foods containing nitrates, tobacco, and strenuous exercise.

Call your doctor if you have weakness, numbness, or tingling in your arms or legs; you have trouble walking or talking; or you have severe vomiting.

How Are Cluster Headaches Treated?

Many treatments exist for cluster headaches. The goal is to help symptoms because cluster headaches cannot be cured. Certain medicines can prevent more headache attacks. For breakthrough headaches (which occur even with preventive medicine), the best treatment is inhaling pure oxygen. The doctor may prescribe oxygen therapy for use at home if breakthrough headaches occur often. If attacks are less frequent, drugs given by mouth, such as verapamil or the steroid methylprednisolone, also work and are more convenient than pure oxygen.

DOs and DON'Ts in Managing Cluster Headaches:

✔ **DO** keep to an adequate and regular sleep schedule.
✔ **DO** take your medicines as prescribed.
✔ **DO** check with your doctor before using over-the-counter pain relievers.
✔ **DO** keep your follow-up doctor appointments.
✔ **DO** call your doctor if you have a fever with your headache.
✔ **DO** call your doctor if you have a headache that is more severe than usual and your usual medicine doesn't help it.
✔ **DO** call your doctor if you have weakness, numbness, or tingling in your arms or legs or you have trouble walking or talking.
✔ **DO** call your doctor if you have severe vomiting that your medicine doesn't control.
✔ **DO** call your doctor if you have problems with your medicine.

⊘ **DON'T** use alcohol, foods containing nitrates, and tobacco.
⊘ **DON'T** expose yourself to oil-based solvents; avoid high altitudes and strenuous exercise. These may start an attack.

FROM THE DESK OF

NOTES

MANAGING YOUR
CONCUSSION

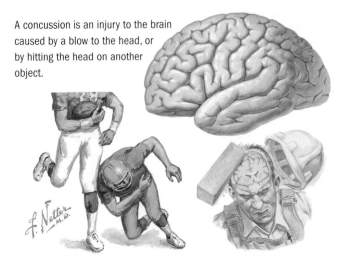

A concussion is an injury to the brain caused by a blow to the head, or by hitting the head on another object.

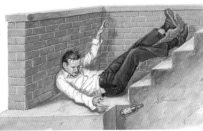

Sudden movement of the brain in the skull can injure the brain. Most concussions result from motor vehicle accidents, industrial accidents, contact sports (such as football and hockey), falls, and physical attacks.

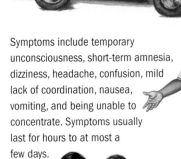

Symptoms include temporary unconsciousness, short-term amnesia, dizziness, headache, confusion, mild lack of coordination, nausea, vomiting, and being unable to concentrate. Symptoms usually last for hours to at most a few days.

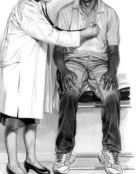

Your doctor makes a diagnosis from a detailed neurological examination and history of loss of consciousness, amnesia, or confusion after a blow to the head. CT or MRI of the brain may be done but usually show normal findings.

What Is a Concussion?

A concussion is an injury to the brain caused by a blow to the head, or by hitting the head on another object. It may result in loss of consciousness or confusion. It may also cause amnesia (loss of memory) about the event related to the concussion as well as time before or after.

What Causes a Concussion?

Sudden movement of the brain in the skull can injure the brain. Most concussions result from motor vehicle accidents, industrial accidents, contact sports (such as football and hockey), falls, and physical attacks.

What Are the Symptoms of a Concussion?

Symptoms include temporary unconsciousness, short-term amnesia, dizziness, headache, confusion, mild lack of coordination, nausea, vomiting, and being unable to concentrate. Symptoms usually last for hours to several days.

How Is a Concussion Diagnosed?

The doctor makes a diagnosis from a detailed neurological examination and history of loss of consciousness, amnesia, or confusion after a blow to the head. The doctor may order computed tomography (CT) or magnetic resonance imaging (MRI) of the brain, but these tests usually show normal findings.

How Is a Concussion Treated?

Treatment consists of rest and careful observation, usually at home. First symptoms of a concussion mimic those of a head injury with bleeding into the brain. If symptoms get worse or don't improve, swelling or bleeding inside the skull needs to be ruled out by your physician with additional tests.

Rest and observation is typical treatment. Drugs such as acetaminophen can help a headache. If symptoms get worse or don't improve, swelling or bleeding inside the skull needs to be ruled out by your physician.

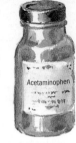

Avoid substances that cause drowsiness, including narcotic pain medicines, alcohol, sleeping pills, muscle relaxants, tranquilizers, and recreational drugs. They may mask important symptoms of worsening condition.

Avoid strenuous activities until the doctor gives an okay. Repeated concussions (especially within 3 months) may cause permanent brain damage and even death. Don't play football, box, or practice martial arts for at least 3 months after a concussion.

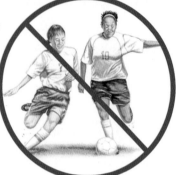

Prevent head injuries: always wear a seat belt in a motor vehicle. Always use helmets when riding motorcycles or bicycles. Use protective gear in sports, and limit contact sports activities.

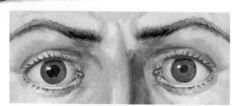

Watch for worsening confusion or headache, drowsiness, loss of memory, nausea, vomiting, muscle weakness, problems walking, unequal pupil size, convulsions, and inability to wake from sleep. They can mean a worsening condition and maybe an emergency.

DOs and DON'Ts in Managing a Concussion:

✔ **DO** take medicines such as acetaminophen for headache.

✔ **DO** eat a light diet. For nausea, eat mostly small amounts of food or fluids.

✔ **DO** get plenty of rest until you feel normal. Ask your doctor about when you may return to work or may exercise. An ice pack to the spot that was hit may help with pain.

✔ **DO** watch for increasing confusion, worsening headache, drowsiness, loss of coordination, loss of memory, nausea, vomiting, muscle weakness, problems walking, unequal pupils, convulsions, and inability to wake from sleep. These signs mean a worsening condition and could mean an emergency.

✔ **DO** call your doctor if you don't improve in about 24 hours.

✔ **DO** prevent head injuries: always wear a seat belt in a motor vehicle. Always use helmets when riding a motorcycle. Use protective gear in sports and limit contact sports activities.

✔ **DO** avoid another concussion. Repeated concussions (especially within 3 months) may cause permanent brain damage and even death. Don't play football, box, or practice martial arts for at least 3 months after a concussion.

🚫 **DON'T** stay alone. Someone should check on you every couple of hours for the first 24 hours or until you feel normal.

🚫 **DON'T** take medicines or substances that cause drowsiness or changes in level of consciousness. These include narcotic pain medicines, alcohol, sleeping pills, muscle relaxants, tranquilizers, and recreational drugs. They may mask important symptoms of a worsening condition.

🚫 **DON'T** eat a heavy diet. It may lead to vomiting.

🚫 **DON'T** do strenuous activities. You may get a more severe headache. Don't operate dangerous machinery. Being dizzy or having decreased muscle coordination, ability to concentrate, or memory may make operation of machinery dangerous.

FROM THE DESK OF

NOTES

FOR MORE INFORMATION

Contact the following sources:

• Brain Injury Association of America (formerly the National Head Injury Foundation)
Tel: (800) 444-6443
Website: http://www.biausa.org

• American Trauma Society
Tel: (800) 556-7890
Website: http://www.amtrauma.org

652   Ferri's Netter Patient Advisor

Copyright © 2010 by Saunders, an imprint of Elsevier, Inc.

CARING FOR YOUR CHILD WITH
DOWN SYNDROME

Down syndrome is a hereditary condition with moderate to severe mental deficiency. Children with Down syndrome are born with extra genetic material on chromosome 21. It occurs in about 1 of 800 to 1000 live births.

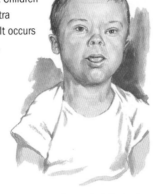

Chromosome

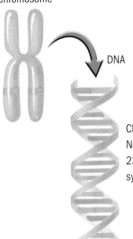

DNA

Chromosomes hold all genetic information. Normally, each person has 46 chromosomes, 23 from each parent. People with Down syndrome have 47 chromosomes.

Children tend to be calm and rarely cry. They have a small head, mental retardation, developmental delays, slanting eyes, short height, and small, low-set ears. The tongue seems too big for the mouth, and muscles seem floppy. Hands are short and broad with one crease in the palm.

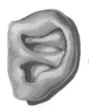
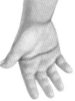
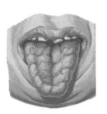

The diagnosis is usually made just after birth, from the physical look of the baby. A blood test to check chromosomes confirms the diagnosis. Two tests done during pregnancy can tell whether the fetus has the syndrome. They are chorionic villus biopsy and amniocentesis. A new genetic test may detect Down syndrome with a blood sample from the mom-to-be.

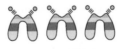

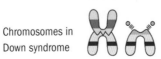

Chromosomes in
Down syndrome

What Is Down Syndrome?

Down syndrome is a hereditary condition with moderate-to-severe mental deficiency. Children with Down syndrome are born with an extra chromosome 21. Other names for this condition are trisomy 21 and mongolism. Dr. John Down, a British doctor, first identified this condition in 1866. Down syndrome occurs in about 1 of 800 to 1000 live births.

The syndrome cannot be cured, but people can live long lives, into their 60s.

What Causes Down Syndrome?

Chromosomes hold all genetic information. Normally, each person has 46 chromosomes, 23 from each parent. People with Down syndrome have 47 chromosomes. The mother's age is important, because the older the mother, the greater the chance of having a child with this syndrome. At age 25 years, the risk is 1 in 1400. At age 40, it's 1 in 100. Down syndrome cannot be prevented. Future parents may want genetic counseling before having a child.

What Are the Symptoms of Down Syndrome?

Children differ mentally and physically from other children their age. They tend to be calm and rarely cry. Other features include a small head, mental retardation, delays in development, slanting eyes, short height, and small, low-set ears. The tongue seems too big for the mouth, and muscles seem floppy. Hands are short and broad with one crease in the palm.

Babies develop language and learning skills (crawling, walking) more slowly than other babies.

How Is Down Syndrome Diagnosed?

The diagnosis is usually made just after birth, from the physical look of the baby. A blood test to check chromosomes will confirm the diagnosis. Two tests done during pregnancy can tell whether the fetus has the syndrome. They are chorionic villus biopsy and amniocentesis. The doctor may also do tests for heart problems. A new genetic test may detect Down syndrome with a blood sample from the mom-to-be

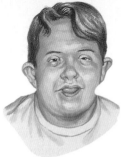

Down syndrome cannot be cured, but many medical and developmental conditions can be helped. Physical therapy and special education can help children control their muscles and develop social skills. Many children can reach a very high level of functioning and be independent.

How Is Down Syndrome Treated?

Many medical and developmental conditions can be helped. For example, in some cases surgery may be used for heart and digestive problems. Physical therapy and special education can help children control their muscles and develop social skills. Many children can reach a very high level of functioning and be independent.

DOs and DON'Ts in Managing Down Syndrome:

✔ **DO** work with your health care team to plan a treatment program for your child.

✔ **DO** consider help from mental health workers, which may help you understand this condition. You may feel guilty, but it's not your fault for having a child with Down syndrome.

✔ **DO** enroll your child in an early intervention program. Look for educational, developmental, and vocational options as your child grows up.

✔ **DO** get help from local and national support groups.

✔ **DO** get genetic counseling.

✔ **DO** call your doctor if you have questions about your child's health or need information about services for your child.

✔ **DO** call your doctor if your child becomes ill or confused or has problems with medicines.

⊘ **DON'T** underestimate your child's ability. Enroll your child in a special teaching program.

Work with your health care team to plan a treatment program for your child. Don't underestimate your child's ability. Enroll your child in a special teaching program.

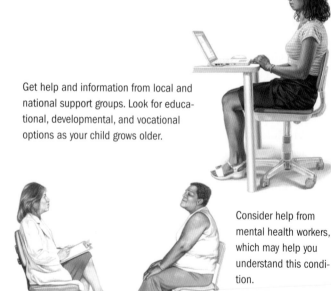

Get help and information from local and national support groups. Look for educational, developmental, and vocational options as your child grows older.

Consider help from mental health workers, which may help you understand this condition.

FROM THE DESK OF

NOTES

FOR MORE INFORMATION

Contact the following source:

• National Down Syndrome Society
  Tel: (800) 221-4602
  Website: http://www.ndss.org

MANAGING YOUR
EPILEPSY

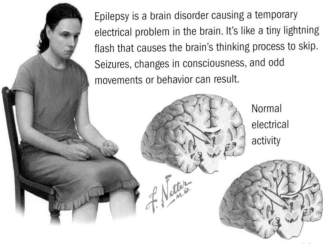

Epilepsy is a brain disorder causing a temporary electrical problem in the brain. It's like a tiny lightning flash that causes the brain's thinking process to skip. Seizures, changes in consciousness, and odd movements or behavior can result.

Normal electrical activity

Electrical activity during seizure

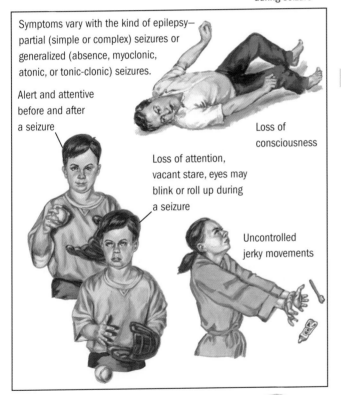

Symptoms vary with the kind of epilepsy—partial (simple or complex) seizures or generalized (absence, myoclonic, atonic, or tonic-clonic) seizures.

Alert and attentive before and after a seizure

Loss of consciousness

Loss of attention, vacant stare, eyes may blink or roll up during a seizure

Uncontrolled jerky movements

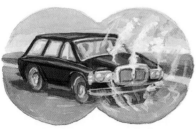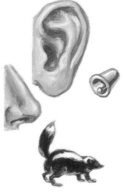

Some people may have warnings of seizures, such as feeling tense, noticing a bad smell, hearing a strange noise, or not seeing right.

What Is Epilepsy?

Epilepsy is a brain disorder causing a temporary electrical problem in the brain. It's like a tiny lightning flash that causes the brain's thinking to start to skip, like a damaged CD. This problem causes seizures (convulsions), changes in consciousness, or odd movements or behavior.

Epilepsy is usually a lifelong condition, but some types, such as seizures caused by brain damage, infections, or tumors, may go away after treatment of the cause.

What Causes Epilepsy?

Causes include brain disorders present at birth, head injuries, infections (meningitis, encephalitis), tumors, poisoning, and drug and alcohol abuse. It isn't contagious but can run in families. Often, the cause is unknown.

What Are the Symptoms of Epilepsy?

Symptoms vary with the kind of epilepsy—partial (simple or complex) or generalized (absence, myoclonic, atonic, or tonic-clonic).

Some people stop what they're doing, stare blankly, and aren't aware of what's happening. Other people lose consciousness, stiffen, twitch, and have uncontrollable jerky movements. They lose bladder control, become violent or angry, laugh for no reason, or make odd body movements. Deep sleep or feelings of confusion follow.

Before a seizure, some people may have warnings such as a tense feeling, bad smell, hearing a strange noise, or not seeing right.

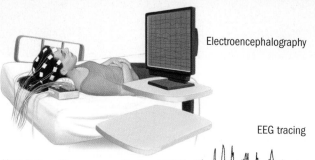
Electroencephalography

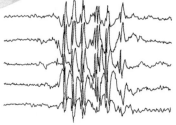
EEG tracing

Your doctor will use your medical history and physical examination for diagnosis as well as check the brain's electrical activity with the EEG. The EEG tracing shows this electrical activity. MRI, CT, or blood tests may be done.

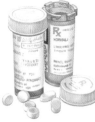

Drugs are the most common treatment to control seizures. Medicine is often changed or adjusted for better control. Surgery may be used if drugs don't help.

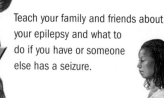

Wear a medical alert bracelet stating that you have epilepsy and listing your medicines.

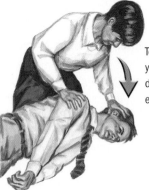

Teach your family and friends about your epilepsy and what to do if you have or someone else has a seizure.

Epilepsy may be a lifelong condition. Learn all you can about your medicines and keep records of your seizures so that you and your doctor can make the best treatment decisions.

How Is Epilepsy Diagnosed?

The doctor will make a diagnosis from a medical history and physical examination. The doctor will check the brain's electrical activity with a test called electroencephalography (EEG). The electroencephalogram tracing shows the electrical activity. Magnetic resonance imaging (MRI) or computed tomography (CT) may be done. Blood tests will be done to check for other causes of seizures.

How Is Epilepsy Treated?

Antiepileptic drugs are the most common treatment to control seizures. Medicine is often changed or adjusted for better seizure control. Surgery may be used if drugs don't help. Other newer treatment options are vagus nerve stimulation and special diets. An electrical device is placed in the shoulder to stimulate a cranial nerve. A high-fat, low-carbohydrate diet may help reduce certain seizures if other treatments don't work.

Medicines can cause side effects, which the doctor will explain.

When someone has a seizure, prevent injuries by cushioning the head, turning the person on their side, and taking away items that could cause injuries. Don't hold the person down, force anything into the mouth, or shout or shake the person. Afterward, let the person rest or sleep if needed.

DOs and DON'Ts in Managing Epilepsy:

✔ **DO** wear a medical alert bracelet or pendant that shows you have epilepsy.
✔ **DO** check with your state about driving. Most states allow people with epilepsy to drive after being seizure-free for 1 year.
✔ **DO** tell your doctor if you have side effects from your medicine.
✔ **DO** tell your doctor if you have new symptoms.
✔ **DO** try to reduce your stress and get adequate sleep.
✔ **DO** keep a record of your seizures. Call your doctor if the pattern or duration of seizures increases.
✔ **DO** have blood tests to make sure that your medicine levels are in the proper range.

⊘ **DON'T** drink alcohol.
⊘ **DON'T** expose yourself to anything that triggered a seizure before.

FOR MORE INFORMATION

Contact the following source:

• Epilepsy Foundation of America
Tel: (301) 459-3700
Website: http://www.epilepsyfoundation.org

FROM THE DESK OF

NOTES

MANAGING YOUR
FRIEDREICH'S ATAXIA

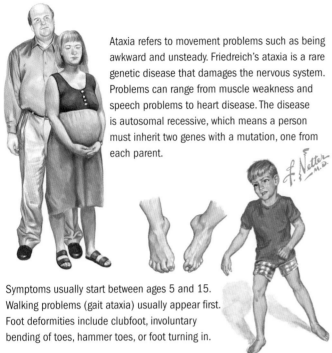

Ataxia refers to movement problems such as being awkward and unsteady. Friedreich's ataxia is a rare genetic disease that damages the nervous system. Problems can range from muscle weakness and speech problems to heart disease. The disease is autosomal recessive, which means a person must inherit two genes with a mutation, one from each parent.

Symptoms usually start between ages 5 and 15. Walking problems (gait ataxia) usually appear first. Foot deformities include clubfoot, involuntary bending of toes, hammer toes, or foot turning in.

Other symptoms include:

Loss of feeling and reflexes

Scoliosis

Rapid, rhythmic, involuntary movements of eyeballs

Some loss of eyesight

Hearing loss

Diabetes

What Is Friedreich's Ataxia?

Ataxia refers to movement problems, such as being clumsy or awkward and unsteady. Friedreich's ataxia is a rare genetic disease that damages the nervous system. The result can range from muscle weakness and speech problems to heart disease and diabetes. The disease progression varies from person to person, but years after first symptoms, people may be confined to a wheelchair. Most people die in early adulthood if they have severe heart disease, a common cause of death in this condition. Some people with less severe symptoms live much longer. Males and females are equally affected.

What Causes Friedreich's Ataxia?

The disease is autosomal recessive, which means a person must inherit two genes with the mutation, one from each parent. Nerve tissue in the spinal cord and nerves controlling muscle movement in arms and legs degenerate and cause the movement problems.

What Are the Symptoms of Friedreich's Ataxia?

Symptoms usually start between ages 5 and 15. They rarely start as young as 18 months or as old as 30 years. The first one is usually walking problems (gait ataxia). It slowly worsens and spreads to the arms and then the trunk. Foot deformities (clubfoot, involuntary bending of toes, hammer toes, or foot turning in) may be early signs. Muscles (especially in feet, lower legs, and hands) weaken and waste away, and deformities develop. Other symptoms include loss of reflexes (in knees and ankles) and loss of feeling in extremities, which may spread to other parts of the body. People get tired easily, and speech gets slurred and slow. Rapid, rhythmic, involuntary movements of eyeballs are common. Most people get scoliosis (spine curves to one side), which can cause breathing problems.

Other symptoms (chest pain, shortness of breath, palpitations, fast heart rate) result from heart disease. Some people get diabetes and some lose hearing or eyesight.

Your doctor will make a diagnosis from your medical history and physical examination. A specialist (neurologist) should confirm the diagnosis. Blood tests, nerve conduction studies, and MRI will be done.

So far, no treatment can cure this condition, but treatment of symptoms and complications can help people function.
Drugs can treat diabetes and heart conditions. Braces or surgery can help scoliosis and foot deformities. Physical therapy can also help.

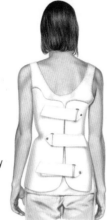

People who were recently diagnosed with the disease and family members can get genetic counseling.

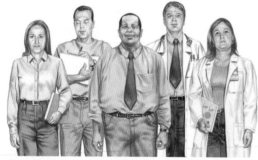

Understand that this progressive disease will need a health care team including doctors, social workers, and physical, occupational, and speech therapists. Look for doctors with experience treating this disease.

FROM THE DESK OF

NOTES

How Is Friedreich's Ataxia Diagnosed?

The doctor will make a diagnosis from the medical history and physical examination. A specialist (neurologist) should confirm the diagnosis.

Blood tests, MRI, and nerve conduction studies will be done.

How Is Friedreich's Ataxia Treated?

So far, no treatment can cure this condition. However, treatment of symptoms and complications can help people function as long as possible.

Drugs can treat diabetes and heart conditions. Braces or surgery can help foot deformities and scoliosis. Physical therapy is helpful to maintain function.

DOs and DON'Ts in Managing Friedreich's Ataxia:

✔ **DO** realize that Friedreich's ataxia is rare. Find doctors with experience with this disease.
✔ **DO** understand that this progressive disease will need services of a health care team, such as physical therapist, occupational therapist, speech therapist, and social workers.
✔ **DO** call your doctor if you fall often or have trouble swallowing, shortness of breath, or chest pain.
✔ **DO** call your doctor if you have symptoms of diabetes (e.g., thirst, increased urination, weight loss).
✔ **DO** call your doctor if you want genetic counseling.

⊘ **DON'T** be afraid to ask for a second opinion.
⊘ **DON'T** forget that Friedreich's ataxia is an inherited genetic disease, and genetic counseling for family members is helpful.

FOR MORE INFORMATION

Contact the following sources:

• Brain Resources and Information Network
National Institute of Neurological Disorders and Stroke
Tel: (800) 352-9424
Website: http://www.ninds.nih.gov

• Friedreich's Ataxia Research Alliance
Tel: (703) 413-4468

• National Ataxia Foundation
Tel: (763) 553-0020
Website: http://www.ataxia.org

• Genetic Alliance
Tel: (800) 336-GENE (336-4363)
Website: http://www.geneticalliance.org

MANAGING YOUR
GENERALIZED TONIC-CLONIC SEIZURES

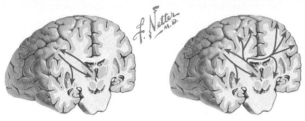

Normal electrical activity

Brain electrical activity during seizures

Generalized tonic-clonic seizures affect the whole body. Abnormal activity of brain nerve cells occurring at the same time in many parts of the brain causes them. People of any age can have them, as a single seizure or part of epilepsy.

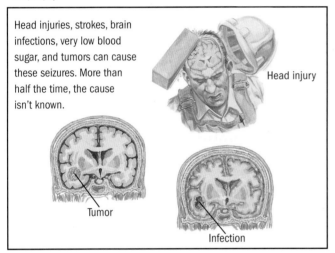

Head injuries, strokes, brain infections, very low blood sugar, and tumors can cause these seizures. More than half the time, the cause isn't known.

Head injury

Tumor

Infection

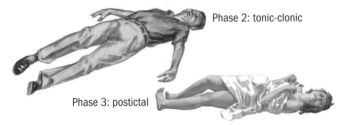

Phase 2: tonic-clonic

Phase 3: postictal

Tonic-clonic seizures involve four phases: 1, auras (odd feeling, strange taste or odor, headache); phase 2, rigid stiffening of the body and fainting. The tonic-clonic phase (3) involves muscle contractions and relaxations, convulsions, loss of consciousness, and loss of bladder and/or bowel control. The postictal phase (4) is a slow return to consciousness.

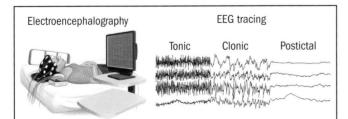

Electroencephalography

EEG tracing

Tonic   Clonic   Postictal

Your doctor will use your medical history and physical examination for diagnosis as well as check your brain's electrical activity with the EEG. The EEG tracing shows this activity. MRI, CT, or blood tests may be done.

What Are Generalized Tonic-Clonic Seizures?

Generalized tonic-clonic seizures, or grand mal seizures, affect the whole body. They usually involve rigid muscles, severe muscle contractions, and loss of consciousness (fainting). People of any age can have them, as a single seizure or part of epilepsy.

What Causes Generalized Tonic-Clonic Seizures?

Abnormal activity of brain nerve cells occurring at the same time in many parts of the brain causes these seizures. Seizures may be brought on by head injuries, strokes, brain infections, very low blood sugar, and tumors. More than half the time, the cause is unknown.

What Are the Symptoms of Generalized Tonic-Clonic Seizures?

These seizures involve four phases. Often signs (auras) warn of a coming seizure. Auras include an odd feeling, strange taste or odor, and headache. Phase 2 (tonic phase) consists of rigid stiffening of the body for a minute or less, and fainting. The tonic-clonic phase (phase 3) appears as strong muscle contractions and relaxations and convulsions and can last several minutes. Loss of consciousness and loss of bladder and/or bowel control may occur. People may have trouble breathing or temporarily stop breathing. Just after a seizure is the postictal phase (phase 4). People slowly return to consciousness.

Lasting tonic-clonic seizures are an emergency called "status epilepticus."

How Are Generalized Tonic-Clonic Seizures Diagnosed?

The doctor will make a diagnosis from a medical history and physical examination. The doctor will do electroencephalography (EEG), a test to check the electrical activity in the brain. Magnetic resonance imaging (MRI) or computed tomography (CT) will be done to get pictures of the brain. Blood tests will also be done to check for other causes of seizures.

The main treatment is medicine. Sometimes more than one anticonvulsant drug is used. Your doctor may get blood samples on a regular basis to make sure that the correct dose is being given.

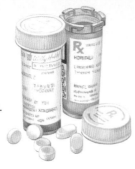

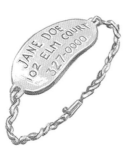

Wear a medical alert bracelet saying that you have a seizure disorder and noting your medicines.

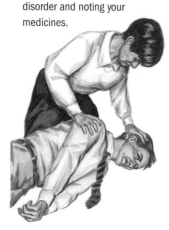

Teach your family and friends about your disorder and what to do if you have or someone else has a seizure.

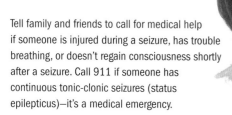

Don't operate dangerous machinery or drive unless your doctor approves. Don't swim alone. Don't climb on ladders or roofs in case you have a seizure.

Tell family and friends to call for medical help if someone is injured during a seizure, has trouble breathing, or doesn't regain consciousness shortly after a seizure. Call 911 if someone has continuous tonic-clonic seizures (status epilepticus)—it's a medical emergency.

How Are Generalized Tonic-Clonic Seizures Treated?

The main treatment is medicine. Sometimes more than one anticonvulsant drug may be used. The doctor may get blood samples periodically to make sure that the correct dose is being used. Often, medicine will reduce the frequency and severity of seizures, but some people may continue to have them.

DOs and DON'Ts in Managing Generalized Tonic-Clonic Seizures:

✔ **DO** take your medicine as prescribed to prevent seizures.

✔ **DO** wear a medical alert bracelet stating that you have a seizure disorder and listing your medicines.

✔ **DO** teach your family and friends about your disorder and what to do if you or someone else has a seizure. Prevent injuries by cushioning the head, turning the person on their side, and taking away items that could cause injuries. Don't hold the person down or force anything into the mouth.

✔ **DO** tell someone near you that you feel a seizure starting, and lie down.

✔ **DO** call for medical help if someone is injured during a seizure, has trouble breathing, or doesn't regain consciousness shortly after a seizure.

✔ **DO** call 911 if someone has continuous tonic-clonic seizures. Status epilepticus is a medical emergency.

✔ **DO** call your doctor if you have any problems with your medicines.

✔ **DO** call your doctor if your seizures become more frequent or severe.

⊘ **DON'T** operate dangerous machinery or drive unless your doctor approves.

⊘ **DON'T** swim alone.

⊘ **DON'T** climb on ladders or roofs in case you have a seizure.

FROM THE DESK OF

NOTES

FOR MORE INFORMATION

Contact the following source:

• Epilepsy Foundation of America
 Tel: (301) 459-3700
 Website: http://www.epilepsyfoundation.org

MANAGING YOUR
GUILLAIN-BARRÉ SYNDROME

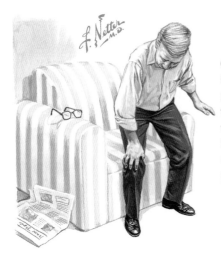

Guillain-Barré syndrome is a rare disorder of the peripheral nerve system that results in muscle weakness. Anyone can get it, at any age. There's no cure, but about 85% of people recover completely.

The exact cause is unknown, but more than two thirds of people have an infection 1 to 3 weeks before the muscle weakness. It's not contagious. Most experts believe that it's an autoimmune disease.

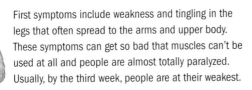

First symptoms include weakness and tingling in the legs that often spread to the arms and upper body. These symptoms can get so bad that muscles can't be used at all and people are almost totally paralyzed. Usually, by the third week, people are at their weakest.

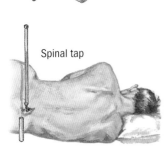

Spinal tap

EMG

Exam

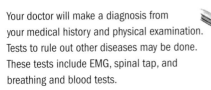

Your doctor will make a diagnosis from your medical history and physical examination. Tests to rule out other diseases may be done. These tests include EMG, spinal tap, and breathing and blood tests.

What Is Guillain-Barré Syndrome?

Guillain-Barré syndrome is a rare disorder of the peripheral nerve system that results in muscle weakness. Peripheral nerves travel to and from the brain. About 3500 cases are diagnosed each year in the United States and Canada. Anyone can get it, at any age, and both sexes equally. There's no cure, but about 85% of people recover completely. It cannot be prevented.

What Causes Guillain-Barré Syndrome?

The exact cause is unknown, but more than two thirds of people have an infection 1 to 3 weeks before the muscle weakness. It isn't contagious. Most experts believe that it's an autoimmune disease. Autoimmune means that the body's own immune (infection-fighting) system attacks the body.

What Are the Symptoms of Guillain-Barré Syndrome?

First symptoms include weakness and tingling in the legs that often spread to the arms and upper body.

These symptoms can get so bad that the muscles cannot be used at all and people are almost totally paralyzed. Then, the disorder can become life-threatening. It can interfere with breathing, blood pressure, or heart rate. Abnormal heartbeat, infections, and blood clots can also occur.

The disorder can develop during hours or days or up to 3 to 4 weeks. Most people have the greatest weakness in the first 2 weeks after symptoms start, so by the third week, 90% are at their weakest.

How Is Guillain-Barré Syndrome Diagnosed?

The doctor will make a diagnosis from the medical history and physical examination. The doctor may want tests to rule out other diseases. These tests include electromyography (EMG) to measure electrical activity of nerves and muscles, lumbar puncture (spinal tap) and analysis of spinal fluid, and breathing and blood tests.

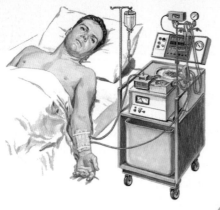

The key to treatment is to prevent complications. Plasmapheresis (shown here) and high-dose immunoglobulin therapy are also used to make the illness less severe and last for a shorter time.

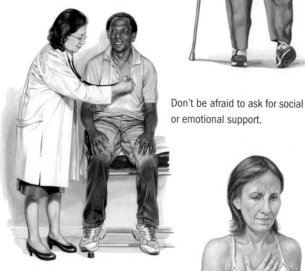

Realize that recovery isn't necessarily quick. Recovery may take a few weeks or as long as months or years. About 30% of people still have weakness after 3 years.

Don't be afraid to ask for social or emotional support.

Call your doctor if you develop numbness or tingling feelings, have trouble swallowing or breathing, feel depressed, or get a fever.

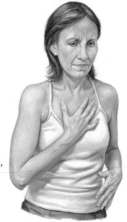

How Is Guillain-Barré Syndrome Treated?

The key to treatment is to prevent complications. Plasmapheresis and high-dose immunoglobulin therapy are also used to reduce the severity and duration of the illness. In plasmapheresis, whole blood is removed from the body, and red and white blood cells are separated from plasma (liquid portion of blood). Blood cells without plasma are then returned to the body. In high-dose immunoglobulin therapy, doctors give intravenous injections of proteins that, in small amounts, the immune system normally uses to attack organisms.

The most critical part of treatment is to keep the body working during recovery of the nervous system. Using a respirator, heart monitor, or another machine that helps the body work may be needed. Usually, people are treated in the hospital, often in the intensive care ward.

DOs and DON'Ts in Managing Guillain-Barré Syndrome:

✔ **DO** understand that Guillain-Barré syndrome can be devastating because of its sudden and unexpected onset.
✔ **DO** realize that recovery isn't necessarily quick. Recovery may take a few weeks or as long as months or years.
✔ **DO** call your doctor if you notice muscle weakness.
✔ **DO** call your doctor if you develop numbness or tingling feelings, have trouble swallowing or breathing, feel depressed, or get a fever.

⊘ **DON'T** be afraid to ask for a second opinion.
⊘ **DON'T** be afraid to ask for social and emotional support.
⊘ **DON'T** miss follow-up appointments after you leave the hospital.

FROM THE DESK OF

NOTES

FOR MORE INFORMATION

Contact the following source:

• GBS/CIDP Foundation International
  Tel: (610) 667-0131, (866) 224-3301
  Website: http://www.gbs-cidp.org/

MANAGING YOUR
HORNER'S SYNDROME

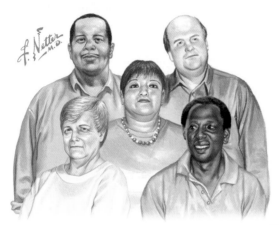

Horner's syndrome is a rare condition affecting nerves to the eye and face. Prognosis and effects depend on the underlying cause.

Some causes are:

Trauma

Drugs

Lung cancer

Herpes infection (shingles)

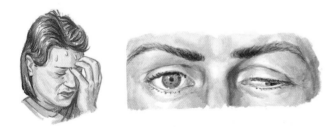

Symptoms are a smaller (constricted) pupil (miosis), drooping eyelid (ptosis), and problems with sweating on the affected side of the face (anhidrosis).

What Is Horner's Syndrome?

The word syndrome means a group of symptoms that together are features of a disease or abnormal condition. Horner's syndrome is a rare condition affecting nerves to the eye and face. It involves a constricted (smaller) pupil, drooping eyelid, and problems with sweating on the affected side of the face.

Prognosis and effects depend on the underlying cause. For example, when it is due to herpes zoster (causing shingles), it is usually not life-threatening and has a good prognosis. However, when due to lung cancer, prognosis is much worse.

What Causes Horner's Syndrome?

Any disease that interrupts nerve fibers to the eye can cause this disorder. Nerve fibers can be damaged from strokes, brain hemorrhage, cerebral aneurysms, or brain tumors. Infections including syphilis, meningitis, and herpes zoster can lead to Horner's syndrome. The disorder can result from blunt trauma injury, motor vehicle accidents, or operations involving the neck, thyroid, lung, aorta, carotid artery, or coronary bypass surgery. Other causes are tumors involving the upper part of the lung or spinal cord in the neck, and drugs including local anesthetics (e.g., lidocaine, bupivacaine), antipsychotics (e.g., thioridazine, chlorpromazine), hypertension medicines (e.g., reserpine, guanethidine), and illicit drugs (e.g., heroin).

Horner's syndrome is not contagious or passed from generation to generation.

What Are the Symptoms of Horner's Syndrome?

Symptoms are a smaller (constricted) pupil (miosis), drooping eyelid (ptosis), and problems with sweating on the affected side of the face (anhidrosis).

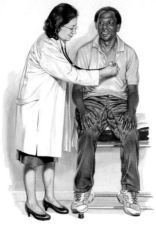

Your doctor will make a diagnosis from your physical examination, as well as x-rays (ultrasonography, angiography, CT, MRI, and magnetic resonance angiography [MRA]).

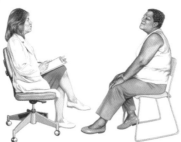

CT of the neck and chest will help rule out head and neck disease, aortic aneurysm, and lung tumors.

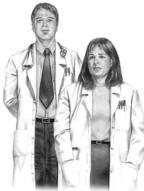

Sometimes, an ophthalmologist or neurologist will be involved in diagnosis. No specific treatment exists for Horner's syndrome. Instead, the underlying cause must be treated (e.g., stopping use of a drug, treating any cancer).

Follow your doctor's recommendations. Be patient. Many tests may be necessary before the cause of the syndrome is found.

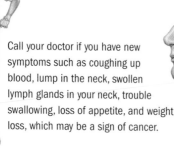

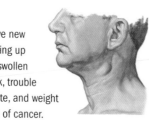

Call your doctor if you have new symptoms such as coughing up blood, lump in the neck, swollen lymph glands in your neck, trouble swallowing, loss of appetite, and weight loss, which may be a sign of cancer.

How Is Horner's Syndrome Diagnosed?

The doctor will make a diagnosis from the physical examination, as well as x-rays (ultrasonography, angiography, computed tomography [CT], magnetic resonance imaging [MRI], and magnetic resonance angiography [MRA]). X-rays help rule out lung cancer. CT of the neck and chest rule out head and neck disease, aortic aneurysm, and lung tumors. Ultrasonography rules out problems with the carotid artery (large artery in the neck taking blood from the heart to the brain).

Sometimes, an ophthalmologist (doctor specializing in eye diseases) or neurologist (doctor specializing in diseases of the brain, spinal cord, and nervous system) will be involved in diagnosis.

How Is Horner's Syndrome Treated?

No specific treatment exists for Horner's syndrome. Instead, the underlying cause must be treated (e.g., stopping use of a drug, treating any cancer).

DOs and DON'Ts in Managing Horner's Syndrome:

✔ **DO** follow your doctor's recommendations. Be patient. Many tests may be needed before the cause of the disorder is found.

✔ **DO** call your doctor if you notice symptoms of Horner's syndrome.

✔ **DO** call your doctor if you are have new signs or symptoms such as coughing up blood, lump in the neck, swollen lymph glands in the neck, trouble swallowing, loss of appetite, and weight loss.

🚫 **DON'T** forget that Horner's syndrome is not a disease. The underlying disease must be treated to correct Horner's syndrome.

FROM THE DESK OF

NOTES

FOR MORE INFORMATION

Contact the following sources:

• NIH/National Eye Institute
  Tel: (301) 496-5248
  Website: http://www.nei.nih.gov

• American Cancer Society
  Tel: (800) 227-2345
  Website: http://www. cancer.org

MANAGING YOUR
HUNTINGTON'S DISEASE

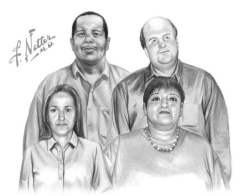

Huntington's disease (or Huntington's chorea) involves degeneration of certain parts of the brain. These parts control movement, thinking, memory, perception, and intelligence. About 30,000 people have this disease in the US. This disease can manifest itself between the ages of 2 and 70 years but is usually diagnosed in early adulthood, at age 30 to 40.

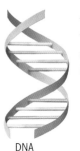

DNA

This inherited disorder is passed from parents to children. The specific cause is a mutation of a gene on chromosome 4. The error in DNA leads to too much protein called huntingtin to be made.

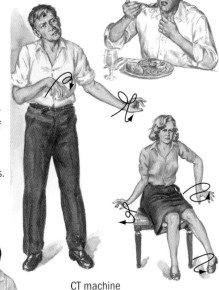

Uncontrolled movements (called chorea), unsteadiness, clumsiness, loss of balance, slurred speech, and trouble swallowing and eating are symptoms.

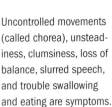

CT machine

CT scan

Your doctor will make a diagnosis from your medical history, physical examination, and laboratory tests. Other tests such as CT (shown here) and MRI may be done.

What Is Huntington's Disease?

Huntington's disease (or Huntington's chorea) involves degeneration of certain parts of the brain. These parts control movement, thinking, memory, perception, and intelligence. About 30,000 people have this disease in the US. At least 150,000 others have a 50% chance of getting the disease.

Today, genetic testing can confirm the diagnosis.

What Causes Huntington's Disease?

This inherited disorder is passed from parents to children. The specific cause is a mutation of a gene on chromosome 4. A mutation means that an error was made in building blocks that make up the DNA (deoxyribonucleic acid). DNA carries genetic information. The mutation leads to too much protein called huntingtin being made. This protein may cause a loss of brain cells and symptoms of the disease.

What Are the Symptoms of Huntington's Disease?

This disease can occur between the ages of 2 and 70 years but is usually diagnosed in early adulthood, at age 30 to 40. Uncontrolled movements called chorea, unsteadiness, clumsiness, loss of balance, slurred speech, and trouble swallowing and eating are symptoms. Chorea is a twisting dance-like motion, usually starting in the feet, fingers, face, or upper chest. Anger, mood swings, irritability, loss of memory, and poor judgment can also occur. Not all people have these exact symptoms. Some may appear rigid, with little movement, or have fine twitching with tremors.

The disease is progressive, meaning slow loss of motor and thinking skills continues. Death can result, most often from pneumonia or complications from injuries.

How Is Huntington's Disease Diagnosed?

The doctor will make a diagnosis from the medical history, physical examination, and laboratory tests. Other tests such as computed tomography (CT) and magnetic resonance imaging (MRI) may be done.

A neurologist (specialist in nervous system diseases) and other specialists may help with diagnosis.

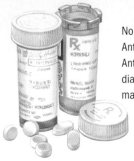

No treatment will reverse Huntington's disease. Antidepressant medicines can help depression. Antipsychotic drugs (haloperidol) or benzo-diazepines (e.g., diazepam or clonazepam) may help the movement problems.

Understand that this disease is inherited. When a family member is diagnosed with this disease, you may have over-whelming anxiety about knowing or not knowing whether you have the gene. Children of a person with the disease have a 50% chance of inheriting the disease gene.

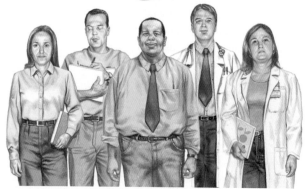

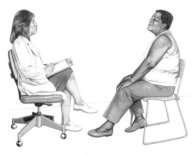

You'll need a team of caregivers. The best person to see for advice is a neurologist, but physical therapists, occupational therapists, psychiatrists, and social workers can all help with treatment.

Don't be afraid to ask for more information. If you're thinking of being tested for the disease, it is important to have pre- and post-test counselings.

How Is Huntington's Disease Treated?

No treatment is available that will reverse Huntington's disease.

Antidepressant medicines can be used for depression. Antipsychotic drugs (haloperidol) or benzodiazepines (e.g., diazepam or clonazepam) may help the problems with movement.

DOs and DON'Ts in Managing Huntington's Disease:

✔ **DO** understand that this disease is inherited. When a family member is diagnosed with Huntington's disease, you may have overwhelming anxiety about knowing or not knowing whether you have the Huntington's disease gene. Children of a person with the disease have a 50% chance of inheriting the disease gene.

✔ **DO** remember that genetic markers or tests can be done to find out whether you carry the Huntington's gene. The decision to have this test won't be easy. Refer to guidelines of the Huntington's Disease Society of America (HDSA).

✔ **DO** call your doctor if a family member has been diagnosed with Huntington's disease.

⊘ **DON'T** forget that people with this disease need a team of caregivers. The best person to see for advice is the neurologist. Physical therapists, occupational therapists, psychiatrists, and social workers can all help with treatment.

⊘ **DON'T** be afraid to ask for more information. If you are thinking of being tested for Huntington's disease, it is important to have pre- and post-test counseling.

FROM THE DESK OF

NOTES

FOR MORE INFORMATION

Contact the following source:

• Huntington's Disease Society of America
Tel: (800) 345-4372
Website: http://www.hdsa.org

Normal pressure hydrocephalus (NPH) is a condition where there is an abnormally high amount of cerebrospinal fluid in the brain's ventricles (cavities). NPH is rare, occurring in 1 of 100,000 people. People of any age can have it, but it occurs most often in elderly people.

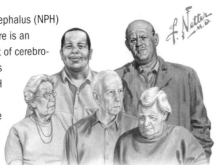

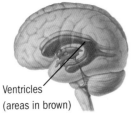
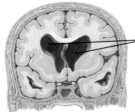

Ventricles (areas in brown)

Ventricles enlarged because of extra CSF

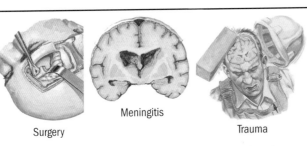

Surgery

Meningitis

Trauma

In almost half of cases, the cause isn't known (idiopathic). The other cases result from trauma, brain surgery, meningitis, infection, or bleeding into the subarachnoid space.

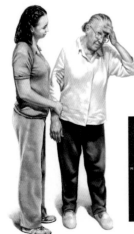

Symptoms often start slowly and progress. They include walking problems, mental impairment (dementia), and problems holding urine in the bladder (incontinence).

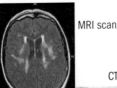

MRI scan

CT machine

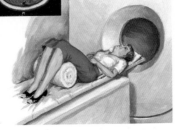

It may be hard to diagnose NPH, because many symptoms may be seen with other diseases (e.g., Parkinson's, Alzheimer's, and other types of dementia). CT and MRI may help with diagnosis.

What Is Normal Pressure Hydrocephalus (NPH)?

Normal pressure hydrocephalus (NPH) is a condition with an abnormally high amount of cerebrospinal fluid in the brain's ventricles (cavities). NPH is rare, occurring in 1 of 100,000 people. People of any age can have it, but it occurs most often in elderly people.

What Causes NPH?

In almost 50% of NPH cases, the cause is unknown. It's called idiopathic. The rest of the cases result from trauma, brain surgery, meningitis, infection, or bleeding into the subarachnoid space, the part between the brain and thin tissues that cover it.

NPH isn't contagious or passed from parents to children.

What Are the Symptoms of NPH?

Symptoms often start slowly and progress. Symptoms include walking problems, mental impairment (dementia), and problems holding urine in the bladder (incontinence).

Most people have a slow, shuffling, and wide-based walk. Many complain of problems starting to walk, with the feeling that the feet are stuck to the floor (called magnet gait).

Dementia involves slowed thinking, memory loss, forgetfulness, problems focusing, and lack of attention.

In early stages of NPH, people need to urinate often and have sudden urges to urinate. Later, incontinence occurs. Incontinence is usually urinary, but people may also have problems with bowel movement (stool) incontinence.

How Is NPH Diagnosed?

The diagnosis may be hard to make, because many symptoms aren't specific and may be seen with other diseases (e.g., Parkinson's, Alzheimer's, and other types of dementia). Imaging studies, including computed tomography (CT) or magnetic resonance imaging (MRI), can help with diagnosis. CT uses special computer x-ray machines to develop pictures of the body. MRI uses radio waves and strong magnetic fields to develop pictures.

Sometimes, lumbar puncture is performed. The doctor puts a needle through the lower back into the space containing cerebrospinal fluid around the spinal cord, and the fluid is removed and sent for study.

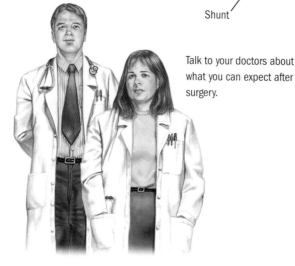

Treatment involves an operation, not medicines. A shunt is put into the brain to drain cerebrospinal fluid through the shunt. The fluid is drained into the abdomen, where it can be absorbed. This draining allows the brain ventricles to return to normal size.

Shunt

Talk to your doctors about what you can expect after surgery.

Call your doctor if you have urinary incontinence, trouble walking, or memory problems.

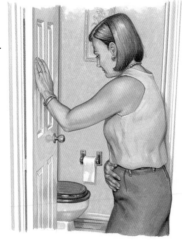

How Is NPH Treated?

No medicines are available for treatment. Treatment involves surgery. A shunt is put into the brain to drain excess cerebrospinal fluid through the shunt. The fluid drains into the abdomen, where it can be absorbed. This draining allows the brain ventricles to return to normal size.

DOs and DON'Ts in Managing NPH:

✔ **DO** realize that about 30% of people with idiopathic NPH have significant improvement after shunts are used. If a cause of NPH is known, 60% will have significant improvement after this operation.

✔ **DO** understand that people with a history of prior strokes have a poor prognosis after treatment compared with those without such a history.

✔ **DO** call your doctor if you have trouble walking.

✔ **DO** call your doctor if you or family members have problems with memory.

✔ **DO** call your doctor if you have urinary incontinence.

⊘ **DON'T** forget that NPH symptoms usually get worse over time if the condition isn't treated, even though some people may show temporary improvements. Some people recover almost completely after treatment and have a good quality of life. Early diagnosis and treatment improve the chance of good recovery.

FROM THE DESK OF

NOTES

FOR MORE INFORMATION

Contact the following sources:

• Hydrocephalus Foundation, Inc.
  Tel: (781) 942-1161
  Website: http://www.hydrocephalus.org/

• Hydrocephalus Association
  Tel: (888) 598-3789
  Website: http://hydroassoc.org/

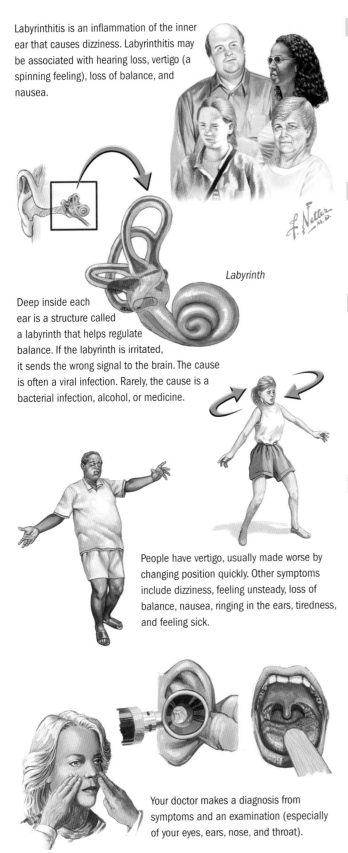

Labyrinthitis is an inflammation of the inner ear that causes dizziness. Labyrinthitis may be associated with hearing loss, vertigo (a spinning feeling), loss of balance, and nausea.

Labyrinth

Deep inside each ear is a structure called a labyrinth that helps regulate balance. If the labyrinth is irritated, it sends the wrong signal to the brain. The cause is often a viral infection. Rarely, the cause is a bacterial infection, alcohol, or medicine.

People have vertigo, usually made worse by changing position quickly. Other symptoms include dizziness, feeling unsteady, loss of balance, nausea, ringing in the ears, tiredness, and feeling sick.

Your doctor makes a diagnosis from symptoms and an examination (especially of your eyes, ears, nose, and throat).

What Is Labyrinthitis?

Labyrinthitis is an inflammation of the inner ear that causes dizziness. Deep inside each ear is a structure called a labyrinth that helps regulate balance. If the labyrinth is irritated, it sends the wrong signal to the brain. Labyrinthitis may be associated with hearing loss, vertigo (feeling of spinning), loss of balance, and nausea.

What Causes Labyrinthitis?

The cause is often a viral infection. Rarely, the cause is a bacterial infection, alcohol, or medicine. Many times the cause is unknown.

What Are the Symptoms of Labyrinthitis?

Symptoms may start suddenly, usually come and go, and last from less than a minute to several hours or days. People have vertigo, usually made worse by changing position quickly. Other symptoms include dizziness, feeling unsteady, loss of balance, nausea, ringing in the ears, tiredness, and feeling sick. Vomiting may occur. Hearing slowly returns to normal in most people, usually within 2 weeks.

How Is Labyrinthitis Diagnosed?

The doctor makes a diagnosis from symptoms and an examination (especially of the eyes, ears, nose, and throat). Mild redness of the nose or throat can occur with a viral infection. Sometimes, the doctor may do special tests for other symptoms such as hearing loss. The doctor may suggest seeing an ear, nose, and throat (ENT) specialist or neurologist (specialist in nervous system diseases). X-rays and laboratory tests are not usually needed.

Labyrinthitis usually goes away by itself, in several days to 2 weeks. For severe dizziness, the doctor may prescribe meclizine. Lying still with eyes closed in a dark room will help severe sickness or dizziness.

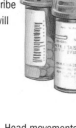

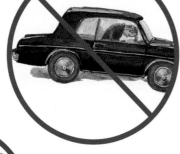

Head movements, called Epley maneuvers, may be prescribed to help relieve the dizziness.

Don't drive until you're symptom free without medicine. Don't use alcohol, tobacco, and caffeine. They may worsen symptoms.

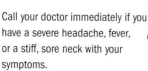

Don't stick anything in your ears, such as cotton swabs.

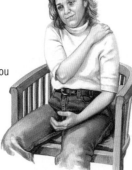

Call your doctor immediately if you have a severe headache, fever, or a stiff, sore neck with your symptoms.

How Is Labyrinthitis Treated?

Labyrinthitis usually goes away by itself, in several days to 1 week. For severe dizziness the doctor may prescribe meclizine. Lying still with eyes closed in a dark room will help severe sickness or dizziness. Change positions, such as getting up from lying down, slowly.

Head movements, called Epley maneuvers, may be prescribed to help relieve the dizziness. Drinking plenty of water or other fluids is important. Dehydration can make symptoms worse.

The doctor may prescribe an antibiotic for a bacterial infection.

DOs and DON'Ts in Managing Labyrinthitis:

✔ **DO** sit or lie down if you're dizzy.
✔ **DO** tell your doctor if your symptoms suddenly worsen.
✔ **DO** drink plenty of fluids.
✔ **DO** tell your doctor about your medical problems and your medicines (including over-the-counter and herbal products).
✔ **DO** call your doctor immediately if you have a severe headache, fever, or a stiff, sore neck with your symptoms.
✔ **DO** call your doctor if you have problems with your medicines.

⊘ **DON'T** stick anything in your ear.
⊘ **DON'T** stop taking your medicine or change your dosage because you feel better unless your doctor tells you to.
⊘ **DON'T** get up from a bed or chair too fast. This may make you more dizzy.
⊘ **DON'T** do activities that require good balance.
⊘ **DON'T** drive until you are symptom free without medicine.
⊘ **DON'T** use alcohol, tobacco, and caffeine. They may worsen symptoms.

FROM THE DESK OF

NOTES

FOR MORE INFORMATION

Contact the following source:

• Vestibular Disorders Association
  Tel: (503) 229-7705
  Website: http://www.vestibular.org

MANAGING YOUR
MÉNIÈRE'S DISEASE

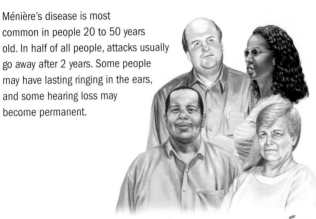

Ménière's disease is most common in people 20 to 50 years old. In half of all people, attacks usually go away after 2 years. Some people may have lasting ringing in the ears, and some hearing loss may become permanent.

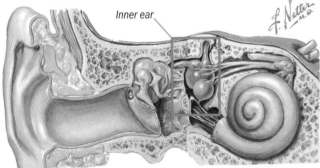

Inner ear

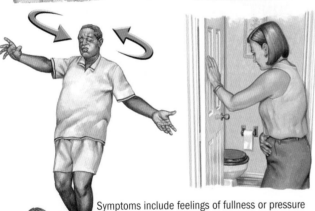

Symptoms include feelings of fullness or pressure in an ear, tinnitus (ringing, buzzing, roaring, or clicking in the ear), dizziness, vertigo, vomiting, sweating, jerky eye movements, loss of balance, and hearing loss.

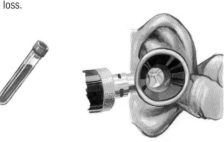

Your doctor will make a diagnosis from your medical history and physical examination. Blood tests, hearing and balance tests, and MRI may be done.

What Is Ménière's Disease?

Ménière's disease is a disorder affecting the inner ear. One in every 1000 people has this disease. It's most common in people 20 to 50 years old, women and men equally. Children rarely get it. In half of all people, attacks usually go away after 2 years. In up to three fourths, attacks go away after 8 years. Some people may have lasting ringing in the ears, and some hearing loss may become permanent.

What Causes Ménière's Disease?

The cause is unknown. Viral infections and autoimmune causes have been suggested.

What Are the Symptoms of Ménière's Disease?

Symptoms include feelings of fullness or pressure in one ear, tinnitus (ringing, buzzing, roaring, or clicking in the ear), dizziness, vertigo (feeling of everything spinning), vomiting, sweating, jerky eye movements, loss of balance, and hearing loss. Some people have all these symptoms, but others have only some. Length and frequency of attacks vary among people. Vertigo is the worst symptom. Vertigo attacks start suddenly, last from a few hours to 24 hours, and go away slowly, leaving a dizzy or unsteady feeling for a few days. Dizziness may occur often and can be severe.

How Is Ménière's Disease Diagnosed?

The doctor will make a diagnosis from the medical history and physical examination. Blood tests, hearing and balance tests, and magnetic resonance imaging (MRI) may be done.

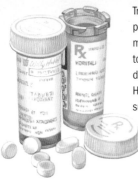

Treatment goals are to reduce symptoms and prevent attacks with medicines. Your doctor may need to prescribe more than one drug to find the best one for you. For frequent and disabling attacks, surgery may be an option. However, most people recover without surgery in a few years.

Don't smoke. Smoking can reduce blood flow to the inner ear. Cut down on caffeine, salt, and alcohol in your diet.

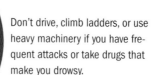

Don't drive, climb ladders, or use heavy machinery if you have frequent attacks or take drugs that make you drowsy.

Don't make sudden changes in position.

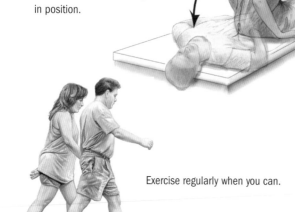

Exercise regularly when you can.

How Is Ménière's Disease Treated?

Treatment goals are to reduce symptoms during an attack and prevent attacks with medications.

For many years, a low-salt diet and diuretics (water pills) have been used for treatment, but their value is unclear.

For frequent and disabling attacks, surgery involving the inner ear may bring permanent relief. However, most people recover without surgery in a few years.

DOs and DON'Ts in Managing Ménière's Disease:

✔ **DO** rest quietly in bed until dizziness and nausea go away.

✔ **DO** exercise regularly when you can.

✔ **DO** ask your doctor about surgery as a treatment option if you have persistent disabling symptoms.

✔ **DO** call your doctor if your attacks become more frequent or last longer than usual.

✔ **DO** call your doctor if you have symptoms that are unlike your usual attack (such as fever or headache).

✔ **DO** call your doctor if your medicine doesn't work or causes other problems.

✔ **DO** cut down on caffeine, salt, and alcohol.

⊘ **DON'T** walk without help if you are dizzy.

⊘ **DON'T** smoke. Smoking can reduce blood flow to the inner ear.

⊘ **DON'T** make sudden changes in position.

⊘ **DON'T** drive, climb ladders, or use heavy machinery if you have frequent attacks or take drugs that make you drowsy.

FROM THE DESK OF

NOTES

FOR MORE INFORMATION

Contact the following sources:

• Deafness Research Foundation
Tel: (866) 454-3924
Website: http://www.drf.org

• Vestibular Disorders Association
Tel: (800) 837-8428
Website: http://www.vestibular.org

MANAGING YOUR MIGRAINE HEADACHE

Migraine headaches are intense headaches affecting one side of the head and are often preceeded by other symptoms. The exact mechanism is unknown, but it is believed that blood vessels in the scalp and brain narrow and then widen. A migraine can last from 2 hours to 3 days.

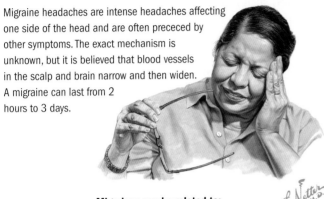

Migraines can be related to:

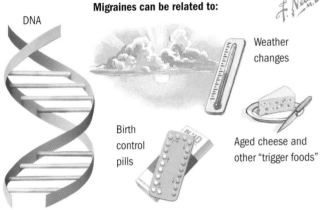

DNA

Weather changes

Birth control pills

Aged cheese and other "trigger foods"

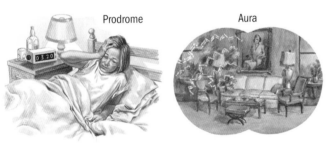

Prodrome

Aura

People with classic migraine often have a prodrome that tells them a headache is starting. Mood changes, hyperactivity, feeling sluggish, fatigue, appetite changes, and nausea do this. Auras (flashes of light, flickering lights, blind spots) come right before a headache.

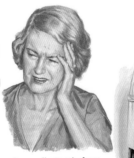

Then, pain becomes intense and throbbing. Nausea and vomiting may occur.

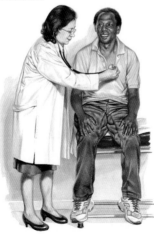

Your doctor makes a diagnosis from your medical history and physical examination. CT or MRI may be done to check for other disorders.

What Are Migraine Headaches?

Migraine headaches are intense headaches that usually affect one side of the head and are often preceded by other symptoms. A migraine can last from 2 hours to 3 days.

What Causes Migraine Headaches?

The cause is unknown, but 60% to 80% of people inherit the tendency to have migraines. Migraines may be associated with alcohol (red wine), foods, fatigue, and weather changes. Other triggers are stress, too little or too much sleep, medicines, menstrual periods, pregnancy, and birth control pills.

What Are the Symptoms of Migraine Headaches?

In classic migraine, hours to days before a headache, people have a symptom (prodrome) that tells them that a headache is starting. These include mood changes, hyperactivity, feeling sluggish, fatigue, appetite changes, and nausea. Auras then come before the headache. They usually last 10 to 30 minutes, then the headache starts and aura symptoms go away. Aura symptoms include hearing and vision problems (flashes of light, flickering lights, blind spots). Dull pain on one side of the head may become intense and throbbing. Nausea and vomiting may occur.

With a common migraine, people don't have an aura, and pain usually occurs on both sides of the head. People have nausea and sometimes numbness or weakness. Some people have vision or stomach problems without the headache.

How Are Migraine Headaches Diagnosed?

The doctor makes a diagnosis from the medical history and physical examination. Computed tomography (CT) or magnetic resonance imaging (MRI) may be done.

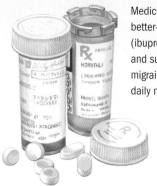

Medicines can be used early—the earlier the better—to reduce or stop symptoms. NSAIDs (ibuprofen, naproxen), as well as ergotamine and sumatriptan, may be prescribed to stop migraines. To prevent frequent migraines, daily medicines may be prescribed.

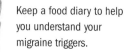

Avoid migraine triggers: chocolate, red wine, cheese, onions, fatty foods, acidic foods (e.g., oranges, tomatoes), stress, and not sleeping.

Keep a food diary to help you understand your migraine triggers.

Lie down in a quiet, dark room, with pillows under your head. Relax and sleep. Minimize noise, light, and odors (especially cooking odors and tobacco smoke).

How Are Migraine Headaches Treated?

Many medicines are prescribed for migraine. Early treatment is best for faster relief. Nonsteroidal antiinflammatory drugs (NSAIDs) such as ibuprofen and naproxen, as well as ergotamine and sumatriptan, may be given to stop migraines.

To prevent frequent migraines, people may use medicine daily. These drugs include beta-blockers, calcium channel blockers, antidepressants, anticonvulsants, NSAIDs, and hormones. Other medicine may be given for long and severe headaches.

Migraine triggers include chocolate, red wine, port wine, cheese, onions, fatty foods, and acidic foods (e.g., oranges and tomatoes) and should be avoided.

DOs and DON'Ts in Managing Migraine Headaches:

✔ **DO** apply a cold cloth or ice pack to your head or splash your face with cold water when you feel a migraine starting.

✔ **DO** lie down in a quiet, dark room, with pillows under your head. Relax and sleep.

✔ **DO** minimize noise, light, and odors (especially cooking odors and tobacco smoke).

✔ **DO** avoid migraine triggers, such as foods, stress, not sleeping, and medicines. Keep a food diary.

✔ **DO** call your doctor if your headache is worse than usual, your usual medicine doesn't work, you have a fever and headache, or you have severe vomiting.

✔ **DO** exercise as much as possible, to be healthy.

⊘ **DON'T** drive or use heavy machinery during an attack.

FOR MORE INFORMATION

Contact the following sources:

• National Headache Foundation
Tel: (888) 643-5552
Website: http://www.headaches.org

• American Headache Society Committee for Headache Education
Tel: (800) 255-2243
Website: http://www.achenet.org

• MAGNUM: Migraine Awareness Group: A National Understanding for Migraine
Tel: (703) 349-1929
Website: http://www.migraines.org

FROM THE DESK OF

NOTES

MANAGING YOUR
MOTION SICKNESS

Motion sickness is a condition in which people become dizzy and feel sick when in a moving vehicle such as a car. It's most common in children 2 to 12 years old, but anyone can have it. Pregnant women are also more likely to have motion sickness.

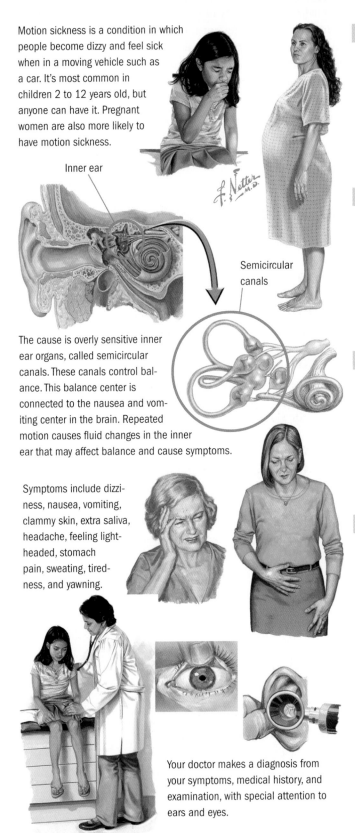

Inner ear

Semicircular canals

The cause is overly sensitive inner ear organs, called semicircular canals. These canals control balance. This balance center is connected to the nausea and vomiting center in the brain. Repeated motion causes fluid changes in the inner ear that may affect balance and cause symptoms.

Symptoms include dizziness, nausea, vomiting, clammy skin, extra saliva, headache, feeling lightheaded, stomach pain, sweating, tiredness, and yawning.

Your doctor makes a diagnosis from your symptoms, medical history, and examination, with special attention to ears and eyes.

What Is Motion Sickness?

Motion sickness is a condition in which people become dizzy and feel sick when in a moving vehicle such as a car. This feeling usually goes away with or without treatment in a few hours.

Motion sickness is most common in children 2 to 12 years old, but anyone can have this problem. Pregnant women are also more likely to have motion sickness.

What Causes Motion Sickness?

The cause is inner ear organs, called semicircular canals, that are too sensitive. These canals deep in the ear control balance. This balance center is connected to the nausea and vomiting center in the brain. Repeated motion causes fluid changes in the inner ear that may affect balance and causing feelings of motion and nausea. Motion sickness isn't contagious.

What Are the Symptoms of Motion Sickness?

Symptoms include dizziness, nausea, vomiting, clammy skin, extra saliva, headache, feeling lightheaded, stomach pain, sweating, tiredness, and yawning. These symptoms usually get worse with longer trips. Motion sickness normally goes away after leaving the moving vehicle (car, plane, or boat). Sometimes, people feel better after throwing up.

How Is Motion Sickness Diagnosed?

The doctor makes a diagnosis from symptoms, a medical history, and examination, with special attention to ears and eyes. Other tests such as computed tomography (CT) and magnetic resonance imaging (MRI) of the brain may be needed.

Prevention is easier than treatment. Some over-the-counter and prescription medicines can prevent motion sickness or help symptoms.

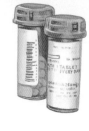

Other things can help:

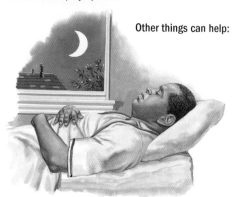

Get plenty of rest before a trip.

Sit in the car's front seat and look out the front window. Sit back and move as little as possible. Get fresh air from an open window.

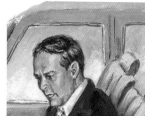

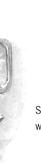

Sit in the middle of a boat or plane where there's less movement.

Don't eat a big high-fat meal, smoke, drink alcohol, write or play games during a trip.

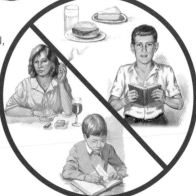

How Is Motion Sickness Treated?

Medicine helps prevent motion sickness. A medicine patch (scopolamine patch) may be put behind the ear. Other things can help: getting plenty of rest before a trip, sitting in the car's front seat and looking out the front window, sitting back and moving as little as possible, sitting in the middle of a boat or plane where there's less movement, getting fresh air from an open window, trying to relax, avoiding reading books or magazines in a moving vehicle, and avoiding spinning amusement park rides.

Prevention is easier than treatment. Some over-the-counter and prescription medicines can prevent motion sickness or help symptoms.

DOs and DON'Ts in Managing Motion Sickness:

✔ **DO** tell your doctor about your medical problems, such as eye, prostate, or breathing problems.

✔ **DO** tell your doctor about your medicines, both prescription and over-the-counter.

✔ **DO** tell your doctor if you're pregnant.

✔ **DO** call your doctor if symptoms persist longer than 24 hours.

✔ **DO** call your doctor if you continue to throw up and become faint or dizzy when you change positions suddenly.

✔ **DO** take medicines prescribed to you by your doctor. Avoid rides that you know will make you sick.

⊘ **DON'T** sit in the back of a car or in a cramped area.

⊘ **DON'T** eat a big, high-fat meal before a trip.

⊘ **DON'T** smoke or drink alcohol before or during a trip.

⊘ **DON'T** read or write during a trip.

⊘ **DON'T** drive if you take medicine for motion sickness, since these medicines can make you very drowsy.

⊘ **DON'T** sit in an area with odors of food or fuel.

FROM THE DESK OF

NOTES

FOR MORE INFORMATION

Contact the following sources:

• MedlinePlus
  Website: http://www.nlm.nih.gov/medlineplus/ motionsickness.html

• Vestibular Disorders Association
  Tel: (800) 837-8428
  Website: http://www.vestibular.org

MANAGING YOUR
MULTIPLE SCLEROSIS

MS is a progressive, lifelong illness that affects nerve cells in the brain and spinal cord. People usually go to the doctor when they are 20 to 40 years old. More women than men have it.

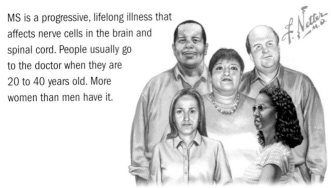

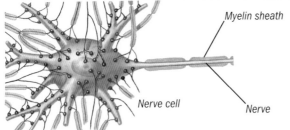

Myelin sheath

Nerve cell

Nerve

Normally, myelin protects nerve cells. It's a fatty substance that acts like electrical wire insulation. Myelin helps signals move along nerves. In MS, myelin becomes damaged or inflamed, interrupts nerve signals, and causes symptoms.

Common symptoms include:

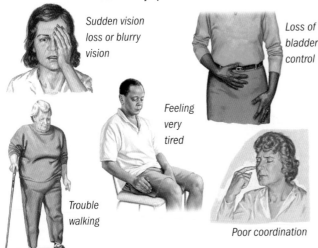

Sudden vision loss or blurry vision

Loss of bladder control

Feeling very tired

Trouble walking

Poor coordination

Your doctor may think of MS because of your age, symptoms, and physical and neurological examinations. Your doctor may order MRI, spinal tap, and visual-evoked response test. You may also see a neurologist.

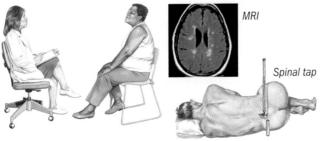

MRI

Spinal tap

What Is Multiple Sclerosis?

Multiple sclerosis (MS) is a progressive, lifelong illness that affects nerve cells in the brain and spinal cord. Normally, myelin protects nerve cells. Myelin is a fatty substance that acts like electrical wire insulation. Myelin helps signals move along nerves. In MS, myelin becomes damaged or inflamed, interrupts nerve signals, and causes symptoms. People can have no symptoms, only one mild symptom, very few symptoms, or many symptoms with severe disability.

MS is more common in women than men and in temperate climates more than the tropics.

What Causes MS?

The cause is unknown, but MS is thought to be an autoimmune illness. That is, the body's own immune system attacks itself. In MS, it attacks the myelin covering.

What Are the Symptoms of MS?

Symptoms improve (during remissions) and then worsen. Symptoms depend on whether the brain or spinal cord is affected. Symptoms of brain involvement include sudden vision loss or blurry vision, clumsiness, slurred speech, tiredness, muscle weakness, and trouble walking. Loss of bladder control and numbness, tingling, weakness, or heavy feelings in arms or legs mean spinal cord involvement.

How Is MS Diagnosed?

The doctor may think of MS because of age, symptoms, and physical and neurological examinations. No one test proves the diagnosis. The doctor will suggest seeing a neurologist (specialist in nervous system diseases). Magnetic resonance imaging (MRI), spinal tap, and visual-evoked response may be done. MRI shows where myelin is inflamed or destroyed. In a spinal tap, the doctor takes a sample of fluid from the spinal cord for study.

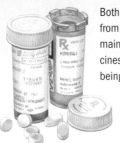

Both the disease process and complications from MS are treated. Corticosteroids are the main treatment for symptoms. Other medicines used depend on the complication being treated.

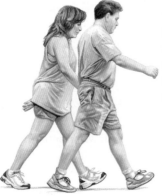

Start physical therapy. It may improve or help maintain your mobility.

Exercises can give you more energy and keep your body fit. You can exercise even if you use a wheelchair. Do regular exercises approved by your doctor or therapist.

Counseling may help you and your family adjust to MS. Contact support groups. You can even find online support groups if you feel more comfortable with that setting. Know that you are not alone and that others can relate to what you're going through.

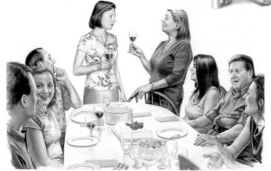

Living with MS can be a challenge because symptoms are unpredictable and variable. Practice a healthy lifestyle and make the most of times of remission.

How Is MS Treated?

MS cannot be cured, but many treatments are available to control the symptoms and slow the progression of the disease. Both the disease and complications (e.g., spastic movements, fatigue, pain, thinking problems, and bladder and bowel problems) are treated.

Corticosteroid drugs are the main treatment to control symptoms. Medicines such as interferon beta-1a and -1b and glatiramer slow MS progress and reduce the number of relapses.

Medicines used for complications include amantadine, baclofen, gabapentin, oxybutynin, propantheline, stool softeners, psyllium, fiber, nonsteroidal antiinflammatory drugs (NSAIDs), and acetaminophen.

Maintaining a healthy lifestyle, getting enough rest and exercise, and keeping to a normal weight are important.

DOs and DON'Ts in Managing MS:

✔ **DO** start physical therapy. It may improve or maintain mobility. Exercises can give you more energy and keep your body fit. Do regular exercises approved by your doctor.

✔ **DO** get counseling. It may help you and your family adjust to MS. Contact support groups.

✔ **DO** call your doctor if you have facial weakness, weakness of a limb, partial blindness, or eye pain.

✔ **DO** use medicines to help prevent or reduce the number of relapses.

✔ **DO** get enough rest and eat a healthy diet for better overall health.

⊘ **DON'T** ignore worsening symptoms, especially visual changes. These can sometimes be stopped if medicine is started promptly.

FROM THE DESK OF

NOTES

FOR MORE INFORMATION

Contact the following sources:

• National Multiple Sclerosis Society
  Tel: (800) 344-4867
  Website: http://www.nationalmssociety.org

• Multiple Sclerosis Association of America
  Tel: (800) 833-4672
  Website: http://www.msassociation.org

MANAGING YOUR
MYASTHENIA GRAVIS

Myasthenia gravis (MG), an autoimmune disease, causes muscles in the eyes, face, throat, arms, and legs to get weak. Muscles that control breathing may also be affected. MG affects both sexes and people of all ages and ethnic groups. Women usually get MG in the late teens and 20s, and men usually get it after age 60.

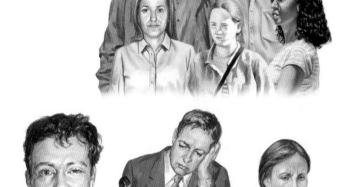

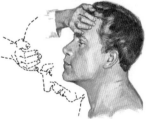

The major symptom is muscle weakness that gets worse with more activity. Temperature, menstrual periods, illness, and stress can affect the weakness. Other symptoms are eye problems (double vision, droopy eyelids); trouble chewing, speaking, or swallowing; drooling; and shortness of breath.

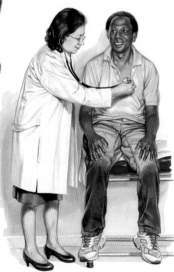

Your doctor will make a diagnosis from a complete physical examination, with tests of lungs, reflexes, and muscle weakness. A specialist may do more tests, including electromyography, Tensilon® test, blood test, and CT.

What Is Myasthenia Gravis (MG)?

Myasthenia gravis (MG) is an illness that causes muscles in the eyes, face, throat, arms, and legs to get weak and tired. Muscles that control breathing may also be affected. The worst weakness usually occurs during the first 3 years.

MG affects people of both sexes, all ages, and all ethnic group. Women usually get MG in the late teens and 20s, and men usually get it after age 60. Progression of MG is extremely slow and most people lead full lives.

What Causes MG?

MG is an autoimmune disease. This means that the body's immune system attacks itself. MG isn't contagious or passed from parents to children.

What Are the Symptoms of MG?

Symptoms may get better (remission) and then worsen (exacerbation). The time between remission and exacerbation varies. The major symptom is muscle weakness that gets worse when people are more active. Temperature, menstrual periods, illness, and stress can affect the weakness. Other symptoms are eye problems (double vision, droopy eyelids); problems chewing, speaking, or swallowing; drooling; and arm and leg weakness. One symptom, shortness of breath, can be very frightening.

How Is MG Diagnosed?

The doctor will make a diagnosis from a complete physical examination, with tests of lungs, reflexes, and muscle weakness. A specialist may do more tests, including electromyography, Tensilon® test, blood test, and computed tomography (CT). Electromyography measures muscle electrical activity as they contract after nerve stimulation. In the Tensilon® test, medicine temporarily improves muscle strength in people with MG. CT will check for a tumor or enlargement of the thymus gland.

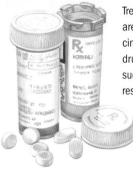

Treatment depends on how severe symptoms are, age, sex, and physical activity level. Medicines such as steroids and anticholinesterase drugs can help symptoms. Lifestyle changes such as eating a good diet and getting enough rest can help.

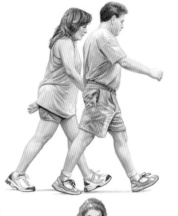

Find a balance between rest and physical activity to prevent muscle weakness. Get physical therapy to keep muscles strong. Try to exercise daily.

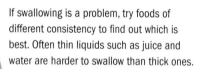

If swallowing is a problem, try foods of different consistency to find out which is best. Often thin liquids such as juice and water are harder to swallow than thick ones.

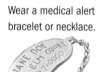

Wear a medical alert bracelet or necklace.

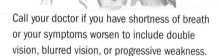

Call your doctor if you have shortness of breath or your symptoms worsen to include double vision, blurred vision, or progressive weakness.

How Is MG Treated?

The treatment depends on how severe symptoms are, age, sex, and physical activity level. Medicines such as steroids and anticholinesterase drugs can help symptoms. Lifestyle changes such as eating a good diet and getting enough rest can also help. Rest briefly during the day (about 10 to 15 minutes), and avoid strenuous work that may make fatigue worse. Try to exercise daily, as advised by the doctor and physical therapist. For double or blurred vision, see an eye doctor, and don't drive or use heavy equipment. If swallowing is a problem, try foods of different consistency to find out which is best. Often thin liquids such as juice and water are harder to swallow than thick ones. Manage stress better. Regular exercise may help with stress management. Avoid smoke and dust.

DOs and DON'Ts in Managing MG:

✔ **DO** try to find a balance between rest and physical activity to prevent muscle weakness.

✔ **DO** get physical therapy to keep muscles strong.

✔ **DO** wear a medical alert bracelet or necklace that says you have myasthenia gravis.

✔ **DO** take medicines as prescribed. Call your doctor if you have problems with your medicines.

✔ **DO** call your doctor if you have shortness of breath or your symptoms worsen to include double vision, blurred vision, or weakness.

⊘ **DON'T** gain weight and become inactive.

⊘ **DON'T** use tobacco. It may worsen shortness of breath.

FROM THE DESK OF

NOTES

FOR MORE INFORMATION

Contact the following source:

• Myasthenia Gravis Foundation of America
Tel: (651)917-6256, (800)541-5454
Website: http://www.myasthenia.org

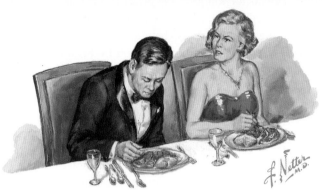

Narcolepsy is a rare condition in which people fall asleep anytime or anywhere without control, regardless of the amount of sleep that they had. The cause is unknown.

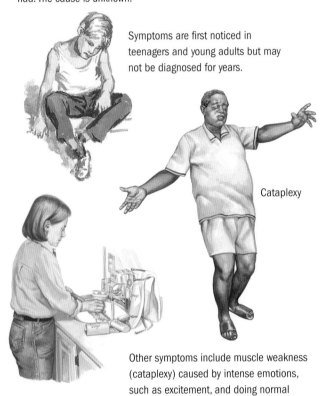

Symptoms are first noticed in teenagers and young adults but may not be diagnosed for years.

Cataplexy

Other symptoms include muscle weakness (cataplexy) caused by intense emotions, such as excitement, and doing normal activities without being aware of it.

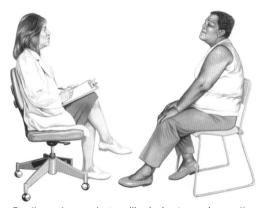

For diagnosis, your doctor will ask about your sleep patterns.

What Is Narcolepsy?

Narcolepsy is a rare condition in which people fall asleep anytime or anywhere without control, regardless of the amount of sleep that they had. People may feel rested after sleeping for 10 or 15 minutes during an attack, but then this rested feeling goes away, and they get sleepy again. These attacks can occur, in men and women equally, when driving, working, or talking. Symptoms are first noticed in teenagers and young adults but may be undiagnosed for years. Narcolepsy is a lifelong condition.

What Causes Narcolepsy?

The cause is unknown. Narcolepsy rarely follows brain trauma but it may occur with nervous system diseases. It tends to run in families.

What Are the Symptoms of Narcolepsy?

Symptoms include daytime sleep attacks lasting from a few seconds to 30 minutes and occurring up to 10 times daily, vivid dreams during attacks, and temporary inability to move before or after the attack.

A common symptom of narcolepsy is partial or complete weakness of muscles (cataplexy) that is caused by intense emotions such as excitement or anger. Other symptoms include doing normal activities without being aware of it and waking often or tossing and turning at night.

Poor nighttime sleeping can lead to tiredness during the day, depression, trouble concentrating or memorizing, vision problems, eating binges, and trouble handling alcohol.

How Is Narcolepsy Diagnosed?

The doctor will do an examination and ask about sleep patterns. The doctor may suggest seeing a doctor who specializes in sleep disorders. Diagnosis may involve spending a night in a sleep laboratory so equipment can be used to find out about sleep patterns.

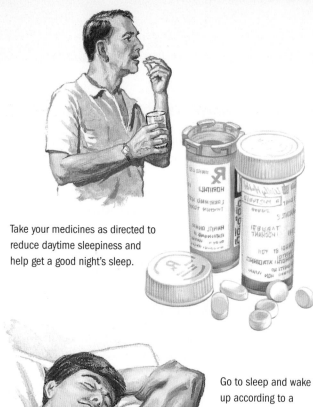

Take your medicines as directed to reduce daytime sleepiness and help get a good night's sleep.

Go to sleep and wake up according to a regular routine.

Wear a medical alert bracelet that notes your condition.

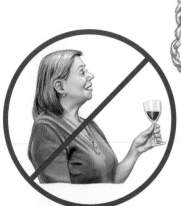

Don't smoke or drink beverages with caffeine or alcohol in the late afternoon or evening.

FROM THE DESK OF

NOTES

How Is Narcolepsy Treated?

No cure is known, and no one therapy will control all symptoms. The doctor will probably prescribe medicines to reduce daytime sleepiness and help get a good night's sleep. Regular naps during the day may also help.

Stimulant medicines combined with 15- to 20-minute naps may improve disabling effects of narcolepsy.

DOs and DON'Ts in Managing Narcolepsy:

✔ **DO** take your medicines as directed.

✔ **DO** take regular naps during the day, if you can.

✔ **DO** go to sleep and wake up according to a regular routine. Try to sleep at least 8 hours a night.

✔ **DO** find a safe, well-lit place to stop and nap if you get sleepy while driving.

✔ **DO** wear a medical alert bracelet that notes your condition.

✔ **DO** educate your friends and family about your disorder.

✔ **DO** call your doctor if you have problems with your medicines or if the number of attacks or their severity increases.

⊘ **DON'T** drive until you control your narcolepsy.

⊘ **DON'T** drive or commute long distances.

⊘ **DON'T** smoke or drink beverages with caffeine or alcohol in the late afternoon or evening.

⊘ **DON'T** use the bed for nonrelaxing activities.

⊘ **DON'T** climb ladders. Don't do things that may be dangerous should you fall asleep or lose muscle control.

⊘ **DON'T** work around dangerous machinery.

FOR MORE INFORMATION

Contact the following sources:

• American Narcolepsy Foundation
Tel: (831) 646-2055
Website: http://www.narcolepsy.com

• Narcolepsy Network, Inc.
Tel: (888) 292-6522, (401) 667-2523
Website: http://www.narcolepsynetwork.org

• National Sleep Foundation
Tel: (202) 347-3471
Website: http://www.sleepfoundation.org

MANAGING YOUR
PARKINSON'S DISEASE

Parkinson's disease is a chronic neurological disorder. It progresses slowly, usually over several years. People gradually lose control of muscle movements. Older people usually get the disease, but people younger than 40 can have early-onset disease.

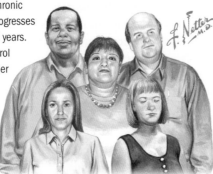

Dopamine area of brain

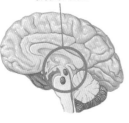

Brain cells that make dopamine start to die, which causes symptoms. It's unclear why this happens, but risk factors include blood vessel problems, infection, toxins (pesticides, carbon monoxide), medicines, head injury or repeated trauma (from sports such as boxing), and tumors. It can run in families.

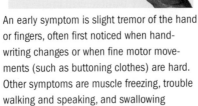

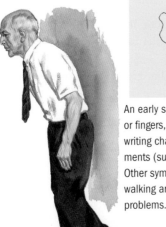

An early symptom is slight tremor of the hand or fingers, often first noticed when handwriting changes or when fine motor movements (such as buttoning clothes) are hard. Other symptoms are muscle freezing, trouble walking and speaking, and swallowing problems.

Your doctor makes a diagnosis from your medical history and physical examination. Laboratory tests, MRI, and CT may be done to rule out other disorders. The doctor may suggest seeing a neurologist.

What Is Parkinson's Disease?

Parkinson's disease is a progressive neurological disorder. It gradually worsens over a period of years with loss of control of muscle movements.

Older people usually get Parkinson's disease, but people younger than 40 can have early-onset disease. Both the actor Michael J. Fox and the boxer Mohammed Ali have Parkinson's.

What Causes Parkinson's Disease?

Brain cells that make the chemical dopamine start to die, which causes symptoms. It's unclear why this happens, but risk factors include blood vessel problems, infection, toxins such as pesticides and carbon monoxide, medicines, head injury or repeated trauma (from sports such as boxing), tumors, water on the brain (hydrocephalus), and thyroid and parathyroid gland problems. Parkinson's disease seems to run in families.

What Are the Symptoms of Parkinson's Disease?

An early symptom is a slight tremor of the hand or fingers. It's often first noticed when handwriting changes or when people have trouble with fine motor movements (such as buttoning clothes). Tremor (called pill rolling) or shaking occurs in one or both hands, especially at rest. Other symptoms are muscle stiffness and freezing, gradual slowing and loss of movement, trouble with walking (especially starting up), swallowing problems, drooling, loss of facial expression, and trouble speaking.

How Is Parkinson's Disease Diagnosed?

The doctor makes a diagnosis from a medical history and physical examination. Laboratory tests, magnetic resonance imaging (MRI), and computed tomography (CT) may be done to rule out other disorders. The doctor may suggest seeing a neurologist (specialist in nervous system diseases).

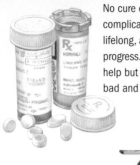

No cure exists, but symptoms can be treated and complications can be prevented. Medicines, taken lifelong, are used to treat symptoms or slow disease progress. Surgery is rarely done and doesn't always help but may be suggested when symptoms get very bad and medicines don't work.

Stereotaxic surgery

Find a support group. These groups can help your sense of well-being and help reduce stress. Get legal, financial, and occupational counseling, especially when you need help with activities of daily living. Support groups are online too.

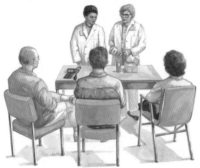

Keep up your exercise program. Daily exercise, such as walking, helps keep muscles limber and strong.

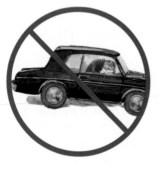

Don't walk on unfamiliar ground without assistance if you have trouble walking. Don't drive or operate dangerous equipment unless your doctor says that you can.

How Is Parkinson's Disease Treated?

No cure exists, but symptoms can be treated and complications can be prevented. Medicines, taken lifelong, are used to treat symptoms or slow disease progress. Surgery is rarely done and doesn't always help, but may be suggested when symptoms get very bad and medicines don't work. Stereotaxic surgery can carefully destroy brain cells causing movement problems. This stops or reduces tremors. Another operation involves transplanting cells from an embryo into the brain. The cells take over the work of the diseased cells. The third operation involves putting small electrodes in the brain to stimulate diseased parts.

People later need help with activities of daily living. An occupational therapist can assist with these.

DOs and DON'Ts in Managing Parkinson's Disease:

✔ **DO** take medicines as your doctor prescribes.

✔ **DO** join a support group. These groups can help your sense of well-being and help reduce stress.

✔ **DO** get legal and financial counseling.

✔ **DO** get occupational therapy and counseling.

✔ **DO** exercise. Daily exercise, such as walking, helps keep muscles limber and strong.

✔ **DO** try to drink thick liquids (nectars, milk shakes) instead of thin ones (apple juice, tea) if swallowing becomes hard.

✔ **DO** call your doctor if you see a change in the severity of your symptoms.

✔ **DO** call your doctor if you fall or become injured.

⊘ **DON'T** forget to take your medicines or change your dosage because you feel better unless your doctor tells you to.

⊘ **DON'T** walk on unfamiliar ground without assistance if you have trouble walking.

⊘ **DON'T** drive or operate dangerous equipment unless your doctor says that you can.

FROM THE DESK OF

NOTES

FOR MORE INFORMATION

Contact the following sources:

• American Parkinson Disease Association
 Tel: (800) 223-2732
 Website: http://www.apdaparkinson.org

• Parkinson's Disease Foundation (PDF)
 Tel: (800) 457-6676
 Website: http://www.pdf.org

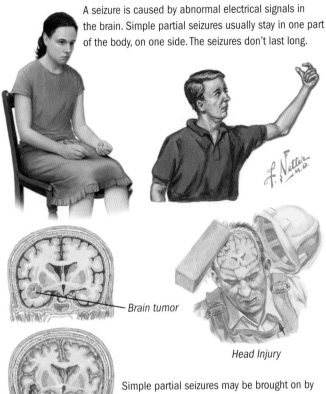

A seizure is caused by abnormal electrical signals in the brain. Simple partial seizures usually stay in one part of the body, on one side. The seizures don't last long.

— Brain tumor

Head Injury

Brain infection

Simple partial seizures may be brought on by a head injury, stroke, brain infection, or tumor, but more than half the time the cause is unknown.

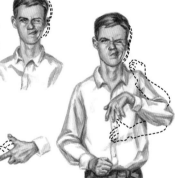

Abnormal movements start in one part of the body, such as a hand or foot, and spread up the limb. These seizures may involve movements such as turning the head, mouth and eye movements, lip smacking, and drooling.

EEG

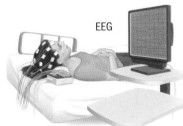

CT

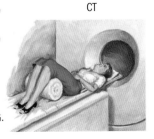

Your doctor will make a diagnosis on the basis of your medical history. Your doctor may also want to order CT or MRI and EEG.

What Are Partial Motor Seizures?

A seizure is caused by abnormal electrical signals in the brain. Simple partial seizures usually stay in one part of the body. This kind of seizure often starts in the arm or leg and then moves upward to other areas on that side of the body. These seizures don't last long.

What Causes Partial Motor Seizures?

Simple partial seizures may be brought on by a head injury, stroke, brain infection, or tumor, but more than half the time the cause is unknown.

What Are the Symptoms of Partial Motor Seizures?

Simple partial seizures usually don't make people unconscious or unaware of what's going on around them. They will be aware of the seizure as it occurs. Abnormal movements start in one part of the body and then spread to another. A hand or foot may be affected first and then spread up the limb. These seizures may involve movements that seem to have a purpose. The movements might be turning the head, mouth and eye movements, lip smacking, drooling, and rhythmic muscle contractions in a part of the body. Abnormal numbness, tingling, and a crawling feeling on the skin may occur.

How Are Partial Motor Seizures Diagnosed?

The doctor will make a diagnosis on the basis of the medical history. The doctor may also want to order computed tomography (CT) of the brain or MRI, and a brain wave study called electroencephalography, or EEG. These tests may tell the doctor whether the seizures have a known cause.

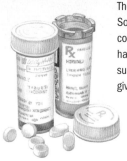

The main treatment for seizures is medicine. Sometimes more than one antiseizure or anticonvulsant drug may be used. The doctor may have to get regular blood samples to make sure that the correct dose of medicine is given.

Wear an ID bracelet saying that you have a seizure disorder and listing the drugs that you take.

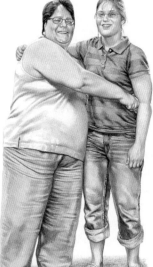

Teach your family and friends about your disorder so they can assist you if needed.

Don't operate complicated machinery or drive unless your doctor has approved. Don't swim alone or climb on ladders or roofs.

How Are Partial Motor Seizures Treated?

The main treatment for seizures is medicine. Sometimes more than one antiseizure or anticonvulsant drug may be used. The doctor may have to get regular blood samples to make sure that the correct dose of medicine is given. The dose schedule may be adjusted to achieve the blood level of medicine that protects against more seizures. Several different medicines may be used, and the doctor will describe the side effects related to each one prescribed. Often, the medicine will reduce the frequency and severity of the seizure. Some people, even though they're taking drugs, continue to have seizures.

People newly diagnosed with epilepsy should take precautions until they are sure that the disorder is controlled. When living alone, they should arrange for someone to stay with them until the doctor believes that it's safe to live alone again.

DOs and DON'Ts in Managing Partial Motor Seizures:

✔ **DO** take your medicine as your doctor prescribed to prevent seizures.

✔ **DO** wear an ID bracelet saying that you have a seizure disorder and listing the drugs that you take.

✔ **DO** teach your family and friends about your disorder and what to do if you have a seizure.

✔ **DO** call your doctor if you have problems with your medicines.

✔ **DO** call your doctor if your seizures become more frequent or severe.

⊘ **DON'T** operate dangerous machinery or drive unless your doctor has approved.

⊘ **DON'T** swim alone.

⊘ **DON'T** climb on ladders or roofs or anything that may be dangerous if you have a seizure.

FROM THE DESK OF

NOTES

FOR MORE INFORMATION

Contact the following source:

• Epilepsy Foundation of America
  Tel: (800) EFA-1000 (332-1000)
  Website: http://www.epilepsyfoundation.org

MANAGING YOUR
POST-CONCUSSION SYNDROME

A concussion results from a head injury. Post-concussion syndrome is a complicated disorder that may follow a concussion. Up to 80% of people who have a concussion will have post-concussion syndrome, usually more women than men.

Symptoms include:

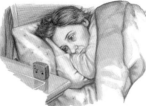

Trouble sleeping, bad dreams

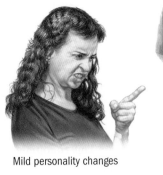

Mild personality changes

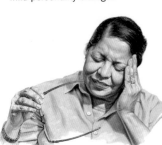

Headache

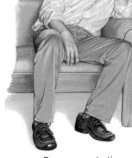

Poor concentration, tiredness

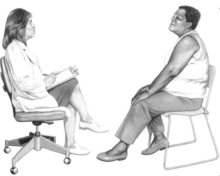

Treatment consists of watchful waiting until symptoms go away. No medicines can shorten recovery time. Most people recover completely. Analgesics such as acetaminophen, aspirin, and ibuprofen usually help the headache.

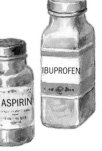

ASPIRIN

IBUPROFEN

What Is Post-Concussion Syndrome?

A concussion is a very brief and temporary loss of consciousness after a head injury. It usually doesn't cause any problems that might be found during a physical examination or tests such as computed tomography (CT) or magnetic resonance imaging (MRI).

Post-concussion syndrome is a complicated disorder that may follow a concussion. It's a collection of different specific symptoms. Up to 80% of people who have a concussion will have post-concussion syndrome, usually more women than men.

What Causes Post-Concussion Syndrome?

The cause is a jarring injury to the brain. The syndrome may also be related to psychological factors.

What Are the Symptoms of Post-Concussion Syndrome?

Symptoms include a headache, poor concentration, mild memory loss, irritability, trouble sleeping, bad dreams, dizziness, tiredness, and sensitivity to noise and light. Sometimes mild personality changes occur. These symptoms go away during weeks to months, but they may last for a year or more. People usually improve slowly during this period.

How Is Post-Concussion Syndrome Diagnosed?

The doctor makes a diagnosis by noting the presence of symptoms in someone who has had a concussion.

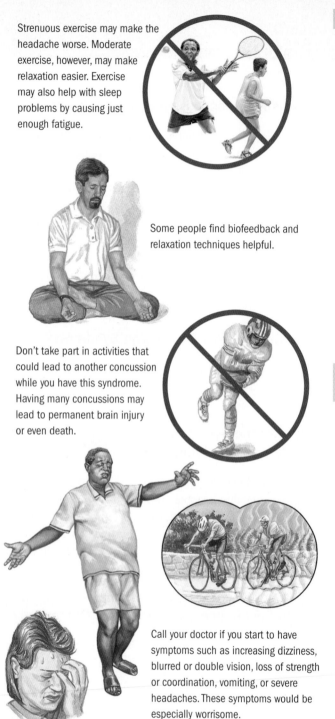

Strenuous exercise may make the headache worse. Moderate exercise, however, may make relaxation easier. Exercise may also help with sleep problems by causing just enough fatigue.

Some people find biofeedback and relaxation techniques helpful.

Don't take part in activities that could lead to another concussion while you have this syndrome. Having many concussions may lead to permanent brain injury or even death.

Call your doctor if you start to have symptoms such as increasing dizziness, blurred or double vision, loss of strength or coordination, vomiting, or severe headaches. These symptoms would be especially worrisome.

How Is Post-Concussion Syndrome Treated?

Treatment consists of watchful waiting until the symptoms go away. Most people recover to their normal pre-injury state, usually without permanent effects.

No medicines will shorten the recovery time. Mild analgesics such as acetaminophen, aspirin, and ibuprofen usually help the headache. Medicines may also be needed for depression or anxiety.

Strenuous exercise may make the headache worse. Moderate exercise, however, may make relaxation easier. Exercise may also help with sleep problems by causing just enough fatigue. Some people find biofeedback and relaxation techniques helpful.

Changing work or school areas to minimize the effects of memory loss or trouble concentrating may also be useful.

Support from friends and family to remind people that the condition is temporary may help in dealing with the symptoms.

DOs and DON'Ts in Managing Post-Concussion Syndrome:

✔ **DO** avoid medicines such as stimulants or decongestants. They may make the irritability worse. This condition will take some time to go away, so avoid medicines that might be habit forming. These drugs include narcotics, sleeping pills, and tranquilizers.

✔ **DO** avoid making life-changing decisions such as quitting school or changing jobs because of your symptoms.

✔ **DO** call your doctor if your symptoms increase over time or if they have not improved in several months.

✔ **DO** call your doctor if you start to have symptoms such as increasing dizziness, blurred or double vision, loss of strength or coordination, vomiting, or severe headaches. These symptoms would be especially worrisome.

🚫 **DON'T** do strenuous exercises. Strenuous activity may make the headache more intense. Even though this condition may last for several months, remember that it will go away.

🚫 **DON'T** take part in activities that could lead to another concussion while you have this syndrome. It may be that having many concussions may lead to permanent brain injury or even death.

FROM THE DESK OF

NOTES

FOR MORE INFORMATION

Contact the following source:

• Brain Injury Association
  Tel: (800) 444-6443
  Website: http://www.biausa.org

MANAGING YOUR
RAMSAY HUNT SYNDROME

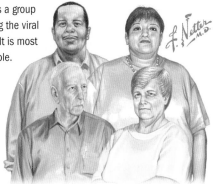

Ramsay Hunt syndrome is a group of symptoms complicating the viral infection called shingles. It is most often seen in elderly people.

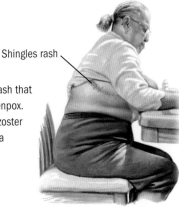

Shingles rash

Shingles is a painful, blistering rash that occurs in people who had chickenpox. The cause is the same varicella-zoster virus that caused chickenpox at a younger age.

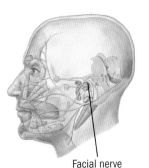

Facial nerve

Ramsey Hunt is an infection of the facial nerve, and symptoms occur around the nerve. Small blisters often seen in shingles occur in and around the ear and along the side of the mouth. Other symptoms are pain, loss of hearing, loss of taste over the front part of the tongue, dizziness, ringing in the ear (tinnitus), and facial paralysis.

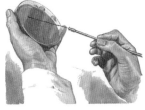

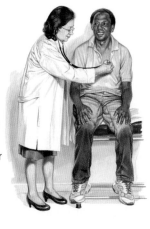

Your doctor makes a diagnosis from your medical history and physical examination. Sometimes, the doctor will peel off the top of a blister and scrape the skin at the bottom for further study.

What Is Ramsay Hunt Syndrome?

Ramsay Hunt syndrome is a group of symptoms complicating the viral infection called shingles. Shingles is a painful, blistering rash. In Ramsay Hunt, the shingles virus attacks the ear, tongue, and facial nerve.

The syndrome is rare in children but is often seen in elderly people, both men and women equally.

Other names for the syndrome are geniculate zoster, herpes zoster oticus, and herpetic geniculate ganglionitis.

What Causes Ramsay Hunt Syndrome?

The cause is the same virus that causes chickenpox (varicella-zoster). The virus was reactivates when the body's immune system weakens and causes shingles. If the infection involves the area near the ear, it can cause the Ramsay Hunt syndrome.

What Are the Symptoms of Ramsay Hunt Syndrome?

Small blisters occur in and around the ear, in the tympanic membrane of the ear, and along the side of the mouth.

Other symptoms are pain, loss of hearing, loss of taste over the front part of the tongue, dizziness, ringing in the ear (tinnitus), and possibly facial paralysis. The facial paralysis is on the same side as the skin lesions. People have difficulty smiling and frowning, and they may have puffy cheeks and trouble closing the eye. The result is drooling, food getting stuck on the affected side, and dry eye. Sometimes, hearing loss and facial paralysis can be permanent.

How Is Ramsay Hunt Syndrome Diagnosed?

The doctor makes a diagnosis from the medical history and physical examination. Sometimes, the doctor will peel off the top of the blister and scrape the bottom. This scraping (called Tzanck smear) will be sent for study. Viral cultures may also be done. A culture involves isolating the virus by growing it on a special culture plate.

Rarely, magnetic resonance imaging (MRI) may be needed to show the facial nerve being affected and to exclude other disorders.

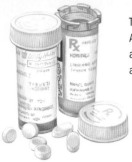

Treatment is with antiviral medicines. Antiinflammatory drugs such as ibuprofen and naproxen and other medications can also ease pain.

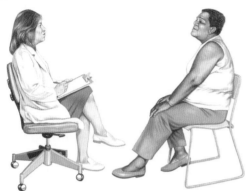

Don't miss follow-up doctor appointments. If facial paralysis continues, a visit to an ear, nose, and throat (ENT) specialist and a specialist of the nervous system (neurologist) may be needed to treat the facial nerve.

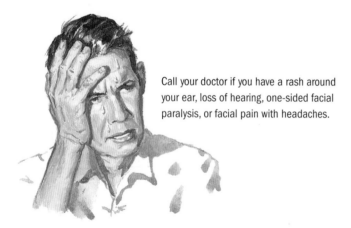

Call your doctor if you have a rash around your ear, loss of hearing, one-sided facial paralysis, or facial pain with headaches.

How Is Ramsay Hunt Syndrome Treated?

Treatment is with antiviral medicines (such as acyclovir, famciclovir, and valacyclovir). These may help skin lesions heal more quickly and reduce pain related to shingles. The doctor will prescribe pain medicines for the acute flare of the rash and for persistent pain after the rash is gone, known as postherpetic neuralgia.

Postherpetic neuralgia is a bothersome effect in some people with shingles and Ramsay Hunt syndrome. After the rash has gone, pain can last for 6 months and maybe longer. Gabapentin or pregabalin may help people with postherpetic neuralgia. Prednisone given early in the course of shingles can in some cases prevent postherpetic neuralgia.

Antiinflammatory drugs such as ibuprofen and naproxen can also help the pain. Sometimes, the doctor may prescribe a short course of narcotic pain medicine for severe pain not controlled by the other medications.

DOs and DON'Ts in Managing Ramsay Hunt Syndrome:

✔ **DO** remember that it takes 2 to 3 weeks for skin lesions to clear up. All symptoms usually go away, but hearing loss or paralysis can sometimes be permanent.

✔ **DO** call your doctor if you have a rash around your ear, loss of hearing, one-sided facial paralysis, or facial pain with headaches.

⊘ **DON'T** miss follow-up doctor appointments. If facial paralysis continues, a visit to an ear, nose, and throat (ENT) specialist and a specialist of the nervous system (neurologist) may be needed to treat the facial nerve.

FROM THE DESK OF

NOTES

FOR MORE INFORMATION

Contact the following source:

• Herpes Resource Center
American Social Health Association
Tel: (919) 361-8400
Website: http://www.ashastd.org/herpes/ herpes_overview.cfm

MANAGING YOUR
RESTLESS LEG SYNDROME

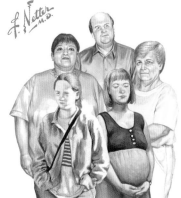

Restless leg syndrome (RLS) is a neurological condition that causes an almost uncontrollable urge to move the legs. It usually occurs in bed at night, or when people lie down and try to relax. This common condition affects up to 10% of the population.

Kidney conditions

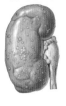

Drugs

Iron deficiency

Pregnancy

The cause isn't known, but diseases such as anemia; drugs; and kidney, nerve, and muscle problems are related to it. Middle-aged people and pregnant women are most likely to get it.

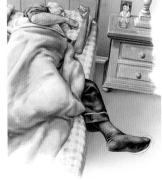

Itching, burning, or crawling feelings deep in the legs make it hard to sleep.

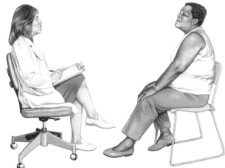

Your doctor can usually make a diagnosis from just your symptoms. Your doctor may order a blood test to rule out other causes, such as iron deficiency.

What Is Restless Leg Syndrome (RLS)?

Restless leg syndrome (RLS) is a neurological condition that causes people to have an almost uncontrollable urge to move their legs. It usually occurs in bed at night, or when people lie down and try to relax. These feelings can also occur in the arms.

This common condition affects up to 10% of the population at some time in their lives. Symptoms can vary from mild to severe, with severe RLS occuring most frequently in people middle-aged or older.

What Causes RLS?

The cause is unknown. It tends to run in families. Middle-aged people and pregnant women are most likely to get it.

Certain medicines such as some antidepressants can cause RLS. People with iron deficiency, anemia, kidney disease, diabetes, Parkinson's disease, nerve damage, muscle problems, or lung disease have greater chances of developing RLS. It has also been related to tobacco, caffeine, and alcohol.

What Are the Symptoms of RLS?

Itching, burning, or crawling feelings deep in the legs make it hard to sleep. Moving the legs temporarily relieves the symptoms. Usually, both sides of the body are affected. Because these feelings can interrupt sleep, people often feel very tired during the day.

Some people also have restless fidgeting in their toes, legs, or feet while they sit.

How Is RLS Diagnosed?

The doctor can usually make a diagnosis from just a description of symptoms. The doctor may order a blood test to rule out other causes, such as iron deficiency. If RLS is severe, the doctor may suggest spending a night in a sleep laboratory where sleeping and symptoms can be monitored.

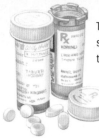

Treatment goals are to reduce symptoms and enable sound sleep. Your doctor may recommend self-help treatment and medicines.

Practice good sleep habits. Go to sleep around the same time every night, get up at the same time every morning, and sleep long enough to feel well rested.

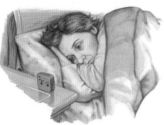

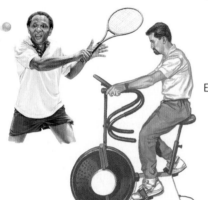

Exercise regularly.

Learn relaxation techniques, such as meditation, yoga, and biofeedback. Ask your doctor where to find classes.

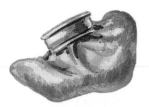

To temporarily relieve restless feelings in your legs, walk or stretch, take a hot or cold bath, massage your legs, or use hot or cold packs.

How Is RLS Treated?

Treatment is aimed at reducing symptoms and enable sound sleep. The doctor may recommend self-help treatment and medicines. Often, a combination of self-help and medicines works well. Some drugs work better than others, so trying different ones to find the best treatment may be needed.

If symptoms are severe and treatment does not work, a visit to a specialist in sleep disorders or a neurologist may be needed. A neurologist is a doctor who specializes in treating disorders of the nervous system.

DOs and DON'Ts in Managing RLS:

✔ **DO** practice good sleep habits. Go to sleep around the same time every night, get up at the same time every morning, and sleep long enough to feel well rested.

✔ **DO** exercise regularly.

✔ **DO** learn relaxation techniques, such as meditation, yoga, and biofeedback. Biofeedback is a method that trains you to control unconscious responses.

✔ **DO** try these methods to relieve the restless feelings in your legs temporarily: walk or stretch, take a hot or cold bath, massage your legs, or apply hot or cold packs.

✔ **DO** call your doctor if your symptoms continue even with medical treatment.

🚫 **DON'T** take herbal products without your doctor's approval. Some of these my affect your sleep cycle.

FROM THE DESK OF

NOTES

FOR MORE INFORMATION

Contact the following sources:

• Restless Legs Syndrome Foundation, Inc.
  Tel: (507) 287-6465
  Website: http://www.rls.org

• American Academy of Sleep Medicine
  Tel: (708) 492-0930
  Website: http://www.aasmnet.org

MANAGING YOUR
SPINAL STENOSIS

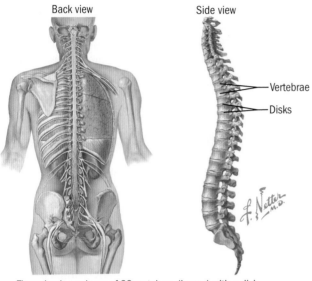

Back view   Side view

Vertebrae

Disks

The spine is made up of 33 vertebrae (bones) with a disk between each one.

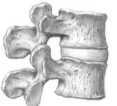

Normal: Disk separates vertebrae (notice height of disk).

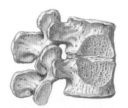

Spinal stenosis: Vertebrae bone "cut-away" to show loss of disk height. Loss of disk deforms the vertebrae, causing pain.

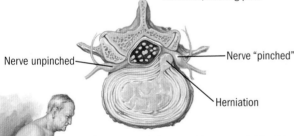

Nerve unpinched

Nerve "pinched"

Herniation

Spinal stenosis is caused by osteoarthritis with aging, wear and tear, or a herniated disk. Disk herniation can "pinch" a nerve, causing pain in the buttocks or lower leg and often leading to a visit to the doctor.

Common posture of someone with spinal stenosis. Flexing the neck, spine, hips, and knees lessens pressure on the spine and reduces pain.

About the Spine

The spine, also called the backbone or spinal column, is made up of 33 bones (vertebrae) from the bottom of the skull to the buttocks. Ligaments connect these bones. Between most vertebrae are flattened, round structures (intervertebral disks) composed of a soft substance in the middle and stronger outer covering. The spinal cord, which holds the nerves, runs through and is protected by vertebrae. Muscles in the back and abdomen support the spine.

What Is Spinal Stenosis?

Spinal stenosis is a narrowing in a part of the spine.

What Causes Spinal Stenosis?

The cause is usually wear and tear, past injury, disk rupture (herniation), or osteoarthritis related to aging. As disks between vertebrae wear out, spaces between vertebrae narrow. Vertebrae become deformed and may develop spurs (bony outgrowths or bulges) that can compress spinal nerves.

What Are the Symptoms of Spinal Stenosis?

Symptoms depend on which area of the spine is narrowed. Narrowing of the lower part produces pain in the lower back, buttocks, and thighs. In severe cases, legs or arms may become numb and weak.

Pinching (compression) of a spinal nerve root may cause intense pain in the buttocks or down the leg. *Sciatica* means pain in the leg caused by pinching, swelling (inflammation), or injury of the sciatic nerve. This nerve runs from the lower spine, down the buttock and back of the knee to the foot. Numbness and pins and needles may also be felt.

Spinal stenosis pain is worse during walking (especially downhill) or standing and gets better by bending forward.

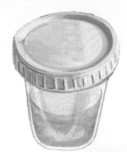

Blood and urine tests may be done to check for any disorders that may be causing the pain.

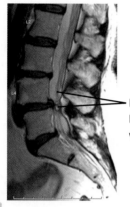

X-rays and MRI may be done to see bones or nerves.

Imaging can show the loss of a disk between vertebrae, as shown here.

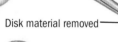

Over-the-counter pain relievers may help, but for more severe pain, stronger narcotic drugs may be needed. Drugs should only be used for a short period of time.

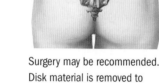

Disk material removed

Incision

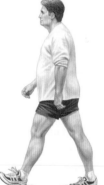

Surgery may be recommended. Disk material is removed to relieve pressure it is putting on a nerve.

Don't stop exercising completely.

How Is Spinal Stenosis Diagnosed?

A medical history and physical examination are used for diagnosis. The doctor may order blood and urine tests to see whether another disorder may be causing symptoms. X-rays of the spine will be done. Magnetic resonance imaging (MRI) bone scan may be done if a better picture is needed of bones, nerves, disks between vertebrae, and other tissues, or if surgery is being considered. A nerve conduction test may tell whether pressure on nerves is causing numbness or tingling in the legs.

How Is Spinal Stenosis Treated?

Physical therapy may help reduce pain and improve mobility.

Over-the-counter pain relievers, such as acetaminophen, or nonsteroidal antiinflammatory drugs (NSAIDs), such as ibuprofen, can help. For really severe pain, stronger narcotic medicines may be used for a short time. All drugs have side effects. NSAIDs may cause stomach upset, rash, and internal bleeding. Narcotic drugs may also cause drowsiness and constipation.

Surgery is used only for pain that doesn't go away. The operation may remove the disk (diskectomy) to relieve pressure on a nerve, or remove part of the bony arch, or lamina, of a vertebra (laminectomy) for a herniated disk.

DOs and DON'Ts in Spinal Stenosis:

✔ **DO** take medicines as prescribed.
✔ **DO** call your doctor if you have drug side effects.
✔ **DO** call your doctor if you have new numbness or tingling in your legs.
✔ **DO** call your doctor if you have trouble urinating or lose control of your bowels or bladder.

🚫 **DON'T** wait for a drug side effect to go away on its own.
🚫 **DON'T** stop exercising completely.

FROM THE DESK OF

NOTES

FOR MORE INFORMATION

Contact the following sources:

• American Academy of Orthopaedic Surgeons
  Tel: (800) 346-AAOS
  Website: http://www.aaos.org

• North American Spine Society
  Tel: (708) 588-8080
  Website: http://www.spine.org

MANAGING YOUR
STROKE

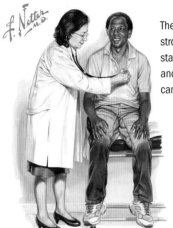

The greatest chance of recovery from a stroke occurs when treatment is started immediately. Quitting smoking and managing high cholesterol levels can help prevent future strokes.

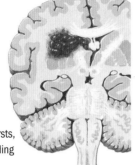

Stroke due to hemorrhage:
If a blood vessel in the brain bursts, blood can spill into the surrounding tissues.

Stroke due to blood clot:
Lack of blood flow and oxygen to the brain occurs when an artery is blocked by debris or a blood clot.

Clots may arise in the fat-rich area of a vessel that supplies blood to the brain.

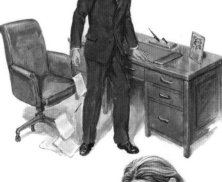

Sudden weakness or paralysis in one arm may be a symptom of stroke or TIA.

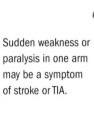

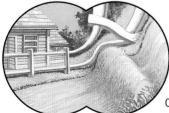

Other symptoms include confusion, vision changes, and dizziness.

What Is Stroke?

A stroke, or cerebrovascular accident (CVA), is an event in which blood flow to the brain stops.

What Causes Stroke?

Most strokes are caused by artery disease and/or high blood pressure. Most often, a blood vessel (artery) taking blood to the brain becomes blocked. This blockage is usually due to a blood clot (thrombus). This type of blockage is an ischemic stroke. A torn or burst blood vessel may also cause bleeding in the brain. This type is called a hemorrhagic stroke.

Plaques or clots in large arteries of the neck may cause warning signs called mini-strokes, or transient ischemic attacks (TIAs), and strokes. Plaque is made of fatty material that sticks to blood vessel walls.

What Are the Symptoms of Stroke?

Symptoms tend to occur suddenly and almost always affect only one side of the body. They are usually worst in the first 24 to 72 hours. Common symptoms include weakness or numbness of face, arm, and leg muscles and difficulty speaking or swallowing. Others are confusion, vision changes, dizziness, and loss of balance. TIA symptoms usually disappear in a few hours. Most last less than 10 minutes. Those lasting longer than 24 hours are called strokes.

The type of symptoms from a stroke depend on the area of the brain that is damaged. Serious strokes can cause paralysis and loss of speech. Less serious strokes may not become apparent for several days.

How Is a Stroke Diagnosed?

Studies used for diagnosis include a physical examination and computed tomography (CT), or magnetic resonance imaging (MRI) of the brain. A study of the heart's electrical activity (electrocardiogram, or ECG) will be done to rule out irregular heartbeat (atrial fibrillation), which may cause a stroke.

An ultrasound of the carotid arteries in the neck may be done to look for a blockage of the arteries supplying blood to the brain.

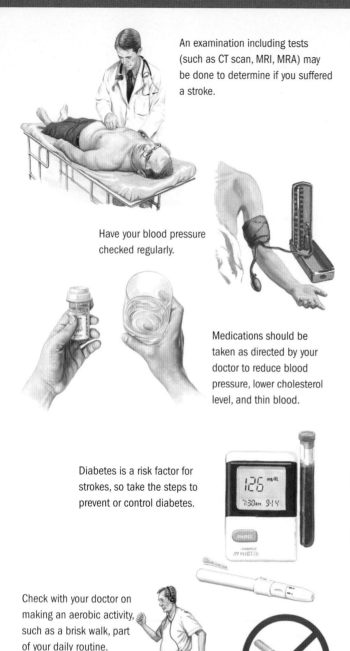

An examination including tests (such as CT scan, MRI, MRA) may be done to determine if you suffered a stroke.

Have your blood pressure checked regularly.

Medications should be taken as directed by your doctor to reduce blood pressure, lower cholesterol level, and thin blood.

Diabetes is a risk factor for strokes, so take the steps to prevent or control diabetes.

Check with your doctor on making an aerobic activity, such as a brisk walk, part of your daily routine.

Don't smoke.

How Is a Stroke Treated?

The type of stroke determines the treatment. However, survival may depend on an immediate visit to the hospital emergency department. There, a potent blood thinner may be given to people with ischemic strokes. This drug, tPA, can dissolve a clot, although certain risks (e.g., bleeding in the brain) are related to it. The emergency room doctor, in consultation with a specialist of the nervous system (neurologist), will determine if this medication is appropriate depending on the type of stroke, elapsed time from beginning of the symptoms, and other criteria.

A stroke may have mild to severely disabling effects. How much ability one can recover may not be known for months or years. Many people need rehabilitation, such as speech therapy, physical therapy, and occupational therapy.

Treatment must also target conditions such as high blood pressure, diabetes, tobacco use, lifestyle, and high cholesterol levels. Also, other strokes must be prevented. Many people can do this by using drugs to prevent blood clots from forming. Often, taking a small amount of aspirin each day will do this. Other people must control high blood pressure and reduce other risk factors for stroke, such as diabetes, high cholesterol levels, smoking, and being overweight.

DOs and DON'Ts in Managing and

Preventing Stroke:

✔ **DO** stop smoking.
✔ **DO** take your medicines.
✔ **DO** exercise according to your doctor's instructions.
✔ **DO** eat a low-fat diet and drink no more than one alcoholic drink a day.
✔ **DO** control your blood pressure, cholesterol level, and diabetes.

⊘ **DON'T** ignore symptoms of stroke. It can be a matter of life or death.

FROM THE DESK OF

NOTES

FOR MORE INFORMATION

Contact the following source:

• American Stroke Association
  Tel: (888) 478-7653
  Website: http://www.strokeassociation.org

MANAGING YOUR
TARDIVE DYSKINESIA

Tardive dyskinesia is a neurological condition caused by long use of medicines called neuroleptics. Neuroleptic drugs are usually given for psychiatric disorders. They are used to make psychotic symptoms, such as delusions, hallucinations, and bizarre behaviors, less intense and occur less often.

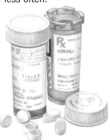

The cause is unknown. Almost half of all people who take neuroleptic drugs for longer than 6 months get it. Older people, especially women, have a greater risk of getting tardive dyskinesia. The occurrence increases with the length of time the medicine is taken.

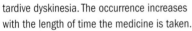

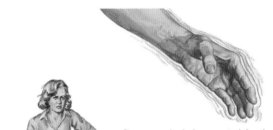

Symptoms include repeated, involuntary, purposeless movements. These include making grimaces; pushing the tongue out; smacking, puckering, and pursing the lips; and rapidly blinking the eyes. People may also have rapid movements of the arms, legs, fingers, and trunk.

Your doctor makes a diagnosis from a detailed medical history and physical examination. Blood tests, CT, and MRI may be done to rule out other causes of tardive dyskinesia.

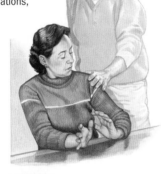

What Is Tardive Dyskinesia?

Tardive dyskinesia is a neurological condition caused by long use of medicines called neuroleptics (antipsychotics). Neuroleptic drugs are usually given for psychiatric disorders. They are used to make psychotic symptoms, such as delusions, hallucinations, and bizarre behaviors, less intense and occur less often.

In the United States, tardive dyskinesia is seen most often in people treated for schizophrenia and bipolar disorder. People who have taken neuroleptics can develop movement disorders while taking the medicine or after stopping the medicine. Older people, especially women, have a greater risk of getting tardive dyskinesia.

What Causes Tardive Dyskinesia?

The cause is unknown. Almost half of all people who take neuroleptics for longer than 6 months will get it. The occurrence increases with the age of the person and the longer the medicine is taken. Tardive dyskinesia isn't contagious or passed from parents to children.

What Are the Symptoms of Tardive Dyskinesia?

Symptoms include repeated, involuntary, purposeless movements. These include making grimaces; pushing the tongue out; smacking, puckering, and pursing the lips; and rapidly blinking the eyes. People may also have rapid movements of the arms, legs, fingers, and trunk. Movements usually get worse with emotional stress and when people move with purpose. They decrease with sedation (calming) and during sleep.

How Is Tardive Dyskinesia Diagnosed?

The doctor makes a diagnosis from a detailed medical history and physical examination. No specific blood tests are used for diagnosis, but the doctor may order blood tests to rule out other causes of the symptoms. The doctor may also order computed tomography (CT) or magnetic resonance imaging (MRI) to make sure that other medical conditions that have symptoms similar to those of tardive dyskinesia aren't causing the symptoms.

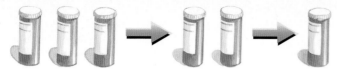

Treatment is mainly directed at prevention by using the lowest possible dose of drug for the shortest time. If tardive dyskinesia does occur, treatment then focuses on reducing the dosage of the medicine or stopping the medicine completely. Don't forget that this dyskinesia can show up after you stop taking the neuroleptic drugs.

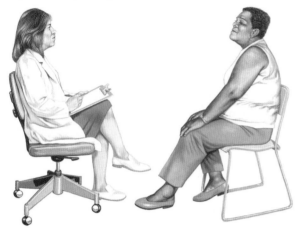

Realize that if you're being treated with neuroleptic drugs and develop tardive dyskinesia, you and your doctor must decide whether you should stop taking the drugs and maybe avoid getting a permanent movement disorder. However, you could then have worse psychotic symptoms.

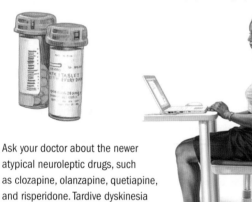

Ask your doctor about the newer atypical neuroleptic drugs, such as clozapine, olanzapine, quetiapine, and risperidone. Tardive dyskinesia may occur less often with these drugs than with the traditional ones.

How Is Tardive Dyskinesia Treated?

Treatment is mainly directed at prevention by using the lowest possible dose for the shortest time. If tardive dyskinesia does occur, treatment then focuses on reducing the dosage of the medicine or stopping the medicine completely. Some drugs, such as levodopa, benzodiazepines, and botulinum toxin, have been used to relieve symptoms of tardive dyskinesia, but with limited success.

DOs and DON'Ts in Managing Tardive Dyskinesia:

✔ **DO** realize if you're being treated with neuroleptics and develop tardive dyskinesia, you and your doctor must decide whether you should stop taking the drugs and maybe avoid getting a permanent movement disorder. However, you could then have worse psychotic symptoms.

✔ **DO** ask your doctor about the newer atypical neuroleptics such as clozapine, olanzapine, quetiapine, and risperidone. All these drugs can be related to tardive dyskinesia, but tardive dyskinesia may occur less often with these atypical neuroleptics than with the traditional neuroleptics.

✔ **DO** call your doctor if you develop involuntary repeated movements and are taking a neuroleptic drug.

✔ **DO** call your doctor if you've reduced your medicine and you notice worsening psychotic symptoms (e.g., delusions and hallucinations).

⊘ **DON'T** forget that tardive dyskinesia can also show up after stopping the use of neuroleptic medicines.

FROM THE DESK OF

NOTES

FOR MORE INFORMATION

Contact the following sources:

• National Institute of Mental Health
Tel: (866) 615-6464
Website: http://www.nimh.nih.gov

• National Alliance on Mental Illness
Tel: (800) 950-6264
Website: http://www.nami.org/

• American Psychiatric Association
Tel: (888) 357-7924
Website: http://www.psych.org

MANAGING YOUR
TENSION HEADACHE

Tension headaches are usually dull, aching, or throbbing headaches that are often related to feelings of fullness, tightness, or pressure (such as feeling as if the head will burst, or as if it's bound or clamped in a vise).

Possible triggers of a tension headache include:

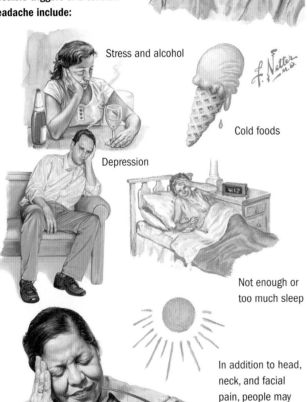

Stress and alcohol

Cold foods

Depression

Not enough or too much sleep

In addition to head, neck, and facial pain, people may have nausea or increased sensitivity to light or sound.

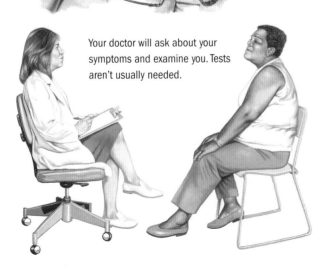

Your doctor will ask about your symptoms and examine you. Tests aren't usually needed.

What Is Tension Headache?

Tension headaches are dull, aching, or throbbing headaches, often with feelings of fullness, tightness, or pressure. A feeling that the head will burst or is bound or clamped in a vise can occur. Both sides of the head and neck are usually affected, especially where neck muscles attach to the skull. These headaches also involve the forehead and temples.

What Causes Tension Headache?

The exact cause of tension headaches is unknown. Possible triggers can be stress, not enough or too much sleep, eating or drinking too much, work, anxiety, depression, eye strain (including sun glare), drugs, alcohol, allergies, food additives, fumes, and chemicals. Women can also get headaches more frequently because of hormone changes.

What Are the Symptoms of Tension Headache?

Symptoms include moderate pain in front or back of the head, neck or scalp tightness, constant pain over sides of the head (like a clamp), throbbing pain all over the face, head pain on awakening, and head pain that interrupts sleep.

How Is Tension Headache Diagnosed?

Tests aren't usually needed. The doctor will ask about headaches and other symptoms and will do a physical examination, especially a neurological examination. More tests such as MRI of the brain may be done to check for other possible problems or when the diagnosis is unclear.

Over-the-counter medications (such as aspirin or acetaminophen) can usually relieve pain. Some people may need prescription drugs.

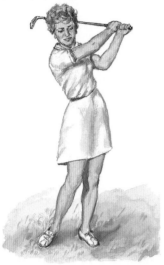

Eat regular meals. Don't eat foods containing nitrates (such as hot dogs) or other additives.

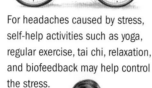

For headaches caused by stress, self-help activities such as yoga, regular exercise, tai chi, relaxation, and biofeedback may help control the stress.

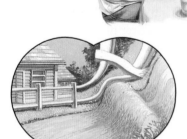

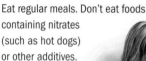

Call your doctor if you have a fever, vomiting, or change in vision.

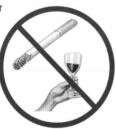

Don't smoke or drink alcohol in excess.

How Is Tension Headache Treated?

The best way to stop these headaches is to avoid the cause if it's known.

Over-the-counter medications (aspirin or acetaminophen) can usually relieve pain.

If headaches are due to stress, self-help activities such as yoga, exercise, tai chi, relaxation, and biofeedback may help control the stress. Counseling may be suggested for emotional problems, anxiety, or depression.

Tension headaches may respond to massage, relaxation, and antianxiety medicines. Some people may need prescription medicine.

DOs and DON'Ts in Managing Tension Headache:

✔ **DO** stop what you're doing and try to relax when a headache occurs.

✔ **DO** massage your shoulders, neck, jaw, or scalp.

✔ **DO** take a hot bath or shower.

✔ **DO** place a warm or cold cloth over your forehead.

✔ **DO** keep a diary of your headaches.

✔ **DO** follow a healthy lifestyle. Eat regular meals. Get enough sleep. Exercise regularly.

✔ **DO** call your doctor if your symptoms are worse or last longer than usual, your usual medicine doesn't work, or you have a fever, vomiting, or change in vision.

✔ **DO** call your doctor if you have problems with your medicine.

⊘ **DON'T** skip breakfast.

⊘ **DON'T** smoke or be in a smoky environment.

⊘ **DON'T** expose yourself to chemicals.

⊘ **DON'T** drink alcohol in excess. Avoid stimulants such as caffeine.

⊘ **DON'T** take drugs not prescribed by your doctor.

⊘ **DON'T** eat foods containing nitrates (such as hot dogs) or other additives that may cause sensitivity.

⊘ **DON'T** overuse prescription or over-the-counter pain pills, which can cause a rebound headache.

FROM THE DESK OF

NOTES

FOR MORE INFORMATION

Contact the following sources:

• National Headache Foundation
Tel: (888) 643-5552
Website: http://www.headaches.org

• American Council for Headache Education
Tel: (800) 255-ACHE (255-2243)
Website: http://www.achenet.org

Tinnitus is a condition that affects hearing. A ringing or buzzing sound is heard in the ears. It causes people to hear noise even when everything around them is silent. The noise may be soft or loud, constant or on and off.

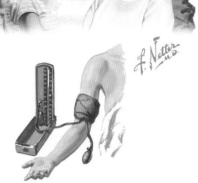

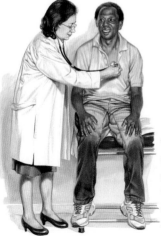

The cause may be an illness or condition, for example, ear infections, thyroid problems, or high blood pressure. An injury to the hearing system from loud noise exposure can also cause tinnitus. In most cases, the cause is unknown.

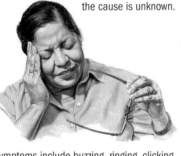

Symptoms include buzzing, ringing, clicking, roaring, and hissing sounds. Other symptoms include hearing loss, dizziness, and vertigo.

Your doctor will do an examination, take a medical history, and maybe order tests. Blood tests may be done to check for other illnesses that may cause tinnitus. Special hearing tests are also done.

What Is Tinnitus?

Tinnitus is a condition that affects hearing. A ringing or buzzing sound is heard in the ears. It causes people to hear noise even when everything around them is silent. The noise may be soft or loud. It could also be a rushing sound that matches the heartbeat. The sounds may be constant or on and off.

Tinnitus may develop in one or both ears. For some people, it's a minor problem. For others, it becomes a serious handicap. Hearing may be lost in the affected ears.

What Causes Tinnitus?

The cause may be an illness or condition, for example, ear infections or very high blood pressure. An injury to the hearing system from loud noise exposure can also cause tinnitus. In most cases, the cause is unknown.

What Are the Symptoms of Tinnitus?

Symptoms include buzzing, ringing, clicking, roaring, and hissing sounds. Other symptoms include hearing loss, dizziness, and vertigo.

How Is Tinnitus Diagnosed?

The doctor will do an examination, take a medical history, and maybe order tests. Blood tests may be done to check for other illnesses that may cause tinnitus. Special hearing tests are also done. The doctor will pay extra attention to the emotional state of mind. Many people with tinnitus are depressed or very anxious and frustrated about their problem. You may be referred to an ear, nose, and throat (ENT) specialist.

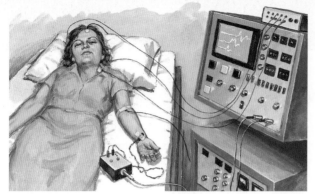

Several treatments can help reduce the noise. More than one treatment may be used at the same time. Biofeedback teaches people how to change the way their bodies respond to stress. Another treatment is tinnitus retraining therapy. People work with experts who help retrain the ear not to hear the noise.

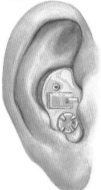

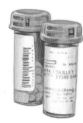

Some medicines may also help. A hearing aid may be needed if hearing loss has occurred.

Masking uses a device that makes soothing background noise (white noise). This noise helps cover up the annoying ringing. Background music or static between stations on a radio can help mask the noise if you have trouble sleeping.

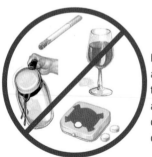

Limit your use of caffeine, tobacco, and alcohol. When possible, avoid medicines that can harm your ears, including aminoglycoside antibiotics and drugs containing salicylates (such as high-dose aspirin).

How Is Tinnitus Treated?

The doctor may prescribe a treatment to reduce the annoying noise. The doctor will also treat any illness or injury causing the tinnitus. For example, medicine may be prescribed to lower high blood pressure.

Several treatments can help reduce the annoying noise. More than one treatment may be used at the same time. Masking uses a device that makes calm, soothing background noise (called white noise). This background noise helps cover up the more annoying noise. Sometimes, soothing background music helps mask the noise. Another treatment is called tinnitus retraining therapy. People work with hearing experts who help retrain the ear not to hear the annoying noise. Biofeedback also teaches people how to change the way their bodies respond to stress. Biofeedback has helped many people with tinnitus. Some medicines may also help. A hearing aid may be needed if hearing loss has occurred.

People with mild tinnitus may not need treatment.

DOs and DON'Ts in Managing Tinnitus:

✔ **DO** try another treatment if one treatment doesn't help. Different people are helped by different treatments.

✔ **DO** try to listen to soothing background music or to the static between stations on a radio if you have trouble sleeping. The static will help mask the noise.

✔ **DO** keep your ears clear of wax.

✔ **DO** limit your use of caffeine, tobacco, and alcohol.

✔ **DO** call your doctor if you feel anxious or depressed.

⊘ **DON'T** listen to loud noises. Wear earplugs whenever you can.

⊘ **DON'T** take medicines that can harm your ears. These medicines include a certain type of antibiotics called aminoglycoside antibiotics and medicines containing salicylates, such as high-dose aspirin.

FROM THE DESK OF

NOTES

FOR MORE INFORMATION

Contact the following source:

• American Tinnitus Association
 Tel: (800) 634-8978
 Website: http://www.ata.org

A transient ischemic attack (TIA), or mini-stroke, is a kind of stroke that lasts less than 24 hours, usually just a few minutes. It occurs when part of the brain doesn't get enough oxygen. People have a higher risk of stroke if they had a TIA before.

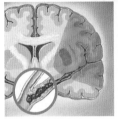

TIAs are caused by clots that get trapped in one of the brain's blood vessels. Clots usually come from the heart or carotid arteries in the neck and are made of blood or fat.

The most common symptom is weakness in any part of the body. Others include:

Vision changes

Trouble walking, dizziness

Memory loss, confusion

CT

Your doctor will make a diagnosis from your medical history, physical examination, and CT or MRI. Other tests may include ultrasonography and angiography.

What Is a Transient Ischemic Attack (TIA)?

A transient ischemic attack (TIA) is a kind of stroke that lasts less than 24 hours, usually just a few minutes. It's also called a mini-stroke. It occurs when part of the brain isn't getting enough oxygen.

TIAs are more common in men older than 60. People have a higher risk of stroke if they had a TIA before.

What Causes a TIA?

Plaques or blood clots in arteries can block blood flow. Most of the time, the body breaks down these plaques, so blood flow begins again and symptoms go away. A TIA is caused by a blood clot that gets trapped in one of the brain's blood vessels. This clot usually comes from the heart or carotid arteries in the neck and is made of blood or fat. The trapped clot stops blood from going to part of the brain, so the brain cannot get the oxygen from the blood.

What Are the Symptoms of a TIA?

The most common symptom is weakness in any part of the body. Other symptoms include confusion, dizziness, double vision, memory loss, numbness, speech and swallowing problems, tingling, vision changes, and trouble walking.

In 70% of cases, symptoms go away in less than 10 minutes, and in 90% they go away in less than 4 hours.

How Is a TIA Diagnosed?

The doctor will make a diagnosis from the medical history, physical examination, and computed tomography (CT) or magnetic resonance imaging (MRI). Other tests may include ultrasonography and angiography.

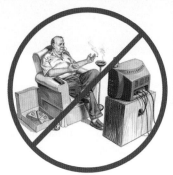

You need to take an active role in your own treatment, because in many cases, underlying conditions (high blood pressure, diabetes, tobacco abuse, inactive lifestyle, and high cholesterol) contribute to the condition.

Medicine may be prescribed to thin your blood so you won't form clots.

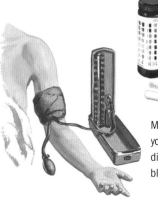

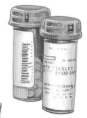

Make sure that your doctor knows about your other medical problems, such as diabetes, high cholesterol level, and high blood pressure.

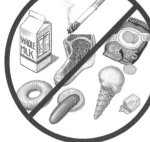

You should not use tobacco products or eat a high-fat diet. These can cause blood vessel disease and increase your risk of having a stroke.

Call your doctor if you have another TIA after starting to take medicine or you have an unusually severe headache.

How Is a TIA Treated?

Treatment depends on the cause. The doctor will be most concerned about preventing a stroke.

Conditions such as high blood pressure, diabetes, tobacco abuse, inactive lifestyle, and high cholesterol level are treated. Aspirin, clopidogrel, and warfarin may be given to thin the blood and prevent clots.

Surgery (carotid endoarterectomy) may be needed to open blocked carotid arteries with big clots.

DOs and DON'Ts in Managing a TIA:

✔ **DO** note the conditions and symptoms when you have a TIA. What were you doing when it occurred? What symptoms did you have? How long did they last? When did they occur?

✔ **DO** take only medicines prescribed by your doctor. Some may mean that you must get regular blood tests.

✔ **DO** make sure that your doctor knows about your other medical problems, such as diabetes, high cholesterol level, and high blood pressure.

✔ **DO** keep follow-up doctor appointments.

✔ **DO** call your doctor if you have another TIA after starting to take medicine.

✔ **DO** call your doctor if you have an unusually severe headache.

✔ **DO** call your doctor if you have problems with your medicines.

⊘ **DON'T** stop taking your medicine or change your dosage because you feel better unless your doctor tells you to.

⊘ **DON'T** use tobacco products. They cause blood vessel disease and increase your risk of having a stroke.

⊘ **DON'T** eat a high-fat diet.

⊘ **DON'T** drive or do any activity that might be dangerous if you have a TIA.

FROM THE DESK OF

NOTES

FOR MORE INFORMATION

Contact the following sources:

• National Institute of Neurological Disorders and Stroke
Tel: (800) 352-9424
Website: http://www.ninds.nih.gov

• National Stroke Association
Tel: (800) 787-6537
Website: http://www.stroke.org

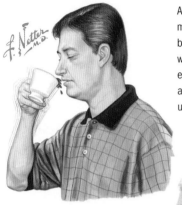

A tremor is a rhythmic, involuntary muscle contraction. A part of the body moves back and forth. Tremor without a known cause is called essential tremor. These tremors affect men and women equally, usually after age 40.

Tremors can affect hands, head, facial structures, vocal cords, trunk, and legs. Most occur in hands and arms. They're worse when limbs are held out or in uncomfortable positions, and they usually stop at rest.

The cause is unknown, but abnormal communications between certain parts of the brain are thought to lead to tremors. They may run in families, with parents having a 50% chance of passing them to their children.

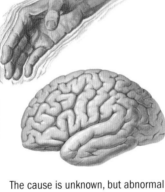

Your doctor makes a diagnosis from a detailed history and physical examination. Tests may be done to rule out other causes (e.g., neurological disorders, thyroid conditions, caffeine use, and medicines).

What Is Essential Tremor?

A tremor is a rhythmic, involuntary muscle contraction. A part of the body moves back and forth. Tremor without a known cause is called essential tremor.

Tremors can be put into five categories: resting, postural, kinetic, task-specific, and psychogenic. Resting tremor occurs when a muscle is at rest, for example, when hands are lying in the lap. People with Parkinson's disease have this type. Postural tremor occurs when people try to hold a position, such as holding the hands out. These tremors include physiological, essential, posttraumatic, and alcoholic tremors. Kinetic tremor occurs during movement with purpose, for example, during finger-to-nose testing. Task-specific tremor appears when doing tasks such as handwriting, speaking, or standing. Psychogenic tremor occurs in older and younger people and can be lessened or can disappear when people get distracted.

Essential tremors affect men and women equally, usually after age 40. These tremors can cause disability and social embarrassment.

What Causes Essential Tremor?

Although the cause is unknown, abnormal communications between certain parts of the brain are thought to lead to tremors. They're not contagious but may run in families, with parents having a 50% chance of passing them to children.

What Are the Symptoms of Essential Tremor?

Essential tremor can affect hands, head, facial structures, vocal cords, trunk, and legs. Most occur in the hands and arms. Tremors usually affect both sides of the body, but may be more noticeable on one side. Tremors are worse when limbs are held out or in uncomfortable positions. They usually stop at rest.

How Is Essential Tremor Diagnosed?

The doctor makes a diagnosis from a detailed history and physical examination. Other causes (e.g., neurological disorders, thyroid conditions, caffeine use, and medicines) must be ruled out. No specific blood tests, genetic testing, or x-ray studies can diagnose essential tremors. However, the doctor might order blood and urine tests, computed tomography (CT), or magnetic resonance imaging (MRI) to find other possible causes of the tremors.

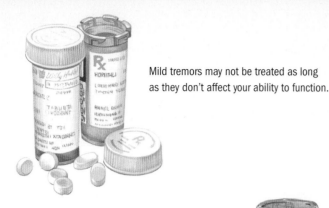

Mild tremors may not be treated as long as they don't affect your ability to function.

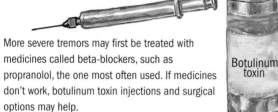

Botulinum toxin

More severe tremors may first be treated with medicines called beta-blockers, such as propranolol, the one most often used. If medicines don't work, botulinum toxin injections and surgical options may help.

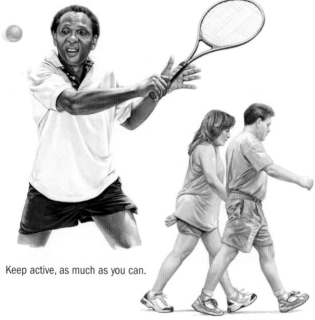

Keep active, as much as you can.

Don't drink caffeine, which may worsen your symptoms. Also, don't use alcohol for treatment.

How Is Essential Tremor Treated?

Mild tremors may not be treated as long as they don't affect the ability to function. More severe tremors may first be treated with medicines called beta-blockers. such as propranolol, the one most often used.

Primidone, gabapentin, clonazepam, diazepam, and alprazolam may also be tried.

If medicines don't work, botulinum toxin injections and surgical options may help.

DOs and DON'Ts in Managing Essential Tremor:

✔ **DO** have an active lifestyle.
✔ **DO** understand that Parkinson's disease causes a tremor at rest and not only with action.
✔ **DO** realize that although alcohol tends to reduce tremors, it shouldn't be used for treatment.
✔ **DO** call your doctor if you have medicine side effects.
✔ **DO** call your doctor if you're worried that you have Parkinson's disease.
✔ **DO** call your doctor if you need a referral to a neurologist (specialist in movement disorders).

⊘ **DON'T** stop medicines without first asking your doctor.
⊘ **DON'T** use caffeine. It may worsen your symptoms.

FROM THE DESK OF

NOTES

FOR MORE INFORMATION

Contact the following sources:

• The National Institute of Neurological Disorders and Stroke
Website: http://www.ninds.nih.gov

• International Essential Tremor Foundation
Tel: (888) 387-3667
Website: http://www.essentialtremor.org

Trigeminal neuralgia is a rare, painful disorder of the trigeminal nerve, a main nerve in the face. Pain can start after a tooth extraction, facial nerve injury, herpesvirus infection, or nerve compression from a blood vessel or tumor. It is more common in women than in men.

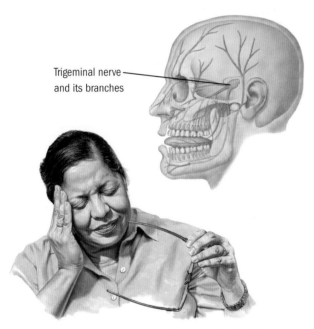

Trigeminal nerve and its branches

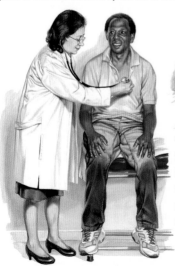

The most common symptom is intense, stabbing, electric shock–like pain in parts of the face affected by the nerve and its branches.

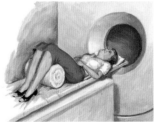

Your doctor makes a diagnosis from your symptoms, medical history, and physical examination. CT (shown here) or MRI may be needed to see whether another medical condition is causing pain.

What Is Trigeminal Neuralgia?

Trigeminal neuralgia is a rare, painful disorder of the trigeminal nerve, a main nerve in the face. Another name for it is tic douloureux. It's a chronic condition with intense pain that can be very debilitating. Episodes can last for days, weeks, or months and then go away for months or years.

Trigeminal neuralgia rarely occurs in people younger than 50, and it's more common in women than in men.

What Causes Trigeminal Neuralgia?

The cause is usually unknown. Sometimes the disorder starts after a tooth extraction, facial nerve injury, herpesvirus infection, or pressing (compression) on the nerve from a blood vessel or tumor.

What Are the Symptoms of Trigeminal Neuralgia?

The most common symptom is intense, stabbing, electric shock–like pain in parts of the face affected by the nerve and its branches. The brief but severe facial pain tends to come and go in the jaw, lips, eyes, nose, scalp, forehead, and face. Pain can start without warning or may be triggered by talking, chewing, putting on makeup, washing the face, or brushing the teeth. Sometimes, even touching a certain part of the face (trigger point) can cause an attack.

How Is Trigeminal Neuralgia Diagnosed?

The doctor makes a diagnosis from symptoms, medical history, and physical examination. Computed tomography (CT) or magnetic resonance imaging (MRI) may be needed to see whether another medical condition is causing pain.

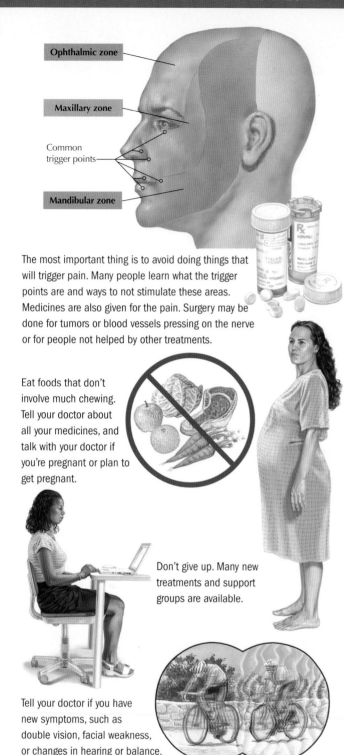

Ophthalmic zone

Maxillary zone

Common trigger points

Mandibular zone

The most important thing is to avoid doing things that will trigger pain. Many people learn what the trigger points are and ways to not stimulate these areas. Medicines are also given for the pain. Surgery may be done for tumors or blood vessels pressing on the nerve or for people not helped by other treatments.

Eat foods that don't involve much chewing. Tell your doctor about all your medicines, and talk with your doctor if you're pregnant or plan to get pregnant.

Don't give up. Many new treatments and support groups are available.

Tell your doctor if you have new symptoms, such as double vision, facial weakness, or changes in hearing or balance.

How Is Trigeminal Neuralgia Treated?

Treatment depends on symptoms. The most important thing is to avoid doing things that will trigger the pain. Many people learn what the trigger points are and ways to not stimulate these areas.

Medicines are also given for the pain.

Surgery is for tumors or blood vessels that press on the nerve or for people who aren't helped by other treatments. These operations include noninvasive radiosurgery (focused radiation therapy), injection or electrical stimulation, and open operation to remove pressure on the nerve.

DOs and DON'Ts in Managing Trigeminal Neuralgia:

✔ **DO** eat foods that don't involve much chewing.
✔ **DO** tell your doctor about your medicines, including prescription and over-the-counter drugs.
✔ **DO** tell your doctor if you're pregnant or plan to get pregnant.
✔ **DO** call your doctor if your symptoms don't get better with the drug that you were prescribed.
✔ **DO** call your doctor if you have side effects with your medicine.
✔ **DO** call your doctor if you have new symptoms, such as double vision, facial weakness, or changes in hearing or balance.

⊘ **DON'T** stop taking your medicine or change your dosage because you feel better unless your doctor tells you to.
⊘ **DON'T** despair. Many new treatments and support groups are available.

FROM THE DESK OF

NOTES

FOR MORE INFORMATION

Contact the following source:

• Trigeminal Neuralgia Association
 Tel: (800) 923-3608, (352) 331-7009
 Website: http://www.fpa-support.org

MANAGING YOUR WHIPLASH

The cervical spine, the part of the spinal column in your neck, has seven bones called cervical vertebrae. Thick fibrous bands called ligaments hold the bones together. Disks between the bones act like shock absorbers. Muscles support and move the neck.

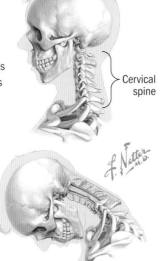

Cervical spine

Whiplash is an injury in which the neck is forced to extend too far back and then quickly go forward. Ligaments, muscles, bone, and disks are injured. More women than men have these injuries.

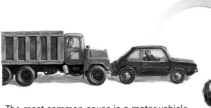

The most common cause is a motor vehicle accident (often a rear-end collision). Trauma from falling, contact sport injury, and physical abuse can also cause whiplash.

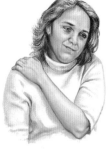

Neck pain is the most common symptom. Neck tightness, stiffness, and headaches over the back of the head occur. You can also have pain over the shoulder and arms, numbness, reduced range of motion, ringing in the ears, and trouble swallowing.

Your doctor makes a diagnosis from your history and physical exam. Sometimes blood tests and x-rays may be done to rule out other causes, such as arthritis, migraine headaches, spinal cord tumor, or cervical disk disease. MRI may also be done to check for nerve injury.

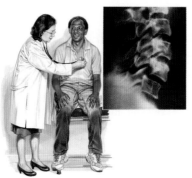

What Is Whiplash?

The part of the spinal column in the neck (cervical spine) has seven bones called cervical vertebrae. Thick fibrous bands called ligaments hold these bones together. Disks between the bones are cushions and act like shock absorbers during normal daily activities. Neck muscles support and move the neck. Whiplash is a neck injury in which the neck is forced to extend too far back and then quickly go forward. Ligaments, muscles, bone, and disks are injured. Whiplash can be uncomfortable and make people miss work. It occurs at any age, more often in women than in men. More than 1 million people a year have whiplash.

What Causes Whiplash?

The cause is usually a motor vehicle accident, trauma from falling, contact sport injury, or physical abuse. Rear-end vehicle collisions account for more than 40% of cases.

What Are the Symptoms of Whiplash?

Neck pain is the most common complaint. Pain usually starts hours to days after the accident. Neck tightness, stiffness, and headaches over the back of the head occur. Pain over the shoulder and arms, numbness, reduced range of motion, ringing in the ears, and trouble swallowing can also be noted in severe cases.

How Is Whiplash Diagnosed?

The doctor makes a diagnosis from the medical history and physical exam. Sometimes blood tests, x-rays, and magnetic resonance imaging (MRI) may be done to rule out other causes. Your doctor may suggest seeing a neurologist (specialist in nervous system diseases) or orthopedic surgeon (specialist in bone diseases).

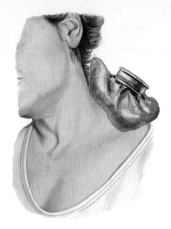

Treatment is usually conservative. First, ice packs are applied to the area, and then heat (as from a heating pad or hot shower) or cold.

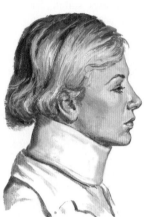

Using a soft cervical collar (usually for no more than 3 days) is usually also recommended.

Pain medicines include antiinflammatory drugs and acetaminophen. Muscle relaxants can also be tried for muscle spasms.

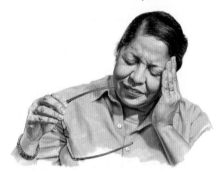

Call your doctor if you have numbness or tingling down your arms, muscle weakness, or headaches or if your symptoms get worse. Don't ignore your symptoms. Many serious conditions can mimic whiplash.

How Is Whiplash Treated?

The goals of treatment are to reduce pain and allow time for the injury to heal. Conservative treatment is usual. Ice packs are applied to the area first, and then heat (heating pad, hot shower) or cold. A soft cervical collar is usually suggested.

For sleeping, a small rolled towel that is 2 inches in diameter or cervical pillow (neck support pillow) should be used. Ultrasound may also help symptoms.

Medicines for pain include antiinflammatory drugs and acetaminophen (alone or with antiinflammatory drugs). Muscle relaxants can also be tried for muscle spasms.

DOs and DON'Ts in Managing Whiplash:

✔ **DO** take muscle relaxants before bedtime. Take medicines as prescribed by your doctor.

✔ **DO** sit in a firm chair and sit against the chair's back.

✔ **DO** remember that most people recover within weeks. However, 20% to 40% of people may develop a chronic syndrome, with headache, neck pain, and anxiety and depression related to the accident.

✔ **DO** wear a seat belt, and drive safely. Raise the padded headrest on the seat so it will protect you.

✔ **DO** wear safety gear if you play contact sports such as football.

✔ **DO** call your doctor if you have numbness or tingling down your arms, muscle weakness, or headaches or if your symptoms get worse.

⊘ **DON'T** stop taking your medicine or change your dosage because you feel better, unless your doctor tells you to.

⊘ **DON'T** lift heavy objects without your doctor's OK.

⊘ **DON'T** miss follow-up doctor appointments.

⊘ **DON'T** ignore your symptoms. Many serious conditions can mimic whiplash.

FROM THE DESK OF

NOTES

FOR MORE INFORMATION

Contact the following source:

• American Academy of Orthopaedic Surgeons
  Tel: (847) 823-7186
  Website: http://www.aaos.org

MANAGING YOUR CATARACTS

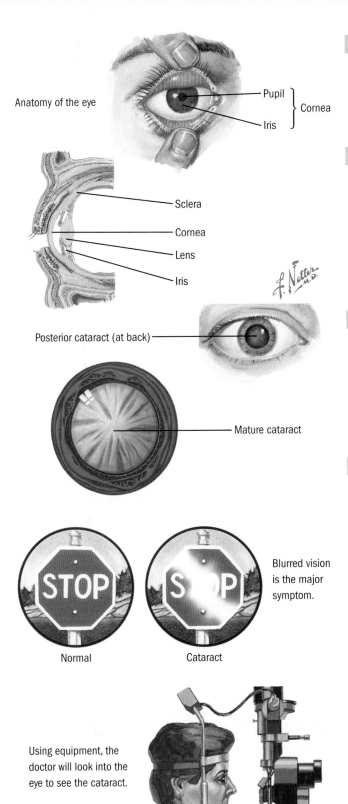

Anatomy of the eye

Pupil
Iris
} Cornea

Sclera
Cornea
Lens
Iris

Posterior cataract (at back)

Mature cataract

Blurred vision is the major symptom.

Normal   Cataract

Using equipment, the doctor will look into the eye to see the cataract.

What Are Cataracts?

A cataract is a clouding of the lens of the eye. The lens is like a glass window that we look through to see. A cataract makes it hard to see clearly.

What Causes Cataracts?

The cause of most cataracts is unknown. However, some cataracts can be caused by long-term use of steroids, redness and swelling (inflammation), infections of the eye, and illnesses such as diabetes.

Most often, cataracts develop with aging. The lens slowly becomes cloudy, thick, hard, and dry and eventually a cataract.

What Are the Symptoms of Cataracts?

The major symptom is blurred vision. At times, distance vision will be blurred more than reading vision, but at other times the reverse is true. Also, poor sight even with eyeglasses or contact lenses, ghost-like images, glare, and a halo around a light may be noticed.

How Are Cataracts Diagnosed?

Your doctor will suspect a cataract based on your history and eye exam. You will be referred to an eye specialist (optometrist or ophthalmologist), who will use equipment to look into the eye to see the cataract. An optometrist is someone who tests for vision defects to prescribe eyeglasses. An ophthalmologist is a medical doctor specializing in eye diseases.

Intraocular lens surgery

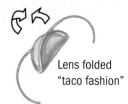
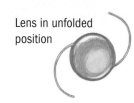

Lens in unfolded position

Lens folded "taco fashion"

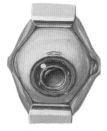

Cloud removed

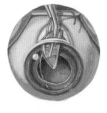
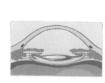
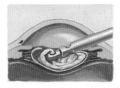

Folded IOL fitted through small incision and inserted into capsular bag → Lens unfolds in capsular bag → Single stitch closure of scleral wound

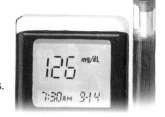

Keep your blood glucose level controlled if you have diabetes.

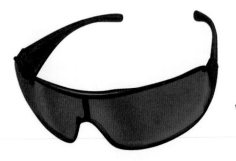

Wear sunglasses.

How Are Cataracts Treated?

Cataracts don't damage the eye. They only cause blurred vision. People who are happy with their overall vision don't need cataract surgery.

Once a person is no longer satisfied with their ability to see, and/or the doctor finds that vision is significantly impaired, cataract surgery should be considered. At times with early cataracts, vision can be improved with glasses. As the cataract progresses, just changing the glasses will not help vision.

Most cataract operations can be performed as outpatient procedures. The eye is numbed with eye drops. Medicine is given to make the person sleepy. In surgery, the clouded lens is removed and usually replaced with a permanent plastic lens, called an intraocular lens. After surgery, there are usually minimal restrictions on activities.

Cataract surgery is never performed on both eyes at the same time. People usually have surgery performed on the weaker eye first, so that they can depend on the stronger eye while the operated eye heals.

DOs and DON'Ts in Managing Cataracts:

✔ **DO** see your doctor right away if you suddenly start to have trouble seeing.

✔ **DO** have another examination if you have a cataract and notice that your vision has gotten worse. Problems other than the cataract may be occurring in the eyes.

✔ **DO** protect your eyes from injury. Wear sunglasses that block 100% of both forms of ultraviolet light, UVA and UVB, especially in sunny climates.

✔ **DO** keep your blood sugar (glucose) level well controlled if you have diabetes. Cataracts grow faster when the blood sugar level is high.

⊘ **DON'T** worry about any restrictions. People with cataracts have no specific restrictions and no specific medicines, diet, or exercises that would help.

FROM THE DESK OF

NOTES

FOR MORE INFORMATION

Contact the following source:

• American Academy of Ophthalmology
  Tel: (415) 561-8500
  Website: http://www.aao.org

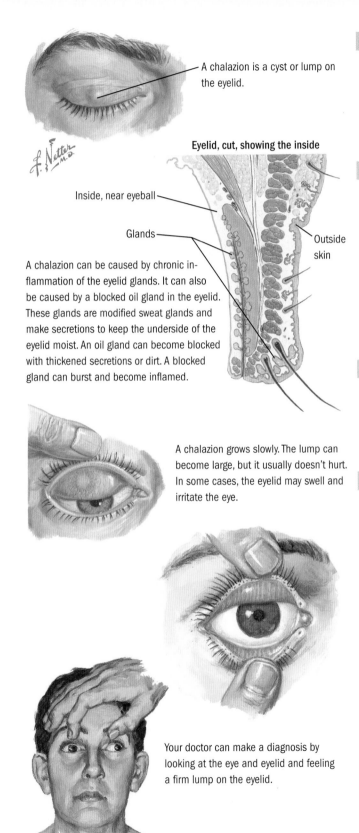

A chalazion is a cyst or lump on the eyelid.

Eyelid, cut, showing the inside

Inside, near eyeball

Glands

Outside skin

A chalazion can be caused by chronic inflammation of the eyelid glands. It can also be caused by a blocked oil gland in the eyelid. These glands are modified sweat glands and make secretions to keep the underside of the eyelid moist. An oil gland can become blocked with thickened secretions or dirt. A blocked gland can burst and become inflamed.

A chalazion grows slowly. The lump can become large, but it usually doesn't hurt. In some cases, the eyelid may swell and irritate the eye.

Your doctor can make a diagnosis by looking at the eye and eyelid and feeling a firm lump on the eyelid.

What Is a Chalazion?

A chalazion is a cyst or lump on the eyelid. Chalazions cannot be prevented. However, using little or no eye makeup, keeping the eyelids clean, and keeping the face, scalp, eyebrows, and hands clean may reduce the chances of having a chalazion.

What Causes a Chalazion?

A chalazion can be caused by chronic inflammation (swelling, redness) of the eyelid glands. It can also be caused by a blocked oil gland in the eyelid. These glands are modified sweat glands and make secretions to keep the underside of the eyelid moist. An oil gland can become blocked with thickened secretions or dirt. When the gland is blocked, it can burst and become inflamed. Sometimes bacteria grow in the blocked gland and cause an infection.

What Are the Symptoms of a Chalazion?

The main symptom is a lump in the eyelid. A chalazion grows slowly. The lump can become large, but it usually doesn't hurt. In some cases, the eyelid may swell and irritate the eye.

How Is a Chalazion Diagnosed?

The doctor can make a diagnosis by looking at the eye and eyelid and feeling a firm lump on the eyelid.

As soon as the painless swelling appears, placing a warm, moist compress on the eyelid will help open the blocked eyelash openings and glands. It also helps reduce redness and swelling. The cloth should be used for up to 10 minutes, four times per day.

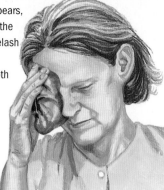

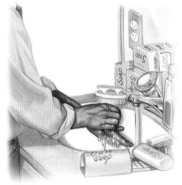

Chalazions cannot be prevented. However, using little or no eye makeup, keeping the eyelids clean, and keeping the face, scalp, eyebrows, and hands clean may reduce the chances of having a chalazion.

Don't use eyedrops or ointment that your doctor has not given to you or prescribed.

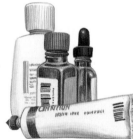

Contact your doctor if the eyelid shows no improvement after a couple of days of self-care. The doctor may remove the chalazion surgically, may inject medicine into it, or may prescribe other medicines to be applied directly to the eyelid.

How Is a Chalazion Treated?

As soon as the painless swelling appears, a warm, moist compress placed over the eyelid will help open the blocked eyelash openings and glands. It also helps reduce redness and swelling. The cloth should be kept in place for up to 10 minutes. It should be used four times per day. Squeezing the chalazion or trying to pop the chalazion should not be done.

Contact the doctor if the eyelid shows no improvement after a couple of days of self-care. The doctor may remove the chalazion surgically, may inject medicine into it, or may prescribe other medicines to be applied directly to the eyelid.

The eyelid must be gently washed with a clean wash cloth or cotton swab.

A chalazion usually goes away after 2 weeks.

DOs and DON'Ts in Managing a Chalazion:

✔ **DO** keep your face, scalp, eyebrows, and hands clean.
✔ **DO** use little or no eye makeup.
✔ **DO** tell your doctor if you don't feel well while you're using the eyedrops or pills.
✔ **DO** call your doctor if your eyelid isn't getting better, hasn't improved in 2 weeks, or is getting worse.
✔ **DO** call your doctor if you get a fever.

⊘ **DON'T** squeeze or try to break open the swollen areas.
⊘ **DON'T** use eyedrops or ointment not given to you by your doctor.
⊘ **DON'T** touch the applicator tip of your eyedrops to any other surface.
⊘ **DON'T** drive, operate machinery, or do anything that could be dangerous if your vision is blurry. Eyedrops and ointment can cause blurred vision.
⊘ **DON'T** wear contact lenses until the chalazion goes away.
⊘ **DON'T** rub your eyes.

FROM THE DESK OF

NOTES

FOR MORE INFORMATION

Contact the following source:

• American Academy of Ophthalmology
Tel: (415) 561-8500
Website: http://www.aao.org

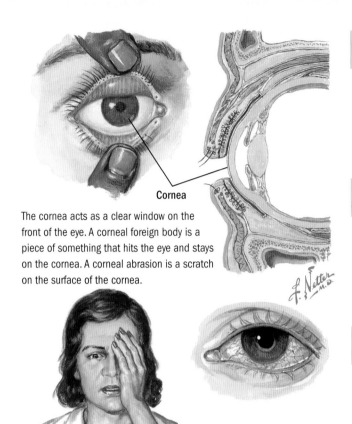

Cornea

The cornea acts as a clear window on the front of the eye. A corneal foreign body is a piece of something that hits the eye and stays on the cornea. A corneal abrasion is a scratch on the surface of the cornea.

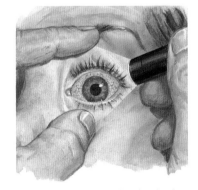

A foreign body—such as a wood sliver, piece of mascara, or damaged contact lens—scratching the cornea usually causes an abrasion. The eye becomes red, painful, and sensitive to light. Vision may be blurred. An abrasion causes redness, tearing, severe eye pain that's worse when blinking, and a feeling that something is in the eye.

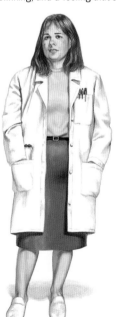

Your doctor will diagnose the abrasion by looking in your eye with a special light. Eye drops containing a dye may first be put into the eye so the doctor can see the abrasion better. The doctor will also check to see whether the foreign body is still in the eye.

What Are a Corneal Foreign Body and Corneal Abrasion?

The cornea acts as a clear window on the front of the eye. A corneal foreign body is something that hits the eye and stays on the cornea. A corneal abrasion is a scratch on the surface of the cornea.

What Causes a Corneal Foreign Body and Corneal Abrasion?

A foreign body scratching the cornea usually causes an abrasion. For example, wood slivers, pieces of mascara, or a damaged contact lens can scratch the cornea. Also, using power tools or hand tools can make something fly into the eye.

What Are the Symptoms of a Corneal Foreign Body and Corneal Abrasion?

A foreign body makes the eye red, painful, and sensitive to light. Vision may be blurred.

Main symptoms of a corneal abrasion are redness, tearing, and severe eye pain. It may be hard to keep the eye open or look at light. It may feel as if something is in the eye. Blinking makes the pain worse.

How Are a Corneal Foreign Body and Abrasion Diagnosed?

The doctor will diagnose the abrasion by looking in the eye with a special light. Eyedrops containing a dye may first be put into the eye so that the doctor can see the abrasion better. The doctor will also check to see whether the foreign body is still in the eye. If a blow to the eye caused the abrasion, a complete eye examination should be done to look for other injuries.

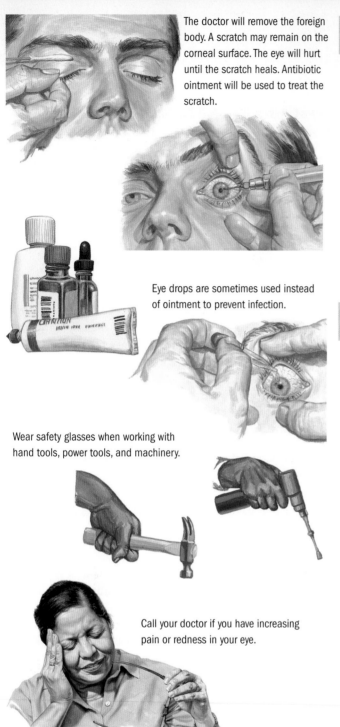

The doctor will remove the foreign body. A scratch may remain on the corneal surface. The eye will hurt until the scratch heals. Antibiotic ointment will be used to treat the scratch.

Eye drops are sometimes used instead of ointment to prevent infection.

Wear safety glasses when working with hand tools, power tools, and machinery.

Call your doctor if you have increasing pain or redness in your eye.

How Are a Corneal Foreign Body and Corneal Abrasion Treated?

The doctor will remove the foreign body. A scratch may remain on the corneal surface for a few days. The eye will hurt until the scratch heals. Antibiotic ointment or eyedrops will be used to treat the scratch. The ointment prevents infection and keeps the corneal surface moist and smooth. It stops the eyelid from rubbing against the irritated area with each blink. Eyedrops are sometimes used instead of ointment to prevent infection.

Oral medicine and moist, cold compresses can help ease pain.

A foreign body that is deeply embedded may need surgery to remove it. Corneal abrasions usually heal in a few days. Larger abrasions may take longer.

DOs and DON'Ts in Managing a Corneal Foreign Body and Corneal Abrasion:

✔ **DO** get treatment as soon as possible.
✔ **DO** use ointment or eyedrops exactly as your doctor tells you.
✔ **DO** rest your eye. Avoid prolonged eye strain.
✔ **DO** have your eye rechecked if doesn't heal after 24 hours or pain gets worse.
✔ **DO** wear safety glasses when working with hand tools, power tools, and machinery.
✔ **DO** call your doctor if you have increasing pain or redness or worsening vision.

⊘ **DON'T** touch or rub your eye, especially when you wake up.
⊘ **DON'T** wear contact lenses until the eye heals and you have finished all ointments or eyedrops for at least 1 day.
⊘ **DON'T** look at bright light.
⊘ **DON'T** use topical anesthetic for pain relief. It may delay the eye from healing.

FROM THE DESK OF

NOTES

FOR MORE INFORMATION

Contact the following sources:

• MedlinePlus
  Website: http://medlineplus.gov

• National Eye Institute, National Institutes of Health
  Tel: (301) 496-5248
  Website: http://www.nei.nih.gov/health/cornealdisease/

• American Academy of Ophthalmology
  Tel: (415) 561-8500
  Website: http://www.aao.org

MANAGING YOUR
DRY EYE

Dry eye is a very common problem. Dry eyes don't make enough tears to keep the eyes moist. Anyone can get it, but if you wear contact lenses, are over 65, or are female, you have greater risk of getting it.

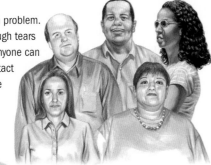

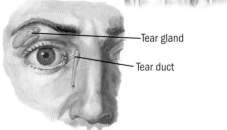

—Tear gland

—Tear duct

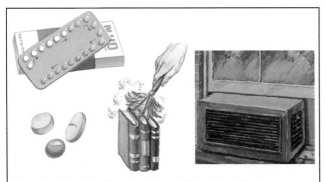

Causes include aging; drugs (such as antihistamines, blood pressure medicines, and birth control pills); living in a dry, dusty, or windy area; air conditioning; and dry heating.

You may have burning, itching, or stinging eyes; feel as if grit is in your eyes; and be sensitive to light. Stringy mucus in or around the eyes, eye fatigue, tearing, and blurred vision are other symptoms.

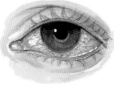

Your doctor makes a diagnosis from your description of symptoms. If an eye disorder or another illness may be causing dry eye, the doctor may suggest seeing an ophthalmologist.

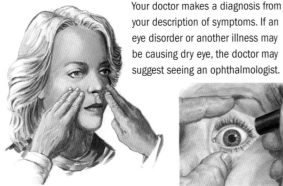

What Is Dry Eye?

Dry eye is a very common problem. Anyone can get it, but people are more likely to get it if they wear contact lenses, are over 65, or are female. Dry eyes don't make enough tears to keep the eyes moist. In time and if left untreated, dry eye can scar the eye's surface.

What Causes Dry Eye?

Usually, no serious medical problem exists. Natural aging, drugs (such as antihistamines, blood pressure medicines, and birth control pills), and living in a dry, dusty, or windy climate can cause dry eye. Other causes are air conditioning, dry heating systems, blinking problems (staring at a computer screen), and wearing contact lenses. Autoimmune diseases, such as rheumatoid arthritis, systemic lupus erythematosus, or Sjögren's syndrome, can rarely cause it. Autoimmune means that the immune system fights itself instead of disease or organisms. Some eye conditions, thyroid disease, and AIDS or HIV can also cause dry eye.

What Are the Symptoms of Dry Eye?

Symptoms include burning, itching, or stinging eyes; feeling as if grit or sand is in the eyes; and sensitivity to bright light. Stringy mucus in or around the eyes, eye fatigue, tearing, and blurred vision are other symptoms.

How Is Dry Eye Diagnosed?

The doctor makes a diagnosis from a description of symptoms. If the doctor thinks that an eye disorder or another illness is causing dry eye, the doctor may suggest seeing an ophthalmologist (specialist in eye diseases).

The specialist may do a Schirmer test. For this simple test, the doctor numbs the eye and puts little paper tabs in the lower lid. After a few minutes, the doctor removes the tabs and measures how damp they are. Tabs with too little moisture mean dry eye.

The eye doctor may also do a slit lamp examination. The slit lamp has a microscope that makes the eye appear larger, so the doctor can see more clearly if the surface of the eye has any damage.

Treatment includes using artificial tears (eye drops) during the day, ointments at night, and hot compresses and eyelid scrubs or massages with baby shampoo.

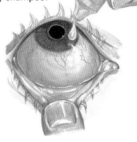

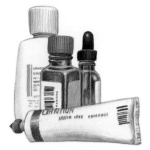

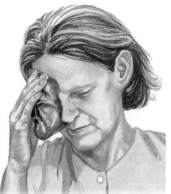

Ask your doctor how to put a hot compress on your eyes and how to do eyelid massage.

Call your doctor if you have eye pain, problems with your vision, or drainage from your eyes.

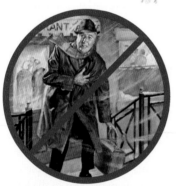

Humidifiers and air filters may help dry eye. Use a humidifier in your house and office to put extra moisture in the air. Don't go out in windy weather if you can help it.

How Is Dry Eye Treated?

Treatment includes using artificial tears, as eye drops, during the day. Ointments can add extra moisture to the eyes at night.

Other treatments include using hot compresses and eyelid scrubs or massages with baby shampoo (to give the eyes a thicker oily layer). Humidifiers, air filters, and slowing fans to stop too much air from moving can also help.

In severe cases, tiny plugs may be put into ducts that drain the tears of the eyes to provide more moisture.

DOs and DON'Ts in Managing Dry Eye:

✔ **DO** use artificial tears regularly and as often as needed to control symptoms.
✔ **DO** use a humidifier in your house and office to provide extra moisture in the air.
✔ **DO** ask your doctor how to put a hot compress on your eye and how to do eyelid massage.
✔ **DO** call your doctor if you have eye pain, problems with your vision, or drainage from your eyes.

⊘ **DON'T** use contact lenses. If you were using them, wear glasses instead.
⊘ **DON'T** use hot air vents to heat your house.
⊘ **DON'T** go out in windy weather if you can help it.

FROM THE DESK OF

NOTES

FOR MORE INFORMATION

Contact the following source:

• American Academy of Ophthalmology
  Tel: (415) 561-8500
  Website: http://www.aao.org

MANAGING YOUR GLAUCOMA

Anatomy of the eye

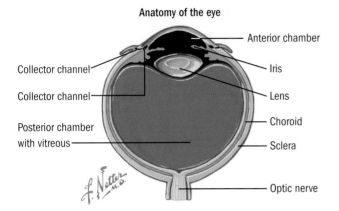

- Anterior chamber
- Iris
- Lens
- Choroid
- Sclera
- Optic nerve
- Collector channel
- Collector channel
- Posterior chamber with vitreous

Aqueous humor flows through the posterior chamber, pupil, anterior chamber, and canal of Schlemm, and leaves by collector channels.

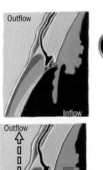

Outflow

Inflow

Normal intraocular pressure

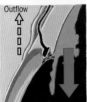

Outflow

Inflow

Increased intraocular pressure

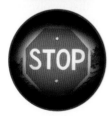

Loss of peripheral vision is a symptom of open-angle glaucoma.

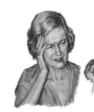

Headache, vomiting, and severe eye pain may occur with closed-angle glaucoma.

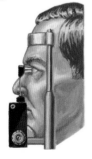

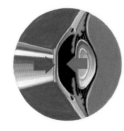

A painless test, called the Goldman tonometry test, measures eye pressure.

What Is Glaucoma?

Glaucoma is an illness caused by too much pressure in the eye (intraocular pressure, IOP). Normally, watery fluid (called aqueous humor) flows into and out of the eye. If this flow becomes blocked, pressure in the eye rises, causing glaucoma. Too much pressure can damage the eye nerve and cause vision loss. Glaucoma must be caught early to prevent this damage.

Average IOP is 16 millimeters of mercury (mm Hg). It's considered to be elevated if it is above 21 mm Hg. Glaucoma is rare before the age of 40 and becomes more common with aging. Women and people who are farsighted may have an increased risk of glaucoma.

The two types of glaucoma are open-angle and closed-angle (angle-closure). In open-angle glaucoma, flow of fluid is blocked slowly (chronic condition). In acute closed-angle glaucoma, fluid flow is blocked suddenly; this is a medical emergency. The causes of open-angle glaucoma, the most common type, are not clear.

What Are the Symptoms of Glaucoma?

Open-angle glaucoma usually produces no symptoms early on. Later, loss of side vision (or peripheral vision) may occur.

Closed-angle glaucoma can cause headache, halos around lights, loss of central vision, severe eye pain, sudden vision change, and vomiting.

How Is Glaucoma Diagnosed?

Glaucoma is easy to diagnose. An eye specialist (optometrist or ophthalmologist) measures eye pressure with a painless test called tonometry. The specialist also tests whether vision is good, especially side vision, and looks inside the eye with an instrument (ophthalmoscope).

The test of side vision is the visual field test. It can show early damage to side vision, the first sign of glaucoma.

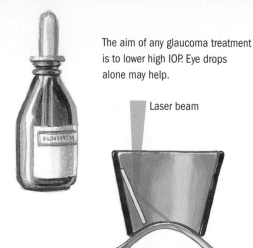

The aim of any glaucoma treatment is to lower high IOP. Eye drops alone may help.

Laser beam

Laser sites

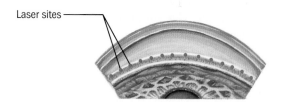

Laser surgery or other operations may be necessary. Often people continue to use eye drops after laser surgery.

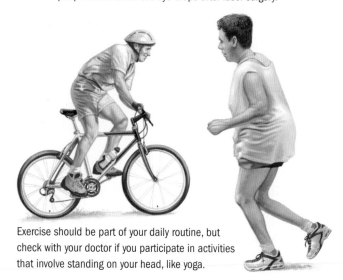

Exercise should be part of your daily routine, but check with your doctor if you participate in activities that involve standing on your head, like yoga.

How Is Glaucoma Treated?

Treatment—eye drops and surgery—is aimed at lowering a high IOP to a more normal IOP.

Some people need only one or two different eye drops. These drops, however, can affect other parts of the body. For example, eye drops that are beta-blockers should be used carefully in people with asthma or breathing or cardiac problems.

Other people need laser surgery or other types of surgery. Laser surgery can be quite effective, but many people will need to continue using eye drops after surgery.

Other operations for glaucoma involve making a new drain to let aqueous fluid flow out faster, so IOP is lowered.

DOs and DON'Ts in Managing Glaucoma:

✔ **DO** take all the medicine prescribed by your doctor. Use it exactly as directed. Once you begin to use the medicine, you will probably use it indefinitely.

✔ **DO** tell your eye doctor if you have another medical illness (e.g., asthma, heart problems, or emphysema) or an allergy to drugs used for glaucoma.

✔ **DO** tell your eye doctor about all medicines you take, because these may interfere with glaucoma medicines.

✔ **DO** call your eye doctor immediately if your symptoms get worse.

⊘ **DON'T** stop taking your medicine or change your dose because you are feeling better.

⊘ **DON'T** use corticosteroids such as prednisone without checking with your eye doctor, because these drugs can raise eye pressure.

⊘ **DON'T** do exercises, such as yoga, that involve standing on the head, but do exercise normally.

FROM THE DESK OF

NOTES

FOR MORE INFORMATION

Contact the following source:

• American Academy of Ophthalmology
Tel: (415) 561-8500
Website: http://www.aao.org

MANAGING YOUR
MACULAR DEGENERATION

Macular degeneration is an eye disease that involves loss of central vision and damage to the macula. It can be wet or dry. It is a main cause of blindness in the United States. It increases with age. Most cases occur between ages 75 and 80.

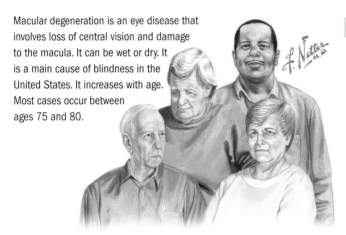

Eyeball

Cornea

Lens

Retina

Retina

Retina

Macula

The macula is in the center of the retina at the back of the eye. It lets you see fine detail.

In wet macular degeneration, abnormal blood vessels at the back of the eye grow and leak blood and fluid. An early symptom is that straight lines look wavy.

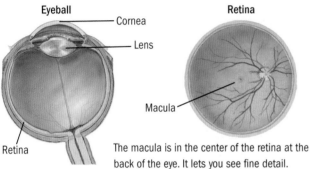

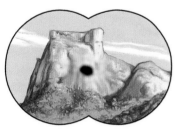

Dry macular degeneration occurs when light-sensitive cells in the macula slowly break down. The most common symptom is blurred vision that leads to central vision loss. As dry macular degeneration gets worse, a blurred spot is seen in the center of vision.

Drusen

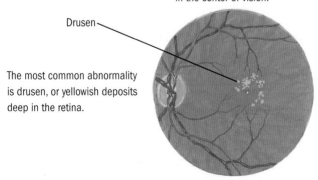

The most common abnormality is drusen, or yellowish deposits deep in the retina.

What Is Macular Degeneration?

The macula is in the center of the retina of the eye. It lets fine detail be seen. The retina is the light-sensitive part at the back of the eye. The retina changes light, or an image, into electrical impulses. These electrical impulses then go to the brain. Macular degeneration is an eye disease that involves loss of central vision and damage to the macula. It has two forms: wet and dry.

Macular degeneration is a main cause of blindness in the United States. It increases with age, with most cases occurring between ages 75 and 80.

What Causes Macular Degeneration?

Wet macular degeneration occurs when abnormal blood vessels behind the retina start to grow under the macula. These new vessels tend to be fragile and leak blood and fluid. The blood and fluid raise the macula from its normal place. Central vision loss tends to occur quickly.

Dry macular degeneration occurs when light-sensitive cells in the macula slowly break down. The loss of central vision is more gradual.

What Are the Symptoms of Macular Degeneration?

The most common symptom of dry macular degeneration is blurred vision that leads to central vision loss. As dry macular degeneration gets worse, a blurred spot is seen in the center of vision. An early symptom of wet macular degeneration is that straight lines look wavy.

The most common abnormality seen on physical exam is drusen, or yellowish deposits deep in the retina.

Unlike wet macular degeneration, dry macular degeneration has three stages, which may occur in one or both eyes. In stage I (early), several small drusen or a few medium-sized drusen are seen. People have no symptoms and no vision loss. In stage II (intermediate), many medium-sized drusen or one or more large drusen are seen. Some people see a blurred central spot. In stage III (advanced), people have drusen and blurred central vision. It's harder to read and recognize faces until they're very close.

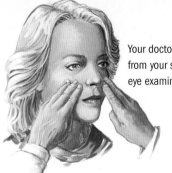

Your doctor makes a diagnosis from your symptoms and a full eye examination.

Early treatment from an ophthalmologist is very important. Treatment can delay and maybe prevent intermediate disease from getting worse. No treatment can stop vision loss in advanced disease. Antioxidants and zinc may slow progression.

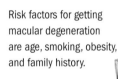

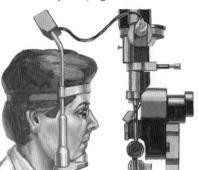

Treatment of wet macular degeneration involves laser surgery or photodynamic therapy. Neither is a cure, but they may slow the rate of vision loss.

Risk factors for getting macular degeneration are age, smoking, obesity, and family history.

Call your doctor if you have blurred vision, you notice that straight lines look wavy, or you have vision changes.

How Is Macular Degeneration Diagnosed?

The doctor makes a diagnosis from symptoms and a full eye examination.

How Is Macular Degeneration Treated?

Early treatment from an ophthalmologist (specialist in eye diseases) is very important. If dry macular degeneration is advanced, no treatment can stop vision loss. Treatment can delay and maybe prevent intermediate disease from getting worse. Antioxidants and zinc may slow progression of ARMD.

Treatment of wet macular degeneration involves laser surgery or photodynamic therapy. Neither is a cure, but they may slow the rate of vision loss.

Newer treatment modalities include injections in the eye (intravenous) of substances known as monoclonal antibodies and antivascular endothelial growth factor. These injections tend to be very expensive.

DOs and DON'Ts in Managing Macular Degeneration:

✔ **DO** realize that an antioxidant-zinc medicine isn't a cure. It won't restore lost vision, but it may delay the start of advanced disease.

✔ **DO** call your doctor if you have blurred vision, you notice wavy lines that should be straight, or you have changes in your vision.

⊘ **DON'T** forget that age is the major risk factor for developing macular degeneration. Other risk factors include smoking, obesity, and family history.

FROM THE DESK OF

NOTES

FOR MORE INFORMATION

Contact the following source:

• National Eye Institute, National Institutes of Health
Tel: (301) 496-5248
Website: http://www.nei.nih.gov/health/maculardegen/ armd_facts.asp

MANAGING YOUR
SJÖGREN'S SYNDROME

Sjögren's syndrome is an autoimmune disease involving inflammation of glands that make tears, saliva, and other substances. It affects more than 1 million adults in the United States; more women than men get it, rarely before age 20.

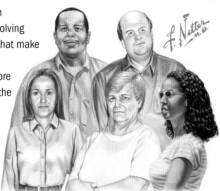

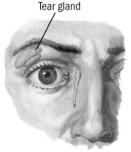

Tear gland

Salivary glands

The tear and salivary glands are most commonly affected, but inflammation of joints, lungs, kidneys, blood vessels, nerves, and muscles can also occur.

The most common symptoms are dry eyes and mouth. Others are dry lips and throat, aches and pains, swollen cheek glands, tiredness, and dry vagina.

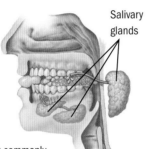

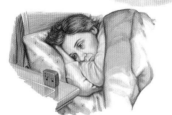

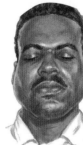

Your doctor will make a diagnosis from your medical history, physical examination, blood tests, and tests for Sjögren's antibodies. Your doctor may do a Schirmer test and lip biopsy.

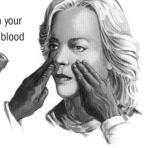

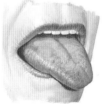

What Is Sjögren's Syndrome?

Sjögren's syndrome is an illness caused by inflammation of glands that make tears, saliva, and other substances. Inflammation of joints, lungs, kidneys, blood vessels, nerves, and muscles can also occur.

This syndrome affects one in every 250 adults in the United States. It occurs nine times more often in women than in men. It rarely develops before age 20.

What Causes Sjögren's Syndrome?

The syndrome occurs when the body's own immune system attacks glands that make saliva and tears and makes them stop working. The cause is unknown, but some hereditary and environmental factors may increase chances having it. The syndrome isn't contagious.

What Are the Symptoms of Sjögren's Syndrome?

The most common symptoms are dry eyes and dry mouth. Dry eyes may cause a sandy feeling under the eyelids, burning eyes, increased sensitivity to light, reduced tears, and eye ulcers. A dry mouth may cause problems chewing and swallowing dry foods and an increased tooth decay, gum disease, and mouth infections. Other symptoms include blurred vision, dry lips and throat, fever, itchy eyes, joint pain, mouth sores, red eyes, rash, shortness of breath, stomach pain, swollen cheek glands, swollen lymph nodes (glands), thirst, tiredness, and dry vagina. Vaginal dryness can cause pain with sex.

How Is Sjögren's Syndrome Diagnosed?

The doctor will make a diagnosis from a medical history, physical examination, and laboratory tests. These tests may include an erythrocyte sedimentation rate (ESR) (to measure inflammation), a complete blood cell count (CBC), and tests for Sjögren's antibodies. The doctor may do a Schirmer test to find out the amount of tears in the eyes and a lip biopsy.

An ophthalmologist (eye doctor) and a rheumatologist (specialist in joint problems) may help with care.

Over-the-counter moisturizers for dry eyes, mouth, and vagina may help. NSAIDs may reduce joint pain and swelling.

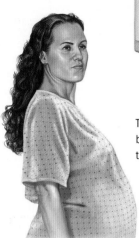

Tell your doctor if you're pregnant or breastfeeding. Use a humidifier at night to prevent dry eyes, mouth, and nose.

Ask your doctor what over-the-counter products you can use for dryness. If an artificial tear medicine burns your eyes, switch to another one or one without a preservative. An eye ointment may help dry eyes at night. Vaginal lubricants used during the day or before sex can also help. Use a cream or ointment for dry skin.

Don't smoke. Smoking can make symptoms worse.

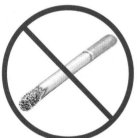

Call your doctor if you have severe stomach pain, eye pain, or sudden vision change.

How Is Sjögren's Syndrome Treated?

There's no cure, but medicines and other therapies can manage the syndrome. Over-the-counter moisturizers for dry eyes, mouth, and vagina may help. Nonsteroidal antiinflammatory drugs (NSAIDs) may help joint pain and swelling. Prednisone and other medicines may be used for severe joint pain or lung, kidney, and blood vessel problems.

DOs and DON'Ts in Managing Sjögren's Syndrome:

✔ **DO** tell your doctor about your medicines, both prescription and over-the-counter.

✔ **DO** tell your doctor if you're pregnant or breastfeeding.

✔ **DO** see your dentist regularly. Brush and floss your teeth after meals.

✔ **DO** ask your doctor what over-the-counter products are available for dryness. If an artificial tear medicine burns your eyes, switch to another one or one without a preservative. If your eyes get dry at night, an eye ointment may help. Vaginal lubricants used during the day or before sex can also help.

✔ **DO** use a cream or ointment for dry skin. These help seal in moisture.

✔ **DO** use a humidifier at night to prevent dry eyes, mouth, and nose.

✔ **DO** call your doctor if you have severe stomach pain, eye pain, or sudden vision change.

⊘ **DON'T** stop taking your medicine or change your dosage because you feel better unless your doctor says to.

⊘ **DON'T** smoke. Smoking can make symptoms worse.

FOR MORE INFORMATION

Contact the following sources:

• Sjögren's Syndrome Foundation
Tel: (800) 475-6473
Website: http://www.sjogrens.org

• American College of Rheumatology
Tel: (404) 633-3777
Website: http://www.rheumatology.org

• The Arthritis Foundation
Tel: (800) 283-7800
Website: http://www.arthritis.org

FROM THE DESK OF

NOTES

MANAGING YOUR
STRABISMUS

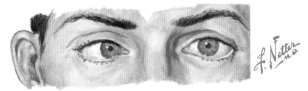

Strabismus is a condition in which the eyes don't move in the same direction. Instead, they point in different directions. One or both eyes may turn either in or out. Over time, the weaker eye becomes "lazier" as the brain uses signals from the stronger eye.

Strabismus runs in some families. Treatment can correct this condition, but without early treatment, some vision may be lost.

Muscles around the eye

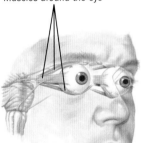

Strabismus has two causes. The first is a difference in strength of muscles around each eye. The second is a difference in each eye's ability to focus.

Strabismus usually appears in early to middle childhood. It can also occur at birth, but it's hard to diagnose it until 3 months of age, because at birth the eyes cannot focus well. In adults, a disease such as diabetes or stroke or an injury to the eye can cause it.

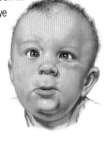

The main symptom is that the eyes seem to look in two different directions. Squinting, frequent eye rubbing, and tilting of the head are common. Double vision and vision in only one eye are other symptoms.

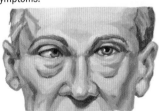

What Is Strabismus?

Strabismus is a condition in which the eyes don't move in the same direction. They appear to point in different directions. One or both eyes may turn either in or out. Over time, the weaker eye becomes "lazier," or less used, as the brain uses signals from the stronger eye.

Strabismus runs in some families. Treatment can correct this condition, but without early treatment, some vision may be lost.

What Causes Strabismus?

Strabismus has two causes. The first is a difference in strength of muscles around each eye. The second is a difference in each eye's ability to focus. If either the muscle strength or focus of one eye is weaker, that eye may start to drift. Strabismus usually appears in early to middle childhood. It can also occur as early as at birth, but it's hard to diagnose strabismus until 3 months of age, because at birth the eyes cannot focus well. Adults can also develop strabismus. In adults, a disease such as diabetes or stroke or injury to the eye can cause it.

What Are the Symptoms of Strabismus?

The main symptom is that the eyes seem to look in two different directions. Squinting, frequent eye rubbing, and tilting of the head are common. Double vision and vision in only one eye are other symptoms.

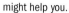

Your doctor will diagnose strabismus by examining your eyes. You may be referred to an eye specialist (ophthalmologist) who will check nerves and muscles around your eyes to see whether surgery might help you.

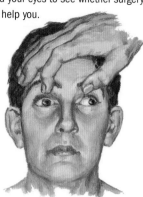

The treatment goal is to make the weaker eye stronger. To do this, you may use glasses or an eye patch over the stronger eye. Your doctor may suggest doing eye muscle exercises. Sometimes, surgery is needed to balance the muscle strength between the two eyes.

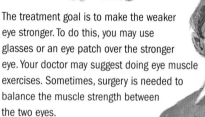

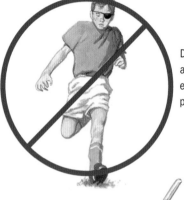

Don't run when you're adjusting to wearing an eye patch. This helps prevent falls and injury.

Call your doctor if you get a fever or pain and redness in the eye after surgery.

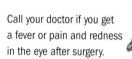

How Is Strabismus Diagnosed?

The doctor will make a diagnosis by doing an eye examination. The examination may include looking through a set of prisms to find the differences between the eyes. The eye exam may also include a visual acuity test, examination of the retina, and a neurological examination. Your doctor may suggest seeing an ophthalmologist (specialist in eye disorders). The specialist will also check nerves and muscles around the eyes. Then, decisions about whether surgery might fix the problem can be made.

Children should usually have their eyes examined every 1 to 4 months until the eyes are stable. After that, they may need examinations every 6 months until the age of 6 years. Annual examinations should follow until age 9 to 11.

How Is Strabismus Treated?

The goal of treatment is to make the weaker eye stronger. To do this, glasses or an eye patch over the stronger eye may be used. This forces the weaker eye to become stronger. The doctor may suggest doing eye muscle exercises. Sometimes, surgery is needed to balance the muscle strength between the two eyes.

DOs and DON'Ts in Managing Strabismus:

✔ **DO** wear the patch or eyeglasses, or both, given to you by your doctor.
✔ **DO** call your doctor if you get a fever or pain and redness in the eye after surgery.

🚫 **DON'T** run when you're adjusting to wearing an eye patch. This will help prevent falls and injury.

FROM THE DESK OF

NOTES

FOR MORE INFORMATION

Contact the following source:

• American Academy of Ophthalmology
  Tel: (415) 561-8500
  Website: http://www.aao.org

MANAGING YOUR
STY

A sty, or hordeolum, looks like a pimple next to an eyelash. It starts when the opening in the eyelid for the eyelash (or root of the eyelash) becomes blocked with oil or dirt. Bacteria then grow and cause an infection. It can form on the inside or outside of the eyelid. People of any age can have one.

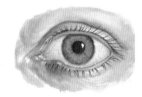

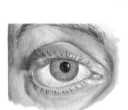

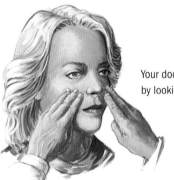

Symptoms are redness, tenderness, and swelling on the eyelid. The eye may water and may be sensitive to light. Sometimes the whole eyelid swells.

Your doctor will make this diagnosis by looking at your eye and eyelid.

A warm, wet compress placed on the eye helps open blocked eyelash holes and oil glands. It also helps reduce redness and swelling.

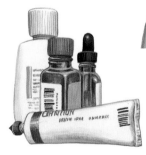

Your doctor may prescribe an antibiotic, as an ointment or eye drops, if an infection is present. Sometimes, over-the-counter pain medicines can help discomfort.

What Is a Sty?

A sty, which is also known by the medical term hordeolum, looks like a pimple next to an eyelash. It starts quickly, when the opening in the eyelid for the eyelash (or root of the eyelash) becomes blocked. It can form on the inside or outside of the eyelid. People of any age can have a sty.

What Causes a Sty?

The opening for the eyelash becoming blocked with oil or dirt will lead to a sty. After the hole is blocked, bacteria grow inside and cause an infection. The kind of bacteria called *Staphylococcus aureus* causes the infection in almost all cases.

What Are the Symptoms of a Sty?

Symptoms are redness, tenderness, and swelling on the eyelid. The eye may water and may be sensitive to light. Sometimes the whole eyelid swells.

How Is a Sty Diagnosed?

The doctor will make this diagnosis by looking at the eye and eyelid.

How Is a Sty Treated?

A warm, wet compress placed on the eye helps open blocked eyelash holes and oil glands. It also helps reduce redness and swelling. The cloth should remain in place for up to 10 minutes. The compress should be applied four times a day.

The doctor may prescribe an antibiotic if an infection is present. Usually, the antibiotic is given in an ointment or eye drops. Rarely, a pill is also given. Other types of eye drops are sometimes used to help take away swelling. Sometimes, over-the-counter pain medicines can help discomfort.

In some cases, the doctor may make a small cut in the swollen area to let the pus drain, or send you to an ophthalmologist to have it lanced.

A sty usually goes away in 5 to 7 days. After that time, the swollen area opens and pus drains out.

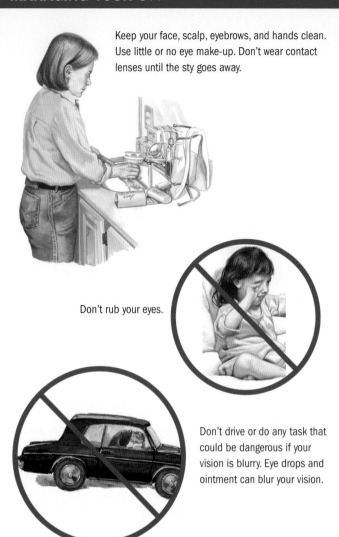

Keep your face, scalp, eyebrows, and hands clean. Use little or no eye make-up. Don't wear contact lenses until the sty goes away.

Don't rub your eyes.

Don't drive or do any task that could be dangerous if your vision is blurry. Eye drops and ointment can blur your vision.

Call your doctor if your eyelid isn't getting better or is getting worse, you develop a fever, the sty bleeds, the bump becomes very large or painful, a blister forms on your eyelid, or your whole eyelid or eye is red.

DOs and DON'Ts in Managing a Sty:

✔ **DO** keep your face, scalp, eyebrows, and hands clean.

✔ **DO** use little or no eye make-up.

✔ **DO** call your doctor if your eyelid isn't getting better or if it's getting worse.

✔ **DO** call your doctor if the sty hasn't improved in 2 weeks.

✔ **DO** call your doctor if you develop a fever.

✔ **DO** call your doctor if you have trouble with your vision.

✔ **DO** call your doctor if the sty bleeds, the bump becomes very large or painful, a blister forms on your eyelid, or your whole eyelid or eye is red.

⊘ **DON'T** squeeze or try to break open the sty.

⊘ **DON'T** use eye drops or ointments not given to you by your doctor.

⊘ **DON'T** touch the eye drop applicator tip to any surface.

⊘ **DON'T** drive, operate machinery, or do any task that could be dangerous if your vision is blurry. Eye drops and ointment can cause blurry vision.

⊘ **DON'T** wear contact lenses until the sty goes away.

⊘ **DON'T** rub your eyes.

FROM THE DESK OF

NOTES

FOR MORE INFORMATION

Contact the following source:

• American Academy of Ophthalmology
Tel: (415) 561-8500
Website: http://www.aao.org

MANAGING YOUR
ACHILLES TENDON RUPTURE

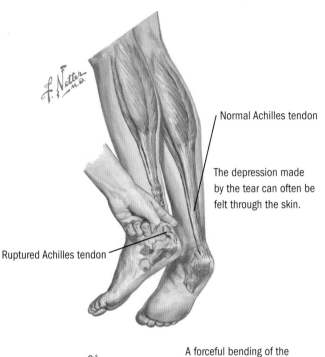

Normal Achilles tendon

The depression made by the tear can often be felt through the skin.

Ruptured Achilles tendon

0°

20°

50°

A forceful bending of the foot toward the shin is often the cause of the tear.

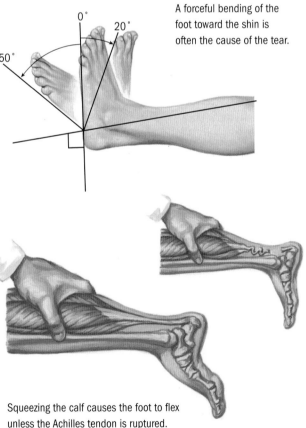

Squeezing the calf causes the foot to flex unless the Achilles tendon is ruptured.

What Is Achilles Tendon Rupture?

A tendon is a band of tough tissue that usually connects muscle to bone. The Achilles tendon is the tendon connecting the calf muscles to the heel. Achilles tendon rupture is a common injury of this tendon. It often occurs in 40- to 50-year-old men who sometimes do athletic activities but can occur at any age.

What Causes Achilles Tendon Rupture?

The tendon can rupture or tear partly or completely by jumping, forcefully bending the foot toward the shin, or receiving a direct hit. Certain medications such as quinolone antibiotics can increase the risk of tendon rupture.

What Are the Symptoms of Achilles Tendon Rupture?

The most common symptom is stabbing pain in the lower calf at the time of injury.

Walking without pain is often impossible, especially when trying to push off the toe. Swelling occurs, and calf muscles may appear bunched up. Standing on tiptoe on the injured foot may also be impossible.

How Is Achilles Tendon Rupture Diagnosed?

The doctor uses a history and physical examination. The doctor will also do a Thompson test, or squeeze test. With a normal or partially torn tendon, squeezing calf muscles causes the ankle to flex. With an Achilles tendon rupture, this squeezing doesn't produce the ankle motion.

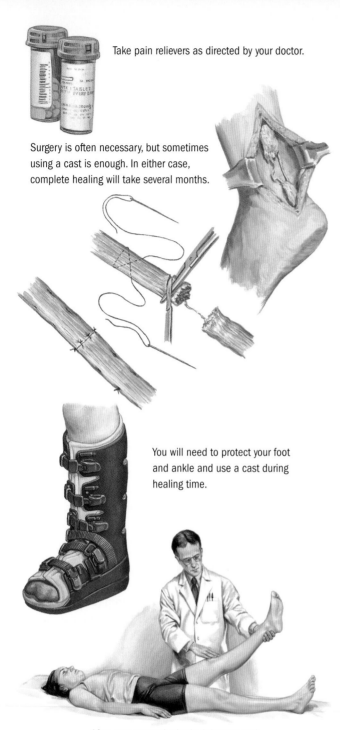

Take pain relievers as directed by your doctor.

Surgery is often necessary, but sometimes using a cast is enough. In either case, complete healing will take several months.

You will need to protect your foot and ankle and use a cast during healing time.

After cast removal, physical therapy and exercise often lead to full recovery.

How Is Achilles Tendon Rupture Treated?

The rupture is sometimes treated with casts but most commonly surgery is used. After surgery, the foot is immobilized with casts in different positions. The doctor will probably suggest using a heel lift or high-heeled shoe for a certain period after the casts are removed.

If the ends of the tendon can reattach without surgery, your doctor may suggest a cast for 10 to 12 weeks, with two cast changes, and then use of a heel lift.

Recovery is slow and may take up to 6 months, but with exercise and physical therapy, most people recover completely.

DOs and DON'Ts in Managing Achilles Tendon Rupture:

✔ **DO** take pain medicines as prescribed.

✔ **DO** protect your cast. It is critical to protect the tendon until it has a chance to heal.

✔ **DO** follow physical therapy and exercise instructions to recover muscle strength and range of motion at the ankle.

✔ **DO** use proper conditioning to prevent another tendon injury. If you have a partial tear, you must follow your rehabilitation program exactly. A complete rupture is possible if the tendon is stressed too much.

✔ **DO** call your doctor if you damage your cast or have another injury.

✔ **DO** call your doctor if you have increasing pain in the calf, cannot rise onto tiptoe or walk, or have increased swelling at the injury site.

⊘ **DON'T** remove or damage your cast. If you tear the repair, treatment starts over again, which will prolong time for complete healing.

⊘ **DON'T** do anything that will cause excessive force on the tendon until healing is complete.

⊘ **DON'T** have cortisone or steroid injections around the Achilles tendon. Such injections have a significant risk for tendon rupture.

FROM THE DESK OF

NOTES

FOR MORE INFORMATION

Contact the following sources:

* American Academy of Family Physicians
  Website: http://www.familydoctor.org

* American Medical Association
  Website: http://www.ama-assn.org

MANAGING YOUR
ANKLE FRACTURE

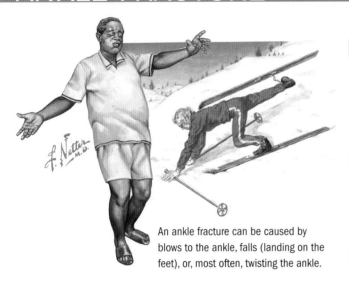

An ankle fracture can be caused by blows to the ankle, falls (landing on the feet), or, most often, twisting the ankle.

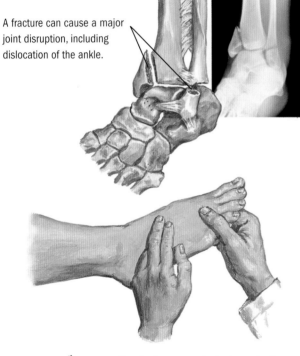

A fracture can cause a major joint disruption, including dislocation of the ankle.

The doctor uses a physical examination and x-rays to diagnose the injury.

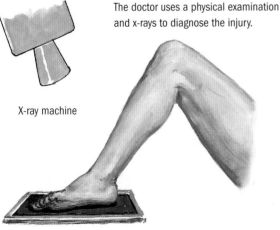

X-ray machine

What Is an Ankle Fracture?

An ankle fracture is a break in any bone of the ankle joint. It may be mild (like a bad sprain) or severe (including joint dislocation). Long-term pain and disability are possible.

What Causes an Ankle Fracture?

Causes include blows to the ankle, falls (landing on the feet), or, most often, twisting the ankle.

What Are the Symptoms of an Ankle Fracture?

Symptoms are pain, especially when putting weight on or moving the ankle, swelling, bruising, and a deformed joint.

How Is an Ankle Fracture Diagnosed?

The doctor uses a physical examination and x-rays.

How Is an Ankle Fracture Treated?

Treatment may be similar to treatment of a sprain (rest, ice, elevation, compression, and using a brace for protection). It may involve surgery and use of screws and plates to hold bones together during healing.

Most often, a cast or removable splint holds bones in position until they heal. If a cast is used, lower leg muscles will be a bit weak after removal of the cast. Physical therapy will help this common side effect. Complications include failure to heal, poor blood flow to the foot or toes (if cast is too tight or swelling occurs in the cast), and infection or bleeding related to surgery.

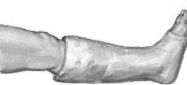

Keep your foot elevated for the first few days to minimize swelling. Using a cast or removable splint that holds bones in a stable position until they heal is the most common treatment.

Don't get a plaster cast wet. Even a fiberglass cast takes a long time to dry. Don't remove your plastic or metal splint unless instructed to. It can't keep your bones in position for healing unless it stays in place.

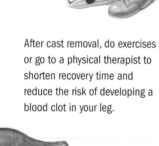

After cast removal, do exercises or go to a physical therapist to shorten recovery time and reduce the risk of developing a blood clot in your leg.

FROM THE DESK OF

NOTES

DOs and DON'Ts in Managing an Ankle Fracture:

✔ **DO** reduce the risk of injury by warming up and stretching before exercising.

✔ **DO** use good running shoes and run on an even surface.

✔ **DO** reduce your weight, if overweight.

✔ **DO** keep fit.

✔ **DO** take pain medicines as prescribed.

✔ **DO** eat a diet with enough calcium to help healing.

✔ **DO** keep your foot raised for the first few days and apply ice to your ankle the first day or so, to minimize swelling.

✔ **DO** exercises or go to a physical therapist after cast removal to shorten recovery time and reduce the risk of developing a blood clot in the leg.

✔ **DO** call your doctor if you notice numbness, tingling, coldness, or darkening of your toes. The cast may be too tight or the ankle may be swollen, reducing blood circulation to your foot.

✔ **DO** call your doctor if you damage your splint or cast so that it is loose or allows your ankle to move more than it should.

✔ **DO** call your doctor if, after surgery, you have fever or you see redness, swelling, or pus at the incision (suggesting infection).

✔ **DO** call your doctor if you have increasing pain or cannot use your ankle at some time after surgery.

✔ **DO** call your doctor if you notice pain or swelling in your calf or leg, which may mean a blood clot.

⊘ **DON'T** spend too much time on your feet or with your foot hanging down. Don't put heat on the ankle. Swelling may hurt circulation.

⊘ **DON'T** get a plaster or fiberglass cast wet.

⊘ **DON'T** stick things such as coat hangers, pencils, or knitting needles down the cast to scratch. If you poke the skin, you may get an infection.

⊘ **DON'T** remove your cast too soon. Early removal may allow another injury.

FOR MORE INFORMATION

Contact the following sources:

• American Trauma Society
Tel: (800) 556-7890
Website: http://www.amtrauma.org

• American Academy of Orthopaedic Surgeons
Tel: (847) 823-7186
Website: http://www.aaos.org

• The American Orthopaedic Society for Sports Medicine
Tel: (847) 292-4900
Fax: (847) 292-4905
Website: http://www.sportsmed.org

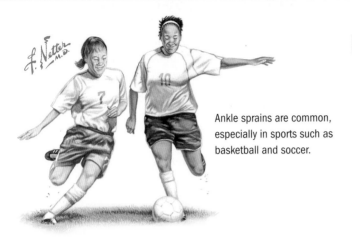

Ankle sprains are common, especially in sports such as basketball and soccer.

Various types of sprains:

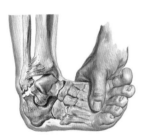

Inversion sprain (calcaneo-fibular and talo-fibular ligaments)

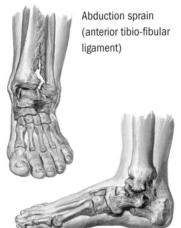

Abduction sprain (anterior tibio-fibular ligament)

Abduction sprain (deltoid ligament)

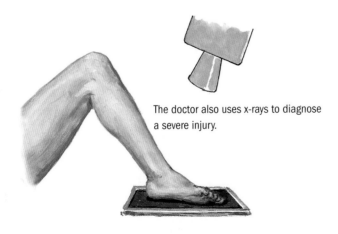

The doctor also uses x-rays to diagnose a severe injury.

What Are Ankle Sprains?

Ankle sprains are injuries resulting from stretching, or partly or completely tearing one or more ligaments holding the ankle joint together. Ligaments are bands of strong, flexible fibers connecting bones. Tendons connect muscles and bones. Ankle sprains are common, especially in sports such as basketball and soccer.

What Causes Ankle Sprains?

Sprains occur when the joint is forced to bend more than normal, thus hurting ligaments. The most common type occurs when the foot turns in (called inversion), and full body weight comes down on the ankle. The foot can also turn too far out (called eversion).

What Are the Symptoms of Ankle Sprains?

Popping or tearing is felt at the time of injury. Pain occurs during the injury and after, when walking or moving the ankle. The ankle may swell and feel stiff. The skin around the ankle may be bruised.

With severe injuries, extreme pain makes weight bearing and moving the ankle hard. Tingling or numbness in the foot may mean nerve or blood vessel damage.

How Are Ankle Sprains Diagnosed?

The doctor will ask about the accident and examine the ankle by moving it to check ligaments and tendons.

For a minor sprain, no more tests are needed. For a severe sprain, the doctor may order x-rays or magnetic resonance imaging (MRI).

At first, treatment includes applying ice to the injury right away, using a compression wrap or air splint on the injured area, and elevating the ankle above the level of the hip. Then, while resting your ankle, stretch it gently to keep it from becoming stiff.

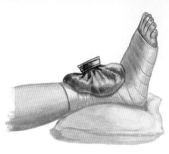

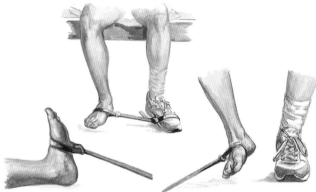

Your doctor may recommend exercises or physical therapy to help you heal, strengthen muscles, and try to prevent future injuries. Over-the-counter pain pills may help.

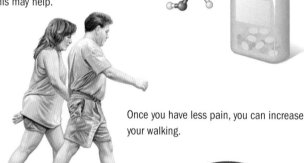

Once you have less pain, you can increase your walking.

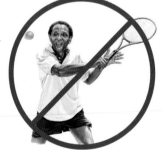

Avoid all activities that will increase swelling, because it will slow your return to complete activity.

How Are Ankle Sprains Treated?

Ice is applied immediately, because swelling starts quickly. The ankle is rested, which may mean using crutches. Walking is kept to a minimum. A compression wrap or splint is put on the ankle. The ankle is elevated above hip level. Remember these by thinking "RICE" (*R*est, *I*ce, *C*ompression, *E*levation). A compression wrap, splint, or brace lets the ankle move without injury. Never use heat before 72 hours after the injury (causes more swelling).

Physical therapy can strengthen muscles, help recovery, and help prevent more injuries.

Over-the-counter pain pills (ibuprofen or acetaminophen) can be taken.

Severe sprains may need surgery and physical therapy.

DOs and DON'Ts in Managing an Ankle Sprain:

✔ **DO** warm up and stretch before exercising.
✔ **DO** wear ankle braces when playing sports if you often get sprains.
✔ **DO** lose weight, if overweight.
✔ **DO** keep fit.
✔ **DO** take medicines and use crutches prescribed by your doctor.
✔ **DO** follow RICE and physical therapy instructions.
✔ **DO** call your doctor if you can't walk on your injured ankle, swelling hasn't left after 2 days or increases, the ankle becomes redder or hot, you have a fever, or you notice popping, catching, or the ankle giving way.
✔ **DO** call your doctor if your foot is numb, tingling, or is a blue or dusky color; or your toes are cold (signs of cut-off circulation).
✔ **DO** call your doctor if you don't see improvement in 7 to 10 days after the sprain.
✔ **DO** call your doctor if you have pain or swelling in the leg (may mean a blood clot).

⊘ **DON'T** do activities that will increase swelling. Avoid early use of heat or too much activity, standing, or sitting with the ankle hanging.
⊘ **DON'T** play sports again until pain and swelling are gone and the ankle is strong.

FROM THE DESK OF

NOTES

FOR MORE INFORMATION

Contact the following sources:

• The American Orthopaedic Society for Sports Medicine
Tel: (847) 292-4900
Fax: (847) 292-4905
Website: http://www.sportsmed.org

• American College of Sports Medicine
Tel: (317) 637-9200
Website: http://www.acsm.org

MANAGING YOUR
ANKYLOSING SPONDYLITIS

Normal vertebal column

Column with ankylosing spondylitis

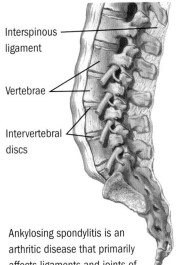

Interspinous ligament

Vertebrae

Intervertebral discs

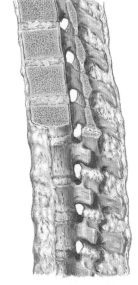

Ankylosing spondylitis is an arthritic disease that primarily affects ligaments and joints of the spine and leads to pain, stiffness, and limited range of motion of the lower back.

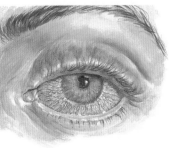

The most common symptom is lower back pain. It can also cause inflammation of the eye, called iritis, and lead to eye pain, redness, and loss of visual sharpness if not treated in a timely fashion.

The doctor uses x-rays for diagnosis.

Radiograph shows ankylosis of sacroiliac joint.

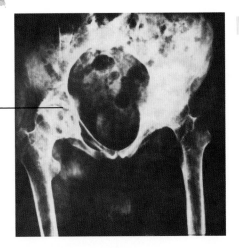

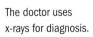

What Is Ankylosing Spondylitis?

Ankylosing spondylitis is a painful, arthritic condition most often found in men younger than 40, although women and children can have it. Ankylosing means joining together, and spondylitis refers to inflammation (swelling) in joints of the spine. Joints of the lower back can fuse, resulting in stooped posture.

Swelling in ligaments attaching to bones causes bone to wear away and then try to heal. New bone replaces elastic tissue called ligaments (ligaments connect bones), and stiffness occurs.

Most often affected are the lower back, chest, and neck. Other affected joints can include hips, shoulders, knees, and ankles. The illness can also affect other organs, such as eyes, heart, and lungs.

What Causes Ankylosing Spondylitis?

The cause is unknown, but it is an autoimmune disease. This means that the body attacks itself, the result being inflammation. People with a gene called HLA-B27 are more likely to get this illness than people without the gene.

What Are the Symptoms of Ankylosing Spondylitis?

The most common symptom is back pain that may start gradually. Early morning stiffness and pain go away during the day with exercise. People lose weight. People feel weak, tired, and feverish and have severe twinges or nagging aches down one leg or through the buttock. People also have night sweats, limited range of motion, stooped posture, and trouble breathing.

How Is Ankylosing Spondylitis Diagnosed?

The doctor takes a medical history, does a physical examination, and gets x-rays of the lower (lumbar) spine. X-rays show inflammation and fusion of the joint (sacroiliac joint) connecting lumbar spine and hip. The doctor may also order MRI.

The doctor may recommend going to a specialist called a rheumatologist.

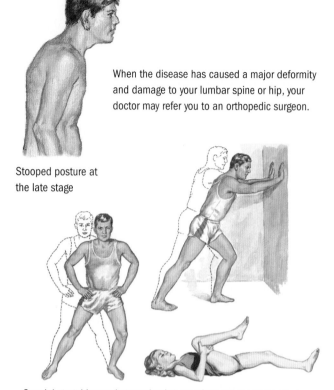

When the disease has caused a major deformity and damage to your lumbar spine or hip, your doctor may refer you to an orthopedic surgeon.

Stooped posture at the late stage

Special stretching and strengthening exercises are recommended to attempt to prevent fusion of joints in bad positions.

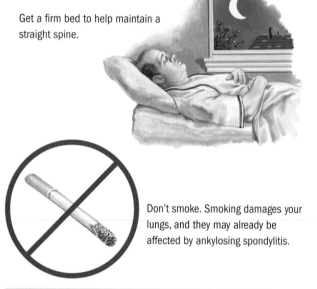

Get a firm bed to help maintain a straight spine.

Don't smoke. Smoking damages your lungs, and they may already be affected by ankylosing spondylitis.

FROM THE DESK OF

NOTES

How Is Ankylosing Spondylitis Treated?

Treatment is mainly for pain and stiffness. Special stretching and strengthening exercises may prevent fusion of joints in bad positions.

A physical therapist can help design an exercise program.

Antiinflammatory drugs, including ibuprofen and naproxen, can help control pain and inflammation. They can have side effects, such as nausea, vomiting, and stomach disorders. Other drugs such as methotrexate and infliximab may slow disease progress.

If the disease caused major deformity and damage to the lumbar spine or hip, an orthopedic surgeon (a specialist in bone diseases) can perform surgery. Other specialists (e.g., ophthalmologist, cardiologist, or pulmonologist (for diseases of the eyes, heart, and lungs) may be needed.

DOs and DON'Ts in Managing Ankylosing Spondylitis:

✔ **DO** take medicines that your physician prescribes.

✔ **DO** begin a daily stretching, strengthening, and movement routine, including breathing exercises.

✔ **DO** use good posture, firm bed, and supportive chair at work help to maintain a straight spine.

✔ **DO** call your doctor if you fall and notice a sudden change in alignment of your neck or back.

✔ **DO** call your doctor if you have drug side effects.

✔ **DO** call your doctor if you need a referral to a specialist.

✔ **DO** call your doctor if you have eye pain, loss of vision, or red eye.

✔ **DO** call your doctor if you have blood in bowel movements.

⊘ **DON'T** smoke.

⊘ **DON'T** drink alcohol if your doctor tells you to stop. Your medicine may react with alcohol.

FOR MORE INFORMATION

Contact the following sources:

• North American Spine Society
Tel: (630) 230-3600
Website: http://www.spine.org/

• Spondylitis Association of America
Tel: (800) 777-8189
Website: http://www.spondylitis.org/

• Arthritis Foundation
Tel: (800) 568-4045
Website: http://www.arthritis.org/

• American College of Rheumatology
Tel: (404) 633-3777
Website: http://www.rheumatology.org/

Avascular necrosis resulting from a hip injury

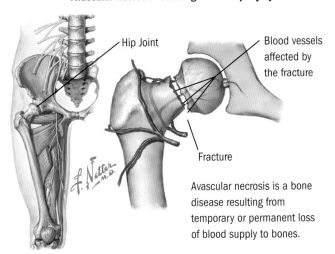

Hip Joint

Blood vessels affected by the fracture

Fracture

Avascular necrosis is a bone disease resulting from temporary or permanent loss of blood supply to bones.

Avascular necrosis resulting from a wrist injury

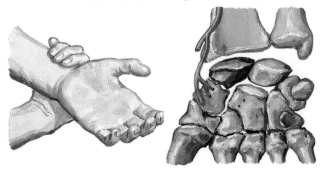

Common causes include:

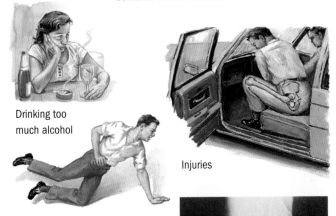

Drinking too much alcohol

Injuries

Your doctor makes a diagnosis by taking a medical history and doing x-rays. The doctor may also recommend MRI.

What Is Avascular Necrosis?

Avascular necrosis is a bone disease resulting from temporary or permanent loss of blood supply to bones. Without blood, bones die. If bones are near a joint, the joint surface often collapses. Avascular necrosis most often affects the ends of long bones, such as the thigh, upper arm, knees, shoulders, ankles, hips, and wrists. The disease may involve one bone, more than one bone at the same time, or more than one bone at different times. Avascular necrosis is also called osteonecrosis, aseptic necrosis, and ischemic bone necrosis.

The disorder affects men and women equally, usually between ages of 30 and 50. Avascular necrosis is not contagious.

What Causes Avascular Necrosis?

Injuries, drinking too much alcohol, blood coagulation disorders, and long-term use of steroids (e.g., prednisone) are common causes.

What Are the Symptoms of Avascular Necrosis?

People may not have symptoms at the start. Later, most people have joint pain, first only with weight bearing and later, pain at rest. Pain usually develops gradually and may be mild or severe. Severe pain can also develop suddenly if the joint surface collapses.

How Is Avascular Necrosis Diagnosed?

The doctor makes the diagnosis by taking a medical history, doing a physical examination, and taking x-rays. The doctor may recommend magnetic resonance imaging (MRI), which is more sensitive for showing avascular necrosis.

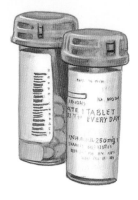

Your doctor may suggest using medicines called nonsteroidal antiinflammatory drugs (e.g., ibuprofen, naproxen) for pain.

Your doctor may do an operation to remove pressure on the bone or to reshape it and improve its blood flow.

Incision site

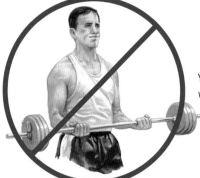

You should avoid weight-bearing activities.

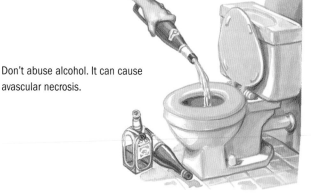

Don't abuse alcohol. It can cause avascular necrosis.

How Is Avascular Necrosis Treated?

The goals of treatment are to prevent further bone and joint damage, reduce pain, improve joint use, and ensure bone and joint survival.

Treatment includes using medicines called nonsteroidal antiinflammatory drugs (e.g., ibuprofen, naproxen), avoiding weight-bearing activities, and using range-of-motion exercises and electrical stimulation. These treatments rarely help for a long time, and most people will need surgery for permanent joint repair.

Surgery may include removing the inner bone layer to reduce the pressure in the bone and increase its blood flow. For advanced necrosis, another operation, osteotomy, reshapes the bone to reduce stress on the affected area. Total joint replacement with artificial parts is used for a destroyed joint in late-stage aseptic necrosis.

DOs and DON'Ts in Managing Avascular Necrosis:

✔ **DO** understand that pain may be severe enough to limit your joint's range of motion.

✔ **DO** remember in some cases, especially those involving the hip, osteoarthritis may develop.

✔ **DO** follow your doctor's instructions about activity limits.

✔ **DO** call your doctor if you have bone or joint pain or if you have drainage, redness, swelling, or pain after surgery.

✔ **DO** call your doctor if you need a referral to a bone specialist (orthopedic surgeon).

✔ **DO** call your doctor if you have a drinking problem.

⊘ **DON'T** abuse alcohol.

⊘ **DON'T** use long-term steroids (e.g., prednisone), if possible.

⊘ **DON'T** miss doctor appointments. Untreated aseptic necrosis will cause severe pain and limited movement within 2 years.

FROM THE DESK OF

NOTES

FOR MORE INFORMATION

Contact the following sources:

• National Institute of Arthritis and Musculoskeletal and Skin Diseases
National Institutes of Health
Tel: (877) 226-4267
Website: http://www.niams.nih.gov

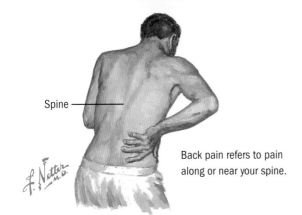

Spine

Back pain refers to pain along or near your spine.

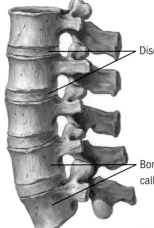

Discs

Causes include strained muscles, pinched nerves, and sometimes a disc (cushion) between the bones that has moved out of place.

Bones of the spine, called vertebrae

Pain, tenderness, and stiffness in the lower back are the most common symptoms. Symptoms may get better after sleep.

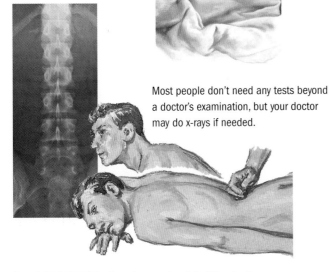

Most people don't need any tests beyond a doctor's examination, but your doctor may do x-rays if needed.

What Is Back Pain?

Back pain refers to pain along or near the spine. Most adults have had back pain at some time. Back pain is usually not serious and often goes away in 1 to 8 weeks, usually less than 1 month.

What Causes Back Pain?

Causes include strained muscles, pinched nerves, and sometimes a disc moving out of place. Discs are cushions between bones of the spine (vertebrae).

Older people may have back pain because of arthritis in joints in the spine. Older women can have weak bones, from osteoporosis, that can develop cracks.

Sometimes pain or disease in another part of the body, such as the hip, causes back pain.

Very few people have serious illnesses (cancer, infection).

What Are the Symptoms of Back Pain?

The most common symptoms are pain and stiffness of the lower back. Certain areas may feel tender. Pain often gets better at night or while resting. Symptoms of pinched nerves are pain going down into the back of the leg (called sciatica), numbness and tingling of the leg, weakness when moving, and pain that worsens while walking or exercising.

How Is Back Pain Diagnosed?

Most people don't need any tests beyond a doctor's examination. The doctor may do x-rays if pain might be due to spinal deformity or medical illness, or if it is long-term.

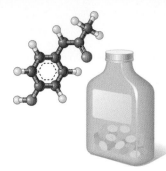

Most back pain just needs pain medicine (e.g., acetaminophen or ibuprofen). Physical therapy may also help. Most people are well within 8 weeks, no matter what treatment they receive.

How Is Back Pain Treated?

Most back pain just needs pain medicine (e.g., acetaminophen or ibuprofen). Physical therapy may help if pain resulted from lifting or pushing done the wrong way. Most people are well within 8 weeks, no matter what treatment they receive. People with long-term pain may need to go to a pain clinic. Surgery and other treatments are needed only rarely.

Take steps for back health: strengthen the back by exercising, quit smoking, keep to a normal weight, learn how to properly move and lift things, and reduce stress.

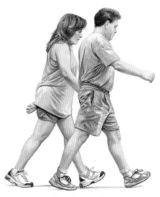
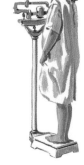

Exercise daily   Maintain a healthy weight

DOs and DON'Ts in Managing Back Pain:

✔ **DO** take pain medicine if needed.

✔ **DO** rest to get past the worst of the pain, and start moving actively after the rest period.

✔ **DO** exercise to strengthen your back.

✔ **DO** see your doctor if pain continues, if you develop weakness or numbness in your legs, or if you have trouble urinating or holding your urine or bowels.

✔ **DO** call your doctor if pain is getting worse, especially if you are older than 50, younger than 20, or you've had cancer.

✔ **DO** call your doctor if pain is from major trauma.

✔ **DO** call your doctor if pain is related to fever, chills, or unexplained weight loss.

✔ **DO** call your doctor if you have severe pain at night or pain travels to your lower belly.

✔ **DO** use good posture and avoid lifting heavy weights. Lift correctly: bend your knees, not your back, and avoid jerking.

✔ **DO** sleep on your side with the legs drawn up toward your chest. Avoid waterbeds and use a stiff mattress.

⊘ **DON'T** rest in bed for more than 48 hours, to avoid blood clots and getting weaker.

⊘ **DON'T** lift or push any heavy objects unless you know how to do so safely.

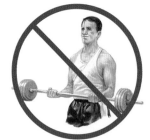

Don't lift or push any heavy objects unless you know how to do so safely.

Do back exercises to strengthen the back.

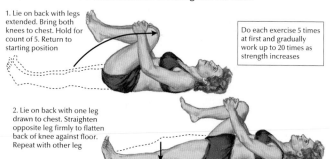

1. Lie on back with legs extended. Bring both knees to chest. Hold for count of 5. Return to starting position

Do each exercise 5 times at first and gradually work up to 20 times as strength increases

2. Lie on back with one leg drawn to chest. Straighten opposite leg firmly to flatten back of knee against floor. Repeat with other leg

FOR MORE INFORMATION

Contact the following sources:

• Spine Health
  Website: http://www.spine-health.com

• American College of Rheumatology
  Tel: (404) 633-3777
  Website: http://www.rheumatology.org

• Arthritis Foundation
  Tel: (800) 283-7800
  Website: http://www.arthritis.org

FROM THE DESK OF

NOTES

MANAGING YOUR
BAKER'S CYST

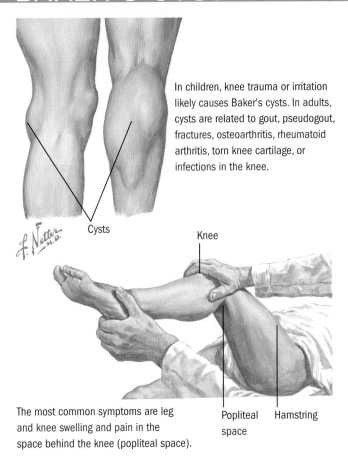

In children, knee trauma or irritation likely causes Baker's cysts. In adults, cysts are related to gout, pseudogout, fractures, osteoarthritis, rheumatoid arthritis, torn knee cartilage, or infections in the knee.

Cysts

Knee

The most common symptoms are leg and knee swelling and pain in the space behind the knee (popliteal space).

Popliteal space   Hamstring

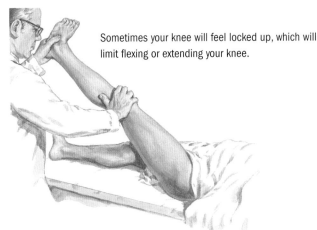

Sometimes your knee will feel locked up, which will limit flexing or extending your knee.

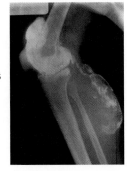

For diagnosis, your doctor may order x-rays (shown here), ultrasound scans, or MRI.

What Are Baker's Cysts?

Baker's cysts are a fluid-filled bursa at the back inner side of the knee. A bursa is a sac that acts like a shock absorber between muscles and bones or muscles and tendons (bands of fibrous tissue that connect muscles to bones). In Baker's cysts, the sac swells, which separates tendons of the hamstring muscles.

Baker's cysts can occur at any age and are curable. They can be uncomfortable and limit movement.

What Causes Baker's Cysts?

In children, trauma or irritation of the knee likely causes these cysts. In adults, they are related to gout, pseudogout, fractures, osteoarthritis, rheumatoid arthritis, torn knee cartilage, and infections in the knee. They cannot be caught or inherited.

What Are the Symptoms of Baker's Cysts?

The most common symptoms are leg and knee swelling and pain in the space behind the knee (popliteal space). Sometimes the knee feels as if it locked up, which limits flexing or extending the knee.

How Are Baker's Cysts Diagnosed?

The doctor diagnoses Baker's cysts by reviewing symptoms, x-rays of the knee, and an ultrasound scan (which uses sound waves to get an image). Sometimes, the doctor will want a sonogram, magnetic resonance imaging (MRI), blood tests, and other imaging studies to rule out other causes of knee pain (e.g., gout, infections, or blood clots in veins of the legs called deep vein thrombosis).

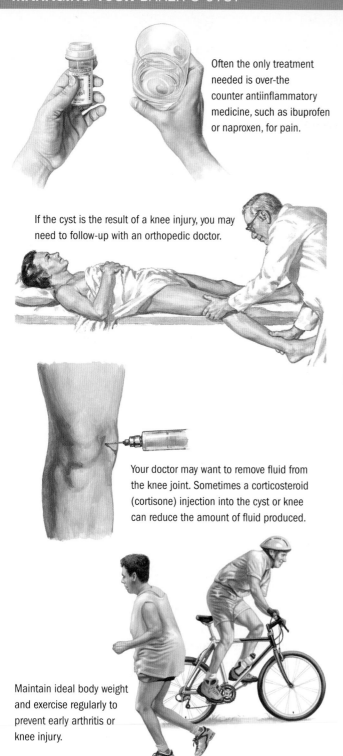

Often the only treatment needed is over-the-counter antiinflammatory medicine, such as ibuprofen or naproxen, for pain.

If the cyst is the result of a knee injury, you may need to follow-up with an orthopedic doctor.

Your doctor may want to remove fluid from the knee joint. Sometimes a corticosteroid (cortisone) injection into the cyst or knee can reduce the amount of fluid produced.

Maintain ideal body weight and exercise regularly to prevent early arthritis or knee injury.

FROM THE DESK OF

NOTES

How Are Baker's Cysts Treated?

Treatment is directed at the cause. Pain and swelling are treated by resting and avoiding stressful activity, and sometimes wearing a knee immobilizer to prevent flexing or extending the knee.

The doctor will usually prescribe antiinflammatory medicine (e.g., ibuprofen, naproxen) to relieve swelling and pain.

If medicines don't help the symptoms, the doctor may suggest a visit with a rheumatologist (a doctor specializing in diseases of joints and soft tissues) or orthopedic doctor (who specializes in bone diseases), for removing (aspirating) fluid from the knee joint or injecting a corticosteroid (cortisone) into the cyst or knee to reduce inflammation and the fluid volume produced.

If these treatments don't work, surgery (to remove the cyst) may be needed, especially if a torn knee cartilage or osteoarthritis is involved.

DOs and DON'Ts in Managing Baker's Cysts:

✔ **DO** take your medicines as prescribed by your doctor.
✔ **DO** realize that sometimes this cyst may get smaller without treatment.
✔ **DO** understand that Baker's cysts can lead to complications including pinched nerve, ruptured cyst, and deep vein thrombosis.
✔ **DO** call your doctor if you have knee pain, leg swelling, or shortness of breath.
✔ **DO** call your doctor if you have side effects from medicines.
✔ **DO** call your doctor if you need a referral to a specialist.
✔ **DO** keep to your ideal body weight and exercise regularly to prevent arthritis or knee injury.

⊘ **DON'T** miss follow-up appointments with your doctor.
⊘ **DON'T** ignore symptoms of knee pain and leg swelling. Baker's cysts can in rare cases lead to serious complications.

FOR MORE INFORMATION

Contact the following sources:

• American College of Rheumatology
  Tel: (404) 633-3777
  Website: http://www.rheumatology.org

• Arthritis Foundation
  Tel: (800) 283-7800
  Website: http://www.arthritis.org

• American Academy of Orthopaedic Surgeons
  Tel: (847) 823-7186
  Website: http://www.aaos.org

MANAGING YOUR BURSITIS

Common locations of bursitis

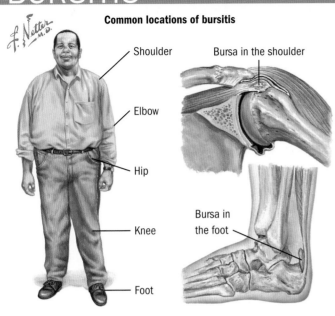

Shoulder

Bursa in the shoulder

Elbow

Hip

Bursa in the foot

Knee

Foot

A bursa is a small fluid-filled sac that cushions muscles and tendons. Bursitis is inflammation (swelling, redness) of a bursa.

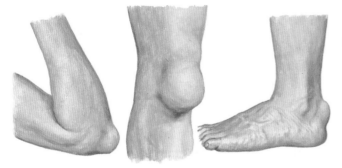

Pain with swelling, redness, and tenderness are usual symptoms.

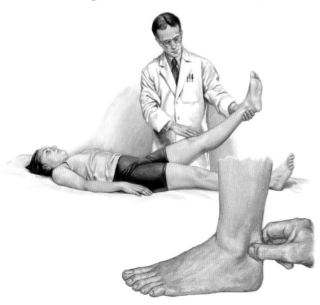

Your doctor will examine you to make a diagnosis. Your doctor may also want x-rays to rule out other conditions.

What Is Bursitis?

Bursitis is inflammation (swelling, redness) of a fluid-filled sac called a bursa. Bursae are found in many parts of the body, usually where muscles and tendons move over bones. Tendons are tough bands of tissue that connect muscles to bones. Bursae help this motion by providing a gliding surface. Bursae are found in and around shoulders, elbows, hips, knees, and feet.

Bursitis can become frustrating. It tends to return, even after treatment, unless the activity causing it is stopped or changed.

What Causes Bursitis?

Injuries from too much use and continued irritation are usual causes. Direct trauma, disorders such as rheumatoid arthritis and gout, and puncture wounds followed by infection may also cause bursitis.

What Are the Symptoms of Bursitis?

Pain with swelling, redness, and tenderness are usual symptoms. Pain usually worsens with pressure against the affected muscle.

How Is Bursitis Diagnosed?

The doctor will diagnose bursitis on the basis of the medical history and physical examination. The doctor may also want x-rays to help rule out other causes of pain, such as a stress fracture.

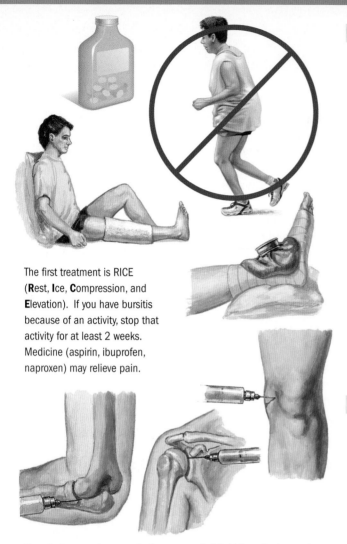

The first treatment is RICE (**R**est, **I**ce, **C**ompression, and **E**levation). If you have bursitis because of an activity, stop that activity for at least 2 weeks. Medicine (aspirin, ibuprofen, naproxen) may relieve pain.

Your doctor may do an aspiration—removal of fluid from the bursa—for temporary relief. This procedure also allows testing the fluid to rule out other causes, such as infection or gout.

If bursitis pain continues after RICE therapy when you start your regular activities, you may want to visit a physical therapist, occupational therapist, or athletic trainer for help.

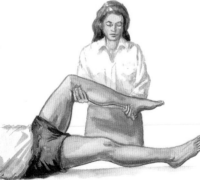

FROM THE DESK OF

NOTES

How Is Bursitis Treated?

RICE (**R**est, **I**ce, **C**ompression, **E**levation) is effective. Resting means stopping the activities for at least 2 weeks. Immobilizing the area with a splint or cast for 7 to 10 days sometimes works. Ice is placed on the area to reduce swelling and relieve pain. Antiinflammatory medications such as aspirin, ibuprofen, and naproxen can manage mild to moderate bursitis. Prescription antiinflammatory drugs are for severe bursitis that didn't respond to other treatments and for extreme pain.

Aspiration, or removing fluid from the bursa, can provide temporary relief and gives the doctor a chance to study the fluid for infection or gout. The fluid may return, however, which may lead to repeated aspiration and possible infection. Steroid injections can sometimes give relief. Infected tissue may need antibiotics or an operation to remove the tissue.

A physical therapist, occupational therapist, or athletic trainer may help retraining for activities to minimize the bursitis. Substituting other exercises for those that cause symptoms is important.

DOs and DON'Ts in Managing Bursitis:

✔ **DO** take over-the-counter antiinflammatory medicines (aspirin, ibuprofen, naproxen) as directed for mild to moderate bursitis. You may need prescription antiinflammatory drugs for severe symptoms.

✔ **DO** stop the problem activity and allow the area to rest for at least 2 weeks. Immobilizing the area may speed recovery.

✔ **DO** substitute the problem activity with those that don't cause symptoms.

✔ **DO** return to activity gradually, as long as you have no pain.

✔ **DO** call your doctor if usual treatments don't work. Your doctor should rule out other more dangerous conditions.

✔ **DO** wear protective gear for contact sports.

✔ **DO** keep to your ideal body weight, avoid strenuous exercises, and don't be a "weekend warrior."

✔ **DO** avoid repeated movements.

⊘ **DON'T** return to activity too soon or too suddenly. Six weeks is the usual time needed for inflammation to stop.

FOR MORE INFORMATION

Contact the following sources:

• American Occupational Therapy Association
Tel: (301) 652-2682
Website: http://www.aota.org

• American College of Rheumatology
Tel: (404) 633-3777
Website: http://rheumatology.org

Cervical disc syndrome refers to pain in the neck part (cervical) of the spine. The cervical part of the spinal column has seven bones (vertebrae) separated by pillow-like discs. These discs are like shock absorbers that cushion the bones and let the head and neck bend.

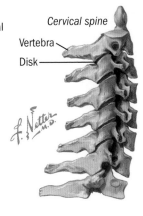

Cervical spine

Vertebra

Disk

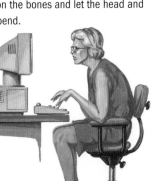

Normal degenerative changes in discs occur with aging. Poor posture and strenuous work with poor lifting methods may make these changes worse.

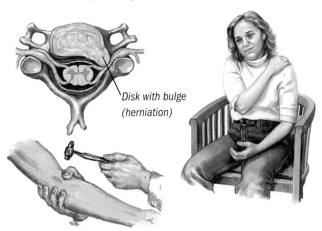

Disk with bulge (herniation)

Neck pain or tingling and numbness may reach the shoulder, upper back, arm, or hand. Disc material may bulge into the spinal canal and compress the spinal cord or nerve root.

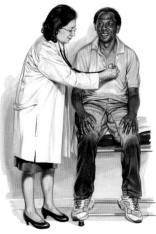

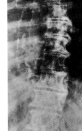

Your doctor makes a diagnosis from a physical examination and x-rays of the cervical spine. MRI of the neck and electromyography or a nerve conduction velocity test (EMG/NCV) may be done.

What Is Cervical Disc Syndrome?

The neck (cervical) part of the spinal column is made of seven bones (vertebrae) separated by pillow-like discs. These discs are like shock absorbers for the head and neck. They cushion the bones and allow the head and neck to bend. Cervical disc syndrome refers to pain in this neck part of the spine.

What Causes Cervical Disc Syndrome?

Many causes include normal degenerative changes in discs with aging. Poor posture and strenuous work with poor lifting methods may make these changes worse. The discs slowly become worn, less plump, and flat. When the disc space becomes narrow enough that vertebrae rub together, edges of the vertebrae have wear-and-tear changes. Then, bone spurs develop that may start to press on the spinal cord or nerve root. As the nerve is irritated, pain, tingling, numbness, or weakness can occur.

Similar changes or trauma may burst the tough cartilage around each disc. Disc material may bulge (herniate) into the spinal canal and press on (compress) the spinal cord or nerve root.

What Are the Symptoms of Cervical Disc Syndrome?

Neck pain or tingling and numbness may reach the shoulder, upper back, arm, or hand. Some people have weakness, clumsiness, and trouble walking. Pain from a bulging disc is worse during movement and during coughing or laughing.

How Is Cervical Disc Syndrome Diagnosed?

The doctor makes a diagnosis from a physical examination and x-rays of the cervical spine. Magnetic resonance imaging (MRI) of the neck and electromyography or nerve conduction velocity test (EMG/NCV), an electrical test of nerves and muscles, may also be done.

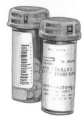

Most cases can be treated with physical therapy, pain control, and antiinflammatory drugs.

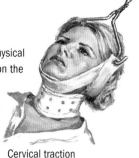

Conservative treatments done by a physical therapist also include local heat put on the area, cervical traction, and special exercises. Symptoms often go away after few weeks. Surgery is usually the final option if other treatments don't work.

Cervical traction

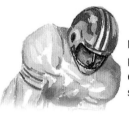

Minimize trauma to your cervical spine. Wear protective gear in contact sports. Do daily exercises approved by your doctor. Gently stretch and bend your neck.

Use good posture while sitting and walking. Put a pillow under your head and neck when lying in bed.

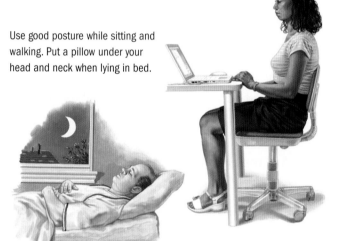

How Is Cervical Disc Syndrome Treated?

Most cases can be treated with physical therapy, pain control, and antiinflammatory drugs. Specialists (orthopedic surgeon, anesthesiologist, or neurosurgeon) may help with treatment. Conservative treatments done by a physical therapist also include local heat put on the area, cervical traction, and special exercises.

Anesthesiologists can inject steroids and anesthetic medicine into the cervical spinal canal to help pain.

Symptoms often go away after few weeks. Surgery is usually the final option if other treatments don't relieve symptoms.

DOs and DON'Ts in Managing Cervical Disc Syndrome:

✔ **DO** use good posture while sitting and walking.
✔ **DO** always wear a seat belt when traveling in a motor vehicle.
✔ **DO** put a pillow under your head and neck when lying in bed.
✔ **DO** daily exercises approved by your doctor. Gently stretch and bend your neck. Keep to your ideal weight.
✔ **DO** call your doctor if your symptoms become much worse or you have new weakness.
✔ **DO** call your doctor if you have trouble walking, have weakness, cannot move your limbs, or lose control of your bowels or bladder.
✔ **DO** minimize trauma to your cervical spine. Wear protective gear in contact sports.

⊘ **DON'T** make a habit of popping your neck.
⊘ **DON'T** return to work until your doctor says you can.
⊘ **DON'T** do strenuous activities until you check with your doctor.
⊘ **DON'T** resume driving until you're pain free without pain medicine.

FROM THE DESK OF

NOTES

FOR MORE INFORMATION

Contact the following sources:

• North American Spine Society
  Tel: (630) 230-3600
  Website: http://www.spine.org

• American Academy of Orthopaedic Surgeons
  Tel: (847) 823-7186
  Website: http://www.aaos.org

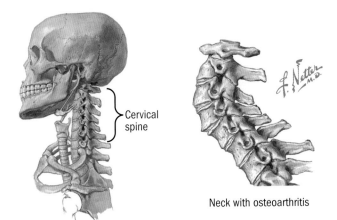

Cervical spine

Neck with osteoarthritis

The neck (cervical) part of the spinal column is made of seven bones called vertebrae. Disks separate the bones and act as shock absorbers to let the neck to bend. Cervical spondylosis is a disorder of these structures. It's also called cervical osteoarthritis.

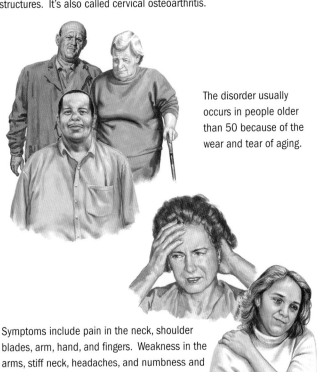

The disorder usually occurs in people older than 50 because of the wear and tear of aging.

Symptoms include pain in the neck, shoulder blades, arm, hand, and fingers. Weakness in the arms, stiff neck, headaches, and numbness and tingling in arms, hands, and fingers also occur.

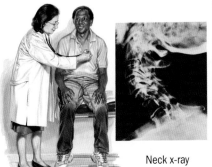

Your doctor will examine you and may order x-rays of the cervical spine. MRI of your neck and an electromyogram/nerve conduction velocity test may also be done.

Neck x-ray

What Is Cervical Spondylosis?

The neck (cervical) part of the spinal column is made of seven bones called vertebrae. Disks separate the bones and act as shock absorbers or cushions to let the neck bend. Cervical spondylosis is a disorder that occurs with aging and causes neck pain. It's also called cervical osteoarthritis.

What Causes Cervical Spondylosis?

The disorder usually occurs in people older than 50 because of the wear and tear of aging. It involves arthritis in the neck and may put pressure on the nerves or spinal cord.

What Are the Symptoms of Cervical Spondylosis?

Symptoms include pain in the neck, shoulder blades, arm, hand, and fingers. Weakness in the arms may develop slowly. Numbness and tingling in arms, hands, and fingers, stiff neck, and headaches in back of the head also occur.

How Is Cervical Spondylosis Diagnosed?

The doctor will make a diagnosis from an examination and x-rays of the cervical spine. Magnetic resonance imaging (MRI) of the neck and an electromyogram/nerve conduction velocity test may also be done. This electrical test of nerves and muscles can help tell how much the nerves are damaged.

How Is Cervical Spondylosis Treated?

A collar or neck brace to limit neck motion usually helps the pain. Using the collar too long will weaken neck muscles, however.

Rest and medicines (analgesics and antiinflammatory drugs) are used for acute pain. Muscle relaxants are used sparingly and only for short periods.

After the pain leaves, neck exercises are started and are used with the collar. Exercises to move the neck help increase motion and strength. Traction may help some people. Spinal manipulation is not suggested for this disorder.

Surgery is rarely needed, after other treatments don't work, to relieve pressure on the nerves or spinal cord.

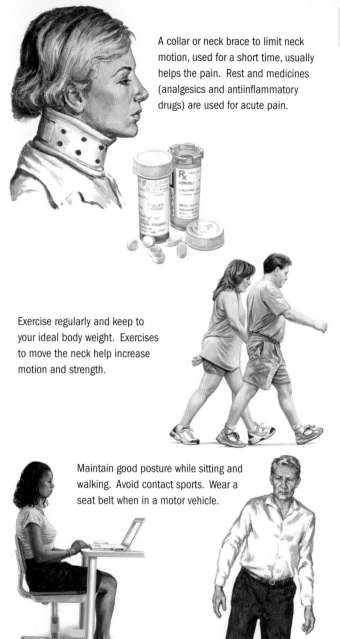

A collar or neck brace to limit neck motion, used for a short time, usually helps the pain. Rest and medicines (analgesics and antiinflammatory drugs) are used for acute pain.

Exercise regularly and keep to your ideal body weight. Exercises to move the neck help increase motion and strength.

Maintain good posture while sitting and walking. Avoid contact sports. Wear a seat belt when in a motor vehicle.

Call your doctor if you have trouble walking, are weak, or cannot move your limbs.

DOs and DON'Ts in Managing Cervical Spondylosis:

✔ **DO** rest, immobilize your neck, and take medicines (analgesics and antiinflammatory drugs) as directed for acute pain.

✔ **DO** exercises that focus on active neck motion and strengthening.

✔ **DO** gently stretch and bend your neck.

✔ **DO** maintain good posture while sitting and walking.

✔ **DO** wear a seat belt when in a motor vehicle.

✔ **DO** minimize trauma to your cervical spine.

✔ **DO** avoid contact sports.

✔ **DO** exercise regularly and keep to your ideal body weight.

✔ **DO** call your doctor if rest and medicine don't help pain. Call immediately if you have sudden muscle weakness or paralysis.

✔ **DO** call your doctor if you have medicine side effects.

✔ **DO** call your doctor if you have trouble walking, are weak, or cannot move your limbs.

⊘ **DON'T** have spinal manipulations if you have acute pain.

⊘ **DON'T** make your neck "pop."

⊘ **DON'T** slouch in a chair or bed.

⊘ **DON'T** do strenuous activities until your doctor says you can.

⊘ **DON'T** resume driving until you're pain free without pain drugs.

FROM THE DESK OF

NOTES

FOR MORE INFORMATION

Contact the following sources:

• North American Spine Society
Website: http://www.spine.org

• American Academy of Orthopaedic Surgeons
Tel: (847) 823-7186
Website: http://www.aaos.org

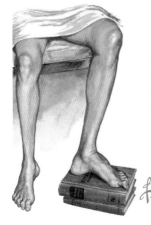

Charcot joint is a chronic condition that mainly affects joints in weight-bearing extremities, such as feet and ankles. It's a process in which joints are destroyed.

The most common cause is diabetes. People with diabetes first have peripheral neuropathy, and then develop Charcot joints. Peripheral neuropathy is a condition that involves problems with nerves that take information to and from the brain and spinal cord.

Symptoms may include swelling and increased skin temperature over the affected joint. Joint instability, loss of sensation, bleeding, and bone changes may also occur.

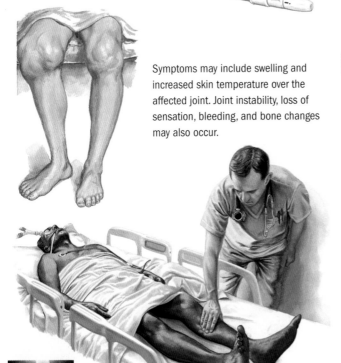

Your doctor can make a diagnosis by doing a physical examination. X-rays will also be done. X-rays can tell the degree of joint destruction. Early diagnosis is critical.

What Is Charcot Joint?

Charcot joint is a chronic condition that mainly affects joints in weight-bearing extremities, such as feet and ankles. It's a process in which joints are destroyed. People with a Charcot joint have reduced sensation in the affected area and problems with nerves that take information to and from the brain and spinal cord (called peripheral neuropathy).

What Causes Charcot Joint?

The most common cause is diabetes. People with diabetes first have peripheral neuropathy, and then develop Charcot joints.

What Are the Symptoms of Charcot Joint?

Symptoms may include swelling, pain, and increased skin temperature over the affected joint. Instability of the joint, loss of sensation, bleeding, and bone changes may also occur.

Charcot joint is relatively painless, often in spite of considerable joint destruction, and people often do not go to the doctor until the deformity is severe.

How Is Charcot Joint Diagnosed?

The doctor can make a diagnosis by doing a physical examination. X-rays will also be done. X-rays can tell the degree of joint destruction and show loss of cartilage, new bone growth, and breaks at the joint.

Sometimes, Charcot joint can be confused with infection, but most people with this disorder have acute inflammation (swelling, redness) but no trauma or cuts or breaks in the skin, which would suggest infection.

Charcot joint is treatable but not curable. Early diagnosis, before the joint becomes badly damaged, is essential.

No drugs can help this condition. Immobilizing the extremity and using crutches, a cane, or a walker help manage the acute condition. These protect the joint by reducing or eliminating weight bearing by the extremity.

Get treatment early. Prevention is key to minimizing joint deformities. Ignoring warning signs may lead to joint destruction with disintegration of the bones and collapse.

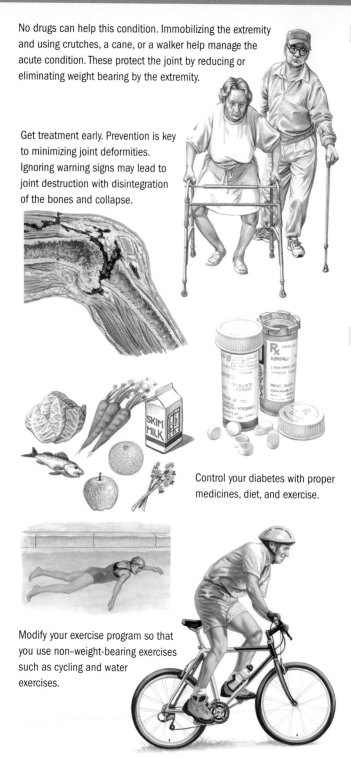

Control your diabetes with proper medicines, diet, and exercise.

Modify your exercise program so that you use non–weight-bearing exercises such as cycling and water exercises.

How Is Charcot Joint Treated?

No drugs are available for treatment. Immobilizing the extremity and using crutches, a cane, or a walker help manage the acute condition. These protect the joint by reducing or eliminating weight bearing by the extremity. Some diseases causing Charcot joint may be treated effectively. However, nerves will not grow back after treatment, and the joint condition may continue to get worse. Surgery is rarely used and is not very successful.

It can take as long as 6 weeks for acute inflammation to go away. Then, joints probably need a brace or other support to prevent flare-ups and joint destruction.

Prevention is key to minimizing joint deformities. Ignoring warning signs may lead to joint destruction with disintegration of the bones and collapse.

DOs and DON'Ts in Managing Charcot Joint:

✔ **DO** control your diabetes with proper medicines, diet, and exercise.
✔ **DO** modify your exercise program. Substitute non–weight-bearing exercises such as cycling and water exercises.
✔ **DO** call your doctor if you notice swelling, heat, or redness around any weight-bearing joint, especially if the joint was treated before.
✔ **DO** call your doctor at the earliest start of swelling, redness, and increased skin temperature over an affected joint.

⊘ **DON'T** begin an aggressive walking or running program right after being fitted with braces or splints.

FROM THE DESK OF

NOTES

FOR MORE INFORMATION
Contact the following sources:
• American Academy of Orthopaedic Surgeons
Tel: (847) 823-7186
Website: http://www.aaos.org
• American Diabetes Association
Tel: (800) 342-2383
Website: http://www.diabetes.org

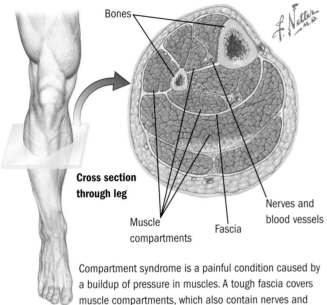

Cross section
through leg

Bones

Muscle
compartments

Fascia

Nerves and
blood vessels

Compartment syndrome is a painful condition caused by a buildup of pressure in muscles. A tough fascia covers muscle compartments, which also contain nerves and blood vessels. Fascia doesn't stretch. If muscles swell, pressure in a compartment can get high and crush blood vessels.

The acute syndrome usually follows injury or surgery. It can happen when an arm or leg swells inside a cast. Chronic compartment syndrome happens after exercise, usually to athletes and soldiers.

Pain is the main symptom. In the chronic syndrome, it starts with exercise and gets worse. In the acute syndrome, severe pain is worst when the muscle is stretched.

Your doctor will take a medical history, do a physical examination, and maybe order x-rays, ultrasonography, or MRI. A specialist may measure pressure inside the muscle compartment with a needle attached to a pressure meter.

What Is Compartment Syndrome?

Compartment syndrome is a painful condition caused by a buildup of pressure in muscles. A tough membrane called a fascia covers groups of muscles. These groupings are called muscle compartments. Compartments also contain nerves and blood vessels. Fascia doesn't stretch. So if muscles inside swell, pressure in a compartment rises. Pressure that gets very high can cause blood vessels to be crushed. Blood cannot pass through the vessels to carry oxygen to muscles and nerves. This is compartment syndrome.

What Causes Compartment Syndrome?

This syndrome can be acute or chronic. The acute type usually follows injury or surgery. It can happen when an arm or leg swells inside a cast. Chronic (or exertional) compartment syndrome happens after exercise, usually to athletes and soldiers.

What Are the Symptoms of Compartment Syndrome?

Chronic compartment syndrome usually causes cramping pain in both legs that begins during exercise and gets worse as exercise continues. Tingling, numbness, or pressure may be felt. The area may be tight but doesn't look swollen. Pain stops after exercise stops. Acute compartment syndrome causes severe pain, which is worst when the muscle is stretched. The area may feel hard.

How Is Compartment Syndrome Diagnosed?

The doctor will probably first test for other, more common causes of pain. The doctor will take a medical history, do a physical examination, and maybe order x-rays, ultrasonography, or magnetic resonance imaging (MRI).

The doctor may suggest seeing a specialist. The specialist will measure pressure inside the muscle compartment with a needle attached to a pressure meter.

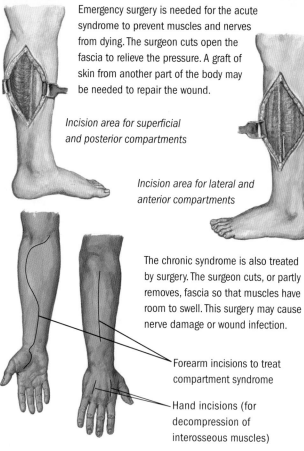

Emergency surgery is needed for the acute syndrome to prevent muscles and nerves from dying. The surgeon cuts open the fascia to relieve the pressure. A graft of skin from another part of the body may be needed to repair the wound.

Incision area for superficial and posterior compartments

Incision area for lateral and anterior compartments

The chronic syndrome is also treated by surgery. The surgeon cuts, or partly removes, fascia so that muscles have room to swell. This surgery may cause nerve damage or wound infection.

Forearm incisions to treat compartment syndrome

Hand incisions (for decompression of interosseous muscles)

Treatments other than surgery include doing different sports (for example, cycling or swimming instead of running), changing the technique for the same sport, taking a complete break from sports, and using painkillers.

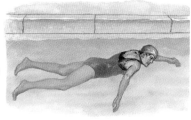

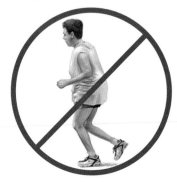

Don't keep exercising through pain. You could damage your nerves or muscles permanently. Call your doctor immediately if you get severe muscle pain after an injury.

How Is Compartment Syndrome Treated?

Emergency surgery is needed for the acute syndrome to prevent muscles and nerves from dying. Treated quickly, they'll likely return to normal. Untreated, people could be disabled or lose a leg or arm. The surgeon will cut open the fascia to relieve the pressure. Often, the wound is left open for 2 to 3 days and then closed in another operation. A graft of skin from another part of the body may be needed to repair the wound.

The chronic syndrome is usually treated by surgery. The surgeon cuts, or partly removes, the fascia so that muscles have room to swell. Most people who have surgery can exercise as before. Muscles may bulge out more, because the fascia doesn't hold them in.

Treatments other than surgery include doing different and various sports (for example, cycling or swimming instead of running), changing the technique for the same sport, taking a complete break from sports, and medications to control the pain. Compartment syndrome often comes back after nonsurgical treatment if the initial cause is untreated.

DOs and DON'Ts in Managing Compartment Syndrome:

✔ **DO** warm up before exercise and cool down after.
✔ **DO** stop exercising if you feel pain.
✔ **DO** follow your doctor's instructions for recovery after surgery.
✔ **DO** call your doctor immediately if you get severe muscle pain after an injury.

⊘ **DON'T** keep exercising through pain. You could damage your nerves or muscles permanently.
⊘ **DON'T** use bandages or supports. They may make pressure in muscle compartments worse.

FROM THE DESK OF

NOTES

FOR MORE INFORMATION

Contact the following source:

• The American Academy of Orthopaedic Surgeons
Tel: (800) 346-2267
Website: http://www.aaos.org

MANAGING YOUR
COSTOCHONDRITIS

The ribs connect to the sternum (breastbone) by cartilage, a thick elastic tissue. This connection is called the costochondral junction, a joining of bone and cartilage. Costochondritis is pain and tenderness in this part of the chest.

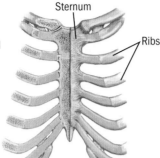

Sternum

Ribs

Costochondral junction

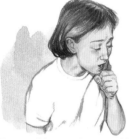

The condition may be caused by exercise, injury, chronic cough, or viral infection, or it may develop for unknown reasons.

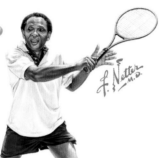

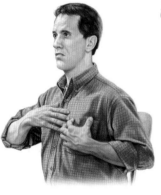

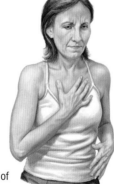

Symptoms include chest pain (often sharp) and tenderness. Some people feel anxious and short of breath. The pain can last from minutes to hours.

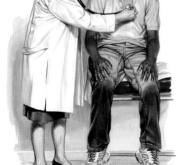

Your doctor makes a diagnosis from a medical history and physical examination, which often shows tenderness over the cartilage.

What Is Costochondritis?

The ribs connect to the sternum (breastbone) by cartilage, a thick elastic tissue. This connection is called the costochondral junction, a joining of bone and cartilage. Costochondritis is pain and tenderness in this part of the chest. Most people get better and are pain free in a few days. It may go away on its own. Costochondritis cannot be prevented.

One type of costochondritis caused by swelling of the cartilage is Tietze's syndrome. It can occur anywhere in the chest but is usually on the left side.

What Causes Costochondritis?

Exercise, injury, chronic cough, or viral infection can cause the cartilage connecting ribs and breastbone to become painful and swollen. The cause can also be unknown.

What Are the Symptoms of Costochondritis?

Symptoms include pain and tenderness in the chest. Pain may be mild or severe and may last for several days or longer. Coughing, sneezing, deep breaths, and certain movements can make the pain worse. Some people feel anxious and short of breath. The pain is often sharp, can last from minutes to hours.

How Is Costochondritis Diagnosed?

The doctor makes a diagnosis from a medical history and physical examination, which often shows tenderness over the cartilage. No specific blood tests or x-rays are needed, but the doctor may order tests to be sure that no other condition is present.

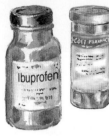

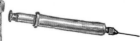

Costochondritis may last several months. It first gets better and then goes away, with or without treatment. NSAIDs such as ibuprofen may be especially helpful. Cortisone injections might be tried if other treatments don't work.

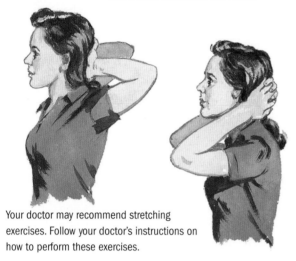

Your doctor may recommend stretching exercises. Follow your doctor's instructions on how to perform these exercises.

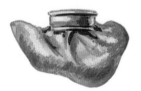

Using a heating pad also helps take the pain away. But don't use a heating pad more than three times a day or for more than 20 minutes at a time. You could get burned.

Don't use oils or creams with a heating pad. The pain could get worse or you could get burned.

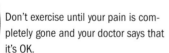

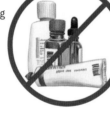

Don't exercise until your pain is completely gone and your doctor says that it's OK.

How Is Costochondritis Treated?

Costochondritis may last several days or weeks. It first gets better and then goes away, with or without treatment. Nonsteroidal antiinflammatory drugs (NSAIDs) such as ibuprofen may be especially helpful. Other treatments include heat and stretching exercises. If these treatments don't work, cortisone injections might be tried but are rarely needed. They usually work quickly.

Using a heating pad also helps to take the pain away. If the condition persists, the doctor may suggest seeing a rheumatologist (a doctor who specializes in joint diseases) or an orthopedist (a doctor who specializes in bone diseases) if the disorder doesn't get better with treatment.

DOs and DON'Ts in Managing Costochondritis:

✔ **DO** follow your doctor's instructions. Finish all your medicine to make sure that the pain and swelling go away completely.

✔ **DO** tell your doctor if you take over-the-counter or prescription medicines.

✔ **DO** make sure your doctor says that it's OK before starting to exercise.

✔ **DO** tell your doctor if pain gets worse even with treatment. Another problem may be causing the pain.

✔ **DO** call your doctor if you have side effects from medicines.

✔ **DO** call your doctor if you have a new, unexplained symptom with your chest pain.

⊘ **DON'T** use a heating pad more than three times a day or for more than 20 minutes at a time. Don't use oils or creams with a heating pad. The pain could get worse or you could get burned.

⊘ **DON'T** exercise until your pain is completely gone and your doctor says that it's OK.

⊘ **DON'T** continue an exercise program that causes pain most of the time.

FROM THE DESK OF

NOTES

FOR MORE INFORMATION

Contact the following source:

• American College of Rheumatology
  Tel: (404) 633-3777
  Website: http://www.rheumatology.org

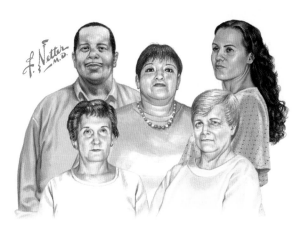

De Quervain's tenosynovitis is inflammation of sheaths around tendons in hand muscles that extend the thumb at the wrist. It can be associated with rheumatoid arthritis.

Tendons are bands of tough fibrous connective tissue that connect muscles to bones. Tendons are protected by sheaths. Inflamed sheaths thicken and cause pain.

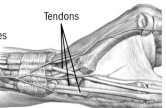

Tendons

The cause is unknown. Repeated use or overuse of the hands can lead to this disorder. It's common in people with clerical, assembly, and manual jobs.

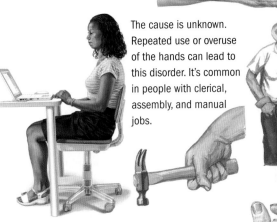

A main symptom is pain over the base of the thumb, near the wrist. This pain occurs slowly and may spread to the thumb or into the forearm.

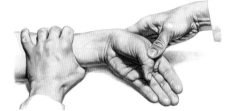

Point of pain

Your doctor will do Finkelstein's test if de Quervain's tenosynovitis is suspected. In this test, your doctor holds the thumb of your hand and pulls the thumb and wrist to stretch the tendon. Pain means de Quervain's tenosynovitis.

What Is De Quervain's Tenosynovitis?

Tendons are bands of tough fibrous connective tissue that usually connect muscles to bones. They transmit forces of muscle contraction to bones. Tendons in the hands are covered and protected by sheaths lined by a membrane called the synovium. When these sheaths are inflamed (swollen, red), they thicken and cause pain. De Quervain's tenosynovitis (or stenosing tenosynovitis) is inflammation of sheaths around tendons of certain muscles in the hand. These muscles work to extend the thumb at the wrist joint.

This disorder is 10 times more common in women than men. It usually occurs between the ages of 30 and 50 and can be associated with rheumatoid arthritis.

What Causes De Quervain's Tenosynovitis?

The cause is unknown. Repeated use or overuse of the hands can lead to this disorder. It's common in people with clerical, assembly, and manual jobs. Direct trauma is another cause. It isn't contagious.

What Are the Symptoms of De Quervain's Tenosynovitis?

A main symptom is pain over the base of the thumb, near the wrist. This pain occurs slowly and may spread to the thumb or into the forearm. It usually involves the dominant hand, which becomes tender when touched or when doing certain movements, such as pinching and grabbing.

How Is De Quervain's Tenosynovitis Diagnosed?

The doctor diagnoses this condition from the medical history and the simple Finkelstein test. In this test, the doctor holds the thumb of the hand and pulls the thumb and wrist to stretch the tendon. Pain means de Quervain's tenosynovitis.

The doctor may order blood tests and x-rays to rule out other causes, such as osteoarthritis, gout, and carpal tunnel syndrome.

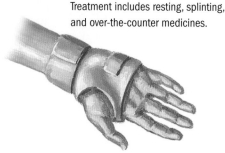
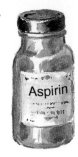

Treatment includes resting, splinting, and over-the-counter medicines.

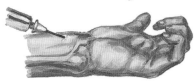

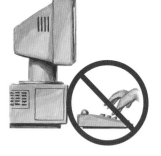
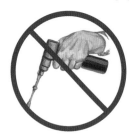

If these treatments don't help, one or more injections of steroids helps relieve pain. When all other treatments don't work, surgery is needed. About 90% of people get help for symptoms by surgery.

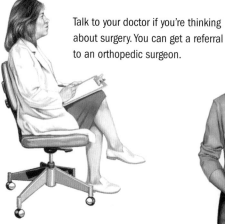
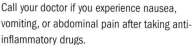

Avoid repetitive movements of the wrist and thumb. Typists, factory workers, and mothers of newborns should be careful of such movements.

Talk to your doctor if you're thinking about surgery. You can get a referral to an orthopedic surgeon.

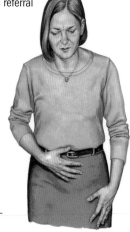

Call your doctor if you experience nausea, vomiting, or abdominal pain after taking anti-inflammatory drugs.

How Is De Quervain's Tenosynovitis Treated?

Treatment includes resting, splinting (prevent friction on tendons), and medicines. Over-the-counter pain medicines include ibuprofen, aspirin, and naproxen. Side effects include upset stomach, heartburn, nausea, and gastrointestinal bleeding. Applying ice or a cold pack over the base of the thumb may also help swelling and pain.

If these treatments don't help, one or more injections of steroids helps pain.

When all these treatments don't work, surgery is needed. About 90% of people get relief of symptoms by surgery.

DOs and DON'Ts in Managing De Quervain's Tenosynovitis:

✔ **DO** remember that repetitive movements are thought to lead to this disorder. Bricklayers, typists, computer keyboard operators, factory workers, concert pianists, and mothers of newborns should be careful to avoid repetitive movements of the wrist and thumb.

✔ **DO** call your doctor if your pain doesn't get better with conservative therapy.

✔ **DO** call your doctor if you see redness or drainage from a surgical or injection site.

✔ **DO** call your doctor if you get heartburn, nausea, vomiting, or abdominal pain after starting antiinflammatory medicines.

✔ **DO** call your doctor if you're thinking about surgery. You can get a referral to an orthopedic surgeon (specialist in hand disorders).

⊘ **DON'T** forget that conservative management (rest, drugs, or both) may be all that's needed to help symptoms.

⊘ **DON'T** miss follow-up doctor appointments.

⊘ **DON'T** be afraid to ask for a second opinion.

⊘ **DON'T** take more than the prescribed dose of antiinflammatory medicine. You might get an upset stomach and other gastrointestinal or kidney or liver problems.

FROM THE DESK OF

NOTES

FOR MORE INFORMATION

Contact the following source:

• National Institute of Arthritis and Musculoskeletal and Skin Diseases
Tel: (877) 226-4267
Website: http://www.niams.nih.gov/

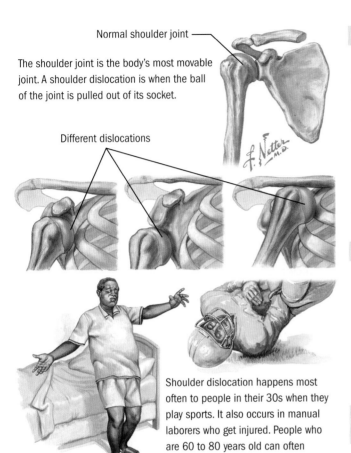

The shoulder joint is the body's most movable joint. A shoulder dislocation is when the ball of the joint is pulled out of its socket.

Normal shoulder joint

Different dislocations

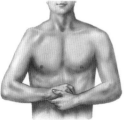

Shoulder dislocation happens most often to people in their 30s when they play sports. It also occurs in manual laborers who get injured. People who are 60 to 80 years old can often dislocate their shoulders in a fall.

Common symptoms include:

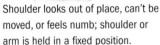

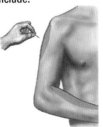

Shoulder looks out of place, can't be moved, or feels numb; shoulder or arm is held in a fixed position.

Pain in the shoulder may travel down the arm and into the hand.

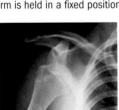

Your doctor will examine you and may order x-rays or MRI to help with diagnosis.

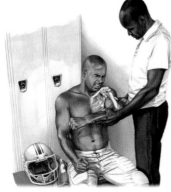

What Is Shoulder Dislocation?

A joint is a point where two or more of bones come together. The shoulder joint is the body's most movable joint. Because of this, it's the most likely one to become dislocated. Dislocation occurs when the ball of the joint (the top rounded part of the upper arm bone) is pulled out of its socket. The two types of shoulder dislocation are atraumatic and traumatic. The atraumatic one often occurs in a teenager who has a loose joint. The traumatic one often results from sporting injuries or using the joint excessively with manual labor.

What Causes Shoulder Dislocation?

Shoulder dislocation happens most often to people in their 30s when they play sports. It frequently occurs in manual laborers who get injured. People who are 60 to 80 years old commonly dislocate their shoulders in a fall. After the first dislocation of a shoulder, the shoulder will be more likely to dislocate again, but this likelihood may decrease with time as the shoulder heals.

What Are the Symptoms of Shoulder Dislocation?

Signs and symptoms include the arm of the affected shoulder looking dislocated or out of place, swelling, bruising or discoloration, holding the shoulder or arm in a fixed position, being unable to move the shoulder, numbness, weakness, and pain in the shoulder. This pain may travel down the arm and into the hand.

How Is Shoulder Dislocation Diagnosed?

The doctor will make a diagnosis from the medical history, and physical examination. You will be asked questions about events leading up to the injury or overuse of the arm. The doctor will do a physical examination and order x-rays. Other imaging tests, such as a magnetic resonance imaging (MRI), may be done.

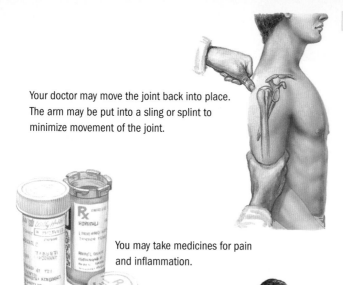

Your doctor may move the joint back into place. The arm may be put into a sling or splint to minimize movement of the joint.

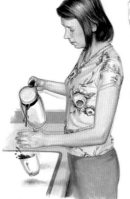

You may take medicines for pain and inflammation.

A physical therapist can help you learn strengthening exercises. Referral to an orthopedist is likely if you dislocated the shoulder before or if it gets harder to use the shoulder and arm.

Call your doctor if you develop weakness in your arm or hand.

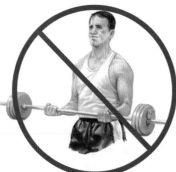

Don't do strenuous activities or lift heavy objects without your doctor's permission.

How Is Shoulder Dislocation Treated?

The doctor may move the joint back into place. The arm may be put into a sling or splint to minimize movement of the joint. The doctor may prescribe medicines for pain and inflammation (swelling, redness).

The doctor may suggest seeing a physical therapist. This health care professional can teach how to reduce the risk of injuring the shoulder again. The therapist may also teach exercises to strengthen the shoulder joint.

Care from another specialist, such as an orthopedist, may be needed. An orthopedist specializes in treating joints and bones. This referral is especially likely if the shoulder was dislocated before or if it becomes increasingly harder to use the shoulder and arm. Surgery may be needed if the shoulder is weak and dislocates often.

DOs and DON'Ts in Managing Shoulder Dislocation:

✔ **DO** tell your doctor about the medicines you take, including prescription and over-the-counter medicines.

✔ **DO** exercises that your doctor, physical therapist, or other health care professional recommends.

✔ **DO** return to your doctor for follow-up care when suggested.

✔ **DO** wear protective clothing and equipment when playing sports.

✔ **DO** call your doctor if your shoulder pain persists after treatment.

✔ **DO** call your doctor if you develop weakness in your arm or hand.

🚫 **DON'T** do strenuous activities or lift heavy objects without your doctor's permission.

FROM THE DESK OF

NOTES

FOR MORE INFORMATION

Contact the following sources:

• National Institute of Arthritis and Musculoskeletal and Skin Diseases
Tel: (877) 226-4267
Website: http://www.niams.nih.gov

• American Academy of Orthopaedic Surgeons
Tel: (800) 346-AAOS (346-2267)
Website: http://www.aaos.org

MANAGING YOUR
ELBOW DISLOCATION

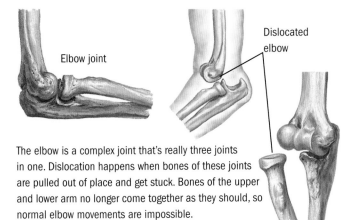

Elbow joint

Dislocated elbow

The elbow is a complex joint that's really three joints in one. Dislocation happens when bones of these joints are pulled out of place and get stuck. Bones of the upper and lower arm no longer come together as they should, so normal elbow movements are impossible.

Elbow dislocation is usually caused by falling on an outstretched arm.

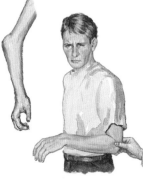

Partial elbow dislocation—nursemaid's elbow—sometimes happens in small children, usually younger than 4. An adult pulling the child up by the arm can cause it.

A dislocated elbow is swollen and very painful and may have a odd shape. Moving it is hard or impossible. The lower arm may look longer or shorter than normal. Nursemaid's elbow usually causes only mild pain and little or no swelling.

Your doctor can usually tell from a physical examination whether the elbow is dislocated. X-rays, CT, or MRI might be needed too.

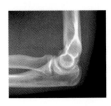

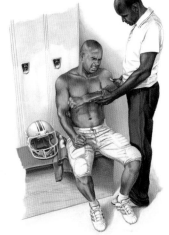

What Is Elbow Dislocation?

The elbow is a complex joint that is really three joints in one. Dislocation happens when bones of these joints are pulled out of place and get stuck. Bones of the upper and lower arm no longer come together as they should, so normal elbow movements aren't possible.

What Causes Elbow Dislocation?

The cause is usually a fall on an outstretched arm. People may also break one or more of the elbow bones, hurt ligaments that hold the bones in place, or hurt nearby nerves or blood vessels.

Partial elbow dislocation (called nursemaid's elbow) sometimes happens in small children, usually younger than 4. An adult pulling the child up by the arm can cause it.

What Are the Symptoms of Elbow Dislocation?

Symptoms include swelling and pain. Moving it is hard or impossible. The elbow may have an unusual shape, or the lower arm may look longer or shorter than normal.

Nursemaid's elbow usually causes only mild pain and little or no swelling.

How Is Elbow Dislocation Diagnosed?

The doctor can usually tell from a physical examination whether the elbow is dislocated. The doctor may also use x-rays, computed tomography (CT), or magnetic resonance imaging (MRI) to look at the elbow.

How Is Elbow Dislocation Treated?

The joint needs to be put back into place. The doctor will do this by placing the arm in position and putting pressure in the right direction. A click can be heard or felt when the joint goes back into place. A complex injury may need surgery to repair it.

After treatment, the elbow will be put in a splint to stop it from moving. Simple dislocations normally need splinting for 5 to 7 days; complicated dislocations may take longer. After this, it's important to get the elbow moving again. Exercises will help, as may sessions with a physical therapist. Playing sports can resume as before, but elbow pads may help protect the joint.

It may be 3 to 6 months before the elbow can move completely freely. Some people have a permanent small loss of movement, especially if the elbow was broken as well as dislocated. The elbow may not extend as far as before, but this shouldn't affect work or everyday tasks.

A partial elbow dislocation (nursemaid's elbow) usually goes back into place easily. X-rays and painkillers aren't usually needed. The child should be able to use the arm freely and painlessly as soon as it's back in place. Some doctors suggest keeping it in a sling for a week. Children can have partial dislocation repeatedly, but usually grow out of this condition. Don't pull hard on a child's arm. Rarely, surgery may be used to stop repeated dislocations.

DOs and DON'Ts in Managing Elbow Dislocation:

✔ **DO** exercises suggested by your doctor or physical therapist. This will help your chances of regaining full movement in your elbow.

⊘ **DON'T** remove the splint before your doctor tells you to.

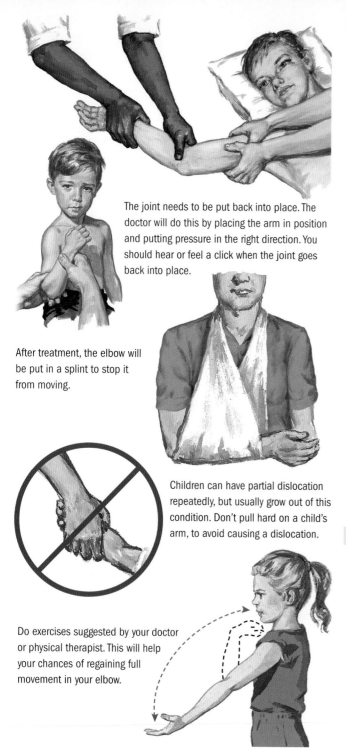

The joint needs to be put back into place. The doctor will do this by placing the arm in position and putting pressure in the right direction. You should hear or feel a click when the joint goes back into place.

After treatment, the elbow will be put in a splint to stop it from moving.

Children can have partial dislocation repeatedly, but usually grow out of this condition. Don't pull hard on a child's arm, to avoid causing a dislocation.

Do exercises suggested by your doctor or physical therapist. This will help your chances of regaining full movement in your elbow.

FROM THE DESK OF

NOTES

FOR MORE INFORMATION

Contact the following source:

• The American Academy of Orthopaedic Surgeons
  Tel: (847) 823-7186
  Website: http://www.aaos.org

MANAGING YOUR
TENNIS ELBOW

Tendons attach muscles to bones. The elbow has an upper arm bone (humerus) and two bones in the forearm (ulna and radius). Bony bulges on the inside and outside of the elbow are the epicondyle part of the upper bone. Tendons of forearm muscles attach to these bulges.

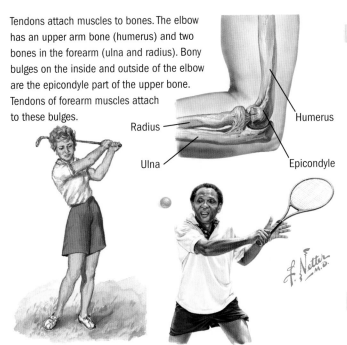

Radius

Ulna

Humerus

Epicondyle

Inflammation of the outer tendons (for extending the wrist), called "tennis elbow," also results from overusing the arm when playing tennis or doing other activities with repetitive motion. Inflammation of the inner tendons (for flexing the wrist), called "golfer's elbow," often results from repeated golf-swing motion or similar motions.

Carpenters, factory workers, musicians, and cashiers, who use their hands repeatedly, can also have this problem. An injury, such as from lifting something that's too heavy, can cause it.

The forearm becomes tender and painful and may have burning feelings. The hand grip may be weak, and it may be hard to lift or grasp objects or to do simple things (writing, brushing teeth).

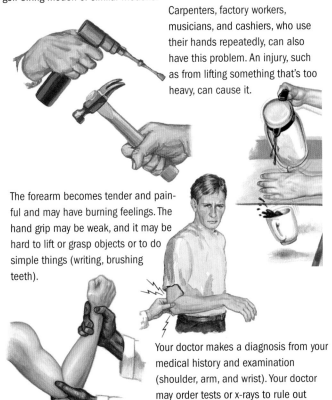

Your doctor makes a diagnosis from your medical history and examination (shoulder, arm, and wrist). Your doctor may order tests or x-rays to rule out conditions (e.g., arthritis, pinched nerve) with similar symptoms.

What Is Tennis Elbow?

Tendons attach muscles to bones. The elbow has an upper arm bone (humerus) and two bones in the forearm (ulna and radius). Bony bulges on the inside and outside of the elbow are the epicondyle part of the upper bone. Tendons of forearm muscles, responsible mainly for flexing and extending the wrist, attach to these bulges.

Inflammation of the outer tendons (for extending the wrist) has the medical name lateral epicondylitis. The common name "tennis elbow" is used because the problem often results from playing tennis or similar repetitive motion. Inflammation of inner tendons (for flexing the wrist) is medial epicondylitis, or "golfer's elbow."

What Causes Tennis Elbow?

The usual cause is overusing the arm, often related to work or sports. Carpenters, factory workers, musicians, and cashiers, who use their hands repeatedly, can have this problem. An injury, such as from lifting something that's too heavy, can also cause it.

What Are the Symptoms of Tennis Elbow?

The forearm becomes tender and painful. Burning feelings going down the arm from the elbow also occur. Pain may first be felt only when using the arm, but later pain may be constant, even at rest. The hand grip may be weak, and it may be hard to lift or grasp objects, or to do simple tasks (writing, brushing teeth).

How Is Tennis Elbow Diagnosed?

The doctor makes a diagnosis by the medical history and physical examination (shoulder, arm, and wrist). Resistance against extending the wrist or flexing it can bring on pain.

The doctor may order other tests or x-rays to rule out other conditions with similar symptoms. These conditions include arthritis, cervical spine disease, neuropathy, and pinched nerve. The doctor may also order magnetic resonance imaging (MRI) to get pictures of inflamed tendons and to rule out a ruptured tendon.

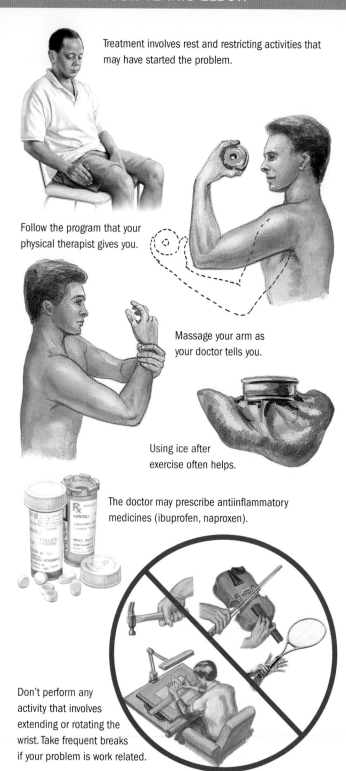

Treatment involves rest and restricting activities that may have started the problem.

Follow the program that your physical therapist gives you.

Massage your arm as your doctor tells you.

Using ice after exercise often helps.

The doctor may prescribe antiinflammatory medicines (ibuprofen, naproxen).

Don't perform any activity that involves extending or rotating the wrist. Take frequent breaks if your problem is work related.

FROM THE DESK OF

NOTES

How Is Tennis Elbow Treated?

Treatment involves rest and restricting activities that may have started the problem. Using ice after exercise and rest and special stretching and strengthening exercises often help.

Wrapping the elbow with an elastic sleeve keeps the arm warm and helps flexibility. A physical therapist may oversee treatment and prescribe ultrasound treatment.

The doctor may prescribe antiinflammatory medicines (ibuprofen, naproxen).

If the pain continues, cortisone injections can be tried.

DOs and DON'Ts in Managing Tennis Elbow:

✔ **DO** stop the activity causing the pain for 1-2 weeks, or maybe longer, depending on your doctor's advice.

✔ **DO** massage your arm as your doctor tells you.

✔ **DO** follow the program that your physical therapist gives you.

✔ **DO** call your doctor if treatment doesn't help symptoms.

✔ **DO** call your doctor if you need a referral to an orthopedic surgeon (a specialist in musculoskeletal diseases).

✔ **DO** call your doctor if you have side effects from medicines.

✔ **DO** take frequent breaks if your problem is work related. Get information about performing tasks safely.

⊘ **DON'T** perform any activity that involves extending or rotating the wrist.

⊘ **DON'T** apply chemical cold packs directly to your skin.

⊘ **DON'T** forget that muscles need to stay warm during sporting events. Always loosen up before activities.

⊘ **DON'T** use sporting equipment that is too large or too small.

⊘ **DON'T** overdo sports or activities.

FOR MORE INFORMATION

Contact the following sources:

• Arthritis Foundation
  Tel: (800) 283-7800
  Website: http://www.arthritis.org

• Nicholas Institute of Sports Medicine and Athletic Trauma
  Website: http://www.nismat.org

• American Academy of Orthopaedic Surgeons
  Tel: (847) 823-7186
  Website: http://www.aaos.org

MANAGING YOUR
FROZEN SHOULDER

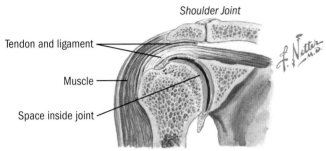

Shoulder Joint

Tendon and ligament

Muscle

Space inside joint

A frozen shoulder is when the shoulder becomes stiff and painful, with limited range of motion. The space inside the shoulder joint slowly gets smaller. Frozen shoulder may take months or years to improve.

The cause of frozen shoulder is not known but risk factors include:

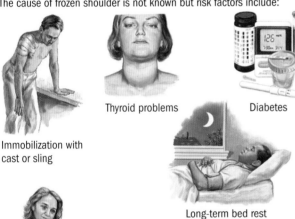

Thyroid problems

Diabetes

Immobilization with cast or sling

Long-term bed rest

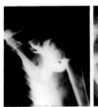

With a frozen shoulder, you have pain throughout your shoulder area, at the front and side. Pain can reach down into upper arm muscles. It's constant, even at rest and at night.

Movement also becomes very limited, and it's very hard to lift your arm.

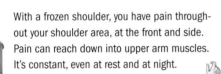

Your doctor makes a diagnosis from a physical examination. Your doctor may order x-rays to rule out other illnesses that may cause symptoms.

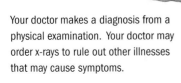

What Is Frozen Shoulder?

A frozen shoulder becomes stiff and painful, with limited range of motion. The space inside the shoulder joint slowly gets smaller. Frozen shoulder may take months to years to improve.

A frozen shoulder develops in stages. In the first stage (freezing), people notice shoulder pain and that it's harder to move that arm. This stage usually lasts about 4 months. In the next 4 months, the shoulder stays very painful. It's possible to move the arm only a little. This is known as being frozen. In the last stage, thawing, pain slowly goes away, and the arm can be moved again. This phase also lasts about 4 months in most cases.

What Causes Frozen Shoulder?

Causes of spontaneous frozen shoulder are unknown. A long period of immobilization, such as with wearing a sling or a cast after an injury, can cause it. Things that can increase chances of getting a frozen shoulder include long-term bed rest, shoulder injury, diabetes, stroke, Parkinson's disease, and thyroid problems.

What Are the Symptoms of Frozen Shoulder?

Pain occurs throughout the shoulder area. The pain is in bones of the shoulder joint. Other nearby bones, including the scapula (shoulder blade) and clavicle (collarbone), can also be painful. Pain can reach down into muscles of the upper arm. The pain occurs at the front and side of the shoulder. It's constant, even at rest and at night.

Besides the pain, movement becomes very limited. It becomes very hard to lift the arm.

How Is Frozen Shoulder Diagnosed?

The doctor makes a diagnosis from a physical examination. The doctor may order x-rays to rule out other illnesses that may cause symptoms. These conditions include degenerative arthritis, tumors, and shoulder dislocation.

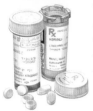

When frozen shoulder occurs without an injury or operation, conservative treatment with physical therapy is best. Your doctor can prescribe different treatments, including nonsteroidal antiinflammatory drugs (NSAIDs) for pain.

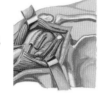

When it develops after shoulder surgery, more aggressive treatment, including more surgery, may be needed.

The key to recovery is to keep moving. Physical therapy, home exercises, and occupational therapy can help relieve pain and maintain arm movement.

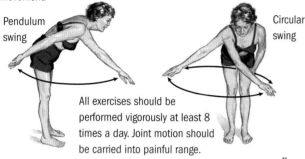

Pendulum swing

Circular swing

All exercises should be performed vigorously at least 8 times a day. Joint motion should be carried into painful range.

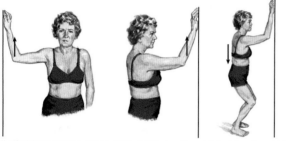

Wall-climbing exercise. Place palm against wall and "climb" wall as high as possible with fingers, first standing with side to wall, then facing wall. Maintain hand in highest position on wall and then bend knees, further stretching shoulder.

Abduction, external rotation (arm pulling)

Adduction, internal rotation (arm pulling)

Pulley exercise

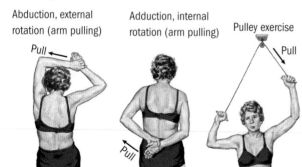

Pull

Pull

Pull

Pull

FROM THE DESK OF

NOTES

How Is Frozen Shoulder Treated?

When frozen shoulder occurs without an injury or operation, conservative treatment with physical therapy is best. When it develops after shoulder surgery, more aggressive treatment, including more surgery, may be needed.

The doctor can prescribe different treatments, including nonsteroidal antiinflammatory drugs (NSAIDs) for pain. Sometimes, stronger pain pills are ordered if NSAIDs don't help.

The key to recovery is to keep moving. Physical therapy, home exercises, and occupational therapy can be prescribed to relieve pain and maintain arm movement. Occupational therapy helps continue normal activities.

The doctor may inject steroids into the joint itself. Very rarely, surgery or manipulation of the shoulder may be needed.

After recovery, frozen shoulder usually won't occur in the same shoulder. Sometimes the other shoulder can become frozen.

DOs and DON'Ts in Managing Frozen Shoulder:

✔ **DO** take pills as your doctor directs.
✔ **DO** follow all instructions from the physical and occupational therapists.
✔ **DO** exercises as instructed.
✔ **DO** call your doctor if you have symptoms that worry you.
✔ **DO** call your doctor if you have shoulder pain that doesn't respond to rest and is related to decreased range of motion of the shoulder joint.
✔ **DO** use and move your shoulder normally. A frozen shoulder often follows periods of lack of use, or immobility, in a shoulder.

⊘ **DON'T** forget to do exercises.
⊘ **DON'T** stop your physical therapy without talking to your doctor.

FOR MORE INFORMATION

Contact the following sources:

• American Academy of Orthopaedic Surgeons
  Tel: (800) 346-AAOS (346-2267)
  Website: http://www.aaos.org

• American Physical Therapy Association
  Tel: (800) 999-2782
  Website: http://www.apta.org

• American College of Rheumatology
  Tel: (404) 633-3777
  Website: http://www.rheumatology.org

• Arthritis Foundation
  Tel : (800) 568-4045
  Website: http://www.arthritis.org

MANAGING YOUR
GANGLIA

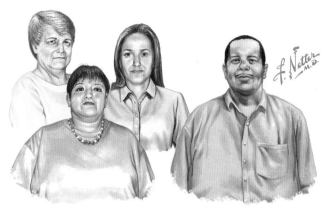

Ganglia are three times more common in women than in men and usually occur in people between 20 and 50 years old.

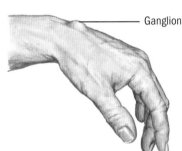

— Ganglion

Ganglia are fluid-filled sacs commonly found on hands or wrists.

Ganglia occur usually as single bumps that are firm, smooth, and round. Some people may have pain, hand numbness, and muscle weakness.

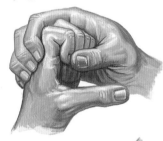

Ultrasonography

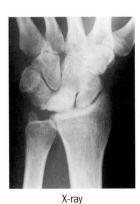

X-ray

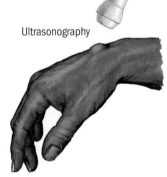

Your doctor usually makes a diagnosis from symptoms. X-rays can rule out other bone or joint problems. Other possible causes of a mass on the hand or wrist include fatty tumor, gout, rheumatoid arthritis, osteoarthritis, and infection. Ultrasonography sometimes helps by showing a smooth wall of a cyst rather than a solid mass.

What Are Ganglia?

Ganglia are fluid-filled sacs commonly found on hands or wrists.

What Causes Ganglia?

The exact cause is unknown, but trauma or degeneration of tissue lining joint covers (capsules) and sheaths (synovium) around tendons can be causes. Synovial tissue makes fluid that lubricates joints, and ganglia are protrusions or expansions of this tissue. Ganglia are three times more common in women than in men. They usually occur in people between 20 and 50 years old. Ganglia aren't contagious.

What Are the Symptoms of Ganglia?

Ganglia occur most often (50% to 70% of cases) on the back of the wrist. The next most common site is over the front of the wrist. Other sites are fingers. They occur on either hand, usually as single bumps that are firm, smooth, and round. When pushed, they may have a wave-like movement.

Ganglia usually develop for months but can arise suddenly. Some people may have pain, because of pressure on nearby structures. Hand numbness and muscle weakness are other symptoms.

How Are Ganglia Diagnosed?

The doctor usually makes a diagnosis from symptoms. The doctor may order x-rays to rule out other bone or joint abnormalities. Other possible causes of a mass on the hand or wrist include lipoma (fatty tumor), gout, rheumatoid arthritis, osteoarthritis, aneurysm of a radial artery, and infection. Ultrasonography sometimes helps by showing a smooth wall of a cyst rather than a solid mass.

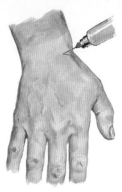

Treatment may not be needed unless pain or muscle weakness is present or cosmetic issues are a concern. Aspiration with a large needle, followed by injection of cortisone, can be tried.

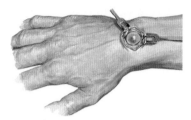

If these treatments don't work or ganglia come back, surgery is the best treatment. The operation, called a total ganglionectomy, usually cures ganglia. It's done with local anesthesia. Remember that ganglia are usually not treated surgically unless certain symptoms occur or cosmetic concerns are an issue.

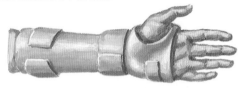

Complications of ganglia include carpal tunnel syndrome, with pain and muscle weakness and pressure on the radial nerve and radial artery.

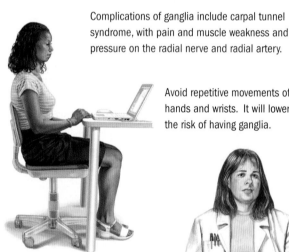

Avoid repetitive movements of hands and wrists. It will lower the risk of having ganglia.

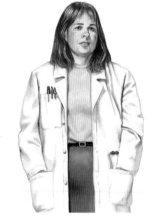

Call your doctor if you have pain, muscle weakness, or numbness near the ganglia. Call your doctor if drainage, redness, fever, chills, or sweats occur after surgery, or if the cyst retuns after treatment.

How Are Ganglia Treated?

Treatment may not be needed unless pain or muscle weakness is present or cosmetic issues are a concern.

Aspiration with a large needle, followed by injection of cortisone, can be tried. Ganglia come back in 35% to 40% of cases.

If these treatments don't work or ganglia come back, surgery is the best treatment. The operation is called a total ganglionectomy and cures ganglia in 85% to 95% of cases.

Complications of ganglia include carpal tunnel syndrome, with pain and muscle weakness and pressure on the radial nerve and radial artery. Complications of ganglion surgery include infection, scar formation, and recurrence.

DOs and DON'Ts in Managing Ganglia:

✔ **DO** understand that ganglia are usually not treated surgically unless certain symptoms appear or cosmetic concerns are an issue.
✔ **DO** tell your doctor about any mass you see on your body.
✔ **DO** go to follow-up appointments with your doctor, especially if the mass changes (e.g., size, redness, warmth, drainage).
✔ **DO** avoid repetitive movements of hands and wrists. It will lower the risk of having ganglia.
✔ **DO** call your doctor if you have pain with ganglia, muscle weakness, or numbness in the area of the ganglia.
✔ **DO** call your doctor if drainage, redness, fever, chills, or sweats occur after surgery.
✔ **DO** call your doctor if the cyst returns after treatment.

⊘ **DON'T** be worried. Ganglia are not cancer or associated with cancer.
⊘ **DON'T** forget that, if surgery is indicated, the operation is usually done with local anesthesia, not general anesthesia. You can expect complete use of the arm and hand by 2 to 6 weeks after surgery, depending on the ganglia location.

FROM THE DESK OF

NOTES

FOR MORE INFORMATION

Contact the following sources:

• American College of Rheumatology
  Tel: (404) 633-3777
  Website: http://www.rheumatology.org

• American Academy of Orthopaedic Surgeons
  Tel: (847) 823-7186
  Website: http://www.aaos.org

MANAGING YOUR GOUT

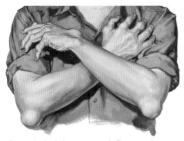

Gout is a kind of arthritis, an illness that causes pain and swelling in joints.

Crystals in joints cause inflammation, pain, and swelling. These crystals are made of uric acid. Either too much uric acid is made, or not enough is removed from the blood by the kidneys. Injuries, surgery, acute illness, aspirin, medicines, some foods (liver and other organ meats, sardines, anchovies), and alcohol can trigger attacks.

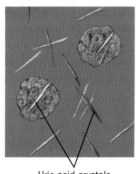

Uric acid crystals in joint fluid

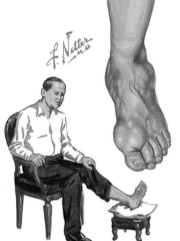

Sudden, intense joint pain and swelling are symptoms. Joints may feel hot and tender and turn red. Even lightly touching the joint can cause severe pain. Feet are most often affected, usually the big toe, but ankles, knees, and hands can also have gout.

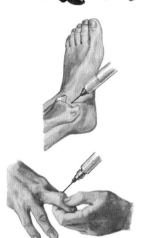

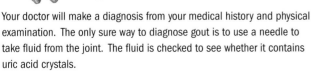

Your doctor will make a diagnosis from your medical history and physical examination. The only sure way to diagnose gout is to use a needle to take fluid from the joint. The fluid is checked to see whether it contains uric acid crystals.

What Is Gout?

Gout is a kind of arthritis, an illness that causes pain and swelling in joints.

What Causes Gout?

Crystals released into a joint cause inflammation, pain, and swelling. These crystals are made of a substance called uric acid. Either too much uric acid is made, or not enough is removed from the blood by the kidneys. Alcohol, aspirin, medicines, and some foods (liver and other organ meats, sardines, anchovies) can cause high uric acid levels. Attacks may occur at any time, but injuries, surgery, acute illness, rich foods, and alcohol can trigger them.

What Are the Symptoms of Gout?

Sudden, intense joint pain and swelling are symptoms. Joints may feel hot and tender and turn red. Even lightly touching the joint can cause severe pain, which is usually continuous and worse if the joint is moved. A sudden attack usually lasts several days. Attacks can happen years apart or occur back to back. Some people can have long-lasting, constant pain. Everyday activities (walking, dressing, lifting) may be hard to do.

Gout can occur in any joint, but most often feet are affected, usually the big toe. Gout can also occur in hands, ankles, insteps, or knees.

How Is Gout Diagnosed?

The doctor will make a diagnosis from the medical history and physical examination. The doctor may do blood tests but they can be unreliable. The only sure way to diagnose gout is to use a needle to take fluid from the joint. The fluid is checked to see whether it contains uric acid crystals.

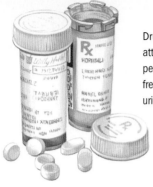

Drugs (NSAIDs) are used to treat attacks. Prevention is needed for people with tophi, kidney stones, and frequent attacks. Medicines can lower uric acid levels and prevent attacks.

Removing fluid from the joint, followed by injecting cortisone into the joint, is another treatment. Cortisone injections usually give the fastest and best relief of pain and swelling.

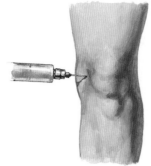

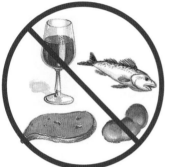

Avoid liver and other organ meats, sardines, and anchovies, which may increase uric acid levels. Stop drinking alcohol.

Make lifestyle changes to prevent attacks. Lose weight if you are overweight.

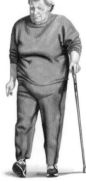

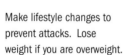

Call your doctor if you begin to lose movement in the joint; you have warmth, redness, or pain after a cortisone injection; you have medicine side effects; or medicine doesn't help your symptoms.

FROM THE DESK OF

NOTES

How Is Gout Treated?

Attacks can be treated and prevented. Nonsteroidal anti-inflammatory drugs (NSAIDs), such as indomethacin and naproxen, are used for treatment. Other drugs include colchicine, another antiinflammatory drug, and prednisone. Removal of fluid from the joint, followed by cortisone injection, is another treatment. Cortisone injections usually give the fastest and best relief of pain and swelling.

After attacks are treated, symptoms usually go away within hours to a few days. Untreated attacks may last several days. People with higher blood uric acid levels are more likely to have many attacks. High uric acid levels for many years can cause deposits of uric acid under the skin, called tophi.

Prevention is needed for people with tophi, kidney stones, and frequent attacks. Lowering uric acid levels prevents attacks. The medicines allopurinol and probenecid can do this.

DOs and DON'Ts in Managing Gout:

✔ **DO** rest the affected joint until symptoms start to improve.

✔ **DO** take your medicines as prescribed.

✔ **DO** ask your doctor which over-the-counter medicines you're allowed to take.

✔ **DO** make lifestyle changes to prevent attacks. Lose weight if you're very overweight. Avoid liver and other organ meats, sardines, and anchovies, which may increase uric acid levels. Stop drinking alcohol.

✔ **DO** call your doctor if you have medicine side effects or medicine doesn't help symptoms.

✔ **DO** call your doctor if you begin to lose movement in the joint.

✔ **DO** call your doctor if you have warmth, redness, or pain after a cortisone injection.

⊘ **DON'T** drink alcohol. Too much alcohol can cause gout.

FOR MORE INFORMATION

Contact the following sources:

• American College of Rheumatology
  Tel: (404) 633-3777
  Website: http://www.rheumatology.org

• Arthritis Foundation
  Tel: (800) 283-7800
  Website: http://www.arthritis.org

• The Arthritis Society
  Website: http://www.arthritis.ca

A femoral neck fracture is a break of the thigh bone (femur) at the hip. Older people, especially women, have these fractures resulting from osteoporosis (thinning of bone) related to aging. If the bone of the hip is thin enough, even twisting can break the bone.

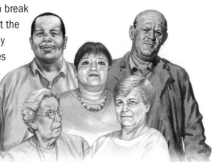

Neck of the femur with fracture   Complete break

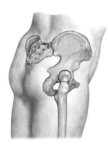

The hip joint is a ball-and-socket joint. The break occurs at the neck, which is the part just below the ball. The blood supply to the broken bone is often interrupted, so these fractures have trouble healing.

The cause can be a severe fall or an auto accident. Osteoporosis related to aging is a risk factor for fractures.

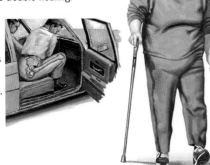

Symptoms are pain in the hip, buttock, or pubic area, especially with movement of the hip or leg. The affected leg is shorter than the other leg, and the foot turns in.

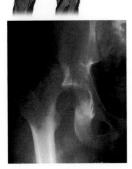

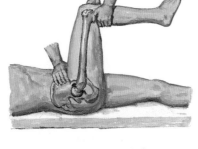

Your doctor makes a diagnosis from a physical examination and x-rays of the hip.

What Is a Hip Fracture?

A femoral neck fracture is a break of the thigh bone (femur) at the hip. The hip joint is a ball-and-socket joint. The break occurs at the neck, which is the part just below the ball. The blood supply to the broken bone is often interrupted, so these fractures have trouble healing. Most people do have a complete recovery after surgery.

What Causes a Hip Fracture?

The cause can be a severe fall or an auto accident. More often, older people, especially women, have these fractures. They result from osteoporosis (thinning of bone) related to aging. If the bone of the hip is thin enough, even twisting can break the bone. People may twist while standing, which breaks the bone, and then they fall. As many as one quarter of all women older than 75 may have severe enough osteoporosis to have a hip fracture.

What Are the Symptoms of a Hip Fracture?

Symptoms are pain in the hip, buttock, or pubic area, especially with movement of the hip or leg. The affected leg is shorter than the other leg, and the foot turns in. Later, bruising on the hip, especially in thin people, can be seen.

How Is a Hip Fracture Diagnosed?

The doctor makes a diagnosis from the physical examination and x-rays of the hip.

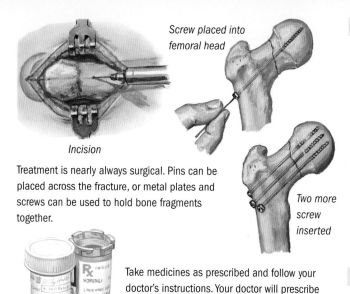

Screw placed into femoral head

Incision

Two more screw inserted

Treatment is nearly always surgical. Pins can be placed across the fracture, or metal plates and screws can be used to hold bone fragments together.

Take medicines as prescribed and follow your doctor's instructions. Your doctor will prescribe pain medicine.

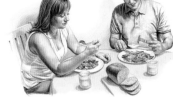

Do your exercises in the form of physical therapy. They are very important for recovery from surgery.

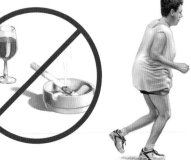

The best ways to prevent hip fractures are to prevent and treat osteoporosis with a good diet (for protein and calcium), exercise, and medicine.

Avoid alcohol and tobacco. They increase the risk of osteoporosis, as does lack of weight-bearing exercise.

How Is a Hip Fracture Treated?

Treatment is nearly always surgical. Pins can be placed across the fracture, or metal plates and screws can be used to hold bone fragments together. Other choices include replacing the ball of the joint with a metal one, and replacing both the socket and the ball. Sometimes, surgery doesn't make the joint stable, usually because the bone that's left is too thin.

For people who are very sick, treatment may be bed rest to try to let the fracture heal.

The best ways to prevent hip fractures are to prevent and treat osteoporosis with diet, exercise, and medicine. Also, make sure that the home environment is safe.

DOs and DON'Ts in Managing a Hip Fracture:

✔ **DO** take medicines as prescribed and follow your doctor's instructions.

✔ **DO** use pain medicines to help recovery.

✔ **DO** eat a good diet to provide protein and calcium. This will help the bone to heal.

✔ **DO** your exercises in the form of physical therapy. They're important for recovery from surgery.

✔ **DO** call your doctor if you have increasing pain in your hip after surgery. This pain could mean infection, bleeding, or loosening of the hip replacement or screws.

✔ **DO** call your doctor if you have trouble walking. It can be a sign of loosening of the hip replacement.

✔ **DO** call your doctor if you have symptoms of infection, such as fever or swelling or redness of the incision line. Tell your doctor about shortness of breath and coughing, which could mean pneumonia or a blood clot to the lungs.

✔ **DO** reduce chances of falls in the home. Use good lighting and avoid tripping hazards such as loose rugs and poor-fitting shoes.

⊘ **DON'T** use alcohol and tobacco. They increase the risk of osteoporosis, as does lack of weight-bearing exercise.

FROM THE DESK OF

NOTES

FOR MORE INFORMATION

Contact the following source:

• American Academy of Orthopaedic Surgeons
  Tel: (847) 823-7186
  Website: http://www.aaos.org

The hip is where the pelvis and leg meet. Hip pain refers to pain affecting any part of this whole area.

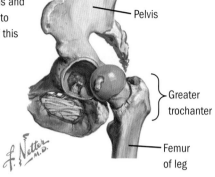

Pelvis

Greater trochanter

Femur of leg

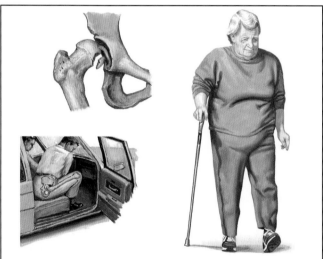

The many causes include injuries, fractures, tumors, or diseases, such as osteoarthritis, rheumatoid arthritis, or ankylosing spondylitis. Inflammation can affect tendons (tendinitis) and the thin, fluid-filled sac (bursa) that protects the joint (bursitis).

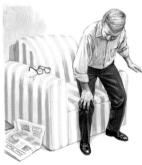

Symptoms depend on the cause. Osteoarthritis may cause mild pain only with activity. Sudden injuries, fractures, and tumors may cause severe pain when trying to walk, make the hip look deformed, and cause bruising in the hip area.

Your doctor makes a diagnosis by taking a medical history, doing a physical examination, and maybe taking x-rays of the joint. The doctor may also order blood tests, MRI, or a bone scan if the diagnosis is unclear or additional treatment is needed.

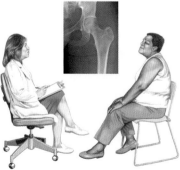

What Is Hip Pain?

The hip is the ball-and-socket joint where the pelvis and leg (femur) meet. Tendons are fibrous tissues that connect muscles to bones. Ligaments join bones (or cartilages) together. Hip pain refers to pain affecting this whole area.

What Causes Hip Pain?

The many causes include injuries, fractures, tumors, or diseases, such as osteoarthritis, rheumatoid arthritis, or ankylosing spondylitis, that affect the hip joint. Inflammation is another cause. It can affect tendons (tendinitis) and the thin, fluid-filled sac (bursa) that protects the joint (bursitis). Problems in sacroiliac joints or low back can also cause hip pain.

What Are the Symptoms of Hip Pain?

Symptoms depend on the cause. Osteoarthritis may cause mild pain only with activity. Sudden injuries, fractures, and tumors may cause severe pain when trying to walk, make the hip look deformed, and cause bruising in the hip area.

How Is Hip Pain Diagnosed?

The doctor makes a diagnosis by taking a medical history, doing a physical examination, and maybe taking x-rays of the joint. The doctor may also order blood tests to see whether the pain is caused by diseases with similar symptoms. Magnetic resonance imaging (MRI) or bone scan may be done if the doctor needs a clearer picture of the bones and structures around them.

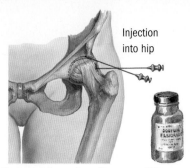

Injection into hip

Treatment depends on the cause. If the cause is osteoarthritis, the doctor may prescribe acetaminophen or an NSAID. For bursitis or tendinitis, the doctor may prescribe an NSAID and suggest physical therapy. Physical therapy usually uses deep heat or ultrasound (or both). For severe bursitis, the doctor may inject an antiinflammatory steroid drug.

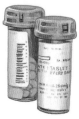

Take your medicines as prescribed. Call your doctor if you have side effects from your medicines. Ask your doctor which over-the-counter pain drugs you may take with your prescription medicines.

Do your prescribed hip exercises daily. Call your doctor if you need a referral to a physical therapist for exercises.

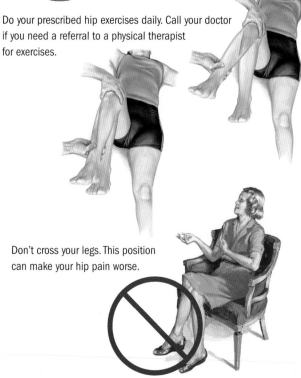

Don't cross your legs. This position can make your hip pain worse.

How Is Hip Pain Treated?

Treatment depends on the cause. If the cause is osteoarthritis, the doctor may prescribe acetaminophen or a nonsteroidal antiinflammatory drug (NSAID). If the cause is bursitis or tendinitis, the doctor may prescribe an NSAID, suggest physical therapy, or do both. Physical therapy usually consists of using deep heat, ultrasound, or both. For severe bursitis, the doctor may inject a steroid-containing medicine (a strong antiinflammatory drug) into the bursa.

More serious causes of hip pain such as a fracture or severe degenerative joint disease may need surgery.

DOs and DON'Ts in Managing Hip Pain:

✔ **DO** take your medicines as prescribed.

✔ **DO** call your doctor if you have side effects from medicines.

✔ **DO** ask your doctor which over-the-counter pain medicines you may take with your prescription drugs.

✔ **DO** your prescribed hip exercises daily.

✔ **DO** call your doctor if medicine and other treatments don't help the pain.

✔ **DO** call your doctor if you need a referral to a physical therapist for exercise.

⊘ **DON'T** wait for a medicine side effect to go away on its own.

⊘ **DON'T** continue an exercise program that causes persistent pain. Pain after exercise usually means that the exercise has to be changed.

⊘ **DON'T** cross your legs. This position can make your hip pain worse.

FROM THE DESK OF

NOTES

FOR MORE INFORMATION

Contact the following sources:

• Arthritis Foundation
  Tel: (800) 283-7800
  Website: http://www.arthritis.org

• American Academy of Orthopaedic Surgeons
  Tel: (847) 823-7186
  Website: http://www.aaos.org

MANAGING YOUR
KNEE PAIN

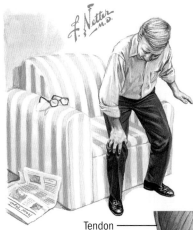

Knee pain is a rather vague diagnosis. It may be pain in the front part of the knee just under the kneecap or deep in the knee joint itself. The location of the pain is important because it will suggest the most likely cause.

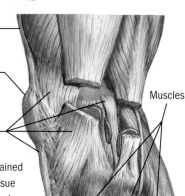

Tendon

Kneecap

Ligaments

Muscles

The many causes include a sprained or torn ligament (connective tissue linking bones), torn cartilage, and arthritis of the kneecap or the whole joint, such as rheumatoid arthritis and osteoarthritis.

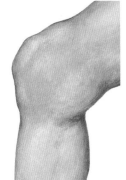

Inside the knee, from the side

Pain and usually swelling and sometimes a clicking or popping feeling are symptoms.

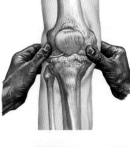

Your doctor will make a diagnosis from your medical history, physical examination, x-rays, and sometimes blood tests.

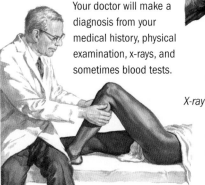

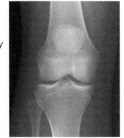

X-ray

What Is Knee Pain?

Knee pain is a rather vague diagnosis. It may be pain in the front part of the knee just under the kneecap or deep in the knee joint itself. The location of the pain is important because it will suggest the most likely cause.

Knee pain is very common and usually goes away by itself after the activity causing it is found and stopped.

What Causes Knee Pain?

The many causes include a sprained or torn ligament, torn cartilage, and arthritis of the kneecap or the whole joint. These inflammatory conditions include rheumatoid arthritis and osteoarthritis.

What Are the Symptoms of Knee Pain?

Pain and usually swelling and sometimes a clicking or popping feeling are symptoms. Sometimes, the knee can catch and lock. In that case, a piece of torn cartilage is trapped in the joint and stops the knee from bending or straightening.

How Is Knee Pain Diagnosed?

The doctor will make a diagnosis from the medical history and physical examination. X-rays of the knees and sometimes blood tests may be done. If fluid is present in the knee (knee effusion), the doctor may put a needle in the knee and take fluid out. The fluid will be sent to a laboratory for study.

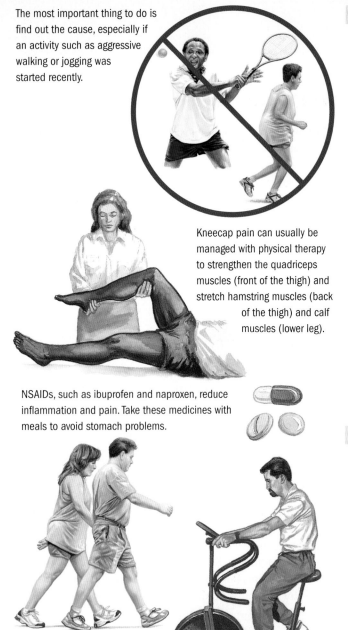

The most important thing to do is find out the cause, especially if an activity such as aggressive walking or jogging was started recently.

Kneecap pain can usually be managed with physical therapy to strengthen the quadriceps muscles (front of the thigh) and stretch hamstring muscles (back of the thigh) and calf muscles (lower leg).

NSAIDs, such as ibuprofen and naproxen, reduce inflammation and pain. Take these medicines with meals to avoid stomach problems.

Talk to your doctor about a time line for resuming activities and which activities they should be. Walking and biking have lower impact on the knee, so it may be better to start with them instead of running or other activities.

FROM THE DESK OF

NOTES

How Is Knee Pain Treated?

The most important thing to do is find out the cause, especially if an activity such as aggressive walking or jogging was started recently. Many people who participate in sports on a court that involve sideways movement have knee symptoms. When these activities are stopped for 2 to 6 weeks, symptoms slowly go away.

Over-the-counter nonsteroidal antiinflammatory drugs (NSAIDs), such as ibuprofen or naproxen, help inflammation (swelling, redness) and pain. These drugs can cause stomach problems and should be taken with meals. People who have ulcers or bleeding ulcers should check with the doctor before using these drugs.

Kneecap pain can usually be managed with physical therapy to strengthen the quadriceps muscles (front of the thigh) and stretch hamstring muscles (back of the thigh) and calf muscles (lower leg). Sprained ligaments often heal with rest and time. Torn ligaments around the knee sometimes need immobilization and then aggressive physical therapy. If the knee pain persists or worsens despite treatment, a surgeon may suggest an operation (arthroscopy) to repair the damage. After symptoms have stopped, activities can be restarted slowly, beginning with activities such as walking or cycling.

DOs and DON'Ts in Managing Knee Pain:

✔ **DO** take your medicines as prescribed.
✔ **DO** stop the activity that causes pain.
✔ **DO** restart activities slowly. Resume very carefully the activity that caused the pain.
✔ **DO** call your doctor if you have tried conservative treatment on your own and you still have symptoms.
✔ **DO** call your doctor if you are doing physical therapy or rehabilitation and your symptoms worsen.
✔ **DO** call your doctor if you have side effects from medicines.

🚫 **DON'T** use NSAIDs if you had bleeding ulcers.
🚫 **DON'T** continue the offending activity, such as running. You can further injure the knee, which may worsen or damage the joint itself.

FOR MORE INFORMATION

Contact the following sources:
- American Academy of Orthopaedic Surgeons
  Tel: (847) 823-7186
  Website: http://www.aaos.org
- American College of Sports Medicine
  Tel: (317) 637-9200
  Website: http://www.acsm.org
- National Athletic Trainers' Association
  Tel: (800) 879-6282
  Website: http://www.nata.org

MANAGING YOUR
KNEE SPRAIN

The knee is a hinge joint that moves forward and backward but doesn't turn in other directions. Two ligaments stabilize it: the medial and lateral collateral ligaments (MCL and LCL). Deep in the joint, the anterior and posterior cruciate ligaments (ACL and PCL) cross each other and attach to the thigh bone and the shinbone. A knee sprain involves damage to these ligaments.

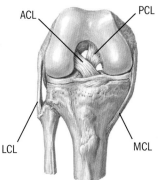

ACL   PCL

LCL   MCL

Knee joint, from the front

Types of sprains and symptoms

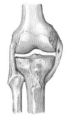 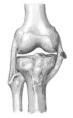 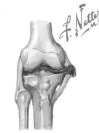

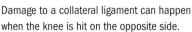

Mild: Stretching of ligament; causes pain and swelling

Moderate: Partial tear of ligament; more pain

Severe: Complete tear of ligament; needs surgery

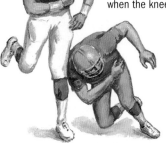

Damage to a collateral ligament can happen when the knee is hit on the opposite side.

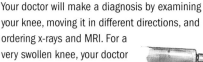

Your doctor will make a diagnosis by examining your knee, moving it in different directions, and ordering x-rays and MRI. For a very swollen knee, your doctor may take fluid from the knee with a needle for study.

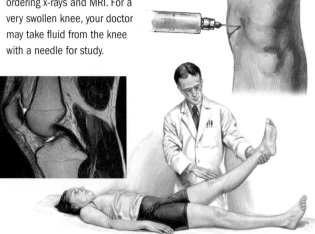

What Is Knee Sprain?

The knee joint is called a hinge joint because it moves forward and backward but doesn't turn in other directions. Ligaments are tough fibrous tissues that connect bones to other bones. Two strong ligaments make this hinge stable: the medial and lateral collateral ligaments (MCL and LCL). Deep in the joint, two more ligaments crisscross each other and attach to the thigh bone at one end and the shinbone at the other. These are the anterior and posterior cruciate ligaments (ACL and PCL).

A knee sprain involves damage to these ligaments. It can be mild, moderate, or severe.

What Causes Knee Sprain?

A sprain occurs when these ligaments stretch or tear. Damage to a collateral ligament can happens when the knee is hit on the opposite side. Damage to a cruciate ligament can occur when the knee joint is twisted or hit directly.

What Are the Symptoms of Knee Sprain?

Symptoms include knee pain and swelling, bruising around the knee, feeling of unsteadiness, knee giving way, and snapping feeling inside the knee.

How Is Knee Sprain Diagnosed?

The doctor will make a diagnosis by examining the knee, moving it in different directions and testing ligaments. The doctor will also order x-rays and magnetic resonance imaging (MRI) of the knee. For a very swollen knee, the doctor may take fluid from the knee with a needle. This may ease pain and helps make the diagnosis.

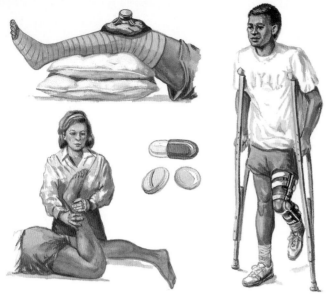

Treatment depends on how severe your injury is. For mild or moderate sprains, raising the leg (higher than the heart) and resting it on a soft pillow and applying ice packs can help. Your doctor may want you to keep weight off your leg by using crutches or a knee brace. Antiinflammatory drugs can help pain and swelling. Physical therapy may also help.

For a severe injury with a fully torn ligament, surgery may be needed to fix the ligament. Recovery may take 2 to 3 months or longer, so be patient. Rushing return to sports or other activities that increase pressure on the knee joint can lead to more injury and delay recovery.

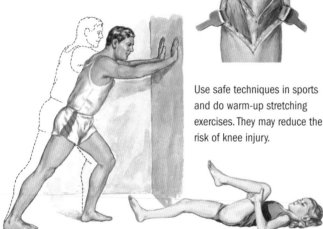

Use safe techniques in sports and do warm-up stretching exercises. They may reduce the risk of knee injury.

FROM THE DESK OF

NOTES

How Is Knee Sprain Treated?

Treatment depends on the severity of the injury. Treatments include putting an ice pack, wrapped in cloth, on the swollen knee. Raising the leg (higher than the heart) and resting it on something like a soft pillow may help swelling go away. The doctor may prescribe antiinflammatory drugs to help pain and swelling. The knee can be wrapped in an elastic compression bandage. Crutches may help until walking is possible without pain. Exercises may reduce stiffness. The doctor may suggest a knee brace to control joint movement.

For a severe injury with a ligament that was completely torn, surgery may be needed to fix the ligament. Recovery may take 2 to 3 months or longer.

A mild sprain may take 2 to 3 weeks for full recovery. A severe sprain may take 6 weeks or longer. Recovery will be slower if sports or other activities that put pressure on the knee joint are restarted too soon.

DOs and DON'Ts in Managing Knee Sprain:

✔ **DO** follow the advice you get about whether to put weight on your leg.
✔ **DO** be patient. You may not be able to do sports for several weeks.
✔ **DO** report continued swelling or pain to your doctor.
✔ **DO** follow instructions for rehabilitation so that you develop good strength and stability and don't injure the knee again. This may prevent another sprain.
✔ **DO** use safe techniques and warm-up stretching exercises. They may reduce the risk of knee injury.
✔ **DO** ask your doctor about taking antiinflammatory medicines regularly.

🚫 **DON'T** return to normal activities or sports if your knee still feels unstable.
🚫 **DON'T** forget to do your rehabilitation exercises.
🚫 **DON'T** try to do activities that cause you pain.

FOR MORE INFORMATION

Contact the following sources:
- American Academy of Orthopaedic Surgeons
  Tel: (847) 823-7186
  Website: http://www.aaos.org/
- American College of Sports Medicine
  Tel: (317) 637-9200
  Website: http://www.acsm.org/
- National Athletic Trainers' Association
  Tel: (800) 879-6282
  Website: http://www.nata.org/

CARING FOR YOUR CHILD WITH
LEGG-CALVÉ-PERTHES DISEASE

Legg-Calvé-Perthes disease involves a loss of the blood supply to the hip joint. This blood supply loss can lead to collapse of the hip joint and early arthritis and stiffness of the hip. This disease usually occurs in children 5 to 12 years old, more often in boys than girls.

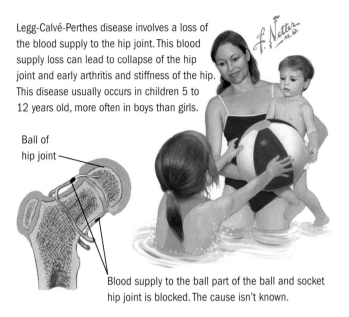

Ball of hip joint

Blood supply to the ball part of the ball and socket hip joint is blocked. The cause isn't known.

This disease usually starts with hip pain, but pain in the thigh or groin or near the knee may occur. The child may limp or have more and more trouble walking because of the pain.

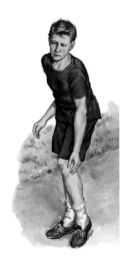

X-ray

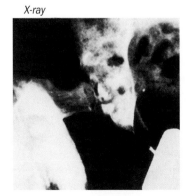

Your doctor makes a diagnosis from a medical history, age of your child, and a physical examination that shows pain when the hip is rotated. X-rays are needed to confirm the diagnosis.

What Is Legg-Calvé-Perthes Disease?

Legg-Calvé-Perthes disease involves a loss of the blood supply to the ball part of the ball and socket hip joint. The ball part is the top (head) of the femur (thigh bone). This loss of blood supply to the femoral head can lead to collapse of the hip joint and early arthritis and stiffness of that joint. This disease usually occurs in children 5 to 12 years old, with more boys affected than girls. The disease isn't very common. If it's found early enough, it can be treated. Usually one hip is affected, but sometimes symptoms can occur in both hips.

What Causes Legg-Calvé-Perthes Disease?

The cause of the loss of blood supply is unknown.

What Are the Symptoms of Legg-Calvé-Perthes Disease?

This disease usually starts with hip pain, but some children report pain in the thigh or groin or near the knee. Usually, the pain starts without a direct injury to the area. The child may limp or have more and more trouble walking because of the pain.

How Is Legg-Calvé-Perthes Disease Diagnosed?

The doctor makes a diagnosis from the medical history, age of the child, and a physical examination that shows pain when the hip is rotated. The child also will have a limp. X-rays are needed to confirm the diagnosis. Magnetic resonance imaging (MRI) will also show how much of the ball of the hip joint is involved.

The goals of treatment are to prevent severe arthritis, have good range of motion of the joint, take weight off the area, and keep the ball of the thigh bone inside the socket.

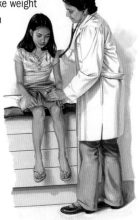

An orthopedic surgeon will use your child's age and the look of the joint on x-rays to decide whether to use casts, braces, or sometimes surgery.

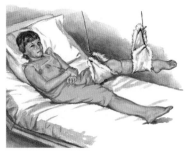

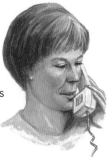

Call your doctor if your child constantly feels pain in one spot under the brace or cast. This spot may be a pressure sore.

How Is Legg-Calvé-Perthes Disease Treated?

The goals of treatment are to prevent severe arthritis, have good range of motion of the joint, take weight off the area, and keep the ball of the thigh bone inside the socket. An orthopedic surgeon (specialist who treats bone and muscle disorders) who has treated children should be involved in care.

The best treatment is to find the disease early. After the orthopedic surgeon confirms the diagnosis, several treatment options are available. The surgeon will use the child's age and the look of the joint on x-rays to decide whether to use casts, braces, or sometimes surgery.

DOs and DON'Ts in Managing Legg-Calvé-Perthes Disease:

✔ **DO** be careful with body casts and long leg braces. They are important for your child to wear but can be troublesome and uncomfortable. To relieve itching, use a hair dryer on a cool setting to blow air into the cast, or tap on the cast directly over the itch. Don't put something into the cast.

✔ **DO** call your doctor if your child constantly feels pain in one spot under the brace or cast. This spot may be a pressure sore.

✔ **DO** call your doctor if redness or swelling occurs, or a foul odor comes from the cast.

✔ **DO** call your doctor if after the treatment plan has been chosen, there are any changes from the program.

✔ **DO** ask your doctor for referrals to specialists who treat this condition.

⊘ **DON'T** put anything inside the cast to scratch. This can cause a skin sore, which can become infected.

FOR MORE INFORMATION

Contact the following sources:

• American Academy of Orthopaedic Surgeons
Tel: (847) 823-7186, (800) 346-2267
Website: http://www.aaos.org

• National Institute of Arthritis and Musculoskeletal and Skin Disease
Tel: (877) 226-4267
Website: http://www.niams.nih.gov

FROM THE DESK OF

NOTES

MANAGING YOUR
LOW BACK PAIN

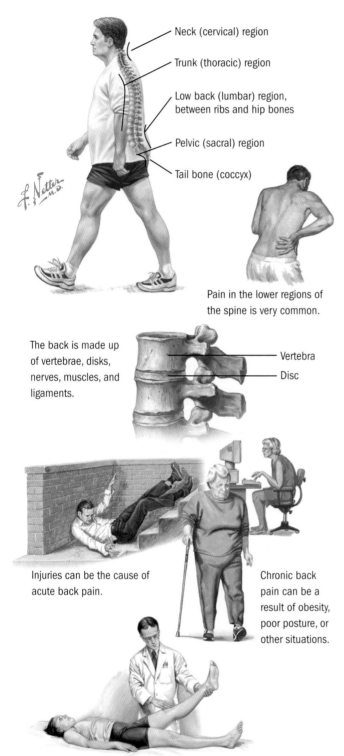

Neck (cervical) region

Trunk (thoracic) region

Low back (lumbar) region, between ribs and hip bones

Pelvic (sacral) region

Tail bone (coccyx)

Pain in the lower regions of the spine is very common.

The back is made up of vertebrae, disks, nerves, muscles, and ligaments.

Vertebra

Disc

Injuries can be the cause of acute back pain.

Chronic back pain can be a result of obesity, poor posture, or other situations.

Physical exam, imaging, and EMG can help in the understanding of an individual's back pain.

What Causes Low Back Pain?

The back is made up of bones (vertebrae) of the spinal column, disks between these bones, the spinal cord (which contains nerves), and muscles and ligaments. Muscles in the back and belly (abdomen) help support the spine. Injury in this area can cause pain. The term low back pain means pain in the lower parts of the spine.

An injury or accident such as a fall can cause *acute* low back pain lasting 1 to 7 days. *Chronic* low back pain lasts longer, for more than 3 months. Many such injuries result from twisting or sudden movement. Obesity, poor posture, and weak back and abdominal muscles may also cause this pain. Some people have pain after sitting for a long time or reaching for something too far away.

Low back pain may also occur with diseases such as arthritis or fibromyalgia and rarely, in more serious conditions such as tumors, kidney disease and blood disorders.

What Are Other Symptoms of Low Back Pain?

Bending at the waist, lifting, walking, and standing may be hard to do. Pain may disturb nighttime sleep. Chronic pain may affect the ability to do a job. If the sciatic nerve is in the injured area, the pain, called *sciatica*, will travel down the leg.

How Is Low Back Pain Diagnosed?

Diagnosis results from taking a medical history, doing a physical, and x-ray studies or magnetic resonance imaging (MRI) may be done if clearer pictures of bones, nerves, disks between the bones, or other areas are needed.

A study using electric current, called an electromyogram (EMG), helps diagnose muscle and nerve problems and may be done if pressure on the nerves may be causing numbness or tingling in the legs.

The doctor may also order blood tests to see whether the pain is caused by another ailment that may have similar symptoms.

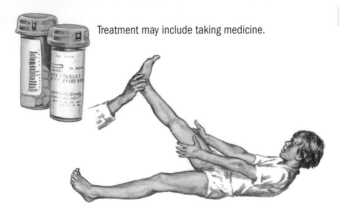

Treatment may include taking medicine.

Physical therapy can also reduce pain and strengthen the back.

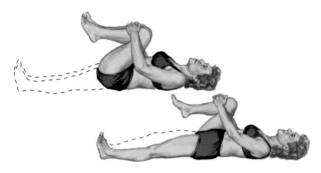

Exercise daily and control your weight. Ask your doctor for examples of more exercises you can do on your own.

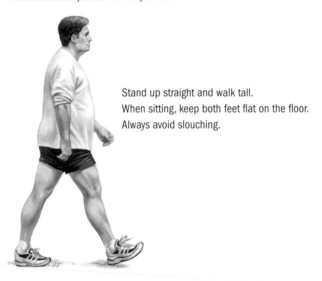

Stand up straight and walk tall.
When sitting, keep both feet flat on the floor.
Always avoid slouching.

How Is Low Back Pain Treated?

Treatment depends on the cause of the pain and how long pain has lasted.

If the pain is due to an injury, the doctor may suggest use of cold compresses. Nonsteroidal anti-inflammatory drugs (NSAIDs) may relieve the pain. Severe pain may require stronger narcotic-containing medicines for a short time. For muscle spasms, a doctor may prescribe a muscle relaxant.

All medicines have side effects. NSAIDs may cause stomach upset, ulcers, rash, and kidney or liver problems. Muscle relaxants may bring about drowsiness, dizziness, or rash.

Physical therapy may help reduce pain. Chronic low back pain can improve with exercises for the lower back and abdomen.

DOs and DON'Ts in Managing Low Back Pain:

✔ **DO** take your medicine as prescribed.
✔ **DO** call your doctor if you have drug side effects.
✔ **DO** lose weight if you are overweight.
✔ **DO** back stretching and strengthening exercises daily.
✔ **DO** use good posture when sitting, standing, or lifting.
✔ **DO** call your doctor if you have difficulty urinating or lose control of your bowels or bladder.

⊘ **DON'T** wait for a drug side effect to go away by itself.
⊘ **DON'T** give up. If you do not feel better, ask your doctor about starting in a special treatment program.
⊘ **DON'T** completely stop exercising.

FOR MORE INFORMATION

Contact the following sources:

• American Physical Therapy Association
  Tel: (800) 999-2782
  Website: http://www.apta.org

• American Academy of Orthopaedic Surgeons
  Tel: (800) 346-AAOS
  Website: http://www.aaos.org

• American Chronic Pain Association
  Tel: (916) 632-0922
  Website: http://www.theacpa.org

• North American Spine Society
  Tel: (708) 588-8080
  Website: http://www.spine.org

FROM THE DESK OF

NOTES

Your lumbar spine is made of five vertebrae separated by discs. These discs are shock absorbers. They cushion the bones and let the lower back be flexible. Lumbar disc syndrome refers to a group of symptoms related to disorders of these lumbar discs.

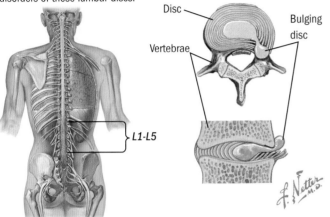

Disc
Bulging disc
Vertebrae
L1-L5

Normal aging causes degenerative changes in discs. Tobacco abuse, poor posture, and poor lifting methods may make these changes worse. Discs slowly become worn, less plump, and flat. Disc spaces become narrow, vertebrae rub together and have wear and tear, and bone spurs may press on the spinal cord or nerve roots.

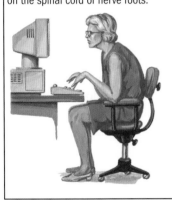

Back pain or tingling and numbness may reach the buttocks, hips, groin, or legs. Pain gets worse while moving, coughing, laughing, or straining.

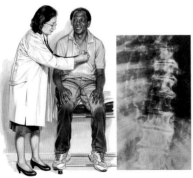

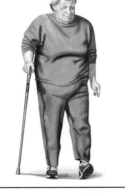

For diagnosis, your doctor may do an examination and order CT, MRI, combined myelography/CT, or EMG/NCV.

What Is Lumbar Disc Syndrome?

The lumbar spine (low back) is made of five vertebrae (bones) separated by cartilaginous discs. These discs are shock absorbers. They cushion the bones and let the lower back be flexible. Lumbar disc syndrome is a group of symptoms related to disorders of these lumbar discs. Degenerative changes or trauma may burst the annulus fibrosus. The annulus fibrosus is the tough band of cartilage around each disc. Disc material may bulge (herniate) into the spinal canal or nerve root canal and cause pain.

What Causes Lumbar Disc Syndrome?

Degenerative changes in discs are due to normal aging. Poor posture and strenuous work with poor lifting methods may make these changes worse. Discs slowly become worn, less plump, and flat. When disc spaces become so narrow that vertebrae rub together, vertebrae edges have wear-and-tear changes. Then bone spurs develop that may press on the spinal cord or nerve roots. As the nerve is irritated, back and leg pain, tingling, and numbness or weakness in the legs or feet can occur. Rarely, with very large, sudden disc bulges, bladder and bowel control may be lost.

What Are the Symptoms of Lumbar Disc Syndrome?

Pain in the back or tingling and numbness may reach the buttocks, hips, groin, or legs. Pain from a bulging disc is worse while moving, coughing, laughing, or straining when having a bowel movement. Some people also have weakness, clumsiness, drop foot, or trouble walking.

How Is Lumbar Disc Syndrome Diagnosed?

The doctor will do an examination and may order x-rays. One or more of the following tests: computed tomography (CT), magnetic resonance imaging (MRI), combined myelography/ CT, and electromyography/nerve conduction velocity test (EMG/NCV), may also be done for persistent pain or if surgery is being considered.

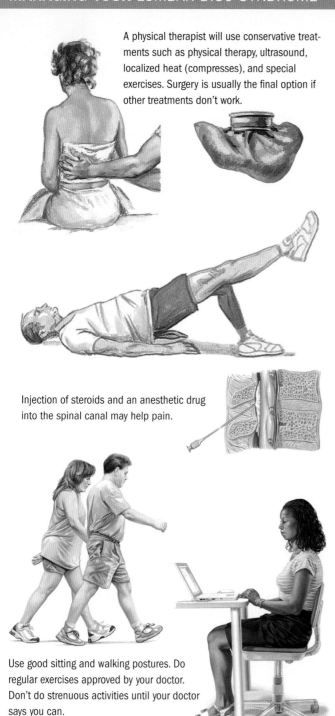

A physical therapist will use conservative treatments such as physical therapy, ultrasound, localized heat (compresses), and special exercises. Surgery is usually the final option if other treatments don't work.

Injection of steroids and an anesthetic drug into the spinal canal may help pain.

Use good sitting and walking postures. Do regular exercises approved by your doctor. Don't do strenuous activities until your doctor says you can.

How Is Lumbar Disc Syndrome Treated?

A trained physical therapist will use conservative treatments, such as physical therapy, ultrasound, localized heat, and special exercises. Injection of steroids and an anesthetic drug into the spinal canal may help pain. Surgery is usually the final option if other treatments don't work.

DOs and DON'Ts in Managing Lumbar Disc Syndrome:

✔ **DO** use good sitting and walking postures.

✔ **DO** always wear a seat belt when traveling in a motor vehicle.

✔ **DO** make a lumbar support, if you sit for long periods. Put a small pillow or rolled towel between your low back and the seat. Stand and walk around often (about every hour).

✔ **DO** always lift heavy objects with the correct straight posture. Hold the object close to your body and use your thigh and leg muscles to lift.

✔ **DO** regular exercises approved by your doctor.

✔ **DO** call your doctor if you have problems with your medicines.

✔ **DO** call your doctor if you have trouble walking, develop weakness or cannot move your limbs, or lose control of your bowels or bladder.

⊘ **DON'T** sit for long periods.

⊘ **DON'T** lift and twist, push, or pull heavy objects. Lift with leg muscles.

⊘ **DON'T** return to work without your doctor's OK.

⊘ **DON'T** do strenuous activities until your doctor says you can.

FOR MORE INFORMATION

Contact the following sources:

- American Physical Therapy Association
  Tel: (800) 999-2782
  Website: http://www.apta.org

- American Academy of Orthopaedic Surgeons
  Tel: (800) 346-AAOS (346-2267)
  Website: http://www.aaos.org

- American Chronic Pain Association
  Tel: (800) 533-3231
  Website: http://www.theacpa.org

- North American Spine Society
  Tel: (630) 230-3600
  Website: http://www.spine.org

- Arthritis Foundation
  Tel: (800) 283-7800
  Website: http://www.arthritis.org

FROM THE DESK OF

NOTES

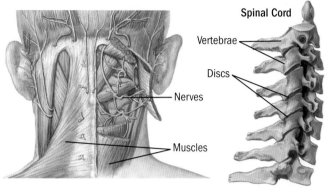

Spinal Cord

Vertebrae

Discs

Nerves

Muscles

The neck is made up of vertebrae, spinal cord with nerves, discs between vertebrae, and tissues such as muscles and ligaments. Neck pain may be caused by an injury or disease affecting this whole area.

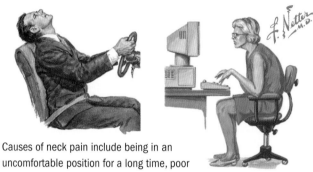

Causes of neck pain include being in an uncomfortable position for a long time, poor posture, diseases such as arthritis and fibromyalgia, and injuries. Stress that causes muscle tension may worsen pain.

People may have problems looking from side to side, driving, reading, and sleeping. Neck pain can cause headaches and may affect your ability to do your job.

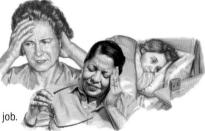

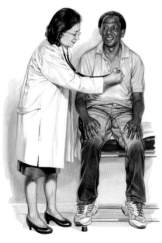

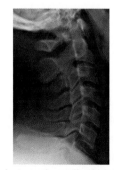

Your doctor makes a diagnosis from your medical history, physical examination, and maybe x-rays. Your doctor may order blood tests, MRI, or EMG.

What Is Neck Pain?

The neck is made up of the vertebrae (bones), spinal cord (which contains nerves), discs between vertebrae, and tissues such as muscles and ligaments. Vertebrae protect the spinal cord. Discs are like shock absorbers for the head and neck. They cushion the bones and allow the head and neck to bend. Ligaments are fibrous bands of tissue connecting bones (or cartilages) together. Neck pain may be caused by an injury or disease affecting this area.

What Causes Neck Pain?

Being in an uncomfortable position for a long time and poor posture can cause neck pain. It may occur with diseases such as osteoarthritis, rheumatoid arthritis, ankylosing spondylitis, and fibromyalgia. It may also result from a neck injury. Stress that causes muscle tension may worsen neck pain.

What Are the Symptoms of Neck Pain?

Symptoms include problems looking from side to side, driving, and reading. Sometimes, pain may prevent sleeping. Neck pain can cause headaches. Neck pain that lasts for months may affect a person's ability to work.

How Is Neck Pain Diagnosed?

The doctor makes a diagnosis from a medical history, physical examination, and maybe x-rays. The doctor may order blood tests to see whether neck pain is due to diseases with similar symptoms.

Magnetic resonance imaging (MRI) may be done if the doctor needs a clearer picture of bones, nerves, discs, and other soft tissues. Sometimes, electromyography (EMG), which helps find muscle and nerve problems, may be done if the neck problem may be causing numbness or tingling in the arms because of pressure on nerves.

Treatment depends on the cause of the pain. If an injury is the cause, using ice on the area and taking NSAIDs and possibly stronger narcotic medicines may help the pain. Muscle spasms may be helped with a muscle relaxant. Physical therapy may reduce pain with deep heat treatments, traction, and exercise.

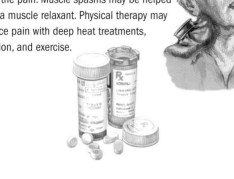

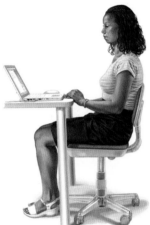

Use good posture when sitting and standing. Do your neck exercises every day.

Call your doctor if you continue to have neck pain or headaches, you have numbness or tingling in your arms, or you need a referral to a physical therapist.

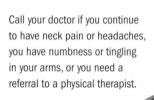

How Is Neck Pain Treated?

Treatment depends on the cause of the pain. If an injury is the cause, the doctor may suggest using ice on the area. Nonsteroidal antiinflammatory drugs (NSAIDs) may help reduce the pain. For especially severe pain, stronger narcotic medicines may be needed for a short time. Muscle spasms may be helped with a muscle relaxant. Physical therapy may reduce pain with deep heat treatments, traction, and exercise. All medicines have side effects. NSAIDs may cause stomach upset, diarrhea, ulcers, headache, dizziness, trouble hearing, or rash. Some side effects of muscle relaxants are drowsiness, dizziness, and rash.

DOs and DON'Ts in Managing Neck Pain:

✔ **DO** take your medicines as prescribed.
✔ **DO** call your doctor if you have side effects from medicines.
✔ **DO** use good posture when sitting and standing.
✔ **DO** ask your doctor about using a cervical pillow for severe pain.
✔ **DO** neck exercises every day.
✔ **DO** call your doctor if you continue to have neck pain or headaches.
✔ **DO** call your doctor if you have numbness or tingling in your arms.
✔ **DO** call your doctor if you need a referral to a physical therapist.

⊘ **DON'T** wait to see whether a side effect of medicine goes away on its own.

FROM THE DESK OF

NOTES

FOR MORE INFORMATION

Contact the following sources:

• National Arthritis Foundation
Tel: (800) 283-7800
Website: http://www.arthritis.org

• American Academy of Orthopaedic Surgeons
Tel: (847) 823-7186
Website: http://www.aaos.org

CARING FOR YOUR CHILD WITH
OSGOOD-SCHLATTER DISEASE

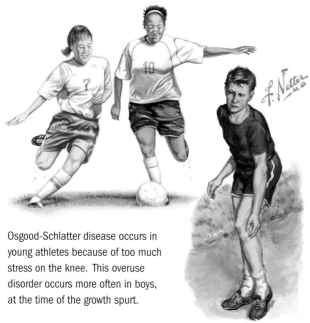

Osgood-Schlatter disease occurs in young athletes because of too much stress on the knee. This overuse disorder occurs more often in boys, at the time of the growth spurt.

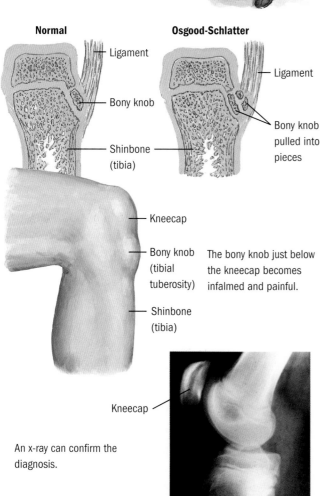

Normal

— Ligament

— Bony knob

— Shinbone (tibia)

Osgood-Schlatter

— Ligament

— Bony knob pulled into pieces

— Kneecap

— Bony knob (tibial tuberosity)

— Shinbone (tibia)

The bony knob just below the kneecap becomes infalmed and painful.

Kneecap —

Shinbone —

An x-ray can confirm the diagnosis.

What Is Osgood-Schlatter Disease?

Osgood-Schlatter disease is a painful condition that usually affects the rapidly growing knee. The bony knob just below the kneecap, where the tendon attaches to the leg bone (shinbone, or tibia), becomes painful.

This overuse disorder occurs more often in boys, usually 11 to 18 years old, at the time of the growth spurt. Girls, usually 8 to 16 years old, can also have it. This problem occurs after they take part in athletics or after a sports-related injury.

This condition usually causes no permanent damage. Most children recover completely.

What Causes Osgood-Schlatter Disease?

The cause is vigorous exercise that may put too much stress on bones and muscles of the knee and lower leg, which are still growing.

Some doctors believe that the bony attachment tries to pull away from the leg bone, which causes inflammation (swelling) and tenderness.

What Are the Symptoms of Osgood-Schlatter Disease?

Pain, tenderness, and swelling below the knee and on the shin are symptoms. They can occur in one or both legs. Pain gets worse when the knee is moved or the bony knob is pressed.

In mild cases, symptoms start to disappear in 6 weeks. After the area is rested, all symptoms should be gone in 1 year. Kneeling may be uncomfortable for 2 to 3 years. Pain usually disappears when the attachment site fuses to the leg bone.

How Is Osgood-Schlatter Disease Diagnosed?

The doctor will examine the area and may order an x-ray of the knee.

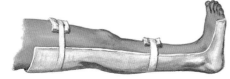

Resting the knee and taking a break from sports for about 6 weeks are usually all that's needed. Remember **RICE**: **R**est, **I**ce, **C**ompression (with an elastic bandage or splint), and **E**levation.

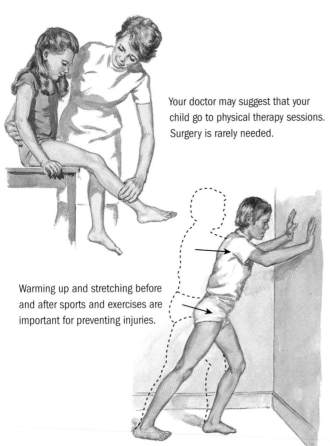

Your doctor may suggest that your child go to physical therapy sessions. Surgery is rarely needed.

Warming up and stretching before and after sports and exercises are important for preventing injuries.

How Is Osgood-Schlatter Disease Treated?

Treatment involves RICE: **R**est, **I**ce, **C**ompressing the area with an elastic bandage or splint, and **E**levating the area. Most children respond to a fairly brief period of rest during the most painful time. If an injury just occurred, the leg should be rested in a raised position for the first day. Ice should be used for the first few days. Not taking part in the sport that caused the injury for a few weeks may help.

Your doctor may suggest seeing a physical therapist for exercises to stretch and strengthen muscles, speed recovery, and increase flexibility. These exercises can prevent the condition from returning.

Your doctor may prescribe pain relievers and antiinflammatory medicines. If treatment doesn't help, a doctor who specializes in bone and muscle disorders (orthopedist) may be seen. Severe cases may need surgery, but this is rare.

DOs and DON'Ts in Managing Osgood-Schlatter Disease:

✔ **DO** encourage your child lose weight if needed.

✔ **DO** have your child do less strenuous activities.

✔ **DO** have your child do exercises prescribed by the physical therapist.

✔ **DO** have your child rest and immobilize the area as needed.

✔ **DO** have your child take medicines as prescribed.

✔ **DO** call your child's doctor if the pain begins to limit activities or returns after treatment.

✔ **DO** have your child warm up and stretch for 15 to 30 minutes before and after activities.

🚫 **DON'T** let your child participate in the sport or activity that caused the injury for 6 weeks.

🚫 **DON'T** let your child do other activities in which the leg is stressed for 6 weeks.

FROM THE DESK OF

NOTES

FOR MORE INFORMATION

Contact the following source:

• American Academy of Orthopaedic Surgeons
  Tel: (847) 823-7186
  Website: http://www.aaos.org

Osteoarthritis is an illness in which joints get inflamed, painful, and stiff. It usually affects the knees, hips, hands, and spine. It's very common when people reach their 70s. It affects both men and women, but women more than men.

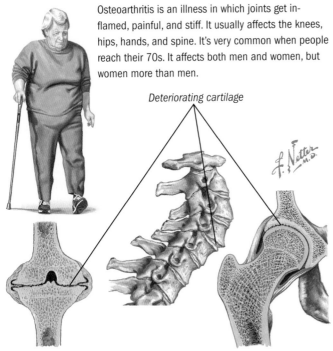

Deteriorating cartilage

These joints contain cartilage, the substance that cushions the place where two bones meet. In osteoarthritis, cartilage loses the ability to cushion the joint and bones rub together. In advanced disease, cartilage completely deteriorates. Causes include aging, injury, trauma, and obesity.

Pain usually gets worse with exercise and stops during rest. Over time, movement is limited and joints are less flexible. Stiffness occurs in the morning but goes away after moving around. Joints become tender and cannot bend.

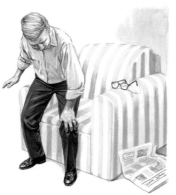

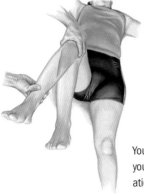
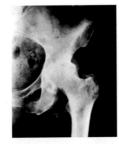

Your doctor makes a diagnosis from your symptoms and physical examination. The doctor may also take joint x-rays to confirm the diagnosis.

What Is Osteoarthritis?

Osteoarthritis (degenerative joint disease) is an illness in which joints get inflamed (swollen, red), painful, and stiff. It usually affects the knees, hips, hands, and spine. These joints contain cartilage, the substance that cushions the spot where two bones meet. As osteoarthritis develops, cartilage loses the ability to cushion the joint and bones rub together. In advanced disease, cartilage completely deteriorates (degenerates).

Osteoarthritis cannot be cured, but keeping to a normal weight and exercising regularly may help delay the start of the disease and improve flexibility. Avoid strenuous activities and contact sports.

What Causes Osteoarthritis?

The causes are aging, injury, trauma, obesity, and other factors. Osteoarthritis is very common when people reach their 70s. It affects both men and women, but women more than men.

What Are the Symptoms of Osteoarthritis?

Osteoarthritis develops slowly. Pain may be the first symptom. It usually gets worse with exercise and stops during rest. Over time, movement is limited and affected joints are less flexible. Stiffness occurs in the morning but goes away after moving around and joints warm up. As osteoarthritis gets worse, joints become tender and lose their ability to bend. People may have a grating feeling when moving.

How Is Osteoarthritis Diagnosed?

The doctor makes a diagnosis from the symptoms and physical examination. The doctor may also take joint x-rays to confirm the diagnosis.

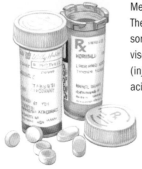

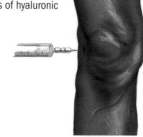

Medicines can help pain and inflammation. They include acetaminophen, NSAIDs, cortisone injections, and viscosupplementation (injections of hyaluronic acid).

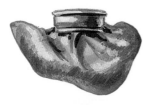

Heating bottles or warm soaks may help early morning stiffness. Cold packs reduce swelling and inflammation and are very useful after physical activity.

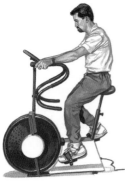

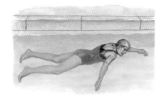

For more severe disease, physical therapy can help maintain use of the joints. Low-impact exercises such as swimming and cycling are good for helping muscle strength and flexibility. Avoid contact sports.

Assistive devices such as canes or braces may be used to minimize stress on knees. Surgery such as joint replacement is used for severe disease that isn't helped by other treatments.

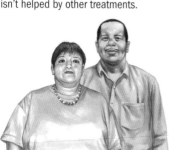

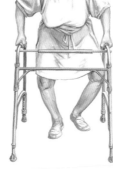

Lose weight if you're overweight.

How Is Osteoarthritis Treated?

Treatment goals are to control pain and prevent more joint degeneration. The kind of treatment depends on the severity of the changes in the joints and lifestyle. Acetaminophen may control symptoms of mild disease. Nonsteroidal antiinflammatory drugs (NSAIDs) may be prescribed for more severe pain. Using heat and cold may help relieve some symptoms. Heating pads or warm soaks may help early morning stiffness. Cold packs reduce swelling and inflammation and are very useful after physical activity.

For a more severe form of osteoarthritis, the doctor may prescribe physical therapy to help maintain use of the joints. Low-impact exercises such as swimming and cycling are good for maintaining muscle strength and flexibility. Lifestyle changes to keep to a healthy weight are very important. Injections of cortisone and other substances into the joints may also be used for mobility. Viscosupplementation involves injecting the substance called hyaluronic acid, which is a natural part of the fluid that lubricates joints. Assistive devices such as canes or braces may be used to minimize stress on knees.

Surgery is used for severe disease that isn't helped by other treatments. It can include joint replacement, cleaning up the area inside near the joint, and fusing bones.

DOs and DON'Ts in Managing Osteoarthritis:

✔ **DO** take your medicines as prescribed by your doctor.
✔ **DO** physical therapy to maintain muscle strength and flexibility.
✔ **DO** make changes to minimize discomfort and stress on your joints. Try swimming, walking, or riding a bicycle rather than running or jogging.
✔ **DO** lose weight if you're overweight.
✔ **DO** call your doctor if your joints are red and swollen.
✔ **DO** call your doctor if you develop a fever or rash with your joint pains.

⊘ **DON'T** participate in contact sports.

FROM THE DESK OF

NOTES

FOR MORE INFORMATION

Contact the following sources:

• American Academy of Orthopaedic Surgeons
  Tel: (847) 823-7186
  Website: http://www.aaos.org

• American College of Rheumatology
  Tel: (404) 633-3777
  Website: http://www.rheumatology.org

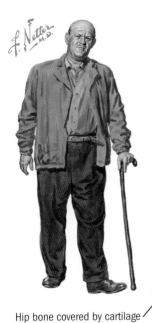

In osteoarthritis of the hip, the protective barrier between the thigh bone (femur) and hip bone is lost. It is very common when people get into their 70s.

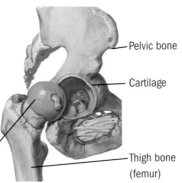

Pelvic bone

Cartilage

Hip bone covered by cartilage

Thigh bone (femur)

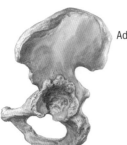

Advanced changes in the hip joint

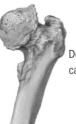

Destruction of cartilage at joint

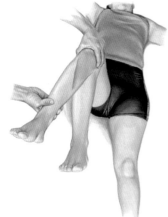

X-rays can show bone damage.

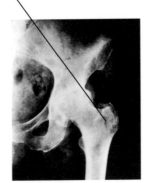

Limited movement of the hip joint points to hip osteoarthritis.

What Is Osteoarthritis?

Osteoarthritis (degenerative joint disease) is an illness in which joints become red and swollen (inflamed), painful, and stiff. Most often, the knees, hips, and spine are involved, but other joints, such as those in the hands, can also show signs. These joints contain cartilage, the substance that cushions bones that touch. During osteoarthritis, cartilage breaks down and loses the ability to cushion the joints. In the hips, the protective barrier between the thigh bone (femur) and the hip bone is lost. The bones rub together, so pain and limited movement result. In advanced osteoarthritis, cartilage in the joints is completely worn away.

What Causes Osteoarthritis of the Hip?

Osteoarthritis is caused by aging, injury, trauma, and other factors. Osteoarthritis is very common when people reach their 70s. It can occur at a younger age in overweight people. It affects both men and women.

What Are the Symptoms of Osteoarthritis of the Hip?

Osteoarthritis develops gradually. The first symptom may be pain, usually in the front part of the thigh or groin. Pain gets worse with exercise and stops during rest. Sometimes, pain travels to the buttocks or lower part of the thigh. Morning stiffness may occur but goes away during the day.

As osteoarthritis gets worse, joints become less flexible. The hips become tender, and a grating sensation may be felt during movement.

How Is Osteoarthritis of the Hip Diagnosed?

The doctor's diagnosis is based on symptoms and a physical examination. The most important sign of early disease is an inability to turn (rotate) the leg toward the center of the body.

The doctor may also take an x-ray of the hip joints or do more tests to rule out other illnesses that can affect joints. Magnetic resonance imaging (MRI) of the hip may be done if surgery is being considered.

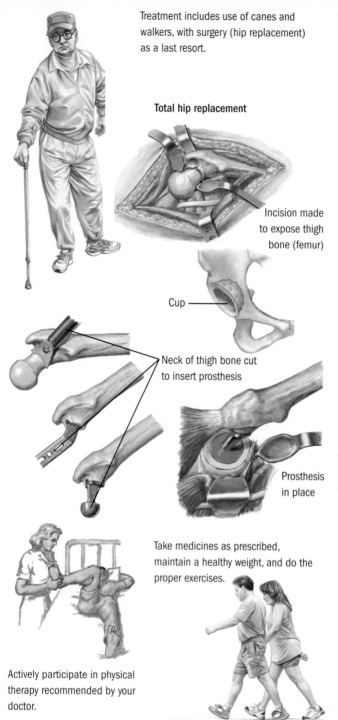

Treatment includes use of canes and walkers, with surgery (hip replacement) as a last resort.

Total hip replacement

Incision made to expose thigh bone (femur)

Cup

Neck of thigh bone cut to insert prosthesis

Prosthesis in place

Take medicines as prescribed, maintain a healthy weight, and do the proper exercises.

Actively participate in physical therapy recommended by your doctor.

How Is Osteoarthritis of the Hip Treated?

Treatment goals are to control pain and preserve mobility. The type of treatment depends on lifestyle and the degree of osteoarthritis. Keeping to a healthy weight is very important. Mild osteoarthritis may need only exercises to protect the hip joints and sometimes medicine for pain.

The doctor may prescribe nonsteroidal antiinflammatory drugs. They reduce pain and swelling (inflammation) but can have side effects (e.g., stomach pain and bleeding, or kidney, liver, and heart problems). Over-the-counter products, such as glucosamine and chondroitin, are popular but have not been proven effective.

Heating pads, warm soaks, and cold packs may help relieve symptoms.

The doctor may prescribe a physical therapy program and medicines (pain relievers and antiinflammatory drugs) for more severe disease. Low-impact exercises, especially swimming, may improve muscle strength.

Devices such as canes or walkers may minimize stress on the hips. Correcting leg length differences with a heel lift may help.

If these approaches don't work, hip replacement surgery may be offered as a last resort.

DOs and DON'Ts in Managing Osteoarthritis of the Hip:

✔ **DO** take your medicines as prescribed.
✔ **DO** use physical therapy to maintain muscle strength and joint flexibility.
✔ **DO** make lifestyle changes to reduce discomfort and stress on affected hip joints.
✔ **DO** lose weight if you are overweight.

⊘ **DON'T** take part in work or sport activities that stress your hips.

FROM THE DESK OF

NOTES

FOR MORE INFORMATION

Contact the following sources:

• American Academy of Orthopaedic Surgeons
Tel: (800) 346-AAOS
Website: http://www.aaos.org

• Arthritis Foundation
Tel: (800) 283-7800
Website: http://www.arthritis.org

MANAGING YOUR
OSTEOARTHRITIS OF THE KNEE

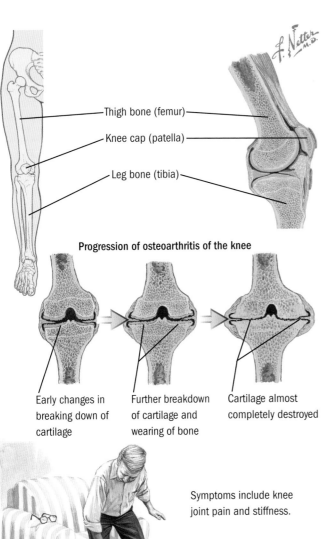

Thigh bone (femur)

Knee cap (patella)

Leg bone (tibia)

Progression of osteoarthritis of the knee

Early changes in breaking down of cartilage

Further breakdown of cartilage and wearing of bone

Cartilage almost completely destroyed

Symptoms include knee joint pain and stiffness.

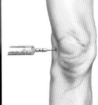

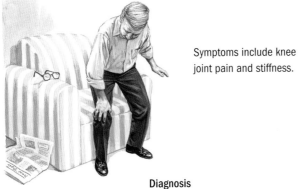

Diagnosis

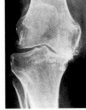

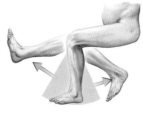

X-rays can show a deformed knee.

Removal of joint fluid for diagnosis

Examination of the knee will show limited movement of the affected knee.

What Is Osteoarthritis?

Osteoarthritis (degenerative joint disease) is an illness in which joints become red and swollen (inflamed), painful, and stiff. Most often, the knees, hips, and spine are involved, but other joints, such as those in the hands, can also show signs. These joints contain cartilage, the substance that provides a cushion where two bones touch. During osteoarthritis, cartilage breaks down and loses the ability to cushion the joints. In the knee, the protective barrier between the thigh bone (femur) and the knee is lost. Bones rub together, and joints swell and become sore and painful. Movement becomes limited. In advanced osteoarthritis, cartilage in the joints is completely worn away.

What Causes Osteoarthritis of the Knee?

Osteoarthritis is caused by aging, injury, trauma, and other factors. Osteoarthritis is very common when people reach their 70s. It can occur at a younger age in overweight patients. It affects both men and women.

What Are the Symptoms of Osteoarthritis of the Knee?

Osteoarthritis develops gradually. The first symptom may be pain. Pain gets worse with exercise and stops during rest. Over time there is limited movement and less flexibility. Morning stiffness may occur but goes away during the day, as the knee warms up.

As osteoarthritis gets worse, the knees lose their ability to bend. They become tender, and a grating sensation may be felt during movement.

How Is Osteoarthritis of the Knee Diagnosed?

The doctor's diagnosis is based on symptoms and a physical examination. An x-ray can confirm the diagnosis.

More tests may be done to rule out other illnesses that can affect joints, such as gout and infections. These tests include blood tests and removing a sample of knee joint fluid. Magnetic resonance imaging (MRI) of the knee may be done if surgery is being considered or if other disorders such as a torn knee ligament are suspected.

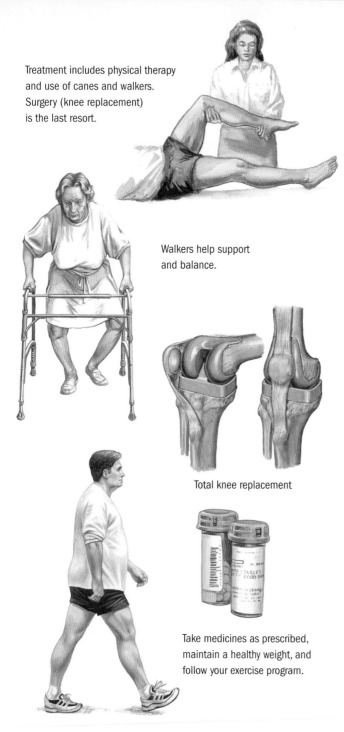

Treatment includes physical therapy and use of canes and walkers. Surgery (knee replacement) is the last resort.

Walkers help support and balance.

Total knee replacement

Take medicines as prescribed, maintain a healthy weight, and follow your exercise program.

How Is Osteoarthritis of the Knee Treated?

Treatment goals are to control pain and prevent joint destruction. The type of treatment depends on lifestyle and the degree of osteoarthritis.

Keeping to a healthy weight is very important. In people with mild osteoarthritis, occasional pain medicine and exercises to protect the knees may be all that is needed. The doctor may prescribe nonsteroidal antiinflammatory drugs. They reduce pain and swelling (inflammation) but can have side effects (e.g., stomach pain and bleeding, or kidney, liver, and heart problems). Over-the-counter products, such as glucosamine and chondroitin, are popular but their effectiveness has not been proven.

Heating pads, warm soaks, and cold packs may help relieve symptoms.

The doctor may prescribe physical therapy and medicines (pain relievers, antiinflammatory drugs, or cortisone injections of the knee) for more severe disease. Low-impact exercises, such as swimming or cycling, may improve muscle strength and flexibility.

Devices such as canes or braces may minimize stress on the knees.

If these approaches don't work, surgery may be offered. Knee replacement surgery is a last resort.

DOs and DON'Ts in Managing Osteoarthritis of the Knee:

✔ **DO** take your medicines as prescribed.

✔ **DO** physical therapy to maintain muscle strength and knee flexibility.

✔ **DO** make lifestyle changes to reduce discomfort and stress on the knees. Try swimming, walking, or riding a bicycle rather than running or jogging.

✔ **DO** lose weight if you are overweight.

⊘ **DON'T** take part in work or sport activities that stress your knees.

FROM THE DESK OF

NOTES

FOR MORE INFORMATION

Contact the following sources:

- American Academy of Orthopaedic Surgeons
  Tel: (800) 346-AAOS
  Website: http://www.aaos.org

- Arthritis Foundation
  Tel: (800) 283-7800
  Website: http://www.arthritis.org

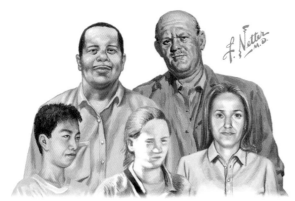

Osteochondritis dissecans is a condition involving the cartilage and underlying bone tissue. It occurs most often in the hip and knee joints, followed by the ankle and elbow. Young (ages 10 to 20) and middle-aged (ages 30 to 60) people most often have it, more males than females.

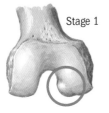 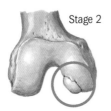 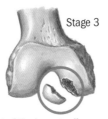

Stage 1   Stage 2   Stage 3

Loss of blood supply in the bone causes a small part of the bone to die. That part may collapse, which makes a notch in the joint surface. Cartilage over dead bone may be damaged, and dead bone may break off and form a loose body that floats around inside the joint.

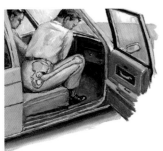

The disorder can occur in people who have an injury or have a history of repetitive trauma.

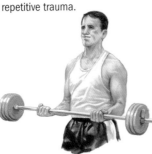

If a part of the joint loosens, the affected joint may lock and swell and become sore. Poor range of motion may be the most important symptom. In time, an affected knee can't hold the body's full weight.

What Is Osteochondritis Dissecans?

Osteochondritis dissecans is a condition in which a portion of cartilage and underlying bone separates from a joint surface and may even become detached. It occurs most often in the hip and knee joints, followed by the ankle and elbow. Young (ages 10 to 20) and middle-aged (ages 30 to 60) people most often have it, more men than women.

Osteochondritis dissecans may cause symptoms only off and on and may not need treatment other than observation. Early diagnosis and treatment are important for the best chances for recovery and return to usual activities, including sports.

What Causes Osteochondritis Dissecans?

The cause remains unclear, but osteochondritis dissecans appears to be related to loss of blood supply in the bone. This loss causes a small part of the bone to die. The affected part of bone may collapse, which makes a notch in the joint surface. Cartilage over this dead bone may become damaged. The dead bone may break off and form a loose body that floats around inside the joint. The disorder can occur in people after an injury or after repetitive trauma to the affected area. Other risk factors are sickle cell anemia and radiation therapy.

What Are the Symptoms of Osteochondritis Dissecans?

Pain may occur, but not always. When pain does occur, it may be vague, mild, and aching and stop and start, which makes diagnosis hard. The symptoms, common in athletes, are similar to those of other knee problems. If a part of the joint loosens, the affected joint may lock and swell and become sore. Poor range of motion may be the most important symptom. In time, an affected knee can't hold the body's full weight.

Your doctor will order x-rays, which show an area in the joint that is either darker or lighter than the bone around it. Sometimes, MRI is needed. Hip, knee, ankle, or elbow pain may occur for different reasons, so your doctor may want other tests to confirm the diagnosis.

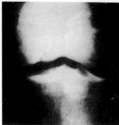

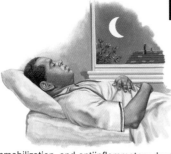

Rest, immobilization, and antiinflammatory drugs usually produce excellent results. Protecting the joint with a cast or brace can help the lesion heal without problems.

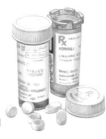

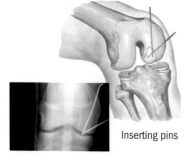

Inserting pins

Arthroscopic removal of loose body

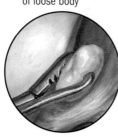

Surgery is rarely needed, especially for young people. If pain worsens and becomes constant or the joint locks and doesn't bend or straighten, surgery, sometimes arthroscopic, may be done.

Don't participate or compete in activities that cause symptoms of osteochondritis dissecans. You may harm the affected joint.

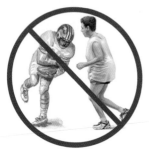

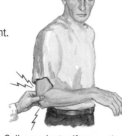

Call your doctor if your pain becomes constant or suddenly changes or if your joint doesn't bend or straighten.

FROM THE DESK OF

NOTES

How Is Osteochondritis Dissecans Diagnosed?

The x-ray shows an area in the joint that is either darker or lighter than the bone around it. Sometimes, MRI is needed to show the extent of the lesion.

Hip, knee, ankle, or elbow pain may occur for different reasons. The x-ray finding of an osteochondritis dissecans lesion doesn't always explain the source of the pain. More tests are often done to confirm the osteochondritis dissecans diagnosis. These may include MRI and nuclear bone scans.

How Is Osteochondritis Dissecans Treated?

Rest, immobilization, and antiinflammatory drugs usually produce excellent results. No diets or exercise programs speed healing. Surgery is rarely needed, especially for young people. Protecting the joint with a cast or brace can let the lesion heal without problems. If pain worsens and becomes constant or the joint locks and doesn't bend or straighten, surgery, sometimes arthroscopic, may be done.

DOs and DON'Ts in Managing Osteochondritis Dissecans:

✔ **DO** rest and immobilize the area as needed.
✔ **DO** take your medicines as prescribed.
✔ **DO** call your doctor if pain becomes constant or suddenly changes.
✔ **DO** call your doctor if the joint locks and doesn't bend or straighten. Your doctor may be able to gently manipulate it or may recommend surgery.

🚫 **DON'T** participate or compete in an activity that causes symptoms of osteochondritis dissecans. You may harm the affected joint.

FOR MORE INFORMATION

Contact the following sources:

• National Institute of Arthritis and Musculoskeletal and Skin Diseases
Tel: (877) 226-4267, (301) 496-8190
Website: http://www.niams.nih.gov

• American Academy of Orthopaedic Surgeons
Tel: (847) 823-7186
Website: http://www.aaos.org

• American College of Rheumatology
Tel: (404) 633-3777
Website: http://www.rheumatology.org

MANAGING YOUR
PLANTAR FASCIITIS

Plantar fasciitis is an inflammation of plantar fascia that causes foot pain.

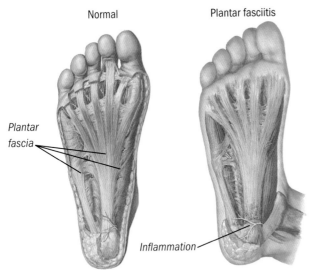

Normal

Plantar fasciitis

Plantar fascia

Inflammation

The plantar fascia is a strong band of tissue, like an elastic band, that runs underneath the bones of the foot. It attaches at one end to the heel bone and at the other, near the toes.

The cause is damage to the plantar fascia. The stress of walking around, running, and being on the feet for long periods can strain and injure the fascia.

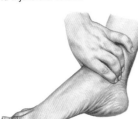

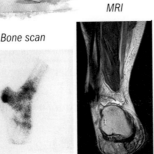

MRI

Bone scan

Your doctor makes a diagnosis from your symptoms and a foot examination, and maybe x-rays of the foot. Bone scan or MRI may be done if the diagnosis is unclear and other diseases such as bone infection are suspected.

What Is Plantar Fasciitis?

The plantar fascia is a strong band of tissue, like an elastic band, that runs underneath the bones of the foot. It attaches at one end to the heel bone and at the other near the toes. Plantar fasciitis is an inflammation (swelling) of plantar fascia. It causes foot pain.

What Causes Plantar Fasciitis?

The cause is damage to the plantar fascia. The stress of walking around, running, and being on the feet for long periods can strain and injure the fascia. Pain results. About half of people with this condition also have a bone spur attached to the heel bone, but the spur itself doesn't cause pain.

What Are the Symptoms of Plantar Fasciitis?

Symptoms include sharp or dull, achy pain in the bottom of the heel. This pain is usually worse during first steps after getting up in the morning or getting up after a rest. Pain usually gets better with walking. In the more severe condition, pain may occur all the time during walking. Sometimes pain spreads from the heel toward the toes, and the heel becomes swollen or bruised.

How Is Plantar Fasciitis Diagnosed?

The doctor makes a diagnosis from the symptoms and a foot examination. Other tests, including x-rays of the foot, bone scan, and magnetic resonance imaging (MRI) may also be done if the diagnosis is unclear and other diseases are suspected.

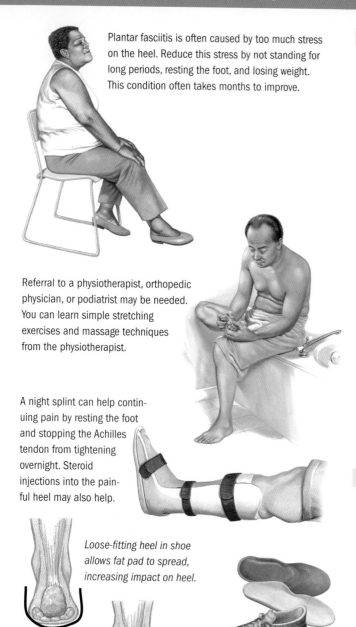

Plantar fasciitis is often caused by too much stress on the heel. Reduce this stress by not standing for long periods, resting the foot, and losing weight. This condition often takes months to improve.

Referral to a physiotherapist, orthopedic physician, or podiatrist may be needed. You can learn simple stretching exercises and massage techniques from the physiotherapist.

A night splint can help continuing pain by resting the foot and stopping the Achilles tendon from tightening overnight. Steroid injections into the painful heel may also help.

Loose-fitting heel in shoe allows fat pad to spread, increasing impact on heel.

Firm, good-fitting heel in shoe keeps fat compacted, cushioning the heel.

Wear good-fitting soft-soled shoes and maybe insoles. Talk to your podiatrist about what you need and follow those instructions.

How Is Plantar Fasciitis Treated?

Stress on the heel may be reduced by not standing for long periods and by resting the foot. Losing weight will also decrease stress on the heel and lessen pain. Painkillers such as acetaminophen and antiinflammatory medicine may help milder symptoms.

If these measures don't work, referral to an orthopedic physician, physiotherapist or podiatrist may be needed. A physiotherapist can teach simple stretching exercises or massage, which are good for a tight Achilles tendon. The physiotherapist may also tape the heel and arch of the foot. A podiatrist can measure the feet for insoles. Insoles can improve problems caused by high arches or flat feet or may just be shock absorbers for the heel.

A night splint can help continuing pain by resting the foot and stopping the Achilles tendon from tightening overnight. Steroid injections into the painful heel may also help. Lasting pain may need other treatments such as a plaster cast over the foot and ankle, transcutaneous nerve stimulation (TENS), and acupuncture.

Surgery is for severe pain that remains. Surgery involves relieving tension of the plantar fascia by detaching it from the heel bone.

DOs and DON'Ts in Managing Plantar Fasciitis:

✔ **DO** rest your foot more, lose weight, and wear the right footwear, such as soft-soled shoes and insoles.

✔ **DO** reduce your exercise for a while. Stop running or run for shorter distances.

✔ **DO** call your doctor if symptoms don't get better with treatment.

✔ **DO** stretching regularly, especially before other exercise. You may be able to help prevent pain from coming back.

⊘ **DON'T** expect an immediate result. This condition often takes several weeks or months to improve.

⊘ **DON'T** do things that you know will make the pain worse.

⊘ **DON'T** walk barefoot on hard surfaces or wear hard-soled shoes.

FROM THE DESK OF

NOTES

FOR MORE INFORMATION

Contact the following sources:

• American College of Foot and Ankle Surgeons
Tel: (800) 421-2237
Website: http://www.acfas.org

• American College of Sports Medicine
Tel: (317) 637-9200
Website: http://www.acsm.org

MANAGING YOUR
ROTATOR CUFF PAIN

Anatomy of the normal shoulder joint

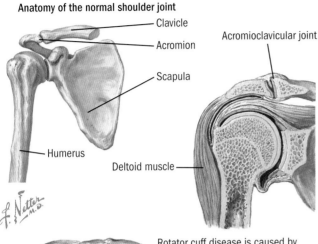

- Clavicle
- Acromion
- Scapula
- Humerus
- Acromioclavicular joint
- Deltoid muscle

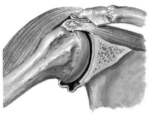

Rotator cuff disease is caused by repeatedly raising the arm, which can lead to inflammation of the tendon and bursa (fluid-filled sac that cushions the joint), and pain.

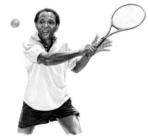

Trauma can be caused by activities, such as swimming, and tennis, in which the arms are repeatedly moved over the head.

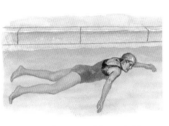

Examination of a man with a rotator cuff injury. The arm and shoulder are moved in specific ways to identify pain/limitations.

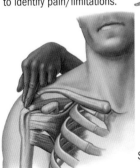

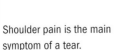

Shoulder pain is the main symptom of a tear.

About the Shoulder

The shoulder area, or girdle, includes bones and joints. The bones are the scapula, clavicle, and humerus. The joints are the glenohumeral, acromioclavicular, and sternoclavicular joints. The shoulder has the greatest range of motion of all joints in the body but is more prone to injury. The large deltoid muscle provides most of the power in shoulder motion. Underneath the deltoid muscle, four rotator cuff muscles fine-tune shoulder movement. Tendons attach these muscles to bones. The rotator cuff is made up of muscles and tendons that hold the upper arm in the shoulder joint.

What Are Common Rotator Cuff Disorders?

Disorders include swelling (inflammation), called tendonitis, and tears of tendons or muscles. Other names for rotator cuff tendonitis include shoulder impingement syndrome, tennis shoulder, and swimmer's shoulder.

What Causes Rotator Cuff Disorders?

Trauma throughout one's lifetime leads to rotator cuff problems. Activities in which the arms are repeatedly moved over the head, such as baseball, swimming, and tennis, cause such trauma. Certain jobs, such as house painting, use similar motions, which stress the shoulders and cause inflammation and pain.

What Are the Symptoms of Rotator Cuff Disorders?

The main symptom is shoulder pain, especially when the arm is moved to the side, up over the head. The arm and shoulder may also feel weak. Other symptoms include pain that worsens with activities, such as brushing hair and lying down to sleep. Pushing objects away from the body with the arm can be painful, but pulling objects is usually not.

Tendonitis can also lead to a tear in the rotator cuff tendon. Then the shoulder becomes weak, and it becomes very hard to do anything with the arm overhead.

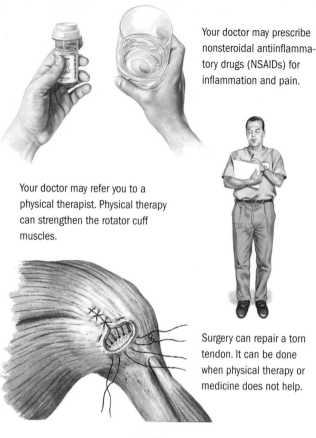

Your doctor may prescribe nonsteroidal antiinflammatory drugs (NSAIDs) for inflammation and pain.

Your doctor may refer you to a physical therapist. Physical therapy can strengthen the rotator cuff muscles.

Surgery can repair a torn tendon. It can be done when physical therapy or medicine does not help.

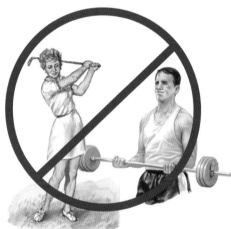

While healing, don't do activities in which your arm goes above your head or that strain your shoulders. Activities such as tennis, golfing, and upper arm weight lifting should be avoided.

How Are Rotator Cuff Disorders Diagnosed?

The doctor uses a medical history and physical examination for diagnosis. The shoulder and arm are moved in specific ways. Magnetic resonance imaging (MRI) helps when a tear is suspected.

How Are Rotator Cuff Disorders Treated?

Rotator cuff tendonitis can usually be treated without surgery.

The doctor may prescribe medicines such as nonsteroidal antiinflammatory drugs (NSAIDs) for inflammation and pain. These drugs, however, can cause stomach pain and bleeding and other problems.

Exercise can help reduce pain. This exercise may include physical therapy to strengthen rotator shoulder tendons. Ice packs applied to the shoulder also help reduce pain and inflammation.

Surgery can repair a torn tendon or can be done when physical therapy does not help. Surgery might be a less invasive arthroscopic operation (inserting a small tool to see the rotator cuff directly and repair any damage).

DOs and DON'Ts in Managing Rotator Cuff Pain:

✔ **DO** take your medicines and perform your exercises as directed.
✔ **DO** rest your arm. Sometimes rest is all that is needed.
✔ **DO** try to do tasks with your unaffected arm.
✔ **DO** call your doctor if pain is bad enough to interrupt sleep at night and can't be controlled with over-the-counter drugs.

⊘ **DON'T** use pain medicine that may be addictive for long-term therapy.
⊘ **DON'T** do activities in which you put your hands above your head. Don't do push-ups, and don't do strenuous sports while healing.

FOR MORE INFORMATION

Contact the following sources:

- American Academy of Orthopaedic Surgeons
  Tel: (800) 346-AAOS
  Website: http://www.aaos.org
- American Physical Therapy Association
  Tel: (800) 999-2782
  Website: http://www.apta.org
- Arthritis Foundation
  Tel: (800) 283-7800
  Website: http://www.arthritis.org

FROM THE DESK OF

NOTES

Muscles and tendons of the normal shoulder joint, back view

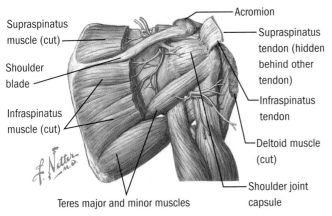

- Supraspinatus muscle (cut)
- Shoulder blade
- Infraspinatus muscle (cut)
- Teres major and minor muscles
- Acromion
- Supraspinatus tendon (hidden behind other tendon)
- Infraspinatus tendon
- Deltoid muscle (cut)
- Shoulder joint capsule

The shoulder has a greater range of motion than any other joint, but it's also more likely to get injured. Four rotator cuff muscles (subscapularis, supraspinatus, infraspinatus, and teres minor) attach to bones by tendons. The common rotator cuff tear is a partial or full tear of one or more tendons.

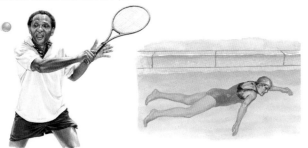

A tear can be caused by regular activities in which the arm must be repeatedly raised and lowered. These include swimming, tennis, house painting, and carpentry. Trauma can also cause it.

The main symptom is shoulder pain, especially when moving the arm sideways up over the head. Pain gets worse with overhead activities such as hair brushing. The arm and shoulder may feel weak.

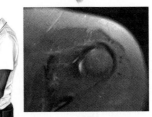

MRI

Your doctor will make a diagnosis from your medical history, physical examination, and maybe MRI. The shoulder is put through ranges of motion that cause pain.

What Is a Rotator Cuff Tear?

The shoulder girdle includes three bones (scapula, clavicle, and humerus) and three joints (glenohumeral, acromioclavicular, and sternoclavicular). The shoulder has a greater range of motion than any other joint. It's also more likely to get injured.

The large, powerful deltoid muscle gives shoulder motion most of the power. Underneath this muscle are four rotator cuff muscles (subscapularis, supraspinatus, infraspinatus, and teres minor). They fine-tune shoulder movement and make the shoulder more stable. These muscles attach to bones by tendons. The rotator cuff is made up of muscles and tendons that hold the upper arm in the shoulder joint. A rotator cuff tear is a partial- or full-thickness tear of one or more rotator cuff tendons. It's fairly common.

What Causes a Rotator Cuff Tear?

The cause is trauma throughout one's lifetime. The tendon touches a bone spur in the shoulder. Tears usually occur during activities or jobs in which the arm is often moved over the head or raised and lowered. Playing baseball, swimming, and tennis are such activities. House painting and carpentry are such jobs.

What Are the Symptoms of a Rotator Cuff Tear?

The main symptom is shoulder pain, especially when moving the arm sideways up over the head. Pain gets worse with overhead activities such as hair brushing. The arm and shoulder may feel weak. Other symptoms include shoulder pain that worsens when lying down. Pushing objects away from the body can hurt, but pulling them does not. A tear in the rotator cuff tendon itself makes the shoulder much weaker, and it's hard to do any overhead activities.

How Is a Rotator Cuff Tear Diagnosed?

The doctor will make a diagnosis from a history and physical examination, especially of the shoulder and back. The doctor puts the shoulder through ranges of motion that cause pain. The doctor will want the arm moved in specific ways. Magnetic resonance imaging (MRI) can help confirm the diagnosis.

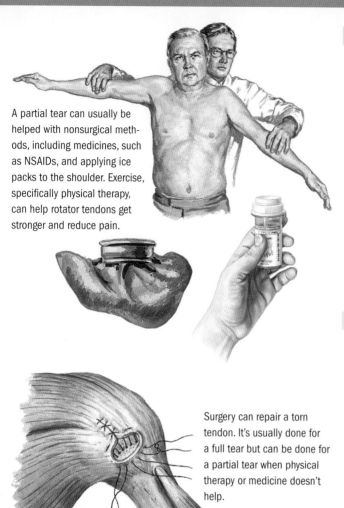

A partial tear can usually be helped with nonsurgical methods, including medicines, such as NSAIDs, and applying ice packs to the shoulder. Exercise, specifically physical therapy, can help rotator tendons get stronger and reduce pain.

Surgery can repair a torn tendon. It's usually done for a full tear but can be done for a partial tear when physical therapy or medicine doesn't help.

How Is a Rotator Cuff Tear Treated?

A partial rotator cuff tear can usually be helped with nonsurgical methods. The doctor may prescribe medicines such as nonsteroidal antiinflammatory drugs (NSAIDs) to help inflammation and pain.

Exercise, specifically physical therapy, can help rotator cuff tendons of the shoulder get stronger and reduce pain. Ice packs put on the shoulder after exercise reduce pain and inflammation.

When physical therapy doesn't work or a full tear is present, surgical decompression may be used. The torn tendon may be fixed with an open or arthroscopic procedure. Surgery involves removing the undersurface of the acromion, fixing other inflamed parts, and repairing the rotator cuff tear.

DOs and DON'Ts in Managing Rotator Cuff Tear:

✔ **DO** take your medications as prescribed.
✔ **DO** try to do tasks with your unaffected arm.
✔ **DO** your exercises as directed.
✔ **DO** call your doctor if pain is bad enough to stop you from sleeping at night and isn't helped with over-the-counter medicines.

⊘ **DON'T** use addictive pain medicines as long-term therapy.
⊘ **DON'T** do activities in which you must use your hands above your head. Don't do pushups. Don't do strenuous sports while your shoulder heals.

While you heal, don't do activities in which you must use your hands above your head. Don't do sports that are strenuous to your shoulder such as tennis, golf, and weight lifting. And don't do pushups.

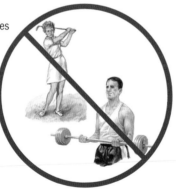

FROM THE DESK OF

NOTES

FOR MORE INFORMATION

Contact the following source:

• American Academy of Orthopaedic Surgeons
Tel: (847) 823-7186, (800) 346-2267
Website: http://www.aaos.org

MANAGING YOUR
ROTATOR CUFF TENDINITIS

Muscles and tendons of the normal shoulder joint, back view

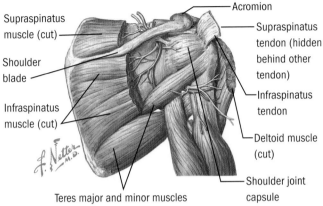

- Supraspinatus muscle (cut)
- Shoulder blade
- Infraspinatus muscle (cut)
- Teres major and minor muscles
- Acromion
- Supraspinatus tendon (hidden behind other tendon)
- Infraspinatus tendon
- Deltoid muscle (cut)
- Shoulder joint capsule

The rotator cuff is made up of muscles and tendons that attach the arm to the shoulder joint and allow arm movement. Rotator cuff tendinitis is inflammation of the tendons of the shoulder.

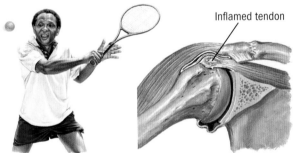

Inflamed tendon

The cause is often participation in sports that involve repeated overhead activities, such as basketball, swimming, lifting weights, and tennis, and doing some jobs, such as house painting and carpentry.

The main symptom is shoulder pain, especially when moving the arm sideways up over the head. The pain gets worse with overhead activities such as hair brushing. The arm and shoulder may feel weak.

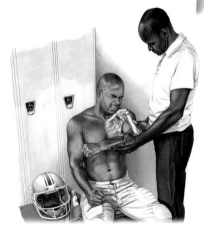

Your doctor can make a diagnosis by a medical history and physical examination. The doctor usually finds the problem by putting the shoulder through motions that reproduce the pain.

What Is Rotator Cuff Tendinitis?

The shoulder has a greater range of motion than any other joint in the body. It's also more likely to get injured.

The large, powerful deltoid muscle gives shoulder motion most of the power. Underneath this muscle are four rotator cuff muscles (subscapularis, supraspinatus, infraspinatus, and teres minor). They attach to bone by tendons. The rotator cuff is made up of these muscles and tendons that attach the arm to the shoulder joint and allow arm movement. Rotator cuff tendinitis is inflammation of the tendons of the shoulder. Long-lasting inflammation or injury can cause rotator cuff tendons to tear. Common names for rotator cuff tendinitis include shoulder impingement syndrome, tennis shoulder, pitcher's shoulder, and swimmer's shoulder.

What Causes Rotator Cuff Tendinitis?

The cause is often participation in sports that involve repeated overhead activities, such as basketball, swimming, lifting weights, and tennis. In some jobs, such as house painting and carpentry, the arm must be raised and lowered often. This motion puts stress on the shoulder that then causes the inflammation of those muscles and tendons. Being older than 40 years is also related to higher risk of having rotator cuff tendinitis.

What Are the Symptoms of Rotator Cuff Tendinitis?

The main symptom is shoulder pain, especially when moving the arm sideways up over the head. The pain gets worse with overhead activities such as hair brushing. The affected arm and shoulder may also feel weak.

How Is Rotator Cuff Tendinitis Diagnosed?

The doctor can diagnose the rotator cuff tendinitis by means of a medical history and physical examination. The doctor usually finds the problem by putting the shoulder through ranges of motion that reproduce the pain. The doctor will examine the shoulder and back and want the arm moved in specific ways.

Magnetic resonance imaging (MRI) of the shoulder can help when the doctor thinks that a rotator cuff tear is present.

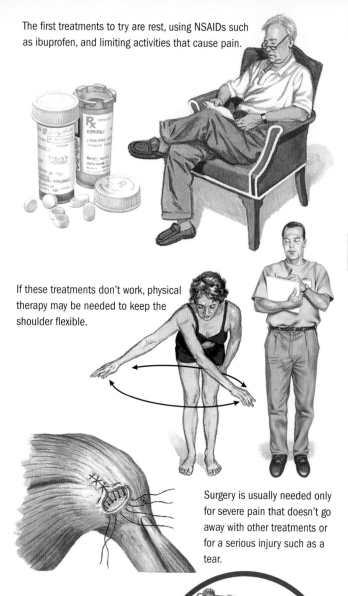

The first treatments to try are rest, using NSAIDs such as ibuprofen, and limiting activities that cause pain.

If these treatments don't work, physical therapy may be needed to keep the shoulder flexible.

Surgery is usually needed only for severe pain that doesn't go away with other treatments or for a serious injury such as a tear.

While you heal, don't do activities in which you must use your hands above your head. Don't do strenuous sports, such as tennis, golf, and weight lifting. And don't do pushups.

How Is Rotator Cuff Tendinitis Treated?

The first treatments to try are rest, using nonsteroidal anti-inflammatory drugs (NSAIDs) such as ibuprofen, and limiting activities that cause pain. If these treatments don't work, physical therapy may be needed to maintain flexibility in the shoulder.

If all these options fail to relieve pain, surgery may be done. Surgery is usually needed only for severe pain that doesn't go away with other treatments or for people who have had a serious injury.

DOs and DON'Ts in Managing Rotator Cuff Tendinitis:

✔ **DO** rest your arm. Sometimes resting the arm and shoulder is all that is needed for healing.

✔ **DO** try to do tasks with your unaffected arm.

✔ **DO** take over-the-counter pain medicine as needed.

✔ **DO** call your doctor if pain is severe enough to stop you from sleeping well at night and isn't helped with over-the-counter medicines.

⊘ **DON'T** participate in strenuous sports while your shoulder is healing.

⊘ **DON'T** involve the affected shoulder in repeated overhead arm movements.

FROM THE DESK OF

NOTES

FOR MORE INFORMATION

Contact the following source:

• American Academy of Orthopaedic Surgeons
Tel: (847) 823-7186, (800) 346-2267
Website: http://www.aaos.org

UNDERSTANDING AND MANAGING YOUR CHILD'S
SCOLIOSIS

Scoliosis is a lateral, or sideways, curving of the spine. It usually begins in childhood or adolescence and may slowly worsen. More girls than boys have severe scoliosis.

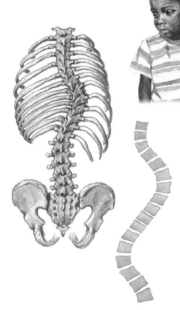

The larger the angle of the curve, the greater the chance that scoliosis will worsen. Curves less than 30 degrees at the end of childhood growth rarely get worse and don't usually need close watching. Curves larger than 50 to 75 degrees may need aggressive therapy.

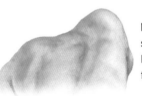

Most children may have a hump, with one side of the back or one shoulder blade higher than the other, when they bend forward, and no other symptoms.

Scoliosis is often found when children have examinations with their family doctor or pediatrician or at school. Your child's doctor makes a diagnosis from a physical examination (with the forward bending test) and x-rays. The doctor can use a scoliometer, a tool to measure spine curvature.

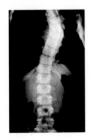
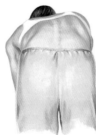
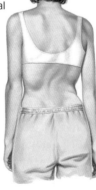

What Is Scoliosis?

Scoliosis is a lateral, or sideways, curving of the spine. It usually begins in childhood or adolescence and may slowly worsen. The younger the age when scoliosis starts, the worse it's likely to become. The degree of curving is measured by angles. The larger the angle, the greater is the chance that scoliosis will worsen. Curves less than 30 degrees at the end of childhood growth rarely get worse and don't usually need close watching. Curves larger than 50 to 75 degrees may need aggressive therapy. More girls than boys have the severe disorder.

What Causes Scoliosis?

The cause is usually unknown. Some cases are due to uneven leg length, congenital (present at birth) spine disorders, or rare neurological disorders. The risk increases with a family history of scoliosis. Backpacks, poor diet, exercising, and bad posture don't cause it.

What Are the Symptoms of Scoliosis?

Most children don't have symptoms such as pain, but may have a hump, with one side of the back or one shoulder blade higher than the other, when they bend forward. Children may have uneven hips and tend to lean to one side.

Emotional aspects of scoliosis may be severe, especially for teenagers. Breathing problems may develop with large curves.

How Is Scoliosis Diagnosed?

Scoliosis is often found when children 10 to 14 years old have examinations with their primary care doctor or at school. The doctor makes a diagnosis from a physical examination (with the forward bending test) and x-ray of the spine. The doctor can use a scoliometer, a tool to measure spine curvature.

A slowly progressive curve may not be painful and not need treatment. Only about 10% of teenagers with scoliosis need treatment, other than regular x-rays to make sure that it's not getting worse.

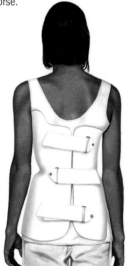
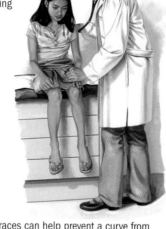

Braces can help prevent a curve from getting worse and can prevent the need for surgery approximately 70% of the time. They don't fix an already developed curve. For more severe scoliosis, surgery (spinal fusion) may be an option.

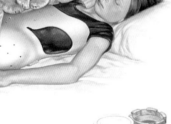
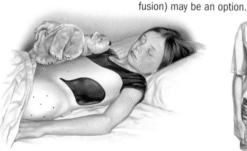

If your child is in pain, the doctor may suggest analgesics or antiinflammatory medicines.

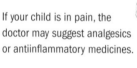
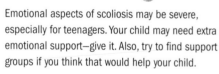
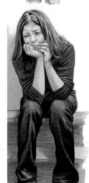

Emotional aspects of scoliosis may be severe, especially for teenagers. Your child may need extra emotional support—give it. Also, try to find support groups if you think that would help your child.

How Is Scoliosis Treated?

A slowly progressive curve may not be painful and not need treatment. Only about 10% of teenagers with scoliosis need treatment, other than x-rays to make sure that it isn't getting worse. A curve that causes pain and deformity may need aggressive treatment.

Analgesics and antiinflammatory drugs may reduce pain. No medicines, injections, diets, or exercises can fix the curve itself.

The doctor will use regular x-rays to watch for progression of the curve. Braces can help prevent a curve from getting worse but don't fix an already developed curve. Braces can prevent the need for surgery approximately 70% of the time. When the curve progresses or causes severe pain, surgery may be an option. The operation involves fusing, or joining, the bones (vertebrae) of the back together.

DOs and DON'Ts in Managing Scoliosis:

✔ **DO** have your child wear a brace as the doctor says.

✔ **DO** encourage your child to exercise. No activities make scoliosis worse. If surgery is needed, talk to your child's doctor about what your child can do safely.

✔ **DO** call your child's doctor if you see a change in the deformity, such as ribs sticking out more, change in leg length, or new pain.

✔ **DO** talk to your doctor about getting emotional support for your child. Look for support groups to help.

🚫 **DON'T** let your child stop wearing the brace unless the doctor tells you to do so.

FROM THE DESK OF

NOTES

FOR MORE INFORMATION

Contact the following sources:

• National Scoliosis Foundation
  Tel: (800) 673-6922
  Website: http://www.scoliosis.org

• American Academy of Orthopaedic Surgeons
  Tel: (847) 823-7186
  Website: http://www.aaos.org

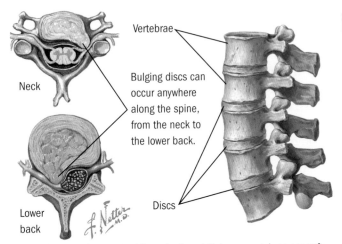

Neck

Vertebrae

Bulging discs can occur anywhere along the spine, from the neck to the lower back.

Lower back

Discs

In the spine, vertebrae protect the spinal cord. Between vertebrae are soft discs that act like shock absorbers. These discs can bulge and press on nerves coming from the spinal cord and cause symptoms. Bulging discs are called slipped discs (or prolapsed intervertebral discs or herniated discs).

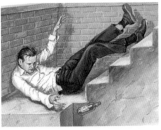

Most slipped discs result from normal wear and tear, but an injury such as a fall can also cause them.

Symptoms depend on where the slipped disc occurs. They may include:

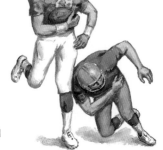

Back pain

Bowel and urinary changes

Headache

Numbness

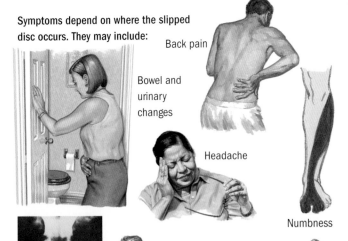

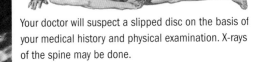
Your doctor will suspect a slipped disc on the basis of your medical history and physical examination. X-rays of the spine may be done.

What Is a Slipped Disc?

In the spine, bones (vertebrae) protect the spinal cord. Between the vertebrae are soft discs that act like shock absorbers. With aging, these discs weaken and can bulge. A bulge may press on nerves coming from the spinal cord and cause symptoms. A bulging disc is called a slipped disc (or a prolapsed intervertebral disc or herniated disc). These bulging discs can occur anywhere along the spine, from the neck to the lower back.

Slipped discs affect men and women and are most common in people between 30 and 50 years old. Most people get better after treatment.

What Causes a Slipped Disc?

Most slipped discs result from normal wear and tear, but an injury such as a fall can also cause them.

What Are the Symptoms of a Slipped Disc?

Most slipped discs don't cause symptoms. Symptoms depend on where in the spine the disc slips. They may include back pain, bowel and urinary changes, headache, neck pain, numbness, tingling, and weakness.

How Is a Slipped Disc Diagnosed?

The doctor will suspect a slipped disc on the basis of the medical history and physical examination. The doctor may order x-rays of the spine to be done. In severe cases, magnetic resonance imaging (MRI) of the spine will be done to confirm the diagnosis and find out the severity of the condition.

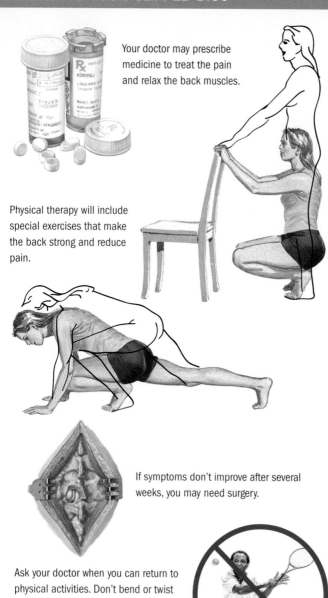

Your doctor may prescribe medicine to treat the pain and relax the back muscles.

Physical therapy will include special exercises that make the back strong and reduce pain.

If symptoms don't improve after several weeks, you may need surgery.

Ask your doctor when you can return to physical activities. Don't bend or twist when you lift something. Ask your doctor about the best way to lift things without hurting your spine.

Call your doctor if you have numbness in your legs, have rectal pain, or have sudden weakness in any part of your body, especially your legs.

How Is a Slipped Disc Treated?

Treatment depends on how severe the symptoms are. Ninety-five percent of people with a lower back slipped disc get better without surgery and return to a normal life within few weeks.

The doctor may prescribe medicine to treat the pain and relax the back muscles. The doctor will also advise to limit days of physical activity. Physical therapy will include special exercises that make the back strong and reduce pain. When a slipped disc doesn't respond to medicines and physical therapy, shots of pain medicine to the affected area may be tried. Surgery is sometimes needed if symptoms don't get better after several weeks of treatment.

DOs and DON'Ts in Managing a Slipped Disc:

✔ **DO** ask your doctor when you can return to work and normal activity.

✔ **DO** call your doctor if your symptoms get worse.

✔ **DO** call your doctor if you have trouble urinating or having a bowel movement or you cannot hold your urine or stool.

✔ **DO** call your doctor if you have numbness in your legs, have rectal pain, or have sudden weakness in any part of your body, especially your legs.

⊘ **DON'T** stop taking your medicine or change your dosage because you feel better unless your doctor says to do so.

⊘ **DON'T** return to work, play sports, or bend forward to pick up your children without your doctor's permission.

⊘ **DON'T** bend or twist when you lift something. Ask your doctor about the best way to lift things without hurting your spine.

FROM THE DESK OF

NOTES

FOR MORE INFORMATION

Contact the following source:

• American Academy of Orthopaedic Surgeons
  Tel: (847) 823-7186, (800) 346-2267
  Website: http://www.aaos.org

CARING FOR YOUR CHILD WITH
SLIPPED FEMORAL EPIPHYSIS

Classification

Grade I (<33%)   Grade II (33% – 50%)   Grade III (>50%)

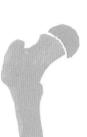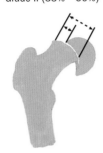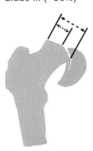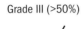

Slipped femoral epiphysis is a hip problem that occurs mainly in older children and teenagers. The femoral epiphysis is the ball part of the hip joint. The growing end of the thigh bone (growth plate) slides off the thigh bone (femur). Twice as many boys as girls have it.

The cause is often unknown, but the condition occurs more often in overweight children.

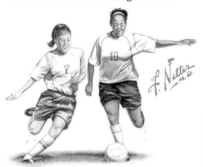

Most of the time, the disorder starts slowly. However, about 10% of the time it can happen suddenly, such as after a fall or injury playing sports.

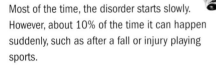

Your child's hip may become stiff and the a limp occurs. Your child can have hip, groin, thigh, or knee pain. Pain worsens with running, jumping, or turning. The affected leg twists out and looks shorter than the other leg.

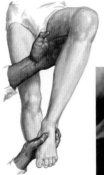

X-ray

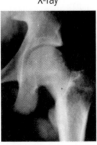

Your child's doctor will take a medical history and do a physical examination. The doctor will rotate your child's hip and check for tenderness. The doctor will also take x-rays of the pelvis and thigh area from different angles.

What Is Slipped Femoral Epiphysis?

Slipped femoral epiphysis is a hip problem that occurs mainly in older children and teenagers. The femoral epiphysis is the ball part (top, or head) of the hip joint, which is a ball and socket joint. The growing end of the thigh bone (femur) is called the growth plate. This problem occurs when the growth plate slides off the thigh bone. Most often, the left hip is affected. Twice as many boys as girls have it.

Children who develop slipped femoral epiphysis in one hip have a 25% to 40% chance of also having it in the other hip.

What Causes Slipped Femoral Epiphysis?

The cause is often unknown, but the condition occurs more often in overweight children. Most of the time, it starts slowly. However, about 10% of the time it can happen suddenly, such as after a fall or injury playing sports.

What Are the Symptoms of Slipped Femoral Epiphysis?

The child's hip may first become stiff. After a while, this stiffness can turn into a limp. Pain can occur in the hip, but it sometimes may be felt in the groin, thigh, or knee. The pain worsens if the child runs, jumps, or turns. As the problem continues, the child may lose some ability to move the hip. The affected leg twists out and looks shorter than the other leg.

If slipped femoral epiphysis occurs after a fall or injury, the pain is sudden and severe, similar to the pain of a broken leg.

How Is Slipped Femoral Epiphysis Diagnosed?

The doctor will take a medical history and do a physical examination. The doctor will rotate the child's hip and check for tenderness. The doctor will also take x-rays of the pelvis and thigh area from several different angles. Other imaging tests may also be done.

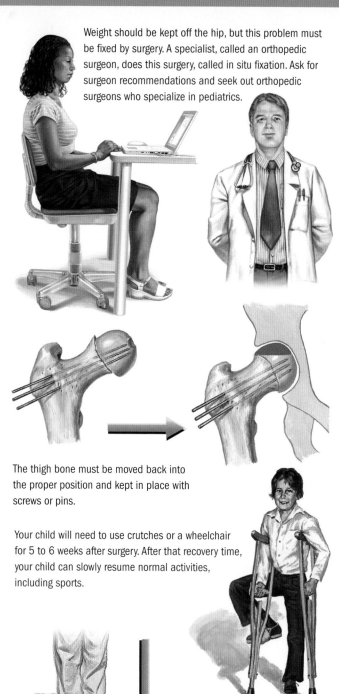

Weight should be kept off the hip, but this problem must be fixed by surgery. A specialist, called an orthopedic surgeon, does this surgery, called in situ fixation. Ask for surgeon recommendations and seek out orthopedic surgeons who specialize in pediatrics.

The thigh bone must be moved back into the proper position and kept in place with screws or pins.

Your child will need to use crutches or a wheelchair for 5 to 6 weeks after surgery. After that recovery time, your child can slowly resume normal activities, including sports.

Encourage your child to have a healthy weight. Overweight children have more risk for having the condition.

How Is Slipped Femoral Epiphysis Treated?

Weight should be kept off the hip, but this problem must be fixed by surgery. The thigh bone must be moved back into the proper position and kept in place with a screw or pin. This operation is called in situ fixation. An orthopedic surgeon does this surgery. An orthopedic surgeon is a doctor specially trained to fix bone problems.

The child will usually need to use crutches or a wheelchair for 5 to 6 weeks after surgery. After that recovery time, the child can slowly resume normal activities, including sports.

The most serious complication is avascular necrosis (osteonecrosis). This disease is caused by loss of blood supply to the bone, so the bone dies and may collapse. Children may need surgery such as hip fusion or total hip replacement earlier as adults or even as teenagers.

DOs and DON'Ts in Managing Slipped Femoral Epiphysis:

✔ **DO** make sure that your child is trained to use crutches.
✔ **DO** watch for symptoms of the disorder starting in the other hip.
✔ **DO** call your doctor if your child complains of hip or knee pains.
✔ **DO** encourage your child to have a healthy weight. Overweight children have more risk for the condition.

⊘ **DON'T** use therapy, such as manipulation or massage, that requires movement of the hip.

FROM THE DESK OF

NOTES

FOR MORE INFORMATION

Contact the following source:

• American Academy of Orthopaedic Surgeons
  Tel: (847) 823-7186, (800) 346-2267
  Website: http://www.aaos.org

The temporomandibular joints (TMJs) are near the ears and let the jaw open and close. TMJ syndrome is a common condition with pain around the TMJ and muscles that control chewing. TMJ syndrome affects 40 to 70 people of every 1000.

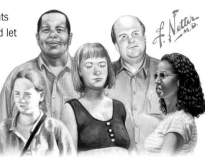

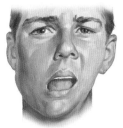

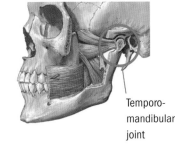

Arthritis of the jaw

Temporo-mandibular joint

Causes include clenching the jaw or grinding the teeth, especially under stress; poorly aligned teeth; badly fitting dentures; and arthritis and injury to the jaw, head, or neck.

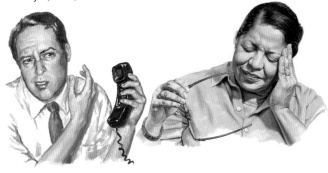

A dull, aching pain in the side of the head, neck, or ear, or on the jaw is most common. Also, tenderness in chewing muscles, clicking or popping sounds when opening the mouth, being unable to open the jaw fully, headache, and earache may occur.

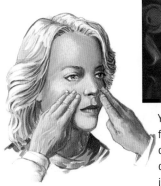

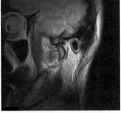

Your doctor will make a diagnosis from symptoms and an examination of your face and jaw. Tests include checking the range of motion of the jaw. Sometimes x-rays, MRI, and arthroscopy may be done.

What Is Temporomandibular Joint Syndrome?

The temporomandibular joints (TMJs) are the two joints near the ears that let the jaw open and close. TMJ syndrome is a common condition with pain around the TMJ and muscles that control chewing. It affects 40 to 70 people of every 1000, women more often than men.

What Causes TMJ Syndrome?

Causes include clenching the jaw or grinding the teeth, especially under stress; poorly aligned teeth; and badly fitting dentures. TMJ syndrome can also be caused by arthritis and injury to the jaw, head, or neck.

What Are the Symptoms of TMJ Syndrome?

The most common symptom is a dull, aching pain that affects the side of the head and along the jawline. Also, tenderness in muscles used to chew, clicking or popping sounds when opening the mouth, and being unable to open the jaw fully may occur. More symptoms include headache, earache, mouth and facial pain, and ringing or buzzing in the ear.

How Is TMJ Syndrome Diagnosed?

The doctor will make a diagnosis from symptoms and an examination of the face and jaw. Tests may include checking the range of motion of the jaw and sometimes x-rays. Other types of imaging such as magnetic resonance imaging (MRI) and arthroscopy may be done. In arthroscopy, the doctor examines the jaw with a lighted tube.

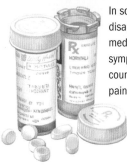

In some people, symptoms of TMJ syndrome disappear on their own. In others, conservative medical treatment and self-help may improve symptoms. Different medicines, both over-the-counter and prescription, can be used for pain relief.

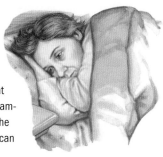

Wearing braces or a splint or bite plate can prevent teeth grinding. The dentist can make a mouthpiece to prevent jaw clenching, especially at night. Some people need a dental examination to see whether alignment of the teeth or jaw is correct. Jaw exercises can help relax the jaw.

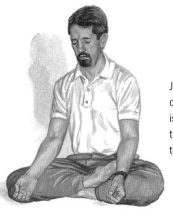

Jaw clenching and teeth grinding can be caused by stress. If stress is causing TMJ, you may need therapy, or you can try relaxation techniques such as meditation.

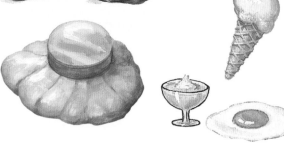

A diet of soft foods may help. Use heating pads or ice packs for discomfort. Avoid excessive chewing (such as chewing gum).

How Is TMJ Syndrome Treated?

In some people, symptoms of TMJ disappear on their own. In others, conservative medical treatment and medications may be effective. Different medicines, both over-the-counter and prescription, can provide pain relief. Antiinflammatory medicine and applying heat or ice will lessen the pain. A soft diet that requires less vigorous chewing will reduce strain and fatigue in jaw muscles.

Teeth and jaw problems can be corrected by braces or wearing a splint or a bite plate to prevent teeth grinding. The dentist can provide a mouthpiece to prevent jaw clenching, especially at night. Some people need a dental examination to see whether alignment of the teeth or jaw is correct. Jaw exercises can help relax the jaw. If stress is part of jaw clenching and teeth grinding, counseling or special therapy may help.

Sometimes pain management methods such as acupuncture and transcutaneous electrical nerve stimulation (TENS) are useful. In TENS, a gentle electrical current is applied to the skin's surface. Acupuncture involves putting tiny needles into special points in the body.

Rarely, for severe pain and treatment failure, jaw surgery may be needed.

DOs and DON'Ts in Managing TMJ Syndrome:

✔ **DO** eat a soft diet if necessary.
✔ **DO** use heating pads or ice packs for discomfort.
✔ **DO** massage the area under your jaw.
✔ **DO** take your medicines as prescribed.
✔ **DO** use your prescribed mouthpiece.
✔ **DO** call your doctor if you have medicine side effects.
✔ **DO** call your doctor if the treatment doesn't help symptoms in a reasonable amount of time.
✔ **DO** call your doctor if your jaw locks open or closed.

⊘ **DON'T** do too much chewing, such as with chewing gum.

FOR MORE INFORMATION

Contact the following sources:

• The TMJ Association
  Tel: (262) 432-0350
  Website: http://www.tmj.org

• National Institute of Dental and Craniofacial Research
  Tel: (301) 496-4261
  Website: http://www.nidr.nih.gov

• American Chronic Pain Association
  Tel: (916) 632-0922, (800) 533-3231
  Website: http://www.theacpa.org

• American Dental Association
  Tel: (312) 440-2500
  Website: http://www.ada.org

FROM THE DESK OF

NOTES

MANAGING YOUR
TENDINITIS

Tendinitis is common in active people. It's irritation, inflammation, pain, and swelling of a tendon. It's a common cause of pain in shoulders, elbows, wrists, and ankles. It occurs in any joint but is most common in the shoulder.

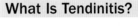

Inflamed shoulder tendon

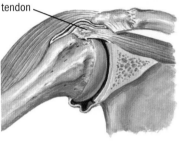

Tendons connect muscles to bones at joints.

Overworking a tendon in a job or injuring it during sports can lead to tendinitis. Other causes are aging-related wear and tear and inflammatory diseases such as arthritis.

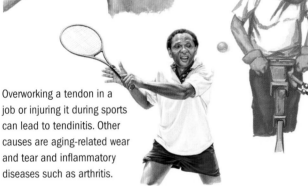

Symptoms include pain, discomfort, trouble using the joint, tenderness, and morning stiffness. The area may be red, swollen, and hot to the touch. In more severe cases, joint movement is restricted.

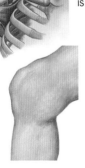

Your doctor makes a diagnosis by taking a medical history and doing a physical examination of the painful area.

What Is Tendinitis?

Tendinitis is irritation, inflammation, pain, and swelling of a tendon. Tendons connect muscles to bones at joints. Injury, trauma, or stress to parts of the body with muscles and tendons can cause tendinitis. It's a common cause of pain in shoulders, elbows, wrists, and ankles in active people. Tendinitis is certain places has specific names, such as tennis elbow, golfer's elbow, rotator cuff tendinitis (shoulder), and Achilles tendinitis (ankle).

What Causes Tendinitis?

Tendinitis usually results from overuse or abnormal use of a tendon or muscle. Overworking the tendon in a job or injuring it during sports can lead to tendinitis. Other causes include aging-related wear and tear, injury, and inflammatory diseases such as arthritis. Most often, tendinitis occurs in the shoulder, but it can occur in any joint, in any tendon.

What Are the Symptoms of Tendinitis?

Symptoms include pain, discomfort, trouble using the involved joint, and tenderness. The area may be red, swollen, and hot to the touch. The area may feel stiff in the morning for a short time. In more severe cases, movement of the joint can be restricted. Pain is worse during activities, and gets better with resting the area. Depending on its location, tendinitis may make it hard to do everyday activities, such as dressing, grooming, reaching, lifting, writing, and walking.

How Is Tendinitis Diagnosed?

The doctor makes a diagnosis by taking a medical history and doing a physical examination of the painful area. X-rays and blood tests are generally not useful.

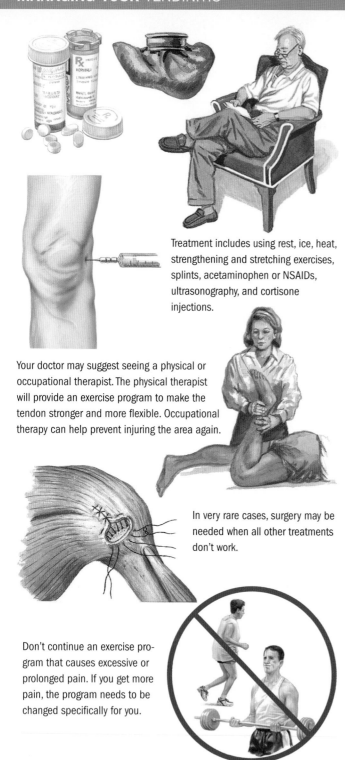

Treatment includes using rest, ice, heat, strengthening and stretching exercises, splints, acetaminophen or NSAIDs, ultrasonography, and cortisone injections.

Your doctor may suggest seeing a physical or occupational therapist. The physical therapist will provide an exercise program to make the tendon stronger and more flexible. Occupational therapy can help prevent injuring the area again.

In very rare cases, surgery may be needed when all other treatments don't work.

Don't continue an exercise program that causes excessive or prolonged pain. If you get more pain, the program needs to be changed specifically for you.

FROM THE DESK OF

NOTES

How Is Tendinitis Treated?

Treatment includes using rest, ice, heat, strengthening and stretching exercises, splints, acetaminophen or nonsteroidal antiinflammatory drugs (NSAIDs), ultrasonography, and cortisone injections. Treatments are often used in combination.

If tendinitis occurred suddenly, within a few hours or days, an ice pack can be used for 15 to 20 minutes at a time, but is usually helpful only during the first few days. The affected area is kept raised, and pressure bandages are applied. The ice pack should not be put directly on the skin. For tendinitis that has lasted for a while, applying heat may help.

The doctor may suggest seeing a physical therapist or an occupational therapist. The physical therapist will provide an exercise program to make the tendon stronger and more flexible. If the problem is work related, an occupational therapist can advise how to prevent injuring the area again.

In very rare cases, surgery may be needed when all other treatments don't work.

DOs and DON'Ts in Managing Tendinitis:

✔ **DO** stop the activity that caused the tendinitis right away.
✔ **DO** rest the affected area.
✔ **DO** take your medicines as prescribed.
✔ **DO** your exercises as prescribed.
✔ **DO** call your doctor if you have side effects from your medicine.
✔ **DO** call your doctor if the treatments don't help the pain.

⊘ **DON'T** put ice or heat directly on the skin.
⊘ **DON'T** stop the treatment prescribed because you feel better unless your doctor tells you to.
⊘ **DON'T** continue an exercise program that causes excessive or prolonged pain. If you get more pain, the program needs to be changed specifically for you.

FOR MORE INFORMATION

Contact the following sources:

• American College of Rheumatology
  Tel: (404) 633-3777
  Website: http://www.rheumatology.org

• Arthritis Foundation
  Tel: (800) 283-7800
  Website: http://www.arthritis.org

• National Institute of Arthritis and Musculoskeletal and Skin Diseases
  Tel: (877) 226-4267
  Website: http://www.niams.nih.gov

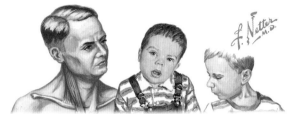

Torticollis is a movement disorder with involuntary muscle contractions. These contractions lead to abnormal movements of neck muscles and cause the head to tilt to one side. Other names for torticollis are twisted neck and wry neck.

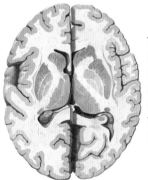

The exact cause is unknown, but torticollis is thought by some to result from a defect in the brain's ability to process chemicals called neurotransmitters. The part of the brain called the basal ganglia is affected. This part takes care of processing messages that start muscle contractions.

Muscle spasms lead to pain and a feeling of a tightly contracted neck muscle. Many people suffer from depression, often from social embarrassment because of body movements and position.

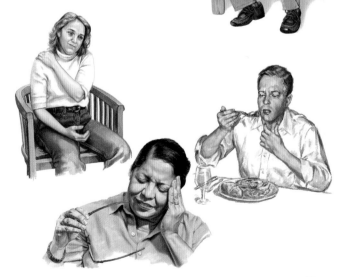

Problems swallowing may occur with pain moving down the arms. The neck position leads to nerves coming from the cervical spine being pinched. People also have tension-type headaches, because of spastic neck muscles.

What Is Torticollis?

Torticollis is a movement disorder (dystonia) with involuntary muscle contractions. These contractions lead to abnormal movements of neck muscles and can cause the head to tilt to one side. Other names for torticollis are twisted neck and wry neck. Torticollis is a focal dystonia. Spasmodic torticollis is the most common focal dystonia.

It can be idiopathic (the cause isn't known) or posttraumatic, after a head injury. Torticollis isn't life-threatening and doesn't shorten life expectancy. Complications of chronic pain and abnormalities of the spine in the neck can occur, however.

What Causes Torticollis?

The exact cause is unknown, but torticollis is thought by some to result from a defect in the brain's ability to process chemicals called neurotransmitters. The part of the brain called the basal ganglia is affected. This part takes care of processing messages that start muscle contractions. Torticollis may be present at birth (congenital torticollis). Posttraumatic torticollis can start suddenly, a few days after head and neck trauma. It can also start months after such trauma.

What Are the Symptoms of Torticollis?

Early symptoms include involuntary contraction of neck muscles, so the head and neck movements and positions aren't normal. The movements may be long lasting and jerky. The movements are described by direction. Anterocollis means forward movement and posture of the head. Retrocollis means backward movement and posture of the head. Laterocollis means sideways head movement.

Muscle spasms lead to pain and a feeling of a tightly contracted neck muscle.

Problems swallowing may occur with pain moving down the arms. The neck position leads to nerves coming from the cervical (neck) spine being pinched. People also have tension-type headaches, because of spastic neck muscles.

Many people suffer from depression, often from social embarrassment because of body movements and position.

Your doctor makes a diagnosis from your medical history and physical examination. X-rays and studies of muscle movements may be done.

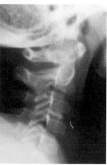
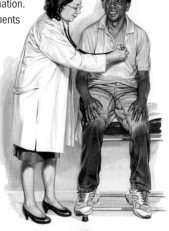

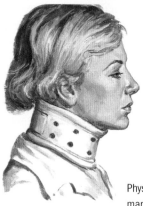
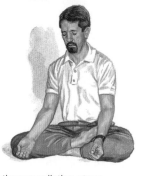

Physical therapy, splinting, stress management, and biofeedback may help.

Medicines may reduce muscle spasms and fix the abnormal amounts of neurotransmitters.

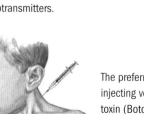

The preferred and best treatment involves injecting very small amounts of botulinum toxin (Botox®) into affected muscles.

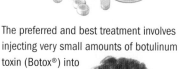

Call your doctor if you have increasing neck pain or spasms or if you get depressed.

How Is Torticollis Diagnosed?

The doctor makes a diagnosis from the medical history and physical examination. X-rays and studies of muscle movements may be done.

The doctor may suggest seeing a specialist who treats the nervous system (neurologist) and a specialist who treats the musculoskeletal system (orthopedist or rheumatologist).

How Is Torticollis Treated?

Various therapies are aimed at reducing or eliminating muscle spasms and pain. Physical therapy, splinting, stress management, and biofeedback may help. Medicines may reduce muscle spasms and fix the abnormal amounts of neurotransmitters. The preferred and best treatment involves injecting very small amounts of botulinum toxin (Botox®) into affected muscles. The toxin stops muscle spasms by stopping the neurotransmitter acetylcholine from being made. The effect lasts several months before more injections are needed.

Surgery may be considered when other treatments don't work.

DOs and DON'Ts in Managing Torticollis:

✔ **DO** take medicines as directed. Don't stop taking medicines even if you feel better without asking your doctor first.

✔ **DO** call your doctor if you have increasing neck pain or spasms.

✔ **DO** call your doctor if you're depressed.

⊘ **DON'T** forget that torticollis can cause wear and tear to the neck and limit the range of motion. Your joints may then be more likely to have arthritis.

FROM THE DESK OF

NOTES

FOR MORE INFORMATION

Contact the following source:

• National Spasmodic Torticollis Association
  Tel: (800) 487-8385
  Website: http://www.torticollis.org

Trigger finger refers to a condition that causes a finger to lock in position. People of all ages get trigger finger, but it's usually seen in those older than 45, more women than men. It's thought to be an occupational risk for dentists, tailors, seamstresses, and meat cutters.

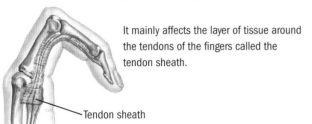

It mainly affects the layer of tissue around the tendons of the fingers called the tendon sheath.

Tendon sheath

The cause is usually unknown, but some conditions have been related to it. These conditions include gout, diabetes, rheumatoid arthritis, and underactive thyroid gland.

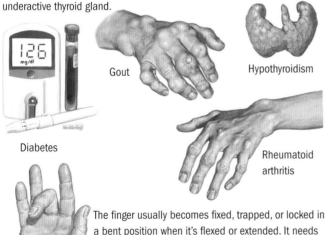

Diabetes

Gout

Hypothyroidism

Rheumatoid arthritis

The finger usually becomes fixed, trapped, or locked in a bent position when it's flexed or extended. It needs someone to help straighten or move it back into its normal spot. Pain and swelling occur.

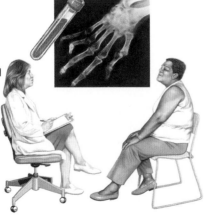

Your doctor usually makes the diagnosis from physical examinations and symptoms. Sometimes blood tests and x-rays may be done to rule out other causes.

What Is Trigger Finger?

Trigger finger refers to a condition that causes a finger to lock in position. It mainly affects the layer of tissue around the tendons of the fingers called the tendon sheath. Tendons are thick fibrous tissues that connect muscles to bones. Inflammation of this sheath prevents the tendon from sliding smoothly through the sheath, so the finger locks in place.

People of all ages get trigger finger, but it's usually seen in those older than 45, and in more women than men. It's thought to be an occupational risk for dentists, tailors, seamstresses, and meat cutters.

What Causes Trigger Finger?

The cause is usually unknown, but some conditions have been related to it. These conditions include gout, diabetes, rheumatoid arthritis, and hypothyroidism (underactive thyroid gland). It's not contagious.

What Are the Symptoms of Trigger Finger?

The finger usually becomes fixed, trapped, or locked in a flexed position when it's flexed or extended. It needs someone to help straighten or move it back into its normal spot. Pain can occur over the tendon area and usually gets worse with movement. Swelling can also be present. In adults, the middle finger is often involved; in children, the thumb is usually affected.

How Is Trigger Finger Diagnosed?

The doctor usually makes the diagnosis from physical examination and symptoms. Sometimes blood tests and x-rays may be done to rule out other causes. These causes include gout, diabetes, fracture, thyroid abnormalities, and carpal tunnel syndrome.

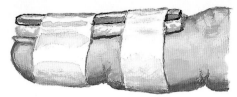

In more minor cases, symptoms may improve by avoiding certain tasks. Resting the finger in a special splint may help.

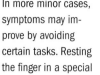

Steroid medicine (cortisone) can be injected into the tendon through the palm. Your doctor can do this in the office. Injections may be needed more than once because the problem may come back. Injections help 65% of people.

If the problem continues, the doctor may suggest surgery. This outpatient operation is done with local anesthetic. A surgeon makes a small cut in the palm and opens up the tight band of tissue around the tendon. Surgery might be done with the tip of a needle, without making a cut.

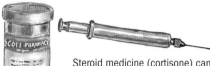

Understand that trigger finger can affect any finger. If it occurs in more than one finger, your doctor should rule out other conditions (e.g., diabetes) before you start treatment.

Call your doctor if you have a fever after surgery or you have drainage from the incision.

How Is Trigger Finger Treated?

The best treatment is to reduce inflammation and bring back the normal sliding movement of the tendon in the sheath. In more minor cases, symptoms may improve by avoiding certain tasks. Resting the finger in a special splint may help.

Otherwise, steroid medicine (cortisone) can be injected into the tendon through the palm. The doctor can do this in the office. Injections may be needed more than once, because the problem may come back. Cortisone injection relieves symptoms in 65% of people. Symptoms usually go away in 3 to 5 days, and the locking goes away in 2 to 3 weeks.

If the problem continues, the doctor may suggest surgery. This outpatient operation is done with local anesthetic. A surgeon will make a small cut in the palm and open up the tight band of tissue around the tendon. Sometimes, surgery can be done with the tip of a needle, without making an incision.

DOs and DON'Ts in Managing Trigger Finger:

✔ **DO** follow the instructions given by your doctor.

✔ **DO** see an orthopedic surgeon (a doctor who specializes in bone and tendon diseases) or rheumatologist (a doctor who specializes in joint and soft tissue diseases) if symptoms continue.

✔ **DO** understand that trigger finger can affect any finger. If it occurs in more than one finger, your doctor should rule out other conditions (e.g., diabetes) before you start treatment.

✔ **DO** call your doctor if you have a fever after surgery or you have drainage from the incision.

⊘ **DON'T** be discouraged if your first cortisone injection didn't work. Repeated cortisone shots improve symptoms in more than 80% of people.

FROM THE DESK OF

NOTES

FOR MORE INFORMATION

Contact the following sources:

• American Academy of Orthopaedic Surgeons
 Tel: (847) 823-7186, (800) 346-2267
 Website: http://www.aaos.org

• American Society for Surgery of the Hand
 Tel: (847) 384-8300
 Website: http://www.assh.org

Trochanteric bursitis is an inflamed bursa over the hip joint. More women than men, usually 40 to 60 years old, have it, but it can occur at any age. It's not a serious problem but can be uncomfortable and limiting.

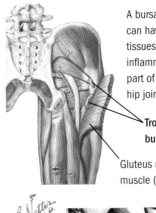

A bursa is a sac that is usually in places that can have friction, such as bones against soft tissues, tendons, or muscles. Bursitis means inflammation of a bursa. The trochanter is a part of the thigh bone (femur) that forms the hip joint.

Trochanteric bursitis

Gluteus maximus muscle (cut)

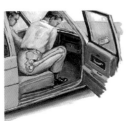

The cause isn't known. Gout, injury, infection, and repeated high-intensity use of the hip joint can trigger it. Other conditions related to it are rheumatoid arthritis and arthritis of the hip and lower back.

The most common complaint is hip pain over the hip surface. Pain is worse when lying down or standing with weight on the affected side for long periods. Walking, climbing, and running make pain worse.

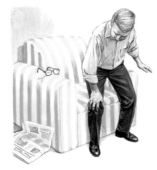

Your doctor makes a diagnosis from your symptoms. Sometimes, the doctor may order blood tests and x-rays to rule out other causes (gout, osteoarthritis, fracture).

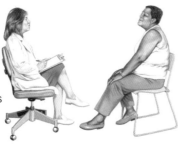

What Is Trochanteric Bursitis?

A bursa is a sac that is usually in places that can have friction, such as bones against soft tissues, tendons, or muscles. Bursitis means inflammation (swelling) of a bursa. The trochanter is a part of the bone called the femur (thigh bone) that forms the hip joint. Trochanteric bursitis is an inflamed bursa over the hip joint. More women than men, usually 40 to 60 years old, have it, but it can occur at any age. It's not a serious problem but can be uncomfortable and limiting.

What Causes Trochanteric Bursitis?

The cause is unknown. Gout, trauma, infection, and repeated high-intensity use of the hip joint can trigger it. Other conditions related to it are rheumatoid arthritis and arthritis of the hip and lower back. It's not contagious or passed from parents to children.

What Are the Symptoms of Trochanteric Bursitis?

The most common complaint is hip pain over the hip surface. Pain is worse when lying down or standing with weight on the affected side for long periods. Walking, climbing, and running make pain worse. Numbness may occur with the pain, and pressing on the area with a finger or hand may reproduce the numbness.

How Is Trochanteric Bursitis Diagnosed?

The doctor makes a diagnosis from symptoms. Sometimes, the doctor may order blood tests and x-rays to rule out other causes such as gout, neuropathy, osteoarthritis, or hip stress fracture.

Treatment is usually conservative. Plenty of rest and heat applied to the area (for 15 to 20 minutes, four to six times per day) are important. Physical therapy exercises can strengthen the hip, knee, and back muscles.

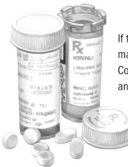

If these measures don't work, your doctor may suggest anti-inflammatory painkillers. Commonly used medicines include ibuprofen and naproxen.

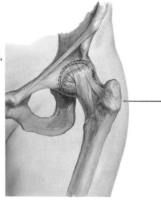

If medicines don't help the pain, you may see a rheumatologist or orthopedist for cortisone injections. Surgery is rarely done, but people who still have problems may have surgery to remove the bursa.

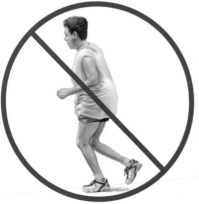

Don't put too much weight on your leg when you have symptoms. Avoid high-intensity exercises such as jumping, running, and climbing.

How Is Trochanteric Bursitis Treated?

Treatment is usually conservative. Plenty of rest and heat applied to the area for 15 to 20 minutes, four to six times per day, are important.

Physical therapy exercises can strengthen the hip, knee, and back muscles. The doctor may also use ultrasonography for treatment.

If these measures don't work, the doctor may prescribe antiinflammatory pain medicines. Commonly used medicines include ibuprofen (800 mg taken orally three times per day) and naproxen (500 mg taken orally twice per day). Acetaminophen can also be used.

If medicines don't help the pain, the doctor may suggest seeing a rheumatologist or orthopedist for cortisone injections. A rheumatologist is a doctor specializing in diseases of joints and soft tissues. An orthopedist is a doctor specializing in bone diseases.

Surgery is rarely done, but people who still have problems after these measures may have surgery to remove the bursa.

DOs and DON'Ts in Managing Trochanteric Bursitis:

✔ **DO** take your medicines as prescribed. Most people get help from antiinflammatory drugs. If cortisone injections are needed, 70% of people respond after the first injection and 90% respond after two injections.

✔ **DO** call your doctor if you have pain and fever after a cortisone injection.

✔ **DO** call your doctor if you have medicine side effects.

✔ **DO** call your doctor if you need a referral to an orthopedist or rheumatologist.

✔ **DO** call your doctor if pain doesn't go away.

🚫 **DON'T** put too much weight on your leg when you have symptoms. Avoid high-intensity exercises such as jumping, running, and climbing.

🚫 **DON'T** ignore symptoms of hip pain, especially if you have a fever. You may have a more serious condition.

FOR MORE INFORMATION

Contact the following sources:

• American Academy of Orthopaedic Surgeons
Tel: (847) 823-7186
Website: http://www.aaos.org

• National Institute of Arthritis and Musculoskeletal and Skin Diseases
Tel: (877) 226-4267
Website: http://www.niams.nih.gov

FROM THE DESK OF

NOTES

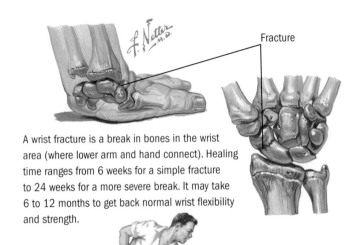

A wrist fracture is a break in bones in the wrist area (where lower arm and hand connect). Healing time ranges from 6 weeks for a simple fracture to 24 weeks for a more severe break. It may take 6 to 12 months to get back normal wrist flexibility and strength.

Falls usually cause these fractures.

Fragile bones of people over 65 and soft bones of children are more likely to break. Playing contact sports (football, soccer), other activities (skating, skateboarding, biking), and vehicular accidents can lead to breaks.

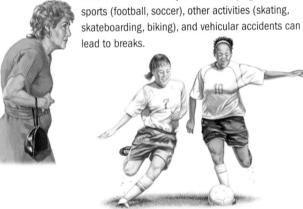

Fractured wrists are painful, bruised, and sore. The wrist often swells and may bend at a strange angle. Trouble holding things and numbness in the wrist and hand are other symptoms.

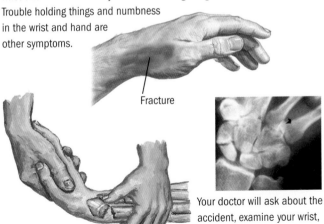

Your doctor will ask about the accident, examine your wrist, and order x-rays.

What Are Wrist Fractures?

The area where the lower arm and hand connect is called the wrist. A fracture is a break in bones in this area. Healing time ranges from 6 weeks for a simple fracture to 24 weeks for a more severe break. It may take 6 to 12 months to get back normal flexibility and strength in the wrist.

What Causes Wrist Fractures?

Falls usually cause these fractures. People almost always put out their hand to break a fall. The impact when hitting the ground with the body's weight on the extended hand can cause breaks.

Several things make wrist fractures more likely. Elderly people may have fragile bones (osteoporosis) that are more likely to break in a fall, even a low-impact fall. Children can break their wrists because they often play sports and their bones are soft. Playing contact sports such as football and soccer and other activities such as skating, skateboarding, and biking can lead to fractures. Breaks can also result from trauma in vehicular accidents.

What Are the Symptoms of Wrist Fractures?

Fractured wrists are painful, bruised, and sore. The wrist often swells and may be bent at a strange angle. People may have trouble holding things and may have numbness in the wrist and hand.

How Are Wrist Fractures Diagnosed?

The doctor will ask about any trauma and will examine the wrist, and maybe other parts of the body if a car accident or severe fall occurred. The doctor will order x-rays to check the bones for breaks. Magnetic resonance imaging (MRI) may be done if the initial x-rays are negative and pain persists or increases after several days of treatment.

A splint or cast is used to treat a fracture. At first, your elbow and fingers may be covered by the splint or cast. As the bone heals, another splint or cast that will allow more movement is put on.

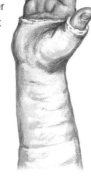

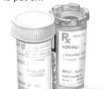

For any wrist fracture, your doctor will prescribe pain medicine for a few days to control your symptoms.

Physical therapy can help you regain movement in your wrist.

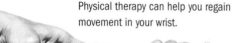

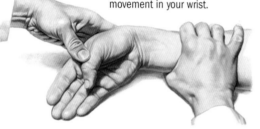

Don't skip follow-up visits with your doctor. They are important for the doctor to watch your progress.

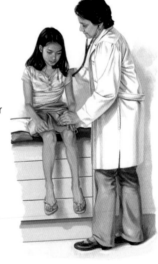

How Are Wrist Fractures Treated?

A splint or cast is used for treatment. The first splint or cast may cover the elbow and fingers. As the bone heals, another one that allows more movement is put on. Weekly x-rays for the first 2 or 3 weeks may be taken to see how the bone heals. A cast is usually worn for 6 to 8 weeks.

For a severe break, surgery may be needed. The surgeon will put pins, screws, and a metal plate into each end of the broken bone to hold pieces together. Metal frames that go outside the body instead of inside are sometimes used.

The doctor may prescribe pain medicine for a few days to control symptoms.

Recovery will depend on how bad the fracture was and which bone or bones were broken. For simple breaks, people recover fully. A serious break may mean that full strength and flexibility in the wrist won't return. Physical therapy can help regain movement in the wrist.

DOs and DON'Ts in Managing Wrist Fractures:

✔ **DO** wear a wrist support device while playing sports.
✔ **DO** call your doctor if you notice loss of feeling or a color change in your hand.
✔ **DO** call your doctor if you develop a fever or pain lasts or gets worse.

🚫 **DON'T** skip follow-up visits with your doctor. They are important so the doctor can watch your progress.

FROM THE DESK OF

NOTES

FOR MORE INFORMATION

Contact the following source:

• American Academy of Orthopaedic Surgeons
  Tel: (847) 823-7186
  Website: http://www.aaos.org

MANAGING YOUR
ALLERGIC RHINITIS

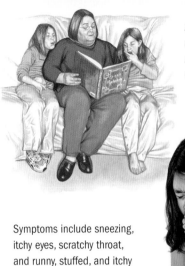

Allergies tends to run in families and affect nearly 25% of Americans. Allergic rhinitis can occur seasonally or year-round.

Symptoms include sneezing, itchy eyes, scratchy throat, and runny, stuffed, and itchy nose.

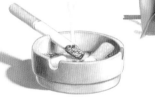

Smoke and smog may cause more problems in people with allergies. Other irritants include mold, pollen, house dust mites, and dust.

— Nasal cavity
— Nose

Lungs

People with allergic rhinitis have nasal cavities that are very sensitive to substances (allergens) in the environment.

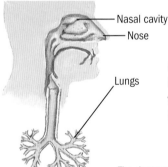

The doctor usually bases the diagnosis on symptoms alone, but may do skin testing to find out which allergens you are sensitive to.

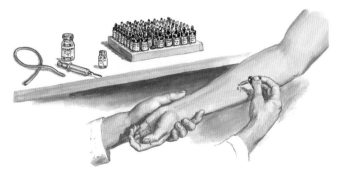

What Is Allergic Rhinitis?

Allergic rhinitis consists of symptoms that occur after exposure to certain substances. This reaction is called an allergy. Allergies can be seasonal (hay fever), especially in spring and fall for a sensitivity to tree and grass pollens. Allergies can also occur year-round (e.g., to pets or house dust mites). Having allergies tends to run in families. Allergies usually occur in people younger than 20 but can develop at any age.

Allergic rhinitis is not contagious and can be controlled.

What Causes Allergic Rhinitis?

Irritants include smoke, smog, pollens, molds, and dust.

What Are the Symptoms of Allergic Rhinitis?

The most common symptoms include sneezing, itchy eyes, scratchy throat, and runny, stuffed, and itchy nose. Other symptoms are headaches and pressure in the front of the face, and difficulty sleeping.

Long-term problems assocated with allergic rhinitis are nasal polyps (growths in the nose) and loss of the sense of smell.

How Is Allergic Rhinitis Diagnosed?

The doctor usually uses symptoms alone for diagnosis. The doctor may do skin tests to see which substances cause the symptoms. A lung function test may help rule out asthma.

How Is Allergic Rhinitis Treated?

The best treatment usually involves reducing or avoiding exposure to substances causing symptoms (allergens), along with using antihistamines, and nasal decongestants. Preventing symptoms with drugs and using a mask may also help. People who respond poorly to drugs may get shots (injections, called desensitization). These injections of an allergen are given in increasing doses to get the body to block the allergic reaction. Possible drug side effects include sleepiness (oral antihistamines), palpitations or changes in blood pressure (oral decongestants), and thinning of tissues in the nose (intranasal steroids).

Treatment by an allergist (a doctor trained in treating allergies) or an ear, nose, and throat specialist may be needed in severe or resistant cases.

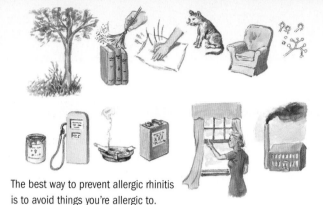

The best way to prevent allergic rhinitis is to avoid things you're allergic to.

Sometimes your doctor will prescribe medicines, such as antihistamines or corticosteroids, or will recommend allergy shots.

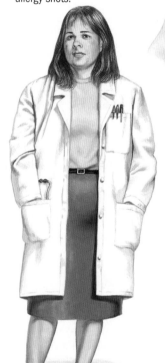

Nasal decongestants can have reverse effects when taken too often. Talk to your doctor about guidelines to follow.

Keep doors and windows closed and use air conditioning or central air with hypoallergenic filters if you have seasonal allergies.

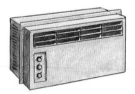

DOs and DON'Ts in Managing Allergic Rhinitis:

✔ **DO** avoid exposure to allergens. Close doors and windows, use air conditioning, and use special filters.

✔ **DO** avoid garden work (or wear a mask) if you are allergic to outdoor molds. Inside the house, use a dehumidifier.

✔ **DO** replace carpets and drapes with flooring and roller blinds, enclose mattresses and pillows in plastic bags, add a HEPA filter to the vacuum cleaner, and wash bedding at high temperatures if you are allergic to dust mites.

✔ **DO** keep the pet outdoors, if possible, if allergic to a pet. Have another household member wash and brush the animal weekly.

✔ **DO** take your medicine as recommended.

✔ **DO** contact your doctor if symptoms become constant and keep you awake, if nasal discharge becomes thick and colored, or you have problems with medicines.

✔ **DO** work with your doctor to identify triggers of symptoms. Your doctor may refer you to an allergist for allergy shots, or to an ear, nose, and throat specialist for advice on long-term management.

⊘ **DON'T** overuse nasal decongestants. These can have a rebound effect that produces the same symptoms as the allergy.

⊘ **DON'T** expose yourself to cigarette smoke or irritating substances.

⊘ **DON'T** forget to review your drugs and options with your doctor and pharmacist, especially if you take other medicines.

FOR MORE INFORMATION

Contact the following sources:

• American Academy of Allergy, Asthma & Immunology
Tel: (800) 822-2762, (414) 272-6071
E-mail: info@aaaai.org
Website: http://www.aaaai.org

• Asthma and Allergy Foundation of America
Tel: (800) 7-ASTHMA (727-8462)
Website: http://www.aafa.org

• American Lung Association
Tel: (800) LUNG-USA (586-4872), (212) 315-8700
Website: http://www.lungusa.org

FROM THE DESK OF

NOTES

CARING FOR YOUR BABY WITH
CLEFT LIP AND PALATE

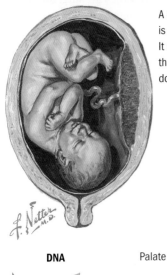

A cleft lip or palate (roof of the mouth) is the most common facial birth defect. It occurs before birth, when the parts that form the baby's face and palate don't come together.

At 8 to 10 weeks of development

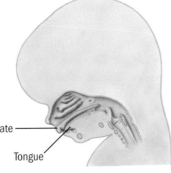

Palate

Tongue

DNA

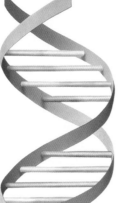

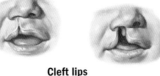

Cleft lips

Cleft palate

The cause of the cleft lip or palate is unknown. Sometimes, this defect runs in families (is genetic).

A cleft may occur on one or both sides of the upper lip and may affect the nose. A cleft palate may affect only the soft part of the palate at the back of the mouth or the bony part of the palate also.

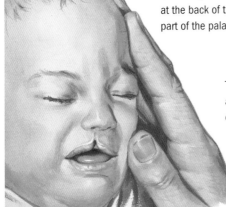

The doctor makes a diagnosis by examining your baby.

What Are Cleft Lip and Palate?

A cleft lip and cleft palate are facial birth defects. Cleft means an opening. These defects affect the upper lip and the roof of the mouth (palate). The parts that form the baby's face and palate don't join before birth.

A cleft lip or palate is the most common facial birth defect. Up to 5000 babies are born in the United States each year with this problem. Clefts occur more often in Asian, Latino, and Native American children.

What Causes Cleft Lip and Palate?

The cause is unknown. The defects sometimes run in families (are genetic). If either parent has a cleft lip or palate, the chance increases that the baby will also. If both parents are normal and have a baby with a cleft lip or palate, chances are higher that babies born later will have it.

What Are the Symptoms of Cleft Lip and Palate?

A cleft may occur on one side or both sides of the upper lip. The split usually affects only the lip but may extend into the nose. For a cleft palate, the soft part of the palate at the back of the mouth may be involved, or the cleft may affect the bony part of the palate (hard palate).

These defects can cause feeding and developmental problems, poor dental development, trouble with speech, and frequent colds, sore throats, and ear infections.

How Are Cleft Lip and Palate Diagnosed?

The doctor makes a diagnosis by a physical examination. The need for more tests depends on the defect's severity.

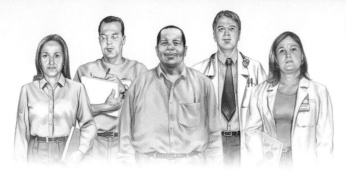

Your doctor will refer you to a team of specialists to help evaluate your baby for problems and suggest treatment, such as surgery to correct the defect. Get help and emotional support from psychologists and social workers if needed.

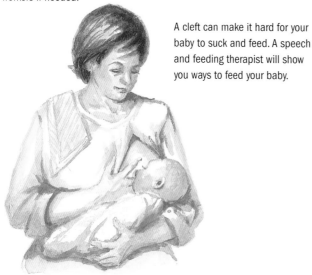

A cleft can make it hard for your baby to suck and feed. A speech and feeding therapist will show you ways to feed your baby.

Your child will need to be watched because frequent ear infections can lead to hearing loss.

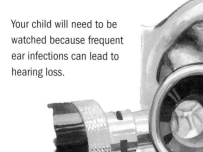

How Is Cleft Lip and Palate Treated?

Surgery can improve a cleft lip or palate. Which type of surgery depends on how bad the defect is. At times the surgeon may be able to fix the baby's lip before sending the baby home. If the baby has a cleft palate, an operation may be done later.

Other treatments depend on which problems the cleft lip or palate causes. A cleft can make it hard for the baby to suck and feed. A speech and feeding therapist will describe ways to feed the baby. The cleft can cause problems in learning to speak. Care of a speech and language therapist will be needed. A cleft may cause frequent ear infections, which can lead to hearing loss.

A team of specialists can help check the baby. This team may include a surgeon who specializes in these defects, hearing specialist, dentist, orthodontist (dentist who straightens teeth), and speech-language specialist (for both speech and feeding problems). Psychologists and social workers may also be involved.

DOs and DON'Ts in Managing Cleft Lip and Palate:

✔ **DO** make sure that your child gets care from doctors who can check for problems with teeth, feeding, hearing, and speaking.

✔ **DO** remember that surgery can correct most defects in 12 to 18 months after birth.

✔ **DO** have a positive attitude and encourage your child to be positive.

🚫 **DON'T** avoid getting help and emotional support from psychologists if needed.

FROM THE DESK OF

NOTES

FOR MORE INFORMATION

Contact the following source:

• Cleft Palate Foundation
  Tel: (919) 933-9044, (800) 242-5338
  Website: http://www.cleftline.org

MANAGING YOUR
HEARING LOSS (DEAFNESS)

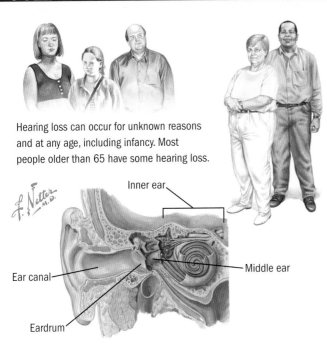

Hearing loss can occur for unknown reasons and at any age, including infancy. Most people older than 65 have some hearing loss.

Inner ear

Ear canal

Middle ear

Eardrum

Hearing loss can result from problems in the ear canal or middle ear that block sound, or in the inner ear or nerves going from the ears to the brain.

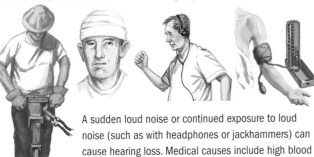

A sudden loud noise or continued exposure to loud noise (such as with headphones or jackhammers) can cause hearing loss. Medical causes include high blood pressure, brain tumors, and head injury

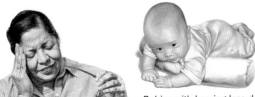

Babies with hearing loss don't respond to sounds. Adults can have ear pain or trouble understanding a conversation. The volume of the television may need to be very high.

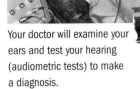

Your doctor will examine your ears and test your hearing (audiometric tests) to make a diagnosis.

What Is Hearing Loss?

Deafness is a decreased ability or complete inability to hear. It may be partial or total and affect one or both ears.

What Causes Hearing Loss?

Hearing loss can occur for unknown reasons and at any age, including in infants. The cause can be a problem in the ear canal or middle ear that blocks sound. The inner ear or nerves that carry sound to the brain can also be damaged. Other causes are sudden loud noise or continued exposure to loud noise (as with earphones), viral or bacterial infection of the ear, certain drugs, and puncture of the eardrum.

Medical causes include high blood pressure, brain tumors, head injury, and Paget's disease. Most people older than 65 have some hearing loss.

Risk factors are a family history of deafness and having a job or hobby with exposure to high noise levels (such as rock musicians or jackhammer operators).

What Are the Symptoms of Hearing Loss?

Infants with hearing loss don't respond to sounds around them, especially startling sounds.

In adults, symptoms include trouble telling the difference among sounds, such as being unable to follow a conversation if there's background noise; turning up the radio or television volume; ringing in the ears; dizziness; and ear pain.

How Is Hearing Loss Diagnosed?

The doctor will examine the ears and test hearing. Audiometry (test of hearing) uses a device that makes tones of different loudness. Other tests involve using a tuning fork, checking the ability to hear differences between words that sound similar, and measuring how loudly words have to be spoken. If hearing loss seems to be related to the brain, magnetic resonance imaging (MRI) may be done.

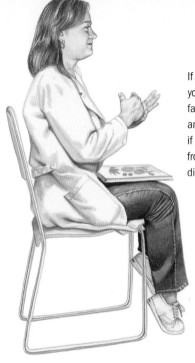

If your hearing loss is permanent, your doctor may send you to a facility to learn sign language and lipreading. Call your doctor if you have pain in or drainage from your ear or you have dizziness, headaches, or fever.

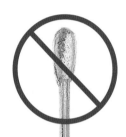

Don't put anything, such as cotton-tipped swabs, in your ears. Wear ear protection to avoid exposure to loud sounds.

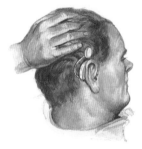

Hearing aids can be helpful. For profound hearing loss (deafness), a cochlear implant, placed inside the ear, can sometimes help.

How Is Hearing Loss Treated?

Treatment depends on the cause. Sometimes, simple earwax removal or eardrum puncture repair may solve the problem. The doctor will prescribe medicine for an infection. Drugs or exposure to loud noise causing hearing loss should be stopped.

Surgery may sometimes restore hearing. For profound hearing loss (deafness), a cochlear implant can sometimes help. This implant, placed inside the ear, is a type of hearing aid that can make sounds louder. Many people learn to rely on hearing aids.

Even if hearing loss is permanent, people can live normally. The important thing is not to become isolated. A local rehabilitation facility may teach sign language and lipreading. Speech therapy may be necessary.

DOs and DON'Ts in Managing Hearing Loss:

✔ **DO** avoid long-term use or overuse of drugs that cause hearing loss. Talk with your doctor about possible problem drugs.

✔ **DO** get treatment for ear infections, allergies, and respiratory problems that could affect the ear.

✔ **DO** avoid long-term exposure to loud noise. If you cannot, wear ear protection (earplugs or earmuffs).

✔ **DO** call your doctor for removal of earwax.

✔ **DO** call your doctor if you have pain in or drainage from your ear or you develop dizziness, headaches, or fever.

⊘ **DON'T** put anything, such as cotton-tipped swabs, in your ears.

⊘ **DON'T** ignore worsening loss of hearing.

FROM THE DESK OF

NOTES

FOR MORE INFORMATION

Contact the following sources:

• National Hearing Aid Helpline
Tel: (800) 521-5247

• National Institute on Deafness and Other Communication Disorders
Tel: (800) 241-1044
Website: http://www.nidcd.nih.gov/health/hearing

Good oral health involves knowing how to brush and floss correctly. Use a soft-bristled brush and fluoride toothpaste to remove plaque. Flossing removes plaque and food that a toothbrush can't reach. If brushing or flossing causes bleeding gums, pain, or irritation, see the dentist.

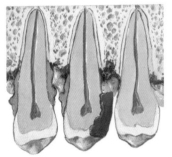

Bacteria that normally live in the mouth cause tooth decay and gum disease. Fluoride is important to prevent tooth decay for all people. Fluoride is in the water supply, toothpastes, and mouth rinses. The dentist or dental hygienist may give fluoride treatments.

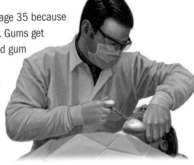

People often lose teeth after age 35 because of gum (periodontal) disease. Gums get inflamed and bleed. Untreated gum disease can cause receding gums, bone loss, loose teeth, and teeth that fall out.

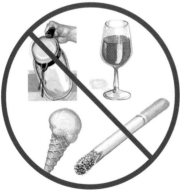

Dry mouth, common in many adults, makes it hard to eat, swallow, taste, and speak. It occurs when salivary glands don't work because of diseases, treatments (chemotherapy, radiation), or medicines (for high blood pressure, allergies). For dryness, drink extra water and avoid sugary snacks, caffeine, tobacco, and alcohol.

Cleaning the Teeth and Gums

Good oral health involves knowing how to brush and floss correctly. Use a soft-bristled brush and fluoride toothpaste to remove plaque. Bacteria on teeth form the sticky, colorless film called plaque. Brush the tongue and along the gum line. Flossing removes plaque and leftover food that a toothbrush cannot reach. If brushing or flossing causes bleeding gums, pain, or irritation, see the dentist. Also, using an antibacterial mouth rinse helps control plaque and swollen gums. People with arthritis or other conditions who have trouble holding a toothbrush can use special devices or an electric toothbrush to help.

Tooth Decay (Cavities)

Bacteria that normally live in the mouth cause tooth decay and gum disease. Fluoride is important to prevent tooth decay for all people. Fluoride is in the water supply, toothpastes, and mouth rinses. The dentist or dental hygienist may give fluoride treatments in the office.

Gum (Periodontal) Disease

People often lose teeth after age 35 because of gum (periodontal) disease. Gums become inflamed (swollen, red) and bleed easily. Untreated gum disease gets worse and causes receding gums and bone loss. Teeth may become loose and fall out. Prevent gum disease by removing plaque by brushing and flossing daily. See the dentist every 6 to 12 months, or right away if these signs are present.

Dry Mouth (Xerostomia)

Dry mouth, common in many adults, may make it hard to eat, swallow, taste, and speak. Dry mouth occurs when salivary glands don't work because of diseases, medical treatments (chemotherapy, radiation), or medicines (for high blood pressure, depression, allergies). For dryness, drink extra water and avoid sugary snacks, caffeinated beverages, tobacco, and alcohol. Before starting cancer treatment, which can cause oral problems, see a dentist.

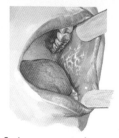
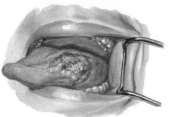

Oral Cancer (Mouth Cancer)

This cancer most often occurs in people older than 40. It often goes unnoticed in early, curable stages, partly because pain isn't usually an early symptom. People who use tobacco products or drink too much alcohol have increased risk for oral cancer. Red or white patches on the gums or tongue, sores that don't heal within 2 weeks, and trouble chewing or swallowing are signals to see a dentist.

Oral cancer most often occurs in people older than 40 who often don't notice it in early, curable stages, partly because pain isn't usually an early symptom. People who use tobacco or drink too much alcohol have higher risk for oral cancer. If you have red or white patches on the gums or tongue, sores that don't heal in 2 weeks, or trouble chewing or swallowing, see a dentist.

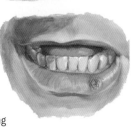

Dentures

Keep false teeth (dentures) clean and free from food that can cause stains, bad breath, and gum irritation. Put dentures in water or a denture-cleansing liquid during sleep. Rinse the mouth with warm salt water in the morning, after meals, and at bedtime. When learning to eat with false teeth, choose soft nonsticky food, cut into small pieces, and chew slowly on both sides of the mouth. Don't fix dentures at home. The dentist should do this.

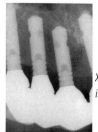

Dental implants hold replacement teeth. The most popular types are metal screws surgically put into jaw bones.

X-ray showing implants

Dental Implants

Dental implants hold replacement teeth. The most popular types are metal screws surgically put into jawbones.

Everyone should use good oral hygiene and have regular checkups by the dentist. Get any special treatments needed, such as using a special toothpaste for a few months if teeth are sensitive because of receding gums. Taking good care of the teeth and gums can protect them for many years.

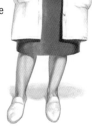

Professional Care

Everyone should use good oral hygiene and have regular check-ups by the dentist. Get any special treatments to have good oral health. For example, if teeth are sensitive because of receding gums, the dentist may suggest using a special toothpaste for a few months. Taking good care of the teeth and gums can protect them for many years.

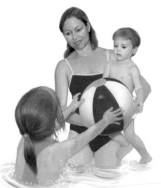

Children learn good oral hygiene from their parents, so take this opportunity to help them develop good habits.

FROM THE DESK OF

NOTES

FOR MORE INFORMATION

Contact the following sources:

• National Institute of Dental and Craniofacial Research
  Tel: (301) 402-7364
  Website: http://www.nidcr.nih.gov/OralHealth/

• American Dental Association
  Tel: (312) 440-2500
  Website: http://www.ada.org

MANAGING YOUR
NOSEBLEEDS

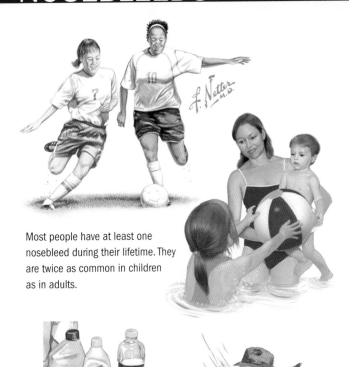

Most people have at least one nosebleed during their lifetime. They are twice as common in children as in adults.

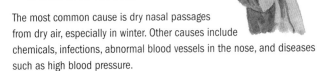

The most common cause is dry nasal passages from dry air, especially in winter. Other causes include chemicals, infections, abnormal blood vessels in the nose, and diseases such as high blood pressure.

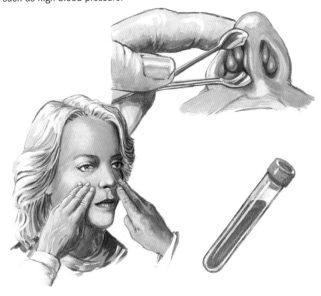

Your doctor will diagnose a nosebleed from a physical examination. Blood work may be done if you lost a large amount of blood or if a blood disorder may be causing the nosebleed.

What Are Nosebleeds?

Epistaxis, or a nosebleed, is the common event of blood draining from the nose. Most people have at least one nosebleed during their lifetime. They are twice as common in children compared with adults. Most stop with direct pressure on the nose, but some may need medical care.

What Causes Nosebleeds?

A break in blood vessels in the nose, such as from an injury (blow to the nose) causes a nosebleed. Other causes include chemicals, infections, abnormal blood vessels in the nose, and diseases such as high blood pressure or bleeding disorders. The most common cause is dry nasal passages from dry air, especially in winter.

What Are the Symptoms of Nosebleeds?

Symptoms include bleeding from one or both nostrils and bleeding down the back of the throat with spitting, coughing, or vomiting of blood.

Prolonged or recurrent nosebleeds may cause anemia.

After a big nosebleed, dark or tarry bowel movements mean that a large amount of blood was swallowed.

How Are Nosebleeds Diagnosed?

The doctor will diagnose the nosebleed from a physical examination. Blood work may be done if a large amount of blood was lost or a blood disorder may be causing the nosebleed.

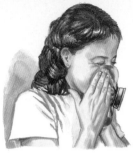

Lean forward so that you can spit out blood running down the throat instead of swallowing it, to help prevent vomiting.

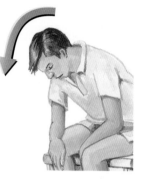

The first treatment is direct pressure on the nose. Putting an ice pack on the neck or the bridge of the nose may help slow blood flow to the nose.

Sometimes, the doctor may pack your nose with absorbent gauze or cauterize (a special kind of burning) the bleeding site.

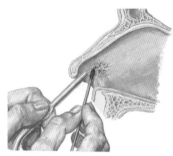

If you get many nosebleeds, avoid aspirin products because they may slow clotting.

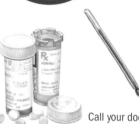

Call your doctor if your nose gushes blood, you vomit repeatedly from swallowed blood, you have a temperature higher than 102°F, or you take blood thinners such as warfarin (Coumadin®).

How Are Nosebleeds Treated?

The first treatment is direct pressure. Grasp the nose firmly between the thumb and forefinger and squeeze it for 10 to 30 minutes without stopping.

Putting an ice pack on the neck or bridge of the nose may help slow blood flow. Leaning forward to spit out blood instead of letting it run down the throat and be swallowed may help prevent vomiting. Using salt water nasal sprays and humidifying the air may help dryness.

Sometimes, packing the nose with absorbent gauze may be needed. The doctor may also cauterize the bleeding site. Some elderly people can have a slowed pulse rate or blood pressure abnormalities from packing and may in some cases need hospitalization.

DOs and DON'Ts in Managing Nosebleeds:

✔ **DO** control your blood pressure. High blood pressure may contribute to nosebleeds.

✔ **DO** avoid aspirin products if you get many nosebleeds. They may slow clotting.

✔ **DO** humidify air in your home and if possible at work, put a little petroleum jelly inside the nostrils, and use a scarf or cloth mask in cold, dry air. Salt water nasal sprays may also help stop nosebleeds caused by dryness.

✔ **DO** avoid chemicals or dusts or wear a filter mask. Your doctor may prescribe a steroid nasal spray if you have infections or allergies.

✔ **DO** call your doctor if blood gushes from your nose or you vomit repeatedly from swallowed blood.

✔ **DO** call your doctor if you cannot control the bleeding or you have repeated nosebleeds in one day.

✔ **DO** call your doctor if you know that high blood pressure or bleeding problems (hemophilia, leukemia) are causing nosebleeds.

✔ **DO** call your doctor if you take blood thinners (warfarin).

✔ **DO** call your doctor if you have a temperature higher than 102° F, especially if your nose was packed or cauterized.

⊘ **DON'T** blow your nose hard or pick at any clots, which may restart the nosebleed.

FROM THE DESK OF

NOTES

FOR MORE INFORMATION

Contact the following sources:

• American College of Emergency Physicians
Tel: (800) 798-1822
Website: http://www.acep.org

• American Academy of Otolaryngology—Head and Neck Surgery
Tel: (703) 836-4444
Website: http://www.entnet.org

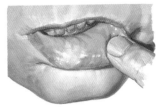

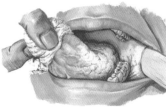

Leukoplakia refers to white spots that occur on the inner lining (mucosa) of the mouth, lips, tongue, or vaginal area. Oral hairy leukoplakia is the mucosal disorder in the mouth. If untreated, up to 20% of cases can become cancer.

Smoking is the most common cause of oral leukoplakia. Other causes are chronic irritation, such as from poorly fitting dental appliances, and mouth infections, such as syphilis, EBV infection, and candidiasis. It's a very common oral viral disease in HIV-positive people.

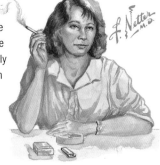

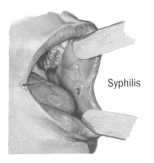
Syphilis

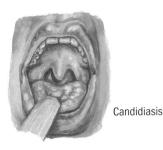
Candidiasis

A small white patch or patches occur inside the mouth or on the tongue or lips. Patches are slightly raised and well defined. The area feels firm and may be more sensitive during eating.

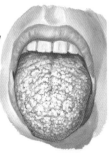

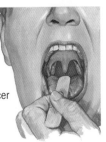

Your doctor makes a diagnosis by an examination. A biopsy is usually needed to find out whether cancer or precancerous lesions are present.

What Is Oral Hairy Leukoplakia?

Leukoplakia refers to white spots that occur on the inner lining (mucosa) of the mouth, lips, or tongue. Oral hairy leukoplakia is the mucosal disorder in the mouth. If untreated, up to 20% of cases can become cancer. Treatment can usually cure leukoplakia, but it often comes back and needs treatment again.

What Causes Oral Hairy Leukoplakia?

Smoking is the most common cause of oral leukoplakia. Chronic irritation, such as from poorly fitting dental appliances, is also related to leukoplakia. Some mouth infections such as syphilis, Epstein-Barr virus (EBV) infection, and candidiasis may also increase the risk of getting leukoplakia. It's one of the most common viral oral diseases of people with human immunodeficiency virus (HIV) infection. It's not contagious.

What Are the Symptoms of Oral Hairy Leukoplakia?

The most common symptom is a small white patch inside the mouth or on the tongue or lips. The patch is slightly raised and well defined. Many patches can occur. The area feels firm and may be more sensitive during eating.

How Is Oral Hairy Leukoplakia Diagnosed?

The doctor makes a diagnosis by examining the area. A biopsy is usually needed to find out whether cancer or precancerous lesions are present. In a biopsy, the doctor removes a small piece of the leukoplakia. The doctor first uses an anesthetic such as lidocaine to numb the area. A sharp sterile knife or biopsy tool is then used to get the sample, which is sent to a laboratory for study with a microscope.

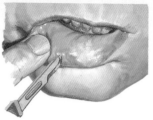

All people should stop smoking, which may help small areas of leukoplakia go away. Sometimes the doctor removes a problem area completely instead of just taking a biopsy sample. Electrosurgery (using an electric needle) and cryosurgery (freezing) can be used for small areas.

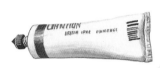

Beta-carotene and isotretinoin are two oral medicines that are sometimes used. Leukoplakia of the lip may be treated with fluorouracil cream.

Don't smoke or use tobacco products. Smoking is the major risk factor for leukoplakia of the mouth and tongue.

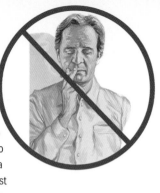

Avoid chronic irritation caused by teeth, dentures, or sharp dental appliances.

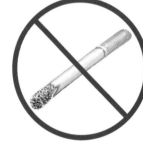

Call your doctor if new white patches occur or if fever or bleeding occurs after treatment.

How Is Oral Hairy Leukoplakia Treated?

All people should stop smoking. Small areas of leukoplakia sometimes go away after smoking stops. Sometimes the doctor removes a problem area completely instead of just taking a biopsy sample. Electrosurgery (using an electric needle) and cryosurgery (freezing) can be used to treat small areas. Beta-carotene (a form of vitamin A) and isotretinoin are two medicines taken by mouth that are sometimes used for treatment. These drugs usually should be taken daily for a few months. Isotretinoin can cause birth defects and shouldn't be taken by pregnant women. Leukoplakia of the lip (and outer vaginal area) can sometimes be treated with fluorouracil cream, applied two times per day for 2 to 3 weeks. This drug causes redness, soreness, and inflammation and actually destroys the involved area.

DOs and DON'Ts in Managing Oral Hairy Leukoplakia:

✔ **DO** tell your doctor about suspicious-looking or unusual areas, including anything on the skin, inside the mouth, or on the tongue.
✔ **DO** call your doctor if leukoplakia doesn't go away after treatment.
✔ **DO** avoid chronic irritation caused by teeth, dentures, or sharp dental appliances.
✔ **DO** call your doctor if new white patches occur.
✔ **DO** call your doctor if fever or bleeding occurs after treatment.

⊘ **DON'T** smoke or use tobacco products. Smoking is the major risk factor for leukoplakia of the mouth and tongue.

FROM THE DESK OF

NOTES

FOR MORE INFORMATION

Contact the following sources:

- American Academy of Otolaryngology—Head and Neck Surgery
  Tel: (703) 836-4444
  Website: http://www.entnet.org
- American Academy of Dermatology
  Tel: (847) 330-0230, (888) 462-3376
  Website: http://www.aad.org

MANAGING YOUR
SALIVARY GLAND INFLAMMATION

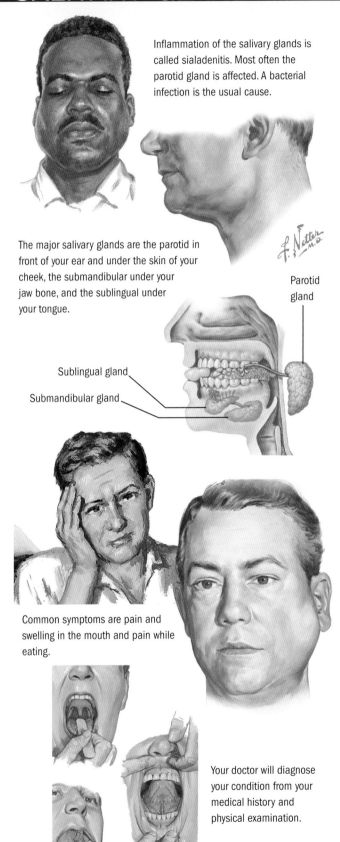

Inflammation of the salivary glands is called sialadenitis. Most often the parotid gland is affected. A bacterial infection is the usual cause.

The major salivary glands are the parotid in front of your ear and under the skin of your cheek, the submandibular under your jaw bone, and the sublingual under your tongue.

Parotid gland

Sublingual gland

Submandibular gland

Common symptoms are pain and swelling in the mouth and pain while eating.

Your doctor will diagnose your condition from your medical history and physical examination.

What Is Salivary Gland Inflammation?

Salivary glands make saliva to keep the mouth moist and to lubricate food being chewed. These glands are divided into major and minor glands. Major glands are the parotid gland in front of the ear and under the cheek, submandibular glands under the jaw bone, and sublingual glands under the tongue. Most of the more than 500 minor salivary glands are in the roof of the mouth. Inflammation (swelling) of the salivary glands is called sialadenitis. Most often the parotid gland is affected. People in their 50s and 60s, chronically ill people with dry mouth, people who had radiation therapy to the mouth, and teenagers and young adults with anorexia have greater chances of getting it.

What Causes Salivary Gland Inflammation?

The cause is usually infection with bacteria, mainly the ones called *Staphylococcus aureus, Pseudomonas, Klebsiella, Enterobacter, Enterococcus,* and *Proteus.* Often, the duct going from the gland under the tongue becomes blocked with mucus or a stone and then becomes infected. Salivary gland inflammation is often related to a chronic illness or dehydration.

What Are the Symptoms of Salivary Gland Inflammation?

Symptoms are pain and swelling in the back of the mouth; pain while eating; redness, irritation, and tenderness where saliva enters the throat from the gland, and the presence of sticky liquid near the salivary gland.

How Is Salivary Gland Inflammation Diagnosed?

The doctor will diagnose this condition from the medical history and physical examination. Usually no tests are needed.

For serious cases that don't get better with medicine, computed tomography (CT) or a special x-ray test called a sialogram may be done.

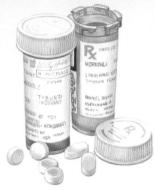

Less serious cases are often treated with methods such as rinsing the mouth, taking antibiotics, and drinking more fluids.

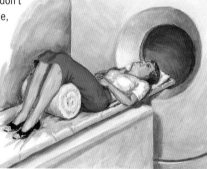

For serious cases that don't get better with medicine, CT or other x-ray tests may be done.

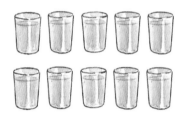

Drink more—about 8 to 10 glasses of water a day. If you can't eat, try a liquid diet (soups, juices, ice cream) and continue to drink water.

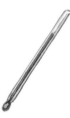

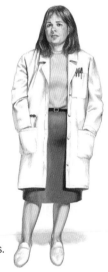

Call your doctor if you get a fever, severe pain that medicine doesn't help, or symptoms that don't get better after 3 days of taking antibiotics.

How Is Salivary Gland Inflammation Treated?

Massaging the salivary gland to relieve pressure from swelling, rinsing out the mouth, applying heat such as warm compresses to the swollen area, and drinking more water are treatments for less serious cases.

Most cases need antibiotics and measures to make more saliva flow, to clear the salivary duct. In addition to the measures noted above, sucking on hard candies and lemon drops helps stimulate saliva production. A liquid or soft diet may help reduce pain during eating. Dilation of the duct may be needed if other things don't work. Your doctor may refer you to a specialist known as an otorhinolaryngologist.

DOs and DON'Ts in Managing Salivary Gland Inflammation:

✔ **DO** take acetaminophen, ibuprofen, or naproxen for minor pain.

✔ **DO** try a liquid or soft diet until the duct is clear.

✔ **DO** drink more (8 to 10 glasses of water daily).

✔ **DO** apply warm compresses to the swollen gland.

✔ **DO** suck on hard candies or lemon drops to help make saliva.

✔ **DO** call your doctor if you get a fever, pain becomes severe and isn't helped by medicine, or your symptoms don't get better after 3 days of taking antibiotics.

⊘ **DON'T** skip doses or stop taking prescribed medication until all medicine is gone.

FROM THE DESK OF

NOTES

FOR MORE INFORMATION

Contact the following sources:

• American Academy of Otolaryngology—Head and Neck Surgery
  Tel: (703) 836-4444
  Website: http://www.entnet.org

• American Dental Association
  Tel: (312) 440-2500
  Website: http://www.ada.org

MANAGING YOUR
SALIVARY GLAND STONES

The major salivary glands are the parotid, submandibular, and sublingual. These glands make saliva to help digest food. Saliva drains into the mouth through salivary ducts. Blockage of these ducts from calcified stones (calculi) is called sialolithiasis.

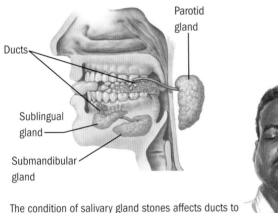

- Ducts
- Parotid gland
- Sublingual gland
- Submandibular gland

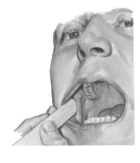

The condition of salivary gland stones affects ducts to the submandibular gland in nearly 80% of cases. It usually affects people 50 to 80 years old. The cause isn't known. The main symptoms are pain and swelling in the cheek and under the tongue. Pain becomes worse during and after eating. Infected glands can cause fever and increased pain.

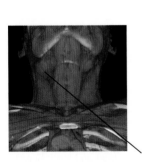

The submandibular gland

Your doctor usually makes a diagnosis from symptoms and physical examination. The stone can sometimes be felt by hand. If the doctor feels a swollen mass, CT may be done. Rarely, x-rays (sialograms) may be taken of the gland.

What Are Salivary Gland Stones?

The major salivary glands are the parotid (on both sides of the face), submandibular (under the jaw), and sublingual (under the tongue). These glands mainly make saliva to help digestion of food. Saliva drains into the bottom of the mouth, next to the upper teeth, and under the tongue through salivary ducts. Blockage of these ducts from calcified stones (calculi) is called sialolithiasis. Most stones are made of chemicals called calcium phosphate and calcium carbonate mixed with cell debris and mucus. Sialolithiasis usually affects people between 50 and 80 years old.

Salivary gland stones affect ducts to the submandibular gland in nearly 80% of cases, the parotid gland in 14%, and the sublingual gland in 6%. Stones in submandibular glands are large and usually occur as one stone when compared with stones in the parotid gland.

What Causes Salivary Gland Stones?

The cause is unknown. It's not contagious or passed from parents to children.

What Are the Symptoms of Salivary Gland Stones?

The main symptoms are pain and swelling in the cheek and under the tongue. Pain becomes worse during and after eating. Other symptoms include salivary gland swelling and tenderness. If the gland becomes infected, fever and increased pain may occur.

How Are Salivary Gland Stones Diagnosed?

The doctor usually makes a diagnosis from symptoms and a physical examination. Symptoms tend to come and go. These periodic painful attacks may be called salivary colic. The stone can sometimes be felt by an examining hand. If the doctor feels a swollen mass, computed tomography (CT) may be done to see the mass and rule out other causes, such as tumors, dental abscesses, swollen lymph glands, lymphoma, sarcoidosis, and sialadenitis (salivary gland infection). Rarely, x-rays may be taken of the gland (sialography), after a dye is injected into the duct to confirm the diagnosis. The doctor may also order blood tests.

The goal of treatment is to reduce pain and swelling. Therapy at first may be conservative, with heat (warm soaks) applied to the area, massage, and increased fluid intake. The doctor may prescribe an antibiotic for infected glands.

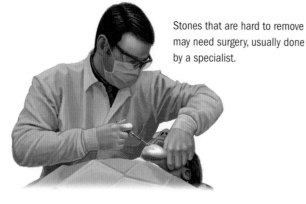

Stones that are hard to remove may need surgery, usually done by a specialist.

Drink plenty of fluids and take care of your mouth. Dehydration puts you at risk for having salivary gland stones.

Don't eat citrus and spicy foods if you think that you have salivary gland stones. Both types of foods increase secretion of saliva and can make the pain caused by a blocked gland worse.

Call your doctor if you have a fever or you see a lump on the side of your mouth or in your neck.

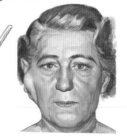

How Are Salivary Gland Stones Treated?

The goal of treatment is to reduce pain and swelling. Therapy at first may be conservative, with heat (warm soaks) applied to the area, massage, and increased fluid intake. The doctor may prescribe an antibiotic for infected glands.

A stone can sometimes be removed by squeezing them out by hand or by making a small cut in the opening to the duct. Stones that are hard to remove may need surgery, usually done by a surgical ear, nose, and throat specialist or a head and neck specialist.

DOs and DON'Ts in Managing Salivary Gland Stones:

✔ **DO** drink plenty of fluids and take care of your mouth. Dehydration puts you at risk for having salivary gland stones.

✔ **DO** call your doctor if you have mouth pain, especially when eating citrus or spicy foods.

✔ **DO** call your doctor if you have a fever or you see a lump on the side of your mouth or in your neck.

⊘ **DON'T** eat citrus and spicy foods if you think that you have salivary gland stones. Both types of foods increase secretion of saliva and can make pain of a blocked gland worse.

⊘ **DON'T** forget that salivary gland stones most often affect the gland under the jaw.

FROM THE DESK OF

NOTES

FOR MORE INFORMATION

Contact the following sources:

• American Academy of Otolaryngology—Head and Neck Surgery
 Tel: (703) 836-4444
 Website: http://www.entnet.org

• American Dental Association
 Tel: (312) 440-2500
 Website: http://www.ada.org

MANAGING YOUR
SLEEP APNEA

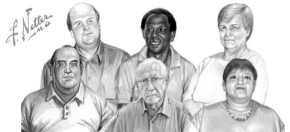

In sleep apnea, breathing stops during sleep. Episodes are usually brief, from 10 to 30 seconds. In severe cases, they occur hundreds of times a night. About 4% of middle-aged men and 2% of women have apnea.

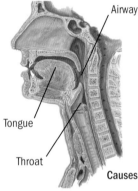

Airway

Obstructive sleep apnea occurs when the muscles in your throat relax too much and block your airway.

Tongue

Throat

Causes of sleep apnea include:

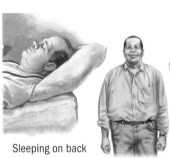

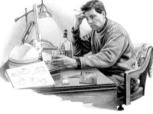

Sleep deprivation and alcohol use

Sleeping on back

Obesity

The most common symptom is loud snoring. Others are breathing pauses with loud snorts or gasps as breathing starts; daytime sleepiness, irritability, or problems concentrating; headache, dry mouth, or sore throat when awakening; and shortness of breath at night.

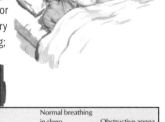

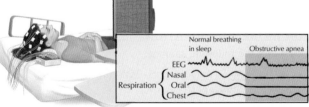

Normal breathing in sleep

Obstructive apnea

EEG

Respiration { Nasal / Oral / Chest

Your doctor will check your medical history and look at your nose and throat for abnormalities. You may have an overnight sleep study done in a sleep disorders clinic. During this test, brain activity, breathing patterns, oxygen levels, and heart rate are recorded.

What Is Sleep Apnea?

Sleep apnea is the condition in which breathing stops during sleep. Apnea episodes are usually brief, from 10 to 30 seconds. In severe cases, they occur hundreds of times a night.

When breathing stops, the oxygen level in the body drops. This tells the brain to signal the body to wake up and take a breath. Most people don't remember waking up, but they have troubled sleep cycles.

Apnea can lead to heart problems and daytime sleepiness.

About 4% of middle-aged men and 2% of women have apnea.

What Causes Sleep Apnea?

The most common cause is obesity (for men, a collar size larger than 17 inches is related to apnea). Very narrow windpipes or very large tonsils can block the throat and cause apnea. Using sleeping pills or alcohol before sleep may increase the chance of having apnea. Other reasons are nasal congestion, sleeping on the back, and sleep deprivation.

What Are the Symptoms of Sleep Apnea?

The most common symptom is loud snoring. Another symptom is breathing pauses during sleep with loud snorts or gasps as breathing starts. Others are daytime sleepiness, irritability, or problems concentrating; headache, dry mouth, or sore throat when awakening; and shortness of breath during the night.

How Is Sleep Apnea Diagnosed?

The doctor will check the medical history and examine the nose and throat for abnormalities. The diagnosis is made by doing an overnight sleep study in a sleep disorders clinic or at home. During this test, called polysomnography, brain activity, breathing patterns, oxygen levels, and heart rate are recorded.

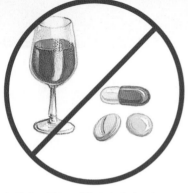

Losing weight, avoiding alcohol and sleeping pills, using nasal decongestants, and not sleeping on the back are usually suggested for mild apnea.

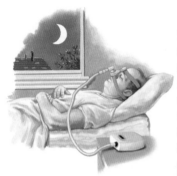

Many people use the system of continuous positive airway pressure (CPAP). CPAP has a mask for the nose connected to a bedside fan with a hose. Air from the fan goes under pressure through the hose and mask and into the throat, to keep lung passages open.

If your partner still hears you snoring while you use CPAP, the pressure may need to be changed.

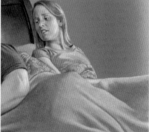

Talk to your doctor if you still feel sleepy even if you use CPAP. You may have another sleep disorder or other medical disorders.

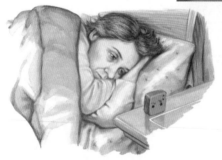

How Is Sleep Apnea Treated?

Treatment and recovery time depend on the severity of apnea. Many people need lifelong treatment. Losing weight, avoiding alcohol and sleeping pills, using nasal decongestants, and not sleeping on the back are usually suggested for mild apnea. Sleeping on the back can be prevented by old-fashioned treatments such as wearing a T-shirt with a pouch in the back filled with tennis balls. Fill a large sock with three or four tennis balls and attach it with a safety pin to the back of the shirt.

Many people use the system of continuous positive airway pressure (CPAP). CPAP has a mask for the nose connected to a bedside fan with a hose. Air from the fan goes under pressure through the hose and mask and into the throat, to keep lung passages open.

Other methods include using an oral appliance that make the jaw move forward during sleep. This helps keep the throat open. Operations to keep airways open are possible but may not work.

DOs and DON'Ts in Managing Sleep Apnea:

✔ **DO** lose weight if you're overweight.
✔ **DO** avoid sleeping pills or alcohol before sleep.
✔ **DO** use CPAP or an oral appliance every night if your doctor prescribes it. Call your doctor if you have problems with CPAP, such as dry nose, congestion, or sneezing.
✔ **DO** talk to your doctor if you still feel sleepy even if you use CPAP. You may have another sleep disorder.

⊘ **DON'T** get sleep deprived. You should sleep 7 to 8 hours each night.

FROM THE DESK OF

NOTES

FOR MORE INFORMATION

Contact the following sources:

• American Sleep Apnea Association
Tel: (202) 293-3650
Website: http://www.sleepapnea.org

• American Lung Association
Tel: (800) LUNG-USA (586-4872)
Website: http://www.lungusa.org

Pharyngitis, the medical term for sore throat, is an infection with throat pain. It usually goes away by itself in a week without causing damage. It is usually caused by a virus.

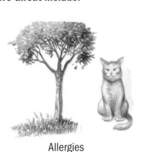

Other causes of a sore throat include:

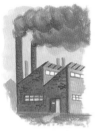

Air pollution

Alcohol

Allergies

Bacteria

Smoking

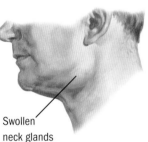

Swollen neck glands

Sore throat is the most common symptom. Others are earache, fever, large tonsils, neck pain, pain when talking or swallowing, red throat, runny nose, snoring and trouble breathing, drooling, and swollen, painful neck glands.

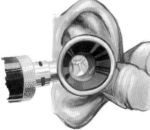

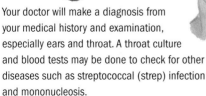

Your doctor will make a diagnosis from your medical history and examination, especially ears and throat. A throat culture and blood tests may be done to check for other diseases such as streptococcal (strep) infection and mononucleosis.

What Is a Sore Throat?

Pharyngitis, the medical term for sore throat, is an infection with throat pain. It usually goes away by itself in a week without causing damage.

What Causes a Sore Throat?

The cause is usually a virus, but air pollution, alcohol, allergies, bacteria, chemicals, and smoking can also cause a sore throat.

What Are the Symptoms of a Sore Throat?

Throat discomfort is the most common symptom. Others, depending on the cause of the sore throat, may be earache, fever, large tonsils, neck pain, pain when talking or swallowing, red throat, runny nose, snoring and trouble breathing, drooling, general aches, and swollen, painful glands in the neck.

How Is a Sore Throat Diagnosed?

The doctor will make a diagnosis from the medical history and examination, especially of the ears and throat. Usually, no other tests are needed. A swab of the throat may also be done if a streptococcal (strep) bacterial infection is suspected to be the cause. Blood tests may be done for other diseases, such as mononucleosis, if these are suspected.

How Is a Sore Throat Treated?

Most cases go away by themselves. Antibiotics are not helpful for viral infections. The doctor will prescribe antibiotics only for a bacterial infection. Drinking warm liquids, eating soft cold food, and gargling with warm saltwater solution may help the pain. Acetaminophen or ibuprofen can also be taken for fever and pain. A cool mist vaporizer may relieve a dry, tight feeling in the throat.

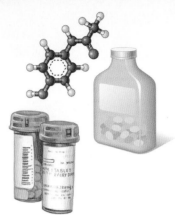

Most cases go away by themselves. Your doctor may prescribe antibiotics for a bacterial infection, but not for a virus. Replace your toothbrush after treatment starts, to prevent reinfection. Take acetaminophen or ibuprofen for fever and pain.

Drinking warm liquids, eating soft cold food, and gargling with warm saltwater solution may help the pain.

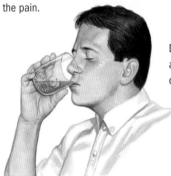

Drink plenty of fluids, but not alcohol. Don't smoke, which can cause or worsen symptoms.

Call your doctor for a severe headache, rash, or cough with thick, yellow-green or bloody sputum. Call your doctor right away or go to the emergency room for breathing or swallowing problems.

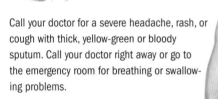

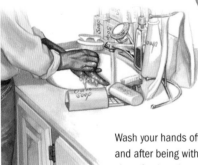

Wash your hands often, especially before you eat and after being with someone who's sick. Don't share food, eating utensils, or drinking glasses.

DOs and DON'Ts in Managing a Sore Throat:

✔ **DO** tell your doctor about your medicines, both prescription and over-the-counter.

✔ **DO** call your doctor if your symptoms get worse or you have a temperature higher than 101° F.

✔ **DO** call your doctor right away or go to the emergency room for breathing or swallowing problems.

✔ **DO** call your doctor if you have joint pain, body swelling, or dark urine.

✔ **DO** call your doctor if you have severe throat pain that stops you from swallowing.

✔ **DO** gargle with a warm saltwater solution.

✔ **DO** use a vaporizer to for a dry, tight feeling in the throat. Clean the vaporizer and change the water daily.

✔ **DO** replace your toothbrush after treatment starts, to prevent reinfection.

✔ **DO** limit activities until symptoms go away.

✔ **DO** increase fluid intake.

✔ **DO** follow a liquid diet (soups, gelatin, ice cream, and juices) if swallowing is hard.

✔ **DO** call your doctor you get a severe headache, rash, or cough with thick, yellow-green or bloody sputum.

✔ **DO** eat a healthy diet and get plenty of sleep to improve your recovery time.

✔ **DO** wash your hands often, especially before you eat and after being with someone who's sick.

✔ **DO** stop smoking and drinking alcohol.

✔ **DO** stay away from cigarette smoke and air pollution.

✔ **DO** get a humidifier if air in your home is very dry.

⊘ **DON'T** give aspirin to a child with fever or sore throat, to avoid the dangerous Reye's syndrome.

⊘ **DON'T** stop taking your medicine or change your dosage because you feel better unless your doctor tells you to.

⊘ **DON'T** share food, utensils, or drinking glasses. Avoid kissing someone who's sick.

FROM THE DESK OF

NOTES

FOR MORE INFORMATION

Contact the following sources:

- Infectious Diseases Society of America
  Tel: (703) 299-0200
  Website: http://www.idsociety.org

- American Academy of Otolaryngology—Head and Neck Surgery
  Tel: (703) 836-4444
  Website: http://www.ent.net

Tonsillitis is infection that causes inflammation of the tonsils. It's very common in children 6 to 12 years old. Most recover quickly, in 4 to 6 days. It's contagious and spreads by direct contact with infected secretions, such as saliva, mucus, and tears.

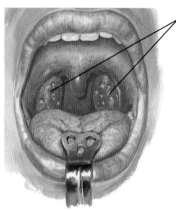

Tonsils are clumps of tissue, one on each side of the throat, that trap bacteria and viruses. Tonsillitis is often caused by a virus, but bacteria can cause it. Tonsils may have a yellow or thin white coating or small white patches.

Symptoms include a sore throat, trouble swallowing, drooling, fever, earache, tender swollen glands in the neck, and tonsils that look swollen and red.

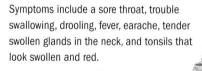

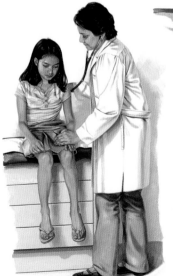

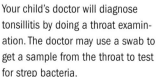

Your child's doctor will diagnose tonsillitis by doing a throat examination. The doctor may use a swab to get a sample from the throat to test for strep bacteria.

What Is Tonsillitis?

Tonsillitis is infection that causes inflammation (swelling and redness) of the tonsils. Tonsils are clumps of tissue, one on each side of the throat, that trap bacteria and viruses.

Tonsillitis is very common in children 6 to 12 years old. Most children recover quickly. The disease usually lasts 4 to 6 days. Tonsillitis is contagious and spreads by direct contact with infected secretions, such as saliva, mucus, and tears.

What Causes Tonsillitis?

The cause is often a virus, but bacteria can also cause tonsillitis. Tonsillitis caused by bacteria is sometimes called strep throat (caused by *Streptococcus* bacteria).

What Are the Symptoms of Tonsillitis?

Symptoms include a sore throat, pain and trouble swallowing, drooling, fever, earache, tender swollen glands in the neck, and tonsils that look swollen and red. Tonsils may have a yellow or thin white coating or small white patches. Some children have a hard time breathing because of very large tonsils.

How Is Tonsillitis Diagnosed?

The doctor will diagnose tonsillitis by examining the throat. The doctor may use a swab to get a sample from the throat to test for strep bacteria. The doctor may also do blood tests if other infections such as mononucleosis are suspected.

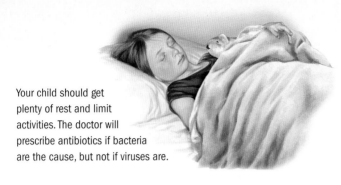

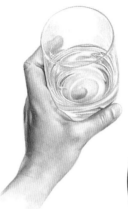

Your child should get plenty of rest and limit activities. The doctor will prescribe antibiotics if bacteria are the cause, but not if viruses are.

Have your child drink plenty of fluids, especially warm liquids.

Don't allow smoking near your child.

Don't give aspirin to children younger than 16. They can get a serious illness called Reye's syndrome. Give acetaminophen instead.

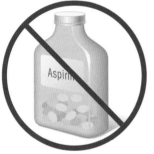

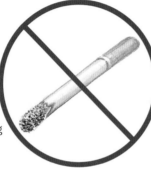

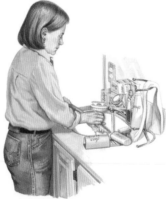

To help prevent spreading the infection, everyone in the household should wash hands regularly. Avoid eating or drinking from the same utensils.

How Is Tonsillitis Treated?

Rest and good fluid intake are the best treatment. If bacteria are the cause, the doctor will prescribe antibiotics. Acetaminophen or ibuprofen can be used for pain and fever. Gargling with a saltwater solution or other soothing liquid may help pain and irritation. A cool mist vaporizer may also help the cough and irritation.

For some children, the doctor may suggest removing the tonsils (tonsillectomy). This surgery is usually done for frequent or long-lasting tonsillitis that causes breathing problems.

DOs and DON'Ts in Managing Tonsillitis:

✔ **DO** make sure that your child drinks plenty of fluids, especially warm liquids.

✔ **DO** have your child gargle with warm saltwater.

✔ **DO** give your child over-the-counter pills or liquids, such as acetaminophen, for pain and fever.

✔ **DO** make sure that your child takes all the antibiotics.

✔ **DO** practice good hygiene to avoid spreading the infection to other family members. Don't let your child eat or drink from the same utensils as other family members.

✔ **DO** let your child increase activity slowly after fever has been gone for 2 to 3 days.

✔ **DO** call your doctor if your child has severe swelling of the tonsils and has trouble breathing.

✔ **DO** call your doctor if your child's fever is gone for a few days and suddenly returns.

✔ **DO** call your doctor if your child gets new symptoms, such as a rash, nausea, vomiting, chest pain, shortness of breath, or cough with thick or discolored sputum.

⊘ **DON'T** give aspirin to children younger than 16. They can get a serious illness called Reye's syndrome.

⊘ **DON'T** smoke or let people smoke around your child. Smoking can worsen the infection and delay recovery.

⊘ **DON'T** let your child stop taking antibiotics until they're all gone.

FROM THE DESK OF

NOTES

FOR MORE INFORMATION

Contact the following sources:

• Infectious Diseases Society of America
Tel: (703) 299-0200
Website: http://www.idsociety.org/

• The American Academy of Pediatrics
Tel: (847) 434-4000
Website: http://www.aap.org

Between 2% and 7% of all children have ADHD. In school-age children, it occurs more in boys than in girls.

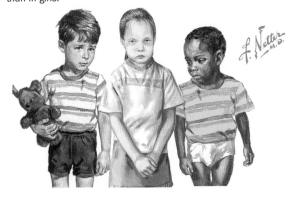

There is no specific test for ADHD. Observations of doctors, parents, teachers, and others are the basis for diagnosis. Depression and anxiety must be ruled out.

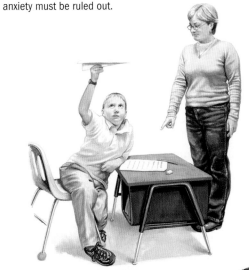

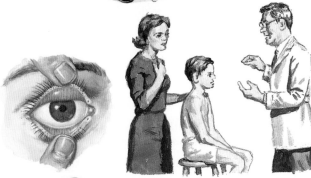

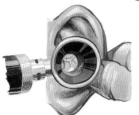

Your doctor will ask about your family history to see if other children also have ADHD. Your child will have a physical examination, including tests of hearing and vision.

What Is Attention Deficit Hyperactivity Disorder (ADHD)?

ADHD is a behavior disorder involving an inability to focus on tasks. Hyperactive behavior is part of ADHD.

Between 2% and 7% of children have ADHD, and in younger children, more boys than girls have it. Some children outgrow ADHD, others control problem behaviors as they grow older, and others may have ADHD into adulthood. Certain children become troubled teenagers and adults with problems such as failure in school, antisocial behavior, and sometimes even criminal behavior.

No ways to prevent ADHD are known. ADHD is not contagious.

What Causes ADHD?

The cause is unknown. It may occur in more than one child in a family.

Environmental factors and hereditary factors may play a role.

What Are the Symptoms of ADHD?

Problem behaviors are the symptoms, usually in a child younger than 7.

Parents, teachers, and doctors may see the behaviors, which include inability to listen, follow instructions, wait turn in games and lines, or pay attention in school or at play; becoming easily distracted; losing things; shifting from one task to another; answering before a question is finished; interrupting or intruding; doing dangerous things without thinking; squirming or inability to stay seated; fidgeting with hands and feet; and talking constantly.

How Is ADHD Diagnosed?

No specific test exists for ADHD. Observations of doctors, parents, teachers, and others are key. Depression and anxiety must be ruled out.

The doctor will ask about the family history, do a physical examination (including hearing and eye tests), and check for learning disabilities and development level. For an ADHD diagnosis, the child must have six or more of eight specific symptoms for at least 6 months, and these must interfere with daily functions.

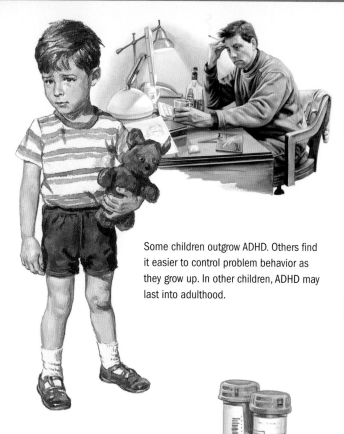

Some children outgrow ADHD. Others find it easier to control problem behavior as they grow up. In other children, ADHD may last into adulthood.

A combination of treatments is often needed. Drugs and behavioral methods are better when used together than when used alone.

Adults with ADHD should consider support groups for anger control. People with ADHD should exercise regularly and try to maintain structure and routine in their lives.

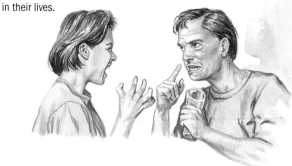

Adults with ADHD often have failed relationships, problems at work, and sometimes alcohol and drug abuse. Many such adults may have been misdiagnosed with anxiety or manic depressive disorders.

How Is ADHD Treated?

The most effective treatment is combination of drugs and behavioral methods used together. Educational, behavioral, and cognitive methods may all be recommended. Drugs used most often are psychostimulants, which help people feel calmer, more relaxed, more focused, and less scattered in thinking.

The doctor may also suggest counseling for child and parents. Support for parents is essential.

DOs and DON'Ts in Managing ADHD:

✔ **DO** set clear behavior limits and reward good behavior.
✔ **DO** use time outs for bad behavior and stop problem behavior before it worsens.
✔ **DO** allow for more activity in safe environments.
✔ **DO** focus on one task at a time.
✔ **DO** try techniques such as anger training, social training, and family therapy, but avoid unproven therapies.
✔ **DO** have realistic expectations.
✔ **DO** talk regularly with your child's teacher.
✔ **DO** call your doctor if symptoms worsen after treatment begins.
✔ **DO** consider support groups for anger control, if you're an adult. Exercise regularly and try to maintain structure and routine.

⊘ **DON'T** forget follow-up appointments.
⊘ **DON'T** self-medicate with drugs or alcohol, or use too much caffeine or sugar as a teenager or adult.
⊘ **DON'T** increase medicine doses unless your doctor says to.

FOR MORE INFORMATION

Contact the following sources:

• CHADD (Children and Adults with Attention-Deficit/Hyperactivity Disorder)
Tel: (301) 306-7070, (800) 233-4050
Website: http://www.chadd.org/

• National Institute of Mental Health
Tel: (866) 615-6464
Email: nimhinfo@nih.gov
Website: http://www.nimh.nih.gov/

FROM THE DESK OF

NOTES

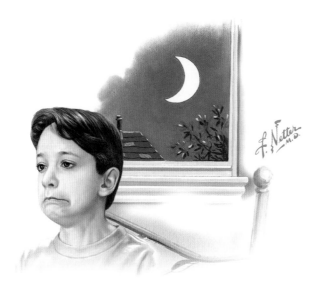

If bedwetting continues in a child 4 years or older, it's important to try to find the physical or emotional causes.

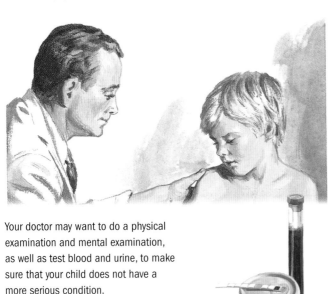

Your doctor may want to do a physical examination and mental examination, as well as test blood and urine, to make sure that your child does not have a more serious condition.

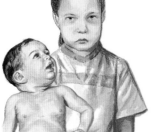

Stress or such changes as the birth of a sibling can contribute to the start or a relapse of bedwetting.

What Is Bedwetting?

Bedwetting, or enuresis, is the unintentional (involuntary) passage of urine into bed or clothes by children aged 4 years or older who have no physical problems.

Having nighttime control of urinating is the final stage of one process of development. Most children can control the bladder at night by age 3 years. Bedwetting is as common in boys as in girls until the age of 5. By age 11, boys who wet the bed outnumber girls by 2 to 1.

What Causes Bedwetting?

The cause is usually unknown. However, emotional problems caused by stress or separation, diabetes, urinary tract infections, family history of bedwetting, and being the firstborn child increase bedwetting risk. Also, stress may play a role in children who have bedwetting after being dry at night. This stress may be the birth of another child, hospitalizations, and head injury. Daytime wetting occurs more in girls than in boys and has more associated emotional problems.

What Are the Symptoms of Bedwetting?

The symptom is losing bladder control, usually in the bed at night, and sometimes during the day in an older child.

How Is Bedwetting Diagnosed?

Because bedwetting may have medical causes, the doctor will look for problems in the urinary tract (e.g., bladder), hormone secretion, sleep patterns, family history, and development of the child. The doctor will do physical and mental status examinations, x-ray studies, and blood and urine tests to be sure that a physical reason is not the cause.

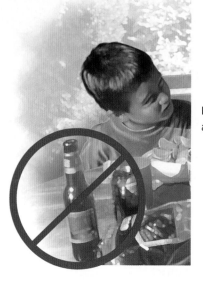

Limiting fluids and caffeine after dinner helps.

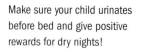

Make sure your child urinates before bed and give positive rewards for dry nights!

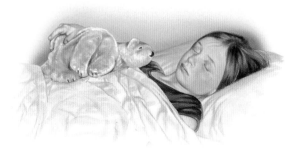

Medications and alarms are available that can help control bedwetting, but if your child has no lasting emotional or medical problems, bedwetting will stop without treatment.

FROM THE DESK OF

NOTES

How Is Bedwetting Treated?

Most children with bedwetting never see the doctor. Most families consider bedwetting part of normal childhood development and try to treat it at home. These attempts include restricting fluids (especially after dinner), and using rewards and punishments. Usually, punishing children makes bedwetting worse and may lead to self-esteem problems.

When initially treating bedwetting, the doctor reassures the child that bedwetting can be treated. About 10% of children who have this first visit improve without treatment. Children with no emotional or medical problems will likely stop bed-wetting on their own. Other treatments involve waking the child to urinate or having the child urinate before going to bed, avoiding liquids at bedtime, and rewards for dry nights. Medicines can also reduce urine output or affect the way the bladder works.

Psychosocial treatments include using a night alarm or a vibrating pad under the pillow. Relapse after successful treatment usually takes place within 6 months after treatment stops (about one third of children relapse).

DOs and DON'Ts in Managing Bedwetting:

✔ **DO** avoid stressful events.

✔ **DO** avoid excessive criticism of your child.

✔ **DO** limit intake of liquids in the evening, and have your child urinate at certain times (e.g., after dinner, before bed).

✔ **DO** give your child positive rewards for dry nights.

✔ **DO** call your doctor if your child previously wet the bed only at night but now has daytime wetting.

✔ **DO** call your doctor if your child's urine smells foul or has blood in it, or if your child has pain when urinating.

✔ **DO** find and treat physical causes promptly.

⊘ **DON'T** baby or smother your child.

FOR MORE INFORMATION

Contact the following sources:

- American Academy of Pediatrics
  Tel: (847) 434-4000
  Website: http://www.aap.org

- American Psychiatric Association
  Tel: (888) 357-7924
  Website: http://www.psych.org

- American Academy of Family Physicians
  Tel: (800) 274-2237
  Website: http://www.aafp.org

PROTECTING CHILDREN FROM ABUSE

Help is available to stop child abuse and neglect:

- **National Child Abuse/Neglect Hotline**
  Tel: (800) 422-4453
  Website: http://childabuseprevention.org

Be aware of signs
of child abuse.

Fractures
from twisting
or sudden jerking

How Common Is Child Abuse?

Child abuse and neglect are major social problems in the United States. The number of alleged abuse incidents reported to state and local child protective services has skyrocketed, and statistics today show that physical abuse is the leading cause of death for children younger than 1 year. The highest incidence of child abuse from birth to 18 years occurs in first year of life, and more than two thirds of victims of physical abuse are younger than 6 years.

What Causes Child Abuse?

Child abuse and mistreatment appear to be associated with poverty, unemployment, child disability, psychiatric problems in parents, substance abuse by parents, parents being abused as children, antisocial behavior of parents, and whether pregnancy was planned. However, these factors alone don't seem to predict the occurrence of abuse. The problem may be more child neglect than abuse. Neglect sometimes results from depression or other mental illness in the parents. Some parents, especially young, first-time parents, may be overwhelmed by caring for a child, become frustrated, and direct anger and frustration at the child.

What Are the Symptoms of Child Abuse?

Children may have orthopedic injuries, bruises, or x-ray evidence of repeated fractures. Shaken infant syndrome is associated with high death rates and physical injury. Child abuse can result in bleeding into the brain, blindness, and injuries to abdominal organs. These injuries account for most of deaths from child abuse.

As many as 30% of cases of failure to thrive in children are thought to be caused by neglect. Failure to thrive may lead to severe behavioral problems later in life. Child abuse may also involve sexual abuse.

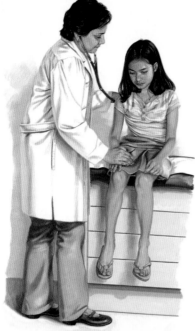

Abused children will need psychological therapy in addition to medical care.

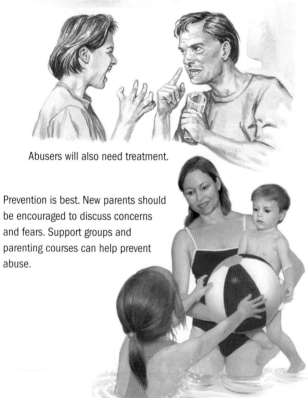

Abusers will also need treatment.

Prevention is best. New parents should be encouraged to discuss concerns and fears. Support groups and parenting courses can help prevent abuse.

How Is Child Abuse Diagnosed?

Abused children have significant problems in emotional, social, and behavioral functioning. They have difficulty trusting others. They may feel guilt and low self-esteem because they believe that they were responsible for the abuse. Abused children have poor social behavior and tend to show anger and aggression toward playmates and schoolmates. They are more likely to have major psychiatric problems such as posttraumatic stress disorder, depression, anxiety, phobias, and personality disorders.

Staff in most emergency departments note children who come in frequently, especially with orthopedic injuries, and who have bruises or on x-ray evidence of old fractures. Physicians and other medical caregivers must report suspected child abuse and can face sanctions for not doing so.

How Is Child Abuse Handled?

Neighbors, family members, or medical personnel who report suspected abuse may prompt treatment.

The primary, most important goal is protection of the child. Medical consequences of abuse must be evaluated and treated, and the child should have psychological therapy. Such treatment often involves using play therapy, including dolls and puppets. Abusers also require treatment, regardless of whether they become involved in the criminal justice system. Support groups for such parents have helped. Many states have a program for monitoring pregnancies to assess whether it is safe for those babies to return home.

Many adults have flashbacks to childhood physical and sexual abuse that make it more likely that they will have psychiatric disorders, including borderline and multiple personality disorder, eating disorders, posttraumatic stress disorder, and alcohol and drug abuse.

The Approach to Child Abuse

The best approach to child abuse is prevention. Evaluating the level of support and the support network for new parents, providing parenting classes, and encouraging new parents to discuss concerns and fears would help. Overwhelmed parents should not be embarrassed to seek medical help and counseling.

FOR MORE INFORMATION

Contact the following sources:

• There are several commercial videos available through your local library or children's hospital. The book entitled *How to Raise a Street Smart Child* is particularly helpful.

• Child Abuse Prevention Association
Tel: (816) 252-8388
Website: http://www.childabuseprevention.org

• Childhelp USA
Tel: (480) 922-8212
Website: http://www.childhelpusa.org

FROM THE DESK OF

NOTES

CARING FOR YOUR INFANT WITH
COLIC

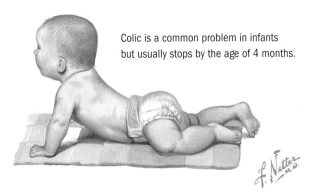

Colic is a common problem in infants but usually stops by the age of 4 months.

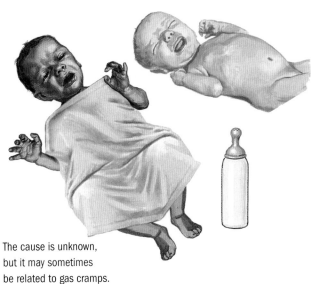

The cause is unknown, but it may sometimes be related to gas cramps. Colic may lead to feeding problems and loss of sleep.

Your doctor will do an examination and tests to make sure that no medical problem is causing your baby's crying.

What Is Colic?

Colic is a term used to describe when a healthy baby cries or screams loudly, often for a long time (sometimes hours), for no clear reason and cannot be soothed. Crying can happen suddenly without warning at any time, but it often occurs at the end of a day. It is common and affects up to one third of babies in their first 3 months of life. No methods for predicting and preventing colic in babies are known.

What Causes Colic?

The cause is unknown. The previous belief was that babies had gas or cramps in the abdomen (belly), but doctors now think that this is not always the case. Experts say colicky babies generally have no pain but don't understand why it occurs.

Colicky crying usually begins in the first couple of weeks after birth. It's often worst at about 6 weeks and usually stops by 4 months. It's not caused by bad parenting, being a single parent, or postpartum depression. It doesn't affect normal development.

What Are the Symptoms of Colic?

Continuous crying or screaming loudly for no clear reason means a colicky baby. Babies may pull up their legs, arch their back, clench their fists, grimace, or look flushed.

Usual soothing methods may not work. Colic can cause babies to have feeding problems and lose sleep.

How Is Colic Diagnosed?

The doctor will take a medical history of the baby to rule out feeding, burping, or bowel problems.

The doctor will also do a physical examination to make sure no medical problem (such as infection, rash, fever, or breathing, skin, or stomach disorders) is the cause. Other tests may also be done.

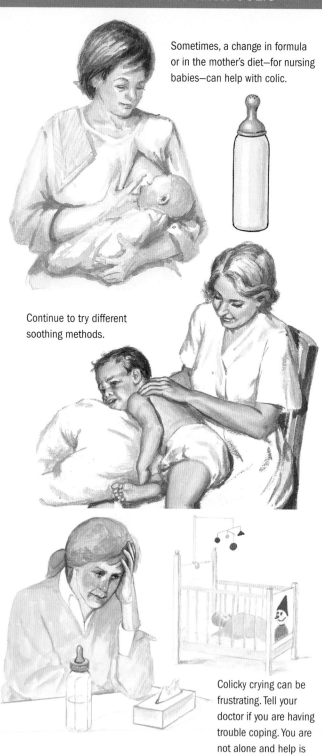

Sometimes, a change in formula or in the mother's diet—for nursing babies—can help with colic.

Continue to try different soothing methods.

Colicky crying can be frustrating. Tell your doctor if you are having trouble coping. You are not alone and help is available.

How Is Colic Treated?

Treating colic can be difficult and frustrating. It mainly involves trying different things that might help. Some of these things include a giving a different type of formula milk or whey-based milk or medicines that calm the stomach or reduce stomach gas. If the baby is breastfed, avoiding foods that could stimulate the baby, such caffeine-containing foods (coffee, tea, chocolate) or foods containing substances that may cause an allergic reaction, such as dairy foods and nuts.

DOs and DON'Ts in Managing Colic:

✔ **DO** try things that usually stop your baby from crying, such as offering a pacifier, singing, walking or driving in the car, or gentle rocking.

✔ **DO** try snug wrapping of your baby (swaddling) and holding your baby in your arms or lap.

✔ **DO** hold your baby upright and walk the baby around.

✔ **DO** put your baby on your lap and gently massage the baby's back.

✔ **DO** ask for help if you feel unable to cope or are about to lose emotional control.

✔ **DO** put your baby in a safe place and let your baby cry for short periods if you can't find a soothing method.

🚫 **DON'T** worry too much about colic. Colic has no effect on a baby's health or development.

🚫 **DON'T** EVER shake a baby!

🚫 **DON'T** ever cover a baby's face with a pillow or other object to quiet the crying!

FROM THE DESK OF

NOTES

FOR MORE INFORMATION

Contact the following sources:

- Colic
  Website: http://familydoctor.org/036.xml

- What to do when your newborn cries
  Website: http://www.mayoclinic.com/health/healthy-baby/PR00037

- Infant and Newborn Care
  Website: http://www.nlm.nih.gov/medlineplus/infantandnewborncare.html

CARING FOR YOUR CHILD WITH
CROUP

A child with croup has a froggy voice and a cough that sounds like a seal bark, because the larynx (voice box) and trachea (windpipe) are swollen.

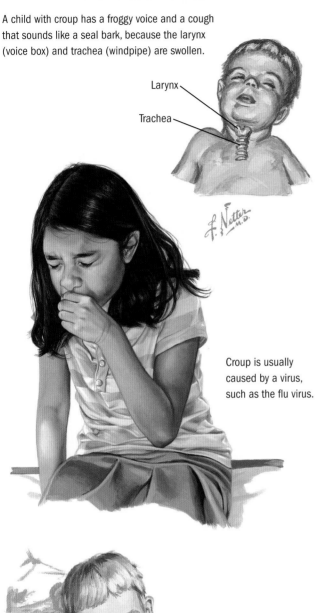

Larynx

Trachea

Croup is usually caused by a virus, such as the flu virus.

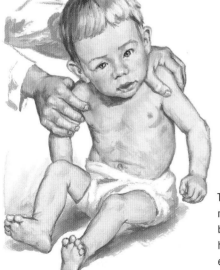

The doctor usually makes a diagnosis by using a medical history and physical examination.

What Is Croup?

Croup (or laryngotracheobronchitis) is a respiratory infection that mainly affects children. The larynx (voice box) and trachea (windpipe) going into the lungs become irritated and swollen. Children have a very hoarse voice and a cough that sounds like a seal barking. Children and parents may be frightened because it is hard for air to go in and out of the lungs and children find it hard to breathe.

Young children between 3 months and 5 years old are more prone to croup. Boys seem to get it more often than girls. Croup is also more likely in children who have at least one parent with asthma or allergies.

Most cases are not serious, and complications are rare. A few children can have pneumonia or serious bacterial infection in the lungs.

What Causes Croup?

An infection in the throat or lungs can lead to croup. The infection is usually due to a virus, such as the flu virus.

What Are the Symptoms of Croup?

Many children have a sore throat, runny nose, or fever before croup. Croup symptoms include a hoarse voice, cough that sounds like a barking seal, fast breathing, and a high-pitched, windy sound while trying to breathe air into the lungs.

Symptoms get worse when the child lies down. Often, symptoms are worse at night.

How Is Croup Diagnosed?

The doctor makes a diagnosis from a medical history and physical examination. X-rays of the child's neck and lungs may be done. X-rays may show swelling of the neck and whether something is stuck or pus or blood in the airway is causing symptoms.

Blood tests may be done if the doctor suspects that the infection could be due to bacteria.

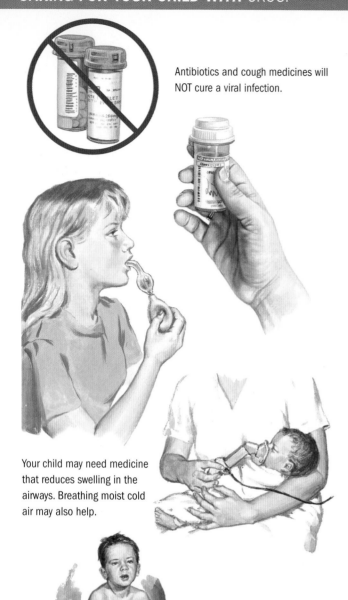

Antibiotics and cough medicines will NOT cure a viral infection.

Your child may need medicine that reduces swelling in the airways. Breathing moist cold air may also help.

Get emergency care if your child has trouble breathing, is pale, or has bluish lips, face, or fingers.

How Is Croup Treated?

Antibiotics don't help because a virus causes croup. Cough medicines also don't help much. Acetaminophen may lower the fever.

Having the child breathe air that is very moist (humid) or very cold may help. Provide moist air by going into a steamy bathroom. For cold air, wrap the child in a warm blanket and stand outside in the cold air for a few minutes.

The doctor may prescribe medicine to reduce airway swelling. In severe cases, the doctor may refer a child who has trouble breathing to the emergency department for oxygen.

Children who don't respond to these treatments may need corticosteroids (injected, by mouth, by nebulizer). Sometimes, children need admission to a hospital.

DOs and DON'Ts in Managing Croup:

✔ **DO** wash hands often, which is the best way to stop the spread of infections.

✔ **DO** keep your children away from children with a sore throat or runny nose.

✔ **DO** get emergency care if your child has trouble breathing and is very pale or has blue lips, face, or fingers. Get emergency care if the child doesn't wake up when you talk to or gently shake the child.

✔ **DO** call your doctor if symptoms don't get better or are getting worse.

✔ **DO** call your doctor if think that your child has side effects from medicine.

⊘ **DON'T** forget to give your child medicine as instructed by the doctor.

⊘ **DON'T** forget follow-up doctor appointments.

FROM THE DESK OF

NOTES

FOR MORE INFORMATION

Contact the following source:
• Website: http://www.familydoctor.org

CARING FOR YOUR CHILD WITH
CYSTIC FIBROSIS

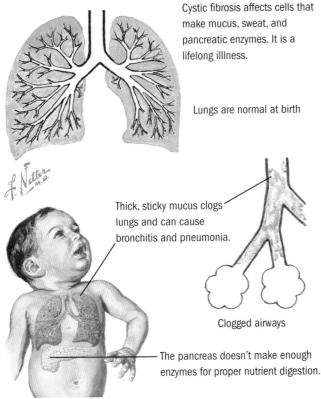

Cystic fibrosis affects cells that make mucus, sweat, and pancreatic enzymes. It is a lifelong illlness.

Lungs are normal at birth

Thick, sticky mucus clogs lungs and can cause bronchitis and pneumonia.

Clogged airways

The pancreas doesn't make enough enzymes for proper nutrient digestion.

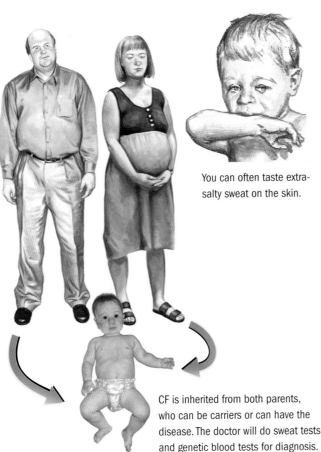

You can often taste extra-salty sweat on the skin.

CF is inherited from both parents, who can be carriers or can have the disease. The doctor will do sweat tests and genetic blood tests for diagnosis.

What Is Cystic Fibrosis?

Cystic fibrosis (CF) is a lifelong illness affecting cells that make sweat and mucus. Mucus is a slippery, somewhat sticky fluid that lubricates and protects mucous membranes. CF mucus is abnormally thick and sticky; it clogs the lungs and causes frequent lung infections.

CF also affects the pancreas, which has trouble making special chemicals called enzymes to digest food. Without enzymes, nutrients can't be absorbed from food.

CF is the most common fatal genetic disease in caucasians in the United States (1 of every 2000 births). People with CF have a shorter life span, but with modern treatments, more people with CF live to middle age or older.

What Causes CF?

CF results from abnormal movement of the chemicals sodium and chloride (salt) in certain cells in mucous and sweat glands.

CF is inherited. A child must inherit a CF gene from each parent (called an autosomal recessive disorder). Both parents can be healthy but are carriers of CF. More than 12 million Americans carry the CF gene but have no symptoms.

What Are the Symptoms of CF?

Children with CF have normal lungs at birth, and symptoms may not appear until later.

Common symptoms are chronic cough and diarrhea, frequent bronchitis and pneumonia, bulky foul-smelling bowel movements (stool), large appetite in spite of poor weight gain, salty skin, and shortness of breath.

The first sign of CF in newborns may be a block of the intestines caused by increased thickness of the first stool.

How Is CF Diagnosed?

The doctor will do a sweat test called pilocarpine iontophoresis. This painless test measures the amount of salt in the child's sweat. A high level can mean CF.

The doctor can do genetic blood tests to look for changes inside cells. The doctor can also do tests on bowel movements (stool) and blood to check effects on the pancreas, and get chest x-rays or do breathing tests to check the lungs.

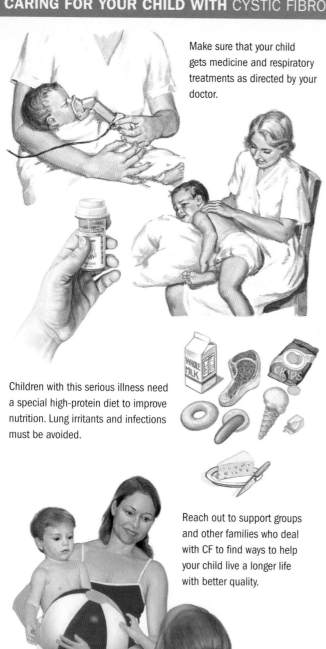

Make sure that your child gets medicine and respiratory treatments as directed by your doctor.

Children with this serious illness need a special high-protein diet to improve nutrition. Lung irritants and infections must be avoided.

Reach out to support groups and other families who deal with CF to find ways to help your child live a longer life with better quality.

How Is CF Treated?

Medicines help thin the mucus and prevent lungs from clogging. Antibiotics are also often given for infections. Enzyme supplements supply missing pancreatic enzymes. A special high-protein, low-fat diet may also improve nutrition.

Respiratory therapy is for the lungs. Thick mucus can be removed from lungs by tapping on the chest (chest percussion). Lying with the head lower than the feet can also help drain mucus. Lung transplantation is a treatment option in some cases and should be discussed with your doctor.

DOs and DON'Ts in Managing CF:

✔ **DO** follow your doctor's instructions and give medicines and treatments as directed. Take your child to the doctor at least three or four times yearly.

✔ **DO** avoid contact with people with respiratory infections.

✔ **DO** get your child a yearly flu shot.

✔ **DO** have your child drink plenty of fluids.

✔ **DO** have your child avoid gas fumes and smoke. These things irritate lungs and make CF worse.

✔ **DO** reach out to support groups.

⊘ **DON'T** neglect respiratory therapy, if advised by your doctor.

⊘ **DON'T** give your child soy protein, which is hard to digest.

⊘ **DON'T** miss doctor appointments.

⊘ **DON'T** stop prescribed antibiotics early or forget to do chest physical therapy.

FROM THE DESK OF

NOTES

FOR MORE INFORMATION

Contact the following source:

• Cystic Fibrosis Foundation
  Tel: (800) 344-4823
  Website: http://www.cff.org

MANAGING YOUR
MARFAN'S SYNDROME

Marfan's syndrome is a rare inherited disorder involving the body's connective tissues. It mainly affects the eyes, heart, blood vessels, and skeleton. It affects females and males equally, of all races.

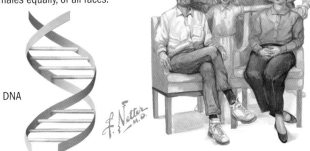

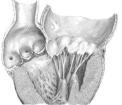

DNA

This syndrome is caused by a genetic defect (gene mutation). Parents pass the gene to their children. No major symptoms are usually seen, so it can be hard to diagnose in children.

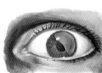

Heart valve abnormalities   Eye conditions

Three of four features are needed for diagnosis: a positive family history; eye conditions such as lens dislocation and nearsightedness; skeletal conditions such as tall height with long spidery fingers, an arm span greater than height, and chest deformities; and heart valve abnormalities.

Skeletal conditions

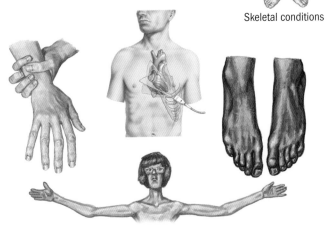

Your doctor may suspect the syndrome from your family history and physical examination showing abnormalities. Diagnosis isn't usually made until early adulthood. An ophthalmologist will do a detailed eye examination. A cardiologist will look for heart problems and do echocardiography. Genetic testing of blood may also be done.

What Is Marfan's Syndrome?

Marfan's syndrome is an inherited disorder involving the body's connective tissues. Connective tissues of the body support and bind other tissues. The syndrome mainly affects the eyes, heart, blood vessels, and skeleton.

This condition is rare. Only 4 to 6 people of 100,000 have it. It affects females and males equally, of all races.

What Causes Marfan's Syndrome?

This syndrome is caused by a genetic defect (gene mutation). In 70% of cases, the genetic defect is passed from parents to children. Each child has a 50% chance of inheriting the disorder from a parent with the syndrome. Approximately 30% of Marfan's cases are due to a new gene mutation.

What Are the Symptoms of Marfan's Syndrome?

No major symptoms are usually seen with Marfan's syndrome, so it can be hard to diagnose in children. Features include eye conditions such as dislocation of the lens and nearsightedness; skeletal conditions such as tall height with long spidery fingers, an arm span greater than height, and chest deformities; heart valve abnormalities; and a positive family history.

How Is Marfan's Syndrome Diagnosed?

The doctor may suspect that the syndrome is present from the family history and a physical examination that shows certain abnormalities. No special test can diagnose the syndrome. Diagnosis isn't usually made until early adulthood. Three of the four features mentioned must be present. An eye doctor (ophthalmologist) will also do a detailed eye examination. A cardiologist (specialist in heart diseases) will look for heart problems and do echocardiography. Echocardiography is a kind of ultrasound that can examine the heart valves. Blood tests may also be done for genetic testing.

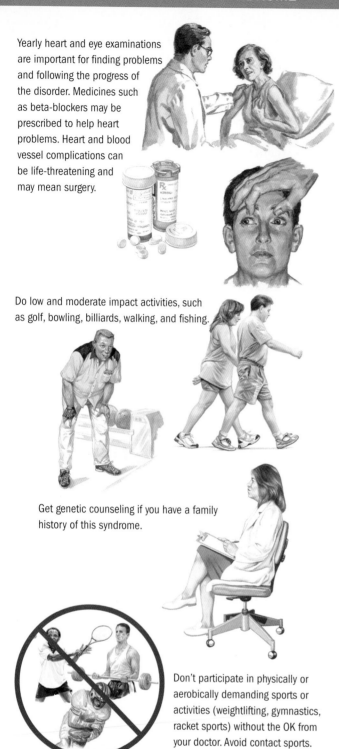

Yearly heart and eye examinations are important for finding problems and following the progress of the disorder. Medicines such as beta-blockers may be prescribed to help heart problems. Heart and blood vessel complications can be life-threatening and may mean surgery.

Do low and moderate impact activities, such as golf, bowling, billiards, walking, and fishing.

Get genetic counseling if you have a family history of this syndrome.

Don't participate in physically or aerobically demanding sports or activities (weightlifting, gymnastics, racket sports) without the OK from your doctor. Avoid contact sports.

How Is Marfan's Syndrome Treated?

The syndrome isn't curable, but diagnosis and proper treatments prolong life. A medical team—geneticist, cardiologist, ophthalmologist, surgeons, and psychologist—will likely be involved in care. Heart and eye examinations done every year are important to both find problems and follow the progress of the disorder. Medicines such as beta-blockers may be prescribed to help the heart problems. Heart and blood vessel complications can be life-threatening and may mean that surgery is needed. Valve surgery may be done for severe disease. With surgery, most patients can live a normal life span. Without treatment, people live an average of about 35 years. The major cause of death is enlargement (dilation) and bursting (rupture) of the aorta, the largest artery carrying blood from the heart to the body.

DOs and DON'Ts in Managing Marfan's Syndrome:

✔ **DO** low and moderate impact activities, such as golf, bowling, billiards, walking, and fishing. Vigorous exercise may lead to serious complications.

✔ **DO** get genetic counseling if you have a family history of Marfan's syndrome.

✔ **DO** call your doctor if you think that you or your family members have symptoms of the syndrome.

⊘ **DON'T** participate in physically or aerobically demanding sports or activities (weightlifting, gymnastics, racket sports) without the OK from your doctor. Avoid contact sports.

FROM THE DESK OF

NOTES

FOR MORE INFORMATION

Contact the following source:

• National Marfan Foundation
  Tel: (800) 862-7326
  Website: http://www.marfan.org

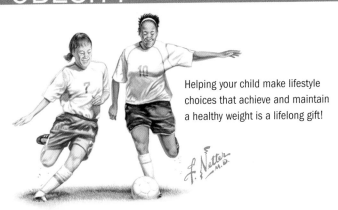

Helping your child make lifestyle choices that achieve and maintain a healthy weight is a lifelong gift!

What Is Obesity?

Childhood obesity means that a child's weight is above the healthy weight range of other children of the same age.

Overweight means that the child's weight is in the upper 15% of that range, and obese means only 5% of children weigh more. This excess weight may cause serious health problems, such as diabetes, orthopedic issues, and emotional problems.

Being overweight as a child often leads to being overweight as an adult. Adults who weigh too much can have serious health problems, such as heart disease, high blood pressure, joint problems, and some cancers.

About 18% to 20% of children in the United States are obese, and an additional 34% to 36% are overweight.

Childhood obesity increases the chance of getting serious diseases:

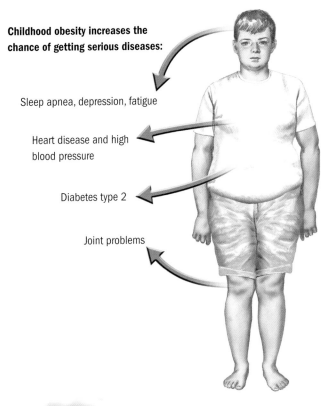

Sleep apnea, depression, fatigue

Heart disease and high blood pressure

Diabetes type 2

Joint problems

What Causes Obesity?

Eating more than the amount of food needed will cause weight gain. Why certain children gain too much weight isn't known. Genetics (parents passing on a tendency to gain weight), eating too much junk food or fast food, being inactive, and living in a society that promotes watching TV and playing video games more than sports and other physical activities.

What Are the Symptoms of Obesity?

There may not be any symptoms. Some children may have a sleep disorder, such as snoring or irregular breathing; feeling tired; being unable to exercise enough; having trouble making friends; and feeling depressed.

How Is Obesity Diagnosed?

The doctor will do a physical examination and will measure height and weigh the child. These results will be compared with those for other children of the same age. The doctor will also take a family medical history and may use other tests (such as of blood and urine) to find out about other health problems and to rule out other causes for weight gain.

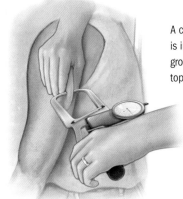

A child is overweight if weight is in the upper 15% of age group; an obese child is in the top 5% of that range.

Take a family approach to healthy eating. Ask your doctor about meal plans. Serve healthy foods and snacks, in correct portion sizes.

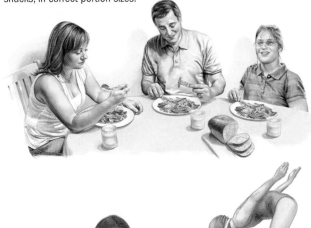

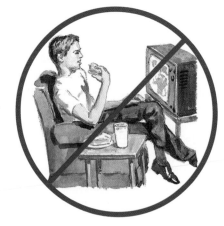

Encourage sports or other physical activities. Exercise as a family.

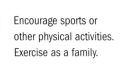

Limit time in front of the TV and computer. Don't allow snacking while watching TV.

FROM THE DESK OF

NOTES

How Is Obesity Treated?

The doctor will set a weight-loss goal and suggest a weight-loss diet and an exercise plan. The doctor may suggest counseling to control impulse eating from stress and depression and help the child reach and maintain the goals. Children need help meeting these goals by having their families eat healthy foods, exercise as a family, and encourage sports activities. Family exercise could be walking and bike riding. It's best to lose weight slowly to keep it off. The earlier a child is treated for obesity, the better the chance for success.

DOs and DON'Ts in Managing Obesity:

✔ **DO** encourage your child to follow the recommended weight-loss diet.

✔ **DO** encourage sports or other physical activities.

✔ **DO** serve healthy foods and snacks, in correct portion sizes.

✔ **DO** eat dinner together, with the TV set off.

✔ **DO** serve lots of fruits and vegetables.

✔ **DO** follow your doctor's suggestions about counseling.

✔ **DO** call your doctor if your child complains of shortness of breath or daytime fatigue.

✔ **DO** call your doctor if your child is following the diet and exercise plans and hasn't lost weight.

⊘ **DON'T** let your child spend too much time watching TV.

⊘ **DON'T** let your child eat after dinner.

⊘ **DON'T** let your child drink soda or eat fast food.

⊘ **DON'T** drive your child everywhere. Walking or bike riding is good.

FOR MORE INFORMATION

Contact the following sources:

• The Endocrine Society
Tel: (301) 941-0200, (888) 363-6274
Website: http://www.endo-society.org

• The National Institutes of Health
Tel: (301) 496-4000
Website: http://www.nih.gov

• The Obesity Society
Tel: (301) 563-6526
Website: http://www.obesity.org

• The American Academy of Pediatrics
Tel: (847) 434-4000
Website: http://www.aap.org

Tourette's syndrome is an illness of the nervous system in which parts of the body move or twitch without control. In these movements, called tics, a part of the body moves repeatedly, quickly, suddenly, and uncontrollably. Sometimes, tics occur often, are severe, and can affect a person's life.

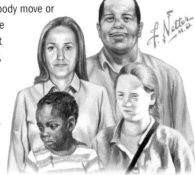

Children and adults can have the syndrome, but it usually starts between the ages of 5 and 15. Many tics may go away as people get older.

The cause is unknown, but it may be inherited with other nervous system problems.

Tics can occur in any body part. Some people also make odd sounds called vocal tics (even cursing). As with body tics, they can't control what they say. Symptoms include barking, blinking, cursing, grunting, head nodding or bobbing, imitating the actions or words of others, licking or smacking the lips, shoulder shrugging, sniffing, snorting, spitting, yelping, and behavior problems.

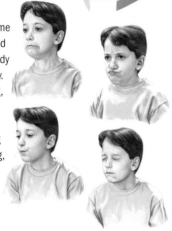

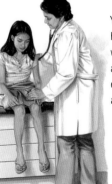

Your doctor makes a diagnosis from a medical history and physical examination. The doctor will ask a child to sit very still to see whether a tic appears. A pediatric neurologist may confirm the illness. The neurologist may want an EEG or MRI.

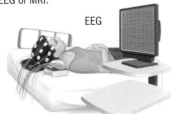

EEG

What Is Tourette's Syndrome?

Tourette's syndrome is an illness of the nervous system in which parts of the body move or twitch without control. In these movements, called tics, a part of the body moves repeatedly, quickly, suddenly, and uncontrollably. Tics can occur in any body part (face, hands, or legs). People can voluntarily stop them for brief periods. Some people also make abnormal sounds called vocal tics. Rarely, they will curse or say bad things to other people. As with body tics, people cannot control what they say. Sometimes, tics occur often, are severe, and can affect a person's life.

Children and adults can have the syndrome, but it usually starts between the ages of 5 and 15. Many tics may go away as a child gets older.

What Causes Tourette's Syndrome?

The cause is unknown, but it may be inherited with other nervous system problems.

What Are the Symptoms of Tourette's Syndrome?

Symptoms are usually mild and hardly noticeable but can be severe. Symptoms often come and go and may go away for a long time. Sometimes old tics go away and new tics appear. Symptoms include barking, behavior problems, blinking, cursing, grunting, head nodding or bobbing, imitating actions or words of others, licking or smacking the lips, shoulder shrugging, sniffing, snorting, spitting, and yelping.

How Is Tourette's Syndrome Diagnosed?

The doctor makes a diagnosis from the medical history and physical examination. The doctor will ask a child to sit very still to see whether a tic appears. A pediatric neurologist may confirm the illness. A neurologist is a doctor who specializes in nervous system problems. The neurologist may want electroencephalography (EEG), a test that measures brain waves. Magnetic resonance imaging (MRI) of the head may also be done. MRI is like an x-ray but uses magnets without x-rays to see inside the body.

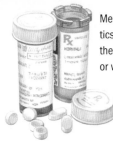

Medicine isn't usually needed for mild tics. For worse tics, medicines called neuroleptics can help control them. The neuroleptics may be prescribed separately or with other medicines to prevent side effects.

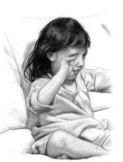

Tell your doctor if you're pregnant or breastfeeding and have Tourette's syndrome.

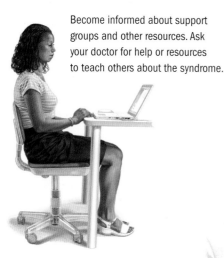

Become informed about support groups and other resources. Ask your doctor for help or resources to teach others about the syndrome.

Don't punish your child for saying bad words. Remember, tics can't be controlled. Call your child's doctor if your child has fever, stiffness, or behavior changes while taking medicine for Tourette's syndrome.

Children may be disruptive in school and have behavior problems. They may see a psychiatrist or psychologist (specialists in behavior problems). Tourette's syndrome is associated with a variety of behavioral symptoms, most often attention deficit hyperactivity disorder and obsessive compulsive disorder.

How Is Tourette's Syndrome Treated?

Medicines called neuroleptics can help control tics. Medicine is usually not needed for mild tics. They may be prescribed separately or with other medicines to prevent their side effects.

The whole family may also go for counseling to help a child and family cope with the disorder.

DOs and DON'Ts in Managing Tourette's Syndrome:

✔ **DO** tell your doctor about your medical problems and medicines, including prescription and over-the-counter drugs.

✔ **DO** tell your doctor if you're pregnant or breastfeeding and have Tourette's syndrome.

✔ **DO** become informed about support groups and other resources.

✔ **DO** call your doctor if you have trouble with your medicines.

✔ **DO** call your doctor if your symptoms get much worse.

✔ **DO** call your doctor if you need help or resources to teach others about the syndrome.

✔ **DO** call your child's doctor if your child has fever, stiffness, or behavior change while taking medicine for Tourette's syndrome.

⊘ **DON'T** stop your medicine or change the dosage because you feel better unless your doctor says to.

⊘ **DON'T** punish your child for saying bad words. Remember, tics cannot be controlled.

⊘ **DON'T** drink alcohol if you take medicine for Tourette's syndrome.

FROM THE DESK OF

NOTES

FOR MORE INFORMATION

Contact the following source:

• Tourette Syndrome Association
Tel: (718) 224-2999
Website: http://www.tsa-usa.org

Rickets is a disease affecting children's bones. Osteomalacia is the same bone disease in adults. The disorder occurs most often in elderly, institutionalized, or hospitalized people, such as those in nursing homes, but can also occur in otherwise healthy adults.

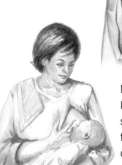

Not enough vitamin D in the diet, medicines, kidney or liver disease, and not enough sunshine can cause the disorder. Vitamin D forms in skin exposed to the sun. Adults with darker skin and babies fed only breast milk also have greater risk of the disorder.

Children grow slower than other children, have bones that break more easily, and have tenderness or pain in arm, leg, back, or hip bones. Their bones can have unusual shapes (such as bowlegs). Other symptoms are teeth problems, poorly developed muscles, and muscle cramps.

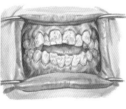

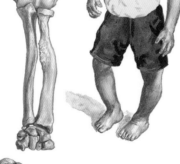

Adults have chronic bone pain, muscle aches, and bones that break easily.

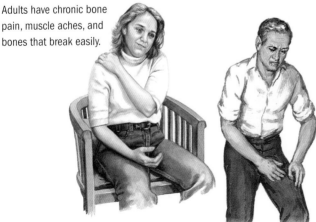

What Is Vitamin D Deficiency?

Rickets is a disease affecting children's bones. Osteomalacia is the same bone disease in adults. In children, bones don't grow as well as they should and become soft and weak. In adults, bones weaken and may break. These disorders start when people don't have enough vitamin D in their diet.

The disorder occurs most often in elderly, institutionalized, or hospitalized people, such as those in nursing homes, but it can also occur in otherwise healthy adults. In the United States, rickets is rare. It occurs most during fast growth periods, when the body needs a lot of calcium and phosphorus (such as children 6 to 24 months old).

What Causes Vitamin D Deficiency?

The cause is a lack (deficiency) of vitamin D. Bones need vitamin D to form properly and be healthy. The vitamin helps the intestines absorb calcium and phosphorus, which are needed to make healthy bones. Vitamin D deficiency can occur because of a poor diet (lack of dairy products, cereals, fish liver oils) or a vegetarian diet. Poor vitamin D absorption can occur because of some seizure medicines, kidney or liver disease affecting metabolism of the vitamin, and not enough sunshine. Vitamin D forms in the skin when it's exposed to the sun. Adults with darker skin have a greater risk of having the deficiency. Also, because breast milk has low amounts of vitamin D, babies fed only breast milk can have the disorder.

What Are the Symptoms of Vitamin D Deficiency?

Adults may have chronic bone pain and muscle aches and tend to break bones easily. Children can grow slower than other children, their bones tend to break more easily, and they can have tenderness or pain in arm, leg, back, or hip bones. Their bones can have an unusual shape. They may have bowlegs, and the spine may have an abnormal curve. They can have problems with teeth, which may appear later and have more cavities. Other symptoms include fever, restlessness (especially at night), poorly developed muscles, and muscle cramps.

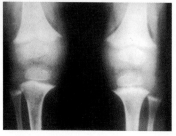

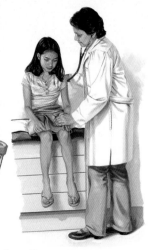

Your doctor makes a diagnosis from a medical history and physical examination. The doctor will test blood and urine samples and take x-rays.

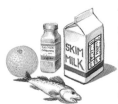

Treatment includes taking supplements of calcium, phosphorous, and vitamin D and eating foods rich in these substances. Good food sources are fish, liver, and fortified milk and orange juice. If you're allergic to milk, use the other sources of calcium and vitamin D.

Children should try to use good posture to correct bone deformities.

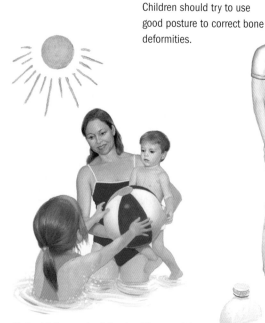

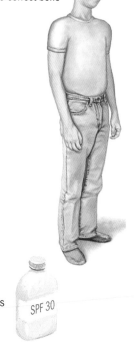

Both children and adults should go outside as often as possible. Sunshine helps vitamin D work well. Remember to use sunscreen!

How Is Vitamin D Deficiency Diagnosed?

The doctor makes a diagnosis from a medical history and physical examination. Blood and urine samples will be tested. X-rays will be done to check bone structure. Rarely, the doctor may take a sample of bone to look at with a microscope.

How Is Vitamin D Deficiency Treated?

Treatment consists of daily supplements of calcium, phosphorous, and vitamin D and eating foods rich in these substances. Good food sources of vitamin D are fish (salmon, mackerel, bluefish), liver, and fortified milk and orange juice.

Both children and adults should go outside as often as possible. Sunshine helps vitamin D work well. Children should try to use good posture to correct bone deformities. Some deformities may need an operation.

DOs and DON'Ts in Managing Vitamin D Deficiency:

✔ **DO** eat a good diet including milk. If you're allergic to milk, find other sources of calcium and vitamin D.

✔ **DO** ask your doctor about vitamin supplements.

✔ **DO** call your doctor if you have bone pain.

⊘ **DON'T** forget to go outdoors as much as possible, but remember to use sunscreen.

FROM THE DESK OF

NOTES

FOR MORE INFORMATION

Contact the following source:

• American Association of Clinical Endocrinologists
  Tel: (904) 353-7878
  Website: http://www.aace.com

MANAGING YOUR
ALCOHOL ADDICTION

Alcohol addiction is a lifelong illness. Such drinking makes you a danger not only to yourself but also to others. Often other addictions, such as to nicotine, are present. Take steps now to cure yourself and regain control of your life.

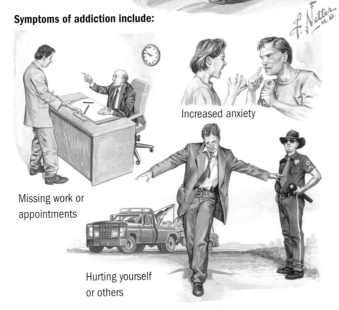

Symptoms of addiction include:

Increased anxiety

Missing work or appointments

Hurting yourself or others

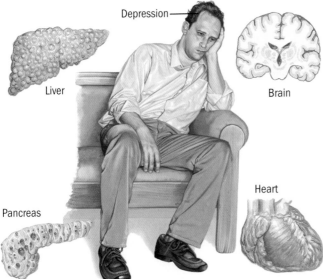

Depression

Liver

Brain

Pancreas

Heart

Your doctor bases the diagnosis on your drinking habits but may also test you for serious diseases and psychiatric problems. Addiction can cause other physical problems, especially liver, pancreas, and heart diseases and neurological disorders (e.g., alcohol dementia, seizures, and DTs [delirium tremens]).

What Is Alcohol Addiction?

Alcohol abuse is one of the four most common causes of death in the United States. Alcohol addiction is a complex disease involving long-term, excessive drinking of alcohol, so that stopping suddenly leads to unpleasant symptoms (withdrawal). Alcoholics are physically addicted to and crave alcohol, become tolerant to alcohol's effects (tolerance), and can relapse. They continue drinking despite serious medical and psychological harm and life disturbances. Over 17 million Americans overuse alcohol, about half being alcoholic (alcohol dependent).

What Causes Alcohol Addiction?

Certain people prone to developing alcohol addiction are more likely to have relatives with alcoholism. They often have other addictions (e.g., to nicotine).

What Are the Symptoms of Alcohol Addiction?

People often deny that they have a problem or try to hide symptoms. Symptoms may be behavioral, physical, or psychological. Behavioral symptoms include being unable to stop drinking after starting, missing work or appointments, hurting themselves or others, and not remembering what was done while drinking. Physical symptoms can be related to long-term alcohol damage and include unsteadiness, nausea, stomach pains, diarrhea, vomiting, sweating, palpitations, blackouts, and jaundice. Psychological symptoms include depression, anxiety, poor sleeping, and forgetfulness.

How Is Alcohol Addiction Diagnosed?

The doctor usually diagnoses alcoholism from the medical history showing behaviors that cause work, social, and psychological problems and signs of tolerance and withdrawal. Blood tests may tell whether alcohol affected the blood, kidneys, liver, and general health.

How Is Alcohol Addiction Treated?

Treatment varies depending on the degree of addiction and how seriously alcohol has affected the body's organs. Brief treatment, including education about dangers of binge drinking and alcohol poisoning, can help alcohol abusers. Alcohol addiction treatment may include detoxification (stopping drinking), medications, counseling, and self-help group support.

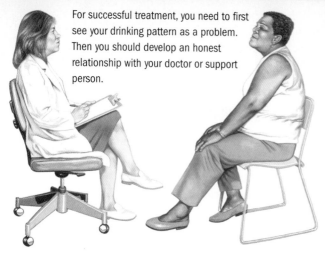

For successful treatment, you need to first see your drinking pattern as a problem. Then you should develop an honest relationship with your doctor or support person.

Successful treatment first requires a belief that a problem exists. Treatment often involves following a 12-step recovery plan (Alcoholics Anonymous) that includes abstinence, education, detoxification, and peer support. Help with housing, jobs, other medical problems, and coping skills is important. Detoxification may cause unpleasant symptoms (e.g., tremors, withdrawal seizures, and even delirium [DTs]), but the doctor can prescribe medicine for withdrawal symptoms. Medicines used for treatment may include benzodiazepines, acamprosate, naltrexone, and disulfiram.

Withdrawal can be very difficult and dangerous but you can work through it! Your doctor can help with this too.

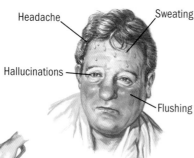

Headache   Sweating

Hallucinations

Flushing

Withdrawal symptoms

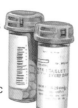

Stop drinking!

Take vitamins and medicines as your doctor suggests, and drink plenty of nonalcoholic beverages.

DOs and DON'Ts in Managing Alcohol Addiction:

✔ **DO** be honest about how much you drink.

✔ **DO** get support from your doctor, self-help groups, counselors, friends, and relatives.

✔ **DO** understand that your attitude toward treatment will make a difference in whether you relapse.

✔ **DO** accept that relapsing after treatment may be part of the illness, and work toward abstinence again.

✔ **DO** call your doctor if you have important medical problems because of alcohol, including vomiting, diarrhea, heartburn, chest tightness, and blood in bowel movements.

✔ **DO** call your doctor if you are depressed.

🚫 **DON'T** drink. Don't see friends who drink. Don't keep alcohol at home.

🚫 **DON'T** lie to your doctor when asked about alcohol abuse. Bring it up if the doctor doesn't.

🚫 **DON'T** give up when you have bad days.

🚫 **DON'T** ever drink and drive.

Alcohol addiction is very common. Many support groups are available—reach out to them. You can learn from others about how to cope, and as you begin to become healthier, you can help others by your example.

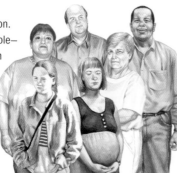

FOR MORE INFORMATION

Contact the following sources:

The best place to get additional information about alcoholism is at your local AA central office. In addition, most mental health centers can also give information, or you can check out the following websites:

• National Association for Children of Alcoholics
  Website: http://www.nacoa.org

• National Institute on Alcohol Abuse and Alcoholism
  E-mail: niaaaweb-r@exchange.nih.gov
  Website: http://www.niaaa.nih.gov

• Alcoholics Anonymous (International Office)
  Tel: (212) 870-3400
  Website: http://www.alcoholics-anonymous.org

• Women for Sobriety, Inc.
  Tel: (215) 536-8026
  Website: http://www.womenforsobriety.org

FROM THE DESK OF

NOTES

MANAGING YOUR
AMPHETAMINE ABUSE

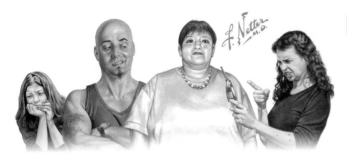

Amphetamines are used legally to treat obesity, sleep disorders, and attention deficit disorder. They act as brain stimulants, provide a "high" that can be addictive, and are now often made in illegal laboratories to be sold to addicts.

The "rush" or "high"

Energetic
Confident
Talkative

After the rush or high wears off

Tired
Depressed
Paranoid
Mood swings

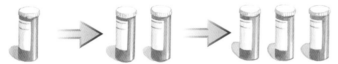

Addicts quickly build up a tolerance to the amphetamine and have to take higher doses to get the same effect.

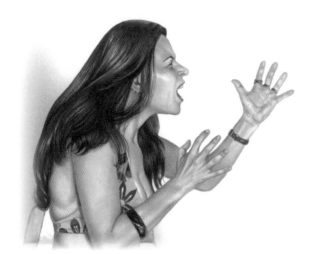

Even small amounts of drug can lead to irritability, insomnia, confusion, anxiety, paranoia, and aggressive behavior.

What Is Amphetamine Abuse?

Amphetamines are drugs that stimulate the brain and nervous system. Methamphetamine is one type of amphetamine with strong, long-lasting effects. Both types can be prescribed, mainly to treat attention deficit disorder, obesity, and narcolepsy (a sleep problem). The legal amphetamine is Dexedrine™. However, most amphetamines are made in illegal laboratories and sold as street drugs.

People smoke, sniff, swallow, or inject amphetamines (called speed, bennies, uppers, A, black beauties). Methamphetamine, a white, bitter powder, is called speed, meth, ice, chalk, glass, crank, and crystal.

Being high on amphetamines impairs judgment. Addicts crave more amphetamines to take away depression and tiredness, and their physical and mental health suffers. Regular users build up a tolerance (need higher doses for the same effect).

What Causes Amphetamine Abuse?

Stimulant drugs activate certain brain systems, which leads to addiction. Methamphetamine releases a chemical (dopamine) that stimulates some brain cells (enhancing mood) but damages others. Over time, methamphetamine reduces dopamine levels, which can cause symptoms like those of Parkinson's disease.

What Are the Symptoms of Amphetamine Abuse?

Effects depend on the amount used and how it is taken. Lower doses make users feel energetic, confident, talkative, and reduce hunger and the need for sleep. Amphetamines also cause anxiety and panic. Higher doses, especially when smoked or injected, give an intense "rush" lasting a few minutes. Extreme tiredness follows the high. Users often have depression, unreasonable mistrust (paranoia), or mood swings.

Central nervous system (CNS) effects of even small amounts include increased wakefulness and physical activity, lower appetite, overheating, and intense happiness (euphoria). Other CNS effects include irritability, insomnia, tremors, convulsions, anxiety, and aggressiveness. Heart rate and blood pressure increase, damaging blood vessels in the brain. Use can cause death.

Long-term users get run-down from lack of food and sleep. Some become seriously mentally disturbed (psychotic).

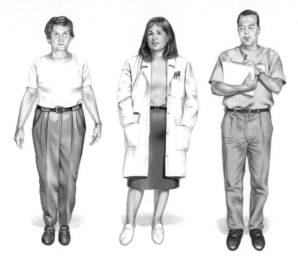

Take steps now to have a healthier lifestyle. Talk to a doctor, drug counselor, or recovery support group. There is no easy way to manage your addiction, but resources are available to help you.

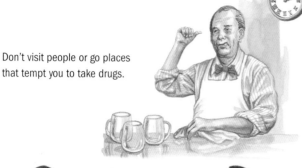

Don't visit people or go places that tempt you to take drugs.

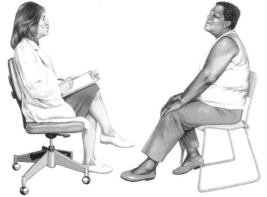

Why did you start taking drugs? Exploring underlying issues with a counselor or trusted friend may help you deal with problems in a different way in the future.

How Is Amphetamine Abuse Diagnosed?

The doctor asks about symptoms and drug use and does an examination. The doctor may test urine for drugs.

How Is Amphetamine Abuse Treated?

The best treatments are behavioral. They help change thinking, expectancies, and behaviors and increase skills for coping with stress. Recovery support groups also seem to help.

No drug treatments are available. Antidepressants can be used to treat the depression often seen in users who abstain.

Emergency room treatment for overdoses focuses on physical symptoms and may include ice baths and anticonvulsant drugs. Antianxiety drugs may help relieve extreme excitement or panic.

DOs and DON'Ts in Managing Amphetamine Abuse:

✔ **DO** get help from your doctor, counselor, support group, or rehabilitation program.
✔ **DO** examine problems and pressures that led to your drug abuse.
✔ **DO** try to stay away from people and places that tempt you to take drugs.
✔ **DO** realize that serious infections (e.g., HIV, hepatitis) are more likely in people injecting drugs and sharing needles.
✔ **DO** call your doctor if you have tremors, irritability, greater wakefulness, reduced appetite, and paranoia.

🚫 **DON'T** forget that help is available. You must recognize the problem and seek help.
🚫 **DON'T** do drugs!

FROM THE DESK OF

NOTES

FOR MORE INFORMATION

Contact the following sources:

- National Institute on Drug Abuse
  Website: http://www.nida.nih.gov
- NIDA for Teens
  Website: http://www.teens.drugabuse.gov
- Narcotics Anonymous World Services
  Website: http://www.na.org

MANAGING YOUR
ANOREXIA NERVOSA

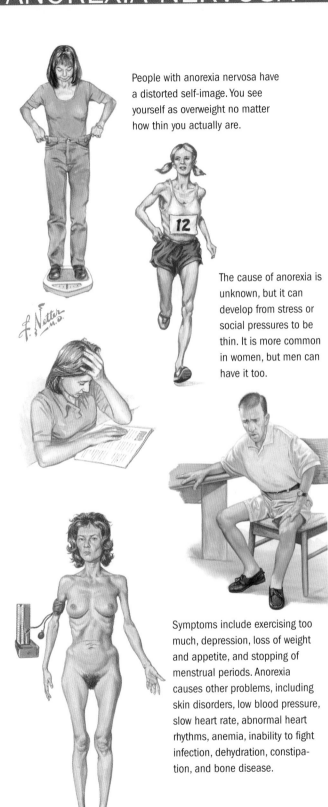

People with anorexia nervosa have a distorted self-image. You see yourself as overweight no matter how thin you actually are.

The cause of anorexia is unknown, but it can develop from stress or social pressures to be thin. It is more common in women, but men can have it too.

Symptoms include exercising too much, depression, loss of weight and appetite, and stopping of menstrual periods. Anorexia causes other problems, including skin disorders, low blood pressure, slow heart rate, abnormal heart rhythms, anemia, inability to fight infection, dehydration, constipation, and bone disease.

What Is Anorexia Nervosa?

Anorexia nervosa, or just anorexia, is an eating disorder in which people have an unreasonable fear of becoming fat. People lose so much weight that they become gaunt. Even then, they still see themselves as fat.

Anorexia nervosa is fairly rare, with groups at highest risk being adolescent girls and young women. It affects women much more than men, and is more common in some jobs (e.g., modeling, ballet dancing). It can be life threatening if untreated.

What Causes Anorexia Nervosa?

The cause is unknown, but anorexia probably results from a combination of factors, such as depression, other psychological problems, intense peer pressure, hormone changes at puberty, and stress. Adolescents may have concerns about sexuality, and these concerns lessen with anorexia because it delays sexual maturity. As children, anorexics were often obedient. As adolescents, they develop anorexia, which becomes their first rebellious act.

What Are the Symptoms of Anorexia Nervosa?

The most common symptoms include loss of weight, exercising too much, menstrual periods that stop, complaints of being fat from someone who is overly thin, depression, and loss of appetite. It can cause medical problems, including skin, heart, blood, bone, and hormone disorders. Dehydration, constipation, and frequent infections may occur.

How Is Anorexia Nervosa Diagnosed?

The doctor makes a diagnosis from the medical history (especially weight and diet), physical examination, and laboratory tests to rule out other conditions. No specific tests exist for anorexia. Extreme weight loss without physical illness, especially in a young woman, is usually an important sign.

Anorexics often deny their illness and may make themselves vomit with syrup of ipecac (causing dental cavities), misuse laxatives and enemas, and use diet and water pills.

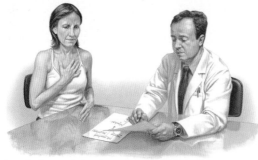

Treatment of anorexia involves counseling for emotional support, education, and reassurance. You may have other health issues that your doctor can help with, such as a proper diet plan.

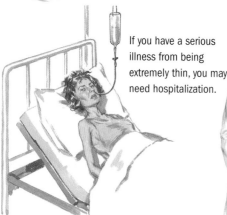

Anorexia doesn't affect just you. It affects all those who care about you. Often, the whole family gets involved in treatment.

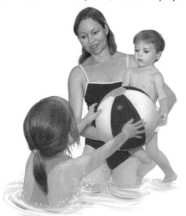

If you have a serious illness from being extremely thin, you may need hospitalization.

To maintain your health, it is vital to have support through an outpatient program after you leave the hospital.

How Is Anorexia Nervosa Treated?

Anorexia requires long-term care, including counseling or psychotherapy. Relapses are common, especially during periods of stress. Recovery depends on the individual.

Treatment first involves working with the person and family. Drugs may be prescribed for depression or anxiety. Programs may use negative and positive feedback, emotional support, education, and reassurance to address fears about gaining weight. Often, the whole family needs counseling. Other medical problems and illness that may have resulted from starvation need treatment, which may mean hospitalization.

Many people remain ill for a long time. Participation in an outpatient program after hospitalization is critical for successful treatment. The death rate associated with anorexia can be rather high.

DOs and DON'Ts in Managing Anorexia Nervosa:

✔ **DO** minimize stress.
✔ **DO** admit that you have an emotional problem.
✔ **DO** eat the diet prescribed by your doctor or nutritionist.
✔ **DO** attend counseling sessions.
✔ **DO** take medicines as directed.
✔ **DO** buy clothes that fit, not clothes that you have to lose weight to get into.
✔ **DO** call your doctor if you have paranoia, hallucinations, depression, or thoughts about suicide.

🚫 **DON'T** vomit food or binge eat.
🚫 **DON'T** skip meals.
🚫 **DON'T** exercise more than what your doctor recommends.
🚫 **DON'T** weigh yourself daily.
🚫 **DON'T** use drugs, diet pills, laxatives, or caffeine to lose weight.
🚫 **DON'T** eat alone, if possible.

FROM THE DESK OF

NOTES

FOR MORE INFORMATION

Contact the following sources:

- Anorexia Nervosa & Related Eating Disorders, Inc. (ANRED)
  Website: http://www.anred.com
- National Association of Anorexia Nervosa (ANAD) and Associated Disorders
  Website: http://www.anad.org
  Hotline: (847) 831-3438

MANAGING YOUR ANXIETY

People who have stress at work or at home can have anxiety. Anxiety affects more women than men. Some medical conditions, including headaches, are highly related to anxiety.

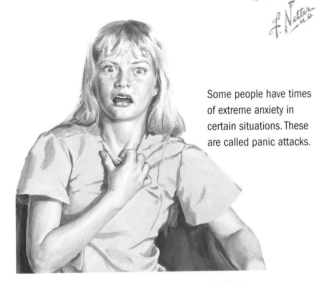

Some people have times of extreme anxiety in certain situations. These are called panic attacks.

Other symptoms include pounding heart, shortness of breath, sweating, muscle tension, trouble sleeping, and shakiness.

What Is Anxiety?

Feeling anxious is normal. However, a continuing problem with anxiety is called generalized anxiety disorder (GAD). People with GAD feel tense and worried much of the time, and some always feel this way.

GAD is fairly common, often occurring before age 18. It affects more women than men and seems more common in some families.

Certain medical conditions, such as colitis, asthma, hypertension, heart disease, ulcers, and headaches, are highly related to anxiety.

What Causes Anxiety?

People stressed at work or at home can have anxiety. GAD is also more likely in people who expect things to be perfect, are tired or overwhelmed, had stressful or harmful experiences, have a medical illness, are withdrawing from alcohol or drugs, or were abused as children.

Some people have panic attacks (extreme anxiety in certain situations) or phobias (anxiety caused by fears, such as of heights, or social situations, such as public speaking).

What Are the Symptoms of Anxiety?

People with GAD feel tense and worried. Other symptoms include restlessness, tiredness, difficulty concentrating, irritability, muscle tension, trouble sleeping, shakiness, headaches, pounding heart, shortness of breath, excessive sweating, and depression. These interfere with daily life.

How Is Anxiety Diagnosed?

The doctor makes the diagnosis after doing an examination and checking symptoms. The doctor may order blood tests or other tests to make sure another illness such as overactive thyroid isn't causing symptoms. People diagnosed with GAD have had tension and worry most days for at least 6 months, and they cannot control worrying even when reassured by others.

Forms of anxiety in addition to GAD, panic attacks, and phobias include obsessive-compulsive disorder, posttraumatic stress disorder, acute stress disorder, anxiety caused by legal drugs (e.g., caffeine) or drugs of abuse (e.g., amphetamines, cocaine), and anxiety caused by medical conditions and medicines.

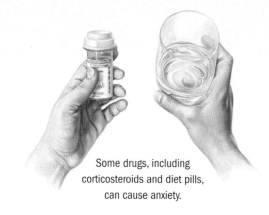

Some drugs, including corticosteroids and diet pills, can cause anxiety.

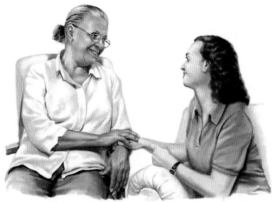

Many people benefit from therapy and can help discover why they are anxious.

Regular exercise, such as walking and swimming, also helps reduce stress and tension.

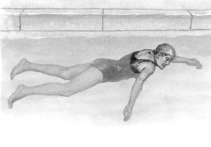

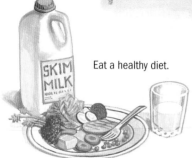

Eat a healthy diet.

How Is Anxiety Treated?

The doctor tries to find out, by taking a medical history, whether a medical condition or substance abuse is the cause. Drugs producing anxiety include corticosteroids (e.g., prednisone), antidepressants (e.g., fluoxetine), inhalers, thyroid medicine, diet pills, and over-the-counter medicines (e.g., antihistamines, cough and cold medicines). Too much caffeine can worsen anxiety.

Medicine to help symptoms include benzodiazepines, such as alprazolam, lorazepam, and clonazepam, and other anti-anxiety medications, such as buspirone. They do have side effects and can be habit forming.

Talk therapy (psychotherapy) and other methods to reduce stress and muscle tension (biofeedback, relaxation) may help symptoms. Regular exercise, such as walking and swimming, can reduce stress and tension.

DOs and DON'Ts in Managing Anxiety:

✔ **DO** tell your doctor about all medicines you take.
✔ **DO** take your medicine as instructed and tell your doctor about side effects.
✔ **DO** exercise regularly.
✔ **DO** tell your doctor or someone you trust if you have suicidal thoughts.
✔ **DO** eat a healthy diet.
✔ **DO** make life changes to reduce stress. Join a support group if you think that may help.
✔ **DO** remember that most drugs for anxiety can sedate you, so avoid drinking alcohol.

🚫 **DON'T** overuse caffeine, alcohol, nicotine, diet pills, and common cold remedies.
🚫 **DON'T** make major decisions while you feel anxious.

FROM THE DESK OF

NOTES

FOR MORE INFORMATION

Contact the following sources:

* Anxiety Disorders Association of America
  Tel: (240) 485-1001
  Website: http://www.adaa.org

* The Anxiety Network International
  Website: http://www.anxietynetwork.com/

* The Anxiety Panic Internet Resource (tAPir)
  Website: http://www.algy.com/anxiety/

MANAGING YOUR
BIPOLAR DISORDER

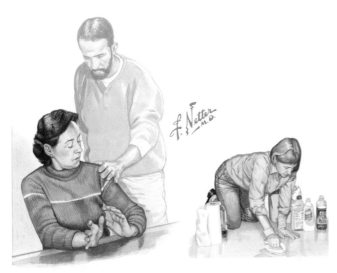

The main symptom of bipolar disorder involves swings between the moods of mania (or hyperactivity) and depression.

People with bipolar disorder in the manic mood feel full of energy and happy and need less sleep.

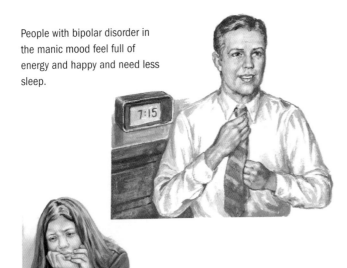

When in a depressed mood, people feel tired and have less energy.

What Is Bipolar Disorder?

Bipolar disorder is a psychiatric condition that was known before as manic depressive disorder. The main symptom involves swings between moods of mania (or hyperactivity) and depression.

It usually occurs by 30 years of age, in both men and women. The disorder seems to run in some families.

What Causes Bipolar Disorder?

The cause is unknown. Stress, drug or alcohol abuse, and use of some prescription drugs may increase the risk.

What Are the Symptoms of Bipolar Disorder?

People in the manic mood feel full of energy and happy. They need less sleep. Speech and thoughts race. Self-esteem is high. Overeating is common. People can have poor judgment and make reckless choices. Manic people can also hear voices or see things that aren't there. Some people do things like clean the house to burn energy.

In a depressed mood, people have less energy, feel sad and cry for no reason, sleep too much or have trouble falling asleep, lose pleasure in life, eat less, and struggle with feelings of worthlessness. Depression may lead to thoughts of death or suicide.

Bipolar disorder often occurs in cycles—an episode once a month, once a week, once a year, once a season, or as often as once a day.

How Is Bipolar Disorder Diagnosed?

The doctor makes the diagnosis after an examination and asking about symptoms. The doctor may order blood tests or other medical tests to make sure another illness isn't causing the symptoms.

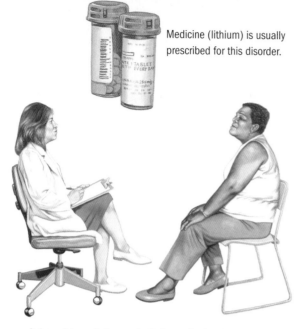

Medicine (lithium) is usually prescribed for this disorder.

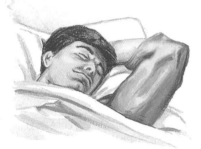

A therapist can help people find out why they have mood swings. Group therapy sessions may also help.

Try to keep to a routine sleep schedule.

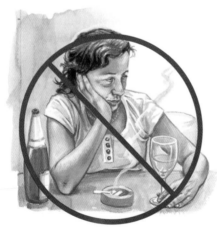

Don't use alcohol or other drugs.

FROM THE DESK OF

NOTES

How Is Bipolar Disorder Treated?

Bipolar disorder is not curable. Medicine (lithium) is the usual treatment to help even out moods. Some people may need to take lithium for a long time, but it isn't addictive.

People are often referred to a psychiatrist or for group therapy. Therapists can help people change behaviors that may make the illness worse.

DOs and DON'Ts in Managing Bipolar Disorder:

✔ **DO** tell your doctor or someone you trust if you have suicidal thoughts.

✔ **DO** talk to your doctor about any herbal remedies and medicines that you're taking.

✔ **DO** try to keep to a routine sleep schedule.

✔ **DO** stay active.

✔ **DO** find a support group if you think that it might help.

✔ **DO** tell your doctor about your medicine's side effects.

✔ **DO** avoid drugs of abuse, especially stimulants such as cocaine, amphetamines, and PCP. They may cause a manic episode.

✔ **DO** call your doctor if you feel that you're getting more energetic or can't relax, or your family members or others describe you as hyper.

✔ **DO** call your doctor if you notice a decreased need for sleep or have trouble sleeping.

🚫 **DON'T** use alcohol or other drugs, such as antihistamines or drugs containing high amounts of caffeine.

🚫 **DON'T** drive when you first start a new medicine.

🚫 **DON'T** make any major decisions during a mood swing.

🚫 **DON'T** stop your medicine or change your dose because you feel better, unless your doctor tells you to.

🚫 **DON'T** change your diet or salt intake while you are taking lithium.

FOR MORE INFORMATION

Contact the following sources:

- Bipolar Disorders Information Center
  Website: http://www.mentalhelp.net/poc/center_index.php?id=4&cn=4

- Depression and Bipolar Aliance
  Tel: (800) 826-3632, (312) 642-0049
  Website: http://www.ndmda.org

- Mood Disorders Support Group of New York City
  Tel: (212) 533-MDSG (533-6374)
  Website: http://www.mdsg.org

MANAGING YOUR
BORDERLINE PERSONALITY DISORDER

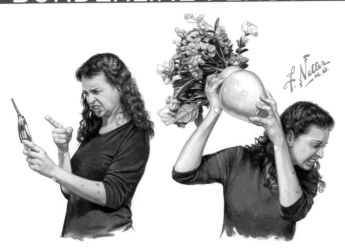

The critical symptom of borderline personality disorder is instability in moods, interpersonal relations, self-image, and behavior.

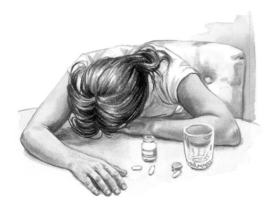

Doing impulsive things, such as over-spending, substance abuse, too much sex, and binge eating, is a sign.

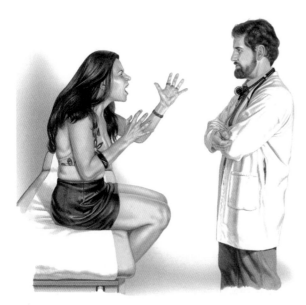

Feeling extreme anger or having trouble controlling anger is also a sign.

What Is Borderline Personality Disorder?

Personality refers to the special traits and behaviors that make up a person. A personality disorder is a behavior pattern that differs from socially acceptable normal behavior. The main characteristic of this disorder is a broad instability in moods, interpersonal relations, self-image, and behavior. This instability often upsets family and work life, long-term planning, and a person's sense of self. People can't regulate emotions normally.

This disorder is common and affects 2% of the general population, usually young women. It accounts for 20% of all hospital stays for mental illness.

The disorder is not contagious.

What Causes Borderline Personality Disorder?

The exact cause is unknown. The cause is thought to be genetic, psychologic, social, and biologic factors that work together. A history of childhood abuse or neglect and abnormal chemicals (serotonin) in brain areas controlling emotion may also be involved.

What Are the Symptoms of Borderline Personality Disorder?

According to a manual from the American Psychiatric Association used for diagnosing mental disorders, people with this disorder must have five or more of certain symptoms. These include unstable and intense personal relations, long-lasting unstable sense of self, impulsive behavior, suicidal or self-destructive behavior, mood problems, feelings of emptiness, intense anger or problems with control of anger, and paranoia (feelings that people are "out to get you").

How Is Borderline Personality Disorder Diagnosed?

A psychiatrist (a doctor specializing in mental and emotional illness) makes a diagnosis on the basis of the symptoms noted above.

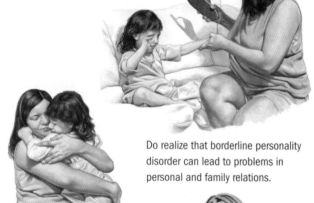

Psychotherapy and cognitive-behavioral therapy are the main treatment methods.

Do realize that borderline personality disorder can lead to problems in personal and family relations.

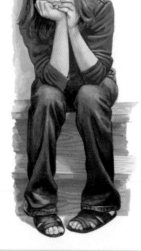

People with borderline personality disorder may have other mental problems as well, such as depression.

How Is Borderline Personality Disorder Treated?

Treatment involves psychotherapy plus cognitive-behavioral therapy. Psychotherapy can be done by a psychiatrist (who can prescribe medicine) or a psychologist (a specialist, not a medical doctor, who diagnoses and treats mental and emotional problems but doesn't prescribe drugs). The goal is to relieve symptoms and change behavior so that relations with family, friends, and co-workers improve.

Cognitive therapy focuses on how certain thinking patterns cause symptoms. Behavioral therapy refers to treatment to break the connection between things that cause stress and reactions to them. The two types of therapy work together to stop symptoms.

Certain medicines may control impulses and brief psychotic events (e.g., hallucinations, delusions), stabilize mood (e.g., lithium), and help with mood swings and depression.

DOs and DON'Ts in Managing Borderline Personality Disorder:

✔ **DO** realize that this disorder can lead to major problems in relations with family and other people.
✔ **DO** understand that people can become suicidal and need monitoring.
✔ **DO** understand that people with this disorder don't get schizophrenia but can have major depression.
✔ **DO** call your doctor if you suspect that a family member may have borderline personality disorder.
✔ **DO** call your doctor if you need a referral to a psychiatrist.
✔ **DO** call your doctor if you feel depressed or are going to harm yourself or others.

⊘ **DON'T** forget that people with this disorder may also have other mental problems (e.g., depression, anxiety, and mood disorders).
⊘ **DON'T** forget that this disorder is chronic, with ups and downs. The most unstable period usually occurs in early adulthood, but most people often continue to have problems with intimate relations.

FROM THE DESK OF

NOTES

FOR MORE INFORMATION

Contact the following sources:

• National Mental Health Association
Tel: (703) 684-7722, (800) 969-6642
Website: http://www.nmha.org/

• Mental Health Resource Center
Tel: (888) 284-3258
Website: http://www.athealth.com/Consumer/rcenter/

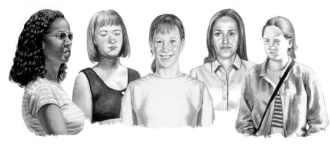

Some people, usually young women, have an abnormal fear of being overweight and make themselves vomit or take drugs to lose weight. They may eat large amounts of food in a short time (binge eating) and then force themselves to vomit or exercise excessively.

Risk factors of bulimia

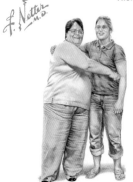

Personal and family history of depression and obesity

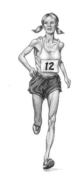

High-pressure sports or careers with weight restrictions

Symptoms of bulimia

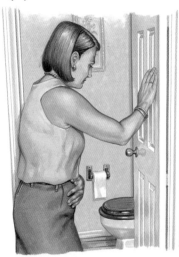

Stomach pain and forced vomiting

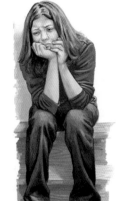

Binge eating

Sadness, guilt after eating

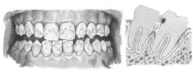

Tooth decay

What Is Bulimia?

Bulimia is an eating disorder. People, usually young women, have an abnormal fear of being overweight and make themselves vomit or take drugs to lose weight. However, most bulimics aren't overweight. They often can't stop eating and secretly eat large amounts of food in a short time, which is called binge eating. Forced vomiting, fasting, and heavy exercise to lose weight follow binge eating. It can be treated, but most people need treatment for several years.

Bulimia is similar to another eating problem, anorexia, but in anorexia, binge eating doesn't occur.

What Causes Bulimia?

The cause is unclear. The disorder is more common in adolescent girls and young adult women. A personal or family history of obesity and depression appears to be a risk factor, as does society's focus on slimness. It occurs more often in people in certain jobs (e.g., modeling) and sports (e.g., running).

What Are the Symptoms of Bulimia?

Symptoms include binge eating, forced vomiting, dieting, eating in secret, fasting, guilt (after eating), nervousness, sadness, stomach pain, tooth decay, and weakness. Others are dehydration, menstrual problems, an enlarged stomach, and slowed stomach emptying.

How Is Bulimia Diagnosed?

After taking a medical history, the doctor does a physical examination, with special attention to feelings and eating habits. The doctor makes a diagnosis on the basis of episodes of binge eating and how often they occur. After overeating, people avoid gaining weight by vomiting or abusing laxatives. Overeating episodes occur at least twice a week for 3 months and are associated with behaviors to avoid weight gain. People are also too concerned with how they look.

The doctor may order electrocardiography (ECG) and blood tests to check for abnormalities of potassium, magnesium, and other chemicals that may be low due to vomiting and that can cause irregular heartbeat. The doctor may also suggest seeing a specialist in eating problems and a dentist (too much vomiting can damage teeth). Bulimics can also have other psychological disorders.

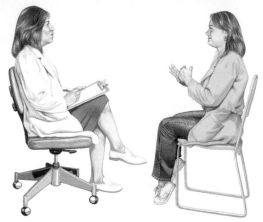

To diagnose bulimia, your doctor will ask questions about your feelings and eating habits and will do a physical examination.

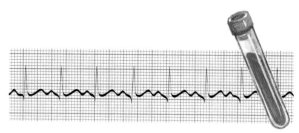

The doctor may order ECG (electrocardiography, a test of the heart's electrical activity) and blood tests.

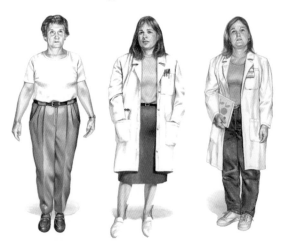

Treatment is often a team approach with your doctor, a psychiatrist, and nutritionist. The doctor may also suggest seeing a specialist in eating problems and a dentist. Understanding your behavior and finding other ways to deal with things will help you recover.

How Is Bulimia Treated?

The treatment goal is to reduce and then end binge eating and behaviors for losing weight, as well as change the basis of self-esteem. People usually admit that they have a problem, which helps treatment. Most often, treatment combines cognitive (deals with abnormal thinking) and behavioral (to change behaviors) therapy. Drugs, especially antidepressants, can also be given.

DOs and DON'Ts in Managing Bulimia:

✔ **DO** be open with your family and doctor about your feelings, eating, forced vomiting, and fasting.
✔ **DO** stay close to friends who support and understand you.
✔ **DO** follow your doctor's directions.
✔ **DO** tell your doctor about other medical problems and medicines you take.
✔ **DO** tell your doctor if you're pregnant.
✔ **DO** eat at regular times.
✔ **DO** reduce stress.
✔ **DO** call your doctor if you notice physical problems related to bulimia or if you feel urges to overeat or binge and cannot control them.

⊘ **DON'T** stop taking medicine or change your dose because you feel better unless your doctor tells you to.
⊘ **DON'T** eat alone.
⊘ **DON'T** take prescription or over-the-counter drugs or exercise without getting your doctor's OK.
⊘ **DON'T** overdo exercise.
⊘ **DON'T** make yourself vomit.
⊘ **DON'T** take diet pills or illegal drugs or drink alcohol in excess.

FROM THE DESK OF

NOTES

FOR MORE INFORMATION

Contact the following source:

• National Eating Disorders Association
Tel: (800) 931-2237
Website: http://www.nationaleatingdisorders.org/

Conversion disorder is defined as findings suggesting a neurological condition (such as paralysis, numbness, or loss of sensation) but without a real neurological problem. They're rare and occur in more women than men. Children younger than 10 and people older than 35 rarely have them. The cause is unknown.

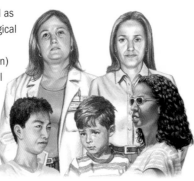

Most symptoms occur suddenly and usually last for a short time. Complaints include

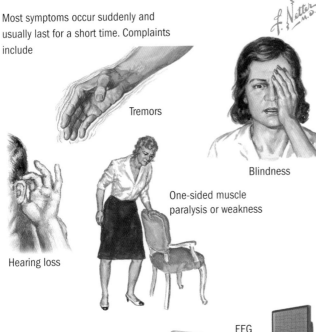

Tremors

Blindness

One-sided muscle paralysis or weakness

Hearing loss

EEG

MRI

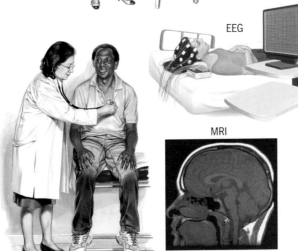

Ultrasound

People with movement or sensing problems but no diagnosis after physical examinations, laboratory tests, EEG, and imaging studies (CT, MRI, ultrasonography) may have this disorder. People must have specific symptoms and psychological problems.

What Is Conversion Disorder?

Somatoform disorders have physical symptoms suggesting that a medical condition exists. However, no medical condition, substance use, or mental disorder can explain them. These illnesses include conversion disorder. This disorder is defined as findings suggesting a neurological condition (such as paralysis, numbness, loss of sensation) but without a diagnosis of a real neurological problem.

Conversion disorders are rare, occurring in 11 of 100,000 people, more women than men. Children younger than 10 and people older than 35 rarely have them.

What Causes Conversion Disorder?

The cause is unknown. It's not contagious or passed from parents to children.

What Are the Symptoms of Conversion Disorder?

Most symptoms occur suddenly and usually last for a short time. They usually go away in 2 weeks. Complaints include one-sided muscle paralysis or weakness, numbness, loss of sensation, loss of voice, blindness, deafness, tremors, and pseudoseizures. Pseudoseizures aren't caused by electrical brain disturbances. Their cause is psychological.

How Is Conversion Disorder Diagnosed?

The doctor does a neurological examination and may refer you to a neurologist. A neurologist is a specialist in nervous system diseases. Imaging tests include computed tomography (CT), magnetic resonance imaging (MRI), and ultrasonography. Electroencephalography (EEG) may also be done. For diagnosis, people must have one or more symptoms, not intentionally produced, that affect movement or senses. These symptoms suggest a neurological or other condition. People must have psychological problems related to these symptoms. Symptoms cannot be explained by actual medical conditions, effects of substances, or behaviors. Symptoms cause distress or inadequacy in social situations or jobs. Symptoms aren't only pain or sexual dysfunction. They aren't explained by another mental disorder.

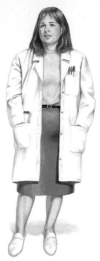
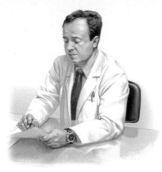

Treatment is hard because people have physical symptoms but test results are normal. A psychiatrist or psychologist may be involved in care. Psychological treatment involves cognitive therapy and behavioral therapy.

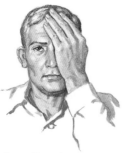
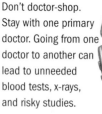

Call your doctor if you develop paralysis, blindness, or loss of sensation. Call if you feel anxious or depressed. Call if you think that you're going to harm yourself or others.

Don't doctor-shop. Stay with one primary doctor. Going from one doctor to another can lead to unneeded blood tests, x-rays, and risky studies.

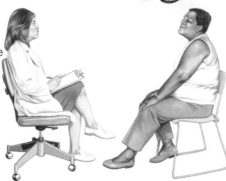
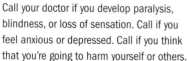

How Is Conversion Disorder Treated?

Treatment is hard because people have physical symptoms but test results are normal. A psychiatrist (a medical specialist) or psychologist (another kind of specialist, for psychological problems) may be involved in care. A psychiatrist can prescribe medicines; a psychologist can treat the patient but cannot prescribe medications.

Psychological treatment involves cognitive and behavioral therapy. Cognitive therapy teaches people how certain thinking patterns cause symptoms. Behavioral therapy breaks the connection between worry about stresses and usual reactions to them.

DOs and DON'Ts in Managing Conversion Disorder:

✔ **DO** realize that a good prognosis is related to a sudden start of the disorder, stress (such as loss or life change) at that time, and a short time between diagnosis and treatment.

✔ **DO** call your doctor if you have paralysis, blindness, or loss of sensation.

✔ **DO** call your doctor if you need a referral to a psychiatrist or psychologist.

✔ **DO** call your doctor if you feel anxious or depressed. Call if you think that you will harm yourself or others.

⊘ **DON'T** forget that this disorder can recur.

⊘ **DON'T** forget this disorder may be triggered by stress that makes the brain unconsciously turn off a body function.

⊘ **DON'T** doctor shop. Stay with one primary doctor. Going from one doctor to another can lead to unneeded blood tests, x-rays, and risky studies.

FROM THE DESK OF

NOTES

FOR MORE INFORMATION

Contact the following sources:

• American Psychiatric Association
Tel: (888) 357-7924
Website: http://www.psych.org

• American Psychological Association
Tel: (800) 374-2721
Website: http://www.apa.org

MANAGING YOUR
DEPRESSION

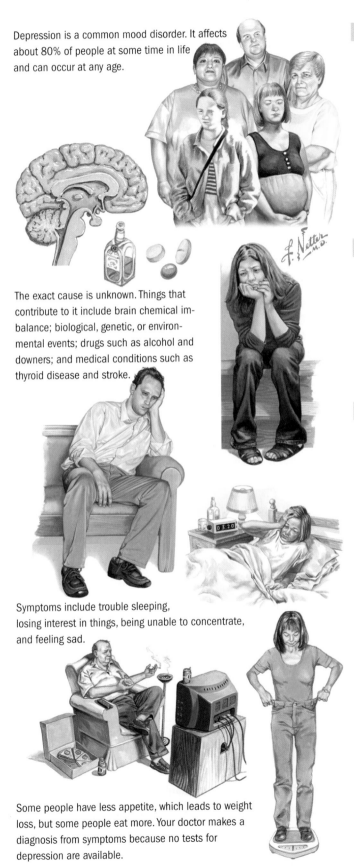

Depression is a common mood disorder. It affects about 80% of people at some time in life and can occur at any age.

The exact cause is unknown. Things that contribute to it include brain chemical imbalance; biological, genetic, or environmental events; drugs such as alcohol and downers; and medical conditions such as thyroid disease and stroke.

Symptoms include trouble sleeping, losing interest in things, being unable to concentrate, and feeling sad.

Some people have less appetite, which leads to weight loss, but some people eat more. Your doctor makes a diagnosis from symptoms because no tests for depression are available.

What Is Depression?

Depression is a very common mood disorder. It's not the same as feeling sad when bad things happen. If sadness lasts for days or weeks, makes it hard to work or do things with family or friends, or involves thoughts of suicide, depression is present.

Depression is treatable but often not preventable. Lifestyle changes such as lowering stress and increasing leisure time and exercise may lower the risk of having depression. It affects about 80% of people at some time in life and can occur at any age. It's more common in women than in men.

What Causes Depression?

The cause is unknown. Probably, many things contribute to it. These include chemicals being out of balance in the brain; genetic, environmental, or developmental events; and biological and psychological factors. Drugs such as alcohol or downers can worsen it. Some medical conditions, such as thyroid disease and stroke, are also often related to depression.

What Are the Symptoms of Depression?

Symptoms include trouble sleeping, such as trouble falling asleep but more likely waking up very early in the morning for no reason. Less often, depression can involve too much sleep (people sleep most of the day).

Some people have less appetite, which leads to weight loss, but some people eat more. Other symptoms include losing interest in things; being unable to concentrate; feeling sad; having crying spells, often for no reason; feeling as if the future won't be better; being agitated or restless; moving and speaking very slowly; and losing interest in sex.

Severe depression involves suicidal or homicidal thoughts or thinking or dreaming about death.

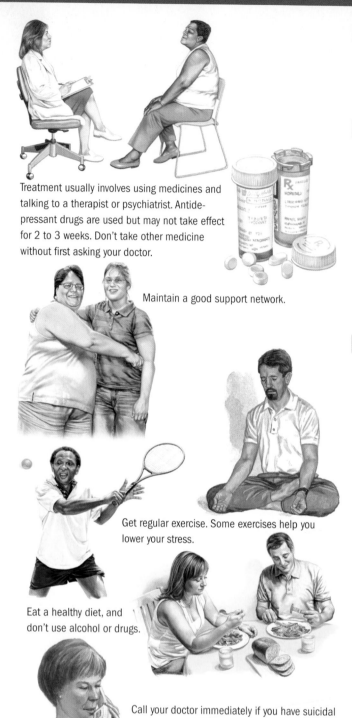

Treatment usually involves using medicines and talking to a therapist or psychiatrist. Antidepressant drugs are used but may not take effect for 2 to 3 weeks. Don't take other medicine without first asking your doctor.

Maintain a good support network.

Get regular exercise. Some exercises help you lower your stress.

Eat a healthy diet, and don't use alcohol or drugs.

Call your doctor immediately if you have suicidal thoughts or thoughts about killing or hurting someone else.

How Is Depression Diagnosed?

No laboratory tests or x-rays can diagnose depression. The doctor makes a diagnosis from symptoms.

How Is Depression Treated?

Treatment usually involves using medicines and talking to a therapist or psychiatrist. Medicines used are antidepressants. Some more common drugs are escitalopram, paroxetine, sertraline, fluoxetine, and citalopram. These are selective serotonin reuptake inhibitors (SSRIs). Others are venlafaxine, duloxetine, and bupropion. Some drugs increase sleep and appetite, but it usually takes 2 to 3 weeks before these drugs help the depression. They also have side effects, such as weight gain, sexual problems, and nausea.

DOs and DON'Ts in Managing Depression:

✔ **DO** lower your exposure to stress.

✔ **DO** make sure you eat a healthy diet.

✔ **DO** exercise regularly.

✔ **DO** call your doctor if your symptoms get worse.

✔ **DO** call your doctor if you have side effects from your medicines.

✔ **DO** call your doctor immediately if you have suicidal thoughts or thoughts about killing or hurting someone else.

✔ **DO** call your doctor immediately if you have psychotic symptoms, such as hearing voices, seeing things that aren't there, or feeling paranoid.

⊘ **DON'T** use alcohol or drugs. These will increase your depression or interfere with certain drugs used to treat depression.

⊘ **DON'T** take any prescription or over-the-counter medicine without first checking with the doctor who prescribed your medicine for depression.

FROM THE DESK OF

NOTES

FOR MORE INFORMATION

Contact the following source:

• Mental Health America
Tel: (800) 969-6642
Website: http://www.nmha.org

MANAGING YOUR
DRUG ABUSE

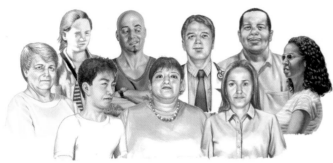

Anyone can be an abuser.

Drug abuse defined

Tolerance:
Abusers need more drug to get the same effect as before.

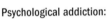

Physical addiction:
Withdrawal symptoms occur when drug use stops.

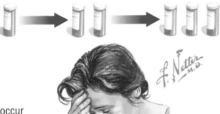

Psychological addiction:
Abusers have severe drug cravings and do things such as forging prescriptions and being violent to get drugs.

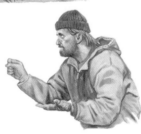

Classifications of drugs

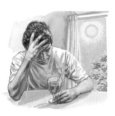

Depressants (alcohol, opiates, painkillers)

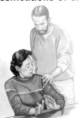

Hallucinogens (LSD)

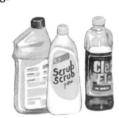

Inhalants (household cleaners, airplane glue)

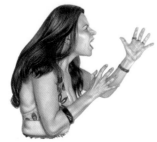

PCP (angel dust)

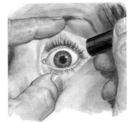

Stimulants (cocaine, crack, amphetamines, caffeine)

What Is Drug Abuse?

Abuse of prescription and illicit drugs is a major problem in the United States. Three terms related to abuse need definitions: tolerance, physical addiction, and psychological addiction.

Tolerance means abusers need more drug to get the same effect as before or to avoid going through withdrawal.

Physical addiction exists with tolerance. People with physical addiction go through withdrawal when they stop using the drug. Symptoms of withdrawal include gooseflesh, nausea, vomiting, abdominal cramps, diarrhea, rapid heartbeat, sweating, insomnia, and severe anxiety. Withdrawal from benzodiazepines, barbiturates, and alcohol can be life-threatening.

Psychological addiction means having a severe drug craving and using drug-seeking behaviors, such as forging prescriptions, faking illnesses, and using violence to get drugs.

What Are the Types of Drug Abuse?

Anyone can be an abuser. Unlike in the past, more women than men today are admitted to drug abuse programs.

Five types of drugs are commonly abused. Depressants make people feel down. They're strongly physically addicting. They include alcohol, barbiturates, opiates, other painkillers, and drugs such as meprobamate. Stimulants produce a high and can cause severe insomnia, restless feelings, and inability to sit still. Stimulants include cocaine (crack), amphetamines (such as methamphetamine), caffeine, over-the-counter drugs with pseudoephedrine, and diet pills. Hallucinogens cause people to see, hear, or feel things that are not actually there, or they make people misinterpret things. They're very dangerous. Hallucinogens include LSD, mescaline, and psilocybin. Inhalants are huffed, snorted, or sniffed. Examples are gasoline, cleaning products, anesthetics (such as nitrous oxide), hair sprays, bug sprays, spray paints, solvents such as toluene, airplane glue, typewriter correction fluid, and kerosene. Teenagers often use these drugs, which are cheap and obtained easily. They can cause serious physical damage and strong drug craving and drug-seeking behaviors. PCP, or angel dust, can cause psychosis or depression, with flashbacks.

Other abused drugs include marijuana, designer drugs, and GHB (date rape drug).

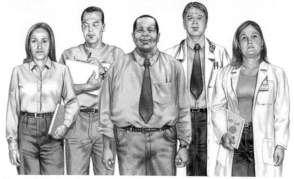

The main point of treatment is to stop the drug abuse. Treatment involves detoxification, education and keeping drug free, and peer support counseling. A team of people can help you, including doctors, therapists, counselors, recovering addicts, friends, and family.

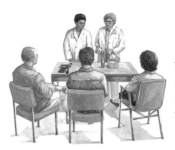

You are not alone. Support groups include AA, CA, and NA. Local and national groups can help you through the recovery process.

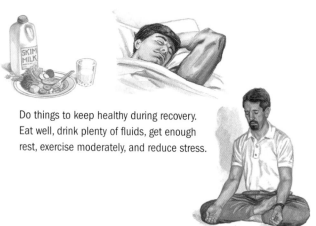

Do things to keep healthy during recovery. Eat well, drink plenty of fluids, get enough rest, exercise moderately, and reduce stress.

How Is Drug Abuse Treated?

Treatment involves detoxification, education and keeping drug free, and peer support counseling. Support groups include Alcoholics Anonymous (AA), Cocaine Anonymous (CA), and Narcotics Anonymous (NA). The main point of treatment is to stop drug abuse. Sometimes, other drugs are used to help stop the abuse. Education is often done in peer support groups with other drug abusers. Abusers need a sponsor, a former abuser who has had years of being clean. People should call their sponsors when they feel that they could relapse.

Some people have both a psychiatric condition and drug abuse. Both need treatment.

DOs and DON'Ts in Managing Drug Abuse:

✔ **DO** tell your doctor or emergency room doctor that you're a recovering drug abuser.
✔ **DO** contact your doctor or support group if you have strong urges to use drugs again (relapse warning signs).
✔ **DO** eat well, drink plenty of fluids, get enough rest, exercise moderately, and reduce stress during recovery.
✔ **DO** call your doctor if you have seizures, psychosis, or suicidal thoughts.

⊘ **DON'T** take other medicines, including over-the-counter drugs, before checking with your doctor.
⊘ **DON'T** see friends and relatives who abuse drugs or remind you of when you did. Socialize with your sponsor and AA or NA members.

FOR MORE INFORMATION

Contact the following sources:

• National Clearinghouse for Alcohol and Drug Information Substance Abuse and Mental Health Services Administration
Tel: (800) 729-6686
Website: http://ncadi.samhsa.gov/

• Habit Smart
Website: http://www.habitsmart.com

• Cocaine Anonymous
Tel: (310) 559-5833
Website: http://www.ca.org

• Narcotics Anonymous
Tel: (818) 773-9999
Website: http://www.na.org

FROM THE DESK OF

NOTES

IDENTIFYING AND UNDERSTANDING
ELDER ABUSE

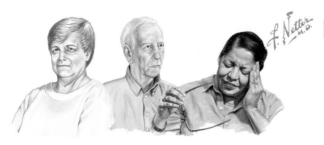

Unfortunately, elder abuse has become more common in the last 20 years. In the United States, about 4% of people older than 65 (about 1 million people) are abused or neglected. Elder abuse can mean abuse of older people in the home, abuse in an institution, and self-neglect or self-abuse.

Abused people are usually older than 75, women, white, and widowed. They have behavioral and physical problems and are socially isolated, so abuse is less likely to be noticed. They likely depend totally on a caregiver.

Types of mistreatment of the elderly

Physical abuse:
Assaults, rough handling, burns, sexual abuse

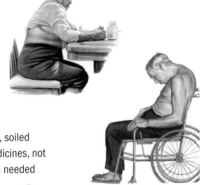

Physical neglect:
Poor hygiene, malnutrition, soiled clothing, giving wrong medicines, not getting medical care when needed

Material abuse:
Withholding, misuse, or theft of money, and withholding means of living

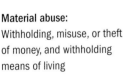

Bank

Psychological abuse:
Verbal or emotional abuse, threats, isolation, or confinement

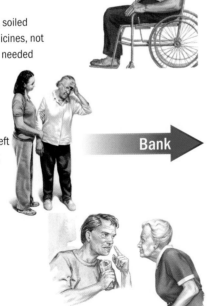

What Is Elder Abuse?

Elder abuse can mean abuse of older people in the home, abuse in an institution, and self-neglect or self-abuse. It can involve physical abuse, physical neglect, psychological abuse, and material abuse. Physical abuse consists of assaults, rough handling, burns, sexual abuse, and confinement. Physical neglect includes dehydration, malnutrition, poor hygiene, letting people wear odd or soiled clothing, giving the wrong medicines, and not getting medical care when needed.

Psychological abuse involves verbal or emotional abuse, threats, and isolation or confinement. Material abuse means withholding, misuse, or theft of money, and withholding means of living.

Elder abuse has become more common in the last 20 years. In the United States, about 4% of people older than 65 (about 1 million people) are abused or neglected. These people are usually older than 75, women, white, and widowed. They have behavioral problems, are incontinent, are very noisy or shout (especially at night), have many physical complaints, and are socially isolated so that abuse is less likely to be noticed. Those more likely to be abused are totally dependent on a caregiver.

How Is Elder Abuse Identified?

Abusers of elderly people are usually married to them. In about 25% of cases, the abuser is an adult child, living in the home, who is dependent on the older person. Elder abuse occurs in all races and economic groups.

To find elder abuse, there should first be a suspicion that it's occurring. People who often have falls and injuries, have many problems with their medicines, and lose weight at home but gain weight in the hospital may be abused. Unexplained leakage of urine (incontinence) and body odor may be signs of elder neglect.

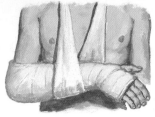

To identify elder abuse, there should first be a suspicion that it's occurring. Signs include numerous falls and injuries, many problems with medicines, and bad body odor and weight loss at home but not in the hospital.

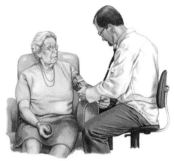

Treatment involves corrective medical problems that may result from abuse. Contacting Adult Protective Services (APS) or hospitalizing for urgent medical care may be needed.

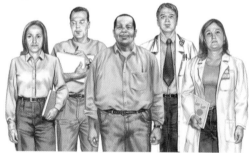

Treatment should be a group effort of doctors, agencies such as APS, therapists, family, and friends.

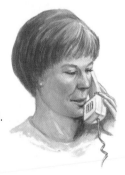

You have a responsibility to get help if you suspect abuse. Call to report abuse.

How Is Elder Abuse Treated?

Treatment involves fixing medical problems that may result from the abuse. Contacting Adult Protective Services (APS) or hospitalizing for urgent medical care may be needed. The abused should be supported and helped, and stress in the environment should be reduced. Sometimes, legal charges must be filed, and the elderly person must be removed from the home.

Elderly people are often vulnerable and dependent and can be abused easily. Abuse can be prevented by being aware that the problem exists, sharing responsibility for caring for an elderly parent, treating medical or psychiatric problems in the elderly person, and having more social contacts for elderly people. Everyone should check on elderly people in neighborhoods and families to prevent mistreatment.

DOs and DON'Ts in Managing Elder Abuse:

✔ **DO** realize that help is available. APS can check into reports of elder abuse and help victims and their families with treatment and protective services.

✔ **DO** call to report abuse. Calls are usually confidential.

🚫 **DON'T** forget that the APS, the Area Agency on Aging, or the county Department of Social Services can investigate elder abuse and neglect. If investigators find abuse or neglect, they can arrange for services to help protect the victims.

FOR MORE INFORMATION

Contact the following sources:

- Often people who want to help older relatives or friends don't live near them. Long-distance caregivers can call a nationwide toll-free Eldercare Locator number (800-677-1116) to locate services in the community in which the elder lives.

- National Center on Elder Abuse
  Website: http://www.ncea.aoa.gov/NCEAroot/Main_Site/Index.aspx

- National Association of Area Agencies on Aging
  Tel: (202) 872-0888
  Website: http://www.n4a.org

FROM THE DESK OF

NOTES

MANAGING YOUR
INSOMNIA

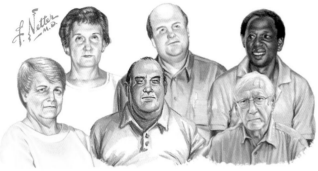

Insomnia is trouble sleeping. It's very common. About 80 million American adults have sleep problems. Anyone can have insomnia but it's more common in older adults. Other conditions affecting sleep include nightmares, night terrors, enuresis (bed-wetting), and sleepwalking.

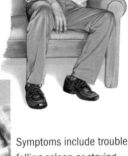

Insomnia may be related to a crisis, medical condition (such as heart disease), emotional or psychiatric problem (such as depression, anxiety, schizophrenia), medicines, and cigarette smoking.

Symptoms include trouble falling asleep or staying asleep, waking very early in the morning, and daytime tiredness.

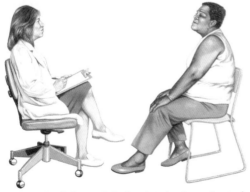

Your doctor can identify insomnia by hearing about symptoms. A sleep study may be done to look at brain waves and sleeping pattern and to rule out other disorders. Both the total amount of sleep and the quality of sleep are important.

What Is Insomnia?

Insomnia is trouble sleeping. It's very common. About 80 million American adults have sleep problems.

Primary insomnia can involve less sleep, less restful sleep, interrupted sleep, and delay in falling sleep. Secondary insomnia is usually related to a psychiatric disorder (depression, anxiety), medical condition, or using alcohol, caffeine, or illicit drugs (amphetamines, cocaine).

Nightmares often occur early in sleep and are usually remembered. Night terrors, which children often have, occur later and aren't remembered. Other conditions affecting sleep include enuresis (bed-wetting) and sleepwalking.

What Causes Insomnia?

Insomnia is most common in elderly people. It may be related to a crisis, a medical condition, such as heart disease, or an emotional or psychiatric problem, such as depression, anxiety, and schizophrenia. Medicines, cigarette smoking, and poor sleep habits lead to insomnia.

What Are the Symptoms of Insomnia?

Symptoms include trouble falling asleep or staying asleep, waking early in the morning, and daytime tiredness.

How Is Insomnia Diagnosed?

The doctor can identify insomnia by hearing about symptoms. Sometimes a sleep study is done to look at brain waves and sleeping pattern and to rule out disorders such as sleep apnea and restless leg syndrome. Measuring the total amount of sleep is not enough to diagnose insomnia. The quality of sleep is also important.

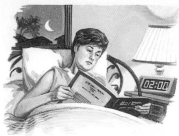

Reducing stress by practicing relaxation may help insomnia. For example, take a warm bath or use soft music, relaxation tapes, earplugs, or eyeshades. Do something relaxing, such as reading, if you cannot sleep after 20 to 30 minutes.

Your doctor may prescribe medicine (sedative and hypnotic drugs), usually used for a short time. Herbal (melatonin and valerian root) and over-the-counter medicines are also used.

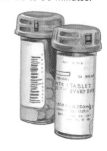

Daily exercise is wonderful for your overall health, but not within 2 hours of your bedtime.

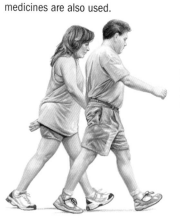

Relaxation methods such as meditation may help. Ask your doctor where you can get more information.

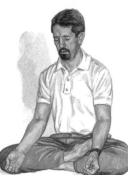

Caffeine and other stimulants shouldn't be taken late in the evening. Don't drink alcohol. It makes sleeping problems worse. Don't smoke.

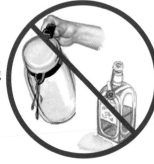

How Is Insomnia Treated?

Treatments include reducing stress, by learning and practicing relaxation. For example, a warm bath, soft music, relaxation tapes, earplugs, eyeshades, and electric blanket may help. The doctor may prescribe medicine, usually used for a short time or just on certain nights. Sometimes, long-term treatment is needed. Prescription medicines include sedative and hypnotic drugs. They include zolpidem and benzodiazepines such as temazepam. They should be used temporarily because of the chance of addiction.

Herbal (melatonin and valerian root) and over-the-counter medicines are also used. Several over-the-counter drugs are available. Over-the-counter sleep aids and some herbal agents may have serious interactions with other drugs. The most commonly used sleep inducer is alcohol, but alcohol makes sleeping problems worse.

Diet is important. Caffeine or other stimulants shouldn't be taken late in the evening.

DOs and DON'Ts in Managing Insomnia:

✔ **DO** have regular bedtime routines. Try to go to bed the same time every night.

✔ **DO** exercise regularly, but not within 2 hours of going to bed.

✔ **DO** get up and do something relaxing if you cannot sleep after 20 to 30 minutes.

✔ **DO** take medicine for severe pain. Pain interferes with sleep.

✔ **DO** call your doctor if you sleepwalk, have night terrors, or snore too much.

✔ **DO** call your doctor if you have side effects from medicines.

✔ **DO** call your doctor if you have depression, anxiety, or mania.

⊘ **DON'T** use sleeping pills given to you by a friend.

⊘ **DON'T** eat within 3 hours or drink liquids within 1 hour of bedtime.

⊘ **DON'T** read or watch TV in bed. Use the bedroom only for sleep.

⊘ **DON'T** go to bed until you feel sleepy.

⊘ **DON'T** take naps after the early afternoon.

⊘ **DON'T** drink alcohol, smoke, or use caffeine. They can disrupt sleep.

FROM THE DESK OF

NOTES

FOR MORE INFORMATION

Contact the following source:

• National Center on Sleep Disorders Research
  Tel: (301) 435-0199
  Website: http://www.nhlbi.nih.gov/about/ncsdr

MANAGING YOUR
OBSESSIVE-COMPULSIVE DISORDER

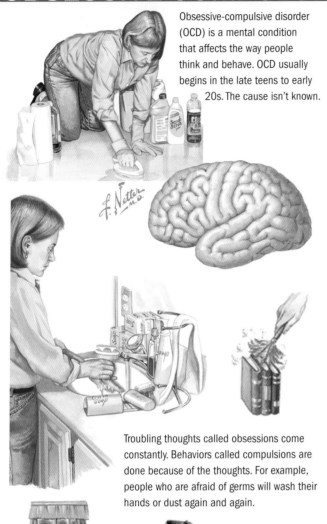

Obsessive-compulsive disorder (OCD) is a mental condition that affects the way people think and behave. OCD usually begins in the late teens to early 20s. The cause isn't known.

Troubling thoughts called obsessions come constantly. Behaviors called compulsions are done because of the thoughts. For example, people who are afraid of germs will wash their hands or dust again and again.

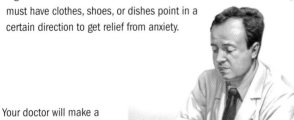

OCD includes checking compulsions. People may get up often during the night to make sure doors were locked and windows were closed. Or people must have clothes, shoes, or dishes point in a certain direction to get relief from anxiety.

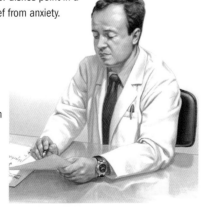

Your doctor will make a diagnosis from a description of your symptoms, not from medical tests.

What Is Obsessive-Compulsive Disorder?

Obsessive-compulsive disorder (OCD) is a psychiatric condition affecting the way people think and behave. Troublesome thoughts called obsessions come constantly. The thoughts may be about violence, fear of something bad happening, or worry about forgetting something. People may feel the need to repeat something. These behaviors, called compulsions, are done because of the thoughts. For example, wondering whether the door is locked may lead to checking the lock several times.

OCD usually begins in the late teens to early 20s. Symptoms may sometimes improve but never really go away.

What Causes OCD?

The cause is unknown.

What Are the Symptoms of OCD?

Common obsessions include aggressive thoughts, such as seeing violent images or having fears of harming others or oneself, of doing something embarrassing, of acting on impulses, of feeling responsible for things going wrong, and of something terrible happening. People with contamination obsessions are excessively focused on body waste, dirt, or germs; are overly concerned with contaminants; and are worried about becoming sick to a degree beyond reasonable expectations. Other obsessions are sexual, hoarding or collecting, and religious. Obsessions involve socially unacceptable behaviors, so people feel guilty and anxious.

The many compulsions include repeating rituals and cleaning or hand washing, counting, checking, and ordering or arranging compulsions. For example, people may get up several times during the night to make sure that appliances were turned off, doors were locked, and windows were closed. Or people must have clothes, shoes, or dishes in a certain order or pointing in a certain direction to get relief from anxiety. People may not want to do these behaviors but often cannot control them. These compulsive behaviors can take up a large part the day and make it hard to complete other more productive activities.

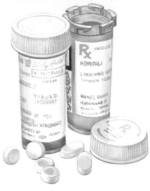

You may need both behavioral treatment and medicines called selective serotonin reuptake inhibitors (SSRIs), such as fluvoxamine, sertraline, and fluoxetine.

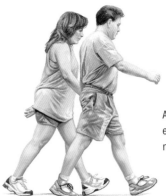

As with any anxiety condition, exercise can often help reduce nervous feelings.

Limit caffeine intake.

Call your doctor if you think of suicide or homicide, or if your obsessions become bizarre. Psychosis can occur. Don't take drugs that overstimulate you or make you nervous, such as PCP or cocaine.

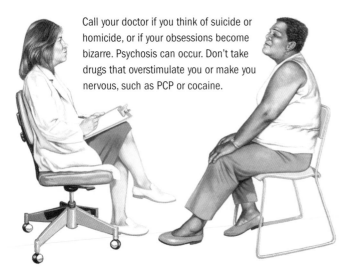

How Is OCD Diagnosed?

The doctor usually bases the diagnosis of OCD on symptoms: feelings of distress plus the problem behaviors. Symptoms usually get worse during stress. People who feel that obsessions and compulsions take up most of their time and are disturbed by this need treatment. Family members or co-workers may point out the symptoms.

How Is OCD Treated?

Treatment goals are to reduce the symptoms and minimize their interference in life. Behavior therapy reduces the compulsions, such as frequent hand washing. People may need a combination of medicines and behavioral treatment. Medicines called selective serotonin reuptake inhibitors (SSRIs), such as fluvoxamine, sertraline, and fluoxetine, are often used.

DOs and DON'Ts in Managing OCD:

✔ **DO** tell your doctor if your symptoms persist or worsen after having treatment for some time.

✔ **DO** tell your doctor if you have new symptoms or you don't feel well from your medicine.

✔ **DO** exercise in moderation.

✔ **DO** call your doctor if you have physical symptoms such as chest pains or palpitations or you have suicidal or homicidal thoughts.

✔ **DO** call your doctor if your obsessions become bizarre. Psychosis may occur with OCD.

⊘ **DON'T** take drugs that stimulate you or make you nervous. These drugs include such illicit drugs as phencyclidine (PCP) and cocaine.

⊘ **DON'T** eat or drink foods and beverages with caffeine.

FROM THE DESK OF

NOTES

FOR MORE INFORMATION

Contact the following sources:

• American Psychiatric Association
Tel: (888) 357-7924
Website: http://www.psych.org

• American Psychological Association
Tel: (800) 374-2721
Website: http://www.apa.org

MANAGING
PARANOID PERSONALITY DISORDER

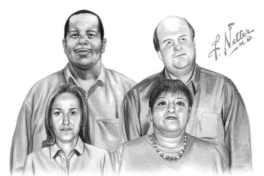

Personality refers to the characteristics and behaviors that make people individuals. A personality disorder is a pattern of behavior that differs from the normal. It leads to problems in relationships with family, friends, and co-workers.

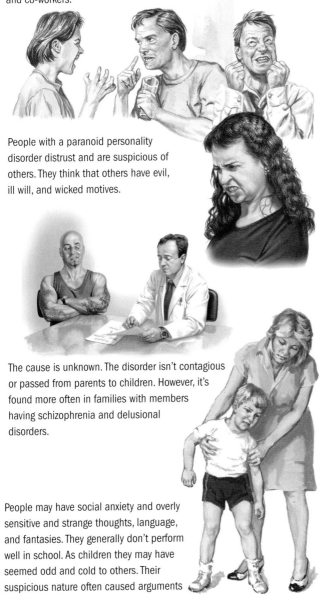

People with a paranoid personality disorder distrust and are suspicious of others. They think that others have evil, ill will, and wicked motives.

The cause is unknown. The disorder isn't contagious or passed from parents to children. However, it's found more often in families with members having schizophrenia and delusional disorders.

People may have social anxiety and overly sensitive and strange thoughts, language, and fantasies. They generally don't perform well in school. As children they may have seemed odd and cold to others. Their suspicious nature often caused arguments and complaints.

What Is a Paranoid Personality Disorder?

Personality refers to the characteristics and behaviors that make people individuals. A personality disorder is a pattern of behavior that differs from the normal of the culture. It leads to many problems in forming relationships with family, friends, and co-workers. People with a paranoid personality disorder distrust and are suspicious of others. It makes them think that others have evil, ill will, and wicked motives. More men than women have this disorder.

What Causes a Paranoid Personality Disorder?

The cause is unknown. The disorder isn't contagious or passed from parents to children. However, it's found more often in families with members having schizophrenia and delusional disorders.

What Are the Symptoms of a Paranoid Personality Disorder?

People may have social anxiety and overly sensitive, peculiar thoughts, language, and fantasies. They don't perform well in school. As children they may have seemed odd. Their suspiciousness often caused arguments and complaints. They misinterpreted actions of others and were often rigid and critical. They were standoffish and seemed cold to others.

How Is a Paranoid Personality Disorder Diagnosed?

A psychiatrist or psychologist usually makes the diagnosis, most often in people in early adulthood. People must have four or more of the following. They falsely think that others are harming or deceiving them. They have unjustified doubts about loyalty or trustworthiness of friends or associates. They don't confide in others because they fear that information will be used against them. They think that innocent remarks or events have hidden threats. They hold grudges. They see attacks on their reputation that others don't see and are quick to get angry. They're suspicious of spouses or sexual partners.

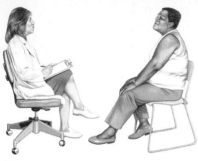

Treatment involves individual psychotherapy and cognitive behavioral therapy. The goal is to help symptoms and change behavior, so relationships with family, friends, colleagues, and co-workers get better.

Although medicines aren't usually given for treatment of paranoid personality disorder, drugs used for psychosis, depression, and anxiety may sometimes help people who also have other mental disorders.

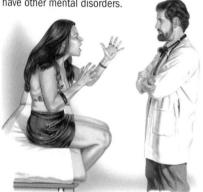

Realize that people may challenge their doctors, which makes treatment difficult.

Don't forget that people with this disorder may frequently have other psychiatric problems. These include depression, anxiety, obsessive-compulsive disorder (OCD), and agoraphobia (fear of crowds).

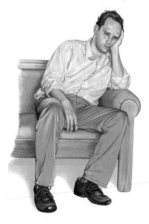

Call your doctor if you think that a family member may have this disorder, you need a referral to a psychiatrist, you feel depressed, or you think that you're going to harm yourself or others.

How Is a Paranoid Personality Disorder Treated?

Treatment involves individual psychotherapy with cognitive behavioral therapy. Psychiatrists and psychologists use psychotherapy. Psychiatrists are specialists in mental and emotional disorders and can prescribe medicines. Psychologists are nonmedical specialists in these problems but don't prescribe drugs. The goal is to help symptoms and change behavior, so relationships with family, friends, colleagues, and co-workers get better.

Cognitive therapy teaches people how certain thinking patterns cause symptoms. Behavioral therapy breaks the connection between worry about stresses and usual reactions to them.

Drugs for psychosis, depression, and anxiety may sometimes help people who also have other mental disorders.

DOs and DON'Ts in Managing a Paranoid Personality Disorder:

✔ **DO** realize that this disorder can lead to problems in relationships.

✔ **DO** realize that people may challenge their doctors, which makes treatment hard.

✔ **DO** call your doctor if you think that a family member may have this disorder.

✔ **DO** call your doctor if you need a referral to a psychiatrist or psychologist.

✔ **DO** call your doctor if you feel depressed.

✔ **DO** call your doctor if you feel that you're going to harm yourself or others.

🚫 **DON'T** forget that people with this disorder may have other psychiatric problems. These include depression, anxiety, obsessive-compulsive disorder, and agoraphobia (fear of crowds).

🚫 **DON'T** forget that this disorder is chronic with lifelong problems with relationships.

FROM THE DESK OF

NOTES

FOR MORE INFORMATION

Contact the following sources:

• Mental Health America
  Tel: (800) 969-6642
  Website: http://www.nmha.org

• American Psychiatric Association
  Tel: (888) 357-7924
  Website: http://www.psych.org

MANAGING YOUR
POSTTRAUMATIC STRESS DISORDER

Posttraumatic stress disorder (PTSD) refers to an anxiety disorder that stems from repeated memories after a stressful event. People can get PTSD after living through or even just seeing an event involving actual or threatened death or serious injury, to themselves or others.

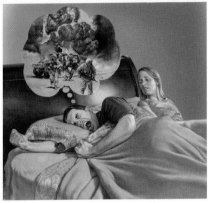

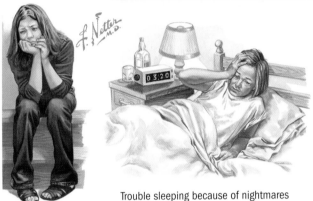

Loss of interest in activities

Trouble sleeping because of nightmares

Withdrawal from others

Symptoms may start right after the event or not for years. Nightmares, traumatic flashbacks, irritable outbursts of anger, feeling emotionally numb, and becoming isolated can occur. Physical symptoms can include sweating, rapid heartbeat, and rapid breathing.

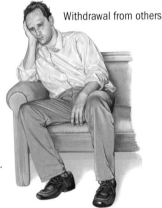

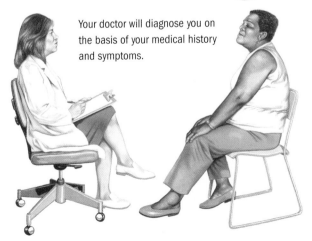

Your doctor will diagnose you on the basis of your medical history and symptoms.

What Is Posttraumatic Stress Disorder?

Posttraumatic stress disorder (PTSD) refers to an anxiety disorder that stems from repeated memories after a stressful event. People can get PTSD after living through or merely seeing a traumatic event that involves actual or threatened death or serious injury, to themselves or others. About half of people with PTSD will recover, and about half have a chronic form that's long-lasting.

What Causes PTSD?

Living through or seeing things that cause fear, horror, or feeling helpless can lead to PTSD. Events that are most often the cause include child abuse, rape, mugging, serious accidents, military combat, earthquakes, plane crashes, and terrorism.

PTSD can occur with other psychiatric disorders, such as phobias, anxiety disorders, and depression.

Lack of family, cultural, or social supports that make it easy to adapt to trauma can also increase the chance of PTSD, such as for Vietnam era veterans.

What Are the Symptoms of PTSD?

Symptoms can begin right after an event but may not start for many years. People can have traumatic flashbacks and nightmares, with the same memories over and over and thoughts that they can't seem to shake. People may relive the event through images or thoughts that can occur at any time.

Physical symptoms, such as sweating, rapid heartbeat, and rapid breathing, can make people avoid thoughts, feelings, and conversations that are related to the trauma. Many people stay away from activities and places that make them remember the event.

People may have hyperarousal and are always waiting to respond to another similar event. They startle easily, cannot sleep or concentrate, become irritable, and have angry outbursts.

People can become numb to emotions. They don't feel connections to others and isolate themselves from friends and family. They lose interest in activities. They can lose contact with reality and their sense of self. They may remember little of the actual event or certain parts of the trauma.

Treatment goals are to help people control their impulses. Peer support groups composed of others who lived through the same kind of trauma can help. In these groups, you talk about experiences and listen to others who had similar traumas.

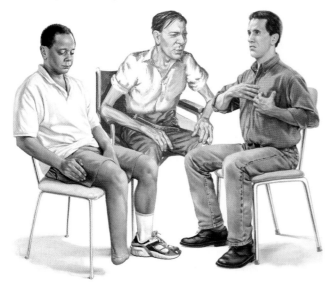

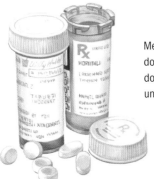

Medicine may be prescribed. If it is, don't stop taking it or change your dose because you feel better or worse unless your doctor says you can.

Minimizing stress and daily exercise can help. Also, avoid drugs such as caffeine and other stimulants.

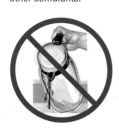

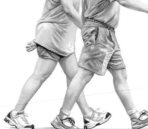

How Is PTSD Diagnosed?

Tests aren't needed. The doctor will diagnose PSTD from the medical history.

How Is PTSD Treated?

Treatment is aimed at helping people control their impulses. Peer support groups composed of others who lived through the same kind of trauma can help. Certain drugs are used for treatment.

Cognitive therapy tries to change the way people think so that they feel better. Usually, it's better to talk about the event (debriefing). Other methods such as meditation, muscle relaxation, imagery, and biofeedback also help.

Anger control training may also help.

DOs and DON'Ts in Managing PTSD:

✔ **DO** take prescribed medicine as directed.
✔ **DO** minimize stress. Exercise is very important, as is avoiding drugs such as caffeine and other stimulants.
✔ **DO** avoid situations that might produce flashbacks.
✔ **DO** call your doctor if you have worse symptoms, feelings of homicide or suicide, uncontrolled rage, or psychotic feelings, especially paranoia.
✔ **DO** call your doctor if you develop physical symptoms, such as asthma or ulcers.

⊘ **DON'T** stop taking medicine or change your dosage because you feel better unless your doctor says to.
⊘ **DON'T** use alcohol or other drugs.

FOR MORE INFORMATION

Contact the following sources:
• National Institute of Mental Health
  Tel: (800) 647-2642
  Website: http://www.nimh.nih.gov
• American Psychiatric Association
  Tel: (888) 357-7924
  Website: http://www.psych.org
• American Psychological Association
  Tel: (800) 374-2721
  Website: http://www.apa.org

FROM THE DESK OF

NOTES

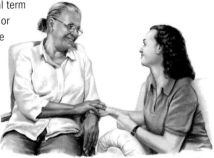

Psychosis is a medical term meaning an impaired or abnormal mental state with delusions or hallucinations. It's a symptom, not a diagnosis.

What Is Psychosis?

Psychosis is a medical term used for an impaired or abnormal mental state with delusions or hallucinations. Delusions are false beliefs. Hallucinations are things that are seen or heard but aren't really there.

What Causes Psychosis?

The cause is unknown. Psychosis is thought to result from a combination of social, genetic, environmental, psychological, and physical factors. It's not contagious. Psychosis is a key symptom of many mental illnesses including schizophrenia, depression, schizoaffective disorder, and bipolar disorder. Psychosis may also be one of the symptoms in many conditions, such as human immunodeficiency virus (HIV) infection, Parkinson's disease, malaria, strokes, brain tumors, and seizure disorders. Medicines, including those for Parkinson's disease and seizures, steroids, and chemotherapy, can cause a psychotic episode. Illicit drugs (e.g., LSD, cocaine, alcohol, amphetamines, marijuana, PCP) can also lead to a psychotic change.

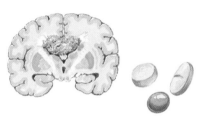

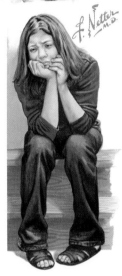

Causes include mental illnesses such as schizophrenia, depression, schizoaffective disorder, and bipolar disorder. Medical conditions, such as HIV infection, Parkinson's disease, malaria, strokes, brain tumors, and seizure disorders, can cause psychosis, as can drugs (prescription and illicit).

What Are the Symptoms of Psychosis?

Psychosis means that people lose contact with reality. A disorganized thought pattern usually results in odd speech (e.g., jumbling words, making no sense with words, thought blocking, and rhyming) and lack of insight. Behavior is bizarre, odd, and unpredictable. People may say that they hear voices telling them to do things (auditory hallucinations). Others may see signs or images telling them to do something (visual hallucinations).

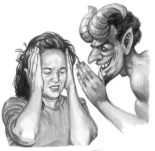

People can have odd speech (e.g., jumbling words, making no sense with words) and lack of insight. Behavior is bizarre, odd, and unpredictable. People may say that they hear voices telling them to do things or see signs or images telling them to do something.

How Is Psychosis Diagnosed?

The doctor makes a diagnosis from a medical history and physical examination. The doctor will do tests to rule out medical illnesses. These include blood tests and imaging studies, such as computed tomography (CT) and magnetic resonance imaging (MRI) of the brain. A spinal tap may also be done. In this procedure, the doctor puts a needle into the spine to collect fluid. This fluid is checked for infection, cancer, and other causes of psychosis.

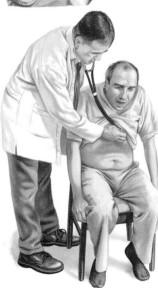

Your doctor makes a diagnosis from your medical history and physical examination. The doctor will do tests to rule out medical illnesses. These include blood tests; imaging studies such as CT and MRI; and a spinal tap.

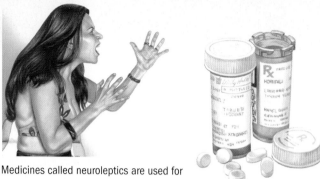

Medicines called neuroleptics are used for acute treatment of bizarre unpredictable behavior.

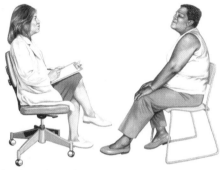

Treatment also depends on the underlying cause. A psychiatrist will treat mental illnesses such as depression or schizophrenia with medicines. Cognitive behavioral therapy may help. People with conditions such as Parkinson's disease and seizure disorders will take drugs for those conditions. For substance abuse, counseling is offered.

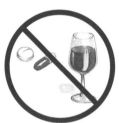

Don't do drugs—prescription, over-the-counter, or illicit. Alcohol, amphetamines, cocaine, sleeping agents (e.g., barbiturates), and medicines for anxiety (e.g., benzodiazepines) can all cause psychosis.

Call your doctor if you feel depressed or anxious, think that you'll hurt yourself or others, or hear or see things that aren't there.

How Is Psychosis Treated?

Medicines called neuroleptics are used for acute treatment of people with bizarre, unpredictable behavior. The aim is to prevent people from hurting themselves or others. These medicines include haloperidol and drugs called benzodiazepines, which are medicines for anxiety (e.g., lorazepam, alprazolam).

Treatment then depends on the underlying cause. For example, for a mental illness such as depression or schizophrenia, a psychiatrist (specialist in mental and emotional disorders) will be involved in treatment with antidepressant or antipsychotic medicines. People with conditions such as Parkinson's disease and seizure disorders will take medicines for those disorders. For substance abuse (e.g., alcohol, narcotics), counseling is offered.

Psychosis often means that a severe mental illness is present. Cognitive behavioral therapy may help. Cognitive therapy teaches people how certain thinking patterns cause symptoms. Behavioral therapy breaks the connection between worry about symptoms and reactions to those symptoms.

DOs and DON'Ts in Managing Psychosis:

✔ **DO** remember that psychosis is a symptom, not a diagnosis.

✔ **DO** call your doctor if you need a referral to a psychiatrist or psychologist.

✔ **DO** call your doctor if you feel depressed or anxious.

✔ **DO** call your doctor if you think that you will harm yourself or others.

✔ **DO** call your doctor if you hear voices or see things that aren't really there.

⊘ **DON'T** do drugs. Alcohol, amphetamines, cocaine, sleeping agents (e.g., barbiturates), and antianxiety medicines (e.g., benzodiazepines) can all cause psychosis.

FROM THE DESK OF

NOTES

FOR MORE INFORMATION

Contact the following sources:

• Mental Health America
  Tel: (800) 969-6642
  Website: http://www.nmha.org

• American Psychiatric Association
  Tel: (888) 357-7924
  Website: http://www.psych.org

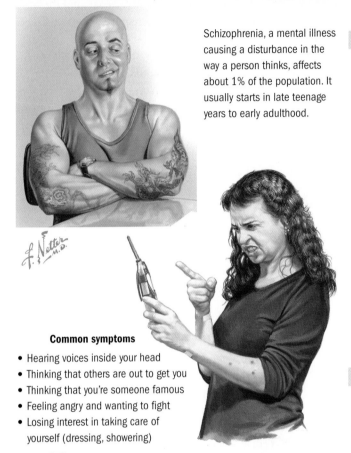

Schizophrenia, a mental illness causing a disturbance in the way a person thinks, affects about 1% of the population. It usually starts in late teenage years to early adulthood.

Common symptoms

- Hearing voices inside your head
- Thinking that others are out to get you
- Thinking that you're someone famous
- Feeling angry and wanting to fight
- Losing interest in taking care of yourself (dressing, showering)

No test is available to diagnose schizophrenia. Usually, a mental health specialist (psychologist or psychiatrist) will make the diagnosis. Blood and urine tests, imaging scans, or x-rays may be done to rule out other causes that have similar symptoms when the diagnosis is unclear.

What Is Schizophrenia?

Schizophrenia is a mental illness causing a disturbance in the way people think. It affects about 1% of the population. It usually starts in late teenage years to early adulthood. It equally affects males and females; however, males usually have a more severe illness with earlier onset.

Thoughts become disordered and out of touch with the real world. Thoughts may race, slow down, or stop, so people talk fast, slowly, or halting. It may be hard for people to think, remember, or understand.

Schizophrenia also causes strange behaviors because of hearing voices inside the head and seeing things that aren't really there. People can have delusions, feel that others are out to get them (paranoia), or act angry or want to fight.

Schizophrenia may also cause people to lose interest in other people and activities and in staying clean, neat, or healthy. People can lose mental abilities and become socially isolated.

What Causes Schizophrenia?

The cause is unknown. It may run in families. First-degree relatives of schizophrenics are 10 times more likely to become schizophrenic than the general population.

What Are the Symptoms of Schizophrenia?

Schizophrenia's main features include ambivalence (e.g., trouble making decisions), problems displaying and expressing emotions, inability to function in social situations, and abnormal thinking.

Abnormal thinking can mean having hallucinations, especially hearing voices of people not actually there. Voices may tell people to do something that they may feel uncomfortable about, such as killing themselves or others. People can also feel paranoid or believe that they have special powers or some medical condition.

How Is Schizophrenia Diagnosed?

No diagnostic tests (blood or genetic testing) exist. A doctor—usually a mental health specialist (psychologist or psychiatrist)—makes the diagnosis from the medical history and physical examination. Blood and urine tests, imaging scans, or x-rays are not needed for diagnosis but may be done to check for other conditions that may cause similar symptoms.

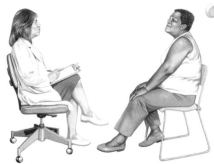

Schizophrenia cannot be cured, but symptoms can be treated. Medicines called antipsychotics and counseling are the most successful treatment tools.

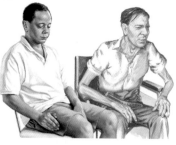

In addition to individual therapy, a support group with other schizophrenic people can help teach social skills and offer support.

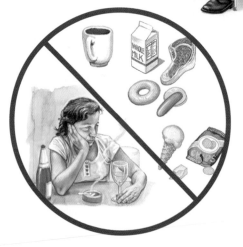

Avoid stress, poor sleep, unhealthy diet, and caffeine, which can make symptoms worse. Don't drink alcohol—it can interact with your medicine.

How Is Schizophrenia Treated?

Schizophrenia isn't curable, but many symptoms can be treated with medicines and counseling (cognitive behavioral therapy). A significant social support system is required by most schizophrenics.

Drugs called antipsychotics can stop hallucinations and paranoia if taken daily. Psychosocial treatment involves having a counselor help with different aspects of daily living, including getting to appointments and helping with medicines. A support group can help teach social skills.

DOs and DON'Ts in Managing Schizophrenia:

✔ **DO** take your medicines every day as prescribed.
✔ **DO** attend programs or participate in activities recommended by your doctor. Consider joining a support group.
✔ **DO** tell your doctor about side effects from medicine.
✔ **DO** avoid alcohol because it may interfere with your medicines.
✔ **DO** avoid stress. Stress, lack of sleep, poor diet, and using caffeine may make psychotic behaviors more likely.
✔ **DO** call your doctor if you hear voices, feel paranoid, or have other odd thoughts.
✔ **DO** call your doctor if you sleep less or if depression or suicidal thoughts occur.

⊘ **DON'T** drive unless your doctor says you can.
⊘ **DON'T** take any recreational drugs.
⊘ **DON'T** use medicines, including over-the-counter drugs, without first checking with your doctor.

FROM THE DESK OF

NOTES

FOR MORE INFORMATION

Contact the following sources:

- National Alliance for the Mentally Ill
  Tel: (800) 950-NAMI (950-6264)
  Website: http://www.nami.org

- National Institute of Mental Health
  Tel: (866) 615-6464
  Website: http://www.nimh.nih.gov

MANAGING YOUR
SEASONAL AFFECTIVE DISORDER

Seasonal affective disorder (SAD) is depression that occurs each year in fall and winter. It stops people from functioning normally. SAD usually occurs between ages 20 and 40, in women more than men, but also affects children and adolescents.

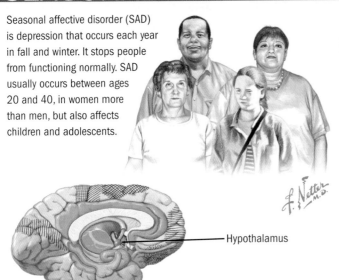

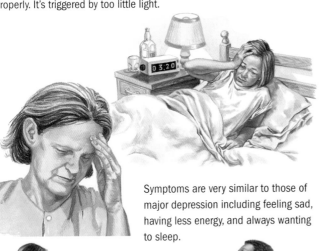

Hypothalamus

The exact cause isn't known, but it's thought to be related to a biochemical problem in part of the brain (hypothalamus) that keeps the body working properly. It's triggered by too little light.

Symptoms are very similar to those of major depression including feeling sad, having less energy, and always wanting to sleep.

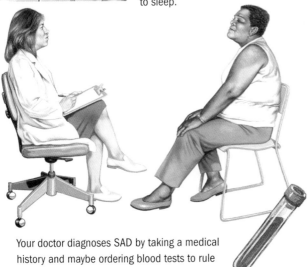

Your doctor diagnoses SAD by taking a medical history and maybe ordering blood tests to rule out conditions that act like SAD.

What Is Seasonal Affective Disorder?

Seasonal affective disorder (SAD) is depression that occurs each year in fall and winter. Symptoms are not present during spring and summer. SAD can be disabling and can stop people from functioning normally.

SAD affects between 4% and 6% of the U.S. population. It usually occurs between ages 20 and 40, in women more than men at a ratio of 4 to 1. SAD also affects children and adolescents but is less likely to affect elderly people. SAD occurs more often in people living in higher latitudes (such as Alaska) where seasonal changes are more extreme.

What Causes SAD?

The exact cause of SAD is unknown. However, it's thought to be related to a biochemical abnormality in the part of the brain that keeps body functions working properly. This part is called the hypothalamus. It controls such functions as blood pressure, body temperature, fluid and electrolyte balance, and body weight. The biochemical problem is thought to be triggered by less sunlight during winter.

What Are the Symptoms of SAD?

Symptoms are similar to those of major depression, including sadness, low energy, trouble concentrating, lack of interest, more appetite leading to weight gain, fatigue, and always wanting to sleep.

How Is SAD Diagnosed?

The doctor diagnoses SAD by taking a medical history. Blood tests to rule out conditions that mimic SAD may also be done when the diagnosis is unclear. These other conditions include hypothyroidism (underactive thyroid gland), abnormal blood calcium levels, conditions caused by medicines, substance abuse (alcohol or recreational drugs), and other psychiatric conditions (e.g., bipolar disorder, major depression).

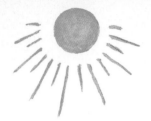
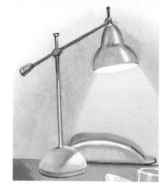

Light therapy is the best treatment. Bright white fluorescent lights can reverse symptoms, as can sunlight.

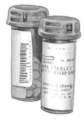

Different treatments may be combined. Three methods—light therapy, medicines, and counseling—can be used together.

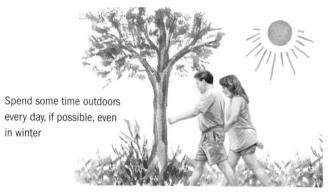

Spend some time outdoors every day, if possible, even in winter

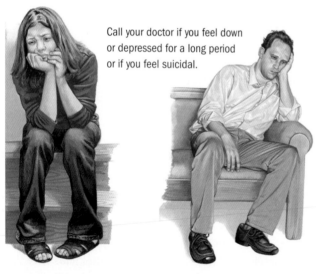

Call your doctor if you feel down or depressed for a long period or if you feel suicidal.

FROM THE DESK OF

NOTES

How Is SAD Treated?

Light therapy is the best treatment. Bright white fluorescent lights can reverse symptoms. Up to 80% of people treated with light therapy have fewer symptoms, sometimes after only 2 to 3 days of treatment. Light therapy is suggested for 30 minutes every day and is used until spring. Tanning booths shouldn't be used to treat SAD.

Different treatments may be combined. Sometimes, medicines are added to light therapy. Antidepressants called selective serotonin reuptake inhibitors (SSRIs) may be used. These drugs include fluoxetine, sertraline, and paroxetine. People can start SSRIs before symptoms begin in the fall and taper them off after symptoms leave in early spring.

Counseling can also help people get through this period. Light therapy can be combined with counseling. All three methods (light therapy, medicines, and counseling) can be used together.

DOs and DON'Ts in Managing SAD:

✔ **DO** tell your doctor about medicines and herbal remedies you take.
✔ **DO** reduce your stress.
✔ **DO** spend some time outdoors every day, if possible, even in winter.
✔ **DO** call your doctor if you feel down or depressed for a long period or if you feel suicidal.

🚫 **DON'T** use tanning beds to get extra light.
🚫 **DON'T** isolate yourself socially. Stay active with exercise, diet, and spending time outdoors during winter.

FOR MORE INFORMATION

Contact the following sources:

• American Psychiatric Association
Tel: (888) 357-7924
Website: http://www.psych.org

• Society for Light Treatment and Biological Rhythms
Website: http://www.sltbr.org

• National Organization for Seasonal Affective Disorder
Website: http://www.nosad.org

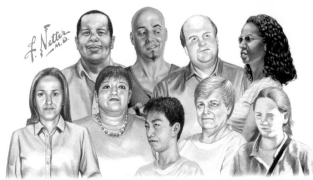

Smoking harms almost every organ in the body. Smokers are generally less healthy than nonsmokers. Take steps now to stop smoking. It's never too late, and you'll feel better and live a healthier life.

Smoking causes serious health problems, including:

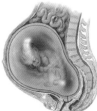

Problems getting pregnant, premature baby, low birth weight, stillbirth

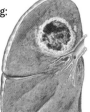

Lung diseases, including cancer, COPD, pneumonia

Cancers of the mouth, stomach, pancreas, bladder, and kidneys

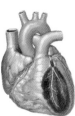

Heart disease and stroke

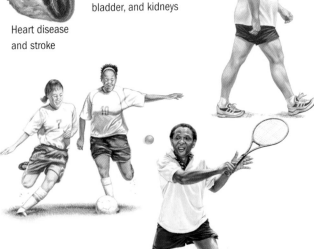

Stop now! Your health will improve and you'll do things you thought you never could! Just 12 hours after stopping, carbon dioxide levels in your blood return to normal. In 2 to 12 weeks, your lungs work better and heart attack risk decreases. Shortness of breath improves in 1 to 9 months. After 1 year, heart disease risk falls by half. After 15 years, heart disease and stroke risks are normal. After 10 years, lung cancer risk is half that of smokers.

What Is Smoking and What Does It Do?

Smoking harms almost every organ in the body. It leads to many kinds of cancer: lung, mouth, esophageal, stomach, pancreas, kidney, and bladder. Smoking damages cells lining the heart and blood vessels and makes blood clots form easily. These effects increase chances of having a heart attack or stroke. Smokers are four times more likely than nonsmokers to die of heart disease. Smoking increases the risk of aortic aneurysm (swelling of a main artery) and circulation problems.

Cigarette smoke damages the lungs and causes chronic obstructive pulmonary disease (COPD, or emphysema and chronic bronchitis). Smokers get colds and chest infections (pneumonia) more often.

Smoking during pregnancy increases the risk of premature birth, low birth weight, stillbirth, and sudden infant death syndrome (SIDS).

Other smoking-related health problems include mouth problems, sexual problems (men), thinning of bones after menopause (women), and stomach ulcers.

Benefits of Quitting

After quitting smoking, the levels of the poisonous gas carbon dioxide in the blood decrease to normal. Between 2 and 12 weeks, lungs start to work better and the risk of heart attack decreases. Coughing and shortness of breath may take 1 to 9 months to improve. After 1 year, heart disease risk falls by half. After 15 years, risks of heart disease and stroke will be normal. After 10 years, the risk of getting lung cancer is half that of a continuing smoker.

Quitting isn't easy, but some methods double your chances of success. Counseling can be individual, group, or telephone-based. Nicotine replacement therapy involves gums, patches, sprays, inhalers, and lozenges with specific amounts of nicotine.

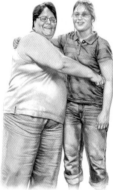

If you find yourself wanting a cigarette, do something to distract yourself. Chew gum or snack on fruit or vegetables. Don't let yourself smoke at all once you've quit, not even just once.

Change your routine to avoid situations that tempt you to smoke. Ask friends and family for support. Think about getting counseling or joining a support program. Relaxation techniques such as meditation may help.

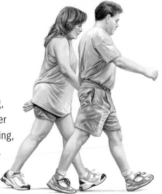

Get moving! By stopping smoking, you've started a path to a healthier you. Get even healthier by exercising, eating right, and avoiding alcohol.

How Do I Quit?

Quitting isn't easy. Nicotine is addictive. People can have withdrawal symptoms (irritability, restlessness, sleep problems), but these go away after a few days.

Certain methods double the chances of success. Counseling can be individual, group, or telephone-based. The doctor, local hospital, or health center can advise about free support programs. Nicotine replacement therapy involves approved gums, patches, sprays, inhalers, and lozenges that have specific amounts of nicotine. Both over-the-counter and prescription preparations are available. Drugs include bupropion, which is a prescription antidepressant, and varenicline, which is an effective prescription pill that can reduce the urge to smoke. It works for 44% of people who take it for the full 12 weeks.

DOs and DON'Ts in Managing Smoking:

✔ **DO** set a date for quitting.
✔ **DO** prepare yourself mentally. Think about how you will deal with cravings and temptation. Focus on why you want to give up.
✔ **DO** throw out all your cigarettes.
✔ **DO** ask friends and family for support.
✔ **DO** change your routine for a while to avoid situations that tempt you to smoke.
✔ **DO** chew gum or eat fruit or vegetables to distract yourself from the urge to smoke.
✔ **DO** think about getting counseling or joining a support program.
✔ **DO** call your doctor if you need a prescription for a smoking cessation product.
✔ **DO** call your doctor if you have medicine side effects.

🚫 **DON'T** let yourself smoke at all once you've quit, not even just one.
🚫 **DON'T** be discouraged if you fail. Most people try several times before they quit successfully.

FOR MORE INFORMATION

Contact the following sources:

• American Lung Association
  Tel: (212) 315-8700, (800) 586-4872
  Website: http://www.lungusa.org

• The American Cancer Society
  Tel: (800) 227-2345
  Website: http://www.cancer.org

• Centers for Disease Control and Prevention
  Tobacco Information and Prevention Source (TIPS)
  Telephone counseling: (800) QUIT-NOW (784-8669)
  Website: http://www.cdc.gov/tobacco/

FROM THE DESK OF

NOTES

Acute respiratory distress syndrome (ARDS) is a life-threatening condition caused by inflammation (swelling) of air sacs in the lung. ARDS occurs in people of any age and in both males and females.

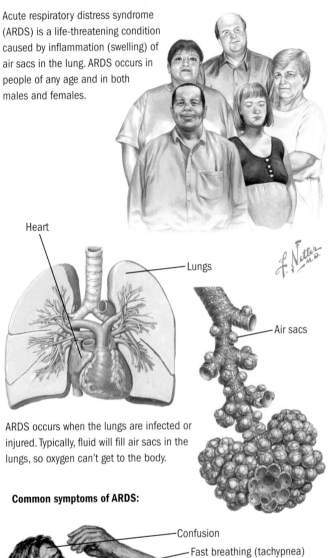

Heart

Lungs

Air sacs

ARDS occurs when the lungs are infected or injured. Typically, fluid will fill air sacs in the lungs, so oxygen can't get to the body.

Common symptoms of ARDS:

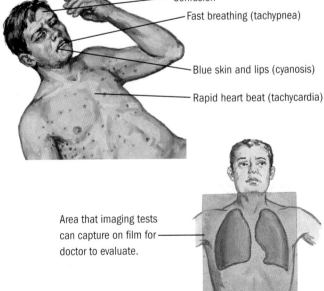

Confusion

Fast breathing (tachypnea)

Blue skin and lips (cyanosis)

Rapid heart beat (tachycardia)

Area that imaging tests can capture on film for doctor to evaluate.

Your doctor will do a chest x-ray and take blood samples for diagnosis.

What Is Acute Respiratory Distress Syndrome?

Acute respiratory distress syndrome (ARDS) is a life-threatening condition caused by inflammation (swelling) of air sacs in the lung. It leads to buildup of fluid in air sacs, which stops oxygen from getting to the bloodstream and the rest of the body. This can cause lung failure resulting in death.

ARDS occurs in people of all ages and equally in men and women. It is not contagious or inherited.

What Causes ARDS?

ARDS often results from infections, trauma, or injury and occurs rapidly (usually within 24 to 48 hours of the cause). Other causes include aspiration of vomit; extensive burns; drug overdose; breathing in of chemicals, smoke, or other toxic fumes; and pancreatitis (inflammation of the pancreas). ARDS can lead to failure not only of lungs but other vital organs including kidneys and liver.

What Are the Symptoms of ARDS?

ARDS symptoms are shortness of breath, low blood pressure, and fever. In early stages of ARDS, a fast heartbeat (tachycardia), fast breathing (tachypnea), and cyanosis (blue skin and lips) are noted. Increasing agitation, lethargy, and confusion follow in later stages.

How Is ARDS Diagnosed?

Laboratory tests and imaging studies help confirm the doctor's belief that ARDS is present. A chest x-ray perhaps provides the first clue. The doctor may order a catheterization (putting a thin catheter, or tube, through a neck vein into the heart) to measure pressures in the heart for diagnosis.

MANAGING YOUR
ASBESTOSIS

Asbestosis is a disease that scars your lungs as a result of breathing in asbestos.

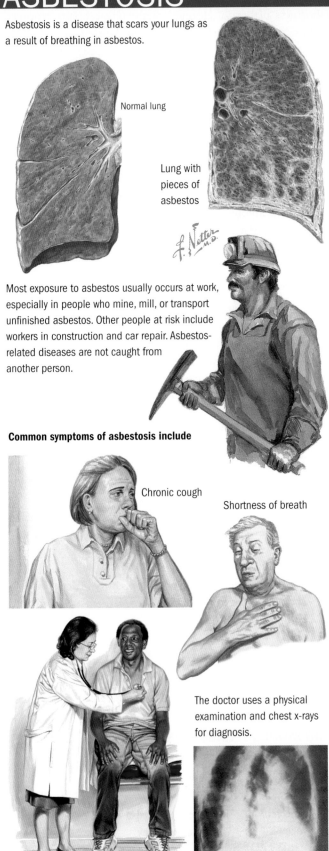

Normal lung

Lung with pieces of asbestos

Most exposure to asbestos usually occurs at work, especially in people who mine, mill, or transport unfinished asbestos. Other people at risk include workers in construction and car repair. Asbestos-related diseases are not caught from another person.

Common symptoms of asbestosis include

Chronic cough

Shortness of breath

The doctor uses a physical examination and chest x-rays for diagnosis.

What Is Asbestosis?

Asbestosis is a disease that scars the lungs as a result of breathing asbestos. Asbestos is a name of a group of natural fibers that were formerly used in various industrial products due to their resistance to burning and for insulation. Up to 20 to 30 years may pass between exposure to asbestos and development of asbestosis.

The probability of developing disease, usually several years after exposure, increases with longer and more intense asbestos exposures. Asbestos-related diseases cannot be caught but can be prevented by avoiding asbestos exposure.

Asbestos can cause diseases of lungs and pleura (layer of tissue covering the lungs), including pleural plaques, pleural effusion, and development of cancer of the lining of the lung (malignant mesothelioma). It can also increase the risk of lung cancer.

What Causes Asbestosis?

Exposure most often occurred at work. Employees at greatest risk included those who mined, milled, or transported asbestos. Others at risk were people such as car repair and construction workers who installed, fixed, or tore down products made with asbestos; people (painters, carpenters) who worked near where asbestos was used; and those living near asbestos factories or mines.

What Are the Symptoms of Asbestosis?

Shortness of breath is the most common symptom because of small, stiff lungs that were scarred by breathing in asbestos fibers. Chronic cough and phlegm (mucus) production are also common.

Pleural plaques (thickened parts of lung linings) generally don't cause symptoms but may be related to a greater risk of developing cancer of the lining of the lung (mesothelioma). Pleural effusion is fluid that collects in the space between the lungs and chest wall. Smaller effusions may cause no symptoms; larger ones can cause shortness of breath.

Symptoms of malignant mesothelioma include chest pain, weight loss, and shortness of breath.

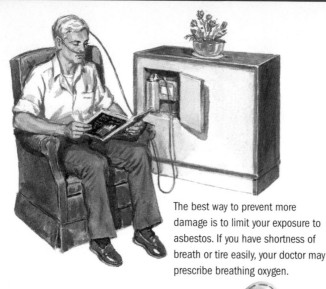

The best way to prevent more damage is to limit your exposure to asbestos. If you have shortness of breath or tire easily, your doctor may prescribe breathing oxygen.

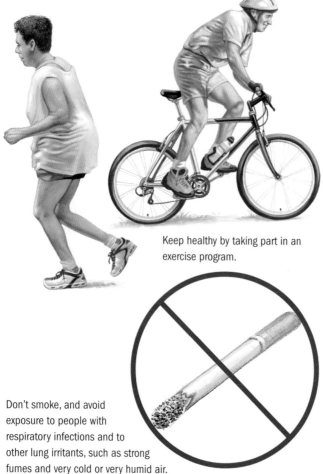

Keep healthy by taking part in an exercise program.

Don't smoke, and avoid exposure to people with respiratory infections and to other lung irritants, such as strong fumes and very cold or very humid air.

How Is Asbestosis Diagnosed?

The doctor makes a diagnosis on the basis of symptoms (shortness of breath, chronic cough) plus asbestos exposure, and findings of lung examinations and chest x-rays.

How Is Asbestosis Treated?

Treatments are limited. None can reverse or prevent lung scarring. Some people with severe progressive disease may benefit from lung transplants. Oxygen may be prescribed to improve shortness of breath and stamina. Inhalers to help breathing may also be prescribed. Further asbestos exposure should be avoided, because more exposure seems to increase risk for additional disease. The amount of safe, low-level exposure isn't clear.

No treatment is needed for pleural plaques, except for follow-up. Prognosis is very poor for mesothelioma because there are no effective treatments.

DOs and DON'Ts in Managing Asbestosis:

✔ **DO** avoid all future asbestos exposures.
✔ **DO** follow all recommended procedures, such as wearing protective masks, when working with asbestos.
✔ **DO** get a yearly flu shot and a pneumococcal pneumonia shot.
✔ **DO** keep your heart healthy by exercising.
✔ **DO** eat a healthy diet.
✔ **DO** call your doctor if you have increased cough, yellow or green sputum, more shortness of breath, fever, or chills.
✔ **DO** call your doctor if you have chest pain, new ankle swelling, weight loss, blood in the sputum, or dusky skin, fingertips, or lips.

⊘ **DON'T** go near people with respiratory infections.
⊘ **DON'T** come in contact with lung irritants such as smoke and very cold or humid air.
⊘ **DON'T** smoke.

FOR MORE INFORMATION

Contact the following sources:
• American Lung Association
 Tel: (800) LUNG-USA (586-4872)
• Agency for Toxic Substances & Disease Registry
 Website: http://www.atsdr.cdc.gov

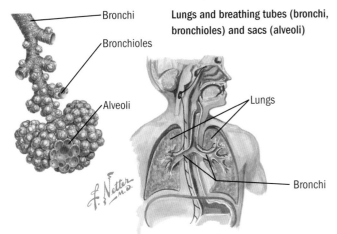

Lungs and breathing tubes (bronchi, bronchioles) and sacs (alveoli)

Bronchi

Bronchioles

Alveoli

Lungs

Bronchi

In asthma, the breathing tubes become clogged.

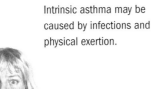

Extrinsic (allergic) reactions may include pollen, dust, and dander.

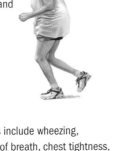

Intrinsic asthma may be caused by infections and physical exertion.

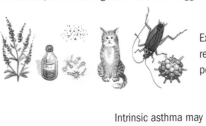

Symptoms include wheezing, shortness of breath, chest tightness, cough, and fast heartbeat.

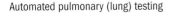

Automated pulmonary (lung) testing

Testing performed before and after breathing in a short-acting drug that dilates bronchi

Printout of results

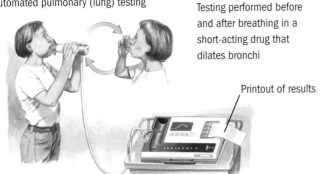

What Is Asthma?

Asthma is a lung disease in which normal airflow into and out of lungs is impaired. Smoke, exercise, cold air, infection, mold, dust, and mites, for example, make lung airway cells produce more mucus. The mucus becomes thicker and more sticky, and breathing tubes (airways) clog up and become very small. Wheezing and shortness of breath result.

Early-onset asthma (extrinsic, or allergic, asthma) has both genetic and environmental causes. Late-onset asthma (intrinsic asthma) in adults older than 35 can be triggered by infections and exercise.

What Are the Symptoms of Asthma?

- Wheezing (a whistling sound as breath is exhaled)
- Shortness of breath
- Chest tightness
- Cough

Emotional stress may also cause an asthma attack and result in a visit to the emergency room and use of oxygen and drugs.

How Is Asthma Diagnosed?

Asthma is diagnosed by reviewing symptoms; doing a physical checkup; and testing lung function, blood, and skin sensitivity. Lung (pulmonary) function tests can tell if breathing is normal and how sensitive airways are. These tests use a peak flow meter to measure air breathed in and out.

How Is Asthma Treated?

Asthma can be mild irregular (intermittent—i.e., symptoms less than two times per week). Or it can be mild long-lasting (persistent—symptoms more than two times per week but less than once daily), moderate persistent (daily symptoms), or severe persistent (constant symptoms). The doctor will base the treatment on asthma's severity.

Drugs, often given by an inhaler, may control asthma. Some work almost immediately and are used during an asthma attack. Others help stop future attacks. Some medications to reduce inflammation, known as leukotriene receptor antagonists (such as Singulair®), can also be given in pill form.

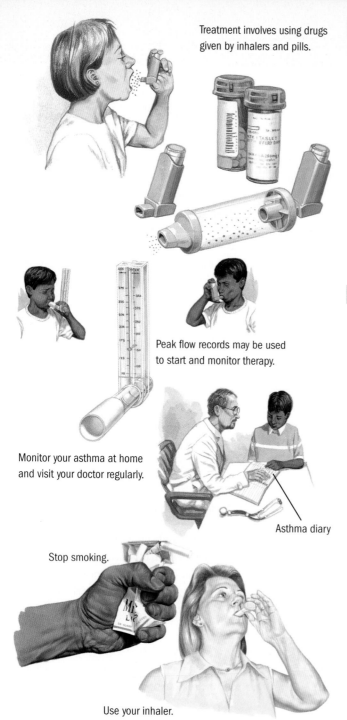

Treatment involves using drugs given by inhalers and pills.

Peak flow records may be used to start and monitor therapy.

Monitor your asthma at home and visit your doctor regularly.

Asthma diary

Stop smoking.

Use your inhaler.

How Is Asthma Treated? (con't)

The three types of common treatments are symptomatic, long-term, and immune therapy. For symptomatic treatment, short-acting drugs in inhalers are used as needed, usually by patients with mild intermittent asthma. Long-acting drugs in inhalers are used every 12 hours.

Long-term treatment involves corticosteroids given in inhalers to reduce lung swelling and redness (inflammation). They are for mild, moderate, and severe persistent asthma.

Immune therapy, often called allergy shots, is for patients who have asthma caused by uncontrolled allergies.

Asthma is treatable, and most flare-ups and deaths caused by asthma can be prevented.

DOs and DON'Ts in Managing Asthma:

✔ **DO** always carry your inhaler with you.

✔ **DO** visit your doctor regularly.

✔ **DO** use the peak flow meter to measure the amount of air you take in when you breathe. Keep records of the amounts and bring them to your doctor appointments.

✔ **DO** get a yearly flu shot and pneumococcal vaccine.

✔ **DO** continue normal activities as tolerated.

✔ **DO** exercise regularly, but make sure your asthma is controlled before starting new exercises.

✔ **DO** reduce the dust mites in your house, e.g., by getting rid of carpets and using special (HEPA) filters.

✔ **DO** talk to your doctor about how pets may affect asthma.

✔ **DO** tell your doctor if your medicines do not control your asthma or have side effects, if your peak flow readings always go down, or if you feel more tired.

⊘ **DON'T** take aspirin and other over-the-counter medicines unless your doctor approves them.

⊘ **DON'T** come into contact with asthma triggers such as cold air or smoke.

⊘ **DON'T** do excessive exercise, especially in cold weather.

FROM THE DESK OF

NOTES

FOR MORE INFORMATION

Contact the following sources:

• American Lung Association
  Tel: (800) LUNG-USA
  Website: http://www.lungusa.org

• National Lung Health Education Program
  Tel: (303) 839-6755
  Website: http://www.nlhep.org

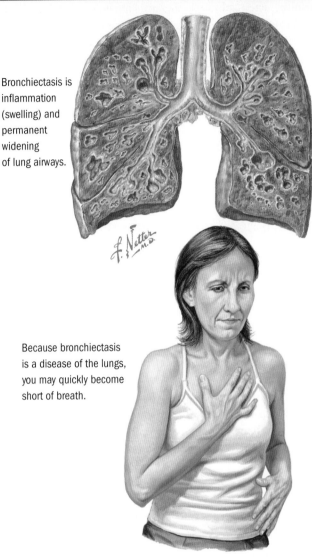

Bronchiectasis is inflammation (swelling) and permanent widening of lung airways.

Because bronchiectasis is a disease of the lungs, you may quickly become short of breath.

What Is Bronchiectasis?

In the lungs, cartilage and muscle support and keep the shape of the airways. Constant irritation of the structures supporting the airways destroys them, causing the airways to get bigger. Bronchiectasis is inflammation (swelling) and widening of lung airways.

Bronchiectasis is not contagious.

What Causes Bronchiectasis?

Severe infection with virus or bacteria, blocked airways, and poor clearing of lung secretions are common causes. Smoking, chronic bronchitis, cystic fibrosis, tuberculosis, pneumonia, and lung cancer increase the chance of getting this disease.

What Are the Symptoms of Bronchiectasis?

People have persistant cough with discolored bad-smelling sputum (lung secretions), wheezing, shortness of breath, tiredness, problems sleeping, and weight loss. Often, sputum contains streaks of blood. Fever may be present.

How Is Bronchiectasis Diagnosed?

Your doctor makes the diagnosis by checking symptoms and ordering tests such as studies of sputum, chest x-rays, lung function tests, and computed tomography (CT). A sputum sample may help tell which organisms are causing the disorder and which antibiotic to use. CT allows the doctor to look at the size of the airways. Bronchoscopy (a test allowing doctors to look into lungs through a lighted tube) may also help diagnosis and help remove mucus plugs.

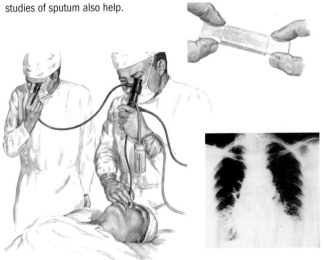

Your doctor can use bronchoscopy (a test in which doctors look into lungs through a lighted tube) to make the diagnosis. Chest x-rays and laboratory studies of sputum also help.

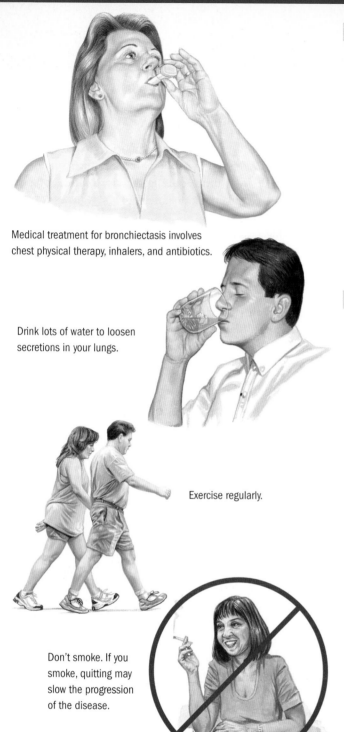

Medical treatment for bronchiectasis involves chest physical therapy, inhalers, and antibiotics.

Drink lots of water to loosen secretions in your lungs.

Exercise regularly.

Don't smoke. If you smoke, quitting may slow the progression of the disease.

How Is Bronchiectasis Treated?

Treatment may be medical or surgical. Medical treatment involves chest physical therapy, inhalers, and antibiotics. Physical therapy uses changes in posture for better drainage of secretions from lungs. Inhalers allow increased airflow through lungs and help clear secretions. Antibiotics reduce inflammation by killing bacteria that infected the airways.

For severe problems that don't respond to other treatments, surgery to remove affected parts of the lung is an option for certain people.

Some people gain back much lung function, but others such as those with bronchiectasis due to cystic fibrosis may have a disease that gets worse and can lead to death.

DOs and DON'Ts in Managing Bronchiectasis:

✔ **DO** make sure that you follow directions for your medicines. They are an important part of helping your lungs work well.

✔ **DO** chest physical therapy to allow your lungs to heal faster so you breathe easier. It is often time-consuming but plays an important role.

✔ **DO** get pneumococcal pneumonia vaccination and flu shots.

✔ **DO** drink lots of water to loosen lung secretions.

✔ **DO** exercise regularly and in moderation. Good exercises are walking, running, swimming, aerobics, and dancing. Exercise helps clear lung secretions.

✔ **DO** call your doctor if treatment doesn't help your symptoms.

✔ **DO** call your doctor if your cough or amount of sputum suddenly increases or if you have a fever.

✔ **DO** call your doctor if you cough up large amounts of blood.

⊘ **DON'T** smoke. Quitting may slow progression of the disease and help symptoms.

FROM THE DESK OF

NOTES

FOR MORE INFORMATION

Contact the following source:

• American Lung Association
  Tel: (800) LUNG-USA (586-4872)
  Website: http://www.lungusa.org

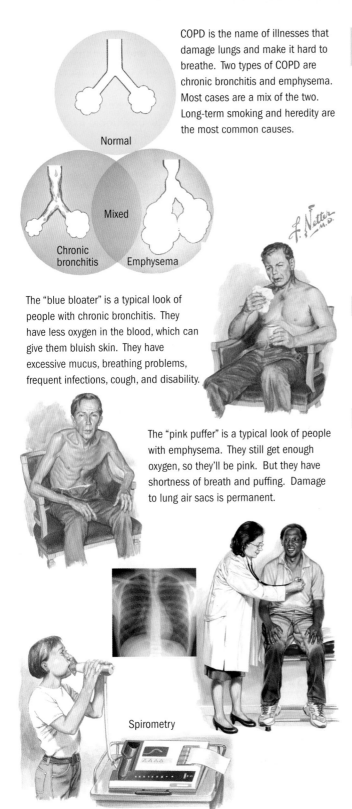

COPD is the name of illnesses that damage lungs and make it hard to breathe. Two types of COPD are chronic bronchitis and emphysema. Most cases are a mix of the two. Long-term smoking and heredity are the most common causes.

The "blue bloater" is a typical look of people with chronic bronchitis. They have less oxygen in the blood, which can give them bluish skin. They have excessive mucus, breathing problems, frequent infections, cough, and disability.

The "pink puffer" is a typical look of people with emphysema. They still get enough oxygen, so they'll be pink. But they have shortness of breath and puffing. Damage to lung air sacs is permanent.

Spirometry

Your doctor makes a diagnosis from your symptoms, complete physical examination, pulmonary (lung) function tests (spirometry), chest x-ray, and levels of oxygen and carbon dioxide in blood in arteries (blood gas levels).

What Is Chronic Obstructive Pulmonary Disease (COPD)?

Chronic obstructive pulmonary disease (COPD) is the name of illnesses that damage lungs and make it hard to breathe. Two common types of COPD are chronic bronchitis and emphysema. Most cases of COPD are a mixture of both diseases. Chronic bronchitis is having excessive mucus (phlegm) for at least 3 months of 2 consecutive years. Emphysema is caused by destruction of air sacs in lungs. Air that's breathed in stays trapped in the lungs, and exchange of oxygen and carbon dioxide doesn't occur in the air sacs.

COPD is usually progressive and not curable, but stopping smoking and drugs can help people live longer.

What Causes COPD?

Long-term smoking and heredity are the most common causes. Others include air pollution, childhood infections, and inhalation injury. COPD isn't contagious.

What Are the Signs and Symptoms of COPD?

Signs and symptoms include shortness of breath that worsens with exercise or frequent upper respiratory infections (such as a cold). As COPD gets worse, people have more trouble breathing, even when resting; lasting cough or need to clear the throat; a lot of mucus; chest tightness; and anxiety. Chronic bronchitis may cause sleep problems from mucus in the airways. Other symptoms are frequent lung infections, wheezing, weight gain, and bluish color of lips or skin. Emphysema causes shortness of breath, barrel-shaped chest, and weight loss, but little cough or sputum production. These diseases can lead to increased strain on the heart.

How Is COPD Diagnosed?

The doctor makes a diagnosis from symptoms, complete physical examination, pulmonary (lung) function tests, chest x-ray, and levels of oxygen and carbon dioxide in blood in arteries.

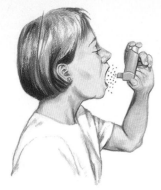

Treatments are aimed at relieving symptoms. They include stopping smoking, exercise, airway dilators, hydration, vaccinations (influenza, pneumonia), oxygen, antibiotics, and decongestants.

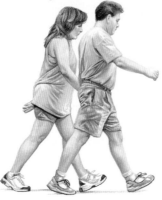

Pursed-lip breathing exercises can help ease breathlessness.

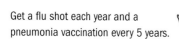

Get a flu shot each year and a pneumonia vaccination every 5 years.

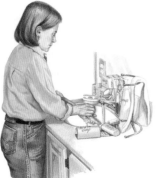

Avoid catching a cold or upper respiratory infection. Wash your hands often, and avoid contact with people who are sick.

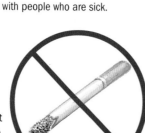

Don't smoke or use tobacco products—this is the most important part of any treatment plan for COPD.

How Is COPD Treated?

Treatment goals are to relieve symptoms. A respiratory doctor (specialist in breathing disorders) may be involved in care.

Treatments include stopping smoking, exercise, air-way dilators, hydration, vaccinations for influenza and pneumonia, oxygen, antibiotics, decongestants, and breathing exercises. Oxygen can be supplied by tank, even a portable one, so people can travel with it. Decongestants help loosen airway mucus. Changes in posture help mucus to drain. Antibiotics and vaccinations reduce the number of infections. In rare cases, lung transplantation is for people with inherited disease.

DOs and DON'Ts in Managing COPD:

✔ **DO** stop smoking. This is extremely important.
✔ **DO** avoid substances that make it hard to breathe, such as chemicals on the job or fumes from heating or cooking.
✔ **DO** avoid catching a cold or upper respiratory infection. Wash your hands often, and avoid contact with people who are sick.
✔ **DO** get a flu shot each year.
✔ **DO** get a pneumonia vaccination every 5 years.
✔ **DO** keep your house well ventilated.
✔ **DO** call your doctor if medicine doesn't help shortness of breath or cough.
✔ **DO** call your doctor if you always feel tired or are losing a lot of weight involuntarily.
✔ **DO** call your doctor if you notice a bluish color in your lips or nails.

⊘ **DON'T** adjust your medicines (including oxygen) without first talking with your doctor.
⊘ **DON'T** go outside or exercise if air is polluted or if the air quality index is poor.
⊘ **DON'T** spend a lot of money on air cleaners. They don't usually help much.

FOR MORE INFORMATION

Contact the following sources:

• National Heart, Lung, and Blood Institute
National Institutes of Health
Tel: (301) 592-8573
Website: http://www.nhlbi.nih.gov

• National Lung Health Education Program
Tel: (972) 910-8555
Website: http://www.nlhep.org

• American Lung Association
Tel: (800) 586-4872
Website: http://www.lungusa.org

FROM THE DESK OF

NOTES

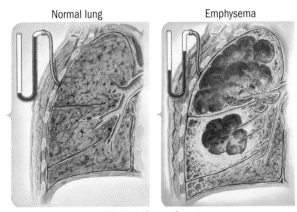

Normal lung   Emphysema

The lung in emphysema

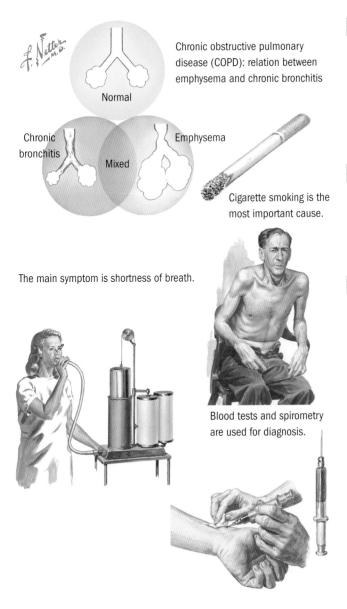

Chronic obstructive pulmonary disease (COPD): relation between emphysema and chronic bronchitis

Normal

Chronic bronchitis

Emphysema

Mixed

Cigarette smoking is the most important cause.

The main symptom is shortness of breath.

Blood tests and spirometry are used for diagnosis.

What Is Emphysema?

Emphysema is a chronic disease of the lungs. It causes decreased lung function and swelling (inflammation) and irritation of airways. Emphysema often occurs with chronic bronchitis (together these two conditions are called *chronic obstructive pulmonary disease*, or COPD).

The lungs consist of two main parts: airways (bronchial tubes) and air sacs (alveoli). During a breath, air passes through airways and into air sacs, where oxygen enters the blood. In emphysema, air sacs become larger, their walls become stiff, and the sacs cannot hold enough air.

What Causes Emphysema?

The main cause is cigarette smoking or exposure to second-hand smoke. Cigarette smoke destroys lung tissue and irritates airways.

Other risk factors include asthma, air pollution, and family history of emphysema.

What Are the Symptoms of Emphysema?

The main symptom is shortness of breath. Others are persistent cough, wheezing, decreased ability to exercise or do usual daily activities, and weight loss.

How Is Emphysema Diagnosed?

The doctor will talk about your symptoms with you and do a physical examination, especially of the chest. He or she will listen to the lungs with a stethoscope to see whether breathing is normal.

A monitor (pulse oximeter) may be used to measure the blood's oxygen level.

Simple blood tests check general health. Some people may need blood tests for levels of oxygen and carbon dioxide in an artery or for alpha-1-antitrypsin enzyme deficiency, a risk factor for emphysema.

A chest x-ray will be done to look at the lungs. Lung function testing (spirometry) may be done to tell whether the disease is emphysema or another lung disorder (e.g., asthma). The testing involves blowing into a tool to measure how much and how fast the lungs blow out air.

Treatment for emphysema

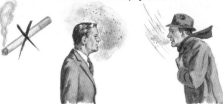

Avoid lung irritation, stop smoking, and avoid air pollution and cold temperatures.

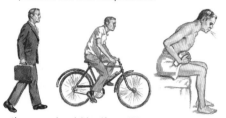

Exercise, continue usual activities if possible, and do breathing exercises.

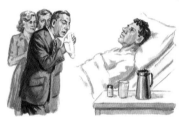

Prevent infections by avoiding sick people and getting flu shots.

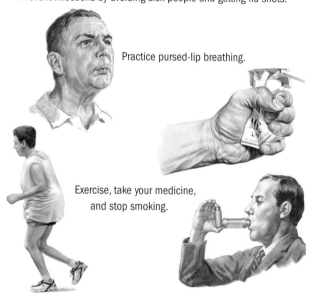

Practice pursed-lip breathing.

Exercise, take your medicine, and stop smoking.

How Is Emphysema Treated?

Treatment depends on the severity of the emphysema. Severe disease may need treatment in the hospital.

The lifestyle change of stopping smoking is the most important step to slow the progress of the disease or even improve it.

Medicines that may help include bronchodilators and corticosteroids. Bronchodilators, usually given by inhalers, cause airways to open. Corticosteroids work by reducing inflammation. They may be given by inhalers or in pill form.

Oxygen may be given in a hospital emergency department. In severe cases, it may be provided in tanks for home use.

Antibiotics may be prescribed if a chest infection is suspected.

Surgery may become an option for advanced emphysema in rare cases.

DOs and DON'Ts in Managing Emphysema:

✔ **DO** quit smoking and avoid a smoky environment.
✔ **DO** ask your doctor and support groups for help with quitting smoking.
✔ **DO** visit your doctor regularly.
✔ **DO** take your medicines as prescribed.
✔ **DO** exercise regularly as tolerated.
✔ **DO** get a flu shot every year and a pneumonia vaccination every 5 years.
✔ **DO** contact your doctor about new or worsening symptoms.

⊘ **DON'T** delay going to the emergency department if you become very short of breath or notice your tongue, fingernails, skin, or lips are turning blue.
⊘ **DON'T** stop taking your medicines without checking with your doctor.

FROM THE DESK OF

NOTES

FOR MORE INFORMATION

Contact the following sources:

• American Lung Association
  Tel: (800) LUNG-USA
  Website: http://www.lungusa.org

• National Lung Health Education Program
  Tel: (303) 839-6755
  Website: http://www.nlhep.org

MANAGING YOUR HYPERSENSITIVITY PNEUMONITIS

Hypersensitivity pneumonitis is an inflammation or irritation of the lungs. It has many other names related to the specific cause, such as farmer's lung (the most common type), air-conditioner or humidifier lung, bird fancier's lung, chemical worker's lung, and wine grower's lung.

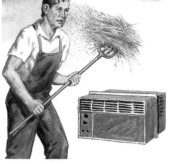

Lungs of workers get irritated by exposure to dust, mold, or fungus. For example, dust may come from moldy hay, straw, and grain (farmer's lung). Bird fanciers are exposed to proteins from feathers and droppings of pigeons and other birds. Particles may move easily through the air because of building air conditioners.

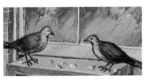

The most common symptoms are fever, chills, cough, shortness of breath, weakness, wheezing, headache and loss of appetite and weight.

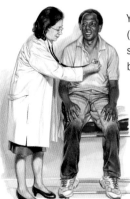

Your doctor may hear certain sounds (crackles, or rales) in your lungs with the stethoscope. The doctor may also order blood tests, chest x-ray, and breathing test.

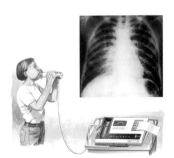

What Is Hypersensitivity Pneumonitis?

Hypersensitivity pneumonitis (or extrinsic allergic alveolitis) is an inflammation or irritation of the lungs due to recurrent exposure to various environmental agents. It has many other names related to the specific cause, such as farmer's lung (the most common type), air-conditioner or humidifier lung, bird fancier's lung, bagassosis, cheese worker's lung, chemical worker's lung, grain handler's lung, wine grower's lung, and mushroom picker's disease.

What Causes Hypersensitivity Pneumonitis?

The cause is exposure to environmental agents in the air. Lungs of workers get irritated by long or repeated exposures to dust, mold, or fungus. For example, dust may come from moldy hay, straw, and grain (farmer's lung). Bird fanciers are exposed to proteins from feathers and droppings of pigeons, parakeets, and other birds. Particles may move easily through the air by air conditioners and heaters in a building.

What Are the Symptoms of Hypersensitivity Pneumonitis?

The most common symptoms are fever, chills, cough, shortness of breath, weakness, wheezing, headache, and loss of appetite. The acute illness may start 4 to 6 hours after exposure to the cause. Symptoms often go away on their own in 12 hours to several days after exposure stops. In time, with repeated exposure, the acute illness may turn into a long-lasting (chronic) lung disease.

How Is Hypersensitivity Pneumonitis Diagnosed?

Diagnosis is based on the physical examination and additional tests. The doctor may hear certain sounds (called crackles or rales) with the stethoscope while you are breathing. These sounds are faint, brief crackling noises. The doctor may also order blood tests, chest x-ray, and breathing test to find out how the lungs are working and to exclude other disorders that have similar symptoms.

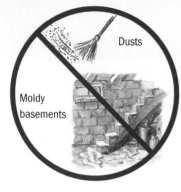

The main treatment is to find the cause of the irritation and try to avoid it. Usually, symptoms go away after the exposure stops.

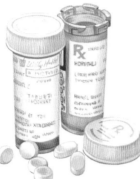

In serious cases, medicines called corticosteroids (prednisone) may be given.

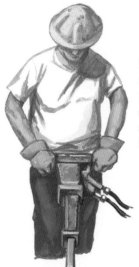

For some people, your work environment may be contributing to your condition. Wear protective masks and use a good ventilation system. These may help prevent becoming sensitized to the irritant and stop of the illness from coming back.

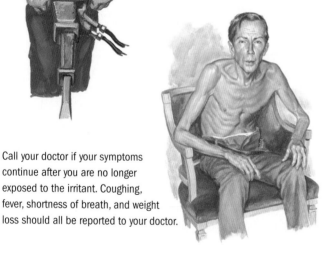

Call your doctor if your symptoms continue after you are no longer exposed to the irritant. Coughing, fever, shortness of breath, and weight loss should all be reported to your doctor.

How Is Hypersensitivity Pneumonitis Treated?

The main treatment is to find the cause of the irritation and try to avoid it, if possible. Usually, symptoms go away after the exposure stops. In serious cases, medicines called corticosteroids (prednisone) may be given.

DOs and DON'Ts in Managing Hypersensitivity Pneumonitis:

✔ **DO** avoid exposure to the irritant if you are diagnosed with hypersensitivity pneumonitis and the irritant is known. Remove or reduce the irritant, such as dust.

✔ **DO** call your doctor if your symptoms last after you are no longer exposed to the irritant.

✔ **DO** wear protective masks and use a good ventilation system. These may help prevent becoming sensitized to the irritant and recurrence of the illness.

⊘ **DON'T** ignore symptoms, especially if they last more than a few days.

FROM THE DESK OF

NOTES

FOR MORE INFORMATION

Contact the following source:

• American Lung Association
  Tel: (212) 315-8700, (800) 586-4872
  Website: http://www.lungusa.org

Idiopathic pulmonary fibrosis (IPF) is a disease of the lungs that causes scarring (fibrosis). Most people are diagnosed at age 40 to 70.

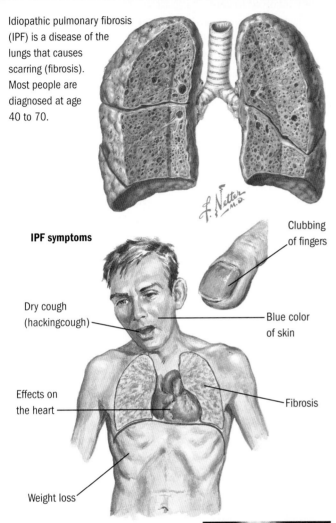

IPF symptoms

Clubbing of fingers

Dry cough (hackingcough)

Blue color of skin

Effects on the heart

Fibrosis

Weight loss

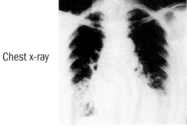

Chest x-ray

Lung biopsy

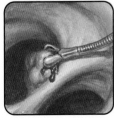

Your doctor can use bronchoscopy (a test to look into lungs through a lighted tube) to make the diagnosis. X-rays and laboratory studies also help. Only an open lung biopsy can confirm the diagnosis.

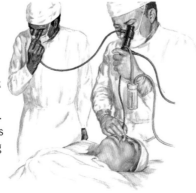

What Is Idiopathic Pulmonary Fibrosis?

Idiopathic pulmonary fibrosis (IPF) is a disease of the lungs that causes scarring (fibrosis). Fibrosis can build up so that lung function is impaired and not enough oxygen can get to body tissues. Men and women are affected equally. Most people are diagnosed at 50 to 60 years old. IPF is not contagious.

What Causes IPF?

The cause is unknown. In a few cases, heredity appears to play a part.

What Are the Symptoms of IPF?

Early symptoms include a dry cough and shortness of breath (dyspnea). Later, dyspnea becomes the major problem. Activities, such as climbing stairs, walking short distances, and dressing, become hard and sometimes almost impossible. Enlargement of the fingertips (clubbing) may develop. The body has difficulty fighting infections. In advanced stages, people may need oxygen constantly. Most people live an average of 4 to 6 years after diagnosis.

How Is IPF Diagnosed?

The doctor may suspect the diagnosis from your symptoms and the physical exam and medical history.

The doctor will order additional tests: chest x-ray, computed tomography (CT) of the chest, blood tests, and pulmonary (lung) function tests. Bronchoscopy and lung biopsy will also be done. In bronchoscopy, the doctor puts a long, narrow, flexible, lighted tube (bronchoscope) into the lungs.

In a biopsy, small pieces of lung are studied to see how much inflammation and fibrosis the lungs have.

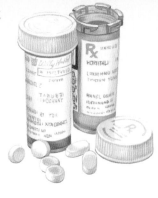

Treatment is aimed at reducing lung inflammation and stopping fibrosis. Drugs used include prednisone and cyclophosphamide.

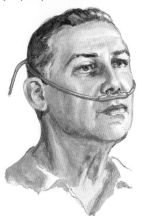

Oxygen improves breathing.

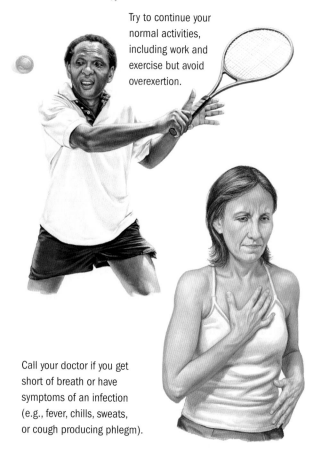

Try to continue your normal activities, including work and exercise but avoid overexertion.

Call your doctor if you get short of breath or have symptoms of an infection (e.g., fever, chills, sweats, or cough producing phlegm).

How Is IPF Treated?

Most people need lifelong treatment, and a lung specialist is usually involved in care.

The goals of treatment are to reduce lung inflammation and stop fibrosis. Once scar tissue forms, the lung cannot return to normal. Drugs are used as treatment. Prednisone and cyclophosphamide, together or alone, are drugs commonly used. Oxygen improves breathing. Lung transplantation is an option in people who do not respond well to other treatments.

DOs and DON'Ts in Managing IPF:

✔ **DO** try to continue your normal activities, including work and exercise but avoid overexertion.

✔ **DO** get emotional and psychological support if you get depressed.

✔ **DO** call your doctor if you get short of breath or have symptoms of an infection (e.g., fever, chills, sweats, cough producing phlegm).

✔ **DO** call your doctor if you have side effects from medicines.

⊘ **DON'T** miss doctor appointments.

⊘ **DON'T** be afraid to ask for second opinions from lung doctors specializing in IPF.

FROM THE DESK OF

NOTES

FOR MORE INFORMATION

Contact the following sources:

• National Heart, Lung, and Blood Institute
  Tel: (800) 575-9355
  Website: http://www.nhlbi.nih.gov

• American Lung Association
  Tel: (212) 315-8700, (800) 586-4872
  Website: http://www.lungusa.org

Diffuse interstitial pulmonary disease is a group of different lung diseases. All cause lung inflammation (swelling) that often leads to scarring (fibrosis).

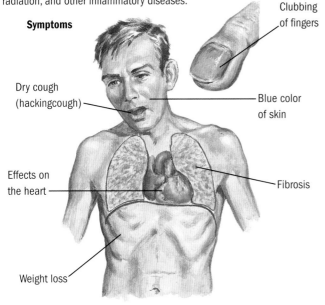

The cause could be unknown but in some cases may be from breathing irritating substances, medicines, radiation, and other inflammatory diseases.

Symptoms

Clubbing of fingers

Dry cough (hackingcough)

Blue color of skin

Effects on the heart

Fibrosis

Weight loss

Your doctor uses a medical and job history (including smoking) and physical examination for diagnosis, as well as x-rays, CT, and bronchoscopy (a test that looks into lungs through a lighted tube).

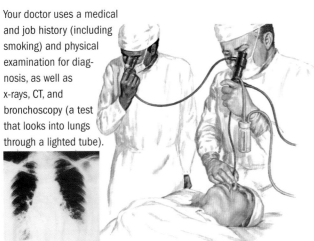

What Is Interstitial Pulmonary Disease?

Diffuse interstitial pulmonary disease is the name of a group of many different lung diseases with different causes and symptoms. However, all these diseases cause inflammation (swelling) of the area around air sacs in the lungs. Inflammation often leads to scarring (fibrosis), and thus the lungs don't work well. These conditions are hard to treat because no cures are usually available. They are not contagious, and no vaccines can prevent them.

What Causes Interstitial Pulmonary Disease?

Often the cause is unknown. Breathing in irritating substances in the environment or workplace, taking certain medicines, radiation exposure, and inflammatory diseases outside lungs may be contributing factors.

What Are the Symptoms of Interstitial Pulmonary Disease?

Symptoms vary, but almost all these diseases cause shortness of breath and a dry cough that usually start slowly and get worse. Fingertips may appear clubbed.

Other symptoms may include chest pain, fever, coughing up blood, fatigue, and weight loss.

How Is Interstitial Pulmonary Disease Diagnosed?

The doctor uses a medical and job history and physical examination for diagnosis.

When severe, lung scarring is present. The doctor may hear crackling breath sounds, like the two pieces of Velcro being pulled apart.

The chest x-rays will show different changes, including a honeycomb-like appearance. Chest computed tomography (CT), lung biopsy, and breathing tests can also be done. The biopsy samples can be obtained by bronchoscopy, a test in which the doctor uses a lighted tube to look into the lungs.

Treatment depends on the specific cause of lung inflammation and fibrosis. The steroid prednisone, inhalers, oxygen, and sometimes lung transplantation are options.

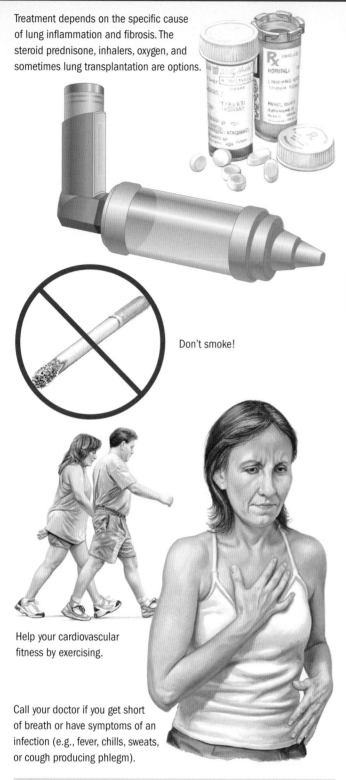

Don't smoke!

Help your cardiovascular fitness by exercising.

Call your doctor if you get short of breath or have symptoms of an infection (e.g., fever, chills, sweats, or cough producing phlegm).

How Is Interstitial Pulmonary Disease Treated?

Treatment depends on the specific cause.

In all cases, smoking should stop.

Inhalers may help for smoking-related lung disease. If the cause is something in the environment, that substance should be avoided. For example, wear protective breathing masks.

Antiinflammatory drugs such as prednisone (a steroid) may be helpful in some cases.

Unfortunately, treatment is not always effective and no drugs reverse lung scarring. Oxygen may help reduce shortness of breath and improve stamina. Lung transplantation is an option in people with progressive disease.

DOs and DON'Ts in Managing Interstitial Pulmonary Disease:

✔ **DO** get a flu shot each fall.
✔ **DO** get a pneumococcal pneumonia vaccination.
✔ **DO** help your cardiovascular fitness by exercising.
✔ **DO** call your doctor if you think that you have a lung infection, because of a sudden worse cough, yellow or green phlegm, fever, chills, or increased shortness of breath.
✔ **DO** call your doctor if you have bloody sputum, chest pain, new ankle swelling, problems with medicines, or dusky-colored skin, fingertips, or lips.

⊘ **DON'T** expose yourself to substances thought to be responsible for your lung disease or environmental pollutants.
⊘ **DON'T** go near people with respiratory infections.
⊘ **DON'T** smoke.

FROM THE DESK OF

NOTES

FOR MORE INFORMATION

Contact the following source:

• American Lung Association
 Tel: (800) 586-4872, (212) 315-8700
 Website: http://www.lungusa.org

Legionnaires' disease is an uncommon type of pneumonia. Elderly people, people with diabetes mellitus or impaired immune systems, and those with organ transplants are most likely to develop legionnaires' disease.

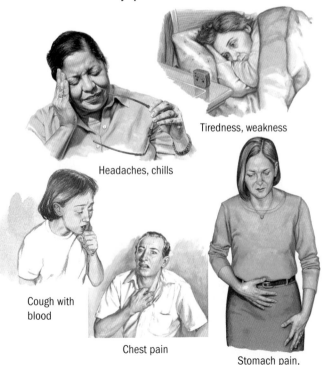

Sometimes the disease affects a group of people, such as passengers on a ship or people staying at a hotel.

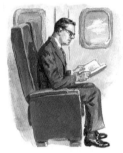

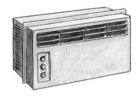

Bacteria

The cause is the kind of bacteria named *Legionella pneumophila.* The bacteria live in water such as parts of air conditioning cooling towers. People are exposed when they breathe in droplets containing *Legionella* bacteria. The organism generally doesn't spread from person to person.

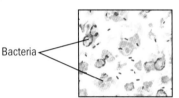

Symptoms include:

Tiredness, weakness

Headaches, chills

Cough with blood

Chest pain

Stomach pain, diarrhea

What Is Legionnaires' Disease?

Legionnaires' disease is an uncommon type of pneumonia (lung infection). It may present as an isolated case, but sometimes the disease spreads through a group, such as passengers on a ship or people staying at a hotel.

Elderly people, people with diabetes mellitus or impaired immune systems, and those who have organ transplants are most likely to develop legionnaires' disease.

What Causes Legionnaires' Disease?

The cause is the kind of bacteria named *Legionella pneumophila.* The disease gets its name because it was first identified when it affected many people attending an American Legion convention in the 1970s. The bacteria normally live in water. Places holding water such as parts of air conditioning cooling towers may be a source of contamination. That's why many people can be affected in one location. People are exposed when they breathe in droplets containing *Legionella* bacteria. The organism generally doesn't spread from person to person. No vaccine is available to prevent the disease.

What Are the Symptoms of Legionnaires' Disease?

First symptoms are headache, muscle aches, tiredness, and weakness. A high temperature (more than 103° F, chills, shortness of breath, cough, and chest pain develop. The fever usually goes down in 3 days, and other symptoms improve in 6 to 10 days. Coughing can bring up blood-streaked sputum or phlegm. People can also have diarrhea, stomach pain, loss of appetite, confusion, and inability to sleep.

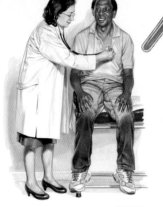

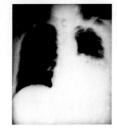

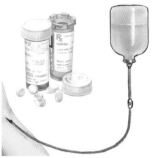

Your doctor examines you and does laboratory tests (of urine and blood) and x-rays. Diagnosis may be hard because symptoms are similar to other infections.

People with legionnaires' disease are usually hospitalized. Antibiotics are given for 14 to 21 days. Treatment in the hospital is initially begun with intravenous antibiotics and then switched to oral antibiotics before discharge.

Take your antibiotics as prescribed and acetaminophen for fever and pain. Drink plenty of fluids (six to eight glasses a day), and breathe moist air to help raise phlegm.

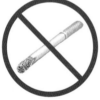

Don't smoke. Smoking can increase your chances of getting legionnaires' disease.

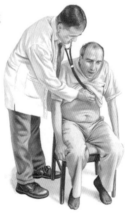

Call your doctor if you don't improve or you become more ill after 48 hours of antibiotic therapy. Some symptoms may last for several weeks, but all should eventually go away.

FROM THE DESK OF

NOTES

How Is Legionnaires' Disease Diagnosed?

The doctor does a physical examination and obtains laboratory tests (of urine and blood). A chest x-ray is also done. Diagnosis may be hard because symptoms aren't specific but are like those of many other forms of pneumonia and some viral infections.

How Is Legionnaires' Disease Treated?

People with legionnaires' disease are usually hospitalized. Antibiotics are given for 14 to 21 days. Intravenous antibiotics are given initially and then switched to oral antibiotics before discharge. Symptoms usually begin to improve within 48 to 72 hours of starting antibiotic therapy.

The disease can be very serious and potentially life threatening in immunocompromised people. Most healthy people usually recover from the disease.

After the first treatment or hospital discharge, people may still feel tired and weak for several months. People with heart and lung diseases, diabetes, or weakened immune system may take longer to recover.

DOs and DON'Ts in Managing Legionnaires' Disease:

✔ **DO** take your antibiotics as prescribed. If you miss a dose, just start again with the next dose and continue to take pills as scheduled until they're gone.

✔ **DO** rest until you feel better. Some symptoms may last for several weeks, but all should eventually go away.

✔ **DO** take acetaminophen for fever and pain.

✔ **DO** drink plenty of fluids (six to eight glasses a day) and breathe moist air to help raise phlegm.

✔ **DO** call your doctor if you don't improve or you become more ill after 48 hours of antibiotic therapy.

⊘ **DON'T** smoke. Smoking can increase your risk of getting legionnaires' disease.

FOR MORE INFORMATION

Contact the following sources:

- Infectious Diseases Society of America
  Tel: (703) 299-0200
  Website: http://www.idsociety.org

- American Thoracic Society
  Tel: (212) 315-8600
  Website: http://www.thoracic.org

- American Lung Association
  Tel: (212) 315-8700, (800) 586-4872
  Website: http://www.lungusa.org

Sarcoidosis is an illness that causes inflammation of many organs. It most often starts in the lungs or lymph nodes. The illness affects both sexes, usually people 15 to 65 years old.

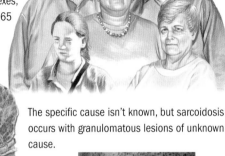

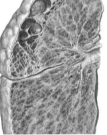

The specific cause isn't known, but sarcoidosis occurs with granulomatous lesions of unknown cause.

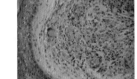

Lung with granulomas

Granuloma seen with a microscope

Some people have one or two symptoms, but others have many, including:

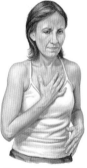

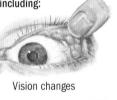

Vision changes

Shortness of breath, chest pain

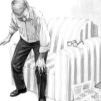

Joint aches and pain, stiff or swollen joints

Swollen lymph glands

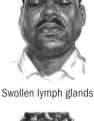

Rash

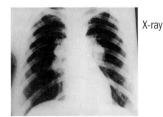

X-ray

Bronchoscopy

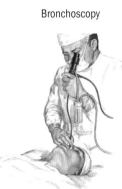

Making a diagnosis is hard. Your doctor will examine you and order a chest x-ray. Blood tests, breathing tests, CT, tissue biopsy, TB tests, and ECG may be done. Bronchoscopy may be done to get a lung sample for study.

What Is Sarcoidosis?

Sarcoidosis is an illness that causes inflammation of many organs. It most often starts in the lungs or lymph nodes (glands). The illness affects both sexes, usually people 15 to 65 years old.

What Causes Sarcoidosis?

The cause isn't known. It is a granulomatous disease. Granuloma means a special kind of tissue inflammation seen with a microscope, and granulomatous means related to granuloma. Sarcoidosis isn't contagious or hereditary.

What Are the Symptoms of Sarcoidosis?

Some people have only one or two symptoms, but others have many. These include shortness of breath, dry cough, joint aches and pain, chest pain, dry eyes, dry mouth, fever, large lymph glands, loss of appetite and weight, palpitations, chronic runny or stuffy nose, rash, and stiff or swollen joints. Others are tiredness, vision changes, and tender red areas over the legs. In complicated cases, eye inflammation, high blood calcium levels, liver and kidney problems, heart rhythm problems, and skin lesions may occur.

How Is Sarcoidosis Diagnosed?

The diagnosis is difficult, because people may not have symptoms, and other disorders can cause similar problems. The doctor will do a physical examination and order a chest x-ray. The x-ray is often abnormal and the physical examination may be normal. The doctor may want blood tests, breathing tests, computed tomography (CT), tissue biopsy, tuberculosis (TB) tests, and electrocardiography (ECG). If the doctor needs a lung sample for diagnosis, a procedure called bronchoscopy will be done by a lung specialist (pulmonologist). The doctor puts a flexible tube through the nose into the lungs. If results are unclear, surgery to open the lungs and get a more extensive piece of tissue (open lung biopsy) may be done.

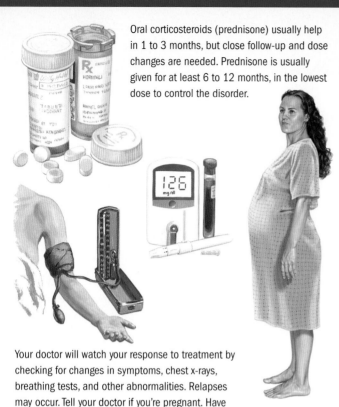

Oral corticosteroids (prednisone) usually help in 1 to 3 months, but close follow-up and dose changes are needed. Prednisone is usually given for at least 6 to 12 months, in the lowest dose to control the disorder.

Your doctor will watch your response to treatment by checking for changes in symptoms, chest x-rays, breathing tests, and other abnormalities. Relapses may occur. Tell your doctor if you're pregnant. Have your blood pressure checked and blood tested for diabetes while you're taking steroids.

Take care of your health. Don't smoke. Smoking makes symptoms worse. Eat a low-salt diet if you take steroids, to avoid fluid gain. Get flu and pneumococcal pneumonia shots. Don't get too much sun.

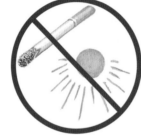

Call your doctor if you have fever, chills, vision changes, chest pain, or palpitations.

How Is Sarcoidosis Treated?

Many people get better without treatment, especially in earlier stages and people without symptoms. However, in people with severe symptoms, treatment may be needed for several weeks to years. Oral corticosteroids (prednisone) usually help in 1 to 3 months, but close follow-up and dose changes are necessary. Prednisone is usually given for at least 6 to 12 months. Usually, the lowest dose to control sarcoidosis is used. Response to treatment is checked by watching for changes in symptoms, chest x-rays, breathing tests, and other abnormalities. Relapses may occur. For severe progressive disease not responding to prednisone, more powerful medications, such as methotrexate, azathioprine, or hydroxychloroquine, may be used.

DOs and DON'Ts in Managing Sarcoidosis:

✔ **DO** tell your doctor about your medicines (prescription and over-the-counter).

✔ **DO** tell your doctor if you're pregnant.

✔ **DO** eat a low-salt diet if you take steroids, to prevent fluid gain.

✔ **DO** have your blood pressure checked and blood tested for diabetes while taking steroids.

✔ **DO** get a flu shot each fall.

✔ **DO** get vaccinated for pneumococcal pneumonia.

✔ **DO** call your doctor if you're very thirsty, urinate a lot, or have weight changes. It could indicate a very high sugar level from prednisone.

✔ **DO** call your doctor if you cough discolored sputum or blood.

✔ **DO** call your doctor if you have fever, chills, vision changes, chest pain, or palpitations.

✔ **DO** call your doctor if your symptoms don't get better or get worse.

⊘ **DON'T** stop taking your medicine or change your dosage because you feel better, unless your doctor tells you to.

⊘ **DON'T** smoke. Smoking makes symptoms worse.

⊘ **DON'T** get too much direct sun exposure. It will make any skin rash from sarcoidosis worse.

FROM THE DESK OF

NOTES

FOR MORE INFORMATION

Contact the following sources:

• National Sarcoidosis Resources Center
  Tel: (732) 699-0733
  Website: http://www.nsrc-global.net

• American Lung Association
  Tel: (800) LUNG-USA (586-4872)
  Website: http://www.lungusa.org

MANAGING YOUR
SILICOSIS

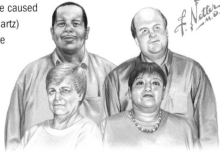

Silicosis is a lung disease caused by breathing in silica (quartz) dust. It can lead to severe respiratory disability.

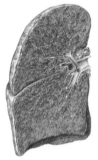

Lung with simple silicosis

Lung with complicated silicosis

In silicosis, first, small rounded nodules develop when silica collects in the lung. Then, the number and size of the nodules may increase. Nodules later join together to make large masses and scar the lungs, which can make the lungs work poorly. This condition is called progressive fibrosis.

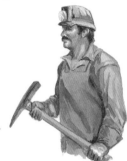

Silica exposures usually occur on the job. Industries in which workers are at risk include metal working (in factories), mining, road and building construction, quarrying, sandblasting, and stone cutting.

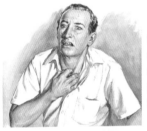

Early silicosis doesn't cause symptoms or significantly hurt lung function. Later, shortness of breath and dry cough are the most common symptoms with progressive fibrosis. Fever and weight loss are others.

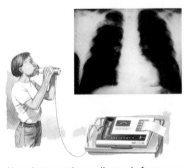

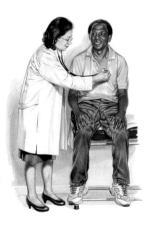

Your doctor makes a diagnosis from your physical exam, job history, and chest x-ray. Breathing tests may be needed to help determine impairment in lung function.

What Is Silicosis?

Silicosis is a lung disease caused by breathing in silica (quartz) dust. Silica is a crystal that occurs naturally, in sand and in rock beds. It becomes dust during mining and working with metal ores. In silicosis, first, small rounded nodules (lumps) develop when the silica collects in the lung. Then, the number and size of the nodules may increase. The nodules later join together to make large masses and scar the lungs, which can make the lungs work poorly. This condition is called progressive fibrosis.

The risk of having silicosis depends mainly on how much and how long people are exposed to silica dust. Years of exposure are usually needed for the illness to develop. However, symptoms may occur in months with shorter but more intense periods of breathing in the silica.

What Causes Silicosis?

Silica exposures usually occur on the job. Industries in which workers are at risk include metal working (in factories), mining, road and building construction, quarrying, sandblasting, stone cutting, and ceramics and abrasives manufacturing.

What Are the Symptoms of Silicosis?

Symptoms may vary. Early in the disease, silicosis doesn't cause symptoms or hurt lung function. With chronic, repeated exposure, the disease progresses and may decrease life span. Some people may have the disease progress, even after silica exposures stop. Shortness of breath and dry cough are the most common symptoms, with progressive, massive fibrosis. Fever and weight loss are others. Severe respiratory disability may lead to early death.

How Is Silicosis Diagnosed?

The doctor makes a diagnosis from the job history, physical examination, and chest x-ray. Breathing tests may be needed to determine the extent of damage. In some cases a lung biopsy may be done. In a biopsy, the doctor removes a small piece of lung for study with a microscope. Having silicosis increases the risk of developing tuberculosis, a serious lung infection. If silicosis is diagnosed, a tuberculin skin test should be done to check for tuberculosis.

If silicosis is diagnosed, a tuberculin skin test should be done. Silicosis increases the risk of TB. A positive test means that exposure to TB bacteria occurred. If the test is positive, medicine is needed to help prevent TB.

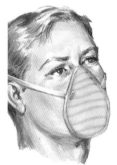

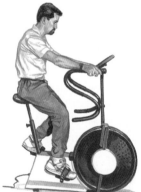

No treatments can reduce the number of lung nodules or prevent progressive fibrosis. More exposure to silica should be avoided. Use special industrial protection measures, such as wearing dust masks and respirators. Some people with severe progressive lung disease may need lung transplantation.

Get a flu shot each fall and get vaccinated for pneumococcal pneumonia.

Maintain good cardiovascular fitness by exercising.

Stop smoking.

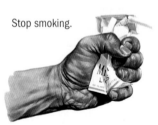

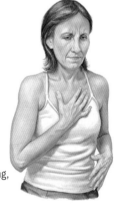

Call your doctor if you have a lung infection, weight loss, chest pain, blood in your sputum, ankle swelling, or dusky skin, fingertips, or lips.

How Is Silicosis Treated?

No treatments are known to reduce the number of silica nodules in the lung or to prevent development of progressive fibrosis. Workers whose chest x-rays show silicosis changes should avoid more exposure to silica. Some people with severe progressive lung disease may need lung transplantation.

DOs and DON'Ts in Managing Silicosis:

✔ **DO** get a flu shot each fall.

✔ **DO** get vaccinated for pneumococcal pneumonia.

✔ **DO** maintain good cardiovascular fitness by exercising.

✔ **DO** call your doctor if you think that you have a lung infection as suggested by symptoms. Such symptoms include a sudden worsening of cough, yellow or green sputum, increased shortness of breath, and fever or chills.

✔ **DO** call your doctor if you have weight loss, chest pain, or blood in your sputum.

✔ **DO** call your doctor if you have dusky skin, fingertips, or lips.

✔ **DO** call your doctor if you have new ankle swelling.

⊘ **DON'T** expose yourself to inhaled silica. Use special industrial protection measures, such as wearing dust masks and respirators.

⊘ **DON'T** expose yourself to smoke, fumes, and very cold or very humid air. These conditions may irritate the lungs.

⊘ **DON'T** smoke.

FROM THE DESK OF

NOTES

FOR MORE INFORMATION

Contact the following source:

• American Lung Association
  Tel: (800) LUNG-USA (586-4872)
  Website: http://www.lungusa.org

MANAGING YOUR
SMOKE INHALATION

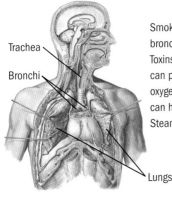

Smoke inhalation occurs when people breathe in soot and toxic fumes, often during a fire. Some fumes given off by substances when they melt or burn are poisonous. They damage the lungs and tubes leading to them.

Trachea

Bronchi

Lungs

Smoke can cause the windpipe and bronchi to swell, so it's hard to breathe. Toxins (cyanide and carbon monoxide) can prevent lungs from absorbing enough oxygen. Without enough oxygen, people can have trouble thinking and pass out. Steam can burn the throat and lungs.

Symptoms include:

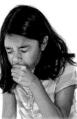

Red, teary eyes

Coughing, wheezing

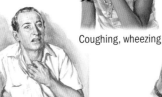

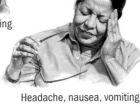

Trouble breathing

Headache, nausea, vomiting

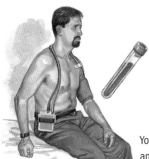

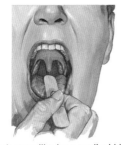

Your doctor will take a medical history and examine you, especially your throat and lungs. Blood (arterial blood gases) and carbon monoxide levels will be tested. A chest x-ray may be done.

What Is Smoke Inhalation?

Smoke inhalation occurs when people breathe in soot and toxic fumes, often during a fire. Some fumes given off by substances when they melt or burn are poisonous. They damage the lungs and tubes leading to them, called the trachea (windpipe) and bronchi.

Smoke can cause the trachea and bronchi to swell, so it's hard to breathe. Toxins (such as cyanide and carbon monoxide) can also hurt the lungs preventing them from absorbing enough oxygen. Without enough oxygen getting to the brain, people can have trouble thinking and pass out. Steam that is breathed in can burn the throat and lungs.

What Causes Smoke Inhalation?

The cause is exposure to fumes during a fire.

What Are the Symptoms of Smoke Inhalation?

Symptoms include coughing, wheezing, or sounding hoarse. Eyes may be red and teary. Soot in and around the mouth, singed nose hairs, and facial burns can be seen.

Poisoning by carbon monoxide can cause headaches, nausea, vomiting, confusion, vision problems, or loss of consciousness.

How Is Smoke Inhalation Diagnosed?

The doctor makes a diagnosis from a medical history and physical examination, especially of the throat and lungs. A chest x-ray may be done to check for fluid accumulations in the lungs and lung damage. A blood test (arterial blood gases) measures levels of oxygen and other gases in the blood. Other tests measure carbon monoxide levels.

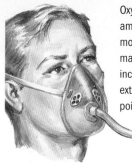

Oxygen treatment may start at the fire or in an ambulance. In the hospital emergency room, more oxygen is given (by mask or nose tube) to make sure breathing is good. Other treatments include suction to remove debris from lungs, extra fluids (for burn victims), and antidotes for poisons such as cyanide.

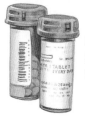

Infection is a risk after smoke inhalation. Antibiotics are given for infections such as pneumonia.

Recovery time depends on how much smoke and poison were inhaled. Minor smoke damage heals in 2 to 3 days with no lasting effects. Go for follow-up appointments as your doctor advises, to avoid serious complications.

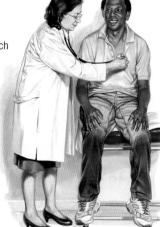

EMERGENCY ROOM

Remember to have fire and carbon monoxide alarms throughout your house. Smoke inhalation is an emergency.

How Is Smoke Inhalation Treated?

Oxygen treatment may be given at the site of the fire or in an ambulance on the way to the hospital. Oxygen is critical. In the hospital emergency room, more treatment is given to make sure that people can breathe well and get enough oxygen. People are usually observed for 4 to 12 hours. If the smoke inhalation is not severe and they do well, they may be able to leave the hospital after a few hours. Some people may need to see their doctor in 12 to 24 hours for a follow-up visit.

For breathing problems, more oxygen may be given at the hospital. A mask or nose tube is used. Sometimes, oxygen under high pressure (hyperbaric oxygen) is given. A special oxygen chamber can take out carbon monoxide from the body faster than regular oxygen can. Sometimes inhalers with bronchodilators are given for easier breathing.

Some people with a swollen windpipe can have a tube placed in the windpipe to help breathing. Other treatments include suction to remove debris from lungs, extra fluids (for burn victims), antidotes for poisons such as cyanide, and antibiotics for infections such as pneumonia.

Recovery occurs in stages. Total recovery time depends on how much smoke and poison were inhaled. People with minor smoke damage recover in 2 to 3 days with no lasting effects. People with severe injuries may need several weeks in the hospital and may have long-lasting breathing problems.

DOs and DON'Ts in Managing Smoke Inhalation:

✔ **DO** call 911 and go to the closest emergency department if you suffer smoke inhalation.

✔ **DO** call your doctor if you have a lasting cough, shortness of breath, or fatigue.

⊘ **DON'T** forget to follow up with your doctor after your discharge from the hospital.

FROM THE DESK OF

NOTES

FOR MORE INFORMATION

Contact the following sources:

• World Burn Foundation
 Tel: (310) 858-1717
 **Website: http://www.burnsurvivorsonline.com/injuries/
 inhalation.asp**

• American Lung Association
 Tel: (212) 315-8700, (800) 586-4872
 Website: http://www.lungusa.org

MANAGING YOUR
WEGENER'S GRANULOMATOSIS

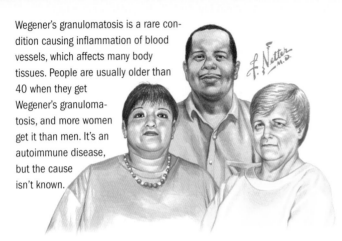

Wegener's granulomatosis is a rare condition causing inflammation of blood vessels, which affects many body tissues. People are usually older than 40 when they get Wegener's granulomatosis, and more women get it than men. It's an autoimmune disease, but the cause isn't known.

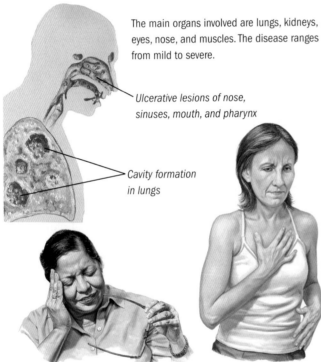

The main organs involved are lungs, kidneys, eyes, nose, and muscles. The disease ranges from mild to severe.

Ulcerative lesions of nose, sinuses, mouth, and pharynx

Cavity formation in lungs

Signs and symptoms include shortness of breath, cough, fevers, weight loss, nosebleeds, chest pain, eye inflammation, weakness, neurological symptoms, and kidney disease (puffy face, swollen legs).

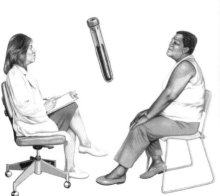

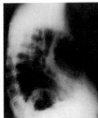

Your doctor will make a diagnosis from your medical history, physical examination, blood tests, x-rays, and biopsy.

What Is Wegener's Granulomatosis?

Wegener's granulomatosis is a rare condition causing inflammation of blood vessels, which affects many body tissues. The main organs involved are the lungs, kidneys, eyes, nose, and muscles. The disease ranges from mild to severe, with kidney failure, shortness of breath with damage to the respiratory system, or eye pain.

People are usually older than 40 when they get it, women more than men.

What Causes Wegener's Granulomatosis?

The cause isn't known. Wegener's is an autoimmune disease, which means that the body's own immune system makes proteins (antibodies) that attack cells and cause damage. It's not inherited or contagious.

What Are the Symptoms of Wegener's Granulomatosis?

Symptoms include shortness of breath, cough, fevers, weight loss, nosebleeds, redness and roughness of the lining of the nose, chest pain, eye inflammation, weakness, neurological symptoms similar to strokes, and kidney disease (puffy face, swollen legs).

How Is Wegener's Granulomatosis Diagnosed?

The doctor will make a diagnosis from a medical history, physical examination, blood tests, x-rays, and biopsy of one or more affected organs.

An antibody (ANCA antibody) can be found in the blood of most affected people and has been linked to Wegener's granulomatosis.

How Is Wegener's Granulomatosis Treated?

Treatment seems to help most symptoms. People can become debilitated and depressed, especially if they don't respond to therapy.

The two main treatments are steroid medicine, such as prednisone, and other medicines called cyclophosphamide or azathioprine. Trimethoprim-sulfamethoxazole may reduce the number of relapses.

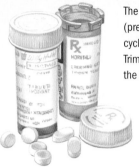

The two main treatments are steroid medicine (prednisone) and another medicine called cyclophosphamide or azathioprine. Trimethoprim-sulfamethoxazole may reduce the number of relapses.

For severe disease, the doctor may give intravenous medicine in the hospital and a special type of blood treatment (plasmapheresis).

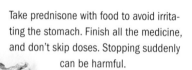

Take prednisone with food to avoid irritating the stomach. Finish all the medicine, and don't skip doses. Stopping suddenly can be harmful.

Exercise. Stay as active as possible to minimize the time spent recovering. But don't overdo it!

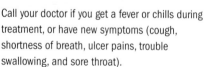

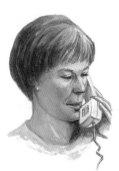

Call your doctor if you get a fever or chills during treatment, or have new symptoms (cough, shortness of breath, ulcer pains, trouble swallowing, and sore throat).

For severe disease, the doctor may give intravenous medicine in the hospital and may order a special type of blood treatment (plasmapheresis). In this treatment, antibodies in the blood are removed quickly, and fresh proteins are given.

DOs and DON'Ts in Managing Wegener's Granulomatosis:

✔ **DO** take prednisone with food to avoid irritating the stomach. Take the full course of medicine because stopping suddenly can be harmful.

✔ **DO** eat well and use supplements as needed, to avoid getting debilitated. Your dietitian can help.

✔ **DO** follow the diet used by diabetic patients, if your blood sugar goes up with prednisone.

✔ **DO** exercise. Stay as active as possible to minimize the time spent recovering. People who are bed bound have a slower recovery.

✔ **DO** keep your doctor appointments. People taking these drugs need close supervision.

✔ **DO** call your doctor if you have symptoms related to treatment, get a fever or chills during treatment, or have any concerns.

✔ **DO** call your doctor if you have new symptoms (cough, shortness of breath, ulcer pains, trouble swallowing, and sore throat).

⊘ **DON'T** take over-the-counter medicines unless your doctor says you can.

⊘ **DON'T** skip doses of prednisone. To do so can be harmful.

⊘ **DON'T** cheat on dietary advice. People with high blood glucose levels (mild diabetes) and kidney problems need to restrict food intake to avoid serious illness.

⊘ **DON'T** overdo work or exercise.

FROM THE DESK OF

NOTES

FOR MORE INFORMATION

Contact the following source:

• National Kidney and Urologic Diseases Information Clearinghouse
Tel: (800) 891-5390
Website: http://kidney.niddk.nih.gov/

Pertussis is also called whooping cough because the cough can sound like a whoop or bark. It's caused by the kind of bacteria named *Bordetella pertussis*.

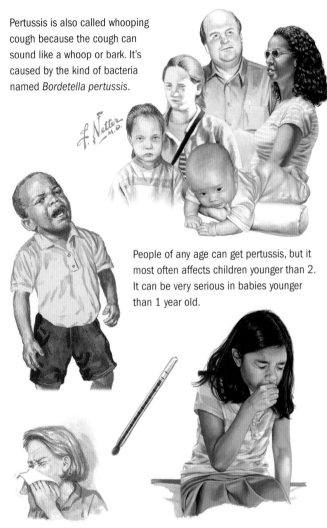

People of any age can get pertussis, but it most often affects children younger than 2. It can be very serious in babies younger than 1 year old.

Symptoms first seem like those of a cold, with a mild cough, but then the cough becomes a dry, severe whooping cough that lasts more than 2 weeks. Other symptoms include slight fever, flushing (red face), loss of appetite, feeling sick, pink eyes, runny nose, and sweating.

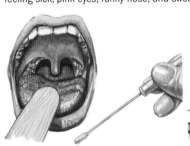

The doctor will examine the ears, nose, and throat. A swab on the throat and nose may be done to take a sample and make sure that another infection is not causing symptoms. Blood tests and chest x-ray may also be needed.

What Is Pertussis?

Pertussis is also called whooping cough because the cough can sound like a whoop or bark. People of any age can get pertussis but it most often infects children younger than 2. It can be very serious in babies younger than 1 year old.

People with pertussis can cough for a long time, to the point of getting exhausted. The infection starts with flu-like symptoms that turn into a severe cough, which can last up to a few weeks.

What Causes Pertussis?

Pertussis is caused by the kind of bacteria named *Bordetella pertussis*.

What Are the Symptoms of Pertussis?

Symptoms first seem like those of a cold, with a mild cough, but then, in 1 week, the cough becomes a dry, severe whooping cough that lasts more than 2 weeks. Long coughing spells occur, and coughing bursts often happening at night, with an average of 15 spells in 24 hours. The whoop isn't always heard. Most children don't have fever during the coughing. Other common symptoms include slight fever, flushing (red face), loss of appetite, feeling sick, pink eyes, runny nose, and sweating.

How Is Pertussis Diagnosed?

The doctor will ask about the medical history and do an examination, paying attention to ears, nose, and throat. The doctor may use a swab on the throat and nose to take a sample and make sure that another infection isn't causing symptoms. Blood tests and chest x-ray may also be needed.

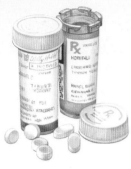

Children and adults can usually be treated at home. The doctor will prescribe antibiotics. Warm fluids such as apple juice can help the cough. Do not self-medicate with regular cough or allergy medicines—these can at times make symptoms worse.

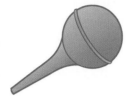

The nose and throat need to be kept clear of thick mucus. You can do this with salt water and a bulb syringe once your doctor shows you how.

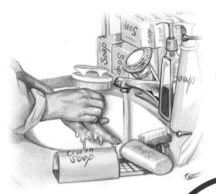

Frequent hand washing is important to avoid spreading the infection.

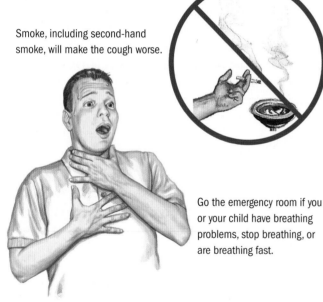

Smoke, including second-hand smoke, will make the cough worse.

Go the emergency room if you or your child have breathing problems, stop breathing, or are breathing fast.

How Is Pertussis Treated?

Children and adults can usually be treated at home. The doctor will prescribe antibiotics. Warm fluids such as apple juice can help the cough. It's important to keep the nose and throat clear of thick mucus to make it easier to breathe. The doctor can show you how to do this with salt water and a bulb syringe. Putting a humidifier in a bedroom can also help breathing.

Pertussis spreads easily, so people who have it should stay away from others. Frequent hand washing is important to avoid spreading the infection. Also, family members and other contacts will need treatment to protect them from infection.

DOs and DON'Ts in Managing Pertussis:

✔ **DO** make sure that your children get vaccinations for pertussis.
✔ **DO** make sure that you or your child drinks plenty of fluids.
✔ **DO** make sure that you or your child stays away from smells or smoke that can make the cough worse.
✔ **DO** use good hand-washing practices, especially after being with someone who's sick. Hand washing is important to avoid spreading infection.
✔ **DO** call your doctor right away or go to the emergency room if you or your child has breathing problems, stops breathing, or is breathing fast; cannot drink; has a high fever; has a seizure; has blue hands, face, or feet; or is very tired or sluggish.

⊘ **DON'T** stop taking medicine or change the dosage because you feel better unless the doctor says to do so.
⊘ **DON'T** try to treat pertussis with cough or allergy medicines. These can at times make symptoms worse.

FROM THE DESK OF

NOTES

FOR MORE INFORMATION

Contact the following source:
• Centers for Disease Control and Prevention
Tel: (800) 311-3435
Website: http://www.cdc.gov

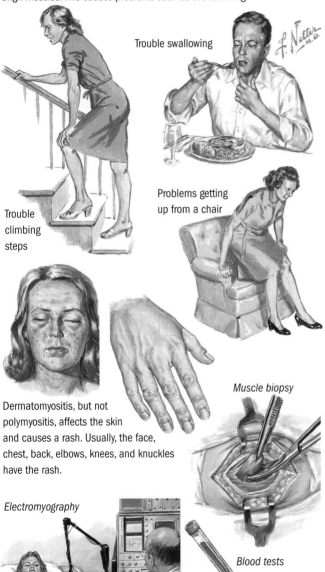

Dermatomyositis and polymyositis are rare diseases that cause inflammation and weakness of the muscles. They affect both adults (ages 45 to 60) and children (ages 10 to 15), more females than males. The cause is unknown, but they are thought to be autoimmune disorders.

Symptoms include weakness of neck, shoulder, upper arm, hip, and thigh muscles. This causes problems such as the following:

Trouble swallowing

Trouble climbing steps

Problems getting up from a chair

Dermatomyositis, but not polymyositis, affects the skin and causes a rash. Usually, the face, chest, back, elbows, knees, and knuckles have the rash.

Muscle biopsy

Electromyography

Blood tests

Your doctor makes a diagnosis with physical examination, blood tests, electromyography, and muscle biopsy.

What Are Dermatomyositis and Polymyositis?

Dermatomyositis and polymyositis are rare diseases that cause inflammation and weakness of muscles. They affect both adults (ages 45 to 60) and children (ages 10 to 15), more females than males.

What Causes Dermatomyositis and Polymyositis?

The cause is unknown, but they are thought to be autoimmune disorders. In autoimmune disorders, the immune system attacks the body's own tissues. Small blood vessels in muscles get damaged, which weakens muscle fibers and makes them break down. The disorders aren't contagious or passed from parents to children.

What Are the Symptoms of Dermatomyositis and Polymyositis?

Symptoms of dermatomyositis are a rash (on the face, chest, back, elbows, knees, and knuckles) and weakness of neck, shoulder, upper arm, hip, and thigh muscles. People may have trouble getting out of chairs, climbing stairs, lifting things, or reaching over their heads. Sometimes, trouble swallowing, sore muscles, tiredness, fever, hard bumps under the skin, and weight loss occur. The disease may also affect the lungs, heart, or gut. No rash occurs in polymyositis, but other symptoms are the same.

How Are Dermatomyositis and Polymyositis Diagnosed?

The doctor makes a diagnosis based on your history, physical examination, blood tests, electromyography, and muscle biopsy. Blood tests can show muscle breakdown, inflammation, or antibodies. Electromyography measures how muscles are working. In a biopsy, the doctor removes a small piece of muscle that is sent for study.

How Are Dermatomyositis and Polymyositis Treated?

Treatments may help the rash and muscle strength improve, but some muscles may be permanently weak. However, treatment may last for months or even years. Sometimes, the disease goes away on its own.

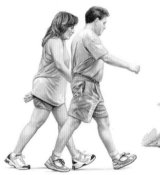

Treatments may help the rash and muscle strength improve. Corticosteroid drugs, especially prednisone, are the main treatment for inflammation. If they don't work, immunosuppressants and immunoglobulins may be tried. You may need to take steroids for a long time, so learn about side effects.

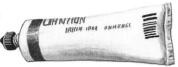

For the rash, hydroxychloroquine and/or medicated skin cream (such as prednisone and tacrolimus) can be used.

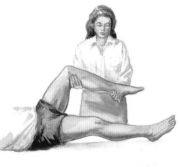

Muscle exercises are an important part of treatment, for flexibility and muscle strength. A physical therapist can create the right exercise program for you. Keeping active will help stop your muscles from getting weaker, but don't push your body too hard. Learn to pace yourself. Rest when you're tired.

Call your doctor or go to the hospital if you have trouble swallowing or breathing.

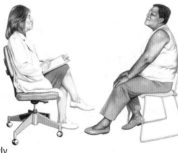

Treatment may last for years. You may need frequent blood tests. Don't stop taking medicines without talking to your doctor when stopping. Prednisone, if used for a long time, must be tapered off slowly.

FROM THE DESK OF

NOTES

Corticosteroid drugs, especially prednisone, are the main treatment for inflammation. If corticosteroids don't work, immunosuppressant drugs and immunoglobulins may be tried. Skin cream (such as prednisone and tacrolimus) may be used for the rash.

Muscle exercises are an important part of treatment. They're for flexibility and help strengthen muscles. A physical therapist can create the right exercise program.

DOs and DON'Ts in Managing Dermatomyositis and Polymyositis:

✔ **DO** get treatment as soon as possible. Early treatment gets better results.

✔ **DO** tell your doctor if you have medicine side effects.

✔ **DO** see your doctor right away if you have trouble swallowing or shortness of breath.

✔ **DO** keep active. This will help keep your muscles from getting weaker. Do your physical therapy exercises.

✔ **DO** cover your skin or wear strong sunscreen when you go out.

✔ **DO** remember that treatments may be needed for years. You may need frequent blood tests to monitor your disease and side-effects of the medications. About half of people have a remission and stop therapy within 5 years of diagnosis. The others will have active disease that needs ongoing treatment or inactive disease with permanent muscle weakness.

✔ **DO** understand that the disease may be related to an increased risk of cancers of the colon, breast, and ovary.

✔ **DO** call your doctor if you have increasing muscle weakness.

⊘ **DON'T** push your body too hard. Learn to pace yourself. Rest when you're tired.

⊘ **DON'T** miss follow-up appointments.

⊘ **DON'T** stop taking medicines without talking to your doctor. Prednisone, if used for a long time, must be tapered off rather than stopped suddenly.

FOR MORE INFORMATION

Contact the following sources:

- The Myositis Association
  Tel: (202) 887-0088, (800) 821-7356
  Website: http://www.myositis.org

- National Organization for Rare Disorders
  Tel: (800) 999-6673, (203) 744-0100
  Website: http://www.rarediseases.org

- National Institute of Arthritis and Musculoskeletal and Skin Diseases
  Tel: (301) 496-8188
  Website: http://www.niams.nih.gov

Dupuytren's contracture is a condition affecting the hands. Tissue inside the palm tightens so fingers curl down toward the palm and stay there. The hands become hard to use. The condition isn't life-threatening, but it can lead to disability.

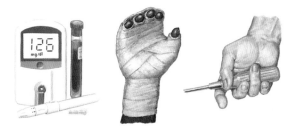

It's more common in older people, manual laborers, and in those who had a hand injury. It's also slightly more common in people who abuse alcohol; smoke; or have HIV infection.

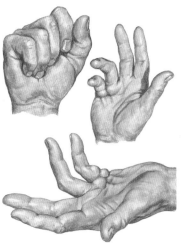

Curling of the fingers toward the palm is the main symptom. People often first notice it when it's hard to reach for something. The little finger and finger next to it (ring finger) are most often affected. The skin on the palm may pucker. One or more lumps may be felt in the palm.

Your doctor makes a diagnosis by looking at your hand. The doctor can find a painless nodule (lump) on the palm. Attempts to extend the finger lead to skin blanching.

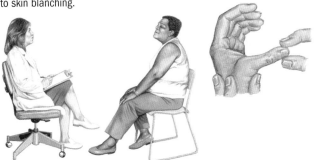

What Is Dupuytren's Contracture?

Dupuytren's contracture is a condition affecting the hands. Tissue inside the palm tightens so fingers curl down toward the palm (contract) and stay there. It may occur in one hand only, but often both hands have this problem. In time, the hands become hard to use. Dupuytren's contracture is most common between ages 40 and 65. The condition isn't life-threatening, but it doesn't go away and can lead to disability.

What Causes Dupuytren's Contracture?

The cause is unknown, but the disorder isn't contagious. It sometimes runs in families. It's slightly more common in people with a history of hand injury and certain conditions such as diabetes, epilepsy, and HIV infection.

What Are the Symptoms of Dupuytren's Contracture?

Curling of the fingers toward the palm and a small painless lump in the middle of the hand are the main symptoms. People often first notice it when it's hard to reach for something. The little finger and finger next to it (ring finger) are most often affected. Eventually, the hand can't be placed flat on a surface. Usually there's no pain, but people may have discomfort when trying to hold something. The skin on the palm may pucker.

How Is Dupuytren's Contracture Diagnosed?

The doctor makes a diagnosis by looking at the hand. The doctor may find a painless nodule (lump) on the palm. The nodule feels hard and ends in a band that goes from the finger to the palm. In time, it's very hard to straighten the finger. The skin over the finger has thin grooves and pits. Attempts to extend the finger lead to skin blanching (whitening).

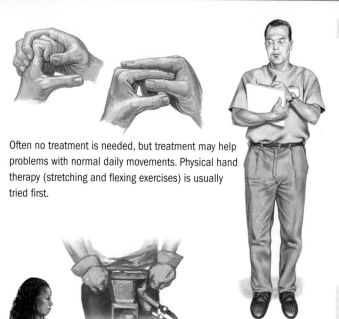

Often no treatment is needed, but treatment may help problems with normal daily movements. Physical hand therapy (stretching and flexing exercises) is usually tried first.

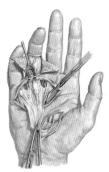

Specially made tools, such as door handles and jar openers, may make daily activities easier. Don't move your hands the same way over and over. Don't put your hands where they get a lot of vibration.

Medicines (collagenase or corticosteroids) can be injected into the hand to slow the disease progress.

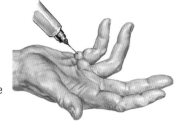

Surgery done by a hand surgeon (orthopedic or plastic surgeon) may help people with significant trouble using their hands. Tissue in the palm is divided or removed, so fingers can return to their normal position.

How Is Dupuytren's Contracture Treated?

Often no treatment is needed, but treatment may help problems with normal daily movements. Physical therapy (stretching and flexing exercises) is usually tried first. Occupational therapy can be used early and after an operation. Specially made tools, such as door handles and jar openers, may make daily activities easier. Splinting of the finger is generally ineffective. Medicines (collagenase or corticosteroids) can be injected into the hand to slow the disease progress. Surgery done by a hand surgeon (orthopedic or plastic surgeon) may help people with significant trouble using their hands. Tissue in the palm is divided or removed. This lets fingers to return to their normal position. The problem can recur, however.

DOs and DON'Ts in Managing Dupuytren's Contracture:

✔ **DO** control contributing factors such as diabetes, epilepsy, and repetitive hand trauma.

✔ **DO** wear protective gloves when doing manual work.

🚫 **DON'T** stop using your hands in a normal everyday way, as much as possible.

🚫 **DON'T** put your hands in a position where they could get injured.

🚫 **DON'T** move your hands the same way over and over. Avoid putting your hands where they get a lot of vibration.

FROM THE DESK OF

NOTES

FOR MORE INFORMATION

Contact the following sources:

• American Academy of Orthopaedic Surgeons
  Tel: (847) 823-7186
  Website: http://www.aaos.org

• Curtis National Hand Center
  Tel: (410) 235-5405
  Website: http://www.unionmemorial.org/hand.cfm

Ehlers-Danlos syndrome is a rare inherited disease that changes connective tissues of the body, which support and bind other tissues. The disorder mainly affects skin and joints but can also affect eyes and blood vessels.

Chromosome with genes

The cause is probably a mutation of a gene. At least 11 different types of the syndrome exist. Types I, II, and III make up almost 90% of the cases.

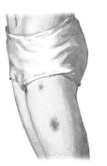

Symptoms are fragile skin that bruises easily and rubbery elastic skin that's very stretchy. Joints are very movable so that a finger can extend back onto the wrist. Hips and other joints can dislocate easily.

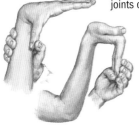

Your doctor makes a diagnosis from a physical examination and family history of the disorder. Genetic and biochemical tests are available for some syndrome types. Sometimes a skin biopsy is done.

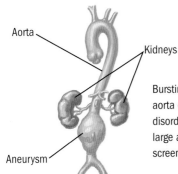

Aorta

Kidneys

Bursting of blood vessels such as the aorta can cause sudden death. The disorder can cause aneurysms, so the large abdominal aorta should be screened yearly.

Aneurysm

What Is Ehlers-Danlos Syndrome?

Ehlers-Danlos syndrome is a rare disease that involves connective tissues of the body, which support and bind other tissues. The disorder mainly affects skin and joints but can also affect the eyes and blood vessels. This disorder is inherited—parents pass it to their children.

No cure exists. Most people have normal life spans, but the type that involves blood vessels could mean a shortened life.

What Causes Ehlers-Danlos Syndrome?

The cause is probably a mutation (change or defect) of a gene. At least 11 different types of the syndrome exist. Types I, II, and III make up almost 90% of the cases.

What Are the Symptoms of Ehlers-Danlos Syndrome?

Symptoms are fragile skin that bruises easily and rubbery elastic skin that's very stretchy. Joints are very movable so that a finger can extend back onto the wrist. Hips and other joints can dislocate easily. Arthritis can occur because of repeated joint dislocations. Other possible manifestations are mitral valve prolapse (leaking of the mitral heart valve), flat feet, and curved spine.

Complications include slow and poor healing of cuts or wounds. In type IV syndrome, muscular walls of the arteries, intestine, and bladder can weaken and burst. Bursting of blood vessels such as the aorta can cause sudden death. The disorder can cause aneurysms (dilations of arteries), so the large abdominal aorta should be screened yearly.

How Is Ehlers-Danlos Syndrome Diagnosed?

The doctor makes a diagnosis by a physical examination and a family history of the disorder. Genetic and biochemical tests are available for some syndrome types. Sometimes a skin biopsy is done. In a biopsy, the doctor gets a small piece of skin with a needle and checks it with a microscope.

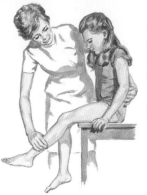

Treatment is supportive and symptomatic, so affected joints are braced, protected, and supported. Exercises and physical therapy are important for stable joints. A physical therapist can teach you muscle-strengthening exercises.

How Is Ehlers-Danlos Syndrome Treated?

Treatment is supportive and symptomatic, so affected joints are braced, protected, and supported. No treatment can reverse the disorder. Surgery must be done carefully, because people heal poorly, and connective tissues that hold the stitches are defective. If an aneurysm is found, the doctor may suggest surgery or close monitoring, depending on its size.

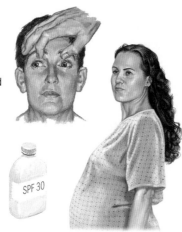

If you have type IV syndrome, pregnancy should be discussed before you try to conceive. Always use sunscreen to protect your skin. Get yearly eye examinations.

SPF 30

DOs and DON'Ts in Managing Ehlers-Danlos Syndrome:

✔ **DO** understand that in type IV syndrome, pregnancy should be discussed before you try to conceive. Bleeding, bursting of the uterus, and tearing of internal tissues can complicate the pregnancy.

✔ **DO** use sunscreen.

✔ **DO** get yearly eye examinations. Nearsightedness is common, and you may need prescription glasses.

✔ **DO** call your doctor if you have a family history of this syndrome.

✔ **DO** call your doctor if you need a referral to specialists in this syndrome.

✔ **DO** call your doctor if you have bleeding, sudden abdominal pain, visual problems, or joint pain, swelling, or deformity.

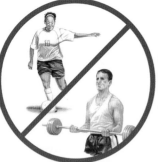

Don't participate in competitive sports. Contact sports, weightlifting, and exerting yourself for long periods can cause joint injury, dislocations, and damage to body structures.

🚫 **DON'T** participate in competitive sports. Contact sports, weightlifting, and exerting yourself for long periods can cause joint injury, dislocations, and damage to body structures. Talk to a physical therapist about muscle-strengthening exercises.

🚫 **DON'T** miss appointments. Don't be afraid to ask your doctor for another opinion from a specialist in this syndrome.

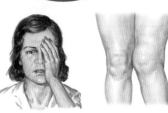

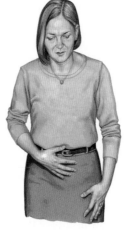

Call your doctor if you have bleeding, sudden abdominal pain, visual problems, or joint pain, swelling, or deformity.

FROM THE DESK OF

NOTES

FOR MORE INFORMATION

Contact the following sources:

- Ehlers-Danlos National Foundation
  Tel: (213) 368-3800
  Website: http://www.ednf.org

- National Organization for Rare Disorders
  Tel: (800) 999-6673
  Website: http://www.rarediseases.org

Erythema nodosum (EN) is a skin condition resulting from inflammation of fat and other tissues under the skin. Large red nodules form, most often on the lower legs, but they can appear on other places. EN is more common in young women, but anyone can get it.

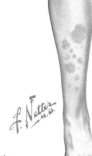

Birth control pills, sulfa drugs, and penicillin are the most common causes. Infections, sarcoidosis, ulcerative colitis, Crohn's disease, thyroid conditions, lupus, and pregnancy are others. Many times, the cause isn't known.

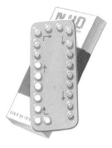

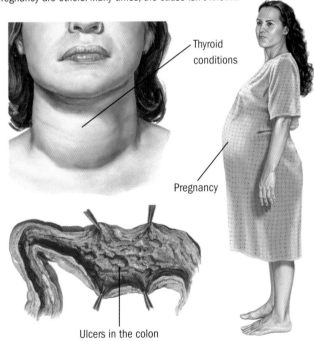

Thyroid conditions

Pregnancy

Ulcers in the colon

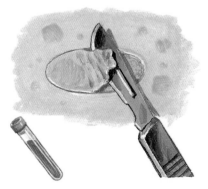

Your doctor may believe that you have EN because of the look of the rash. The nodules look like bruises and change color. A skin biopsy and blood tests may be done to confirm the diagnosis.

What Is Erythema Nodosum?

Erythema nodosum (EN) is a skin condition involving inflammation (swelling) of fat and other tissues under the skin. Red nodules (small round masses) form on the legs, thighs, lower arms, and other parts of the body. EN is more common in young women, but anyone can get it.

What Causes EN?

The most common causes are drugs (especially birth control pills, penicillin, and sulfa medicines) and infections. Sarcoidosis, ulcerative colitis, Crohn's disease, thyroid conditions, lupus, and pregnancy are other causes. Many times, the cause is unknown.

What Are the Symptoms of EN?

The main symptom is large red nodules on lower legs. The nodules are usually painful or tender, are warm to touch, and appear suddenly. Nodules look like bruises and slowly change from pink to red to bluish to brown over 7 to 10 days. The nodules usually go away within 8 weeks, but new ones may form, so recovery may take several weeks or months. Fever and swollen ankles and knees often occur.

How Is EN Diagnosed?

The doctor makes a diagnosis by the look of the nodules. Sometimes, a skin biopsy sample is needed. In a biopsy, a small piece of skin is removed and studied with a microscope. A medical history, physical examination, chest x-ray, and blood tests may help find out whether something specific is the cause.

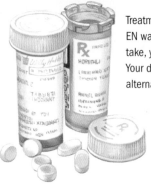

Treatment depends on the cause. If EN was caused by medicine that you take, you may need to stop taking it. Your doctor will work with you to find alternatives.

Taking aspirin or other over-the-counter medicine and NSAIDs may help pain and inflammation.

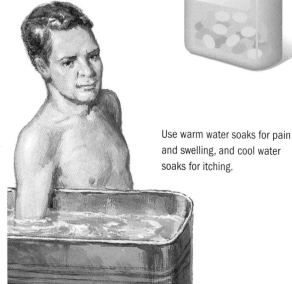

Use warm water soaks for pain and swelling, and cool water soaks for itching.

Reduce swelling by keeping your legs raised as much as possible.

How Is EN Treated?

Treatment depends on the cause. For example, if a drug is the cause, it may have to be stopped. If an infection is found, medicine will be used to treat it.

Some things can ease pain and discomfort. These include keeping the legs raised as much as possible and wearing support stockings (for swelling). Taking aspirin or other over-the-counter medicine and nonsteroidal antiinflammatory drugs (NSAIDs) may help reduce pain and inflammation. Use warm water soaks for pain and swelling, and cool water soaks for itching. Severe cases may need steroid drugs such as prednisone.

DOs and DON'Ts in Managing Erythema Nodosum:

✔ **DO** take your medicines as prescribed.
✔ **DO** follow your doctor's treatment instructions.
✔ **DO** ask your doctor which over-the-counter medicines you may take with your prescription drugs.
✔ **DO** call your doctor if you have side effects from your medicines.
✔ **DO** call your doctor if treatment isn't improving your symptoms in a reasonable amount of time.
✔ **DO** call your doctor if you get new, unexplained symptoms.

🚫 **DON'T** use drugs and other substances that may have caused EN.

FROM THE DESK OF

NOTES

FOR MORE INFORMATION

Contact the following sources:
- American Academy of Dermatology
  Tel: (866) 503-7546
  Website: http://www.aad.org
- Arthritis Foundation
  Tel: (800) 283-7800
  Website: http://www.arthritis.org.

Giant cell arteritis is a condition that causes arteries to become inflamed or swollen. The cause is unknown. It almost always occurs in people older than 50, more women than men.

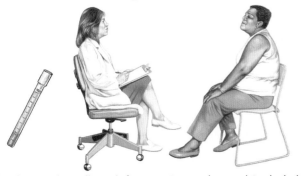

It's also called temporal arteritis because the temporal arteries, which are at the temples on both sides of the head, are the ones usually affected, but any arteries can be inflamed.

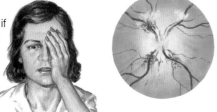

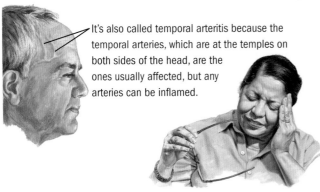

Most symptoms are related to the head and face: headaches; scalp tenderness, especially over the temples; pain in the jaw or tongue when chewing or talking; blurred or double vision; and flu-like symptoms.

Blindness can result if arteries taking blood to the eyes are involved.

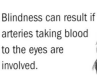

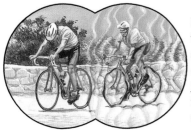

Your doctor makes a diagnosis from symptoms and a complete physical. A special blood test called the erythrocyte sedimentation rate, which measures inflammation, will be done.

What Is Giant Cell Arteritis?

Giant cell arteritis is a condition that causes arteries to become inflamed or swollen. It's also called temporal arteritis because the temporal arteries, which are at the temples on both sides of the head, are the ones usually affected. However, arteries in any part of the body can be inflamed. Inflammation can lead to narrowing of an artery, which sometimes becomes completely blocked. This then reduces the blood supply to nearby tissues and organs. Blindness can result if arteries taking blood to the eyes are involved.

What Causes Giant Cell Arteritis?

The cause is unknown. It almost always occurs in people older than 50, more women than men. Another disorder called polymyalgia rheumatica often occurs with giant cell arteritis. Polymyalgia rheumatica causes stiffness and aching in the back, shoulders, and hips.

What Are the Symptoms of Giant Cell Arteritis?

Most symptoms are related to the head and face. They include headaches; scalp tenderness, especially over the temples; pain in the jaw or tongue when chewing or talking; blurred or double vision; and flu-like symptoms (muscle aches, joint stiffness, fever, fatigue, and loss of appetite).

How Is Giant Cell Arteritis Diagnosed?

The doctor makes a diagnosis from symptoms and a complete physical examination. A special blood test (erythrocyte sedimentation rate), which measures inflammation, will be done. This rate is very high in this disorder. The doctor may also do a biopsy of the temporal artery. The doctor will remove a small piece of artery and check it with a microscope for signs of inflammation. A chest x-ray may also be done since giant cell arteritis carries an increased risk of aneurysm (abnormal enlargement) of the aorta, the main artery that brings blood to body parts.

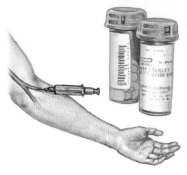

A corticosteroid such as prednisone is given, usually at the same dose for the first month. With improvement, the dose can slowly be reduced. Treatment will probably last 1 to 2 years. People with vision loss or impairment can receive corticosteroids intravenously.

Understand the side effects from prednisone. Long-term use can cause cataracts, peptic ulcer disease, osteoporosis, diabetes, and hypertension.

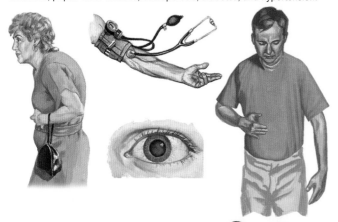

Don't miss follow-up doctor visits. Your doctor must monitor your symptoms and do periodic blood tests (sedimentation rate).

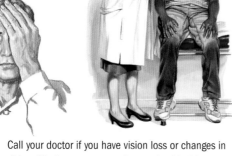

Call your doctor if you have vision loss or changes in vision. Blindness can occur in people with this disorder. Also call your doctor if you have new headaches with fever or pain when chewing food.

How Is Giant Cell Arteritis Treated?

A corticosteroid such as prednisone is given, usually starting at 40 to 60 mg per day. The same dose is continued for the first month. If symptoms and sedimentation rate improve, the dose can slowly be reduced (tapered). The treatment will probably last 1 to 2 years.

People with vision loss or impairment at the time of diagnosis may be given intravenous methylprednisolone for the initial 3 to 5 days of treatment.

DOs and DON'Ts in Managing Giant Cell Arteritis:

✔ **DO** take medicines as prescribed. Symptoms usually improve after a few days, but continuing your medicine as directed is important. Don't change your dosage or stop the medicine unless your doctor tells you to.

✔ **DO** report medicine side effects to your doctor.

✔ **DO** see your doctor if you don't see improvement in a week or so.

✔ **DO** understand the side effects from prednisone. Long-term use can cause cataracts, peptic ulcer disease, osteoporosis, diabetes, and hypertension.

✔ **DO** call your doctor for vision loss or changes in vision.

✔ **DO** call your doctor if you have new headaches with fever or pain when chewing food.

🚫 **DON'T** miss follow-up doctor visits. Your doctor must monitor your symptoms and do periodic blood tests (sedimentation rate).

🚫 **DON'T** forget that prednisone therapy may be needed for 1 to 2 years to prevent the disease from coming back.

🚫 **DON'T** ignore visual problems. Blindness can occur in people with giant cell arteritis.

FROM THE DESK OF

NOTES

FOR MORE INFORMATION

Contact the following sources:

• American College of Rheumatology
  Tel: (404) 633-3777
  Website: http://www.rheumatology.org

• National Institute of Arthritis and Musculoskeletal and Skin Diseases
  Tel: (301) 496-8188
  Website: http://www.niams.nih.gov

CARING FOR YOUR CHILD WITH
JUVENILE RHEUMATOID ARTHRITIS

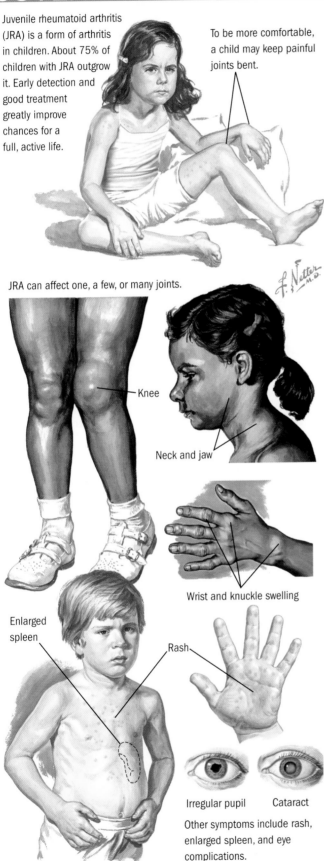

Juvenile rheumatoid arthritis (JRA) is a form of arthritis in children. About 75% of children with JRA outgrow it. Early detection and good treatment greatly improve chances for a full, active life.

To be more comfortable, a child may keep painful joints bent.

JRA can affect one, a few, or many joints.

Knee

Neck and jaw

Wrist and knuckle swelling

Enlarged spleen

Rash

Irregular pupil   Cataract

Other symptoms include rash, enlarged spleen, and eye complications.

What Is Juvenile Rheumatoid Arthritis?

Juvenile rheumatoid arthritis (JRA) is a form of arthritis in children. It is also known as "juvenile idiopathic arthritis" and "Still's disease." JRA differs from adult rheumatoid arthritis. It is a chronic disease and last for months or years, but about 75% of children outgrow it. No cure exists, but earlier detection, better drugs, and good treatment greatly improve chances for a full, active life.

JRA can make it hard to do daily activities such as writing, dressing, and carrying things (hands, wrists); walking, playing, and standing (hips, knees, feet); and turning the head (neck).

What Causes JRA?

JRA is an autoimmune disorder but its cause is unknown. Autoimmune means that the body's infection-fighting (immune) system attacks its own tissues. Genetic and environmental factors may increase chances of getting JRA. JRA cannot be caught from another person.

What Are the Symptoms of JRA?

Symptoms include joint pain and stiffness that are usually worse in the morning but get better toward the end of the day. Children may hold painful joints close to the body or bent. The three JRA types are pauciarticular, polyarticular, and systemic.

Pauciarticular JRA affects only a few joints (normally less than four: knees, elbows, and ankles) and occurs in 50% of children with JRA, more often in girls. Eye disease (inflammation, or swelling) can develop.

Polyarticular JRA affects many joints and occurs in about 30% of children with JRA, more commonly in girls. Neck, knees, ankles, feet, wrists, and hands are affected. Children with this type may also have eye inflammation.

Systemic JRA occurs in about 20% of children with JRA, boys and girls equally. It often starts with fever, rash, changes in blood cells, and joint pain.

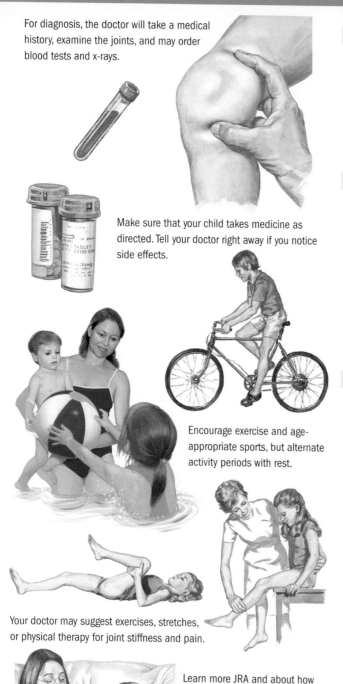

For diagnosis, the doctor will take a medical history, examine the joints, and may order blood tests and x-rays.

Make sure that your child takes medicine as directed. Tell your doctor right away if you notice side effects.

Encourage exercise and age-appropriate sports, but alternate activity periods with rest.

Your doctor may suggest exercises, stretches, or physical therapy for joint stiffness and pain.

Learn more JRA and about how you can help your child. Talk with teachers and school nurses about available services. Local or online support groups can also help.

How Is JRA Diagnosed?

The doctor takes a medical history, examines the joints, and may order laboratory tests and x-rays. Testing for the specific blood proteins rheumatoid factor (RF) and antinuclear antibody (ANA) may help diagnosis. Systemic JRA may be hard to diagnose because inflammation may not start right away.

How Is JRA Treated?

A combination of medicines, therapies, exercise, education, and pacing activities to prevent tiredness is best. A doctor who treats arthritis should care for your child.

Medicines for inflammation include nonsteroidal antiinflammatory drugs (NSAIDs). Disease-modifying drugs (such as methotrexate) can also be tried.

Exercise is important for joint movement and muscle strength. Splints can help rest painful, swollen joints.

DOs and DON'Ts in Managing JRA:

✔ **DO** have your child take prescribed medicines.
✔ **DO** call the doctor if your child has medicine side effects.
✔ **DO** encourage exercising.
✔ **DO** encourage your child to participate in many of the same activities as other children, but alternate activities with rest.
✔ **DO** speak to your child's teachers and school nurse. Ask about school services to help your child.
✔ **DO** call your child's doctor if medicines don't help or if you need referrals to physical or occupational therapists.

⊘ **DON'T** give up. If one drug doesn't work, talk with your child's doctor about changing to a different one.
⊘ **DON'T** have your child continue with exercises that make the symptoms worse. Speak with the doctor about alternate exercises.
⊘ **DON'T** forget to have your child get regular eye examinations. Some drugs can affect the eyes.

FROM THE DESK OF

NOTES

FOR MORE INFORMATION

Contact the following source:

• Arthritis Foundation
  Tel: (800) 283-7800
  Website: http://www.arthritis.org

CARING FOR YOUR CHILD WITH KAWASAKI DISEASE

Kawasaki disease (KD) is a rare condition that causes inflammation of blood vessels and several other manifestations. KD usually occurs in children younger than 5, more boys than girls. It's the leading cause of acquired heart disease in children.

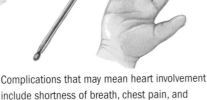

Symptoms include fever that lasts for more than 5 days; red swollen eyes; cracked lips; strawberry-colored tongue; red, swollen, sore throat; swollen neck lymph glands; and rash on the trunk and limbs.

Complications that may mean heart involvement include shortness of breath, chest pain, and symptoms of congestive heart failure, including leg swelling.

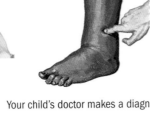

Your child's doctor makes a diagnosis from the symptoms and physical exam. The doctor may also order blood tests, x-rays, echocardiography, and cardiac catheterization.

Cardiac catheterization

Echocardiography, a kind of ultrasonography, uses sound waves to examine the heart. In catheterization, the doctor puts a tube into the leg artery and moves it up into heart arteries. Dye is then injected and can show blocked arteries.

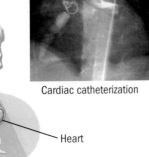

Heart

Echocardiography

What Is Kawasaki Disease?

Kawasaki disease (KD) is a rare condition that causes inflammation of blood vessels (vasculitis) and several other manifestations noted below. KD usually occurs in children younger than 5, more often in boys than girls. In the United States, about 4000 new cases are diagnosed each year. It's the leading cause of acquired heart disease in children.

What Causes KD?

The cause is unknown, but an infectious agent may trigger the inflammation. KD isn't contagious, however. It is not a hereditary disorder.

What Are the Symptoms of KD?

Symptoms include fever that lasts for more than 5 days, and is associated with red swollen eyes (conjunctivitis); cracking lips; strawberry-colored tongue; red, swollen, sore throat; swollen lymph glands in the neck; and rash on the trunk and limbs. Complications that may mean heart involvement include shortness of breath; chest pain; and symptoms of congestive heart failure, such as leg swelling, being unable to lie flat in bed, suddenly waking up short of breath, and shortness of breath with exertion.

How Is KD Diagnosed?

The doctor makes a diagnosis from physical examination and symptoms: fever lasting more than 5 days plus four of five other features. These features include inflammation of the whites of the eyes (conjunctivitis) and swollen eyes; mucous membrane changes (red tongue and dry, cracked lips); swollen hands and feet; swollen neck lymph glands; and rash on the trunk of the body.

The doctor may order blood tests and x-rays, but no specific blood test can diagnose KD.

For suspected heart involvement, echocardiography (a sonogram of the heart) and cardiac catheterization can be done. In catheterization, the doctor puts a tube into the leg artery and moves it up into heart arteries. Dye is then injected to show blockages in coronary (heart) arteries.

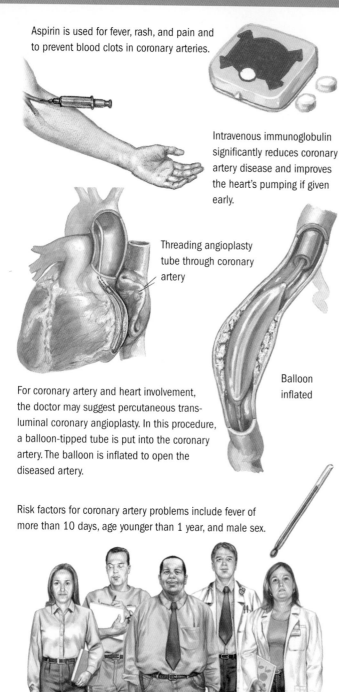

Aspirin is used for fever, rash, and pain and to prevent blood clots in coronary arteries.

Intravenous immunoglobulin significantly reduces coronary artery disease and improves the heart's pumping if given early.

Threading angioplasty tube through coronary artery

Balloon inflated

For coronary artery and heart involvement, the doctor may suggest percutaneous trans-luminal coronary angioplasty. In this procedure, a balloon-tipped tube is put into the coronary artery. The balloon is inflated to open the diseased artery.

Risk factors for coronary artery problems include fever of more than 10 days, age younger than 1 year, and male sex.

Don't forget that KD is a rare disease that needs a medical team who have experience with this condition.

FROM THE DESK OF

NOTES

How Is KD Treated?

Aspirin is used for fever, rash, and pain and to prevent blood clots in coronary arteries. Intravenous immunoglobulin can significantly reduce coronary artery disease and improve the heart's pumping if given early. For coronary artery and heart involvement, the doctor may suggest percutaneous transluminal coronary angioplasty. In this procedure, a balloon-tipped tube is put into the coronary artery. The balloon is inflated to open the diseased artery. A child with many diseased vessels may have coronary artery bypass surgery. Heart transplant may sometimes be considered.

DOs and DON'Ts in Managing KD:

✔ **DO** remember that nearly 20% of children may have heart damage.
✔ **DO** understand that risk factors for coronary artery problems are fever of more than 10 days, age younger than 1 year, and male sex.
✔ **DO** call your child's doctor if your child has a fever, rash, or shortness of breath.
✔ **DO** call your child's doctor if you see swollen lymph glands in the neck.
✔ **DO** call your child's doctor if you need a second opinion.

🚫 **DON'T** forget that KD is a rare disease that requires care from a team of doctors who have experience with this condition.
🚫 **DON'T** be afraid to ask for a second opinion.
🚫 **DON'T** ignore symptoms.

FOR MORE INFORMATION

Contact the following sources:

• Kawasaki Disease Foundation
  Tel: (978) 356-2070
  Website: http://www.kdfoundation.org

• American Heart Association
  Tel: (800) 242-8721
  Website: http://www.americanheart.org

• American College of Cardiology
  Tel: (800) 253-4636
  Website: http://www.acc.org

Polymyalgia rheumatica (PMR) is an inflammation of the muscles. Muscles around the neck, shoulders, buttocks, hips, and thighs get painful and stiff. It usually affects people older than 50.

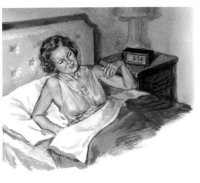

Many people have trouble rolling over in bed or getting out of bed. The cause is unknown, but it may be an autoimmune condition.

Muscle stiffness and pain, worse in the morning, most often affect the hips, neck, arms, shoulders, back, and thighs. Other symptoms are fever, poor appetite, tiredness, weight loss, and joint pain, stiffness, and swelling.

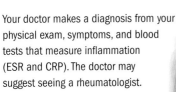

Your doctor makes a diagnosis from your physical exam, symptoms, and blood tests that measure inflammation (ESR and CRP). The doctor may suggest seeing a rheumatologist.

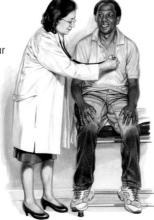

What Is Polymyalgia Rheumatica (PMR)?

Polymyalgia rheumatica (PMR) is an inflammation of the muscles. Muscles around the neck, shoulders, buttocks, hips, and thighs get painful and stiff. Many people have trouble rolling over in bed or getting out of bed. It usually affects people older than 50.

What Causes PMR?

The cause is unknown, but it may be an autoimmune condition. In an autoimmune disorder, the body's immune system attacks the body itself. PMR isn't contagious or hereditary.

What Are the Symptoms of PMR?

Muscle stiffness and pain most commonly affect the hips, neck, arms, shoulders, back, and thighs. Symptoms are worse in the morning and tend to get better during the day. Other symptoms include poor appetite, sadness and depression, tiredness, weight loss, fever, sweats, and restless and disturbed sleep. Joint pain, stiffness, and swelling may occur. Some people also have a condition called giant cell arteritis (temporal arteritis), which may cause headaches and sudden vision changes.

How Is PMR Diagnosed?

The doctor makes a diagnosis from the physical examination, symptoms, and blood tests that measure inflammation. Two blood tests commonly performed are erythrocyte sedimentation rate (ESR) and C-reactive protein (CRP) level. Other blood tests may be done to be sure that another problem isn't present. The doctor may suggest seeing a rheumatologist (specialist in joint and muscle disorders).

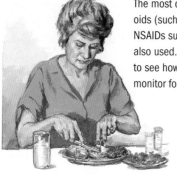

The most common treatment is corticosteroids (such as prednisone), taken with food. NSAIDs such as ibuprofen are sometimes also used. Regular blood tests are needed to see how the treatment is working and to monitor for medicine side effects.

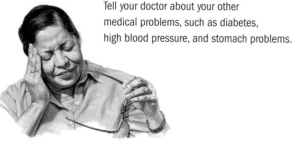

Exercise at least 30 minutes daily. Exercise can help ease the pain. Ask your doctor which exercise is best for you.

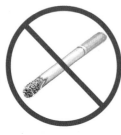

Tell your doctor about your other medical problems, such as diabetes, high blood pressure, and stomach problems.

Call your doctor if your pain or stiffness returns during treatment. Call if you have new headaches, cramping in your tongue or jaw, or sudden changes in vision.

Keep healthy: stop smoking. Try to control your weight. See your eye doctor yearly.

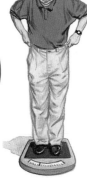

How Is PMR Treated?

Treatment leads to improvement in almost all symptoms in a few days. Treatment may be necessary for several months or often up to 2 to 3 years. The most common treatment is corticosteroids (such as prednisone), taken with food. Nonsteroidal antiinflammatory drugs (NSAIDs) such as ibuprofen are sometimes also used. Corticosteroids can cause increased appetite, weight gain, trouble sleeping, easy bruising, and stomach upset. Longer term use can lower resistance to infection and cause stomach ulcers and bone thinning (osteoporosis). Regular blood tests are needed to see how the treatment is working. People should receive enough calcium and vitamin D to prevent osteoporosis.

A regular exercise program can help ease the pain.

DOs and DON'Ts in Managing PMR:

✔ **DO** tell your doctor about your other medical problems (diabetes, high blood pressure, stomach problems).

✔ **DO** tell your doctor about your medicines, including prescription and over-the-counter drugs.

✔ **DO** take your steroid medicine with food.

✔ **DO** ask your doctor about how to keep your bones strong.

✔ **DO** have your blood pressure checked and blood tested for diabetes while you take prednisone.

✔ **DO** see your eye doctor yearly.

✔ **DO** exercise, at least 30 minutes daily. Ask your doctor which exercise is best for you.

✔ **DO** try to control your weight.

✔ **DO** stop smoking.

✔ **DO** call your doctor if you have medicine side effects.

✔ **DO** call your doctor if your pain or stiffness returns during treatment.

✔ **DO** call your doctor if you have new headaches, cramping in your tongue or jaw, or sudden changes in vision.

⊘ **DON'T** stop taking your medicine or change your dosage because you feel better unless your doctor tells you to.

FROM THE DESK OF

NOTES

FOR MORE INFORMATION

Contact the following sources:

• American College of Rheumatology
  Tel: (404) 633-3777
  Website: http://www.rheumatology.org

• Arthritis Foundation
  Tel: (800) 283-7800
  Website: http://www.arthritis.org

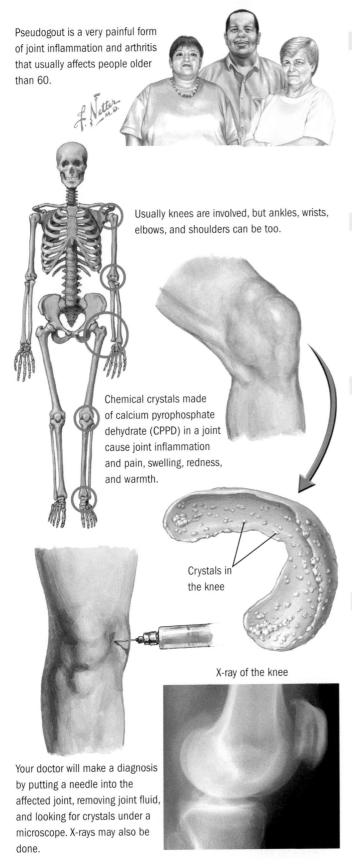

Pseudogout is a very painful form of joint inflammation and arthritis that usually affects people older than 60.

Usually knees are involved, but ankles, wrists, elbows, and shoulders can be too.

Chemical crystals made of calcium pyrophosphate dehydrate (CPPD) in a joint cause joint inflammation and pain, swelling, redness, and warmth.

Crystals in the knee

X-ray of the knee

Your doctor will make a diagnosis by putting a needle into the affected joint, removing joint fluid, and looking for crystals under a microscope. X-rays may also be done.

What Is Pseudogout?

Pseudogout is a very painful form of joint inflammation and arthritis that usually affects people older than 60. Normally only one joint at a time, usually knees, is involved. Other joints affected are ankles, wrists, elbows, and shoulders. Because it's similar to gout but has a different cause, it's called pseudogout, meaning false gout.

About 5% of people over age 60 get pseudogout.

What Causes Pseudogout?

Release and accumulation of chemical crystals into a joint causes the attacks. These crystals, made of calcium pyrophosphate dehydrate (CPPD), cause joint inflammation (redness, swelling). Why some people get pseudogout and others don't isn't clear. It's not caused by an infection and is not contagious.

What Are the Symptoms of Pseudogout?

Symptoms are joint pain, swelling, warmth, and redness that start quickly. Pain is often constant and gets worse if the joint is moved. Activities such as walking, dressing, and lifting may be hard. Sometimes, more than one joint is involved.

Attacks may occur at any time, but certain events such as surgery or an illness can trigger them. Symptoms usually go away within days after treatment; untreated they may last for several weeks or more. Between attacks, most people have no symptoms.

How Is Pseudogout Diagnosed?

The only way to be certain of the diagnosis is to put a needle into the affected joint, remove joint fluid, and look for pseudogout crystals under a microscope.

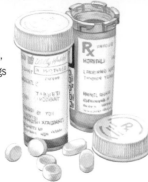

There's no way to get rid of the crystals, but medicine can help symptoms. Drugs include NSAIDs, such as ibuprofen, naproxen, or indomethacin, or stronger medicines, such as prednisone or colchicine.

Removal of joint fluid and then cortisone injection into the joint is another common treatment.

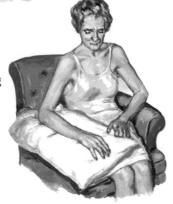

Regardless of the treatment, resting the affected joint is important until symptoms go away.

How Is Pseudogout Treated?

There's no way to get rid of the crystals, but medicine can help symptoms. Nonsteroidal antiinflammatory drugs (NSAIDs), such as ibuprofen, naproxen, or indomethacin, are used for treatment.

Sometimes, stronger antiinflammatory medicines, such as prednisone or colchicine, are needed.

Removal of joint fluid followed by cortisone injection into the joint is another common treatment. Cortisone injections usually give the fastest and most complete relief of pain and swelling.

Regardless of the treatment, it is important to rest the affected joint until symptoms start to go away.

DOs and DON'Ts in Managing Pseudogout:

✔ **DO** rest the affected joint until you start to get better.

✔ **DO** take your medicines as prescribed.

✔ **DO** call your doctor if treatment isn't improving symptoms, you start to lose full motion in the affected joint, or you have worsening warmth, redness, or pain after a cortisone injection.

⊘ **DON'T** wait to see whether side effects of medicine will go away. Call your doctor.

FROM THE DESK OF

NOTES

FOR MORE INFORMATION

Contact the following sources:

• The Arthritis Foundation
Tel: (800) 283-7800
Website: http://www.arthritis.org

• American College of Rheumatology
Tel: (404) 633-3777
Website: http://www.rheumatology.org

MANAGING YOUR
RAYNAUD'S PHENOMENON

Raynaud's phenomenon is a condition causing reduced blood flow to the fingers, toes, ears, and tip of the nose. It usually occurs with exposure to cold temperatures. It may happen at any age, but usually people 20 to 40 years old have it, more women than men.

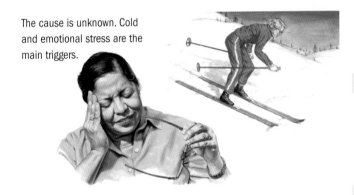

The cause is unknown. Cold and emotional stress are the main triggers.

Skin on fingers turns white, then blue, and then purple or red. Attacks may last a few minutes to hours. Sores or ulcers may develop. With low blood flow for a long time, skin could turn black and die. Pain, tingling, and numbness can occur when areas turn white. Swelling, warmth, or throbbing can occur when areas turn purple or red. Some cases are mild.

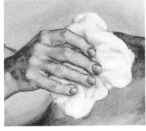

Your doctor makes a diagnosis from your medical history and examination. The doctor may do blood tests to find out about other conditions.

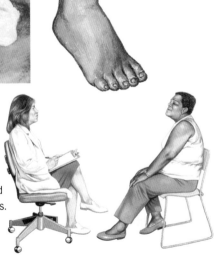

What Is Raynaud's Phenomenon?

Raynaud's phenomenon is a condition causing decreased blood flow to the fingers, toes, ears, and tip of the nose. It usually occurs with exposure to cold temperatures. Skin in the area first turns white, then blue, and then purple or red. These attacks may last from a few minutes to several hours. Without treatment, sores or ulcers may develop. With low blood flow for a long time, skin in affected areas could be permanently damaged.

Raynaud's phenomenon may occur at any age, but usually people 20 to 40 years old have it, more women than men.

What Causes Raynaud's Phenomenon?

The cause is unknown. Cold and emotional stress are the main triggers. It's not contagious. Raynaud's phenomenon may be associated with more severe diseases such as scleroderma.

What Are the Symptoms of Raynaud's Phenomenon?

Fingers lose color (turn white) when exposed to cold. Pain, tingling, and numbness can occur when the areas turn white. Areas later turn bluish and then red. Some people have swelling, warmth, or throbbing when the areas turn purple or red. Toes, nose, and ears can also be affected.

How Is Raynaud's Phenomenon Diagnosed?

The doctor makes a diagnosis from a medical history and physical examination. Blood tests may be done to find out whether other conditions are present. The doctor may put a person's hands in cold water to test the body's reaction to cold.

You must keep warm. Dress in layers, wear lined mittens instead of gloves, wear a hat and scarf, and always carry a sweater. To avoid exposure to cold, have someone warm the car in the winter, and use an oven mitt to get items out of the refrigerator and freezer.

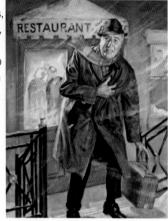

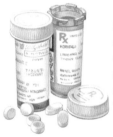

For a severe condition, the doctor may prescribe calcium channel blockers (such as amlodipine) to decrease spasm in arteries on the surface of the skin and improve blood flow. If these treatments don't help, surgery may be done to cut nerves that cause blood vessels to spasm and close.

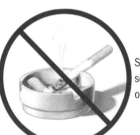

If emotional stress causes attacks, relaxation and biofeedback may help.

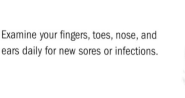

Stop smoking! Smoking worsens circulation so less blood flows to affected areas. Sores or infections can develop in those areas.

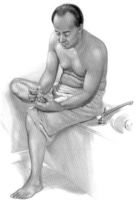

Examine your fingers, toes, nose, and ears daily for new sores or infections.

How Is Raynaud's Phenomenon Treated?

The best way to manage the phenomenon is by a combination of therapies and prevention. To keep the body warm, dress in layers, wear lined mittens rather than gloves, wear a hat and scarf, and always carry a sweater. To avoid exposure to cold, have someone warm the car in the winter, use an oven mitt to get items out of the refrigerator and freezer, and warm the bathroom by letting warm water run before taking a shower or bath.

Smoking impairs circulation so less blood flows to affected areas. Sores or infections have a greater chance of developing in those areas. People with this condition must stop smoking.

If emotional stress seems to cause an attack, relaxation and biofeedback may help.

For a severe condition, the doctor may prescribe calcium channel blockers (such as amlodipine) that can improve blood flow by decreasing spasm. If these medicines don't help and symptoms are severe, surgery called sympathectomy may be suggested. This surgery involves cutting nerves that cause blood vessels to contract and decrease blood flow.

Most people lead fairly normal lives by following the doctor's advice. People who work outside or have jobs exposing the body to cold temperatures should try to modify the job or look for another job.

DOs and DON'Ts in Managing Raynaud's Phenomenon:

✔ **DO** wear gloves if you're exposed to cold.
✔ **DO** stop smoking. Smoking further impairs circulation.
✔ **DO** check your fingers, toes, nose, and ears daily for new sores or infections.
✔ **DO** call your doctor if treatments don't help your symptoms.
✔ **DO** call your doctor if you need a referral to a smoking cessation program.

⊘ **DON'T** get too nervous; emotional stress may trigger attacks.

FROM THE DESK OF

NOTES

FOR MORE INFORMATION

Contact the following sources:

• National Heart, Lung, and Blood Institute
Tel: (301) 592-8573
Website: http://www.nhlbi.nih.gov

• Arthritis Foundation
Tel: (800) 283-7800
Website: http://www.arthritis.org

MANAGING YOUR
RHEUMATOID ARTHRITIS

Rheumatoid arthritis (RA) is a disease that causes joint inflammation. The cause isn't known, but it's an autoimmune disorder, meaning that the body's own defense system against disease attacks healthy cells. Two to three times more women than men have RA.

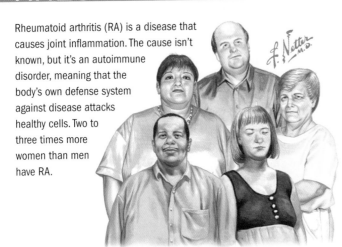

Joints affected most are in the hands, wrists, feet, and knees. Inflammation leads to pain, stiffness, and swelling. Stiffness is usually worse in the morning or after sitting still for a long time.

Other symptoms include dry, burning, or itching eyes; skin nodules; tiredness; leg ulcers; decreased appetite; shortness of breath; and fever.

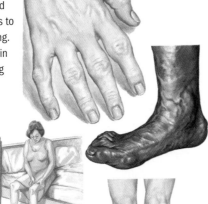

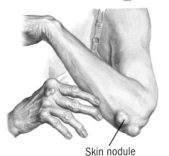

Skin nodule

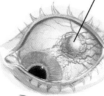

Eye nodule

Your doctor takes your medical history, examines your joints, and orders blood tests and maybe x-rays. Tests may include ESR (to measure inflammation), CBC, and a test called rheumatoid factor.

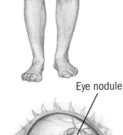

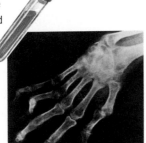

What Is Rheumatoid Arthritis?

Rheumatoid arthritis (RA) is a disease that causes inflammation (swelling, redness) leading to pain, stiffness, and swelling in joints. Affected most often are hands, wrists, feet, and knees. Less common are affects in other body parts, including lungs, eyes, heart, blood vessels, skin, and nerves. RA can affect the ability to do daily activities. RA of hands can affect writing, opening jars, dressing, and carrying items. Arthritis affecting hips, knees, or feet can make it hard to walk, bend, or stand.

RA affects 1% to 5% of adults worldwide. Two to three times more women than men have RA. It's more common during a woman's childbearing years.

There is no cure for RA, but with treatment people with RA can lead full lives.

What Causes RA?

RA is an autoimmune disorder. Autoimmune means that the body's own immune (disease-fighting) system attacks healthy cells. Some inherited and environmental factors may increase a person's chance of getting RA, but the exact cause is unknown. RA is not contagious.

What Are the Symptoms of RA?

The most common symptoms are joint pain and stiffness that is worse in the morning after waking up and after sitting still for a long time. Stiffness usually gets better after movement. Symptoms tend to come and go and can be mild to severe. Other symptoms include burning or itching eyes, tiredness, leg ulcers, reduced appetite, numbness and tingling, shortness of breath, skin nodules, weakness, and fever. Joints can be red, swollen, tender, deformed, and warm.

How Is RA Diagnosed?

The doctor takes a medical history, examines the joints, and orders tests and maybe x-rays. Tests may include erythrocyte sedimentation rate (ESR), which measures inflammation; complete blood cell count (CBC); and a test called rheumatoid factor (RF). Sometimes, fluid from a joint is tested.

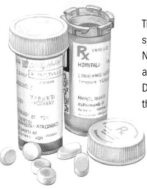

The goal of treatment is to control symptoms. Medicines such as NSAIDs help reduce inflammation and control pain and swelling. Disease-modifying drugs may slow the RA process.

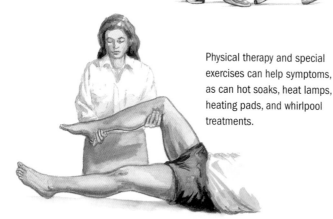

Exercise to maintain joint movement and muscle strength. Talk to your doctor about ways to do this while managing fatigue. If you're overweight, exercising will also help you lose weight.

Physical therapy and special exercises can help symptoms, as can hot soaks, heat lamps, heating pads, and whirlpool treatments.

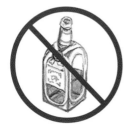

While being treated, don't drink alcohol in excess.

How Is RA Treated?

The best way to manage RA is to use medicines, different therapies, exercise, education, and pacing of activities to prevent fatigue. Medicines called nonsteroidal antiinflammatory drugs (NSAIDs), such as naproxen and ibuprofen, reduce pain and swelling. Disease-modifying drugs may slow the RA process and should be started early.

Learning about RA is essential. Exercise is important for joint movement and muscle strength. Being active plus resting helps fatigue. Physical therapy and special exercises can help symptoms, as can hot soaks, heat lamps, heating pads, and whirlpool treatments. Splints may protect joints. Sometimes surgery is needed to fix a joint.

DOs and DON'Ts in Managing RA:

✔ **DO** tell your doctor about your other medical problems.
✔ **DO** take your medicines as prescribed.
✔ **DO** tell your doctor if you're pregnant or plan to get pregnant.
✔ **DO** lose weight if overweight.
✔ **DO** talk to someone to help with stress.
✔ **DO** exercise.
✔ **DO** call your doctor if you have side effects from medicines or if treatments aren't helping pain, swelling, or fatigue.
✔ **DO** call your doctor right away or go to the emergency room if you have fever with a red, warm joint.

⊘ **DON'T** stop taking your medicine or change your dosage because you feel better unless your doctor says to.
⊘ **DON'T** let yourself get run-down.
⊘ **DON'T** drink alcohol in excess while being treated.

FROM THE DESK OF

NOTES

FOR MORE INFORMATION

Contact the following sources:

• Arthritis Foundation
 Tel: (800) 283-7800
 Website: http://www.arthritis.org

• American College of Rheumatology
 Tel: (404) 644-3777
 Website: http://www.rheumatology.org

MANAGING YOUR
SYSTEMIC LUPUS ERYTHEMATOSUS

Systemic lupus erythematosus (SLE) is a disease that causes inflammation in connective tissue (or collagen) and damage to several organs. SLE can affect joints, skin, lungs, heart, blood vessels, kidneys, nervous system, and blood cells. SLE occurs more frequently in people 15 to 40 years old.

Symptoms depend on which organ is involved. First ones may be fatigue and pain, swelling, or stiffness of joints, usually in hands, wrists, and knees. Joint pain can be severe. A rash may occur on sun-exposed parts of the body, often the face (cheeks and nose), called a butterfly rash because it looks like the wings of a butterfly.

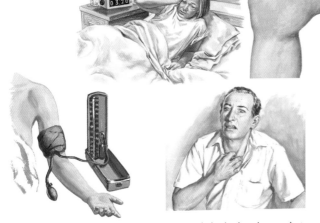

Other symptoms are spasms in the blood vessels in the hands, causing painful fingers and color changing to white and blue (Raynaud's phenomenon), painful breathing with shortness of breath (pleurisy), high blood pressure, and confusion.

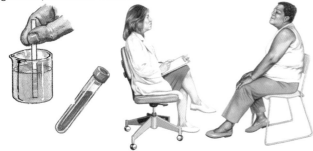

Your doctor makes a diagnosis from your medical history, physical examination, and laboratory tests. X-rays may also be done. Laboratory tests include ESR, CBC, ANA, urinalysis, and anti-DNA test, which is specific for SLE. The doctor may suggest seeing a rheumatologist.

What Is Systemic Lupus Erythematosus (SLE)?

Systemic lupus erythematosus (SLE) is a disease that causes inflammation in connective tissue and can damage several organs. It can affect joints, skin, lungs, heart, blood vessels, kidneys, nervous system, and blood cells. Some people also have Raynaud's phenomenon, which causes spasms in blood vessels, and pain and discoloration in the fingers, toes, ears, and nose.

SLE affects about 1 in 2000 people, five times more women than men; it is most often diagnosed in people 15 to 40 years old. African Americans and people of Asian and Hispanic ancestry get SLE more often than Caucasians.

No cure exists.

What Causes SLE?

The cause is unknown, but hereditary and environmental factors may increase the risk of having SLE. SLE isn't contagious or transmitted from parent to offspring.

What Are the Symptoms of SLE?

Symptoms depend on which organ is involved. The first ones may be fatigue and joint pain, and swelling or stiffness, usually in hands, wrists, and knees. Joint pain can be severe and interfere with activities and work. People may have a rash on sun exposed parts of the body, often the face (cheeks and nose). This is called a butterfly rash. Raynaud's phenomenon makes fingers change color and become painful when exposed to cold. Some people have pleurisy (inflammation of the lining of lungs), which can make breathing painful, with shortness of breath. Affected kidneys may lead to high blood pressure and kidney failure. SLE may affect memory and mood and cause stress or confusion.

How Is SLE Diagnosed?

The doctor makes a diagnosis from a medical history, physical examination, and laboratory tests. X-rays may be done. Laboratory tests include an erythrocyte sedimentation rate (ESR), complete blood cell count (CBC), antinuclear antibody (ANA), and urinalysis. The ESR measures inflammation. The CBC counts blood cells and platelets. The doctor may order an anti-DNA test, which is more specific for SLE. The doctor may suggest seeing a rheumatologist (specialist in joint problems).

Treatment depends on symptoms and which organs are involved. Medicines reduce inflammation. NSAIDs are often given first. Prednisone may also be used. If these don't help, disease-modifying medicines can slow the disease. These include hydroxychloroquine, methotrexate, azathioprine, and cyclophosphamide. If one medicine doesn't work, talk to your doctor about others.

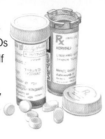

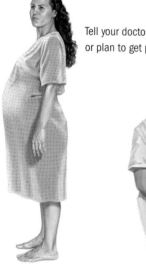

Tell your doctor if you're pregnant or plan to get pregnant.

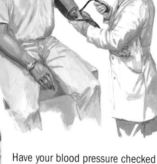

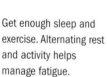

Have your blood pressure checked and blood tested for diabetes while you're taking prednisone. See your eye doctor yearly.

Get enough sleep and exercise. Alternating rest and activity helps manage fatigue.

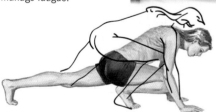

How Is SLE Treated?

Treatment depends on symptoms and which organs are involved. Medicines help reduce inflammation. Nonsteroidal anti-inflammatory drugs (NSAIDs) are often given first. The doctor may also prescribe prednisone, which works quickly. If they don't help enough, disease-modifying medicines can slow the disease. These include hydroxychloroquine, methotrexate, azathioprine, and cyclophosphamide.

Exercise is important for joint movement and muscle strength.

DOs and DON'Ts in Managing SLE:

✔ **DO** tell your doctor if you're pregnant or plan to get pregnant.
✔ **DO** have your blood pressure checked and blood tested for diabetes while you're taking prednisone.
✔ **DO** see your eye doctor yearly.
✔ **DO** get sleep and exercise. Alternating rest and activity helps manage fatigue.
✔ **DO** take your medicines as prescribed. Call your doctor if you have medicine side effects.
✔ **DO** call your doctor if you have a temperature higher than 101° F, blood in urine or stool, shortness of breath, chest pain, or severe stomach pain.

⊘ **DON'T** stop taking your medicine or change your dosage because you feel better unless your doctor tells you to.
⊘ **DON'T** give up. If one medicine doesn't work, talk to your doctor about others.

FROM THE DESK OF

NOTES

FOR MORE INFORMATION

Contact the following sources:

• The Arthritis Foundation
  Tel: (800) 283-7800
  Website: http://www.arthritis.org.

• Lupus Foundation of America
  Tel: (301) 670-9292, (800) 558-0121
  Website: http://www.lupus.org

MANAGING YOUR APPENDICITIS

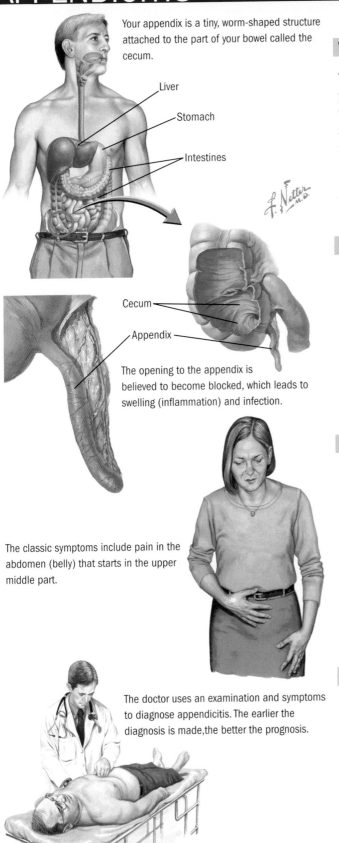

Your appendix is a tiny, worm-shaped structure attached to the part of your bowel called the cecum.

Liver

Stomach

Intestines

Cecum

Appendix

The opening to the appendix is believed to become blocked, which leads to swelling (inflammation) and infection.

The classic symptoms include pain in the abdomen (belly) that starts in the upper middle part.

The doctor uses an examination and symptoms to diagnose appendicitis. The earlier the diagnosis is made, the better the prognosis.

What Is Appendicitis?

The appendix is a tiny, worm-shaped structure attached to the part of the bowel (large intestine) called the cecum. Appendicitis is swelling (inflammation) and infection of the appendix. Although the appendix has no real purpose in the body, an infected appendix can be life-threatening.

Appendicitis occurs in up to 10% of the population, most often in people between 10 and 30 years old. With prompt treatment, appendicitis has an excellent prognosis.

What Causes Appendicitis?

The exact cause is unclear. The opening from the cecum to the appendix becomes blocked (obstructed), which leads to inflammation and growth of bacteria. Infection prevents blood flow, gangrene begins, and the appendix can burst open (rupture, or perforate).

Things that can obstruct the appendix include fecoliths (tiny pieces of undigested vegetable surrounded by stool) and enlarged lymph nodes caused by viruses, parasites, or tumors.

What Are the Symptoms of Appendicitis?

The classic symptom is pain in the abdomen (belly) that starts in the upper middle part. The pain then usually moves down to the right lower corner of the abdomen.

Movement, coughing, and straining make the pain worse. Nausea, vomiting, abdominal swelling, and low-grade fever also occur. Waiting too long before seeking medical care can result in a burst appendix.

A burst appendix is a medical emergecy and can produce an abdominal mass with pain, and a temperature higher than 102° F.

How Is Appendicitis Diagnosed?

The doctor makes a diagnosis by checking symptoms and doing a physical examination. Blood tests may help, but no specific blood tests can diagnose appendicitis. X-rays including ultrasound (using sound waves to view abdominal organs) and computed tomography (CT) may help in some cases to rule out other diseases.

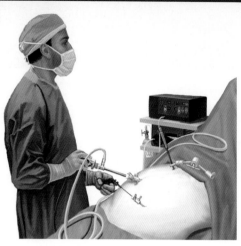

Surgery to remove the appendix is the treatment. Laparoscopy (using a lighted tube passed into the abdomen) is the preferred method.

How Is Appendicitis Treated?

Treatment is removal of the appendix, an operation called an appendectomy. An appendectomy is the most common emergency abdominal operation done in the United States. The preferred operation is by laparoscopy (laparoscopic appendectomy). A lighted tube (scope) is passed into the abdomen to see and remove the appendix. Another operation involves making a cut in the lower right side of the abdomen to remove the appendix (open appendectomy). Antibiotics for infection and drugs for pain, and maybe stool softeners, are usually prescribed.

In simple cases, most people will be in the hospital for 1 day or may go home the same day of surgery. For a ruptured appendix, the hospital stay will be longer, to give intravenous antibiotics and monitor for complications.

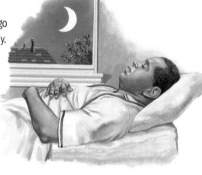

In simple acute appendicitis, most people will be in the hospital for 1 day or may go home on the day of surgery.

DOs and DON'Ts in Managing Appendicitis:

✔ **DO** report your symptoms. The earlier the diagnosis is made, the better the prognosis. Delays can lead to a burst appendix.

✔ **DO** call your doctor if you have vomiting, diarrhea or blood in your stool, a mass in your abdomen, or abdominal pain with fever.

✔ **DO** call your doctor if you need a referral to a surgeon.

⊘ **DON'T** miss follow-up appointmnets.

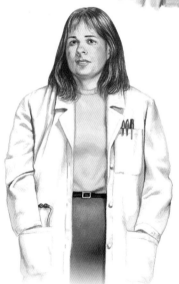

Don't delay seeking medical care when you have abdominal pain.

FROM THE DESK OF

NOTES

FOR MORE INFORMATION

Contact the following sources:

• MedlinePlus Health Information
  U.S. National Library of Medicine
  Website: http://www.nlm.nih.gov/medlineplus/appendicitis.html

• American College of Surgeons
  Tel: (800) 621-4111, (312) 202-5000
  Website: http://www.facs.org

MANAGING YOUR
FEMORAL HERNIA

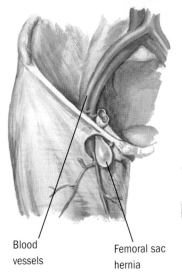

A femoral hernia is a bulge of intestine or fatty tissue pushing through a weak muscle in the groin. It occurs near the thigh, usually on the right side. More women than men tend to have these hernias.

Blood vessels

Femoral sac hernia

Two-sac hernia

Contributing factors:

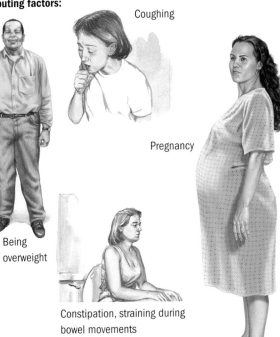

Coughing

Pregnancy

Being overweight

Constipation, straining during bowel movements

Your doctor will make a diagnosis by examining you.

What Are Femoral Hernias?

A femoral hernia is a bulge of intestine (bowel) or fatty tissue pushing through a weak muscle in the groin. It occurs near the thigh, usually on the right side. More women than men tend to have them. It can't be entirely prevented.

What Causes Femoral Hernias?

Contributing factors include being overweight, pregnancy, coughing a lot, constipation, straining to have a bowel movement (stool), and heavy lifting. Getting older, smoking, being born prematurely or having a low birth weight, illness, and using steroid medicines tend to increase chances of having a femoral hernia.

What Are the Symptoms of Femoral Hernias?

Very small hernias may cause no symptoms. The main symptom is a bulge in the groin. It gets bigger on standing and smaller when lying down. It may cause an aching pain that might be felt in the inner part of the thigh.

A bulge that gets bigger and starts to hurt more can mean an incarcerated or strangulated hernia. With an incarcerated hernia, bowel or fat became stuck in the hernia. With a strangulated hernia, blood flow is blocked. Other symptoms of these hernias include nausea, vomiting, and severe constipation. Also, the hernia won't get smaller when lying down.

How Are Femoral Hernias Diagnosed?

The doctor will make a diagnosis by doing a physical examination. If surgery is suggested, blood and urine tests, electrocardiography (ECG) (a record of the heart's electrical activity), and chest x-ray may be done before the surgery.

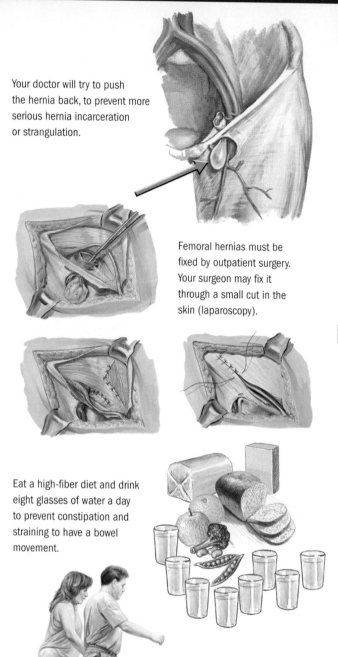

Your doctor will try to push the hernia back, to prevent more serious hernia incarceration or strangulation.

Femoral hernias must be fixed by outpatient surgery. Your surgeon may fix it through a small cut in the skin (laparoscopy).

Eat a high-fiber diet and drink eight glasses of water a day to prevent constipation and straining to have a bowel movement.

Keep your weight down and follow safety instructions about lifting heavy objects.

How Are Femoral Hernias Treated?

First, the doctor will try to push the hernia back, to prevent incarceration and strangulation.

However, femoral hernias must be fixed by outpatient surgery. The operation used depends on the hernia size and general health. The surgeon may fix it through a small cut in the skin (laparoscopy). The surgeon repairs the hernia by using a lighted tube that is put through a very small hole in the skin. A mesh material may be put over the hernia to add strength, so that the hernia won't occur again.

The doctor will prescribe pain pills and may suggest using a mild laxative to avoid straining when moving the bowels. After surgery, sudden and severe twisting and turning and driving a car should be avoided to prevent loosening the stitches or incision.

DOs and DON'Ts in Managing Femoral Hernias:

✔ **DO** follow your doctors instructions about taking pain pills, returning to work, and resuming sex after surgery.
✔ **DO** eat a high-fiber diet and drink eight glasses of water a day to prevent constipation and straining to have a bowel movement.
✔ **DO** call your surgeon if the incision gets red or swells or fluid seeps from it. Also call your surgeon if your temperature gets higher than 100° F.
✔ **DO** reduce your chance of getting femoral hernias by keeping your weight down, eating a high-fiber diet, drinking enough water, and following safety instructions about lifting heavy objects.

⊘ **DON'T** forget follow-up appointments.
⊘ **DON'T** lift heavy objects or drive until your surgeon says you can.

FROM THE DESK OF

NOTES

FOR MORE INFORMATION

Contact the following sources:

• American Gastroenterological Association
Tel: (301) 654-2055
Website: http://www.gastro.org

• Society for Surgery of the Alimentary Tract
Tel: (978) 526-8330
Website: http://www.ssat.com

MANAGING YOUR CHOLECYSTITIS

Cholecystitis (also known as a gallbladder attack) is an inflammation of the gallbladder causing severe pain. It occurs most often in women over 40.

Liver

The gallbladder is a small sac located under the liver. It stores bile that the liver makes and squirts it into the bowel when meals are eaten. Bile helps digest fats.

Gallbladder

Gallstone

The usual cause is gallstones getting stuck in the duct. Problems not related to stones (acalculous cholecystitis) can also cause it, such as sickle cell disease, infections, bile storage trouble, and diabetes. Other risks for cholecystitis are like those for gallstones.

Inflamed gallbladder

Duct

Signs and symptoms

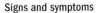

The skin and whites of the eyes may look yellow if the main duct bringing bile to the intestines is blocked by a stone.

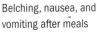

Belching, nausea, and vomiting after meals

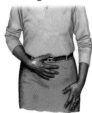

The most common symptom is pain (area of pain indicated by black circles). The pain is worse upon breathing in or moving, or when pressing on the area.

Your doctor makes a diagnosis from your medical history and physical examination. X-rays, blood tests, and ultrasonography will confirm it.

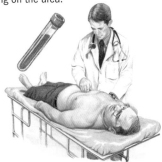

What Is Cholecystitis?

The gallbladder is a small sac located under the liver. It stores bile that the liver makes and squirts bile into the bowel (intestine) when a meal is eaten. Bile helps digest fats in the food. Cholecystitis is inflammation of the gallbladder. It's often called a gallbladder attack. Cholecystitis is usually caused by gallstones that get stuck in the duct (tube) that takes bile from the gallbladder to the bowel.

What Causes Cholecystitis?

Cholecystitis is usually caused by gallstones (called cholelithiasis) but it can also be related to problems with bile being made or stored in the gallbladder. This other type is called acalculous, meaning without calculi (stones). Other causes are sickle cell disease, infections, and diabetes. The acalculous type is found more often in older men, very sick people, or bedridden elderly people. Other risk factors for cholecystitis are like those for gallstones. They include age, female sex, certain ethnic groups (such as Native Americans), obesity, fasting, high-fat diet, losing and gaining weight excessively, drugs, and pregnancy.

What Are the Symptoms of Cholecystitis?

The most common symptoms are pain and cramping in the upper right side of the abdomen (belly). Pain in the chest, upper back, or right shoulder may also occur. Pain is worse with breathing in or moving or when pressure is on the area. Belching, nausea, and vomiting can occur, usually after eating high-fat foods. Low temperature, yellow skin and whites of the eyes, pale stools (bowel movements), and itchy skin may occur if the main duct bringing bile to the intestines is blocked by a stone. An infected gallbladder may cause high temperature and chills.

How Is Cholecystitis Diagnosed?

The doctor makes a diagnosis from a medical history and physical examination. X-rays, blood tests, and ultrasonography will confirm it. When ultrasonography shows unclear results, the doctor uses a special x-ray test (HIDA scan).

The doctor may observe, not treat, people with no symptoms. People needing treatment have the gallbladder removed by surgery (cholecystectomy). Laparoscopic removal, which uses four tiny cuts instead of one big one, is usual. It allows shorter recovery and can be an outpatient surgery.

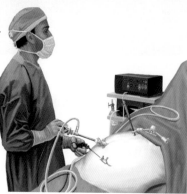

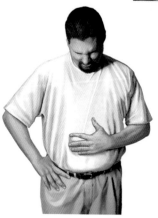

Removing the gallbladder doesn't affect normal living, except for occasional indigestion when eating fatty foods for 6 to 12 months after removal. This problem usually goes away.

Don't eat high-fat foods, extra large meals, and foods that cause symtoms. Don't fast for long periods or go on crash diets.

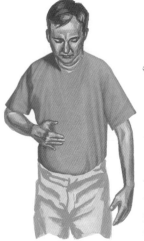

Tell your doctor if you have pain that you think may be caused by gallstones. Call your doctor right away if you get a fever with abdominal pain.

How Is Cholecystitis Treated?

For treatment, the gallbladder and gallstones are removed by surgery (cholecystectomy). Laparoscopic removal is the usual method. It allows shorter recovery and can be an outpatient surgery. For laparoscopic removal, the surgeon makes four tiny cuts in the abdomen. The surgeon uses instruments through these cuts to remove the gallbladder. If laparoscopic surgery cannot be used, standard surgery is done, which will require a prolonged hospital stay.

Removing the gallbladder doesn't affect normal living, except for occasional indigestion when eating fatty foods for 6 to 12 months after gallbladder removal. This problem usually goes away.

Drugs can also be used to dissolve stones, but medicines can take months or years to work and are only rarely used.

DOs and DON'Ts in Managing Cholecystitis:

✔ **DO** tell your doctor if you have pain that you think may be caused by gallstones.
✔ **DO** call your doctor right away if you get a fever with abdominal pain.
✔ **DO** maintain a normal weight.

🚫 **DON'T** eat meals high in fat, extra large meals, and foods that cause symptoms. Fatty foods make the gallbladder contract and may squeeze a stone into the duct. Avoid high-fat meals.
🚫 **DON'T** fast for long periods or go on crash diets.

FOR MORE INFORMATION

Contact the following sources:

• National Digestive Diseases Information Clearinghouse
  Tel: (301) 654-3810, (800) 891-5389
  Website: http://www.niddk.nih.gov/health/digest/nddic.htm

• MedlinePlus
  Website: http://www.nlm.nih.gov/medlineplus/gallbladderdiseases.html

• American Gastroenterological Association
  Tel: (301) 654-2055
  Website: http://www.gastro.org

• American College of Gastroenterology
  Tel: (703) 820-7400
  Website: http://www.acg.gi.org

• American College of Surgeons
  Tel: (312) 202-5000, (800) 621-4111
  Website: http://www.facs.org

FROM THE DESK OF

NOTES

MANAGING YOUR GALLSTONES

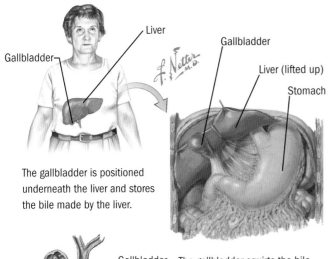

Gallbladder · Liver

The gallbladder is positioned underneath the liver and stores the bile made by the liver.

Gallbladder
Liver (lifted up)
Stomach

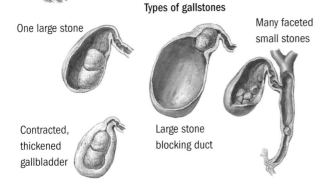

Gallbladder
Bile duct
Intestine

The gallbladder squirts the bile through the bile ducts into the intestine to help with digestion of food. Sometimes bile fluid contains solid clumps (stones), which can clog the passageways.

Types of gallstones

One large stone

Many faceted small stones

Contracted, thickened gallbladder

Large stone blocking duct

Risk factors that can cause gallstones

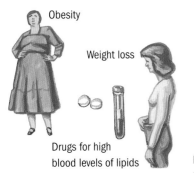

Obesity

Weight loss

Drugs for high blood levels of lipids

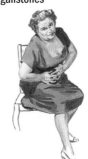

Pain caused by a gallstone typically occurs after meals.

What Are Gallstones?

Gallstones are solid deposits of cholesterol and other substances in bile that develop because the levels of these chemicals become unbalanced. The gallbladder is a small sack located underneath the liver. It stores bile that the liver makes and squirts the bile into the bowel (intestine) when a meal is eaten. Bile helps digest fats in the food. Under certain conditions, the gallbladder can form gallstones (cholelithiasis).

Gallstones are common: up to 20% of men and 40% of women get gallstones. More women get gallstones because of the effects of estrogen (a female hormone) on bile. Being overweight, aging, and fasting for a long time increase the risk of getting gallstones.

What Are the Symptoms of Gallstones?

Most gallstones produce no symptoms and may never lead to trouble, but they can cause intense pain. If a gallstone gets stuck in the tube (duct) that takes bile to the bowel, the gallbladder will squeeze harder, and the duct may tighten around the stone. Severe cramps in the belly (abdomen), or maybe between the shoulder blades, will result. Feeling sick to the stomach and vomiting are likely. Symptoms go away if the stone falls back into the gallbladder or moves through the bile duct into the bowel. A gallstone stuck at the end of the duct may cause swelling (inflammation) in the pancreas, and the skin and eyes may turn yellow (jaundice) if the bile ducts are blocked and there is a backup of bile.

How Are Gallstones Diagnosed?

Ultrasound (a special x-ray machine that uses sound waves to get pictures of body organs) can be used to find almost all gallstones and is usually the first test ordered. When ultrasound shows unclear results, the doctor can use a special x-ray test (HIDA scan).

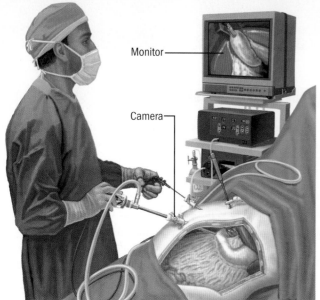

Treatment may include an operation (laparoscopic cholecystectomy) to remove gallbladder and gallstones.

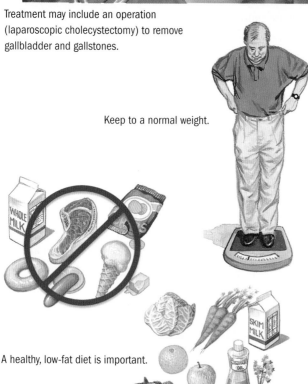

Keep to a normal weight.

A healthy, low-fat diet is important.

How Are Gallstones Treated?

Gallstones can be cured by surgically removing the gallbladder and gallstones (cholecystectomy). This is usually done with a laparoscopic method using only tiny cuts, instead of one large cut, for the doctor to insert instruments into the belly to remove the gallbladder. This operation allows a shorter recovery time and can be an outpatient surgery.

Treatment of gallstones in people without symptoms (asymptomatic) remains unclear. Many doctors suggest surgery because of possible complications, but the risk of complications from surgery is generally small. You should discuss the situation with your doctor, because you may have a higher risk (e.g., if you have diabetes, heart disease, emphysema).

In rare cases when surgery is too dangerous, your doctor may suggest drugs to dissolve the gallstones, but medicines may not work and must be used for a long time.

DOs and DON'Ts in Managing Gallstones:

✔ **DO** maintain a normal weight. If you are overweight, ask your doctor to help you with slow, steady weight loss.

✔ **DO** notify your doctor if you have pain that you think may be related to gallstones. Call your doctor immediately if you have a fever with the pain.

🚫 **DON'T** eat meals high in fat, extra large meals, and foods that cause stomach upset. Fatty foods make the gallbladder tighten and it may squeeze a stone into the duct. Even more important, avoid high-fat meals after following a low-fat diet.

🚫 **DON'T** fast for long periods or go on a crash diet.

FROM THE DESK OF

NOTES

FOR MORE INFORMATION

Contact the following sources:

• American College of Surgeons
  Tel: (312) 202-5000
  Website: http://www.facs.org

• American College of Gastroenterology
  Tel: (703) 820-7400
  Website: http://www.acg.gi.org

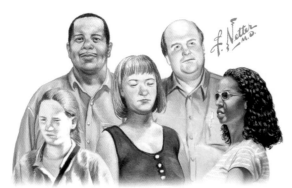

An ingrown nail occurs when a toenail (or fingernail) has a sharp end that grows down and burrows into the flesh of the finger or toe. Any finger or toe can have an ingrown nail, but usually big toes are affected. Untreated, ingrown toenails can lead to serious infections.

Causes of an ingrown toenail include:

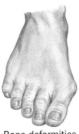

Wearing shoes that are too small

Diabetes

Bone deformities or toe injuries

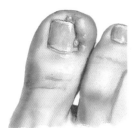

Symptoms include a hard, swollen, and tender toe around the nail. This area becomes red and very sore and feels warm. Skin grows over the ingrown nail.

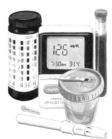

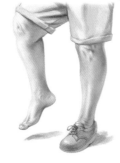

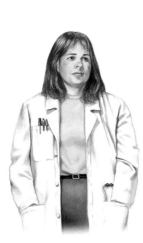

Your doctor makes a diagnosis by looking at and examining your nail and toe. If the toe area with the ingrown nail is infected, the doctor may take a sample of pus or fluid to determine which type of bacteria is causing the infection.

What Is an Ingrown Toenail?

An ingrown nail occurs when a toenail (or fingernail) has a sharp end that grows down and burrows into the flesh of the finger or toe. Any finger or toe can have an ingrown nail, but usually the big toes are affected. Untreated, ingrown toenails can lead to serious skin and bone infections.

What Causes an Ingrown Toenail?

Causes include wearing shoes that are too small, using the wrong method to trim the nail, bone abnormalities, or a toe injury such as stubbing the toe. People who are elderly, who have diabetes, or who have problems with blood circulation in their legs have greater chances of having ingrown toenails. This is also true of children and teenagers who may outgrow their shoes. Nails tend to thicken with age, which leads to elderly people having ingrown toenails.

What Are the Symptoms of an Ingrown Toenail?

Symptoms include a hard, swollen, and tender toe around the nail. This area becomes red and very sore and feels warm. Skin grows over the ingrown nail. If the toe becomes infected, pus or fluid may drain from the toe.

How Is an Ingrown Toenail Diagnosed?

The doctor makes a diagnosis by looking at and examining the nail and toe. If the ingrown nail is infected, the doctor may take a sample of pus or fluid and send it for study to find out which bacteria is causing the infection.

For a mild problem, soaking the foot or hand in warm, soapy water several times daily may solve the problem. Lifting the edge of the ingrown nail gently and putting some cotton under the nail to separate it from the toe may help. For a severely infected toe or ingrown toenails that keep coming back, the doctor may remove part of the nail.

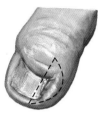 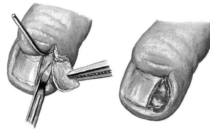

Dashed line shows incision line.

Part of nail and nail bed is removed.

After surgery

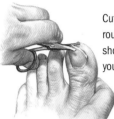

Cut your toenails properly: straight across with no rounded corners or sharp edges. Don't cut them too short. If you don't want to or can't cut your toenails yourself, go to a podiatrist.

Clean and dry areas around your nails after a bath or shower. Always keep your feet clean. Check them daily, especially if you have diabetes.

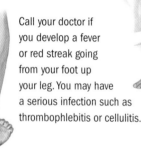

Call your doctor if you develop a fever or red streak going from your foot up your leg. You may have a serious infection such as thrombophlebitis or cellulitis.

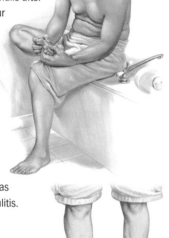

Wear clean socks and open-toed shoes while your toe heals. Wear shoes that fit well—not too tight or too short.

How Is an Ingrown Toenail Treated?

If the problem isn't severe, soaking the foot or hand in warm, soapy water several times each day may solve the problem. Lifting the edge of the ingrown nail gently and putting some cotton under the nail to separate it from the toe may help. For a severely infected toe or ingrown toenails that keep coming back, the doctor may remove part of nail. The doctor will numb the toe and use scissors to cut away the ingrown part of the toenail. A podiatrist, a doctor who specializes in foot problems, can also remove the toenail.

The doctor will prescribe antibiotic medicine for an infected toe with an ingrown nail. People with diabetes can have serious complications from ingrown toenails, such as sores (foot ulcers), which could need surgery.

DOs and DON'Ts in Managing an Ingrown Toenail:

✔ **DO** wear clean socks and open-toed shoes while your toe heals.

✔ **DO** clean and dry the areas around your nails after a bath or shower. Always keep your feet clean.

✔ **DO** call your doctor if you develop a fever or red streak going from your foot up your leg. You may have a serious infection such as thrombophlebitis or cellulitis.

✔ **DO** wear shoes that fit well (not too short or too tight).

✔ **DO** cut your toenails properly. Cut straight across with no rounded corners. Don't cut them too short. If you don't want to or can't cut your toenails yourself, go to a podiatrist.

🚫 **DON'T** cut into your nails on the side so that you have a sharp edge. The edge may grow into the toe around the nail.

🚫 **DON'T** pick at your toenails or tear them off.

FROM THE DESK OF

NOTES

FOR MORE INFORMATION

Contact the following sources:

• American Academy of Family Physicians
  Tel: (800) 274-2237
  Website: http://familydoctor.org

• American College of Foot and Ankle Surgeons
  Tel: (800) 421-2237
  Website: http://www.acfas.org

MANAGING YOUR
INGUINAL HERNIA

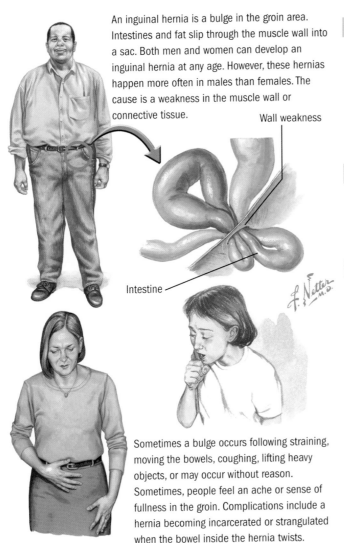

An inguinal hernia is a bulge in the groin area. Intestines and fat slip through the muscle wall into a sac. Both men and women can develop an inguinal hernia at any age. However, these hernias happen more often in males than females. The cause is a weakness in the muscle wall or connective tissue.

Wall weakness

Intestine

Sometimes a bulge occurs following straining, moving the bowels, coughing, lifting heavy objects, or may occur without reason. Sometimes, people feel an ache or sense of fullness in the groin. Complications include a hernia becoming incarcerated or strangulated when the bowel inside the hernia twists.

Affected babies will have a bulge that comes and goes with straining, crying, coughing, or standing.

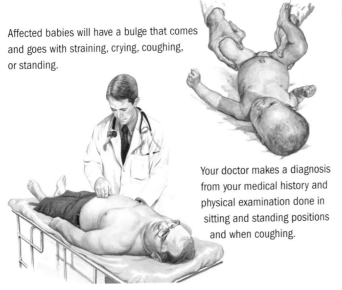

Your doctor makes a diagnosis from your medical history and physical examination done in sitting and standing positions and when coughing.

What Is an Inguinal Hernia?

An inguinal hernia is a bulge in the groin area. Intestines and fat slip through the muscle wall into a sac formed by the hernia. Both men and women can have an inguinal hernia, and at any age. However, these hernias happen more often in males than females.

What Causes an Inguinal Hernia?

The cause is a weakness in the muscle wall or connective tissue.

What Are the Symptoms of an Inguinal Hernia?

Sometimes a bulge occurs without other symptoms. Sometimes, people feel an ache or sense of fullness in the groin. Usually, people can push the bulge back in. Bulges might go back in on their own when people lie down. Babies have a bulge that comes and goes with straining, crying, coughing, or standing. The bulge can be pushed back into the baby's stomach. Complications include a hernia becoming incarcerated or strangulated. Incarcerated hernias have part of the intestine, some fat, or an ovary stuck in the sac. Strangulated means that tissues in the hernia become twisted. It can lead to gangrene, which means that tissues in the hernia die because they have no blood supply.

If a hernia becomes incarcerated, it can't be pushed back. It's an emergency.

How Is an Inguinal Hernia Diagnosed?

The doctor makes a diagnosis from a medical history and physical examination done in sitting and standing positions and when coughing.

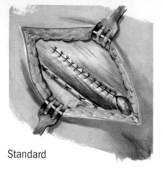

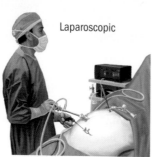

Laparoscopic

Standard

Surgery is the treatment. It should be done as soon as possible, even in very young babies, if the hernia is painful or cannot be pushed back in. The operation can be standard (with a regular incision) or laparoscopic (with a tiny incision).

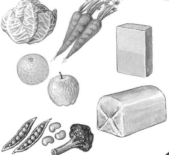

Use pain medicine after surgery as directed by your doctor. If your doctor approves, walk around and even climb stairs, but don't overdo it.

Be careful that you don't get constipated. Eat enough high-fiber foods and drink eight glasses of liquids daily. You may need a mild laxative.

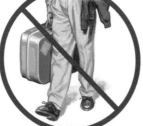

Don't lift anything heavier than 5 pounds after surgery. Ask someone to do it for you.

How Is an Inguinal Hernia Treated?

Surgery is the treatment of choice. It should be done as soon as possible, even in very young babies, if the hernia is painful or cannot be pushed back in. The operation can be standard (with a regular incision) or laparoscopic. In laparoscopic surgery, the doctor uses a thin tube that goes through a small cut in the skin. The doctor can see through the tube, which has a light at its tip, to the inside of the body.

DOs and DON'Ts in Managing an Inguinal Hernia:

- ✔ **DO** use pain medicine after surgery as directed by your doctor.
- ✔ **DO** walk around and even climb stairs if your doctor approves, but don't overdo it.
- ✔ **DO** be careful that you don't get constipated. Eat enough high-fiber foods and drink eight glasses of liquids daily. You may need a mild laxative (such as milk of magnesia).
- ✔ **DO** shower if you wish, with dressings on or off after your doctor says that it's OK. The strips of tape across the incision can get wet. After you dry yourself, replace dressings with clean, dry ones.
- ✔ **DO** have sex when your doctor says you can.
- ✔ **DO** call your doctor if you have unusual symptoms or if your scrotum swells.
- ✔ **DO** call your doctor if the incision becomes red, swollen, or has drainage. Call if you have a temperature higher than 100° F.
- ✔ **DO** keep your weight down.
- ✔ **DO** follow safety instructions when you do heavy lifting.
- ✔ **DO** see your doctor if you have a long-lasting cough or allergies.

- ⊘ **DON'T** lift anything heavier than 5 pounds after surgery. Ask someone to do it for you.

FOR MORE INFORMATION

Contact the following sources:

- American Gastroenterological Association
  Tel: (301) 654-2055
  Website: http://www.gastro.org
- American Pediatric Surgical Association
  Tel: (847) 480-9576
  Website: http://www.eapsa.org
- Society for Surgery of the Alimentary Tract
  Tel: (978) 526-8330
  Website: http://www.ssat.com

FROM THE DESK OF

NOTES

MANAGING YOUR LIPOMA

Lipomas are deposits of fatty material that grow slowly under the skin, between skin and muscle. They occur on the neck, back, shoulders, arms, and thighs. They are harmless. They aren't cancerous and are the most common benign tumors in adults. They can affect both sexes and all ages, but are more common in middle-aged women than other people.

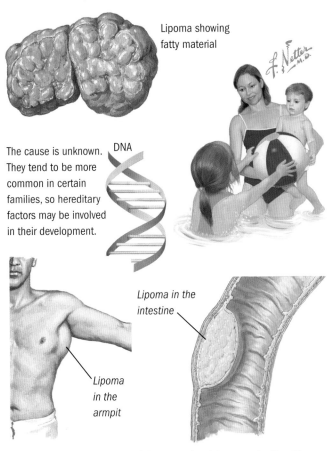

Lipoma showing fatty material

The cause is unknown. They tend to be more common in certain families, so hereditary factors may be involved in their development.

DNA

Lipoma in the intestine

Lipoma in the armpit

A lipoma usually starts as a painless, round, soft bump under the skin. Most feel doughy or rubbery and can usually be moved easily. They are usually asymptomatic but can be painful if they press on nerves.

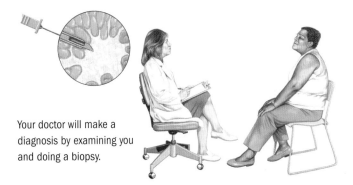

Your doctor will make a diagnosis by examining you and doing a biopsy.

What Is a Lipoma?

A lipoma is a deposit of fatty material that grows slowly under the skin, between the skin and muscle layer. They occur most often on the neck, back, shoulders, arms, and thighs; they may also grow in other parts of the body such as the intestine. Lipomas are harmless. They are not cancerous and are the most common benign tumors in adults. Lipomas can affect both sexes and all ages, but are more common in middle-aged women than other people.

What Causes a Lipoma?

The cause is unknown. Lipomas tend to be more common in certain families, so hereditary factors may be involved in their development.

What Are the Symptoms of a Lipoma?

A lipoma usually starts as a painless, round, soft bump under the skin. People may not know that they have a lipoma. Most feel a bit doughy or rubbery, but they range in firmness from soft to hard. They can usually be moved around easily. More than one may be present. They can be painful if they press on nerves or if they have many blood vessels inside them. They vary in size but are rarely larger than 3 inches across. They occur most often on the forearms, legs, torso, and neck area. Lipomas can occur in other parts of the body, such as the lungs, intestines, and breasts, and their symptoms depend on the location.

How Is a Lipoma Diagnosed?

The doctor will suspect the diagnosis from a physical examination. However, the diagnosis can be confirmed only by a biopsy. In a biopsy, the doctor removes a piece of the tissue and looks at it with a microscope.

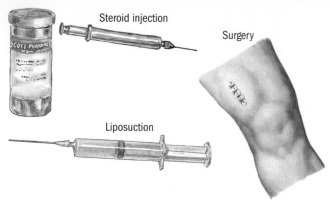

Steroid injection

Surgery

Liposuction

Lipomas are harmless lumps that don't need treatment. Lipomas that are bothersome for cosmetic reasons or because they're very large are usually removed by surgery or liposuction. Liposuction often cannot remove the whole lipoma.

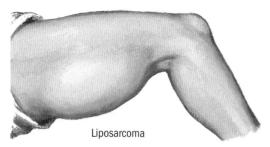

Liposarcoma

Have a doctor check any lump that may appear on your body. Lipomas are harmless, but other lumps may be more serious, such as liposarcomas, and may need treatment.

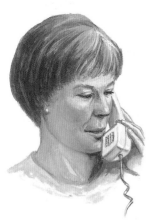

Call your doctor if you see a significant increase in the size, such as doubling, of your lipoma in a 12-month period. Because lipomas grow slowly, the size increase could be a sign of another problem.

How Is a Lipoma Treated?

Lipomas are harmless lumps that usually don't need any treatment. Lipomas that bother people because of cosmetic reasons or because they are extremely large are usually removed by surgery. Lipomas don't usually recur after surgery. They can also be removed by liposuction, but liposuction often cannot remove the whole lipoma.

Lipomas are harmless, but the doctor should make sure that the lump isn't another kind of lump such as a cyst, abscess, or liposarcoma. Liposarcomas are cancers that grow in fatty tissues. However, they grow quickly (instead of slowly, like lipomas), don't easily move under the skin, and can be painful.

DOs and DON'Ts in Managing a Lipoma:

✔ **DO** have any lump that may appear on your body checked. Lipomas are harmless, but other lumps may be more serious and may need treatment.

✔ **DO** call your doctor if you see a significant increase in the size, such as doubling, of your lipoma in a 12-month period. Because lipomas grow slowly, the size increase could be a sign of another problem.

✔ **DO** call your doctor if you see redness or swelling and warmth at the site of surgery for the lipoma.

✔ **DO** call your doctor if the lipoma becomes painful.

⊘ **DON'T** ignore lumps that you find on your body. Have your doctor check them.

FROM THE DESK OF

NOTES

FOR MORE INFORMATION

Contact the following sources:

• American Academy of Dermatology
 Tel: (847) 330-9239, (866) 503-7546
 Website: http://www.aad.org

• American College of Surgeons
 Tel: (312) 202-5000
 Website: http://www.facs.org

MANAGING YOUR
PNEUMOTHORAX

Pneumothorax is a condition in which air leaks from a hole in a lung and gets trapped in the space between the lung and chest wall. When air gets into this space, the lung collapses.

An opening letting air leak out can be caused by injury (traumatic) such as a puncture or by bursting of a lung bleb (spontaneous pneumothorax) from hard coughing or unknown reason.

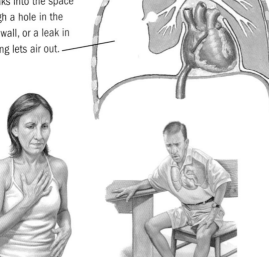

Lung collapse because air leaks into the space through a hole in the chest wall, or a leak in the lung lets air out.

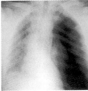

The most common symptoms are shortness of breath and sharp chest pain. Others are fainting and fatigue.

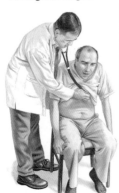

Your doctor will take your medical history and examine you. The doctor can hear decreased loudness of breath sounds on one side of the chest with a stethoscope. A chest x-ray can confirm pneumothorax and exclude other causes of shortness of breath.

What Is Pneumothorax?

Pneumothorax is a condition in which air leaks from a hole in a lung and gets trapped between the lung and the chest wall (the pleural space). A small amount of fluid in this space normally keeps the outside of the lung from getting stuck against the inside of the chest. This keeps the lung expanded. When air gets into the pleural space, the lung partly or completely collapses.

What Causes Pneumothorax?

Air leaking into the pleural space through a hole in the chest wall or a leak in the lung that lets air escape causes pneumothorax. Traumatic pneumothorax results from an injury such as a puncture of the chest wall or a broken rib that punctures the lung.

Spontaneous pneumothorax can occur in people with emphysema and in tall, very thin people. A hard cough makes part of the lung burst and air leak from the lung. Spontaneous pneumothorax may run in families. About 9 of 100,000 people in the United States have this condition each year.

What Are the Symptoms of Pneumothorax?

The most common symptoms are shortness of breath and sharp chest pain, especially when inhaling and exhaling. Others are fainting and fatigue.

How Is Pneumothorax Diagnosed?

The doctor will take a medical history and do a physical examination. The doctor will hear decreased loudness of breath sounds on one side of the chest with a stethoscope. A chest x-ray can confirm pneumothorax. The doctor will check the oxygen level in the blood and check the heart with electrocardiography (ECG). The ECG measures the heart's electrical activity.

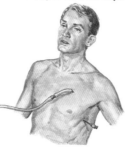

Treatment depends on the degree of pneumo-thorax and the cause. A small pneumothorax can be treated by letting the body absorb the air by itself. With a slightly larger pneumothorax, a needle can be put into the chest to remove the air, so the lung expands. A larger pneumothorax may need to have a chest tube placed to remove the air. A machine draws out the air so the lung expands. For a large leak, the tube may need to stay in for a few days.

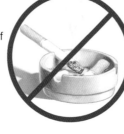

Don't smoke. Smoking increases your risk of pneumothorax and may cause coughing.

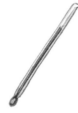

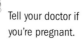

Tell your doctor if you're pregnant.

Call your doctor if you have a temperature higher than 101° F or see pus coming from your chest tube. You could have an infection.

Call your doctor right away if you have shortness of breath. Your lung could be collapsing.

How Is Pneumothorax Treated?

Treatment depends on the degree of pneumothorax and the cause. A small pneumothorax can be treated by letting the body absorb the air by itself. For a larger pneumothorax, a needle can be put into the chest to remove the air so the lung expands. A large pneumothorax may need to have a chest tube put into the chest to remove the air. A suction machine connected to the tube draws out the air so the lung expands. If the leak is large, the tube may need to stay in for a few days to keep the lung expanded until the leak heals.

DOs and DON'Ts in Managing Pneumothorax:

✔ **DO** tell your doctor about your other medical problems.
✔ **DO** tell your doctor about your medicines, both prescription and over-the-counter.
✔ **DO** tell your doctor if you're pregnant.
✔ **DO** call your doctor if your symptoms get worse.
✔ **DO** call your doctor if you have a fever (temperature higher than 101.0° F) or see pus coming from your chest tube. You could have an infection or pneumonia.
✔ **DO** call your doctor if your symptoms come back, if you had pneumothorax before. Up to 50% of people with spontaneous pneumothorax have another pneumothorax.
✔ **DO** call your doctor right away if you have sudden onset of shortness of breath. Your lung could be collapsing.

⊘ **DON'T** try to remove the chest tube by yourself.
⊘ **DON'T** exert yourself or cough too much, which can lead to air leaks.
⊘ **DON'T** smoke. Smoking increases your risk of pneumothorax and may cause coughing.

FROM THE DESK OF

NOTES

FOR MORE INFORMATION

Contact the following sources:

• American Lung Association
  Tel: (800) LUNG-USA (586-4872)
  Website: http://www.lungusa.org

MANAGING YOUR
RECTAL CANCER

Rectal cancer is cancer that grows in the rectum. The cause isn't known. It tends to happen more with older age, especially in men, and usually grows slowly. Most of the time, it starts as a small growth called a polyp.

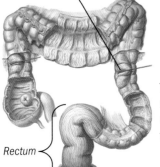

Colon (large intestine)

Rectum

The rectum is the last 10 inches or so of the colon in the digestive tract. It ends at the anus, which is the opening to the outside.

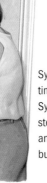

Symptoms may not occur for a long time, especially if a growth is small. Symptoms include blood in the stools, thinner stool than usual, and an urge to have a bowel movement but nothing comes out.

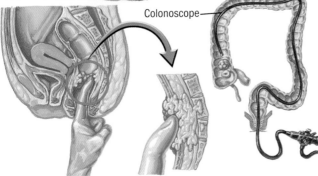

Colonoscope

Your doctor makes a diagnosis from your medical history, physical examination, laboratory tests, and colonoscopy. The doctor inserts a small, flexible, lighted tube into the anus to see inside the whole colon. The doctor can also use the tube to do a biopsy. If cancer is found, the doctor will stage it with CT, x-rays, and blood tests.

What Is Rectal Cancer?

The rectum is part of the colon (large intestine) in the digestive tract. It's the last 10 inches or so of the colon and ends at the anus, which is the opening to the outside. Rectal cancer is cancer that grows in the rectum. It tends to happen more with older age, especially in men, and usually grows slowly. Most of the time, it starts as a small growth called a polyp.

What Causes Rectal Cancer?

The cause is unknown.

What Are the Symptoms of Rectal Cancer?

People may not have symptoms for a long time, especially if the growth is small. Sometimes, people have blood in the stools (bowel movements). The stool may be thinner than usual, because it squeezes past the cancer. People may also feel urges to have bowel movements, but nothing comes out.

How Is Rectal Cancer Diagnosed?

The doctor makes a preliminary diagnosis from a medical history, physical examination, and laboratory tests. The doctor will do a colonoscopy. The doctor puts a small flexible tube into the anus. The tube has a light at the tip, so the doctor can see inside the rectum and colon. It's long enough to go into the whole colon. It also has a tool at the tip so the doctor can take a small sample of tissue (biopsy) to be checked with a microscope to see if it has cancer cells.

If cancer is found, the doctor will do other tests to see if the cancer has spread. This is called staging. These tests include computed tomography (CT) of the abdomen (belly) and pelvis, x-rays, and blood tests.

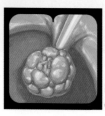

Polyp removal
during colonoscopy

Chemotherapy

Small polyps and very small rectal cancers may be removed during colonoscopy. Larger cancers will be removed by surgery. The type depends on the size and location of the cancer and how far it has spread. Anticancer medicines (chemotherapy) and radiotherapy may also be used to shrink the cancer.

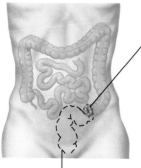

Dashed line shows part removed

Pouch made for stool

If the cancer is large, the doctor may remove the whole rectum and anus. If this happens, the doctor will perform a colostomy. In this procedure, a pouch is made from the colon and comes out through the skin. Stool will come out into a small bag.

Understand the importance of colon screening with colonoscopy for everyone, starting at age 50, or earlier for family members of people with colon cancer.

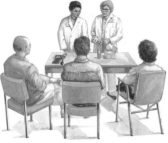

Don't be afraid to ask your primary doctor about support groups. In these groups, you can share your concerns with others who have also been diagnosed and treated for rectal cancer.

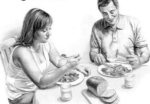

After surgery, make sure that you have a healthy diet. Ask your doctor for guidelines.

How Is Rectal Cancer Treated?

Small polyps and very small rectal cancers may be removed during colonoscopy. Larger cancers will be removed by surgery. The type depends on the size and location of the cancer and how far it has spread. Anticancer medicines (chemotherapy) and radiotherapy may also be used to shrink the cancer. If the cancer is large, the doctor may have to remove the whole rectum and anus. If this happens, the doctor will do a colostomy. In this procedure, a pouch is made from the colon and comes out through the skin. Stool will come out into a small bag.

DOs and DON'Ts in Managing Rectal Cancer:

✔ **DO** understand the importance of colon screening for everyone starting at age 50, and earlier for family members of people with colon cancer.

✔ **DO** make sure that you have a colonoscopy generally 1 year after surgery and regularly after that, or as recommended by your doctor, to screen for return of cancer.

✔ **DO** call your doctor if you have trouble moving your bowels, abdominal pain, or blood in the stool.

⊘ **DON'T** miss follow-up appointments with your primary doctor and specialists who treated you for rectal cancer.

⊘ **DON'T** be afraid to ask your primary doctor about support groups. In these groups, you can share your concerns with others who have also been diagnosed and treated for rectal cancer.

⊘ **DON'T** forget the importance of good nutrition after surgical treatment.

⊘ **DON'T** delay telling your doctor about new symptoms or concerns.

FROM THE DESK OF

NOTES

FOR MORE INFORMATION

Contact the following sources:

• American Cancer Society
  Tel: (800) 227-2345
  Website: http://www.cancer.org

• American College of Surgeons
  Tel: (312) 202-5000, (800) 621-4111
  Website: http://www.facs.org

MANAGING YOUR VARICOSE VEINS

Blood travels in arteries and veins. Arteries take blood with oxygen and nutrients away from the heart to body cells. Veins carry blood back to the heart from the cells. Varicose veins are enlarged, twisted-looking veins close to the skin's surface. They occur most often in legs.

Normal leg veins

Leg muscles help support veins and push blood up toward the heart. Valves in veins help stop blood from falling down or pooling in the legs. If valves stop working, blood flows back down and pools in the legs instead of moving up toward the heart. Varicose veins result.

Symptoms include legs that ache or feel heavy. Others are bulging, bluish veins along the thigh or ankles or across the knees; swelling; and dry, itchy skin. Skin color changes, thin skin, ulcers, and soft tissue infections can occur.

Your doctor makes a diagnosis from a leg examination and symptoms. If a blood clot is possible, the doctor may order an ultrasound scan.

Ultrasound scan

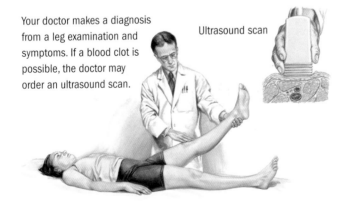

What Are Varicose Veins?

Blood travels in vessels called arteries and veins. Arteries take blood with oxygen and nutrients away from the heart to body cells. Veins carry blood back to the heart after cells get the oxygen and nutrients. Varicose veins are enlarged, twisted-looking veins that lie close to the skin's surface. They occur most often in the legs. Leg muscles help support veins and push blood up toward the heart. Valves in veins help stop blood from falling down or pooling in the legs.

For many people, varicose veins are mostly a cosmetic problem. For others, they cause symptoms and more serious problems, such as blood clots, skin ulcers, or blood circulation disorders.

What Causes Varicose Veins?

The cause is weakening or failure of valves in veins to stop blood from pooling in the legs. They aren't contagious or inherited but do run in families. They're more common in older people, women, overweight people, and people who stand in one place for long periods.

What Are the Symptoms of Varicose Veins?

Symptoms include legs that ache or feel heavy, especially after standing or sitting for long periods. Others are bulging, bluish veins along the thigh or ankles or across the knees; swelling; and dry, itchy skin. Skin color changes, thin skin, ulcers, and infection of soft tissue (cellulitis) can occur near the ankles.

How Are Varicose Veins Diagnosed?

The doctor makes a diagnosis from a leg examination and symptoms. If a blood clot is possible, the doctor may order ultrasonography.

Your doctor may suggest wearing elastic pressure stockings. They will stop blood from pooling in your legs. Stockings come in different pressures and lengths. Sclerotherapy and surgery to remove large veins can also be used.

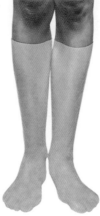

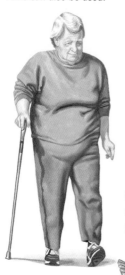

Lose weight if you're overweight. The extra weight puts more pressure on your veins. Exercise and raising the legs will help too.

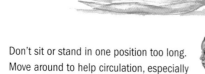

Don't sit or stand in one position too long. Move around to help circulation, especially on airplanes.

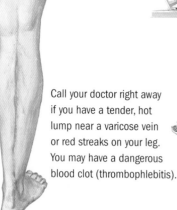

Call your doctor right away if you have a tender, hot lump near a varicose vein or red streaks on your leg. You may have a dangerous blood clot (thrombophlebitis).

How Are Varicose Veins Treated?

Treatment includes staying off your feet as much as possible, wearing elastic support stockings, having sclerotherapy, and having surgery. For people without symptoms and no ulcers or skin breakdown, observation, exercise, losing weight, raising the legs, and elastic stockings are used. Stockings can be knee-high, thigh-high, or pantyhose length and should cover the veins.

In sclerotherapy, the doctor injects solutions into a small dilated vein that's causing symptoms. The solutions make the veins collapse and scar.

Surgery is usually used if other treatments don't help symptoms; if ulcers, leg swelling, skin breakdown, and leg clots occur; and if people have cosmetic concerns. The most common surgery is called ligation (tying) and stripping. A certain large vein is tied and pulled out of the leg. Many smaller varicose veins are branches of this large vein. The smaller veins are injected with sclerosing solution. The leg is then wrapped with elastic bandages.

DOs and DON'Ts in Managing Varicose Veins:

✔ **DO** exercise (walk) regularly and lose weight.
✔ **DO** raise your legs, and avoid standing in one place for long periods.
✔ **DO** wear compression stockings daily for them to work properly.
✔ **DO** call your doctor if your varicose veins cause pain, you have skin breakdown or ulcers, or you're bleeding from a varicose vein.
✔ **DO** call your doctor if you have a tender, hot lump near a varicose vein. It can be a dangerous blood clot (thrombophlebitis).

🚫 **DON'T** stand or sit for long periods; this helps prevent blood from pooling in the legs.

FROM THE DESK OF

NOTES

FOR MORE INFORMATION

Contact the following sources:

• American College of Phlebology
  Tel: (510) 346-6800, (866) 634-8346
  Website: http://www.phlebology.org

• The American Society for Dermatologic Surgery (ASDS)
  Tel: (800) 441-2737
  Website: http://www.asds-net.org

MANAGING YOUR ENLARGED PROSTATE

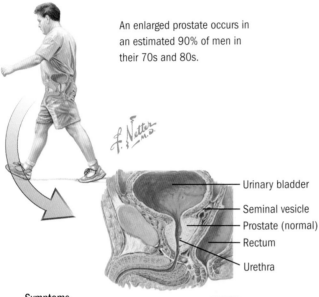

An enlarged prostate occurs in an estimated 90% of men in their 70s and 80s.

- Urinary bladder
- Seminal vesicle
- Prostate (normal)
- Rectum
- Urethra

Symptoms

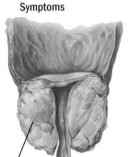

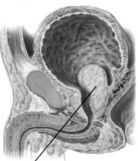

Enlarged prostate causing a narrow urethra

Enlarged prostate pressing into the bladder

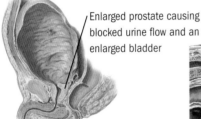

Enlarged prostate causing blocked urine flow and an enlarged bladder

A rectal exam is usually the first step toward diagnosis.

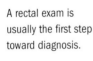

Low urine flow suggests BPH. Urine tests and blood tests will be done to rule out cancer and other disorders.

About the Prostate

The prostate is a walnut-sized reproductive gland in men. It produces a fluid that is a major part of the semen. It lies in front of the large intestine and below the urinary bladder (which stores urine). It surrounds the urethra, the tube that carries urine out of the body. The prostate often enlarges as a man ages.

What Is Benign Prostatic Hyperplasia (BPH)?

BPH is the common condition of enlargement of the prostate gland. Benign means that BPH is not cancer. It is also not contagious or sexually transmitted.

What Causes BPH?

The cause is unknown, but aging and male hormones are related to BPH.

What Are the Symptoms of BPH?

Symptoms are rare before age 40 but occur in more than half of men in their 60s and as many as 90% in their 70s and 80s. Symptoms are related to difficulty urinating, including weak urine stream, urgency (need to urinate quickly), leaking or dribbling urine, and more frequent urination, especially at night.

Severe BPH can cause serious problems, such as infections, bladder or kidney damage, and incontinence. If bladder damage is permanent, BPH treatment may not work. When BPH is found earlier, it is less likely to cause serious complications.

How Is BPH Diagnosed?

Diagnosis begins with a medical history and doctor's examination of the prostate with the finger (digital rectal examination). Blood and urine tests and a sonogram (ultrasound) may be done to evaluate for incomplete bladder emptying due to obstruction from an enlarged prostate and to ex-clude other causes of the symptoms. A blood test called prostate-specific antigen (PSA) may be used to rule out prostate cancer. The doctor should review risks and benefits of this controversial test.

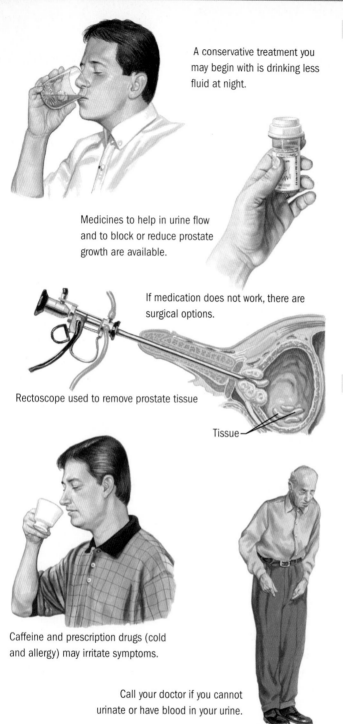

A conservative treatment you may begin with is drinking less fluid at night.

Medicines to help in urine flow and to block or reduce prostate growth are available.

If medication does not work, there are surgical options.

Rectoscope used to remove prostate tissue

Tissue

Caffeine and prescription drugs (cold and allergy) may irritate symptoms.

Call your doctor if you cannot urinate or have blood in your urine.

How Is BPH Treated?

Most people with symptoms require treatment at some point. Effective treatments range from conservative, which means simply drinking less fluid at night, to taking medicines or having surgery.

Medicines include alpha-blockers such as tamsulosin to help urine flow and reduce blockage in the bladder. Other medications, such as finasteride, inhibit production of the hormone testosterone, so the prostate shrinks or stops growing. Over-the-counter drugs include saw palmetto, but their effectiveness has not been proven.

If drugs don't work, surgery can be tried. These operations range from slightly invasive to very invasive. The operation called TURP (transurethral resection of the prostate) is used for 90% of all surgeries for BPH. Other operations include transurethral microwave therapy (uses microwave heat), transurethral needle ablation (radiofrequency therapy, uses radio waves), and laser surgery.

DOs and DON'Ts in Managing BPH:

✔ **DO** understand that common drug side effects include lightheadedness and dry mouth.

✔ **DO** tell your doctor about any over-the-counter medicines, herbs, or supplements you take. These may cause symptoms.

✔ **DO** realize that surgical complications may include urinary incontinence, erection problems, and bleeding.

✔ **DO** understand that 10% to 30% of men with BPH also have prostate cancer.

✔ **DO** call your doctor if you cannot urinate or have blood in your urine.

⊘ **DON'T** forget that caffeine and certain prescription drugs (e.g., for colds and allergy) may cause irritating prostate symptoms.

⊘ **DON'T** forget to discuss with your doctor the risks and benefits of operations and use of the PSA blood test for diagnosing prostate cancer.

FROM THE DESK OF

NOTES

FOR MORE INFORMATION

Contact the following sources:

• American Urological Association
  Tel: (401) 727-1100
  Website: http://www.auanet.org

• National Kidney and Urologic Diseases
  Information Clearinghouse
  Website: http://www.niddk.nih.gov

MANAGING YOUR HYDROCELE

A hydrocele is a sac of clear fluid that forms in the scrotum. Hydroceles are most often found in newborn babies, on one side or both sides of the scrotum. Also, men, usually older than 40, can have hydroceles.

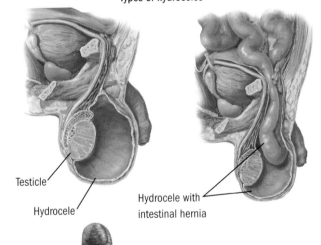

In babies, hydroceles are usually caused during development. Testicles don't move properly from the lower abdomen down into the scrotum.

Hydroceles can also be caused by infections, inflammation, radiation therapy, and injuries. They're not contagious.

Types of hydroceles

Testicle

Hydrocele

Hydrocele with intestinal hernia

Hydroceles generally don't cause pain. They cause the scrotum to swell on one or both sides. This swelling makes the scrotum feel like a water-filled balloon. Your doctor makes a diagnosis from a physical examination. Ultrasonography may be done if the diagnosis is unclear.

What Is a Hydrocele?

A hydrocele is a sac of clear fluid that develops in the scrotum, the loose pouch of skin that holds the testicles. Hydroceles are most often found in newborn babies. They can be on one side or both sides of the scrotum. In babies, most hydroceles go away on their own. Also, men, usually older than 40, can have hydroceles. No way to prevent hydroceles is known.

What Causes a Hydrocele?

In babies, hydroceles are usually caused during the baby's development. As babies develop, the testicles should move from the lower abdomen (belly) into the scrotum. Each testicle moves in a sac with fluid around it. Usually, the sac closes and the fluid moves back into the body. If fluid remains after the sac closes, one type of hydrocele forms. Sometimes, the sac may not close completely, and another type of hydrocele forms. Hydroceles can also be caused by infections, inflammation, radiation therapy, and injuries. Hydroceles aren't contagious or hereditary.

What Are the Symptoms of a Hydrocele?

Hydroceles generally don't cause pain. They do cause the scrotum to get swollen on one or both sides. This swelling makes the scrotum feel like a balloon filled with water.

How Is a Hydrocele Diagnosed?

The doctor will make a diagnosis from a physical examination of the scrotal area. Sometimes, the doctor will order ultrasonography of the scrotum to diagnose a hydrocele. Ultrasonography is a test that uses sound waves to get pictures of inside the body. It's important to find out whether a hydrocele or another more serious problem (such as testicular torsion or a tumor) is present.

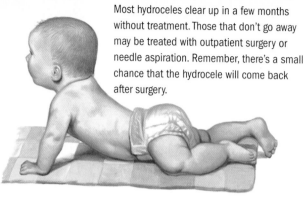

Most hydroceles clear up in a few months without treatment. Those that don't go away may be treated with outpatient surgery or needle aspiration. Remember, there's a small chance that the hydrocele will come back after surgery.

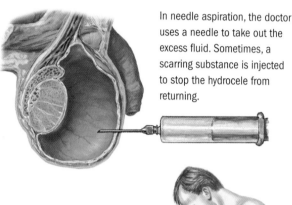

In needle aspiration, the doctor uses a needle to take out the excess fluid. Sometimes, a scarring substance is injected to stop the hydrocele from returning.

Hydroceles don't affect how the testicles work and won't make you impotent or unable to have an erection.

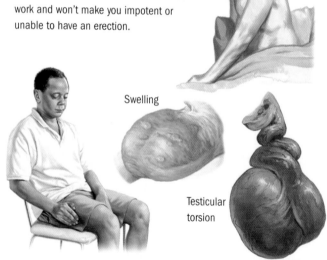

Swelling

Testicular torsion

Call your doctor if you have pain or swelling of a testicle or feel a lump on a testicle. The doctor should check for other causes of lumps, including spermatoceles, testicular torsion, and testicular cancers.

How Is a Hydrocele Treated?

Most hydroceles clear up in a few months with no treatment. Those that don't go away in that time may be treated with surgery. Surgery can be done as an outpatient operation. Either spinal or local anesthesia may be needed. Another treatment possibility is aspiration. In this procedure, the doctor sticks a needle into the scrotum and takes out the excess fluid. A urologist (doctor specializing in the genital and urinary system) can do this. Some urologists use aspiration along with injection of scarring agents to prevent the hydrocele from returning. As with any operation, complications of bleeding and infection can occur.

DOs and DON'Ts in Managing a Hydrocele:

✔ **DO** call your doctor if you have swelling in the scrotal area.

✔ **DO** get the opinion of a urologist if you're thinking of surgery.

✔ **DO** remember there's 2% chance that the hydrocele will come back after surgery.

✔ **DO** call your doctor if you notice pain or swelling of a testicle or feel a lump on the testicle.

✔ **DO** call your doctor if you need a referral to a surgeon (urologist).

✔ **DO** call your doctor if you have pain, bleeding, or fever after surgery for a hydrocele.

⊘ **DON'T** forget that hydroceles don't affect how the testicles work and won't make you impotent or make you unable to have an erection.

⊘ **DON'T** forget to report lumps or swelling to your primary doctor. Other causes of lumps include spermatoceles, testicular torsion, and testicular cancers.

FROM THE DESK OF

NOTES

FOR MORE INFORMATION

Contact the following source:

• American Urological Association
Tel: (866) 746-4282
Website: http://www.auanet.org

Hypospadias is a condition, present at birth, that occurs when a boy's urethra is too short. The urethra opens along the shaft of the penis (usually underneath) instead of at the tip of the penis. It can also open at the scrotum.

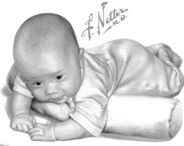

The urethra is the tube that takes urine from the bladder out of the body through the penis.

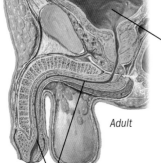

Adult

Urethra

Bladder

Types of hypospadias

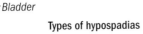

Glandular

Penile

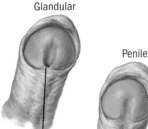

Openings

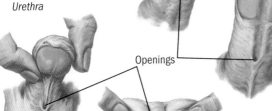

Penoscrotal

Scrotal

Hypospadias can be mild to severe and cause a curved erect penis and abnormal spraying of urine. The cause isn't known.

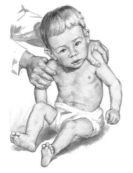

Your child's doctor makes a diagnosis from a medical history and physical examination. The doctor may suggest seeing a urologist.

What Is Hypospadias?

The urethra is the tube that takes urine from the bladder out of the body through the penis. Hypospadias is a condition, present at birth, that occurs when a boy's urethra is too short. The urethra opens along the shaft of the penis (usually underneath) rather than at the tip (head) of the penis. Hypospadias can be mild to severe, depending on where the urethra opens.

It's fairly common, occurring in about 1 in 250 to 300 male babies in the United States and in more white than black babies.

What Causes Hypospadias?

The cause is unknown, but genetic, endocrine, and environmental factors may be involved.

What Are the Symptoms of Hypospadias?

The opening of the urethra isn't at the head of the penis. It's usually near the head but can be at the middle or bottom of the penis. Some males also have a curved penis when erect, have abnormal spraying of urine, and may need to sit down to urinate.

How Is Hypospadias Diagnosed?

The doctor makes a diagnosis from a medical history and physical examination. The doctor may suggest seeing a urologist (specialist in urinary problems).

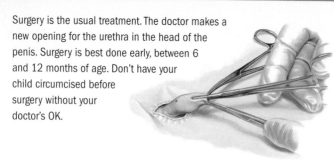

Surgery is the usual treatment. The doctor makes a new opening for the urethra in the head of the penis. Surgery is best done early, between 6 and 12 months of age. Don't have your child circumcised before surgery without your doctor's OK.

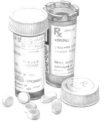

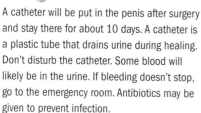

A catheter will be put in the penis after surgery and stay there for about 10 days. A catheter is a plastic tube that drains urine during healing. Don't disturb the catheter. Some blood will likely be in the urine. If bleeding doesn't stop, go to the emergency room. Antibiotics may be given to prevent infection.

Call your child's doctor right away if after surgery your child has fever, pus coming from the penis, no urine coming from the penis for more than 1 hour, or urine squirting from any part on the penis.

After surgery, your child should grow to have a normal sex life and be able to father children when he's an adult.

How Is Hypospadias Treated?

Surgery is the usual treatment. The doctor makes a new opening for the urethra in the head of the penis. Surgery is best done early, between 6 and 12 months of age. However, surgery can also be done on adults.

Surgery isn't major. Most boys go home the day they have the surgery. They will have a catheter in the penis. A catheter is a plastic tube that drains urine. The urine normally has blood in it. The doctor may prescribe medicine for pain and antibiotic medicine to prevent infection.

Most catheters are removed in 10 days. Usually two checkups are needed after surgery. After surgery, a normal future sex life and the ability to father children are expected.

If hypospadias isn't treated, problems with toilet training, sex in adulthood, and urethral strictures and fistulas may occur.

DOs and DON'Ts in Managing Hypospadias:

✔ **DO** tell your doctor about your child's medical problems.
✔ **DO** use two diapers after surgery, one to collect stool and one to collect urine from the catheter.
✔ **DO** keep your child's penis clean. If stool gets on the wound, rinse the area with clear water.
✔ **DO** call your child's doctor right away if after surgery your child has fever, pus coming from the penis, no urine coming from the penis for more than 1 hour, or urine squirting from any part on the penis.
✔ **DO** call your doctor right away or go to the emergency room if after surgery your child has bleeding from his penis that doesn't stop.

🚫 **DON'T** have your child circumcised without your doctor's OK.
🚫 **DON'T** let your child straddle toys such as a tricycle or bouncer without your doctor's OK.
🚫 **DON'T** give your child a bath without your doctor's OK.
🚫 **DON'T** try to move your child's catheter.

FROM THE DESK OF

NOTES

FOR MORE INFORMATION

Contact the following sources:

• Hypospadias and Epispadias Association
 Website: http://www.heainfo.org

• American Society for Reproductive Medicine
 Tel: (205) 978-5000
 Website: http://www.asrm.org

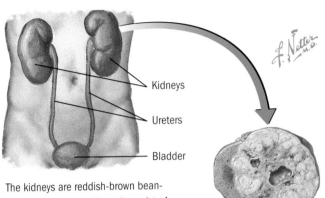

Kidneys

Ureters

Bladder

The kidneys are reddish-brown bean-shaped organs just above the waist. As part of the urinary system, they filter blood and make urine to get rid of body wastes. Renal cell carcinoma accounts for 90% to 95% of all kidney cancers, but it's rare.

Renal cell carcinoma

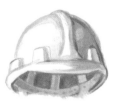

The cause isn't known, but risk factors include cigarette smoking, radiation, and on-the-job exposure to petroleum products and asbestos.

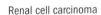

Early disease may cause no symptoms. As the tumor grows, symptoms include:

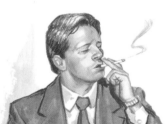

Bloody urine

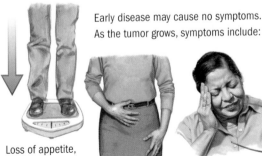

Loss of appetite, weigh loss

Abdominal pain

Tiredness, fevers

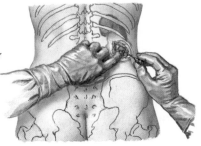

Your doctor may order CT, MRI, and ultrasonography for diagnosis, but the only way to confirm the diagnosis is with a biopsy, shown here.

What Is Kidney Cancer?

The kidneys are reddish-brown bean-shaped organs located just above the waist, one on each side of the spine. As part of the urinary system, their main jobs are filtering blood and making urine to get rid of body wastes. Renal cell carcinoma is a certain type of kidney cancer. It accounts for 90% to 95% of kidney cancers, but it's not very common (occurs in 1 of 10,000 people yearly). Twice as many men as women have it, usually between 50 and 70 years old.

What Causes Kidney Cancer?

The cause is unknown. However, risk factors include cigarette smoking, radiation, and on-the-job exposure to petroleum products, asbestos, or steel plant emissions. People with von Hippel-Lindau disease, tuberous sclerosis, and polycystic kidney disease have an increased risk for this cancer.

What Are the Symptoms of Kidney Cancer?

Early disease may cause no symptoms. As the tumor grows, symptoms may include blood in the urine, lump or mass in the kidney area, tiredness, loss of appetite, weight loss, fevers, and pain in the abdomen (belly).

How Is Kidney Cancer Diagnosed?

The doctor makes a diagnosis by special x-rays including computed tomography (CT), magnetic resonance imaging (MRI), and ultrasonography. The only way to confirm the diagnosis is with a biopsy. For a biopsy, the doctor removes a small piece of the kidney and checks it with a microscope. CT or MRI is also used to learn the stage or extent of disease, which helps plan treatment. Staging tells the doctor whether the cancer has spread and if so how far, such as to lymph nodes (glands) or lungs.

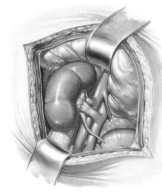

Diagnosis and treatment of your cancer will need a team of doctors including your primary care doctor, surgeon, oncologist, and maybe radiation oncologist.

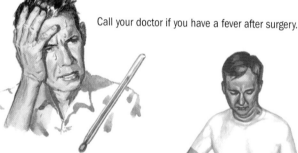

The most common treatment is an operation to remove the kidney (nephrectomy). Radiation therapy can relieve pain when the cancer spreads to bones.

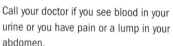

Call your doctor if you have a fever after surgery.

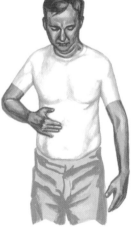

Call your doctor if you see blood in your urine or you have pain or a lump in your abdomen.

How Is Kidney Cancer Treated?

The most common treatment is an operation to remove the kidney (nephrectomy). The whole kidney, adrenal gland, tissue around the kidney, and lymph nodes may be removed. A procedure called arterial embolization may be used to shrink the tumor. It blocks the main blood vessel to the kidney so the tumor doesn't get the oxygen-carrying blood and other substances that it needs to grow.

Radiation therapy (or radiotherapy) uses high-energy radiation to kill cancer cells. It can also be used to relieve pain (as palliative therapy) when kidney cancer spread to bones.

Chemotherapy (drugs for killing cancer cells) is generally not very helpful against kidney cancer. Immunotherapy involves the use of biological agents such as interferon, sunitinib, and bevacizumab. It is a newer treatment modality that has shown some success in the treatment of advanced kidney cancer.

DOs and DON'Ts in Managing Kidney Cancer:

✔ **DO** understand that diagnosis and treatment of this cancer will need a team of doctors including your primary care doctor, surgeon, oncologist (specialist in cancer), and maybe radiation oncologist (specialist in use of radiation to treat cancer).

✔ **DO** call your doctor if you see blood in your urine or you have pain or a lump in your abdomen.

✔ **DO** call your doctor if you have fever after surgery.

✔ **DO** call your doctor if you see drainage from the surgical incision site.

⊘ **DON'T** forget that all treatments have side effects. For example, surgery can cause pain and infection. Radiation can cause dry, red, itchy skin. Chemotherapy can cause nausea, vomiting, hair loss, easy bruising, easy bleeding, and infections.

⊘ **DON'T** be afraid to ask for a second opinion.

FROM THE DESK OF

NOTES

FOR MORE INFORMATION

Contact the following sources:

• National Cancer Institute
  Tel: (800) 422-6237
  Website: http://www.cancer.gov

• American Cancer Society
  Tel: (800) 227-2345
  Website: http://www.cancer.org

MANAGING YOUR
PEYRONIE'S DISEASE

Peyronie's disease is a disorder involving the penis. It's seen in about 1% of men, usually 45 to 60 years old. It's less common in men of African or Asian heritage. It's not serious but can be embarrassing and lead to erectile dysfunction.

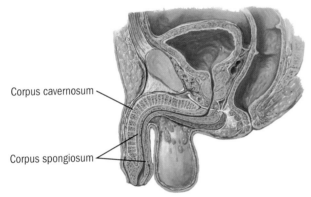

Corpus cavernosum

Corpus spongiosum

The penis has spongy tissues called the corpus cavernosum and corpus spongiosum. With sexual arousal, these tissues fill with blood, so an erection occurs. An erect penis is normally straight. In Peyronie's disease, the erect penis curves abnormally and gets shorter.

Cross section of penis

Normal

Scar tissue

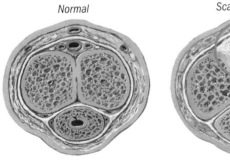
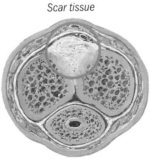

The exact cause is unknown, but scar tissue may make a hard lump or plaque on the penis. Scar tissue pulls that side of the penis so it can't expand right during arousal, and the penis curves. Injury from sex, accidents, medicines, or surgery may cause scar tissue.

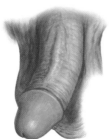

Your doctor makes a diagnosis from a physical examination, especially of the penis, and medical history. Blood tests and ultrasonography may be done.

What Is Peyronie's Disease?

Peyronie's disease is a disorder involving the penis. The penis is made of spongy tissues called the corpus cavernosum and corpus spongiosum. With sexual arousal, these tissues fill with blood, so an erection occurs. The penis is normally straight in an erection. In Peyronie's disease, the penis curves abnormally and gets shorter during an erection.

This disease is seen in about 1% of men, usually 45 to 60 years old. It's less common in men of African or Asian heritage. It's not serious but can be embarrassing and uncomfortable and can lead to erectile dysfunction.

What Causes Peyronie's Disease?

The exact cause is unknown. However, scar tissue may make a hard lump or plaque on one side of the penis. The scar tissue pulls that side of the penis so it cannot expand properly during arousal. This makes the penis curve. Trauma caused by vigorous sex, accidents, medicines, or previous surgery on the penis may cause the scar tissue to form. The disease isn't contagious or hereditary.

What Are the Symptoms of Peyronie's Disease?

The most common symptoms are painful erections and curvature (bending) of an erect penis. The penis curves up if scar tissue is on top, and it curves down if the plaque is under the penis. These symptoms can occur slowly, usually during 2 years. Other symptoms include impotence (cannot get an erection), no pleasure with sex, pain without an erection, problems with sex (penetration), and penis shortening. One side or more of the penis may have a thick band of hard tissue.

How Is Peyronie's Disease Diagnosed?

The doctor makes a diagnosis from a physical examination, especially of the penis, and medical history. The doctor may order blood tests to rule out other causes and ultrasonography to look for scar tissue. Ultrasonography uses sound waves to make pictures of inside the body and is painless and harmless.

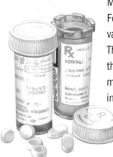

Men with mild symptoms may need no treatment. For mild to moderate symptoms, medicine or a vacuum device may be used to help get erections. This device stops blood from leaving the penis, so the penis stays erect. Medicine may be taken by mouth, put on the penis, or given as an injection into the penis.

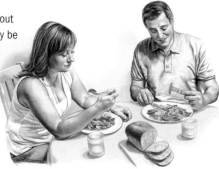

Talk to your partner about your condition. You may be embarrassed by it, but talking with your partner may help relieve stress and make your partner aware that your condition isn't about a loss of attraction.

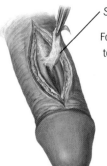

Scar tissue removed

For severe symptoms, surgery may be needed to remove scar tissue, remove tissue from the side opposite the plaque (cancels the bend), or implant a device to help rigidity. Surgery often offers the best results. Sex can resume 6 weeks after surgery.

Call your doctor if pain or curvature of the penis is getting worse or if after surgery you have a fever or foul-smelling drainage.

How Is Peyronie's Disease Treated?

Very mild symptoms may not need treatment. Peyronie's disease often goes away on its own. For mild to moderate symptoms, medicine or a vacuum device may be used to help get erections. A vacuum device stops blood from leaving the penis too early, so the penis stays erect. Medicine may be taken by mouth, put on the penis, or given as a shot in the penis. For severe symptoms, surgery may be needed to remove scar tissue, remove tissue from the side opposite the plaque (cancels the bend), or implant a device to help rigidity. Surgery often offers the best results, and sex can be resumed 6 weeks after surgery. Many men have a tender midline scar, which often goes away without treatment in 6 to 15 months.

DOs and DON'Ts in Managing Peyronie's Disease:

✔ **DO** tell your doctor about your other medical problems.

✔ **DO** tell your doctor about your medicines, both prescription and over-the-counter.

✔ **DO** call your doctor if pain or curvature of the penis is getting worse.

✔ **DO** call your doctor after surgery if you have a fever or foul-smelling drainage.

⊘ **DON'T** stop taking your medicine or change your dosage because you feel better unless your doctor tells you to.

FROM THE DESK OF

NOTES

FOR MORE INFORMATION

Contact the following source:

• American Urological Association
  Tel: (866) 746-4282
  Website: http://www.auanet.org

When a baby boy is born, the foreskin over the penis is usually too tight to show the head of the penis. Then, the foreskin slowly loosens. Phimosis is an inflammation of the foreskin that occurs when the foreskin stays too tight. Paraphimosisoccurs when the foreskin is so tight that, after it's pulled back, it gets stuck behind the head of the penis.

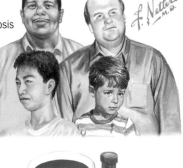

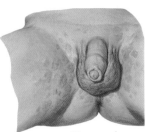

Diaper rash

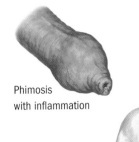

Catheter use

Long-term irritation or inflammation or repeated infections of the head of the penis (including diaper rash) can cause these disorders. They may occur more often in babies and teenagers. Diabetic males who use catheters can get it.

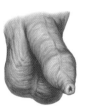

Phimosis

Phimosis with inflammation

Symptoms of phimosis are trouble urinating, problems pulling the foreskin back, repeated infections, and problems having sex.

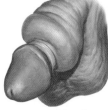

Paraphimosis

Paraphimosis can occur after pulling the foreskin back when cleaning the penis, after an erection, or after sex. It's an emergency and can cause severe pain and swelling of the penis.

What Are Phimosis and Paraphimosis?

When a baby boy is born, the foreskin over the penis is usually too tight to show the head (tip) of the penis. During the first year or two of life, the foreskin slowly loosens. Phimosis is an inflammation (swelling, redness) of the foreskin. It occurs when the foreskin doesn't loosen but stays too tight. Phimosis can also develop in babies and teenagers because of infections (including diaper rash) or irritation. Phimosis can occur in males with diabetes if they use catheters.

Paraphimosis occurs when the foreskin is so tight that, after it's pulled back, it becomes stuck behind the head of the penis. It cannot be pulled forward again. This condition can occur after pulling the foreskin back when cleaning the penis. It can also happen after an erection or after sex.

These disorders can occur at any age, but a higher occurrence is seen in babies and teenagers.

What Causes Phimosis and Paraphimosis?

Phimosis and paraphimosis are usually due to irritation that is present for a long time, chronic inflammation, or repeated infections of the head of the penis.

What Are the Symptoms of Phimosis and Paraphimosis?

Symptoms of phimosis are trouble urinating, problems pulling the foreskin back, repeated infections, and problems having sex. Symptoms of paraphimosis are being unable to pull the foreskin forward, severe pain in the penis, and swelling of the penis.

Your doctor will make a diagnosis by examining the penis. No tests are needed, but the doctor may suggest seeing a urologist.

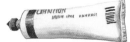

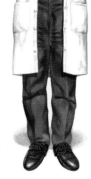

Phimosis can get better without treatment or can be treated with gentle stretching of the foreskin by hand. A special medicated cream can also be used. If this treatment doesn't work, the foreskin can be surgically loosened or removed (circumcision).

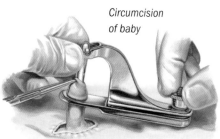

Circumcision of baby

Paraphimosis is a serious medical emergency. It must be treated quickly because it can hurt the penis. The doctor makes small cuts into the foreskin to loosen it and release the penis. Circumcision will cure paraphimosis.

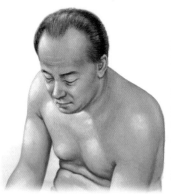

Keep your foreskin clean if you have phimosis. Phimosis can be caused by infection. Don't try to loosen the foreskin yourself if it gets stuck. Make sure that if you use a catheter you pull your foreskin forward again after using the catheter. If you don't, you may get paraphimosis.

Don't use creams or lotions on your penis unless your doctor prescribes them.

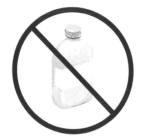

How Are Phimosis and Paraphimosis Diagnosed?

The doctor will make a diagnosis by examining the penis. No tests are needed, but the doctor may suggest seeing a urologist. A urologist is a doctor who specializes in treating the urinary system and male reproductive organs.

How Are Phimosis and Paraphimosis Treated?

Phimosis is not usually a medical emergency. It can get better without treatment. It can often be treated with gentle stretching of the foreskin by using the hands. A special medicated cream can also be applied. This procedure is repeated at regular times for 2 to 4 weeks. If this treatment doesn't work, the foreskin can be surgically loosened or removed (circumcision).

Paraphimosis is a serious medical emergency. It must be treated quickly because this condition can hurt the penis. The procedure involves making small cuts into the foreskin to loosen it and release the penis. Circumcision will cure paraphimosis.

DOs and DON'Ts in Managing Phimosis and Paraphimosis:

✔ **DO** learn to keep your foreskin clean if you have phimosis. Phimosis can be caused by infection.

✔ **DO** ask your doctor for advice if you are diabetic and use a catheter. A catheter that is causing irritation or infections can lead to phimosis.

✔ **DO** make sure that if you use a catheter you remember to pull your foreskin forward again after using it. If you don't, you may get paraphimosis.

✔ **DO** get to a doctor right away for treatment if you have paraphimosis.

⊘ **DON'T** try to loosen the foreskin yourself if it gets stuck. You can make your symptoms worse.

⊘ **DON'T** use creams or lotions on your penis unless your doctor has prescribed them.

FROM THE DESK OF

NOTES

FOR MORE INFORMATION

Contact the following source:

• American Academy of Family Physicians
  Tel: (800) 274-2237
  Website: http://www.aafp.org

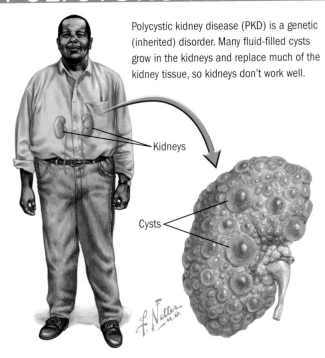

Polycystic kidney disease (PKD) is a genetic (inherited) disorder. Many fluid-filled cysts grow in the kidneys and replace much of the kidney tissue, so kidneys don't work well.

Kidneys

Cysts

DNA

The two major inherited forms are autosomal dominant PKD and autosomal recessive PKD. The first is most common and manifests in adults; the second is rare and usually affects young children.

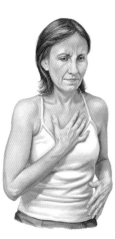

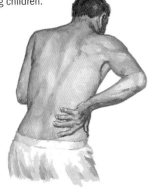

Early manifestations may be kidney infections and high blood pressure. Later symptoms include dull pain in the back and sides; shortness of breath; and swollen ankles.

Your doctor diagnoses PKD by checking your family history for PKD and finding three or more kidney cysts with ultrasonography.

What Is Polycystic Kidney Disease?

Polycystic kidney disease (PKD) is a genetic disorder. In PKD, many fluid-filled cysts grow in the kidneys. These cysts can slowly replace much of the kidney tissue, so kidneys don't work well. After many years, kidney failure can result. About half of people with the major type of PKD have kidney failure (also called end-stage renal disease, ESRD).

In the United States, about 500,000 people have PKD. It's the fourth leading cause of kidney failure. No cure is known.

What Causes PKD?

The two major inherited forms are autosomal dominant PKD and autosomal recessive PKD. The first is most common (about 90% of all cases) and initially manifests in people 30 to 40 years old. Autosomal recessive PKD is rare and usually affects young children.

What Are the Symptoms of PKD?

Most people have no symptoms until adulthood. Then symptoms appear and slowly worsen. Early manifestations are frequent kidney infections and high blood pressure. Symptoms when cysts get larger are dull pain in the back and sides (between ribs and hips); fatigue; weakness; swelling (especially around ankles or eyes); shortness of breath; and itching skin.

Autosomal dominant PKD can also cause hematuria (blood in urine) and kidney stones. Cysts in the liver and pancreas, abnormal heart valves, kidney stones, brain aneurysms (bulges in blood vessel walls), and diverticulosis (small sacs on the colon) occur more frequently in people with PKD.

How Is PKD Diagnosed?

The doctor diagnoses PKD by checking the family history for PKD and finding three or more kidney cysts with ultrasonography. Ultrasonography uses harmless sound waves to get pictures of the cysts.

The doctor may suggest consultation with a nephrologist, a doctor who specializes in kidney diseases, because of increased risk of kidney failure with PKD.

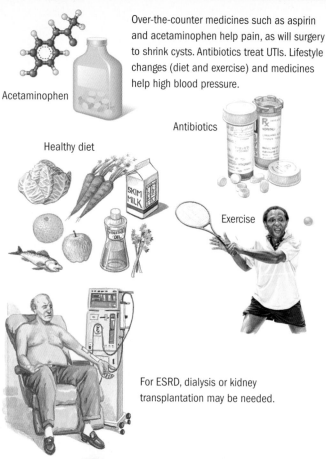

Over-the-counter medicines such as aspirin and acetaminophen help pain, as will surgery to shrink cysts. Antibiotics treat UTIs. Lifestyle changes (diet and exercise) and medicines help high blood pressure.

Acetaminophen

Antibiotics

Healthy diet

Exercise

For ESRD, dialysis or kidney transplantation may be needed.

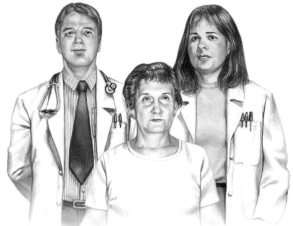

Don't forget that PKD treatment will need a team approach involving several doctors such as your primary care doctor, a kidney specialist (nephrologist), and a surgeon if surgery is needed for large painful, cysts or kidney transplant.

FROM THE DESK OF

NOTES

How Is PKD Treated?

Treatment focuses on treating high blood pressure and preventing complications such as kidney stones, urinary tract infections (UTIs), and renal failure.

Over-the-counter medicines such as aspirin and acetaminophen help pain. Surgery to shrink cysts can relieve severe back and side pain. Antibiotics treat UTIs. Lifestyle changes (diet and exercise) and medicines help high blood pressure.

For ESRD, dialysis or transplantation may be used. In hemodialysis, blood goes through a machine that cleans it and is returned to the body. In peritoneal dialysis, fluid is put into the abdomen where it picks up wastes and is then removed. New kidneys (transplants) don't develop cysts.

DOs and DON'Ts in Managing PKD:

✔ **DO** call your doctor if you get a fever or other signs of infection.

✔ **DO** call your doctor if you pass less urine, have blood in your urine, feel burning during urination, need to urinate more often, or feel greater urgency to urinate.

✔ **DO** call your doctor if you have abdominal pain.

✔ **DO** understand that severe or unusual headaches may be caused by brain aneurysms or high blood pressure.

✔ **DO** get counseling with a genetics expert if you're thinking of becoming pregnant.

🚫 **DON'T** forget that PKD will need a team approach involving several doctors.

🚫 **DON'T** be afraid to ask for a referral to a doctor or institution experienced with kidney transplantation or dialysis.

FOR MORE INFORMATION

Contact the following sources:

• PKD Foundation
  Tel: (800) 753-2873
  Website: http://www.pkdcure.org

• National Kidney Foundation
  Tel: (800) 622-9010
  Website: http://www.kidney.org

• National Kidney and Urologic Diseases
  Information Clearinghouse
  Tel: (800) 891-5390
  Website: http://www.kidney.niddk.nih.gov/

MANAGING YOUR
TESTICULAR TORSION

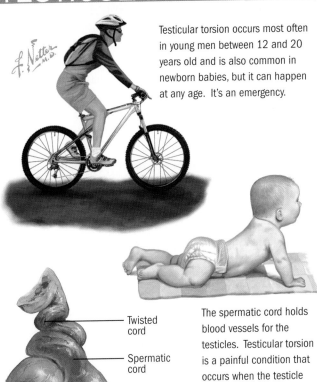

Testicular torsion occurs most often in young men between 12 and 20 years old and is also common in newborn babies, but it can happen at any age. It's an emergency.

Twisted cord

Spermatic cord

Testicle

The spermatic cord holds blood vessels for the testicles. Testicular torsion is a painful condition that occurs when the testicle twists on the end of the spermatic cord cutting off the testicle's blood supply.

Symptoms are sudden severe pain in the testicle and sometimes lower abdominal pain with nausea. The testicle can be swollen and tender.

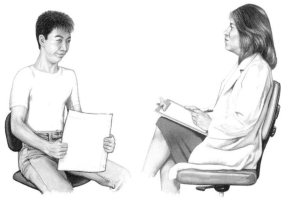

Your doctor will take a medical history and do a physical examination. Ultrasonography or a nuclear scan will be done to confirm the diagnosis and rule out other disorders.

What Is Testicular Torsion?

Testicular torsion is a painful condition that occurs when the testicle twists on the end of the spermatic cord. This cord holds blood vessels that supply the testicle with blood. This corkscrew-like twisting cuts off the testicle's blood supply. If the testicle stays tightly twisted, it will be damaged and could die.

Testicular torsion occurs most often in young men between 12 and 20 years old and it's also common in newborn babies, but it can happen at any age. It's rare, occurring in 1 in 5000 males. It can occur suddenly, for no reason, or following trauma, and is a medical emergency.

What Causes Testicular Torsion?

Before birth, testicles start to develop inside the abdomen (belly). As the fetus grows, testicles move down until they are inside the scrotum. Testicles stay attached to the abdomen by the spermatic cord and are fixed to tissues around them. Sometimes, the attachment is too loose and the testicle hangs too freely on the spermatic cord. Testicular torsion is more common in men with this problem, but it can occur without any abnormality.

What Are the Symptoms of Testicular Torsion?

Symptoms are sudden severe pain in the testicle and sometimes lower abdominal pain with nausea. The testicle can be swollen, tender to touch, and drawn up toward the abdomen.

How Is Testicular Torsion Diagnosed?

The doctor will take a medical history and do a physical examination. Ultrasonography or a nuclear scan will be done to confirm the diagnosis and rule out other disorders. The scan shows low blood flow to the testicle if torsion exists.

To prevent permanent damage or loss of testicle, surgery must be done right away. If the testicle has been permanently damaged, it's removed (orchiectomy). Remember, losing one testicle doesn't mean loss of erections, orgasms, or ability to father children.

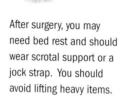

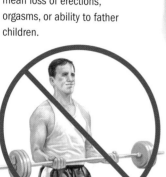

After surgery, you may need bed rest and should wear scrotal support or a jock strap. You should avoid lifting heavy items.

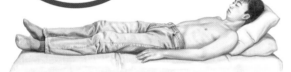

You should also avoid playing contact sports, especially if you have a testicle removed.

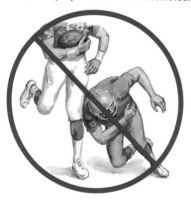

Don't ignore a painful testicle, delay getting medical advice, or be embarrassed! This condition is a medical emergency and needs surgery very quickly.

FROM THE DESK OF

NOTES

How Is Testicular Torsion Treated?

Immediate surgery must be done to prevent permanent damage to or loss of the testicle. Surgery untwists the testicle and the spermatic cord and puts them back in their normal positions. If surgery is delayed longer than 4 to 6 hours after the pain started, the testicle may not survive. The other testicle is often fixed to prevent similar torsion. If the testicle hasn't survived, it's removed (called orchiectomy). If the other testicle is healthy and not removed, sex life and the ability to father children won't be affected.

After surgery, bed rest and wearing scrotal support or a jock strap (for swelling or discomfort) may be needed. Lifting heavy items or playing contact sports should be avoided. Sex can be resumed when it's comfortable.

DOs and DON'Ts in Managing Testicular Torsion:

✔ **DO** get medical help right away if you have sudden severe pain or swelling in the testicles or if your symptoms come back after surgery. The testicle can twist again.

✔ **DO** call your doctor if you feel a lump on your testicle.

✔ **DO** call your doctor if you have fever, bleeding, or pain after surgery.

🚫 **DON'T** ignore a painful testicle, delay getting medical advice, or be embarrassed! This condition is a medical emergency and needs surgery quickly, within several hours, or the testicle may die. The surgeon will take your condition seriously.

🚫 **DON'T** miss follow-up appointments with the urologist (specialist in urinary problems) after surgery.

🚫 **DON'T** be misled. The loss of one testicle does not mean loss of erections, orgasms, or ability to father children.

FOR MORE INFORMATION

Contact the following sources:

• American Urological Association
 Tel: (866) 746-4282
 Website: http://www.urologyhealth.org/

• National Institutes of Health
 Tel: (301) 496-4000
 Website: http://www.nih.gov

• American Academy of Family Physicians
 Tel: (800) 274-2237
 Website: http://www.familydoctor.org/

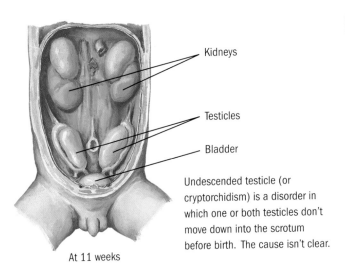

Undescended testicle (or cryptorchidism) is a disorder in which one or both testicles don't move down into the scrotum before birth. The cause isn't clear.

At 11 weeks

This condition occurs in about 3% of male babies who are born at term and about 30% of premature babies.

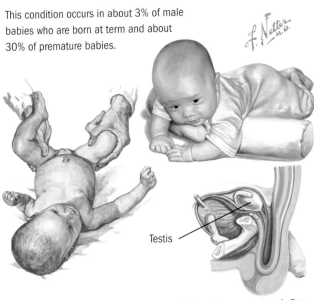

Testis

The doctor usually finds undescended testicles during a newborn's first physical examination. In about 80% of cases, the doctor can feel them further up in the inguinal canal. There are no other symptoms.

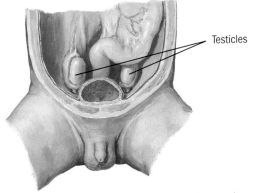

Testicles

If the doctor cannot feel them in the inguinal canal, an ultrasound examination, CT, or laparoscopy may be done.

What Is an Undescended Testicle?

Undescended testicle or testis (also called cryptorchidism) is a disorder in which one or both testicles don't move into the scrotum before birth. Shortly before birth, the testicles usually move through a space from the abdomen (belly) down into the scrotum. When a testicle doesn't drop down, it's undescended.

This condition occurs in about 3% of male babies who are born at term and about 30% of premature babies. In fact, almost 100% of all boys who weigh less than 2 pounds at birth will have undescended testis.

What Causes an Undescended Testicle?

The reasons for undescended testicles aren't clear. Perhaps not enough hormones from the mother or from developing testicles were present to cause normal growth. Some blockage may have prevented descent. Hormones taken during pregnancy may also have affected the testicles.

What Are the Symptoms of an Undescended Testicle?

The testicle cannot be seen or felt in its normal location of the scrotum. Usually the baby has no other symptoms.

How Is an Undescended Testicle Diagnosed?

The doctor usually finds undescended testicles during a newborn's first physical examination. In about 80% of cases, the doctor can feel them further up in the inguinal canal (a passage in the lower abdominal wall).

If the doctor cannot feel them in the inguinal canal, an ultrasound examination may be done. This test uses sound waves to look inside the body.

The doctor may order other tests if the ultrasound doesn't show the testicles. Computed tomography (CT) can make images of the inside of the body more clearly. Sometimes an operation called laparoscopy needs to be done. In laparoscopy, the doctor uses a small, flexible, lighted tube (laparoscope) to see into the abdomen.

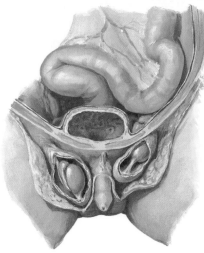

In some cases, treatment is not necessary—the testicles often descend on their own by the child's first birthday. If they haven't moved on their own by then, surgery (orchiopexy) will be done to move the testicles down into the scrotum.

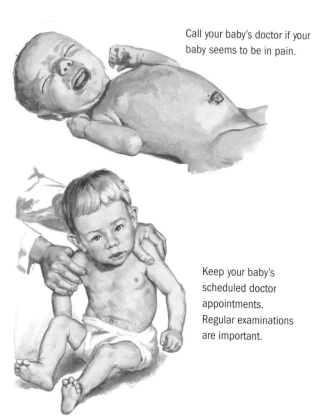

Call your baby's doctor if your baby seems to be in pain.

Keep your baby's scheduled doctor appointments. Regular examinations are important.

How Is Undescended Testicle Treated?

If the testicles can be felt up in the inguinal canal, they often descend on their own, without any treatment, usually by the baby's first birthday. If they haven't moved down on their own by that time, some treatment will be needed. Surgery, called orchiopexy, will be done to move the testicles into the scrotum.

Undescended testicles that aren't corrected may cause fertility problems, such as low sperm counts, later in life. Men who had an undescended testicle, either fixed by surgery or not, have a greater risk of getting testicular cancer.

DOs and DON'Ts in Managing an Undescended Testicle:

✔ **DO** keep your baby's doctor appointments. Regular examinations are important.

✔ **DO** call your baby's doctor if your baby seems to be in pain.

🚫 **DON'T** panic. In most cases, the testicles will descend on their own without treatment.

FROM THE DESK OF

NOTES

FOR MORE INFORMATION

Contact the following source:

• American Urological Association
Tel: (866) 746-4282
Website: http://www.auanet.org

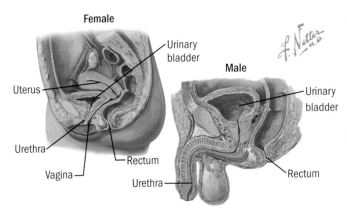

F. Netter M.D.

Female

- Uterus
- Urethra
- Vagina
- Urinary bladder
- Rectum

Male

- Urinary bladder
- Rectum
- Urethra

Urinary incontinence is a very common disorder where one is unable to control urine flow in certain situations.

Types of incontinence

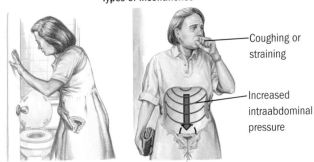

- Coughing or straining
- Increased intraabdominal pressure

Urge incontinence: Losing urine on the way to the bathroom or going to the bathroom too often

Stress incontinence: Loss of urine in a gush or spurt from certain activities (coughing, sneezing, lifting, etc.)

Urodynamic test (simple cystometry)

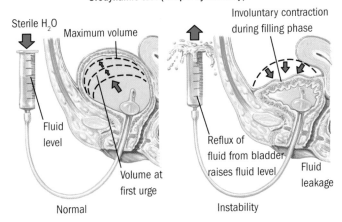

- Sterile H$_2$O
- Maximum volume
- Fluid level
- Volume at first urge
- Involuntary contraction during filling phase
- Reflux of fluid from bladder raises fluid level
- Fluid leakage

Normal

Instability

Urodynamic tests measure pressure in the bladder, urine flow, and the amount of urine left in the bladder after urination.

What Is Urinary Incontinence?

Urinary incontinence is the uncontrollable loss of urine. It is very common, especially in women. Up to 60% of women have incontinence.

What Are the Causes of Urinary Incontinence?

The two most common types are stress incontinence and urge incontinence. Stress incontinence is losing urine in a spurt or gush with certain activities (e.g., coughing, sneezing, lifting, exercising). It can be caused by childbirth or growing older. Urge incontinence is losing urine on the way to the bathroom. It can be caused by drugs, caffeine, alcohol, or growing older. Many bladder problems worsen during menopause.

What Are the Symptoms of Urinary Incontinence?

In very mild incontinence, a small amount of urine sometimes leaks (dribbles) during a cough or sneeze, or on the way to the bathroom. In mild to moderate incontinence, urine leaks daily and/or a pad is needed for protection. In severe incontinence, urine soaks a pad several times each day. Incontinence may limit daily activities.

How Is Urinary Incontinence Diagnosed?

Diagnosis involves taking a medical history, x-rays, blood tests, urinalysis, and other tests to see how the bladder works. These tests, called urodynamic tests, measure pressure in the bladder, urine flow, and the amount of urine left in the bladder after urination.

Treatment Options

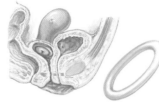

Kegel exercises strengthen the pelvic floor muscles. You contract the muscles that prevent urination, holding for 10 seconds, then relaxing. Try doing three sets of 10 each day. They can be done anywhere: while sitting, standing, or lying down.

A pessary is a plastic device used for multiple gynecologic problems, including stress incontinence. The pessary helps support the bladder.

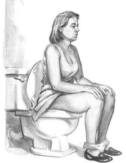

Bladder training can be helpful in treating urge incontinence.

If exercise and bladder training don't work, there are various operations that may help.

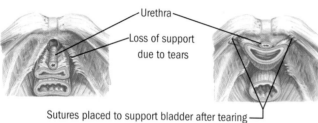

Urethra

Loss of support due to tears

Sutures placed to support bladder after tearing

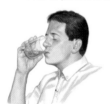
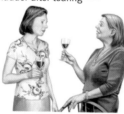

Don't drink fluids in excess. Alcohol and liquids containing caffeine are diuretics and will make your incontinence worse. Space fluid intake throughout the day.

How Is Urinary Incontinence Treated?

Strengthening pelvic floor muscles is usually the first step in managing stress incontinence. Tightening these muscles is called a Kegel exercise. If Kegel exercises do not help, special physical therapy may improve bladder control. This therapy includes biofeedback and electrical stimulation.

Special devices, called pessaries, are also available to treat stress incontinence. These devices can be used to support organs such as the bladder. Sometimes pessaries are useful when urine is lost only during certain activities, such as jogging, aerobics, and horseback riding.

The first step in treating urge incontinence is usually training the bladder to empty (void) at certain times. The goal is for 3 hours to pass before the need to void during the daytime without any leaking. Sometimes medicines can help with bladder training. These drugs may cause dry mouth or eyes but are generally well tolerated. Various operations can also be used for stress incontinence. Specialists such as gynecologists or urologists do these operations.

DOs and DON'Ts in Managing Urinary Incontinence:

✔ **DO** your Kegel exercises as directed.
✔ **DO** take your medicine as directed.

🚫 **DON'T** drink lots of liquids containing caffeine (e.g., coffee, black tea, sodas). Caffeine can make the kidneys produce more urine faster than normal. Both stress and urge incontinence will get worse, and you will void more often.
🚫 **DON'T** drink excessive amounts of alcohol. Alcohol is also a diuretic.
🚫 **DON'T** drink large amounts of fluids during the day or at one time.
🚫 **DON'T** drink liquids after 7 to 8 pm if you get up more than twice during the night to urinate.

FOR MORE INFORMATION

Contact the following sources:
- National Association for Continence
  Tel: (800) 252-3337
  Website: http://www.nafc.org
- American Urological Association
  Tel: (866) 746-4282
  Website: http://www.urologyhealth.org
- Simon Foundation for Continence
  Tel: (800) 237-4666
  Website: http://www.simonfoundation.org

FROM THE DESK OF

NOTES

A varicocele is an enlargement of veins inside the scrotum, similar to a varicose vein in the leg. A varicocele can form in one or both sides of the scrotum. They're usually harmless but can affect fertility. Some 40% of infertile men have a varicocele.

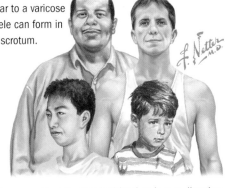

One-way valves in veins let blood go in one direction, toward larger veins. When valves inside veins in the testicles and scrotum don't work properly, blood backs up and causes the veins to swell. A varicocele results.

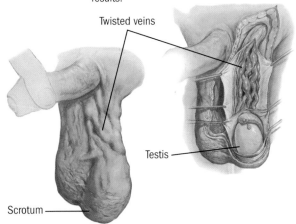

Twisted veins

Testis

Scrotum

Usually, men have no symptoms. If symptoms occur, they can include a larger, painless scrotum and a dull pain or a heavy, dragging feeling in the scrotum. The testicle on the affected side may shrink. The scrotum may feel like a bag of worms because of the enlarged veins.

Ultrasound

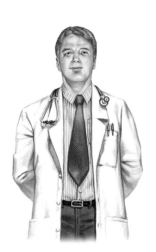
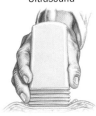

Your doctor makes a diagnosis by examining the scrotum. If the diagnosis is unclear, the doctor may order ultrasonography. This test can rule out other causes of swelling of the scrotum.

What Is a Varicocele?

A varicocele is an enlargement of veins inside the scrotum, similar to a varicose vein that can appear in the leg. The scrotum is the pouch that hangs below the penis and holds the testicles. Veins carry blood from tissues and cells back to the heart, where the blood cells get oxygen. The scrotum has two sides, the right and the left. A varicocele can form in either side or both sides. It often forms on the left because these veins are normally under more pressure than the ones on the right. A varicocele may result in an enlarged scrotum.

Varicoceles are common. About 15% of all men get them. They can develop in childhood, but most often they occur in teenage boys and young men. Varicoceles are usually harmless, but they can affect fertility (the ability to make a woman pregnant). About 40% of infertile men have a varicocele.

What Causes a Varicocele?

Veins contain one-way valves that push blood in one direction, toward larger veins. When valves inside the veins in the testicles and scrotum don't work properly, blood backs up and causes these veins to swell. A varicocele is the result.

What Are the Symptoms of a Varicocele?

A varicocele usually causes no symptoms. People don't know that it exists until a doctor examines the scrotum. Sometimes a man or boy becomes aware of a larger scrotum, but this is painless. There may be a dull pain or a heavy, dragging feeling in the scrotum. A varicocele may also cause the testicle on the affected side to shrink because of the pressure. People may notice a painless swelling in the scrotum that feels like a bag of worms. The enlarged veins make the scrotum feel like this.

How Is a Varicocele Diagnosed?

The doctor will diagnose a varicocele by examining the scrotum. If the diagnosis is unclear, the doctor may order an imaging test called ultrasonography. This test can get pictures of the veins with the scrotum. Other causes of swelling of the scrotum can be ruled out.

No treatment is needed unless pain, other symptoms, or fertility problems occur or if the testicle shrinks. Treatment, if needed, involves a minor operation called a varicocelectomy, done by a urologist. Veins may be taken out or tied so that the blood supply is stopped. This surgery may help fertility. There's about a 15% chance that the problem will return, but the surgery can be done again.

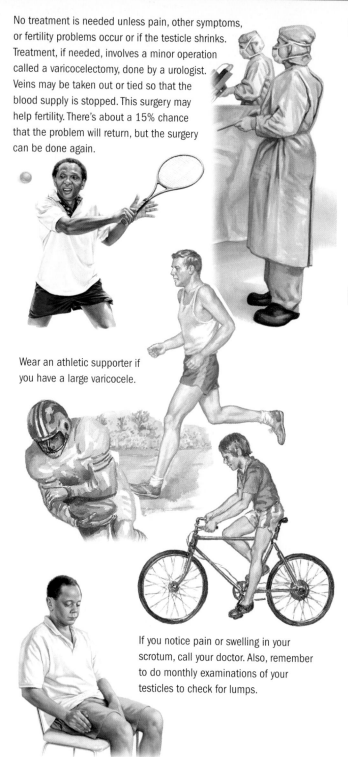

Wear an athletic supporter if you have a large varicocele.

If you notice pain or swelling in your scrotum, call your doctor. Also, remember to do monthly examinations of your testicles to check for lumps.

How Is a Varicocele Treated?

No treatment is needed unless pain or other symptoms occur, the testicle shrinks, or fertility problems appear. Treatment, if needed, involves an operation called a varicocelectomy. In this operation, veins may be taken out or tied so that the blood supply is stopped and the veins collapse. A doctor called a urologist will do this surgery. A urologist specializes in treating the male and female urinary system and male reproductive system. This procedure may help fertility. Surgical removal of the veins is a minor operation, and 1 to 7 days off work will be needed. Discomfort or bruising may occur. There's about a 15% chance that the problem will return. If it does, the surgery can be done again.

DOs and DON'Ts in Managing a Varicocele:

✔ **DO** wear an athletic supporter if you have a large varicocele.
✔ **DO** call your doctor if you have symptoms.
✔ **DO** call your doctor if you have fertility problems.

⊘ **DON'T** ignore pain or swelling in your scrotum.

FROM THE DESK OF

NOTES

FOR MORE INFORMATION

Contact the following source:

• American Urological Association
Tel: (866) 746-4282
Website: http://www.auanet.org

FERRI'S NETTER PATIENT ADVISOR
INDEX

 Spanish translation available online at www.netterreference.com
(see inside front cover for PIN code)

 Available online at www.netterreference.com
(see inside front cover for PIN code)

 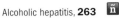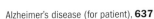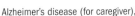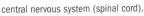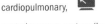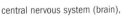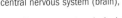